Medical Microbiology

Medical Microbiology

SECOND EDITION

Patrick R. Murray, PhD
Professor, Departments of Pathology and Medicine,
Washington University School of Medicine;
Director, Clinical Microbiology Laboratory,
Barnes Hospital,
St. Louis, Missouri

George S. Kobayashi, PhD
Professor, Departments of Medicine and Microbiology,
Washington University School of Medicine;
Associate Director, Clinical Microbiology Laboratory,
Barnes Hospital,
St. Louis, Missouri

Michael A. Pfaller, MD
Professor and Vice-Chairman,
Department of Pathology,
Oregon Health Sciences University,
Portland, Oregon

Ken S. Rosenthal, PhD
Professor,
Department of Microbiology and Immunology,
Northeastern Ohio Universities College of Medicine,
Rootstown, Ohio

with 505 *illustrations*

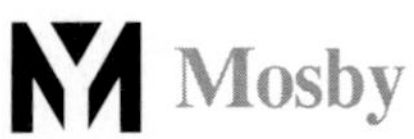

St. Louis Baltimore Boston Chicago London Madrid Philadelphia Sydney Toronto

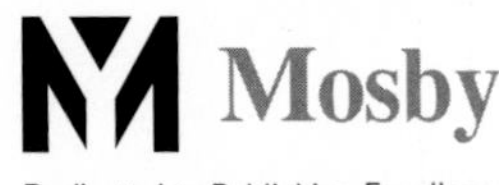

Dedicated to Publishing Excellence

Editor: Robert Farrell
Developmental Editor: Emma D. Underdown
Project Manager: John Rogers
Production Editor: Chris Murphy
Designer: Julia Taugner
Front cover photos: top two photos courtesy Dr. Patrick Murray, bottom right © Dr. Dennis Kunkel/Phototake
Back cover photos: center photo © Dr. Dennis Kunkel/Phototake, top right and bottom right courtesy Dr. Patrick Murray

SECOND EDITION

Printed in the United States of America
Composition by Graphic World, Inc.
Printing/binding by Von Hoffmann Press

Mosby–Year Book, Inc.
11830 Westline Industrial Drive
St. Louis, Missouri 63146-3318

Library of Congress Cataloging in Publication Data
Medical microbiology/Patrick R. Murray . . . [et al.]. – 2nd ed.
p. cm.
Includes bibliographical references and index.
ISBN 0-8016-7634-7
1. Medical Microbiology. I. Murray, Patrick R.
[DNLM: 1. Microbiology. 2. Parasitology. QW 4 M4862 1994]
QR46.M4683 1994
616′ .01 – dc20
DNLM/DLC
for Library of Congress

93-11644
CIP

93 94 95 96 97 / 9 8 7 6 5 4 3 2 1

Contributing Authors

Julius M. Cruse, MD, PhD

Professor of Pathology
Associate Professor of Medicine and of Microbiology
University of Mississippi Medical Center;
Director of Immunopathology and Transplantation Immunology
University Hospital
Jackson, Mississippi

Chapter 9
Natural Immunity and Physiological Defense Mechanisms

Chapter 10
Acquired Immunity

Chapter 11
Microbial Virulence Factors

Guylaine Lépine, MS

Department of Oral Biology
University of Florida College of Dentistry
Gainesville, Florida

Chapter 2
Bacterial Structure

Robert E. Lewis, Jr, PhD

Professor of Pathology
University of Mississippi Medical Center;
Co-Director of Immunopathology and Transplantation Immunology
University Hospital
Jackson, Mississippi

Chapter 9
Natural Immunity and Physiological Defense Mechanisms

Chapter 10
Acquired Immunity

Chapter 11
Microbial Virulence Factors

Ann Progulske-Fox, PhD

Associate Professor
Department of Oral Biology
University of Florida College of Dentistry
Gainesville, Florida

Chapter 2
Bacterial Structure

Chapter 3
Bacterial Metabolism

Chapter 4
Bacterial Genetics

Venkatarama K. Rao, MD, PhD

Resident in Internal Medicine
Barnes Hospital
St. Louis, Missouri

Chapter 3
Bacterial Metabolism

Chapter 4
Bacterial Genetics

Jon B. Suzuki, DDS, PhD

Professor, Department of Microbiology and Periodontics
Dean, School of Dental Medicine
University of Pittsburgh;
Chief, Hospital Dentistry
Presbyterian and Montefiore University Hospitals
Pittsburgh, Pennsylvania

Chapter 40
Oral Microbiology

To our families, students, and colleagues
who have provided the inspiration and motivation
to make this undertaking a reality

Preface

THE increasing complexity of microbiology poses a challenge for both the teacher and the student. The teacher must present a broad array of facts as coherent intellectual concepts, while the student must be able to assimilate this information. This educational process should be guided by a contemporary, informative textbook. Unfortunately, most textbooks are either a compendium of information or a philosophical treatise on pathogenesis. In the former case, presentation of information in a reference book format does not aid the student in distinguishing between what he or she needs to know and what is informative but excessive; in the latter situation the foundation of basic knowledge for understanding the biology of the pathogens is frequently not established.

In the first edition of ***Medical Microbiology*** we attempted to provide a balanced, comprehensive presentation of medically important information that we felt every student would need to know. For this goal we adopted a format of concise presentations supplemented with numerous tables, color illustrations, and summary boxes. From the comments of the students and teachers who have used this book, the approach was successful. But like good teachers and students, we also have learned. The comments and suggestions from students, teachers, and invited reviewers have formed the foundation of this second edition of ***Medical Microbiology***.

This new edition represents a dramatic expansion of topics, with the addition of three new sections and 13 additional chapters. The chapters covering bacterial structure (Chapter 2), metabolism (Chapter 3), and genetics (Chapter 4) have been greatly expanded in Section I. An increased emphasis on the role of immunity in disease and prevention has been introduced throughout the text and is emphasized in Section II. For example, a discussion of the role of the normal microbial flora in health and disease (Chapter 8) is followed by two chapters that examine natural (Chapter 9) and acquired (Chapter 10) immunity, and one chapter (Chapter 11) that explores the interaction between host immunity and microbial virulence factors. Section III introduces the topics of antisepsis, sterilization, and disinfection (Chapter 12), followed by a comprehensive discussion of chemotherapy for all major groups of microorganisms (Chapters 13 through 16), and a discussion of the utility of vaccines for controlling bacterial and viral diseases (Chapter 17).

The organism-oriented sections (Section IV through VII) have also been updated extensively. In addition to supplementing the information presented in the first edition, we have expanded the use of summary boxes and color illustrations to help emphasize important concepts and facts for the student. We have also introduced the use of clinical cases and summary questions at the end of each chapter, with the goal that these will help orient the student and emphasize how the presented information can help with the clinical management of a patient. Each section starts with a chapter that discusses the laboratory diagnosis of infections (Chapters 18, 42, 46, and 52). Finally, summary chapters have been added to the Bacteriology (Chapter 41) and Virology (Chapter 70) sections, which we hope the student will find helpful for integrating the concepts presented in the preceding chapters.

In the first edition we asked for comments from students and educators and were pleased with the positive, constructive response we received. We have tried to develop this second edition of ***Medical Microbiology*** to satisfy these needs. We realize that all efforts in education represent a progression of learning, so please let us know if this new edition has been successful. As educators, our goal is to convey information in a coherent, concise fashion. If this textbook accomplishes that goal, then we will be satisfied. If our efforts fall short in some area, tell us.

As is true with all projects of this nature, the successful progression from conception to fruition involves many individuals. We are grateful to Dr. Julius Cruse, Dr. Robert Lewis, Dr. Ann Progulske-Fox, Dr. Ram Rao, Dr. Jon Suzuki, and Ms. Guylaine Lépine for contributing their special expertise. We would also like to thank the staff at Mosby for their invaluable help. Particular thanks go to Bob Farrell, Emma Underdown, Andrea Whitson, Chris Murphy, and John Rogers. Finally, we wish to thank all of the students and educators who kindly reviewed the chapters in this edition and helped refine the final product.

P.R. Murray
G.S. Kobayashi
M.A. Pfaller
K.S. Rosenthal

Reviewers

David Abraham, PhD
Associate Professor
Department of Microbiology and Immunology
Jefferson Medical College
Philadelphia, Pennsylvania

John H. Cross, PhD
Professor
Department of Preventive Medicine and Biometrics
Uniformed Services University of the Health Sciences
Bethesda, Maryland

John A. Edwards
University of Wisconsin Medical School
Madison, Wisconsin

Robert P. Ellis, PhD
Professor
Department of Microbiology
Colorado State University College of Veterinary Medicine and Medical Science
Fort Collins, Colorado

Steven Glenn, MS, SM (AAM/ASCP)
Assistant Director
Clinical Microbiology Laboratory
The University Hospital
Cincinnati, Ohio

Brian D. Heim
Northeastern Ohio Universities
College of Medicine
Rootstown, Ohio

Wai L. Lee
Washington University School of Medicine
St. Louis, Missouri

Jonathan D. Martin, PhD
Associate Professor of Microbiology
Division of Basic Medical Sciences
Mercer University School of Medicine
Macon, Georgia

John A. Mihok, MT(ASCP), SM, CLS
Director, Medical Technology Program
Monmouth Medical Center
Long Branch, New Jersey

Gary V. Paddock, PhD
Associate Professor
Department of Microbiology and Immunology
Medical University of South Carolina
Charleston, South Carolina

Neil J. Sargentini, PhD
Assistant Professor
Department of Microbiology and Immunology
Kirksville College of Osteopathic Medicine
Kirksville, Missouri

John E. Sippel, PhD
Associate Professor of Microbiology
Division of Basic Medical Sciences
Mercer University School of Medicine
Macon, Georgia

N. N. Sjak-Shie, PhD
Washington University School of Medicine
St. Louis, Missouri

Martin D. Skipper
Northeastern Ohio Universities
College of Medicine
Rootstown, Ohio

Bonnie Smith, PhD
Department of Microbiology
The University of Health Sciences
Kansas City, Missouri

Joel D. Stone
University of California, Davis, School of Medicine
Davis, California

Dixie D. Whitt, PhD
Lecturer, Department of Microbiology
University of Illinois at Urbana-Champaign
Urbana, Illinois

Contents

SECTION V
MYCOLOGY

George S. Kobayashi

SECTION VI
PARASITOLOGY

Michael A. Pfaller

SECTION VII
VIROLOGY

Ken S. Rosenthal

CHAPTER 1

Introduction to Microbiology

THE true complexity of our surroundings was unappreciated until the existence of microorganisms was first revealed with the microscope. Indeed, the use of microscopy has helped to define the relationships among a diversity of organisms, ranging from the smallest viruses consisting of a few proteins and minimal genetic information to multicellular parasites almost 10 meters in length.

Microbiology, the study of living organisms, is traditionally subdivided into the examination of viruses, bacteria, fungi, and parasites. Although each group of organisms represents an increase in size and structural complexity, all groups are fully capable of significant disease. **Viruses** are the smallest known organisms (generally less than 1 μm). They consist of either DNA or RNA (but not both), surrounded with a protein coat and, in some but not all viruses, a lipid envelope. Because these particles have limited genetic information and metabolic capabilities, they are strict intracellular parasites. **Bacteria** are larger, ranging in size from 0.1 μm to 5 or more μm in length. The organisms contain both DNA and RNA, although the genetic information is not organized within a nucleus. Most bacteria can freely divide; however, some remain strict intracellular parasites (e.g., *Chlamydia*, some rickettsia). **Fungi** are larger and more complex than bacteria. Their genetic material is organized within a nuclear structure, and protein synthesis is regulated on a complex membrane framework, the endoplasmic reticulum. **Parasites** vary enormously in their complexity, ranging from simple single-cell organisms such as amoeba to highly complex multicellular organisms such as worms and insects.

As the science of **microbiology** increased in sophistication, the characterization of organisms evolved from morphological descriptions to analysis of their phenotypical and genotypical properties. Despite these advances, the initial recognition and identification of organisms are still determined most commonly by the morphological appearance of the microscopic cells and macroscopic colonies.

MICROSCOPY

Microscopy maximizes the principles of enlargement and **resolution** (i.e., the ability to distinguish that two objects are separate and not one). Three general approaches have been used to accomplish these goals: brightfield microscopy, fluorescent microscopy, and electron microscopy.

Brightfield Microscopy

Two lens systems are used to magnify the specimen: an **objective lens** and an **ocular lens**. Three different objective lenses are commonly used: low-power (×10), which can be used to scan a specimen; high-dry (×40), which is used to look for large microbes such as parasites and filamentous fungi; and oil immersion (×100), which is used to observe bacteria, **yeasts** (single cell stage of fungi), and the morphological details of larger organisms. Additional magnification of the specimen is accomplished with ocular lenses (generally ×10). The total magnification of the specimen is the product of the magnifications of the objective and ocular lenses.

The resolving power of a microscope is determined by the wavelength of light used to illuminate the subject and the angle of light entering the objective lens (referred to as the **numerical aperature**). The best brightfield microscopes have a resolving power of approximately 0.2 μm, which is the lower limit for seeing most bacteria.

Although most bacteria and larger microorganisms can be seen with brightfield microscopy, the refractive indices of the organisms and background are similar. Thus organisms must be stained with a dye to be observed. A variation of brightfield microscopy is **darkfield microscopy**, in which the specimen is illuminated with light directed from the periphery. This procedure is useful for observing organisms between 0.1 and 0.2 μm in width (e.g., *Treponema pallidum* [etiological agent of syphilis], *Borrelia burgdorferi* [Lyme disease], and *Leptospira* [leptospirosis]). Another approach is **phase-contrast microscopy**, which uses a filtering system to visualize phase differences in light as it passes through objects of different densities. This type of microscopy gives the organisms a three-dimensional appearance.

Fluorescent Microscopy

Some compounds called **fluorochromes** are able to absorb short-wavelength ultraviolet or ultrablue light and emit energy at a higher wavelength. Although some compounds and microorganisms demonstrate natural or autofluorescence, this microscopic technique generally

TABLE 1-1 Common Microbiological Stains

Stain	Principle	Application
Acridine orange	Fluorochrome that intercalates with nucleic acid, changing the dye's optical characteristics; fluoresces orange under UV light	Primarily to detect bacteria and fungi, although any cell containing nucleic acids will fluoresce
Auramine rhodamine	Nonspecific fluorochrome that binds mycolic acids in cell walls of acid-fast organisms; fluoresces orange-yellow under UV light	Detection of acid-fast organisms such as mycobacteria, nocardia, and some parasites
Calcofluor white	Fluorochrome that binds to cellulose in fungal cell walls; fluoresces blue-white under UV light	Detection of fungi in clinical specimens
Capsule stain	Name is a misnomer; dye such as crystal violet is used to stain the bacterium and background, whereas the surrounding capsule is unstained	Demonstrate bacterial capsules
Flagella	A variety of dyes are used to stain bacterial flagella	Demonstrate arrangement of flagella; useful for identification of some organisms
Gram	Differential bacterial stain; gram-positive bacteria retain crystal violet-iodine complex; this washes out of gram-negative cells during decolorization; the latter group of bacteria are stained with the red counterstain, safranin	Differential bacterial stain
India ink	Contrasting dye that stains organisms and background material but not capsule	Demonstrates capsule surrounding fungus *Cryptococcus*
Kinyoun	Basic dye carbolfuchsin stains mycolic acids in cell wall of acid-fast organisms; organisms appear pink-red	Detection of acid-fast organisms such as mycobacteria, nocardia, and certain parasites
Lactophenol cotton blue	Strongly acidic dye that is a good counterstain for tissues, bacteria, and protozoa	Primarily to stain filamentous fungi and their characteristic fruiting structures
Ludol iodine	Nonspecific contrast dye	Primarily to detect parasites
Toluidine blue O	Stains fungi and *Pneumocystis* lavender, background material blue	Detection of *Pneumocystis*
Trichrome	Contains chromotrope 2R and light green SF as primary stains	Useful for studying morphology of protozoa and other parasites
Wright-Giemsa	Consists of methylene blue and eosin dyes	Detection of blood parasites such as malaria
Ziehl-Neelsen	Acid-fast stain (see Kinyoun stain)	Detection of mycobacteria, nocardia, and some parasites

involves staining organisms with fluorescent dyes and examining them with a specially designed fluorescent microscope. This microscope utilizes a mercury vapor lamp that emits a shorter wavelength of light compared with traditional brightfield microscopy. This procedure is particularly sensitive because organisms will appear as brightly fluorescing particles against a black background.

Electron Microscopy

In contrast with brightfield and fluorescent microscopy, electron microscopy utilizes magnetic coils (rather than lenses) to direct a beam of electrons from a tungsten filament through a specimen and onto a screen. Because this process uses a much shorter wavelength of light, magnification and resolution are dramatically improved. Viral particles can be seen only by electron microscopy. Two types of electron microscopes are used: **transmission electron microscopy**, in which particles pass directly through the specimen, and **scanning electron microscopy**, in which particles pass through the specimen at an angle, producing a three-dimensional picture.

Staining Procedures

Since microorganisms are difficult to detect by brightfield microscopy, a number of staining procedures have been developed for the detection of specific organisms (e.g., bacteria, mycobacteria, fungi, parasites) or organelles (e.g., capsule, flagella). For additional technical information, see the Bibliography at the end of this chapter. The principles and applications of the most commonly used stains are summarized in Table 1-1.

TABLE 1-2 Medically Important Gram-Positive Bacteria

Shape of cell	Family/group	Genus
Cocci	Micrococcaceae	*Staphylococcus*
		Micrococcus
		Planococcus
		Stomatococcus
	Streptococcaceae	*Streptococcus*
		Enterococcus
	Miscellaneous	*Aerococcus*
		Gemella
		Lactococcus
		Leuconostoc
		Pediococcus
		Peptostreptococcus
		Sarcina
		Coprococcus
Bacilli	Spore-formers	*Bacillus*
		Clostridium
	Lactobacillaceae	*Lactobacillus*
	Actinomycetaceae	*Actinomyces*
		Bifidobacterium
	Nocardiaceae	*Nocardia*
		Rhodococcus
	Mycobacteriaceae	*Mycobacterium*
	Miscellaneous	*Propionibacterium*
		Eubacterium
		Corynebacterium
		Arcanobacterium
		Listeria
		Gardnerella
		Erysipelothrix

IDENTIFICATION AND CLASSIFICATION OF MICROORGANISMS

Detailed information about the methods used to identify microorganisms is presented throughout this text. However, note that a number of techniques are used to identify an isolated organism. As discussed previously, the microscopic and macroscopic morphological characteristics of an organism are particularly useful. In fact, most **molds** (filamentous fungi) and parasites are identified primarily by their morphological appearance. In contrast, a preliminary classification of a bacterium can be obtained by observing the microscopic appearance of the organism (e.g., staining characteristics with the Gram stain [**gram-positive** or **gram-negative**]), as well as the size and shape of the macroscopic colony. However, definitive identification requires additional testing. Likewise, the morphology of a viral particle as seen by electron microscopy may be useful for a preliminary identification. However, the expense of this procedure precludes its use for most laboratories.

TABLE 1-3 Medically Important Gram-Negative Bacteria

Shape of cell	Family/group	Genus
Cocci	Neisseriaceae	*Neisseria*
	Moraxellaceae	*Moraxella*
		Branhamella
		Acinetobacter
	Anaerobes	*Veillonella*
		Acinominococcus
		Megasphaera
Bacilli	Enterobacteriaceae	*Escherichia*
		Edwardsiella
		Citrobacter
		Salmonella
		Shigella
		Klebsiella
		Enterobacter
		Serratia
		Proteus
		Providencia
		Morganella
		Yersinia
	Vibrionaceae	*Vibrio*
		Aeromonas
		Plesiomonas
	Spirillaceae	*Campylobacter*
		Helicobacter
	Pseudomonadaceae	*Pseudomonas*
		Xanthomonas
	Pasteurellaceae	*Pasteurella*
		Haemophilus
		Actinobacillus
	Miscellaneous	*Brucella*
		Bordatella
		Francisella
		Cardiobacterium
		Kingella
		Eikenella
		Flavobacterium
		Calymmatobacterium
		Streptobacillus
		Spirillum
		Afipia
		Bartonella
	Legionellaceae	*Legionella*
		Tatlockia
		Fluoribacter
	Bacteroidaceae	*Bacteroides*
		Prevotella
		Porphyromonas
		Fusobacterium
		Bilophora
		Leptotrichia
		Wolinella

TABLE 1-4 Medically Important Miscellaneous Bacteria

Family/order	Genus
Spirochaetales	*Treponema*
	Borrelia
	Leptospira
Chlamydiaceae	*Chlamydia*
Mycoplasmataceae	*Mycoplasma*
	Ureaplasma
Rickettsiaceae	*Rickettsia*
	Coxiella
	Rochalimaea
	Ehrlichia

Measurement of specific metabolic pathways and the resultant by-products is the most important means for identifying bacteria and yeasts. During the past 25 years, this biochemical testing has increased in sophistication, utilizing a large battery of tests and computer analysis of test results. This process has increased our understanding of the diversity of microbes capable of producing human disease.

Other techniques that have been used to characterize organisms include analysis of their susceptibility to antibiotics, **bacteriocins** (small-molecular–weight proteins capable of killing specific bacteria), and viruses (also called **bacteriophages**). Although these procedures were used extensively in the past, they are technically difficult and have a limited ability to discriminate among organisms. More recently nucleic acid analysis has proved to be a powerful tool for microbial identification. Whereas this procedure was used initially for the taxonomic classification of organisms, the current ability to detect localized genes or specific genetic sequences has assumed increasing importance for the direct detection of organisms in clinical specimens. Over the next decade sophisticated techniques to amplify genetic sequences should allow rapid detection of a multitude of organisms that laboratories either cannot detect at all or cannot do so in a clinically useful, timely fashion.

Bacteria are one of the largest, most diverse groups of clinically important microbes. In Chapters 2 through 4 the molecular structure, metabolic properties, and genetic properties of this group of organisms are presented. A detailed description of specific bacteria is presented in Chapters 18 through 41. As an overview, the taxonomic classification of the major, medically important bacteria is summarized in Tables 1-2 through 1-4. Similar taxonomic summaries for fungi, parasites, and viruses are presented in Chapters 5 through 7, respectively.

QUESTIONS

1. Name the four major groups of microorganisms and their general distinguishing features.
2. Describe three microscopic procedures.
3. What microbiological stains are used to detect acid-fast organisms? fungi?

Bibliography

Balows A, Hausler W, Herrmann K, Isenberg H, Shadomy HJ, editors: *Manual of clinical microbiology*, ed 5, Washington, DC, 1991, American Society for Microbiology.

Baron E, Finegold S: *Bailey and Scott's diagnostic microbiology*, ed 8, St. Louis, 1991, Mosby.

SECTION I

MICROBIAL PHYSIOLOGY

CHAPTER 2

Bacterial Structure

CELLS are the fundamental units of living forms; they comprise all living creatures, from the smallest bacterium to the largest of the plants and animals. In all bacteria, as well as in the simplest, unicellular plants, protozoans, and fungi, each cell exists as an independent unit and must be capable of carrying out all the processes necessary for cellular survival. Other organisms, including all higher plants and animals, are composed of many cells of various types. There is a division of labor among these types, in which each is dedicated to carrying out a different set of functions necessary for the existence of the organism as a whole. The process whereby a cell becomes specialized is known as **cellular differentiation,** and the resulting cell is called a **differentiated** cell. Examples of differentiated cells include myocytes (muscle cells) specialized for contractile function and intestinal brush border cells specialized for the efficient absorption and processing of nutrients. All cells, regardless of extent of differentiation, share a common overall structure.

Our understanding of cell structure and architecture has grown as the techniques by which we can look at cells have improved in precision and sensitivity. Cells come in a wide range of sizes. Bacteria are the smallest cells and are visible only with the aid of the microscope. The smallest bacteria are only 0.1 to 0.2 μm in diameter. Larger bacteria may be many microns in length. Interestingly, a new species of bacteria has recently been described that is several hundred times larger than the average bacterial cell and is visible to the naked eye. Most species, however, are approximately 1 μm in diameter and are therefore visible using the light microscope, which has a resolution of 0.2 μm. Animal and plant cells are in general much larger and range from 7 μm (the diameter of a red blood cell) to several feet (the length of certain nerve cells).

When bacteria were discovered in the seventeenth century by Antony van Leeuwenhoek, the inventor of the microscope, the available technology allowed only a gross description of cellular shape. Even with improved optics, analysis of subcellular structure even of the larger plant and animal cells was not possible. Not until the advent of the electron microscope in the twentieth century could cell structure be analyzed in detail. The electron microscope allowed classification of cells into two major groups, based on the presence or absence of a true nucleus. Animals, plants, and fungi belong to the eukaryotes (Greek for "true nucleus"), whereas bacteria and the blue-green algae belong to the prokaryotes (Greek for "primitive nucleus"). Besides the presence of a nucleus, several other features distinguish prokaryotes and eukaryotes, as outlined in Table 2-1.

CELLULAR MEMBRANE

All cells, both prokaryotic and eukaryotic, are surrounded by the cellular or **cytoplasmic membrane** (Figure 2-1). This membrane is composed primarily of phospholipids arranged in two layers. It functions as a barrier to the leakage of substances out of the cell or entry of unwanted materials. Embedded in this **lipid bilayer** are multiple proteins, which facilitate transport of substances across the membrane and also carry out various metabolic reactions. Prokaryotic cells do not contain any internal membranes and therefore rely on the cytoplasmic membrane for carrying out all membrane-localized functions. The most important of these is aerobic respiration by which metabolic energy is produced. In contrast, eukaryotic cells contain multiple internal membrane-bound **organelles** within which different cellular processes occur (Figure 2-2). Examples of eukaryotic membrane-bound organelles include the mitochondria, endoplasmic reticulum, and Golgi apparatus.

NUCLEUS

A cell's content of genetic material (deoxyribonucleic acid or DNA) is known as its **genome.** The basic molecular structures of prokaryotic and eukaryotic DNA are indistinguishable. Both are composed of two helical chains of purine and pyrimidine nucleotides associated with one another by hydrogen bonding to form a double helix. In eukaryotes, the genetic material is enclosed within a lipid bilayer known as the **nuclear membrane.** This membrane is similar in structure to the cytoplasmic membrane except that it is interrupted at regular intervals to form openings called **nuclear pores.** These pores enable substances to pass in and out of the nucleus, allowing communication between this organelle and the cytoplasm. Within the nucleus, the eukaryotic DNA is associated with several highly basic proteins known as **histones.** The DNA

TABLE 2-1 Major Characteristics of Eukaryotes and Prokaryotes

Characteristic	Eukaryotes	Prokaryotes
Major groups	Algae, fungi, protozoa, plants, animals	Bacteria
Size (approximate)	>5 μm	1 × 3 μm
Nuclear structures		
Nucleus	Classic membrane	No nuclear membrane
Chromosomes	Strands of DNA	Single, closed strand of DNA
Cytoplasmic structures		
Mitochondria	Present	Absent
Golgi bodies	Present	Absent
Endoplasmic reticulum	Present	Absent
Ribosomes (sedimentation coefficient)	80S	70S
Cytoplasmic membrane	Contains sterols	Does not contain sterols*
Cell wall	Absent or composed of cellulose or chitin	Complex structure containing protein, lipids, and peptidoglycans
Reproduction	Sexual and asexual	Asexual (binary fission)
Movement	Flagella, if present, are complex	Flagella, if present, are simple
Respiration	Via mitochondria	Via cytoplasmic membrane

From Holt S. In Slots J, Taubman M, editors: *Contemporary oral microbiology and immunology*, St Louis, 1992, Mosby.
*Except in *Mycoplasma*.

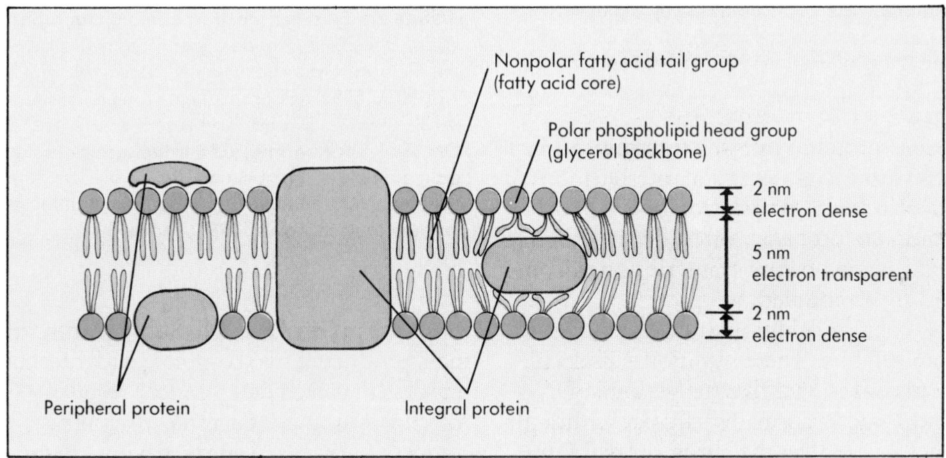

FIGURE 2-1 A diagram of classic unit membrane as visualized in both prokaryotes and eukaryotes. Hydrophilic proteins enclose a hydrophobic lipid layer. Peripheral and integral proteins are intercollated into the entire membrane. The integral proteins function to transport material from the outside to the inside of the cell and to provide structural integrity. The phospholipid head groups are embedded in the protein layers and the fatty acid tails extend into the central region of the membrane. (Modified from Newman MG, Nisengard R: *Oral microbiology and immunology*, Philadelphia, 1988, WB Saunders.)

becomes tightly wound around the histone particles, allowing the DNA strands to be organized into a compact package known as a **chromosome.**

Whereas eukaryotic DNA is organized into several individual molecules (chromosomes), the prokaryotic genome normally consists of a single circular molecule. Prokaryotic DNA is not wound with histone proteins and is not organized into discrete chromosomes. Furthermore, the prokaryotic DNA molecule is found within the cytoplasm of the cell in a discrete area known as the **nucleoid.** The absence of a nuclear membrane in prokaryotes has great functional significance. Because eukaryotic DNA is surrounded by a membrane, messenger RNA (mRNA) must be transported out of the nucleus and into

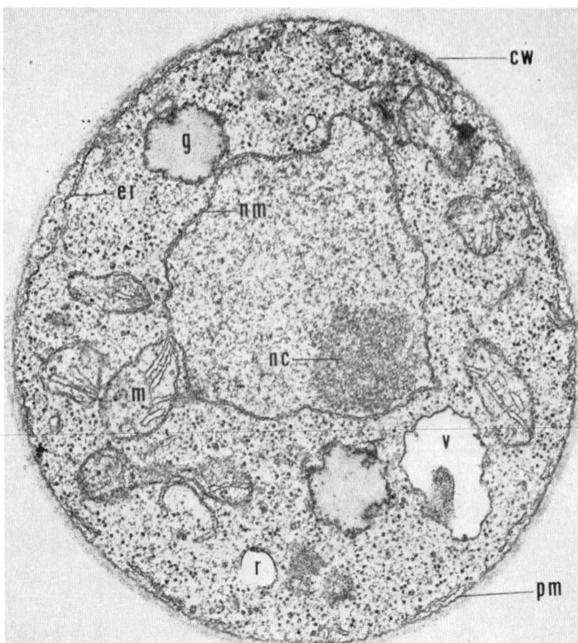

FIGURE 2-2 Electron micrograph of eukaryotic cell, the fungus *Cryptococcus neoformans.* Note the complexity of this cell, with a well-defined nucleus containing a nucleolus *(nc)* and bounded by a nuclear membrane *(nm)*. The cytoplasm contains ribosomes *(r)*, mitochondria *(m)*, vacuoles *(v)*, storage granules *(g)*, and endoplasmic reticulum *(er)*. The cell is bounded by a plasma membrane *(pm)* and a cell wall *(cw)*. (From Emmons CW et al.: *Medical mycology,* ed 2, Philadelphia, 1970, Lea & Febiger.)

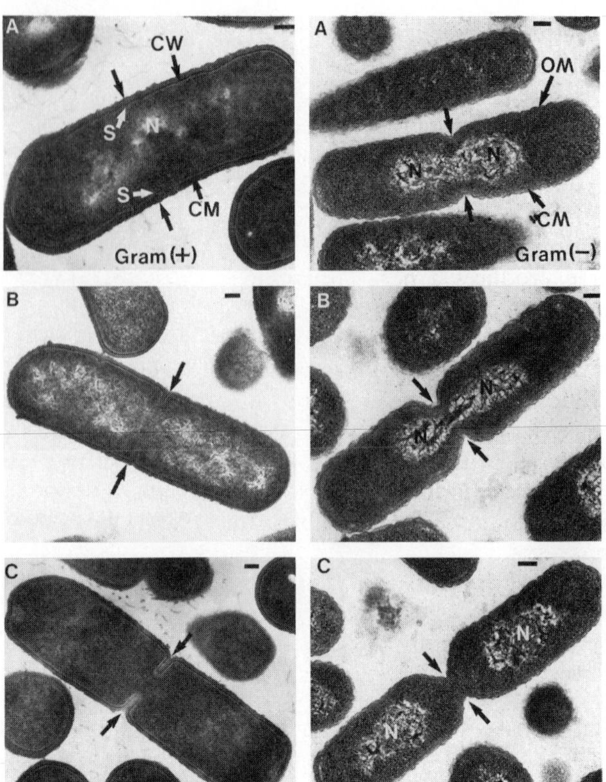

FIGURE 2-3 Selected electron photomicrographs of gram-positive *(Bacillus subtilis) (left)* and gram-negative *(Escherichia coli) (right)* cell division. Gram-positive cell division occurs by septum formation, whereas gram-negative cell division occurs by constriction. **A, B,** and **C** represent a progression in cell division. *OM,* Outer membrane; *CM,* cytoplasmic membrane; *CW,* cell wall; *S,* septum; *N,* nucleoid. Bar = 0.1 μm. (From Slots J, Taubman MA, editors: *Contemporary oral microbiology and immunology,* St. Louis, 1991, Mosby.)

the cytoplasm before protein synthesis (translation) can begin. Because this physical separation of the mRNA synthesis **(transcription)** and **translation** does not occur in prokaryotes, the two processes often occur simultaneously (translation begins before transcription is complete) and are said to be **coupled.**

Some bacteria contain additional DNA molecules beyond the genomic DNA. These additional molecules are referred to as **plasmids** and, like the genomic DNA, are double stranded and normally circular although significantly smaller in size than the chromosomal DNA. Plasmids are most commonly found in gram-negative bacteria, and although not usually essential for cellular survival, they often provide a selective advantage. Many plasmids confer resistance to one or more antibiotics. Because they can be spread from cell to cell, they contribute to proliferation of multidrug-resistant bacterial strains, making treatment of infections caused by these organisms very difficult.

Processes of cellular division are very different in prokaryotes and eukaryotes. Eukaryotic cell division occurs via a complex process known as **mitosis.** DNA synthesis occurs, and the chromosomes are each doubled, forming two sister **chromatids.** The nuclear membrane then dissolves, and a scaffolding known as the spindle apparatus is formed. The chromosomes line up on this apparatus, and the sister chromatids are pulled to opposite poles of the cell. Subsequently, the cell divides in half, producing two complete daughter cells. This process ensures that each daughter cell receives a full complement of chromosomes. Bacteria, in contrast, reproduce by a process known as **binary fission.** Because there is only one molecule of DNA, a spindle apparatus and the other components of the mitotic cycle are not necessary. Instead, the bacterial cell grows to a genetically predetermined length at which point a cross-wall is formed and two new cells are produced (Figure 2-3). Coupled with this process is the replication of the chromosome and any plasmid DNA so that the daughter cell contains a duplicate of the parental genome.

EUKARYOTIC ORGANELLES

Protein synthesis in both bacteria and eukaryotic cells takes place on **ribosomes,** which are a complex of protein and ribonucleic acid (rRNA). Eukaryotic ribosomes are somewhat larger and heavier than their prokaryotic counterparts. The former is referred to as 80S, whereas the latter is termed 70S based on this size difference and resultant differences in migration in a centrifugal field. This difference in ribosome structure is the mechanism by which certain antibiotics selectively inhibit protein synthesis by prokaryotic but not eukaryotic ribosomes. In eukaryotes, the ribosomes become associated with a complex membranous network known as the **rough endoplasmic reticulum** (see Figure 2-2). As the ribosome produces a new protein it is extruded into the endoplasmic reticulum (ER), where it may be sequestered from the remainder of the cytoplasmic components. Once within the ER the new protein may be modified by the addition of carbohydrate groups and ultimately packaged for export out of the cell. Additional eukaryotic organelles that participate in this protein modification process include the **smooth endoplasmic reticulum** (referred to as smooth since it lacks ribosomes) and the **Golgi apparatus.**

Eukaryotic cells also contain organelles, known as **mitochondria** (see Figure 2-2), which are dedicated to energy production. Mitochondria contain two lipid bilayer membranes, the more internal of which is folded numerous times to form **christae.** Embedded within the christae are components of the electron transport chain by which usable energy is produced. Bacteria, in contrast, do not possess mitochondria but instead rely on cytoplasmic and cell-membrane–localized enzymes to carry out these same functions. Interestingly, the eukaryotic mitochondria contain a genome of their own, as well as ribosomes. Mitochondrial ribosomes resemble prokaryotic ribosomes in size and structure. These similarities have led to speculation that mitochondria were derived from bacteria, which became incorporated into a eukaryotic progenitor. Moreover, the similarities between bacteria and eukaryotes often make antibiotics directed against prokaryotic ribosomes toxic to eukaryotic cells as well.

In addition to the differences just discussed, ultrastructurally, the prokaryotes differ considerably from eukaryotic cells. For example, several cell wall components are unique to bacteria in that they are found nowhere else in nature. Indeed, the presence of certain of these are the basis for classifying organisms as prokaryotes.

CELL WALLS

One of these structures unique to bacteria and upon which classification is based is the **peptidoglycan** of prokaryotic cell walls. With the exception of the Archaeobacteria (which contain a pseudoglycan or pseudomurein related to peptidoglycan) and mycoplasmas (which have no cell walls at all) the cytoplasmic membranes of all prokaryotes are surrounded by a rigid peptidoglycan layer. Since the peptidoglycan provides rigidity, it also determines the shape of the particular bacterial cell. Chemically, peptidoglycan is a regular heteropolymer of alternating molecules of *N*-acetylglucoseamine (GlcNAc) and *N*-acetylmuramic acid (MurNAc) (Figure 2-4). The GlcNAc and MurNAc sugars alternate in B,1-4 glycosidic bonds to a length of 10 to 65 disaccharide residues. The individual chains are cross-linked via short peptides consisting of L-alanine, D-glutamic acid, meso-diaminopimelic acid (DAP) or lysine, and D-alanine. Usually the covalent cross-linking occurs between the DAP and the lactyl groups of the MurNAc. The degree of cross-linking can vary considerably, with very few to many of the MurNAc moieties cross-linked. This cross-linking of the long individual chains forms a strong, rigid network providing an integral component of bacterial cell walls. The β-lactam antibiotics (penicillins and cephalosporins) inhibit peptidoglycan synthesis. Thus the interruption of the integrity of the peptidoglycan usually results in death of the bacterial cell.

Biologically, peptidoglycan interferes with phagocytosis, is **mitogenic** (stimulates mitosis of lymphocytes), and has **pyrogenic** activity (induces fever). The peptidoglycan of some streptococcal species contributes to the establishment of the chronic inflammatory response in a rheumatoid arthritis model system, as well as in a rheumatic fever model.

Gram-positive Cell Wall

Although both gram-positive and gram-negative bacteria contain peptidoglycan in their cell walls, the two types of cell walls are very different (Figure 2-5). First, the amount of peptidoglycan is quite different in that the peptidoglycan of gram-positive cell walls is usually 30 to 200 molecules thick, providing 40% to 80% of the total cell wall dry weight (Figure 2-6). These multiple layers are often cross-linked in three dimensions, providing a very strong, rigid cell wall. In contrast, the peptidoglycan in gram-negative cell walls is usually only one molecule (layer) thick (Figure 2-7). Gram-positive cell walls are usually devoid of lipids and proteins. However in unusual cases such as *Corynebacterium diphtheriae, Mycobacterium tuberculosis,* and *Nocardia asteroides,* long-chain fatty acids are components of the cell wall. Gram-positive cell walls also contain water-soluble polymers of polyol phosphates called **teichoic acids,** which are common surface antigens and function as structures that attach to other bacteria, as well as to specific receptors on mammalian cell surfaces. These teichoic acids thus are important factors in virulence. Carbohydrates present on gram-positive cell walls may be covalently bound to the peptidoglycan on the external surface and constitute an integral component of the cell wall. Alternatively, carbohydrates may be loosely bound and compose a **capsule** or **slime** layer (see the following).

Gram-negative Cell Wall

Gram-negative cell walls are much more complex, both structurally and chemically (see Figure 2-7). Structurally, the gram-negative cell wall contains two layers external to the cytoplasmic membrane. Immediately external to the cytoplasmic membrane is a thin peptidoglycan layer, which accounts for only 5% to 10% of the gram-negative cell wall by weight. It is unusual for this gram-negative

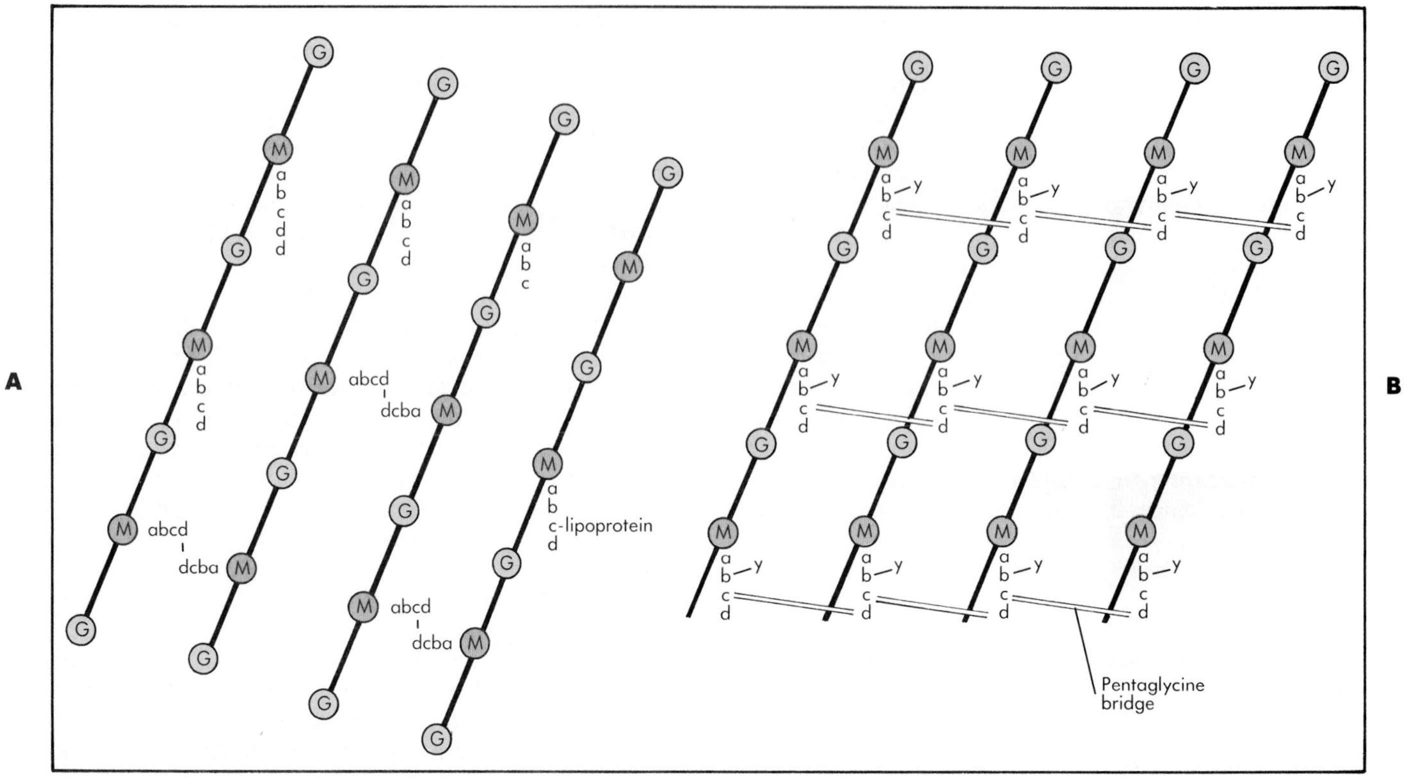

FIGURE 2-4 A, *Escherichia coli* peptidoglycan structure. **B,** *Staphylococcus aureus* peptidoglycan structure. *M,* N-acetylmuramic acid; *G,* N-acetylglucosamine; *a,* L-alanine; *b,* D-glutamic acid; *c,* either *meso*-diaminopimelic acid in **A,** or 1-lysine in **B;** *d,* D-alanine; *X,* pentaglycine bridge; *Y,* $-NH_2$. (Modified from Joklik KJ, Willet HP, Amos DB, Wilfert CM, editors: *Zinsser microbiology,* Norwalk, Conn, 1988, Appleton & Lange.)

peptidoglycan layer to contain interpeptide bridges; thus it is much less rigid than the gram-positive peptidoglycan. External to the peptidoglycan layer is the **outer membrane,** which is unique to gram-negative prokaryotes. The area between the external surface of the cytoplasmic membrane and the internal face of the outer membrane is referred to as the **periplasmic space.** This space is actually a compartment containing a variety of hydrolytic enzymes, which are important to the cell for the breakdown of large macromolecules into smaller products that the cell uses for metabolism. The composition of these enzymes varies from species to species, depending on the nutritional requirements of the cell. These enzymes typically include proteases, phosphatases, lipases, nucleases, and carbohydrate-degrading enzymes. In the case of pathogenic gram-negative species, many of the lytic virulence factors such as collagenases, hyaluronidases, and proteases are compartmentalized here. The periplasmic space also contains a variety of binding proteins, which bind specific molecules such as penicillin for transport into the cytoplasm. Some binding proteins are also components of the chemotaxis system, which senses the external environment of the cell.

Outer Membrane

As mentioned previously, the outer membrane (see Figure 2-7) is unique to gram-negative prokaryotes and functions as a molecular sieve by regulating the passage of molecules greater than 700 daltons (d) into the cell. This membrane is a typical **lipid bilayer** but differs from any other biological membrane in its lipid composition and number of proteins. The inner lipid leaflet contains phospholipids that are normally found in bacterial membranes. However, the outer leaflet is composed primarily of an amphipathic molecule (meaning it has both hydrophobic and hydrophilic ends) called the **lipopolysaccharide** (LPS). Because of its toxic and other biological properties (see the following) this molecule was originally named the **endotoxin.** Except for those LPS molecules that are in the process of synthesis, the outer leaflet of the outer membrane is the only location where LPS molecules are found, as they are never translocated to the inner leaflet of the outer membrane. Thus this membrane is asymmetrical, with phospholipids located in the inner leaflet and the LPS substituting for the phospholipids in the outer leaflet.

The array of proteins found in gram-negative outer

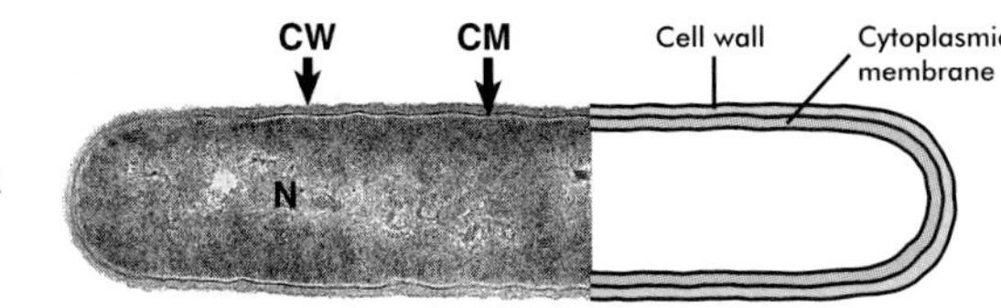

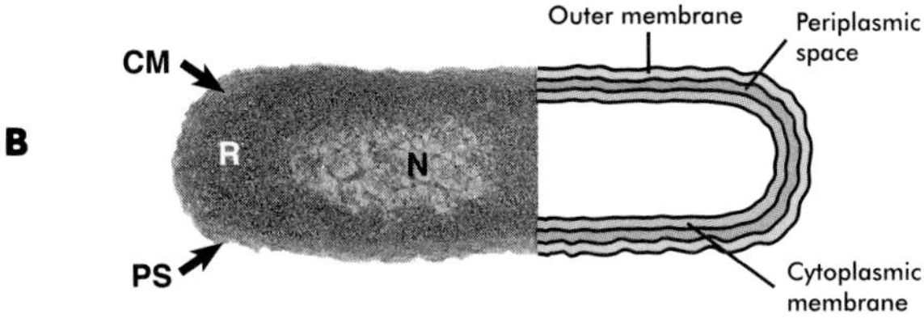

FIGURE 2-5 Transmission electron photomicrograph of the prokaryotic cells **(A)** *Bacillus subtilis* and **(B)** *Escherichia coli.* The bacteria are bound by a cell wall *(CW)* and internal cytoplasmic membrane *(CM).* A periplasmic space *(PS)* is seen between the outer membrane *(OM)* and the cytoplasmic membrane in the gram-negative *E. coli.* Ribosomes *(R)* and nucleoid *(N)* fill the cytoplasmic region. *PP,* Pyrophosphate storage granule. (From Slots J, Taubman MA, editors: *Contemporary oral microbiology and immunology,* St. Louis, 1991, Mosby.)

membranes is quite limited. However, the few proteins are present in high numbers, resulting in a total protein content higher than that of the cytoplasmic membrane. Importantly, many of the proteins of the outer membrane traverse the entire lipid bilayer and are thus **transmembrane proteins.** A group of these proteins are known as **porins** because they form pores through the membrane that allow the diffusion of hydrophilic molecules less than 700 d in size through the membrane (Figure 2-8). The outer membrane also contains **integral proteins,** which help maintain the integrity of the outer membrane, as well as peripheral proteins or surface proteins, some of which are receptor molecules for bacteriophages. The association between the outer membrane and the peptidoglycan is maintained by a **lipoprotein,** which is an intrinsic protein of the outer membrane and is linked to the peptidoglycan through DAP or lysine residues.

Lipopolysaccharide

The amphipathic LPS molecule is composed of three main regions: (1) the hydrophobic **lipid A,** (2) the **core polysaccharide,** and (3) the hydrophilic **O-antigen** or O-specific polysaccharide (see Figure 2-8). With respect to the outer membrane, the lipid A portion of the molecule is embedded in the outer leaflet, with the O-antigen extending distally from the surface of the membrane. Thus the hydrophobic portion of the molecule takes the place of phospholipids in the outer leaflet of the membrane bilayer. This portion of the LPS

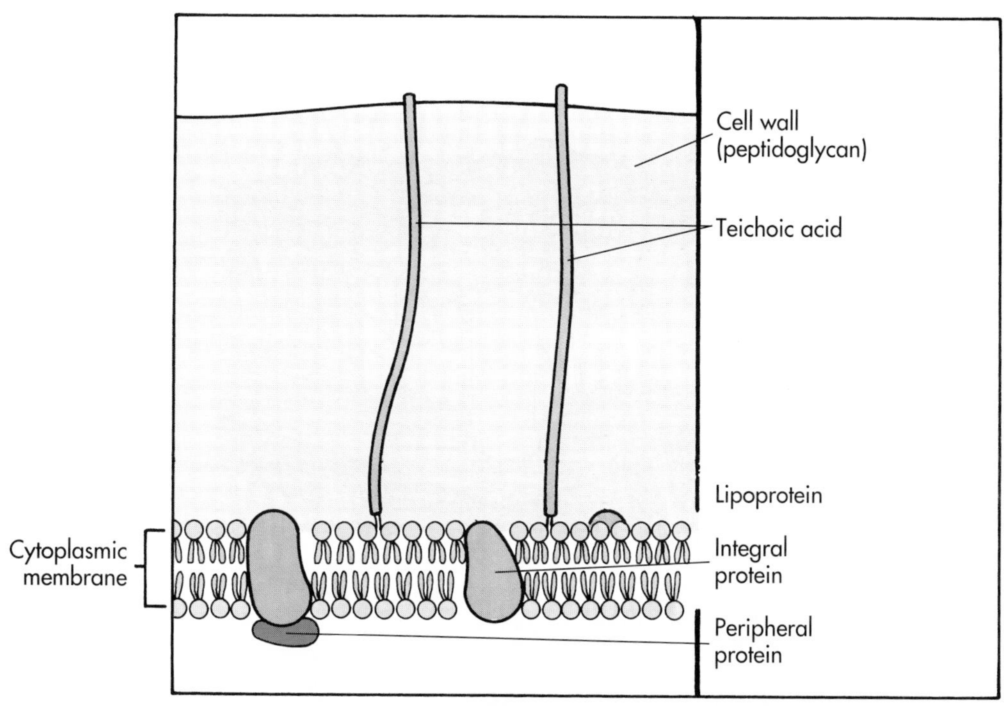

FIGURE 2-6 Three-dimensional representation of the cell wall of a gram-positive bacterium. (Modified from Newman MG, Nisengard R: *Oral microbiology and immunology,* Philadelphia, 1988, WB Saunders.)

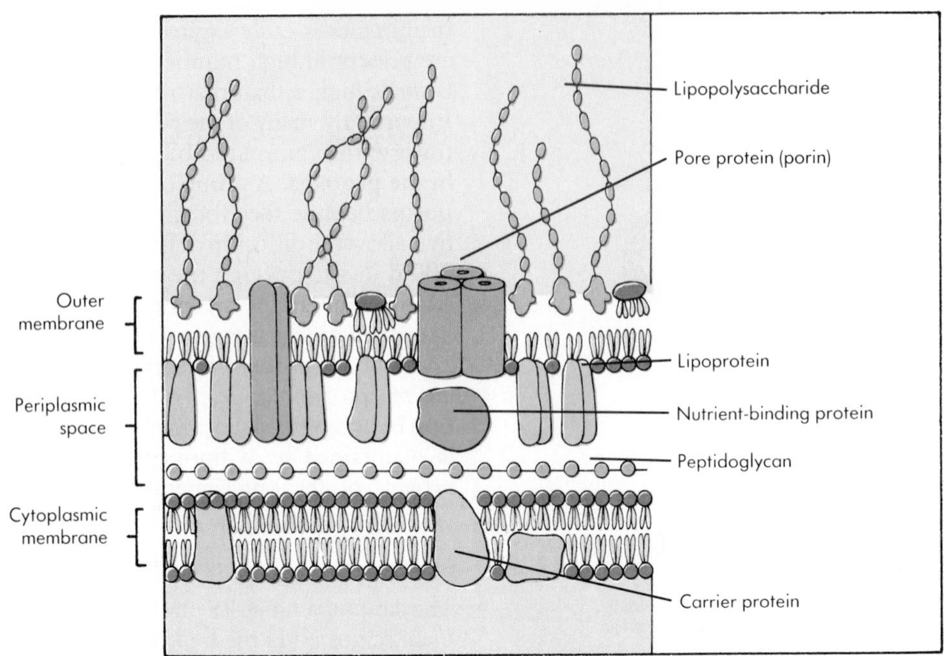

FIGURE 2-7 Three-dimensional structure of the gram-negative cell envelope. The innermost layer surrounding the cell cytoplasm is the cytoplasmic membrane. Carrier proteins embedded in the membrane facilitate transport of solutes through the membrane barrier. Outside the cytoplasmic membrane is a thin peptidoglycan layer and an outer membrane. The area between the cytoplasmic membrane and the outer membrane is referred to as the periplasmic space and is filled with hydrated peptidoglycan and binding proteins for nutrients. Within the outer membrane porin proteins and other membrane proteins are present. A lipoprotein layer binds the outer membrane to the peptidoglycan layer. Finally, a complex lipopolysaccharide is attached to the outer layer of the outer membrane. (Modified from Newman NG, Nisengard R: *Oral microbiology and immunology,* Philadelphia, 1988, WB Saunders.)

molecule consists of a glucosamine disaccharide whose hydroxyl groups are esterified with β-hydroxy fatty acids, the only β-hydroxy acids found in prokaryotes. Also attached to the disaccharide is a trisaccharide of 2-keto-3-deoxyoctonoic acid (KDO), which is an eight carbon sugar unique to LPS and thus also unique to gram-negative prokaryotes. The short outer core polysaccharide links the lipid A region to the O-antigen polysaccharide. The O-specific polysaccharide consists of repeating units of a tetrasaccharide or pentasaccharide subunit. The specific composition of these repeating units varies tremendously, producing the O-somatic antigen on which serotyping of many different gram-negative species is based. For example, there are hundreds of different serotypes of *Salmonella* based on the O-antigen composition.

In addition to O-antigen composition, variation occurs with respect to the number of repeating units in an LPS molecule. Whereas most gram-negative bacteria synthesize LPS molecules with a full length O-antigen, some species make only short molecules of O-antigen or in a few cases almost no O-specific polysaccharide at all. In addition, mutant cells that are defective in synthesizing O-antigen have been isolated and studied. All chemical forms of LPS that have very little (perhaps one unit of the tetrasaccharide) or no O-antigen are called "rough" LPS molecules, as opposed to the full size "smooth" molecules. This terminology is based on the colonial morphology of each cell type, with those bacterial cells that have a truncated LPS appearing as colonies with rough edges when grown on agar plates and those with the full length LPS molecules appearing as normally smooth colonies. The bacterial mutants in LPS biosynthesis that have been isolated have proved that the presence of the O-antigen is not essential for cell viability, but that the presence of the lipid A is essential. It should be understood, however, that the presence of the O-antigen is important in resistance to certain antibiotics and may be important for survival in the host.

LPS is a heat stable toxin (even stable to autoclaving), which is liberated from gram-negative bacteria upon lysis and cell death. This endotoxic activity is associated with the lipid A component and elicits a broad spectrum of pathophysiological effects. When present in sufficient quantities in the blood, LPS will cause death within 1 or 2 hours because of irreversible shock and cardiovascular collapse. In lesser amounts, LPS functions as an activator of a variety of inflammatory mediators including activation of the complement cascade by the alternate pathway, and activation of tumor necrosis factor, interleukin-1, and

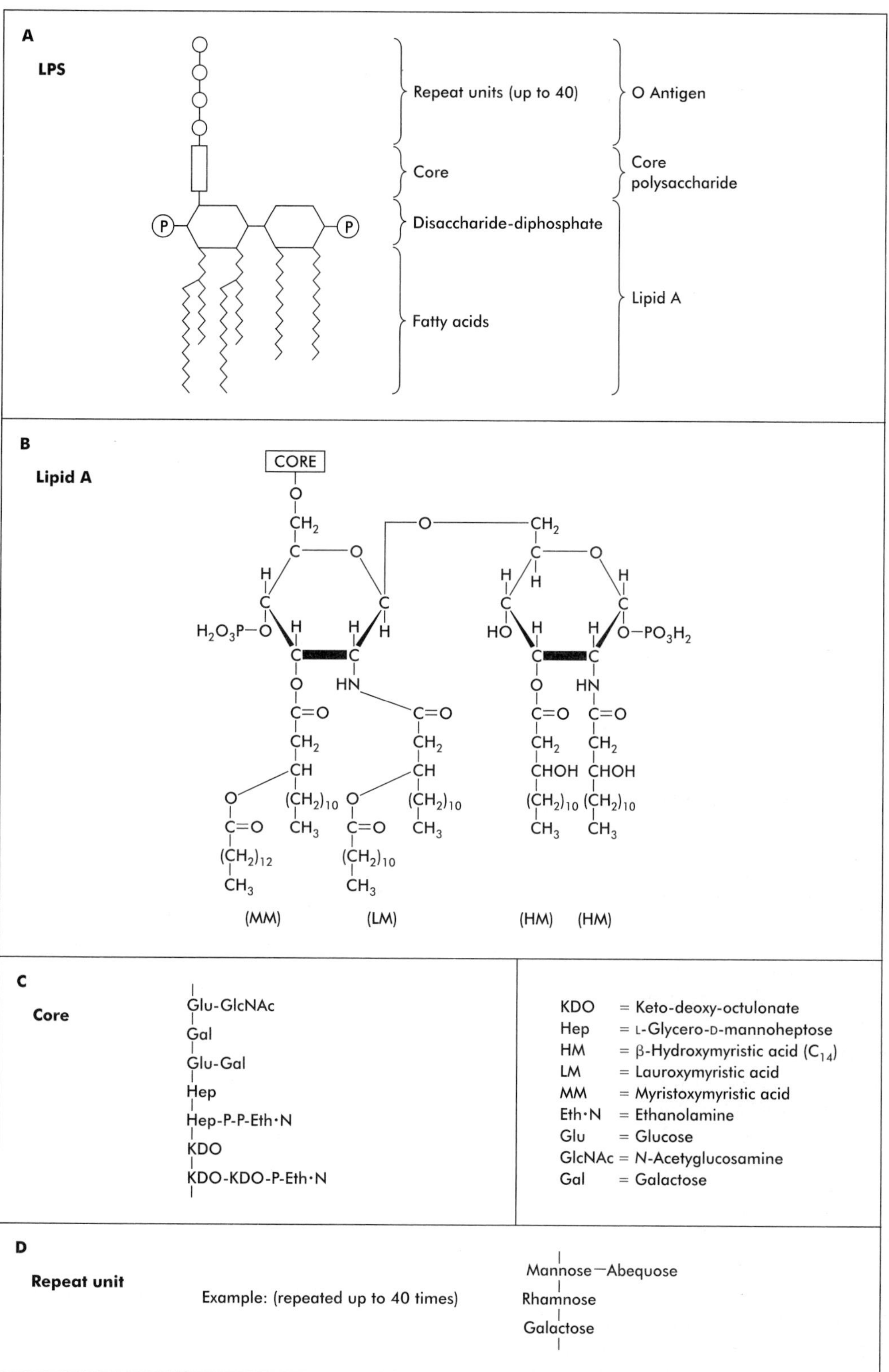

FIGURE 2-8 The lipopolysaccharide *(LPS)* of the gram-negative cell envelope. **A,** Segment of the polymer showing the arrangements of the major constituents. **B,** Structure of lipid A of *Salmonella typhimurium.* **C,** Polysaccharide core. **D,** Typical repeat unit *(Salmonella typhimurium).* (Redrawn from Brooks GF, Butel JS, Ornston LN, editors: *Jawetz, Melnick and Adelberg's medical microbiology,* ed 19, Norwalk, Conn, 1991, Appleton & Lange.)

prostaglandins. In cell culture, LPS is toxic to fibroblasts and other cell lines. In addition, it is pyrogenic, causes platelet aggregation, increases resistance to certain antibiotics, causes resistance to phagocytosis, and plays a role in bone resorption. Thus on biological terms, the LPS of gram-negative bacteria is among the most active components of prokaryotes.

Capsules and Slimes

Almost without exception, pathogenic and commensal bacteria are capable of producing copious amounts of extracellular slime or capsular material. When this material is closely associated with the cell surface, it is referred to as a **capsule** (Figure 2-9). In cases when it is loosely adherent and nonuniform in density or thickness, the material is referred to as a **slime layer.** Except for the case of *Bacillus anthracis,* which produces a polypeptide capsule, all other host-associated bacteria studied to date produce polysaccharide capsules or slimes. These capsules and slimes are extremely hydrated; preparation of capsules or slimes by normal electron-microscopic techniques produces images of capsules that actually represent only 3% to 5% of their size in vivo because the processing of the specimens for electron microscopy requires that the sample be dehydrated.

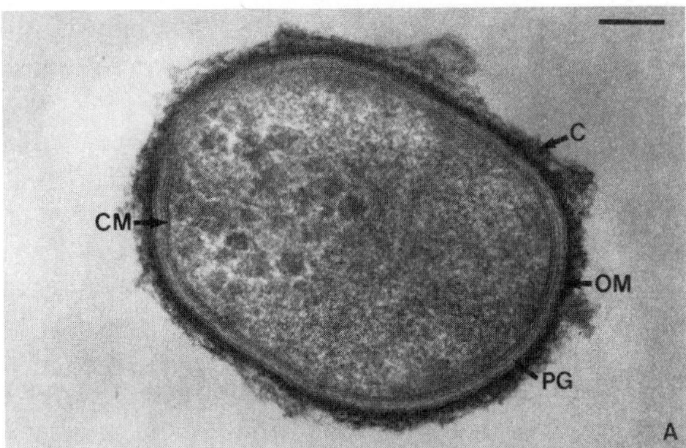

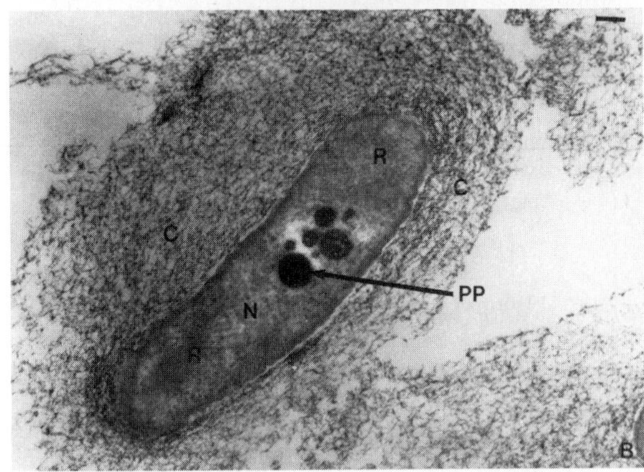

FIGURE 2-9 Transmission electron photomicrograph of *Porphyromonas* (formerly *Bacteroides*) *gingivalis* and *Pseudomonas aeruginosa* revealing the surface-associated capsule. Both strains were isolated from human patients; *P. gingivalis* from an adult periodontis patient and *P. aeruginosa* from a cystic fibrosis patient. *C,* Capsule; *OM,* outer membrane; *PG,* peptidoglycan; *CM,* cytoplasmic membrane; *PP,* polyphosphate; *R,* ribosome. Bar = 0.1 μm. (From Slots J, Taubman MA, editors: *Contemporary oral microbiology and immunology,* St. Louis, 1991, Mosby.)

Capsules and slimes are known as accessory structures because they are not required for cell growth in vitro. Interestingly most bacterial species produce capsules or slimes when first cultured from a host. However, upon successive transfers, many of the isolates will no longer produce these materials, possibly because the presence of the capsule on the cell surface offers no selective advantage in normal in vitro situations. In the host, capsule and slime synthesis is regulated, with the bacterial cells producing the extracellular materials when necessary for survival in the host but turning off the formation when the presence of a capsule would be a disadvantage.

The primary function of most capsules and slime layers is to serve as antiphagocytic structures. Importantly, in mixed infections, the presence of a capsule or a slime layer on one bacterial species may protect neighboring unrelated bacteria from phagocytosis. Capsules may also protect the cell from other hazards of the environment including the presence of antibiotics. For example, the strains of *Pseudomonas aeruginosa* found in the lungs of cystic fibrosis patients produce unusually large amounts of capsular material. Because of the presence of this material, normal concentrations of antibiotics cannot penetrate to the bacterial cell wall. Thus higher than normal concentrations of antibiotics are often required for treatment.

In some cases bacterial capsules also function as adhesins and thus provide the specific adherence interactions between the bacterial cell and the host tissues or between the bacterial cell and other bacterial cells. The most completely studied example of this is *Streptococcus mutans,* which is the etiological agent of dental caries. The dextran and levan capsules of this group of bacteria are the means by which these bacteria attach and stick to the tooth enamel. Because this tight adherence to the tooth surface is required for caries formation, the capsules are considered virulence factors.

SURFACE APPENDAGES

Flagella

Bacterial **flagella** are proteinacious, helically coiled organelles of motility that extend outward from the cell surface. Bacterial species may have one or several flagella on their surface (Table 2-2). Since the arrangement and number of flagella on the bacterial surface is characteristic of a particular species, flagellar arrangement is often used as a means of taxonomic classification. Until recently, no relationship between motility and virulence was known. Although not all bacteria produce flagella, it is now apparent that motility and thus the presence of functioning flagella is a virulence factor for some bacteria.

Fimbriae and Pili

Fimbriae (Latin for "fringe"), or the original term **pili,** are hairlike projections on the bacterial cell surface. Pili were originally described as protein projections on gram-negative cell surfaces. However, because gram-positive bacteria may also have hairlike projections and these may also contain carbohydrates, the term *fimbriae* is now used to denote any nonflagellar hairlike projection. The term *pili* is presently reserved for the appendages of gram-negative bacterial species involved in the formation of conjugal pairs for the transfer of DNA between bacterial cells via conjugation. Fimbriae can be distinguished from flagella morphologically because they are smaller in diameter (3 to 8 nm vs 15 to 20 nm) and usually not coiled in structure. There are generally several hundred fimbriae arranged peritrichously (uniformly) over the entire surface of the bacterial cell. They may be as long as 15 to 20 μm, or many times the length of the cell.

The primary function of fimbriae is to mediate adherence of the bacterial cell to other bacteria, to mammalian cells, or to hard and soft surfaces. Fimbriae are very specific in their attachment to other surfaces because they interact with only certain sugars. Since fimbriae are organelles responsible for adherence, they are often considered virulence factors. The presence of fimbriae is a characteristic most common among pathogenic bacteria of the mucosal surfaces. As such, urinary tract pathogens such as *Escherichia coli* typically are fimbriated. In some cases a direct and required aspect of virulence is the presence of fimbriae. One of the strongest cases for the direct relationship of fimbriation and virulence is *Neisseria gonorrhoeae.* Virulent strains of *N. gonorrhoeae* are fimbriated and are able to adhere to genital tract mucosal surfaces. However, avirulent *N. gonorrhoeae* do not have fimbriae and are unable to adhere to the host tissue. The presence of specific fimbriae is also a requirement for *E. coli* to colonize and infect the urinary tract.

TABLE 2-2 Taxonomic Descriptions of Prokaryotes Based on Numbers and Arrangements of Flagella

Terminology	Flagellum arrangement
Atrichous	No flagella
Monotrichous	One flagellum at one end
Amphitrichous	One or more flagella at each end
Lophotrichous	Two or more flagella at one or both ends
Peritrichous	Flagella surrounding the cell
Polar	*Monotrichous,* a single flagellum at one or both ends of the cell *Multitrichous,* two or several flagella at one or both ends of the cell
Lateral	Flagella arise predominantly from the middle pole of the cell *Monotrichous,* one flagellum Multitrichous, several flagella in the form of a tuft originate from the midportion of the cell
Peritrichous	Random, haphazard arrangement of flagella scattered around the bacterial cell
Mixed	The presence of two or more flagella exhibiting distinctly different physical properties in different regions of the bacterial cell

Modified from Wistreich and Lechtman: *Microbiology and human disease,* ed 2, Mission Hills, Calif, 1976, Glencoe Press.

SPORES

Some pathogenic, gram-positive bacteria such as members of the genera *Bacillus* and *Clostridium* are spore-formers. Under harsh environmental conditions such as the loss of a nutritional requirement, they can convert from the **vegetative state** to a **dormant state** or **spore.** The conversion process includes the formation of numerous spore coats and the uptake of calcium with the synthesis of dipicolinic acid. At the end of this process the spore is a dehydrated, highly refractile particle containing the genomic DNA. This DNA is resistant to desiccation, intense heat, radiation, and attack by most enzymes and chemical agents. In fact, bacterial spores are so resistant to environmental factors that they can exist for centuries as viable spores. The germination or transformation of spores into the vegetative state is stimulated by either mild heating or the presence of certain amino acids such as alanine. Once the germination process has begun, the spore will take up water, swell, shed its coats, and produce one new vegetative cell identical to the original vegetative cell, thus completing the entire cycle.

Clearly, the structural components of bacterial cells are not inert structures but interact in various ways with the host tissues. Many of these components contribute significantly to the virulence of pathogenic genera.

QUESTIONS

1. Compare the peptidoglycan layers of gram-negative and gram-positive bacterial cell walls.
2. What are the structural differences between gram-positive and gram-negative cell walls?
3. List the components that are unique to lipopolysaccharide.
4. Contrast eukaryotic and prokaryotic cell structure.
5. What prokaryotic structures are targets of antimicrobial agents?

Bibliography

Gunsalus IC, Sokatch JR, and Ornston LN, editors: *The bacteria,* vol 7, New York, 1979, Academic Press.

Joklik KJ, Willet HP, Amos DB, and Wilfert CM, editors: *Zinsser microbiology,* Norwalk, Conn, 1988, Appleton & Lange.

Slots J and Taubman MA, editors: *Contemporary oral microbiology,* St. Louis, 1992, Mosby.

Stanier RY, Doudorodd M, and Adelberg EA: *The microbial world,* ed 4, Englewood Cliffs, NJ, 1976, Prentice Hall.

CHAPTER 3

Bacterial Metabolism

ALL living cells require water as well as certain nutrients to grow and divide (Table 3-1). Among the inorganic substances (trace elements) are ions such as Mg^{2+}, Zn^{2+}, Mn^{2+}, Co^{+}, and Fe^{3+}, which function as cofactors in a variety of enzyme systems. Similarly, Na^{+} is essential for certain nutrient transport systems. Phosphorous (as PO_4) is an essential constituent of nucleotides and phospholipids, whereas sulfur is found in certain coenzymes (e.g., acetyl-CoA) as well as in two of the amino acids. Similarly, a source of nitrogen (either as NH_4^{+} or organic nitrogen compounds) is essential for the synthesis of amino acids and nucleotides. Finally, oxygen is a component of a variety of essential compounds and, in addition, functions in its elemental form as the terminal electron acceptor in aerobic respiration, the process by which energy in the form of adenosine triphosphate (ATP) is produced.

Among the organic compounds necessary for growth are carbohydrates, which function in cellular structure and energy production; amino acids and nucleotides, which represent the building blocks for proteins and nucleic acids, respectively; and lipids, which are the major component of the cellular membrane. Finally, the vitamins, like the trace elements described above, are required in small quantities and function as cofactors for certain enzymatic reactions.

Although all living cells share the same basic nutritional needs, different cells or cell types have different specific requirements depending on their biosynthetic repertoire. For example, human cells are incapable of synthesizing certain amino acids and certain types of lipids. Since these substances are necessary for cellular survival, they must be provided exogenously. A great diversity exists within the prokaryotic kingdom in specific growth requirements. For example, certain strains of *Escherichia coli* (a member of the intestinal flora), when provided with the inorganic nutrients listed previously plus a simple source of carbon, such as glucose, can synthesize all of the amino acids, nucleotides, lipids, and carbohydrates necessary for growth and division. At the other extreme are bacteria such as the causative agent of syphilis, *Treponema pallidum,* whose growth requirements are so complex that a defined laboratory medium that can support its growth has yet to be found.

Because of this diversity, growth requirements may be used as a convenient means of classifying different bacteria. For example, unlike animal cells, not all bacteria require oxygen for growth. Some organisms such as *Clostridium perfringens,* which causes gas gangrene, are unable to grow in the presence of oxygen. Such bacteria are referred to as **obligate anaerobes.** Other organisms such as *Mycobacterium tuberculosis,* which causes tuberculosis, require the presence of molecular oxygen for growth and are hence referred to as **obligate aerobes.** The vast majority of bacteria, however, fall in between and will grow in either the presence or the absence of oxygen. These bacteria are referred to as **facultative.** One may also classify bacteria on the basis of the predominant source of carbon. Those that utilize CO_2 as the predominant source of carbon for the synthesis of organic compounds are referred to as **autotrophs (lithotrophs),** whereas cells, like animal cells, that utilize organic carbon sources are known as **heterotrophs (organotrophs).**

METABOLISM AND THE CONVERSION OF ENERGY

All cells require a constant supply of energy to survive. This energy, typically in the form of ATP, is derived from the ordered breakdown of various organic substrates (carbohydrates, lipids, and proteins). This process of substrate breakdown and conversion into usable energy is known as **catabolism.** The energy produced may then be used in the synthesis of cellular constituents (cell walls, proteins, fatty acids, and nucleic acids), a process known as **anabolism.** Together these two processes, which are interrelated and tightly integrated, are referred to as **intermediary metabolism.**

The specific metabolic pathways used by bacteria for the breakdown and synthesis of organic substrates are, for the most part, shared by all living cells (prokaryotic and eukaryotic). These similarities form the basis for the concept of the **unity** of biochemistry (i.e., the chemistry of all life forms is essentially the same, and the mechanisms for the synthesis of energy as ATP, the synthesis and functioning of the genetic code, and the identification of the metabolic pathways for degrading carbohydrates, proteins, and lipids are essentially identical). This com-

TABLE 3-1 Essential Elements, Their Sources, and Functions in Prokaryotes

Element	Source	Function in metabolism
MAJOR ESSENTIAL ELEMENTS		
C*	Organic compounds, CO_2	Major components of cellular material
O*	O_2, H_2O, organic compounds	
H*	H_2, H_2O, organic compounds	
N*	NH_4^+, NO_3, N_2, organic compounds	
S*	$SO^{2}/_{4}^{-}$, HS^-, S_0, $S_2O^{2}/_{3}$, organic sulfur compounds	Constituent of S-containing amino acids, cysteine, methionine, thiamine pyrophosphate, coenzyme A, biotin, and α-lipoic acid
P*	HPO, $HPO^{2}/_{4}^{-}$	Constituent of nucleic acids, phospholipids, nucleotides
K*	K^+	Major inorganic cation, cofactor (e.g., pyruvate kinase)
Mg*	Mg^{2+}	Cofactor of many enzymes (e.g., kinases); component of cell walls, membranes, ribosomes, and phosphate esters
Ca*	Ca^{2+}	Component of exoenzymes (amylases, proteases) and cell walls: major component of endospores as Ca-dipicolinate
Fe*	Fe^{2+}, Fe^{3+}	Present in cytochromes, ferredoxins, and other iron-sulfur proteins; cofactor (dehydratases)
Na	Na^+	Transport
Cl	Cl^-	Important inorganic anion
MINOR ESSENTIAL ELEMENTS		
Zn	Zn^{2+}	Component of the enzymes alcohol dehydrogenase, alkaline phosphatase, aldolase, RNA and DNA polymerase
Mn	Mn^{2+}	Present in superoxide dismutase; cofactor of the enzymes PEP carboxykinase, isocitrate synthase
Mo	$MoO^{2}/_{4}$	Present in nitrate reductase, nitrogenase, xanthine dehydrogenase, and formate dehydrogenase
Se	$SeO^{2}/_{3}$	Component of glycine reductase and formate dehydrogenase
Co	Co^{2+}	Required element in coenzyme B_{12}-containing enzymes (glutamate mutase, methylmalonyl-CoA mutase)
Cu	Cu^{2+}	Present in cytochrome oxidase and nitrite reductase
Ni	Ni^{2+}	Present in urease, hydrogenase, and in factor F_{430}
W	$wo^{2}/_{4}$	Present in some formate dehydrogenases

Modified from Gottschalk E: *Bacterial metabolism*, ed 2, New York, 1985, Springer-Verlag.

monality has practical significance: Since bacteria are often more suitable for manipulation in the laboratory than plant or animal cells are, they provide excellent models by which to study metabolism. Indeed many of the metabolic pathways were initially elucidated based on early studies with bacteria.

The metabolic process generally begins with the hydrolysis of large macromolecules in the external cellular environment by specific enzymes or exoenzymes. The small subunit molecules produced (monosaccharides, short peptides, and fatty acids) may then be transported into the cytoplasm where they may be converted by one or more pathways to one common universal intermediate, pyruvic acid. From pyruvic acid the carbons derived from the imported nutrients may be channeled toward either energy production or the synthesis of new carbohydrates, amino acids, lipids, and nucleic acids.

Metabolism of Glucose

The current level of knowledge of bacterial metabolism is very extensive. For the sake of simplicity, this section will present an overview of the pathways by which the model carbohydrate, glucose, is metabolized to produce energy or other usable substrates. For a discussion of metabolism of other organic compounds including proteins and lipids, see a textbook of biochemistry such as listed in the Bibliography.

Embden-Myerhof-Parnas (EMP) Pathway

Bacteria utilize three major metabolic pathways in the catabolism of glucose. Most common among these is the glycolytic or Embden-Myerhof-Parnas (EMP) pathway (Figure 3-1). This pathway represents the primary means in both bacteria and eukaryotic cells for the conversion of glucose to pyruvate, which, as noted previously, is central

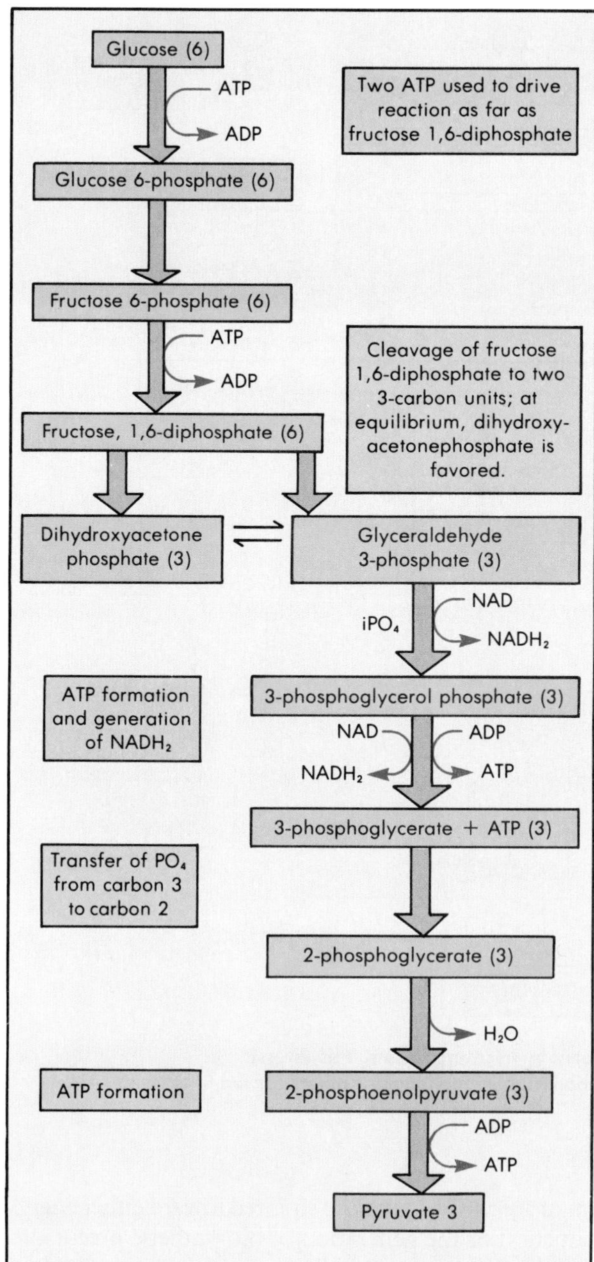

FIGURE 3-1 Embden-Meyerhof-Parnas (EMP) glycolytic pathway results in the conversion of glucose to pyruvate. Sum of glucose + 2 ADP + 2 Pi + 2 NAD → 2 pyruvate + 4 ATP + 2 NADH + 2 H^+. Double arrows denote 2 moles reacting per mole of glucose.

to a variety of other cellular metabolic pathways. These reactions, which occur under both aerobic and anaerobic conditions, begin with the "activation" of glucose to form glucose-6-phosphate. This reaction, as well as the third reaction in the series, in which fructose-6-phosphate is converted to fructose-1,6-diphosphate, requires one mole of ATP per mole of glucose and represents an initial investment of cellular energy stores.

Energy is produced during glycolysis in two different forms. In the first, the high energy phosphate group of one of the intermediates in the pathway is utilized under the direction of the appropriate enzyme (a **kinase**) to generate ATP from ADP. This type of reaction is termed **substrate level phosphorylation** and occurs at two different points in the glycolytic pathway (i.e., conversion of 3-phosphoglycerol phosphate to 3-phosphoglycerate and 2-phosphoenolpyruvic acid to pyruvate). Four ATP molecules are produced in this manner per molecule of glucose. Accounting for the two ATP molecules consumed in the initial reactions, the glycolytic conversion of glucose to two molecules of pyruvic acid results in the net production of two molecules of ATP. The NADH produced represents the second form of energy, which may then be converted to ATP in the presence of oxygen.

In the absence of oxygen, substrate level phosphorylation represents the primary means of energy production. The pyruvic acid produced from glycolysis is then converted to a variety of end products characteristic of the bacterial species in question in a process known as **fermentation.** Many bacteria are identified on the basis of their fermentative end products (Figure 3-2). This process also allows the recycling of the oxidized nicotinamide-adenine dinucleotide (NAD) from the reduced form produced during glycolysis. In yeast, fermentative metabolism results in the conversion of pyruvate to ethanol. Alcoholic fermentation is uncommon in bacteria, which most commonly employ the one step conversion of pyruvic acid to lactic acid. This process is responsible for making milk into yogurt and cabbage into sauerkraut. Other bacteria utilize more complex fermentative pathways, producing various acids, alcohols, and often gases. These products lend flavors to various cheeses and wines.

Tricarboxylic Acid Cycle

In the presence of oxygen, the pyruvic acid produced from glycolysis, as well as from metabolism of other substrates, may be completely oxidized to CO_2 using the tricarboxylic acid (TCA) cycle (Figure 3-3), which results in the production of additional energy. The process begins with the oxidative decarboxylation of pyruvate to the high energy intermediate, acetyl-CoA; this reaction also produces NADH. The two remaining carbons derived from pyruvate then enter the TCA cycle by condensation with oxaloacetate, with the formation of citrate. In a stepwise series of oxidative reactions, the citrate is converted back to oxaloacetate, with the net production of 2 moles of CO_2, 3 moles of NADH, 1 mole of FADH, and 1 mole of GTP. The latter is produced via substrate level phosphorylation in a reaction in which succinyl-CoA is converted to succinate.

The TCA cycle allows the organism to generate substantially more energy per mole of glucose than is possible with glycolysis alone. In addition to the GTP (an ATP equivalent) produced by substrate level phosphorylation, the NADH and FADH produced may enter the

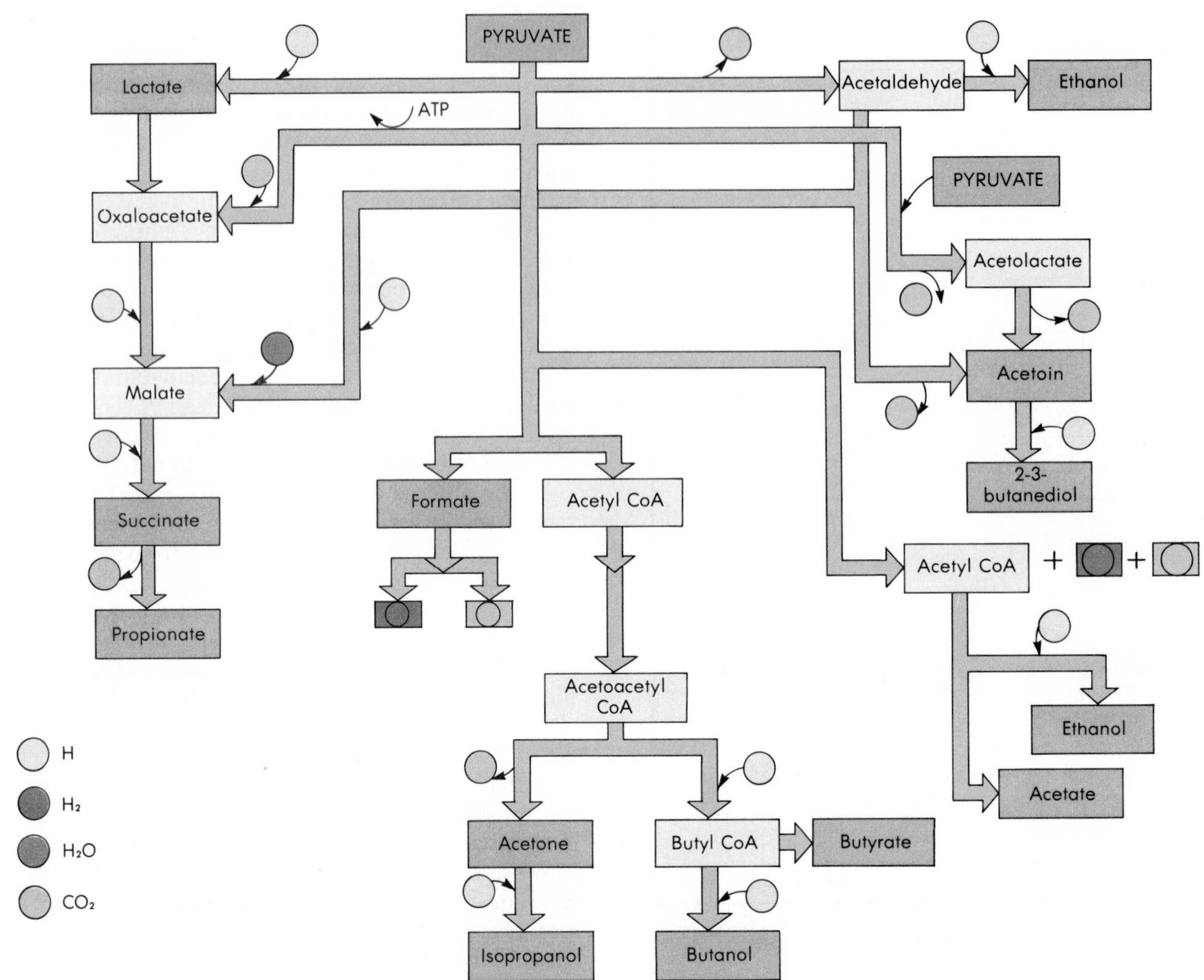

FIGURE 3-2 Diversity of pyruvate metabolism demonstrated by microorganisms. This diversity of metabolic products has been exploited in the clinical laboratory as phenotypic markers for the differential classification of microbial isolates.

electron transport chain. In this chain, the electrons carried by **NADH** (or FADH) are passed in a stepwise fashion through a series of donor/acceptor pairs and ultimately to oxygen (Figure 3-4). This process, known as **aerobic respiration,** results in the generation of 3 moles of ATP per mole of NADH and 2 moles of ATP per mole of FADH. The energetics of aerobic glucose metabolism are depicted in Figure 3-5.

Note that in anaerobic organisms in which there is no aerobic electron transport and no complete TCA cycle, only the first conversion occurs. Thus, in comparison with the 2 ATPs per glucose produced via glycolysis in these organisms, organisms capable of aerobic metabolism can generate 19 times more energy from the same starting material as anaerobic organisms can.

In addition to the efficient generation of ATP from glucose (and other carbohydrates), the TCA cycle represents a means by which carbons derived from lipids (in the form of acetyl-CoA) may be shunted toward either energy production or the generation of biosynthetic precursors. Similarly, the cycle includes several points at which amino acid skeletons may enter (see Figure 3-3). For example, deamination of glutamic acid yields alpha-ketoglutarate, whereas deamination of aspartic acid yields oxaloacetate, both of which are TCA cycle intermediates. The TCA cycle therefore serves several functions: (1) it is the major mechanism for the generation of ATP; (2) it serves as the final common pathway for the complete oxidation of amino acids (Figure 3-6), fatty acids, and carbohydrates; and (3) it supplies key intermediates (i.e., alpha-ketoglutarate, succinyl-CoA, and oxaloacetate) for the ultimate synthesis of amino acids, lipids, purines, and pyrimidines. The last two functions make the TCA cycle a so-called **amphibolic** cycle (i.e., it may function in both the anabolic and the catabolic functions of the cell.

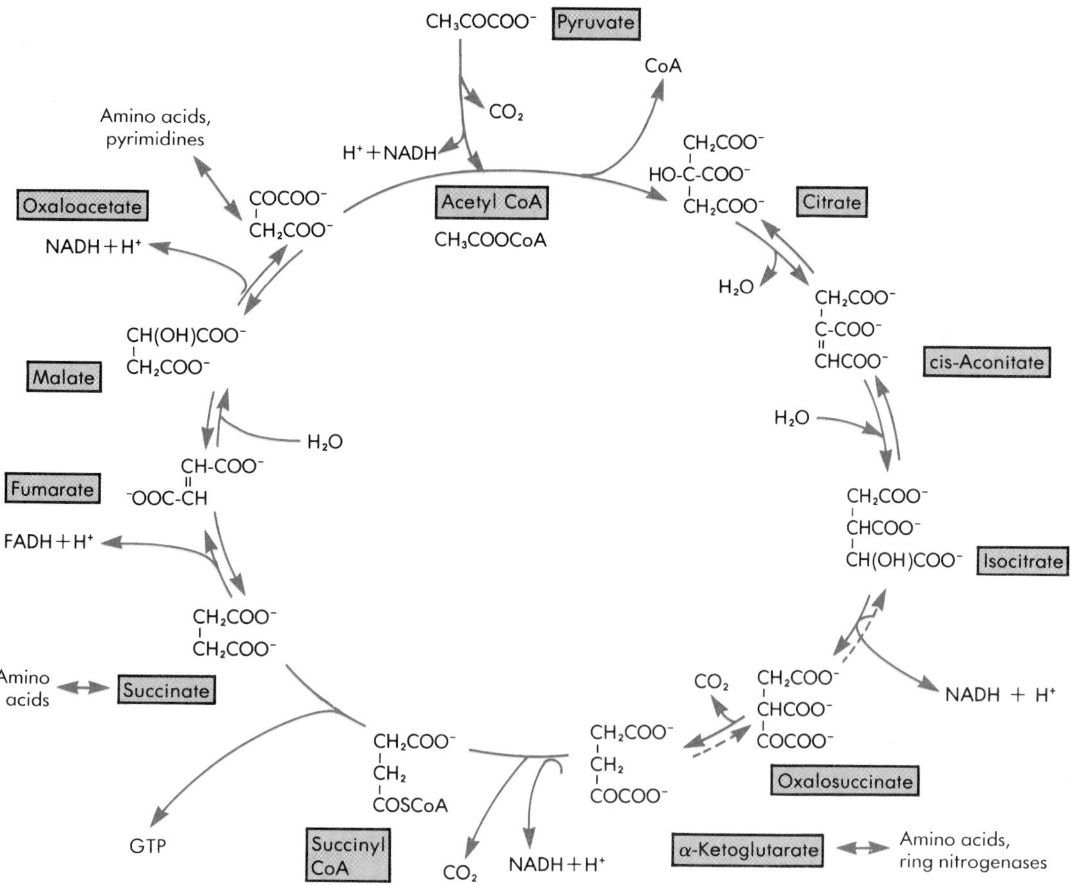

FIGURE 3-3 Tricarboxylic acid (TCA) cycle occurs in aerobic conditions and is an amphibolic cycle.

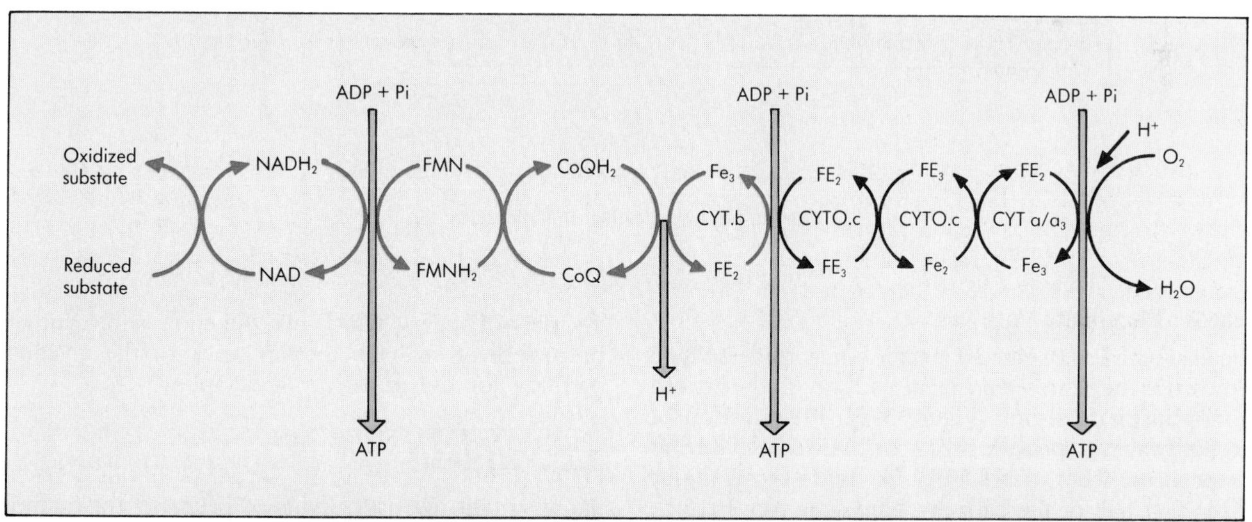

FIGURE 3-4 Electron transport chain, showing sequential oxidation steps and energy-generating steps. Electron transfer is accompanied by a flow of protons (H^+) from $NADH_2$ through coenzyme Q but not in later steps involving cytochromes. Three ATPs are formed per molecule of $NADH_2$ reoxidized but only two ATPs are formed per molecule of $FADH_2$ reoxidized. (Redrawn from Slots J, Taubman MA, editors: *Contemporary oral microbiology and immunology,* St. Louis, 1992, Mosby.)

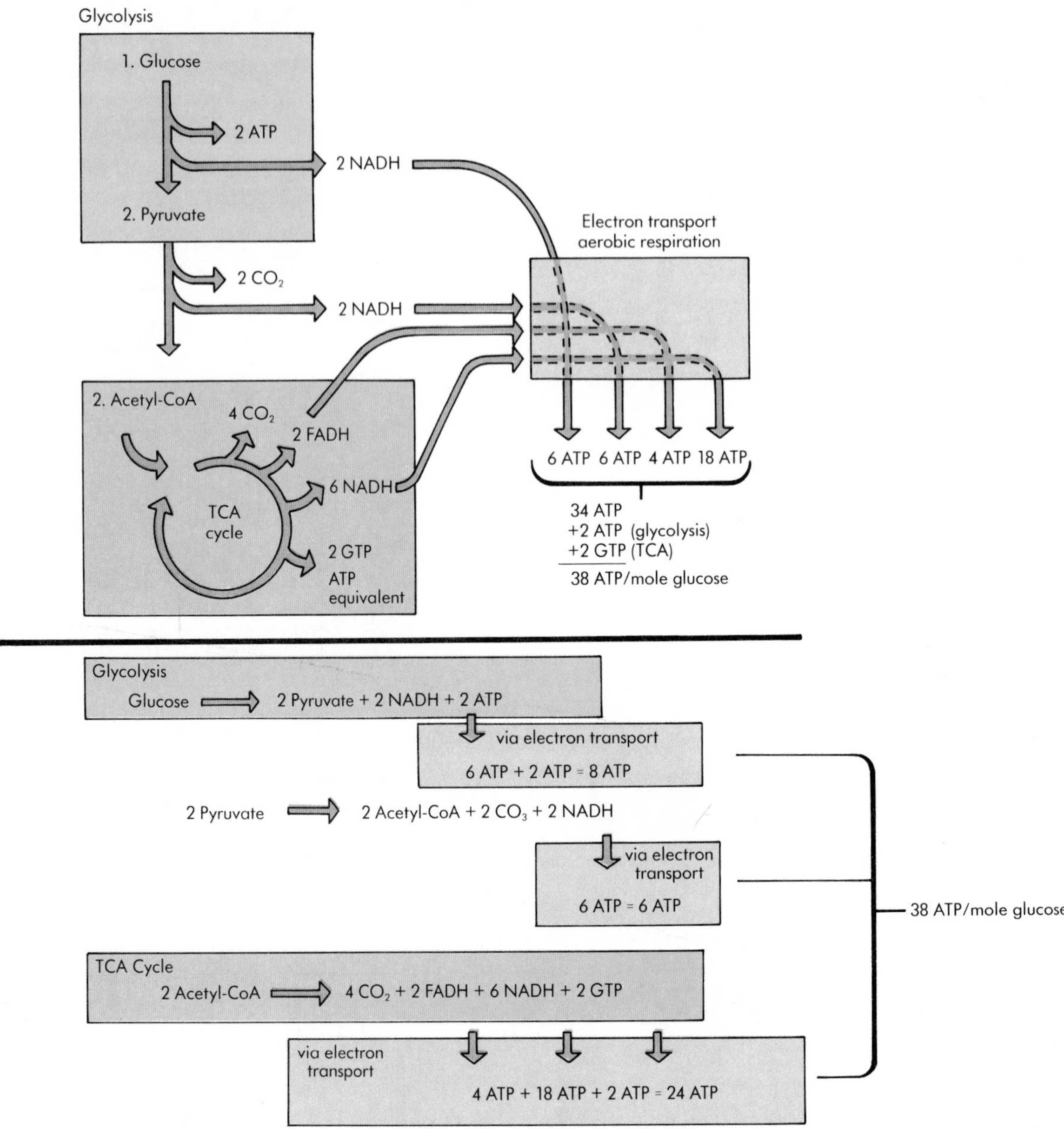

FIGURE 3-5 Aerobic glucose metabolism.

Pentose Phosphate Pathway

The final pathway of glucose metabolism considered here is known as the pentose phosphate pathway, or the **hexose monophosphate shunt** (Figure 3-7). The function of this pathway is to provide precursors, as well as reducing power in the form of **NADPH** for use in biosynthesis. In the first half of the pathway, glucose is converted to ribulose-5-phosphate, with consumption of 1 mole of ATP and generation of 2 moles of NADPH per mole of glucose. The ribulose-5-phosphate may then be converted to ribose-5-phosphate, a precursor in nucleotide biosynthesis or alternatively, xylulose-5-phosphate. The remaining reactions in the pathway employ enzymes known as transketolases and transaldolases to generate a variety of sugars, which may function as biosynthetic precursors or may be shunted back to the glycolytic pathway for use in energy generation.

BIOSYNTHESIS

To this point, we have discussed primarily the catabolic pathways of the bacterial cell, pathways that result in the generation of ATP, NAD(P)H, and a variety of chemical intermediates. These products may then be used for the synthesis of the major cellular constituents (i.e., peptidoglycan, LPS, proteins, and nucleic acids). The following describes the highpoints of the synthesis of each of these macromolecules from component sub-

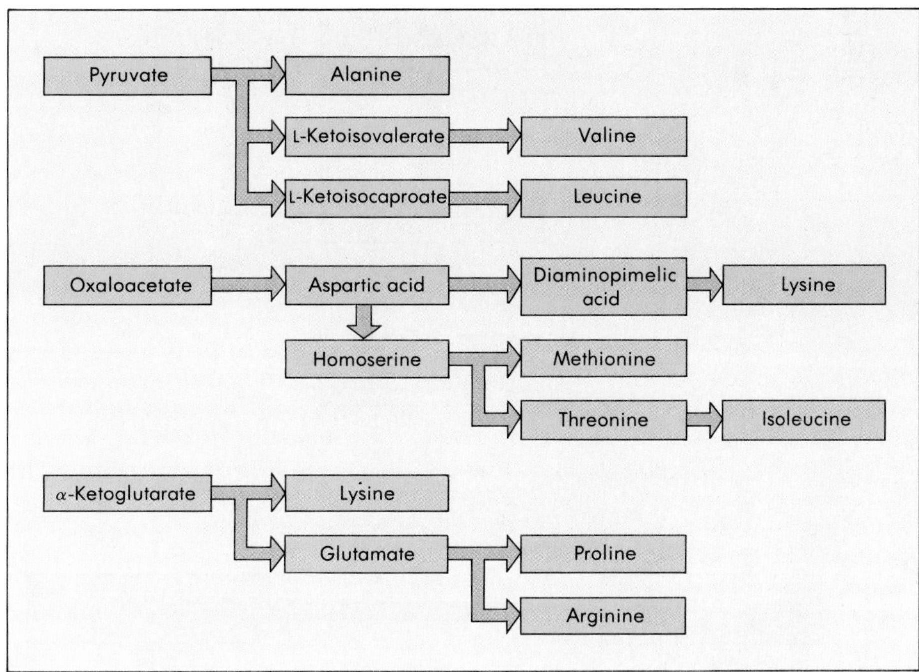

FIGURE 3-6 Examples of amino acids derived from intermediates of the TCA cycle.

units. DNA and RNA are discussed more fully in Chapter 4.

Peptidoglycan

Peptidoglycan consists of polymeric backbones of repeating *N*-acetylglucosamine-*N*-acetylmuramic acid disaccharide units that are linked via tetrapeptide bridges into a macromolecular network (see Chapter 2). Peptidoglycan biosynthesis occurs in four distinct stages (Figure 3-8). Stages 1 and 2 occur in the cytoplasm and involve the synthesis of soluble precursors. Beginning with glucose, a series of reactions are carried out resulting in the synthesis of *N*-acetylglucosamine-1-phosphate. This product is then "activated" by reaction with UTP to form UDP-*N*-acetylglucosamine. In the next series of reactions this compound is modified first to UDP-*N*-acetylmuramic acid followed by the stepwise addition of amino acids to form UDP-*N*-acetylmuramic acid-pentapeptide. This pentapeptide is unique in that it contains both L- and D-form amino acids, ending in the sequence, D-alanine-D-alanine. Indeed, this represents one of the few places in nature that D-amino acids are found. In stage 3, the *N*-acetylmuramyl-pentapeptide unit is then transferred to a lipid carrier, **undecaprenol** (bactoprenol), a high molecular weight lipid component of the cell membrane. The *N*-acetylglucosamine residue is then added, followed in gram-positive bacteria by addition of a pentaglycine chain. In gram-negative bacteria, this pentaglycine chain is absent. The isoprenoid carrier with attached subunit is then translocated to the outer surface of the cytoplasmic membrane, where it is incorporated into the growing polymer of the cell wall. In stage 4, the individual chains of the gram-positive wall are cross-linked by reaction of the terminal amino group of the pentaglycine chain and the fourth D-alanine residue of a neighboring chain, with release of the terminal D-alanine. In gram-negative cell walls, which are thinner and have fewer cross-links, a direct bond occurs between adjacent tetrapeptides without an intervening pentaglycine bridge.

An understanding of the biosynthesis of peptidoglycan is essential in medicine since these reactions are unique to bacterial cells and hence can be inhibited with little or no adverse effect on host (human) cells. A number of antibiotics currently in use target one or more steps in this pathway (see Chapter 13).

Lipopolysaccharide

Like that of peptidoglycan, the synthesis of lipopolysaccharide (LPS), which is present only in gram-negative bacteria, consists of both cytoplasmic and extracytoplasmic phases. The lipid A moiety is synthesized by addition of fatty acids, as well as one or more molecules of the unusual sugar residue, 2-keto-3-deoxyoctulonic acid (KDO) to the glucosamine disaccharide unit. A unique feature of the lipid A is the presence of β-hydroxy fatty acids esterified to the disaccharide. The hydrophobic nature of the lipid A-KDO complex allows it to become dissolved in the cytoplasmic membrane. Within the membrane, additional sugars may be added to complete the lipid A-core polysaccharide complex. Meanwhile, additional sugars are polymerized on a carrier molecule (undecaprenol phosphate) identical to that used in peptidoglycan synthesis. When a polysaccharide of the appropriate length is achieved, the entire complex is

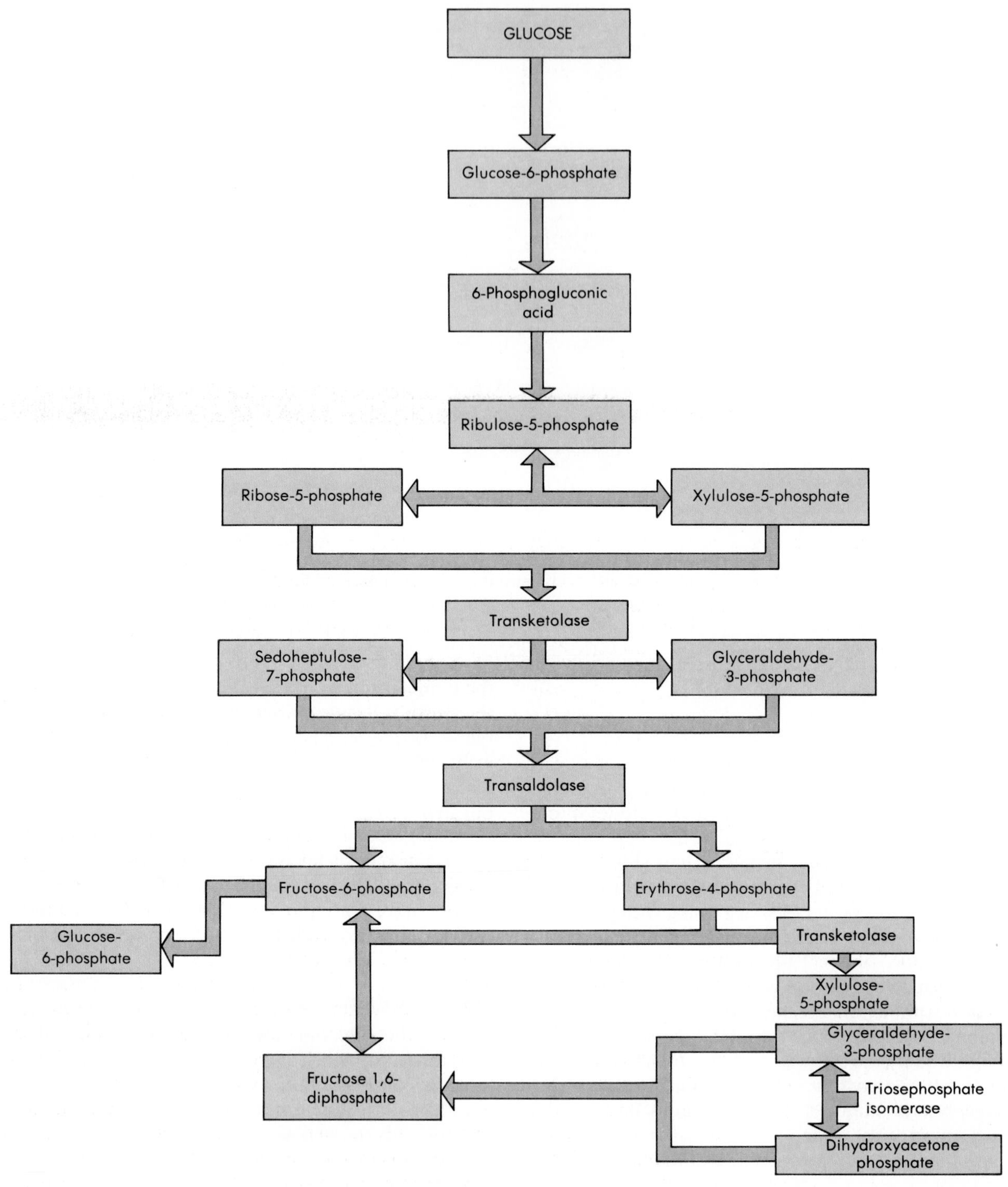

FIGURE 3-7 Pentose phosphate cycle, or hexose monophosphate pathway. The enzymes transketolase and transaldolase are central to the cycle's activity.

joined to the core polysaccharide-lipid A moiety embedded in the outer surface of the inner membrane. Once formed, the completed LPS subunits are transported to the outer surface of the outer membrane, probably through small areas known as Bayer's junctions where the inner and outer membranes are contiguous.

Nucleic Acid Synthesis

Before synthesis of nucleic acids may proceed, the cell must have adequate supplies of the component nucleotides. As we have already seen, nucleotides not only serve as components of DNA and RNA but also are crucial in all of the biosynthetic reactions in the growing cell by

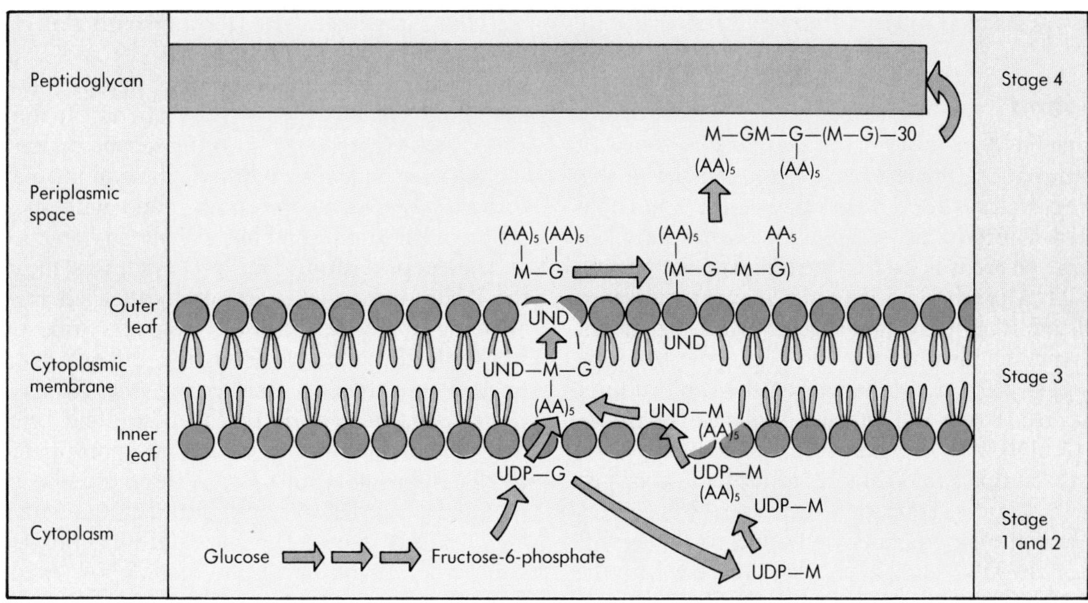

FIGURE 3-8 Synthesis and translocation of the peptidoglycan molecule. **Stage 1 and 2,** Cytoplasm: formation of *N-acetylglucosamine (G)* and attachment to nucleotide *(UTP)* to form UDP derivative. Subsequent synthesis results in formation of UDP-*N*-acetylmuramic acid *(M)* plus a pentapeptide *(AA)*5. **Stage 3,** Inner aspect of cytoplasmic membrane: UDP-M-*(AA)*5 is transferred to a lipid carrier, undecaprenol *(UND)* with release of UDP. Release of UDP results in addition of *N*-acetylglucosamine. Outer leaflet of cytoplasmic membrane: peptidoglycan monomer und–M-*(AA)*5–G migrates to outer leaflet of cytoplasmic membrane for peptidoglycan polymerization. In the periplasmic space, at approximately 30 disaccharide units, polymer is released from UND. **Stage 4,** Polymer migrates to nascent peptidoglycan to be incorporated by cross-linkage. (Redrawn from Slots J, Taubman MA, editors, *Contemporary oral microbiology and immunology,* St. Louis, 1992, Mosby.)

serving as activators of specific molecules in synthesis of polysaccharides, including LPS and peptidoglycan. In addition, nucleotides serve as a usable form of metabolic energy. Synthesis of the purine nucleotides (AMP and GMP) begins with ribose-5-phosphate formed as a product of the pentose monophosphate shunt. The bicyclic purine ring system is constructed in a stepwise fashion on the sugar phosphate moiety. The product of this series of reactions is the purine nucleotide, inosine monophosphate, which may then be converted to either guanosine or adenosine monophosphate. In contrast, the pyrimidine nucleotides are produced by synthesis of the pyrimidine, orotate, which is then attached to the ribose phosphate forming orotidine monophosphate. This nucleotide may then be converted alternately to either cytidine monophosphate or uridine monophosphate. The corresponding deoxynucleotides for use in DNA are synthesized by direct reduction at the 2′ carbon atom of the sugar portion of the ribonucleotide.

DNA Replication

The bacterial chromosome represents a storehouse of information that defines the characteristics of the cell and by which all cellular processes are carried out. It is therefore essential that this molecule be duplicated in an error-free manner. The process begins with unwinding of the double helix at a defined point known as the *origin of replication.* DNA synthesis, with specific DNA polymerase and the two parental DNA strands as templates, occurs in both directions around the circular chromosome. The localized area where the DNA is unwound and DNA synthesis is occurring is known as the *replication fork,* which contains, in addition to the polymerase, several other proteins essential to the process. These proteins include DNA-binding proteins, which help to keep the parental strands separated, as well as gyrases, which assist in the unwinding of the parental helix. Bacterial gyrases are the targets of a new class of antibiotics known as the *fluoroquinolones,* of which ciprofloxacin is an example. In this process the polymerase moves down the DNA strand, incorporating the appropriate (complementary) nucleotide at each position. Replication is complete when the two replication forks meet 180 degrees from the origin. Because the two DNA molecules that result consist of one parental strand and one newly replicated strand, this form of replication is described as **semiconservative.** To maintain the high degree of accuracy required for replication, the DNA polymerases possess "proofreading" functions, which allow the enzyme to confirm that the appropriate nucleotide was inserted and to correct any errors that were made.

Transcription

Because the DNA represents the permanent record of cellular information, the cell cannot risk damage to this copy during routine use. A working copy, known as mRNA, is thus produced, which is then transported to the ribosome where it is used as the template for protein synthesis. RNA synthesis occurs in a manner similar to DNA replication, employing a specific DNA-dependent RNA polymerase instead of a DNA polymerase. The process begins when a component of the multisubunit polymerase recognizes a particular sequence of nucleotides in the DNA (the **promoter,** see Chapter 4) and binds tightly to this site. Promoter sequences occur just before the start of the sequence, which actually encodes a protein. Once the polymerase has bound to the appropriate site on the DNA, RNA synthesis proceeds with the sequential addition of ribonucleotides complementary to the sequence in the DNA. Once an entire gene or group of genes (**operon,** see Chapter 4) has been transcribed, the RNA polymerase dissociates from the DNA, a process mediated by signals within the DNA. The bacterial DNA–dependent RNA polymerase is inhibited by rifampin, an antibiotic that is often used in the treatment of tuberculosis. Both transfer RNA (tRNA), which is used in protein synthesis, and ribosomal RNA (rRNA), a component of the ribosomes, are produced in a similar manner.

Translation

Translation represents the process by which the genetic code, in the form of the mRNA, is converted into a sequence of amino acids, the protein product. For the purposes of translation, the nucleotide sequence of the mRNA is divided into groups of three consecutive nucleotides. Each set of three nucleotides is known as a **codon** and encodes a particular amino acid. Since there are four different nucleotides, 4^3 or 64 combinations of 3 are possible, each codon coding for only a single amino acid (or termination signal). However, since there are only 20 amino acids, each may be encoded by multiple triplet codons. This feature is known as the **degeneracy** of the genetic code and may function in protecting the cell from the effects of minor mutations in the DNA or mRNA (see Chapter 4). The tRNA molecules each contain a three nucleotide sequence complementary to one of the codon sequences. This tRNA sequence is known as the **anticodon** and is designed to be able to base pair and bind to the codon sequence on the mRNA. Attached to the opposite end of the tRNA is the amino acid that corresponds to the particular codon/anticodon pair.

The process of protein synthesis begins with the formation of the so-called initiation complex in which the two ribosomal subunits, mRNA, and initiator tRNA with attached amino acid corresponding to the first codon are bound together. The ribosome contains two tRNA binding sites, the A (aminoacyl) site and P (peptidyl) site, each of which allows base pairing between the bound tRNA and the codon sequence in the mRNA. The tRNA corresponding to the second codon occupies the A site. The amino group of the amino acid attached to the A site forms a peptide bond with the carboxyl group of the amino acid in the P site in a reaction known as **transpeptidation.** This process leaves the tRNA in the P site uncharged (without an attached amino acid), allowing it to be released from the ribosome. The ribosome then moves down the mRNA exactly three nucleotides, thereby transferring the tRNA with attached nascent peptide to the P site and bringing the next codon into the A site. The appropriate charged tRNA is brought into the A site, and the process is repeated. Translation continues until the new codon in the A site is one of the three termination codons, for which there is no corresponding tRNA. At that point the translation complex is disassembled, and the new protein is released to the cytoplasm.

The process of protein synthesis represents an important target of antimicrobial action. The aminoglycosides (e.g., streptomycin, gentamicin), as well as the tetracyclines, act by binding to the small ribosomal subunit and inhibiting normal ribosomal function. Similarly, the macrolide and lincosamide groups of antibiotics (e.g., erythromycin, clindamycin) act by binding to the large ribosomal subunit.

SECONDARY METABOLISM

Although bacteria and animal cells share most of the pathways of intermediary metabolism, certain bacteria carry out additional series of reactions by which various unique compounds are produced. These reactions are said to comprise the secondary metabolism, and their products are referred to as **secondary metabolites.** The most important examples of secondary metabolites are the antibiotics, which are produced by members of a limited number of bacterial genera including *Bacillus, Streptomyces,* and *Nocardia.* The reaction pathways of secondary metabolism are often very complex and since they are not essential for cellular division, they are usually expressed during stationary phase, after productive growth has ceased. Secondary metabolism analogous to that in bacteria occurs in plants but is as yet undescribed in animal cells.

QUESTIONS

1. List the biosynthetic reactions that are inhibited by antibiotics. Give an example of each.
2. What are the four steps in peptidoglycan synthesis, and where in the cell do they occur?
3. How many moles of ATP are generated per mole of glucose in glycolysis, the TCA cycle, and electron

transport? Which of these occur in anaerobic and which in aerobic conditions?

4. Why is DNA replication considered semiconservative?

Bibliography

Davis BD, Dulbecco R, Eisen HN, and Ginsberg HS, editors: *Microbiology,* ed 4, Philadelphia, 1990, J.B. Lippincott.

Jawetz E, Melnick JL, and Adelberg EA: *Review of medical microbiology,* ed 16, Los Altos, Calif., 1984, Lange Medical Publications.

Lehninger AL: *Principles of biochemistry,* New York, 1982, Worth Publishers.

Mandell GL, Douglas RG, and Bennett JE, editors: *Principles and practice of infectious diseases,* ed 3, New York, 1990, Churchill Livingstone.

Slots J and Taubman M: *Contemporary oral microbiology and immunology,* St. Louis, 1992, Mosby.

CHAPTER 4

Bacterial Genetics

DNA: THE GENETIC MATERIAL

The bacterial cell is the smallest self-contained living entity governed by genetic information, deoxyribonucleic acid (DNA). Bacteria do not possess a nucleus like eukaryotes, but a structure called a nucleoid, which lacks a nuclear membrane and appears by electron microscopy to be free of ribosomes. Genetic studies, as well as electron microscopic analysis, have shown that most prokaryotes possess one giant, covalently closed, circular chromosome. The *Escherichia coli* genome consists of 4.2×10^3 kilobases (kb), which implies a length of 1.3 mm (i.e., about 1000 times the diameter of the cell).

In all bacterial genomes, replication of DNA occurs at a growing point called the fork, which moves linearly from an origin to a terminus. The *E. coli* chromosomal DNA is replicated bidirectionally from a point of origin called OriC. A population of *E. coli* cells can double in number every 18 to 180 minutes. Cells may thus divide in less time than is required for replication of the chromosome (40 minutes); thus multiple sites of initiation of replication occur at the origin of the partially replicated chromosome. This multiforked chromosome allows the initiation of multiple growth forks. The frequency of initiation of replication at the origin is related to the growth rate of the bacteria. Unidirectional replication can also occur, as is the case for some plasmids and during conjugation. In general, bacterial genes are present as a single copy. For a more complete description of DNA replication, transcription, and translation, see the biochemistry textbooks in the Bibliography.

Plasmids

Plasmids are a diverse group of extrachromosomal genetic elements. Like the bacterial chromosomal DNA, they can autonomously replicate and as such are referred to as **replicons.** Plasmids are usually circular double-stranded molecules of DNA varying from 1.5 to 400 kd. However, *Borrelia burgdorferi,* the causative agent of Lyme disease, and the related *B. hermsii* are unique among all eubacteria in that they possess linear plasmids. Plasmids usually do not encode essential functions for bacteria and are thus unnecessary for the growth of the microorganism. Plasmids do, however, carry additional genetic information that is responsible for the appearance of new phenotypic properties in a bacterial cell. For example, plasmids may confer high levels of antibiotic resistance and encode the production of bacteriocins or toxins, as well as contain genes that may provide the bacteria a unique advantage in metabolizing some substrates.

Each plasmid is maintained at a specific number of copies per chromosome. There may be as few as one copy in the case of large plasmids, or as many as 50 of smaller plasmids. Plasmids are often classified according to their **incompatibility group.** Plasmids are part of the same incompatibility group if they are unable to coexist in the same bacterial cell. Plasmids from the same incompatibility group are undistinguished from each other during DNA replication and partitioning between daughter cells.

Large plasmids (20 to 120 kb) such as the fertility factor F found in *E. coli* or the resistance transfer factor (RTF) (80 kb) are often able to mediate their own transfer from one cell to another by a process called conjugation (see the following). These conjugative plasmids encode all the necessary factors for their transfer. Some smaller plasmids that are not conjugative can, however, be mobilized, meaning that they possess the necessary sequences to allow their transfer but they do not themselves encode for the necessary transfer proteins. Finally, some plasmids are more sedentary and do not transfer at all. Plasmids can be transferred into a bacterial cell by means other than conjugation, such as transformation, transduction, or incorporation in the cellular chromosome as discussed later.

Regulation of Gene Expression

Bacterial cells must be able to adapt very quickly to any change in concentration of nutrients in their environment. A fundamental concept in bacterial genetics concerns the elementary regulatory mechanisms: to minimize the requirement for energy, a system is turned on only when it is needed. Thus bacteria avoid making the enzyme(s) of a pathway when the substrate is absent, but they are always ready to produce these enzymes if the substrate should appear in the environment. The primary mechanism that bacteria have evolved to minimize the energy cost for this type of on-and-off regulation is the grouping of the genes that encode enzymes of a particular pathway. Such a structural organization is called an

operon and consists of only one promoter, which is the target for regulation, adjacent genes coding for each enzyme, and one terminator of transcription. Thus all the genes coding for the enzymes of a particular pathway are usually coordinately regulated and transcribed as a polycistronic (multigene) messenger ribonucleic acid (mRNA), which is in turn translated sequentially into proteins by the ribosome machinery.

Bacterial gene expression can be regulated in this manner at the initiation or termination of both transcription and translation. Examples of such regulation mechanisms follow.

Transcriptional Regulation

Initiation of transcription may be under either positive or negative control. Genes under **negative control** are expressed, unless they are switched off by a repressor protein. This **repressor protein** will prevent gene expression by binding to a specific DNA sequence, called the **operator,** making it impossible for the RNA polymerase to initiate transcription at the promoter. Inversely, genes whose expression is under **positive control** will not be transcribed unless an active regulator protein, called **apoinducer,** is present. The apoinducer will bind to a specific DNA sequence and will assist the RNA polymerase in the initiation steps by a still unknown mechanism.

Operons can be either **inducible** or **repressible.** Operons are considered to be inducible when the introduction of a substrate into a growth medium leads to the increase of the expression of the enzymes necessary for its metabolism. These inducible operons function only in the presence of a small molecule called the **inducer.** Biosynthetic enzymes whose amount is reduced by the presence of their end products are called repressible enzymes. Those end-product metabolites are usually small molecules known as **corepressors.**

The lactose (*lac*) operon responsible for degradation of the sugar lactose is an inducible operon under negative regulation (Figure 4-1). In the absence of lactose, the operon is repressed by the binding of the repressor protein to the operator sequence, thus impeding the RNA polymerase function. The addition of lactose will, however, reverse this repression. Full expression of the *lac* operon also requires a protein-mediated positive control mechanism. In *E. coli,* a protein called the catabolite gene activator protein (CAP) forms a complex with cAMP, acquiring the ability to bind to a specific DNA sequence present in the promoter. The CAP-cAMP complex enhances binding of the RNA polymerase to the promoter, thus allowing an increase in the frequency of transcription initiation. The CAP-cAMP complex may increase the operon transcription by protein-protein interaction with the RNA polymerase or by protein-DNA interaction.

The tryptophan operon (Figure 4-2), which contains the structural genes necessary for tryptophan biosynthesis, is under dual transcription control mechanisms. The tryptophan operon is a repressible operon under negative control that is also controlled by an antitermination mechanism.

Posttranscriptional or Translational Regulation

Translational control has been found to occur with both monocistronic and polycistronic mRNA. With polycistronic mRNA, **translational control** refers to differences in the copy number of each protein expressed from each gene. For example, for the *lac* operon, β-galactosidase, galactoside permease, and acetylase are produced at a ratio of 10:5:2, respectively. The translational process may also be regulated by factors other than their intrinsic structures. In other words, translational initiation may be controlled by a regulator molecule, which will act either directly or indirectly to determine if an initiation site for a coding region is available to the ribosomes.

Damage to DNA

Since DNA conveys genetic information, there is no molecule in a living organism whose integrity is as vital to the cell as is its DNA. Cells must be able to replicate DNA very accurately. Furthermore, accidental damage to DNA must be minimized by the elaboration of efficient DNA repair systems. These damage-containment systems are so important for the life of a cell that a bacterium may devote a large percentage of its genome to specify and control the enzymes involved.

Mutations Affecting the DNA

A **mutation** can be defined as any change in the base sequence of the DNA. Many types of mutations affect a single base. Such mutations have no effect on the replication and transcription processes. However, base substitutions responsible for DNA sequence changes exert damaging effects on the next generation, since any changes in the DNA sequence are transferred from parent to daughter cell. A single base change can result in a **transition,** where one purine is replaced by another purine, or a pyrimidine by another pyrimidine. A **transversion** can also result, where a purine is replaced by a pyrimidine and vice versa. To give rise to a protein, the DNA is first transcribed into mRNA by the RNA polymerase, then this single-strand template is translated into a protein. In the translation process, a **transfer RNA (tRNA)** loaded with a specific amino acid recognizes a set of three nucleotides, defined as a **codon,** on the mRNA. The protein is elongated by the concerted action of the ribosomes until a stop codon is encountered, wherein the final protein is released.

A **silent mutation** is a change at the DNA level that does not result in any change of amino acid in the encoded protein. Such silent mutations have no demonstrable phenotypic effect. This type of mutation occurs because of the degeneration of the genetic code, as many codons code for the same amino acid. A **missense mutation** results in a different amino acid being inserted in the protein. Such missense mutations may or may not change

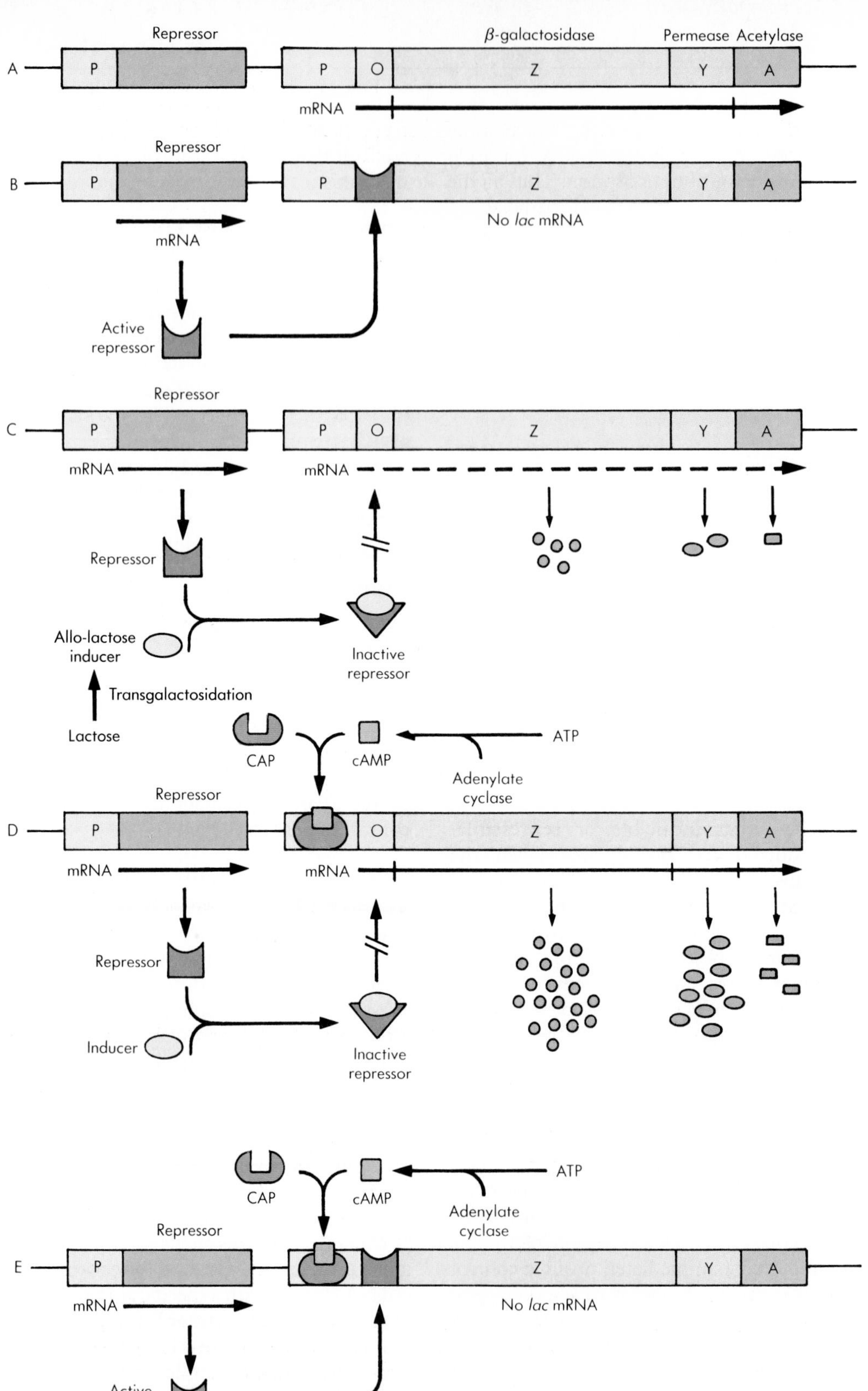

FIGURE 4-1 The lactose operon. **A,** The lactose operon is transcribed as a polycistronic mRNA from the promoter *(P)* and translated into three proteins: β-galactosidase *(Z)*, permease *(Y)* and acetylase *(A)*. The *lacI* gene encodes the repressor protein. **B,** The lactose operon is not transcribed in the absence of allolactose inducer, as the repressor competes with the RNA polymerase at the operator site *(O)*. **C,** The repressor, complexed with the inducer, does not recognize the operator because of a conformation change in the repressor. The *lac* operon is thus transcribed at a low level. **D,** *E. coli* is grown in a poor medium in presence of lactose as the carbon source. Both the inducer and the CAP-cAMP complex are bound to the promoter, which is fully "turned on," and a high level of *lac* mRNA is transcribed and translated. **E,** Growth of *E. coli* in a poor medium without lactose will result in the binding of the CAP-cAMP complex to the promoter region and binding of the active repressor to the operator sequence, as no inducer is available. The result will be that the *lac* operon will not be transcribed.

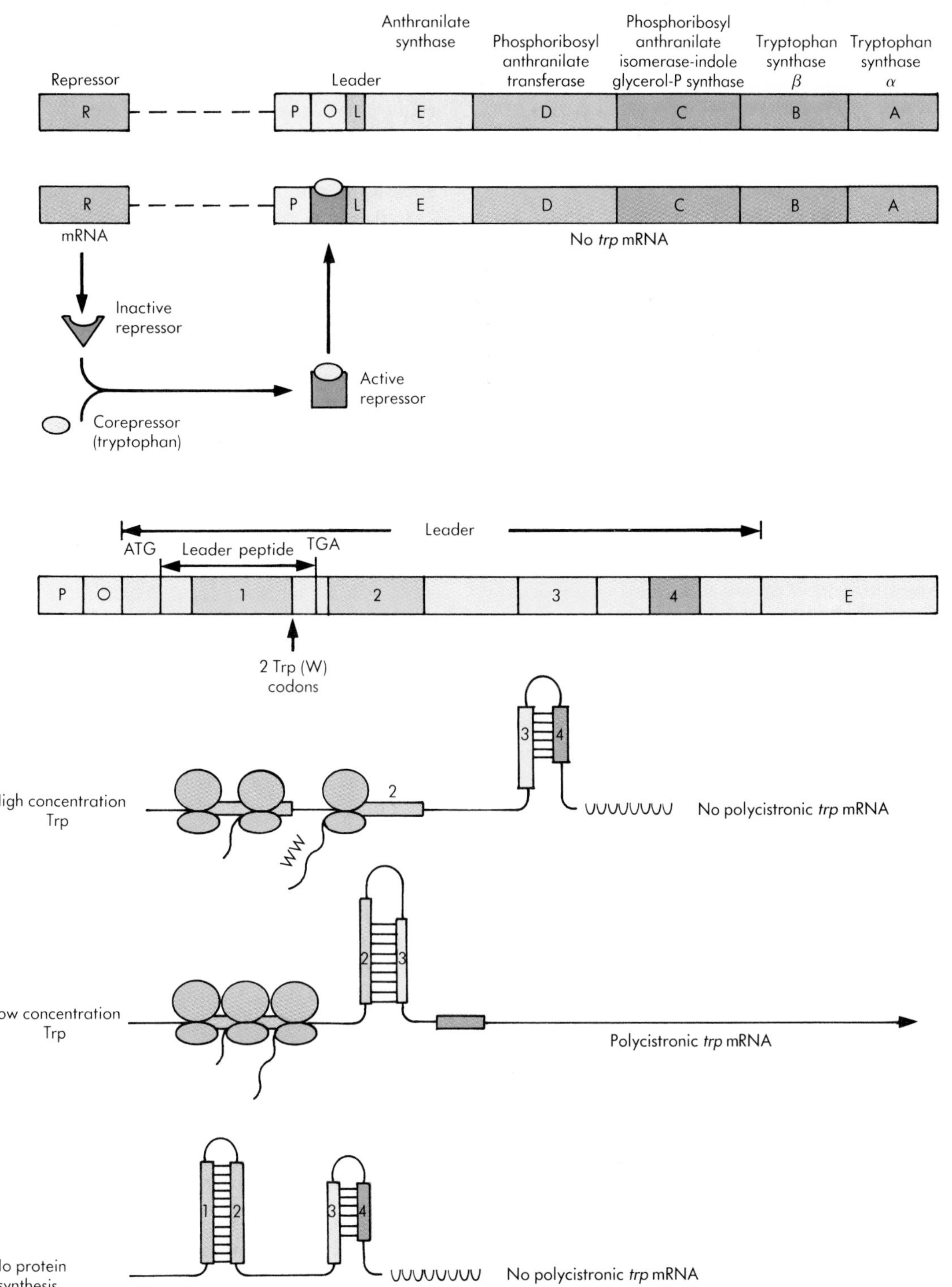

FIGURE 4-2 Regulation of the tryptophan operon. **A,** The *trp* operon encodes the five enzymes necessary for tryptophan biosynthesis. This *trp* operon is under dual control. **B,** The conformation of the inactive repressor protein is changed following its binding by the corepressor, tryptophan. The resulting active repressor binds to the operator *(O)*, blocking any transcription of the *trp* mRNA by the RNA polymerase. **C,** The *trp* operon is also under the control of an attenuation-antitermination mechanism. Upstream the structural genes are the promoter *(P)*, the operator, and a leader (L) which can be transcribed into a short peptide containing 2 tryptophans (W) near its distal end. The leader mRNA possesses 4 repeats (1, 2, 3, and 4), which can pair differently according to the tryptophan availability, leading to an early termination of transcription of the operon or its full transcription. In the presence of a high concentration of tryptophan, regions 3 and 4 of the leader mRNA can pair, forming a terminator hairpin, and no transcription of the *trp* operon occurs. However, in the presence of little or no tryptophan, the ribosomes stall in region 1 when translating the leader peptide because of the tandem of tryptophan codons. Then regions 2 and 3 can pair, forming the antiterminator hairpin, and leading to transcription of the *trp* genes. Finally, the regions 1 : 2 and 3 : 4 of the free leader mRNA can pair, also leading to a stop of transcription before the first structural gene *trpE*.

the phenotype. Finally, a **nonsense mutation** changes a codon encoding an amino acid to a stop codon. For example, a change to the codon TAG will make the translation stop abruptly before reaching the end of the transcript.

More drastic changes can occur in proteins when multiple bases are involved. For example, **frameshift mutations** occur when a small deletion or insertion, which is *not* in multiples of three, arises. This results in a change in the reading frame, usually leading to premature truncation of the protein. **Null mutations,** which completely destroy gene function, arise when there is an extensive insertion or deletion or gross rearrangement of the chromosome structure. The interruption of a gene by transposition (see the following), which may be many thousands of base pairs long, and the aberrant action of cellular recombination processes are two mechanisms that may give rise to null mutations.

Many mutations occur spontaneously in nature; however, mutations can also be induced by physical or chemical agents. Among the physical agents used to induce mutations in bacteria are (1) heat, which results in deamination of nucleotides, (2) ultraviolet light, which causes pyrimidine dimer formation and, (3) ionizing radiation such as x-ray, which may be responsible for opening a ring of a base or single- or double-strand breaks in the DNA.

Chemical agents that also are mutagens can be grouped into three classes. The first class consists of **nucleotide base analogues.** Such chemicals are incorporated into the DNA during replication because of their structural similarity to the normal four bases. These base analogues, however, lead to a base-pair formation that is not as strong as normal, leading to mispairing and frequent mistakes during DNA replication. One of the most powerful base analogues known is 5-bromouracil. Because of its similarity with thymidine, this mutagen can easily be introduced into the replicating DNA. After tautomerization (i.e., structural rearrangement of the molecule) from the keto to the enol state, 5-bromouracil can pair to the guanine nucleotide instead of adenine. This mispairing will then have repercussions on the next generation, where G will be changed to an A. Thus the tautomerization of 5-bromouracil within DNA causes replication errors, which are expressed as mutations with the next generation, changing a U-A base pair to a G-C base pair.

A second class of chemical mutagens includes the **frameshift mutagens,** which usually cause the addition or deletion of a single base. These polycyclic flat molecules, such as ethidium bromide or acridine derivatives, are able to insert between the bases (intercalate) as they stack with each other in the double helix. These intercalating agents increase the spacing of successive base pairs, destroying the regular sugar-phosphate backbone and decreasing the pitch of the helix. These changes lead to frequent mistakes during DNA replication. These mutations affect replicating DNA and also seem to require the presence of short runs of the same base pair. Finally, some mutagens will act directly on the DNA, resulting in a modification of the normal base into a chemically different structure. The modified bases may base-pair abnormally, may not pair at all, or the damage may cause the removal of the base from the DNA backbone. **DNA-reactive chemicals** include products such as nitrous acid (HNO_2), as well as alkylating agents including nitrosoguanidine and ethyl methane sulfonate, which are known to add methyl or ethyl groups to the rings of the DNA bases.

Mutations can also occur in other genes to eliminate the effects of a mutation in the original gene. Such a phenomenon is termed **suppression.** An extragenic suppressor usually involves a mutation in an anticodon of tRNA. This mutated tRNA will read a mutated codon either in the sense of the original codon or give an acceptable substitute. Intragenic suppression is achieved by a second compensating mutation within the gene, which will restore the original reading frame of a gene containing a frameshift mutation.

Repair Mechanisms of DNA

Bacterial cells have evolved a number of different repair mechanisms to minimize damage to their DNA. These repair mechanisms can be divided into five groups: (1) **Direct DNA repair** involves the enzymatic removal of damages such as pyrimidine dimers and alkylated bases. (2) **Excision repair** involves the excision of a DNA segment containing the damage followed by synthesis of a new DNA strand (Figure 4-3). Two types of excision repair mechanisms, generalized and specialized, exist. (3) **Recombinational** or **postreplication repair** mechanisms retrieve missing information by genetic recombination when both DNA strands are damaged. (4) The **SOS response** involves the induction of many genes (approximately 15) following DNA damage or interruption of DNA replication. (5) The **error-prone repair** mechanism is used when a DNA template is not available for directing an accurate repair. This system constitutes the last resort for a bacterial cell before dying.

GENE EXCHANGE IN PROKARYOTIC CELLS

The exchange of genetic material between bacterial cells may occur by one of three mechanisms: (1) **transformation,** which results in the acquisition of new genetic markers by the incorporation of exogenous or foreign DNA; (2) **transduction,** which is the transfer of genetic information from one bacterium to another by a bacteriophage; and (3) **conjugation,** which is the mating or quasi-sexual exchange of genetic information from one bacterium (the donor) to another bacterium (the recipient). Conjugation occurs with most, if not all, eubacteria. Conjugation usually occurs between members of the same species but has also been demonstrated

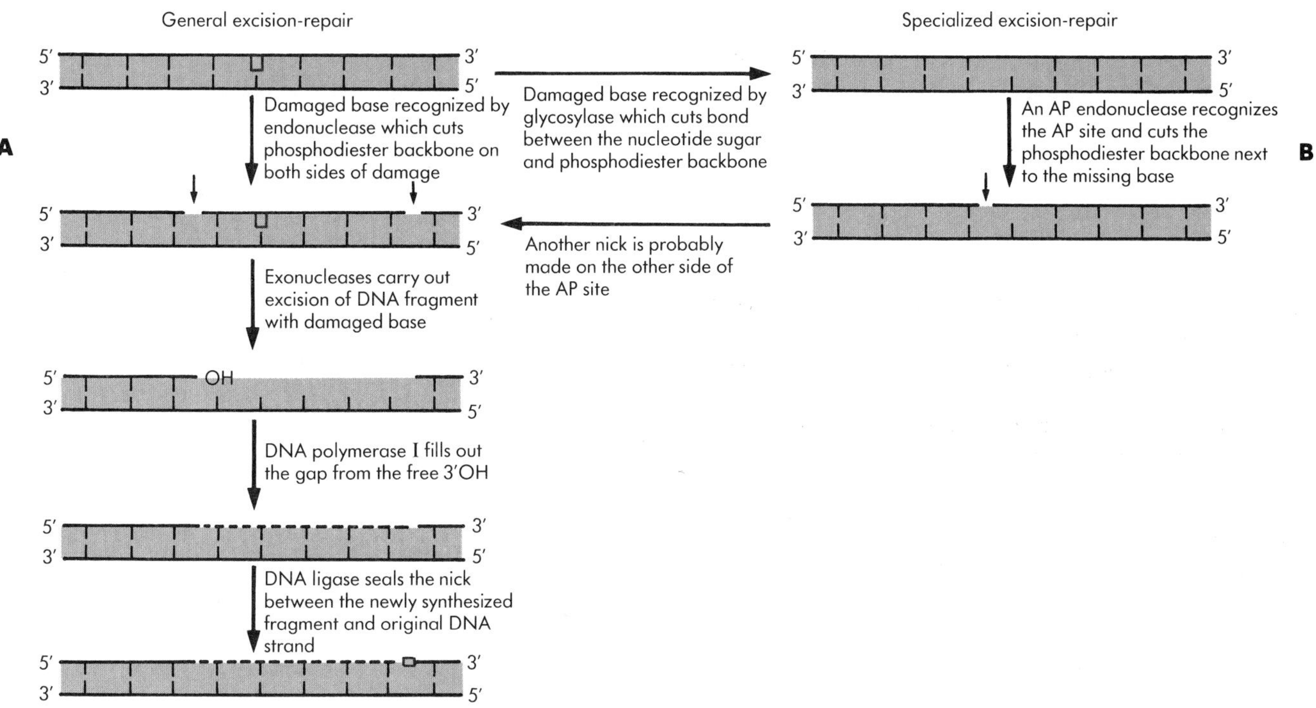

FIGURE 4-3 **A,** Generalized and **B,** specialized excision repair mechanisms.

to occur between prokaryotes and cells from plants, animals, and fungi.

Many bacteria, especially many pathogenic bacterial species, are quite promiscuous, meaning that the bacteria frequently exchange DNA. This genetic information exchange produces additions to the recipient genome. The transferred DNA can be either integrated into the recipient chromosome or stably maintained as an extrachromosomal element (plasmid) and passed on to daughter bacteria as an autonomously replicating unit.

Transformation

Transformation was the first mechanism of genetic transfer to be discovered in bacteria. In 1928 Frederick Griffith first observed transformation in the study of pneumococcal infection of mice. Griffith, an English microbiologist, made the observation that pneumococcus virulence was related to the presence of a surrounding polysaccharide capsule. The bacteria possessing a polysaccharide capsule appeared smooth (S) when grown on agar plates and possessed the ability to kill mice. In comparison, colonies appearing with rough edges (R) were unencapsulated and nonlethal. He then discovered that a mixture of killed S plus live R bacteria was lethal. When bacteria were isolated from this lethal mixed infection, it was found that the R bacteria had been replaced or "transformed" to S bacteria, now able to make a virulent capsular polysaccharide. His studies led to the identification of DNA as the transforming principle some 15 years later by Oswald Avery, Colin MacLeod, and Maclyn McCarty.

Both gram-positive and gram-negative bacteria can take up and stably maintain exogenous DNA. Transformation systems can be classified in two groups. The first group includes those systems in which competence occurs naturally, **competence** being the ability of a cell to interact with exogenous DNA, leading to its uptake. Naturally occurring competence has been described for bacteria, including *Haemophilus influenzae, Streptococcus pneumoniae, Bacillus* species, and *Neisseria* species. Thus genetic manipulation in these species has been relatively easy. The competence of bacteria is not, however, a permanent feature but represents a transient state in the life of a population. This transitory phase of competence usually develops toward the end of logarithmic growth, some time before a population enters the stationary phase. The mechanisms leading to DNA uptake in gram-positive and gram-negative bacteria are different. In gram-negative bacteria such as *Neisseria* and *Haemophilus,* DNA uptake depends on a short specific sequence approximately 10 nucleotides long. This sequence is recognized and bound by a membrane protein. Duplex DNA then enters the competent cells. In gram-positive bacteria such as *Streptococcus* and *Bacillus* species, the double-stranded DNA is nonspecifically bound and cut on the surface of the cells, yielding double-stranded fragments varying from 7 to 10 kb in size. From these duplex DNA fragments, only one strand will enter the bacterial cell. A delay of approximately 5 minutes occurs between the moment following single-stranded DNA uptake and the actual integration of the DNA into the recipient genome. This phenomenon is called the **eclipse** because the transforming DNA is actually protected from external deoxyribonucleases (DNAses, enzymes that degrade DNA) inside the cell, but it cannot be recovered as an active form.

Most bacteria do not exhibit a natural ability for DNA uptake. In such cases, chemical methods have been developed to artificially induce competence. Plasmid transformation of *E. coli* was first demonstrated by Cohen and collaborators in 1972. They applied the technique of Mendel and Higa, who observed transfection (i.e., infection of *E. coli* by a bacteriophage in the presence of $CaCl_2$ at 0° C followed by a brief heat pulse at 37° C to 42° C). These conditions were shown to induce a general state of competence for DNA uptake. Since this first demonstration of artificially induced competence, many studies have addressed the process of plasmid transformation to increase the frequency of resulting transformants. A recently developed alternative method for transformation makes use of high-voltage pulses, which generate membrane distortions and allow DNA uptake. This method, known as **electroporation,** has been effective with a wide variety of both gram-positive and gram-negative microorganisms.

Conjugation

Genetic transfer in *E. coli* was first reported by Lederberg and Tatum in 1946, when they observed sexlike exchange between two mutant strains of *E. coli* K12 ([biotin$^-$ methionine$^-$ threonine$^+$ phenylalanine$^+$] and [biotin$^+$ methionine$^+$ threonine$^-$ phenylalanine$^-$]). It was later demonstrated that conjugation requires cell-to-cell interaction and that the exchange of genetic material is always unidirectional, with the genetic information moving from male to female cells. Many different conjugative plasmids have been found in several gram-negative bacterial species such as *E. coli* and *Bacteroides* species, as well as in some gram-positive bacteria including *Streptococcus, Streptomyces,* and *Clostridium.* Many of these large conjugative plasmids specify colicins or antibiotic resistances. One of the best known conjugative plasmids, called the fertility factor or F, is 94 kb in size and is found in *E. coli.* The male donor is defined as F^+; the female recipient cell is termed F^-. Many of the F-like plasmids that are found in gram-negative bacteria exhibit a conjugative mechanism very similar to the F plasmid.

The conjugation process, as described here for the F plasmid, can be divided into four stages (Figure 4-4). Conjugation initiates with contact between the donor (F^+) and recipient cells (F^-). The F plasmid is responsible for the synthesis of sex-specific pili; these pili are probably involved in the recognition of suitable recipient cells and thus allow a close interaction between donor and recipient cells. The F pilus may also cause wall-to-wall contact between the pairs by retraction, leading to the formation of a cytoplasmic bridge. These extensive surface contacts may generate a signal that results in the initiation of plasmid replication and DNA transfer. The proteins necessary for this transfer are encoded by 19 genes, representing one third of the F DNA. The DNA that is transferred by conjugation is not a double helix but a single-stranded molecule. **Mobilization** begins when a plasmid encoded protein makes a single-stranded site-specific cleavage at the transfer origin called OriT. The nick initiates rolling circle replication, and the displaced linear strand is probably the intermediate structure directed to the recipient cell. Little is known, however, about how the DNA or DNA-protein complex leaves the donor and enters the recipient cell. Finally, the transferred single-stranded DNA is recircularized and its complementary strand synthesized. The F plasmid is defined as conjugative because it carries all the genes necessary for its own transfer. However, some plasmids such as ColE1 and ColK are not conjugative plasmids, but they are mobilizable. These plasmids may be mobilized by some conjugative plasmids cohabiting the same cell.

An important property of F is its ability to integrate into the bacterial chromosome, generating a **Hfr cell** or a high frequency of recombination. Such integration of the F plasmid involves breakage and rejoining of both molecules of DNA. Many sites of exchanges exist in both F and an *E. coli* chromosome, leading to Hfr strains. Analysis of some of the Hfr strains indicated that they result from a recombination process between a homologous insertion sequence present on both the F plasmid and the chromosome. Indeed, three types of insertion sequences, IS2, IS3 and γδ, have been found in the F plasmid. In Hfr strains, the F plasmid ceases its autonomous replication, but its genes involved in mobilization and transfer are still expressed. Thus conjugation can still be initiated by a nick at the OriT site. However, since F is integrated into the chromosome, only part of the plasmid sequence is initially transferred, followed by chromosomal DNA and sometimes, but only rarely, the remainder of the F plasmid. It would take 100 minutes at 37° C to transfer the complete male genome to the female recipient. However, the fragile connection between the mating pairs is usually broken and the transfer aborted before being completed—explaining why, usually, only the chromosomal sequences adjacent to the integrated F are transferred. Therefore a mating between a Hfr strain and a F^- strain usually leaves the recipient F^-. Artificial interruption of a mating between a Hfr and a F^- pair has been helpful in constructing a consistent map of the *E. coli* chromosomal DNA. In such maps the position of each gene is given in minutes according to its time of entry into a recipient cell in relation to a fixed origin (Figure 4-5).

Conjugative R (antibiotic resistance) plasmids have been found in gram-positive bacteria such as *Streptococcus, Streptomyces,* and *Clostridium.* However, conjugation in gram-positive bacteria does not seem to rely on the presence of pili. Instead, the mating pair is brought together by the presence of an adhesin molecule present on the surface of the donor cell. Moreover, some bacteria, such as *Streptococcus faecalis,* produce a peptide sex pheromone, which is thought to elicit a mating response leading to the expression of the adhesin in the donor cells.

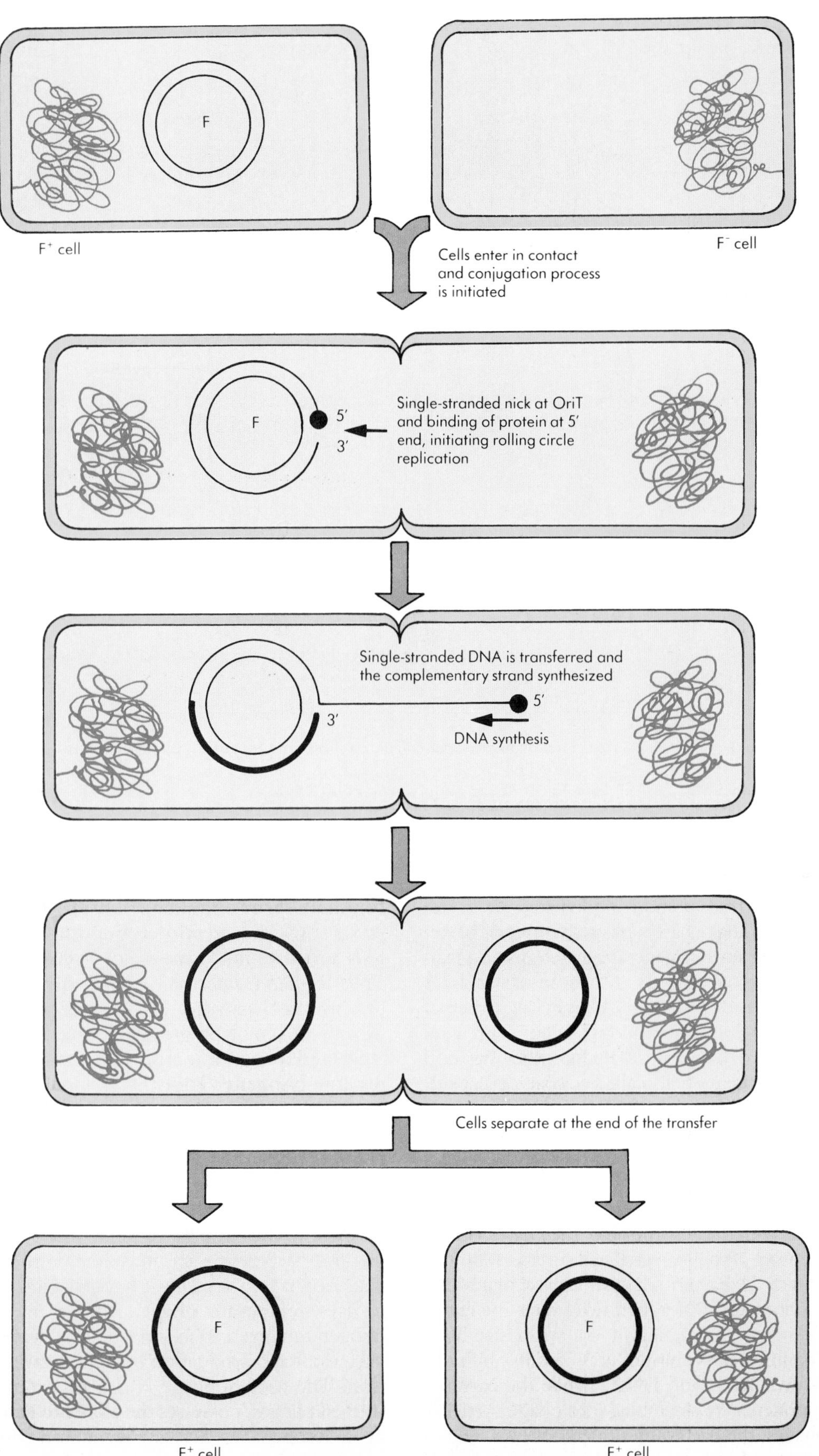

FIGURE 4-4 Genetic transfer of the F plasmid by conjugation.

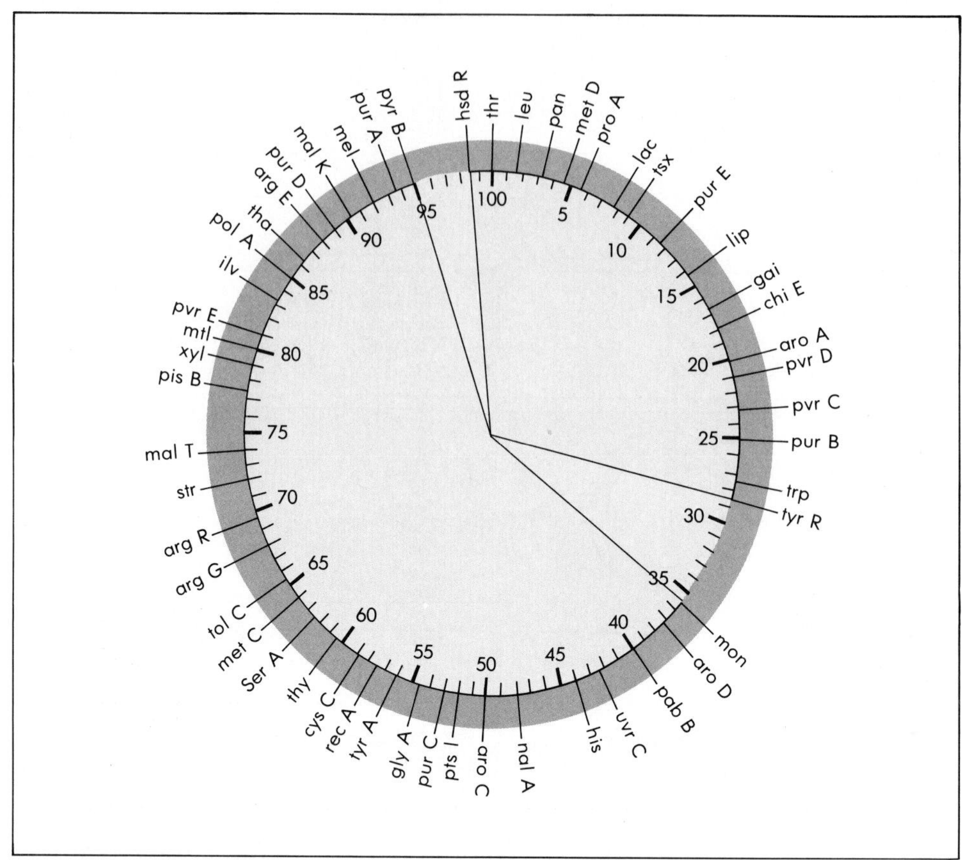

FIGURE 4-5 Chromosomal map of *Escherichia coli* genes. The time (minutes) to transfer DNA segments from the origin of the first Hfr strain is represented by the numbers. (Redrawn from Bachmann BJ, Low KB, and Taylor AL: *Bacteriol Rev* 40:116, 1976.)

Transduction

Genetic transfer by transduction is mediated by bacteriophages. **Bacteriophages** are parasitic viruses of bacterial cells, using their energy-generating systems and protein synthesizing factors, as well as their amino acids. A bacteriophage genome can be DNA or RNA, either of which may be single- or double-stranded. The viral genome is protected from nucleases or other harmful substances by a protein shell, called a coat or **capsid.** During the process of bacterial infections, only the nucleic acid component is introduced into the bacterium, with the capsid remaining outside the microorganism. Bacteriophage life cycles are either lytic or lysogenic. The **lytic cycle** results in lysis of bacterial cells (Figure 4-6). The lytic cycle begins with the adsorption of the phage particle to specific receptors on the bacterial cell surface, followed by the injection of the bacteriophage nucleic acid into the cell. The bacteriophage DNA then takes over the entire bacterial machinery, instructing it to synthesize viral structures. The infected bacterium may lose its ability to synthesize its own RNA and DNA. Inside the bacterial host, the components are assembled into phage particles. With most phages, the bacterium undergoes lysis, releasing mature bacteriophages into the surrounding medium. However, a few filamentous phages release progeny continuously by outfolding of the bacterial cell wall. This process, which is defined as **budding,** does not result in lysis and does not cause major damage to the host cell. Thus bacteria infected with filamentous phages can produce viral particles for very long periods. A phage capable of only lytic growth is called a **virulent phage.**

Bacteriophage infection by certain phages may also result in **lysogeny** (Figure 4-7). Under these conditions, bacteriophage entry does not result in bacterial cell lysis. As with the lytic process, the infection is initiated with the phage binding to specific receptors on the cell surface and injecting its DNA through the cell wall. However, instead of turning the cell into a "phage factory," the phage DNA inserts into the bacterial genome, where it replicates as an integral part of the chromosome as the cell grows. A bacteriophage possessing a lysogenic life cycle is referred to as a **temperate phage.** After many generations, a lysogen can revert to its virulent state, leading to lysis and bacteriophage production by a mechanism called **induction.** The bacteriophage λ, one of the most extensively studied phages, possesses the ability to enter either a lytic or a lysogenic cycle. Lysogeny can also result in a phenotypic change in the bacterial host. For example,

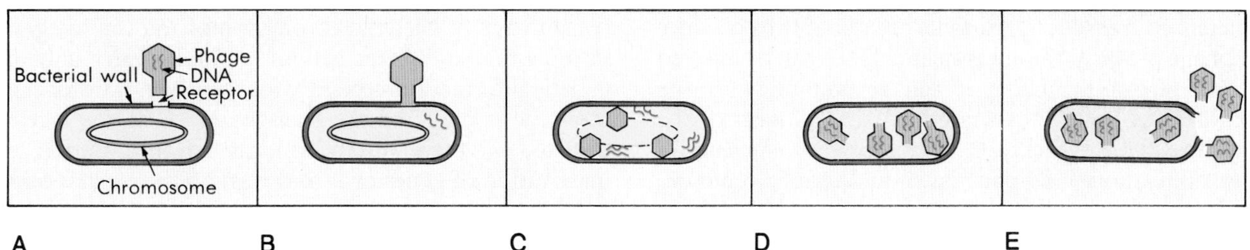

FIGURE 4-6 Bacterial transduction with release of mature bacteriophages following cell lysis. **A,** The phage tail combines with a specific receptor site in the bacterial cell wall. **B,** The phage DNA is injected into the bacterium. **C,** Replication of the bacterial chromosome is disrupted, and phage DNA codes for formation of phage components. **D,** The components are assembled into phage particles. **E,** The cell lyses and releases the mature phage particles.

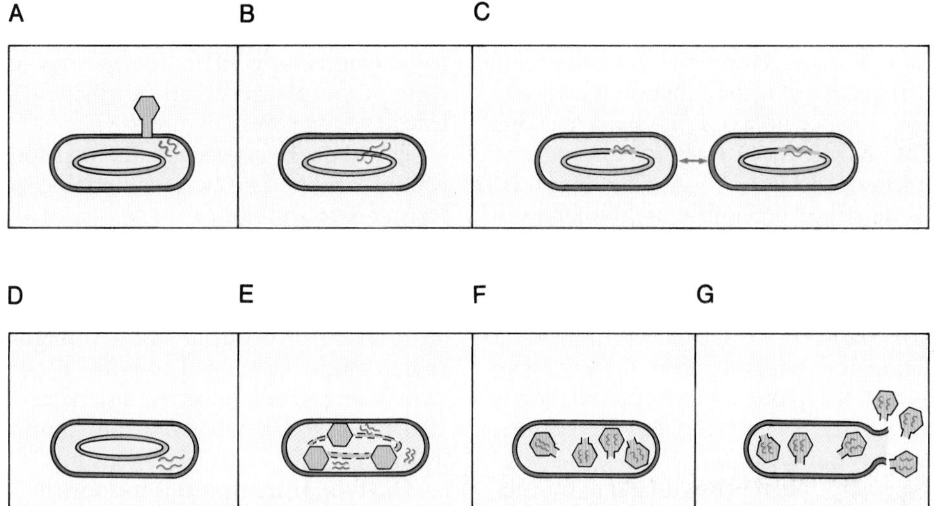

FIGURE 4-7 Lysogenic infection of bacterium with temperate bacteriophage. **A,** The phage infects a sensitive bacterium, and the phage DNA is injected. **B,** The phage DNA becomes integrated with the bacterial chromosome. **C,** The bacterium multiplies, apparently unaffected by the infection. It has been lysogenized. **D,** Occasionally, the phage DNA becomes detached from a bacterial chromosome and takes control. **E,** An individual cell (or by induction all the cells) produces phage components. **F,** The components are then later assembled into phage particles. **G,** Ultimately, the cell lyses and releases mature phage particles.

only those strains of *Corynebacterium diphtheriae* that are lysogenic for a β-prophage or related temperate phages produce the diphtheria toxin. The expression of the toxin is induced under certain nutritional conditions. A lysogenic phage is also responsible for toxin production in some strains of *Clostridium botulinum.*

Several phages are known in which host DNA can be packaged into the viral capsid. These phages are called **transducing phages.** Transduction is defined as the transfer of bacterial DNA from one cell to another by means of a bacteriophage infection. Transduction processes fall broadly into two classes: specialized and generalized. In **specialized transduction,** a hybrid phage–bacterial genome is generated when a prophage genome is improperly excised from its host chromosome, dragging along some adjacent bacterial genes. The generation of specialized transducing particles is rare, occurring only in about 1 per 10^6 to 10^7 cells. The λ phage mediates specialized transduction. **Generalized transduction** results from a random and accidental packaging of host DNA into the phage capsid. Thus generalized transducing particles should contain all or nearly all bacterial DNA and little or no phage DNA.

One of the best studied phages that produces generalized transducing particles is phage P1, which infects *E. coli.* This phage has both a lytic and a lysogenic cycle. The P1 phage infects its *E. coli* host as described previously. However, once the P1 genome is inside the cell, a gene encoding a nuclease is expressed. This nuclease is responsible for the degradation of the *E. coli* host chromosomal DNA; and in about 1% of the infected cells these bacterial fragments are packaged into P1 capsids. Even if these generalized transducing particles are not able to produce P1 phage progeny, the encapsulated DNA can be injected into a new host where it can recombine with the homologous host DNA. Assuming that all parts of the chromosome are packaged with the same efficiency, a large population of P1 particles should contain representatives from each infected host gene.

Generalized transducing particles have proved valuable in genetic mapping of bacterial chromosomes, since the distance between two mutational sites that can cotransduce into (be transduced by) the same particle can be estimated. For example, the P1 phage can grow on a leucine (leu^+) lactose (lac^+) *E. coli* strain. The resulting lysate will contain a small number of P1/leu^+ lac^+ transducing particles. The lysate is then used to transduce a leu^- lac^- *E. coli* strain to leu^+ lac^+. The transduced *E. coli* cells may be selected on agar plates containing leucine and lactose, and their number determined. In such a joint transduction, the frequency of recombination is inversely proportional to the distance between two markers. This can be explained by the fact that P1 capsids can package only a maximum length of DNA. Thus if two markers, such as leu and lac described previously, are too far away from each other on the donor bacterial chromosome, the probability for them to be cotransduced falls rapidly.

The second way to estimate the distance between two mutational sites is by transductional recombination. Such type of recombination deals with mutations present in the same gene. In this case, the frequency of recombination is directly proportional to the distance between the mutated positions. Generalized transduction can also be used to modify the genotype of recipient plasmids and to transfer a variety of extrachromosomal factors. For example, P1 phage has been used to transfer the F factor, R factors, and colicin factors in *E. coli.* PBS1, PBP1, and PMB1 can transduce the plasmid pBL10 in *Bacillus pumilus* and P22 transfers R factors and colicin factors in *Salmonella typhimurium.*

Conjugative Transposons

Transposons are segments of DNA able to move from one position to another in the genome or from the chromosomal DNA to a plasmid or the reverse. They were first discovered in *E. coli* during a study of a class of highly polar mutations in the galactose and the lactose operons. It was noticed that these mutations could not be simply reverted by base substitutions or frameshift mutagens but only by excision of a large DNA fragment. Since then, many transposable elements have been characterized. The transposons found in bacteria can be divided into three classes: insertion sequences, complex transposons and phage-associated transposons.

Insertion Sequences

The **insertion sequence (IS)** elements are the simplest transposons. They range in length from 150 to 1500 base pairs and possess inverted repeats of 15 to 40 base pairs at their ends (Figure 4-8). The IS elements are normal constituents of bacterial chromosomes and can integrate into plasmid and phage genomes. The ISs carry only the genetic information necessary for their own transfer (i.e., the gene coding for the transposase). The ISs can be detected if their insertion leads to interruption or inactivation of genes or if they turn on the expression of adjacent genes.

Complex Transposons

The group of conjugative plasmids known as R factors has received considerable attention from the medical community. The R plasmids are composed of two functionally distinct parts: the resistance transfer factor and the transposon carrying genes for various kinds of drug resistances. These resistance plasmids are the most common cause of acquired antibiotic resistance in infecting bacteria and therefore represent a considerable threat to chemotherapy. The transposons carried by these conjugative plasmids can be divided into two general categories or types (Figure 4-8).

The type I, or **composite transposons,** contain a central region that carries selectable genes such as for resistance to antibiotics, for resistance to toxic substances, or even genes for prototrophy. This central region is flanked on either side by two identical or nearly identical IS elements. The IS elements can be positioned in either an inverted or a direct repeat configuration. Tn903, a representative of a type I composite transposon, contains two identical and inverted insertion sequences of the element IS903 at its ends. This transposon carries the gene encoding resistance to kanamycin.

The type II transposons include the **TnA transposon family.** These transposons are quite large (approximately 5 kb) and are not considered as composite transposons because they do not rely on the presence of IS modules for transposition. Instead, each transposon member is bound by two short repeats varying from 30 to 40 base pairs long. The central region usually contains three genes. One gene encodes an antibiotic resistance or resistance to toxic substances, and two other genes encode proteins involved in the transposition process: the transposase and the resolvase. The members of the TnA family transpose only by a replicative pathway (discussed later). The Tn3 transposon, which contains the genes necessary for ampicillin resistance, is an example of a type II transposon.

Phage-associated Transposons

An additional class of transposons includes the **transposable phages** such as Mu and D108, which use transposition as their normal mode of reproduction. Phage Mu is a temperate phage whose DNA is integrated almost at random into the genome of its host following infection. The insertion of the prophage usually inactivates the bacterial gene into which it is inserted by interrupting its coding sequence and by terminating transcription. It can also inactivate distal genes in the same operon. Induction of the Mu prophage, however, does not lead to its excision from the host DNA. Instead, it undergoes repeated

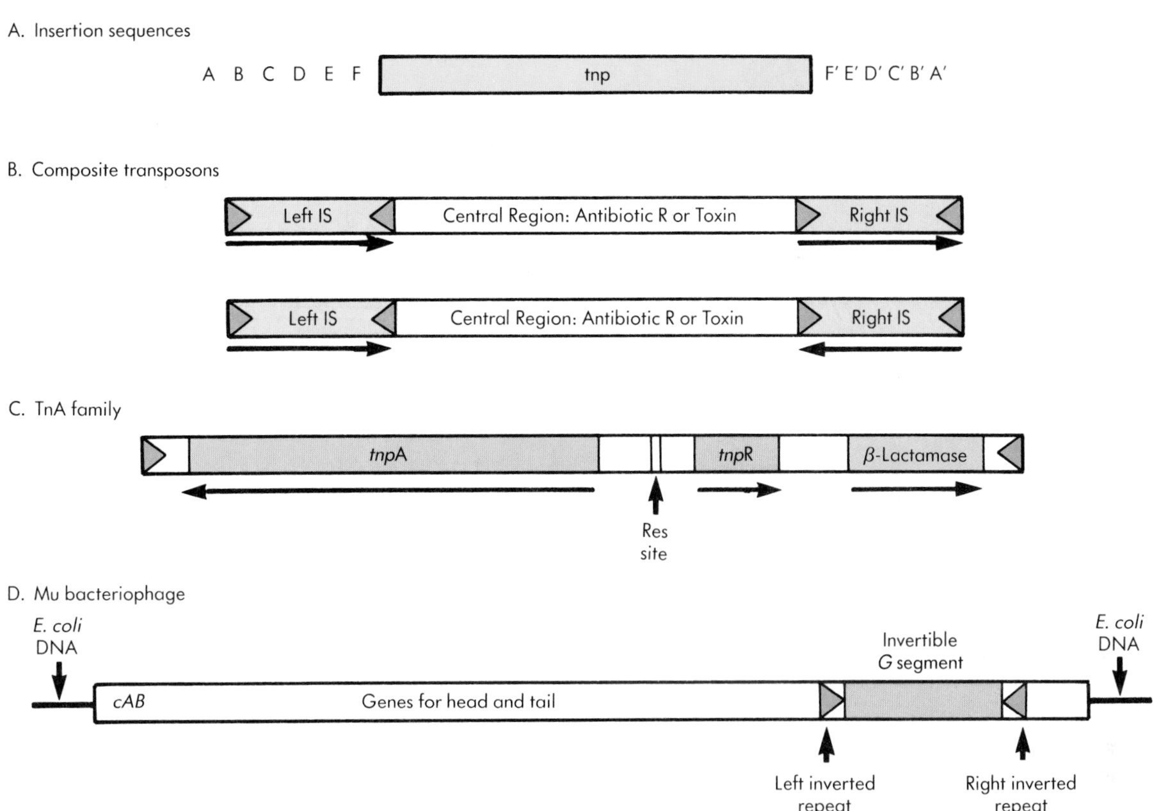

FIGURE 4-8 Transposons. **A,** The insertion sequences code only for a transposase ***(tnp)*** and possess inverted repeats (15 to 40 bp) at each end. **B,** The composite transposons contain a central region coding for antibiotic resistances or toxins, flanked by 2 ISs, which can be either directly repeated or reversed. **C,** Tn3, a member of the TnA transposon family. The central region encodes three genes: a transposase ***(tnpA)***, a resolvase ***(tnpR)*** and a β-lactamase, conferring resistance to ampicillin. A Resolution site **(Res site)** is used during the replicative transposition process. This central region is flanked on both ends by direct repeats of 38 bp(▶◀). **D,** Phage-associated transposon exemplified by the bacteriophage Mu.

replicative transposition to many different target sites on the chromosome. Packaging of the phage genome ultimately occurs from these chromosomally located units.

Replication Process of the Transposons

One common characteristic of transposition is that transposons do not move randomly but seem to prefer certain target sequences. The length of these target sequences varies among the transposons, and the target sequence is different for each insertion or a particular transposon. During the insertion process of a transposon, this target sequence is duplicated, flanking the transposon on both sides.

Transposition may occur by one of two mechanisms. In **conservative transposition,** the transposing element is displaced from its original site of insertion to a new location. Some elements such as IS10 and IS50, as well as the composite transposons containing these modules, are known to move only by conservative transposition. With **replicative transposition,** the transposing element is duplicated, resulting in two complete copies integrated in direct orientation and separated by bacterial host DNA. Transposon members of the TnA family move only by replicative transposition. In all cases, deletions, as well as inversions, can be caused by the presence of a transposon following an aberrant excision.

CONTRIBUTION OF GENETIC ENGINEERING TO MEDICINE

One of the most important contributions of prokaryotic genetic engineering is the development of vectors or vehicles allowing the cloning of any DNA sequence. Cloning vectors must allow the insertion of foreign DNA in them but still be able to replicate normally in the bacterial host. Many types of vectors are currently used: (1) **plasmid vectors** such as pBR322 and pUC, (2) bacteriophages such as λ, or more recently (3) **cosmid vectors,** which combine some of the advantages of plasmids and phages. To clone a foreign piece of DNA or **complementary DNA (cDNA),** DNA obtained by

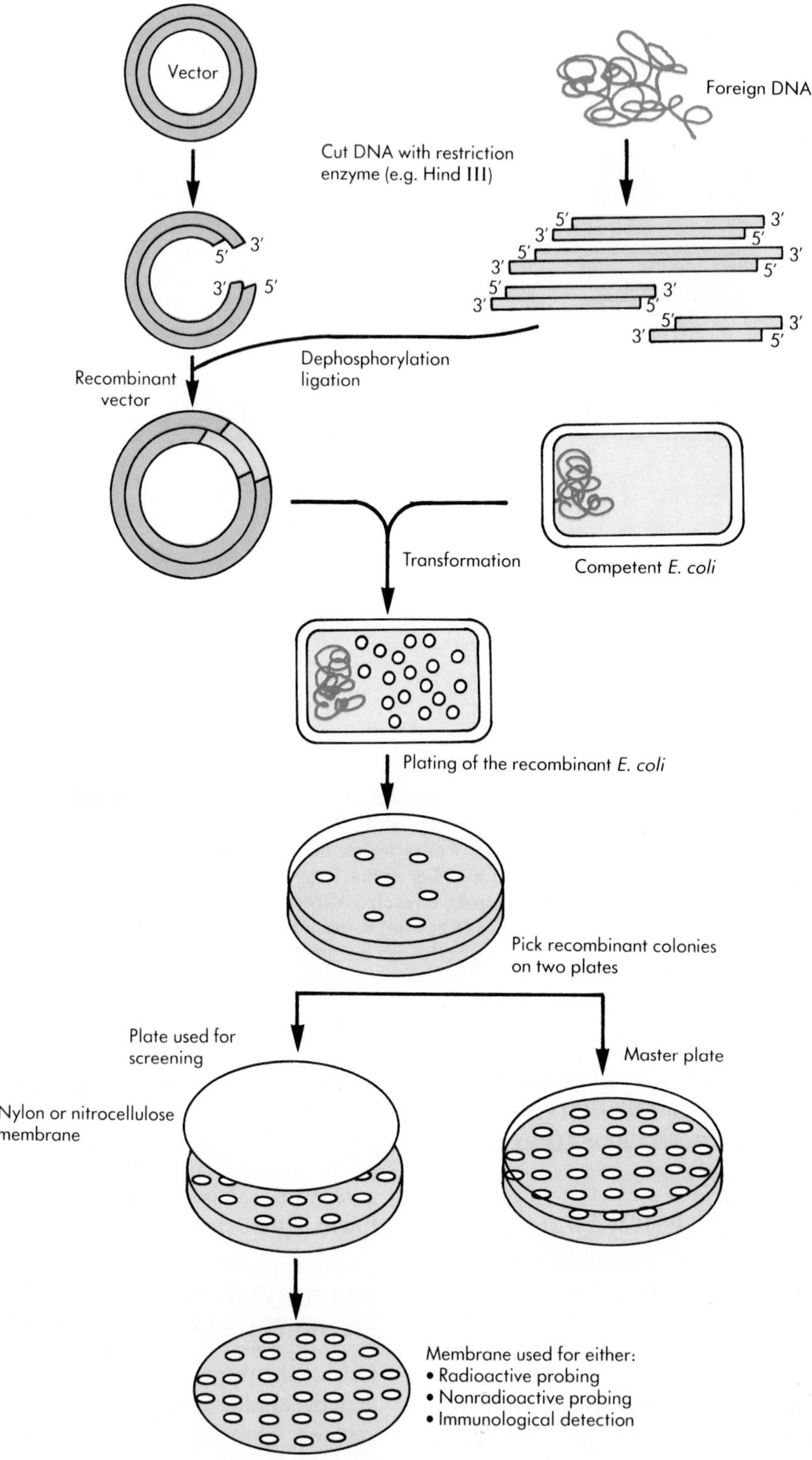

FIGURE 4-9 Cloning of foreign DNA in vectors. The vector and the foreign DNA are first digested by a restriction enzyme. The vector DNA is usually dephosphorylated using calf intestine alkaline phosphatase (CIAP) or bacterial alkaline phosphatase (BAP). The vector is then ligated to the foreign DNA using T4 DNA ligase. The recombinant vectors are transformed into *E. coli* cells made competent by one of the techniques described in the text. The recombinant *E. coli* are plated, and each clone is picked onto 2 different agar plates, one of which is kept as a master plate. Colonies are then transferred to nylon or nitrocellulose membranes, which are used with detection techniques such as dot blot analysis with radioactive or nonradioactive probes as well as immunoscreening.

TABLE 4-1 Common Restriction Enzymes Used in Molecular Biology With Their Origin and Recognition Sites

Microorganism	Enzyme	Recognition site
Acinetobacter calcoaceticus	*Acc* I	5′ G T ↓ (A/C) (G/T) A C C A (T/G) (C/A) ↑ T G
Bacillus amyloliquefaciens H	*Bam*H I	5′ G ↓ G A T C C C C T A G ↑ G
Escherichia coli RY13	*Eco*R I	5′ G ↓ A A T T C C T T A A ↑ G
Haemophilus influenzae R_d	*Hind* III	5′ A ↓ A G C T T T T C G A ↑ A
Haemophilus influenzae Serotype c, 1160	*Hinc* II	5′ G T (C/T) ↓ (G/A) A C C A (G/A) ↑ (C/T) T G
Providencia stuartii 164	*Pst* I	5′ C T G C A ↓ G G ↑ A C G T C
Serratia marcescens S_b	*Sma* I	5′ C C C ↓ G G G G G G ↑ C C C
Staphylococcus aureus 3A	*Sau*3A I	5′ ↓ G A T C C T A G ↑
Xanthomonas malvacearum	*Xma* I	5′ C ↓ C C G G G G G G C C ↑ C

reverse transcription of the mRNA, both the vector and the DNA must be cleaved with restriction enzymes (Figure 4-9). Restriction enzymes recognize a site-specific sequence and make either a staggered cut, generating sticky ends, or a blunt cut with blunt ends (Table 4-1). The ligation of the vector with the DNA fragments generates a chimeric molecule called **recombinant DNA** (Figure 4-9). The total number of recombinant vectors obtained when cloning chromosomal DNA is known as a **genomic library** because there should be at least one representative of each gene in the library. The recombinant DNA is then transformed into a bacterial host, usually *E. coli,* which can generate an almost infinite amount of the desired DNA fragment. The library can then be screened to find an *E. coli* clone possessing the desired DNA fragment. Various screening techniques can be used such as the dot blot or the immunoscreening procedures, which both include transferring the bacterial colonies to a solid support called a membrane. The positive clones can be discovered using a labeled DNA fragment as a probe in the dot blot technique or for the immunoscreening method, specific polyclonal or monoclonal antibodies. The DNA sequence from the chosen clone can be determined and oftentimes the cloned protein purified.

Eukaryotic genes may be expressed in prokaryotic systems by using an expression cloning vector. With some modification of the previously described scheme, an expression library can be constructed. Such a vector system will provide the foreign (eukaryotic) DNA with a promoter and a ribosome binding site. The only disadvantage of the expression of eukaryotic genes in prokaryotic cells is that the mRNA will not be processed. This problem, however, can be overcome by cloning the cDNA, which eliminates the splicing step necessary for eukaryotic gene expression being synthesized from the already processed mRNA. In humans, many genetic diseases are caused by the lack of a single protein. With the recent developments in genetic engineering, therapy is now possible for some of these diseases. For example, useful proteins such as insulin, interferon, growth hormones, and interleukin can now be produced in recombinant bacteria in sufficient quantities to allow their isolation and use in therapy.

The production in bacteria of recombinant vaccines for viral or parasitic infections represents an additional application of molecular biology. This new technology is based on the expression in microorganisms of genes from pathogens that encode surface antigens capable of inducing neutralizing antibodies in the host. The major purpose of cloning the relevant genes into suitable organisms is to make large amounts of pure antigens. Such an approach also possesses the advantage of eliminating the need to work with the intact disease organisms. The development of a vaccine against hepatitis B represents the first success of recombinant DNA vaccines approved for human use by the U.S. Food and Drug Administration. This vaccine is produced by the yeast *Saccharomyces cerevisiae,* which has been transformed with the recombinant vector containing the cloned viral gene encoding a surface protein. A second hepatitis B antigen has also been cloned and expressed in *E. coli.* This antigen, called the **core antigen,** represents one of the major components of the viral nucleocapsid. This core antigen is part of a widely distributed diagnostic kit used to detect antibodies to this immunogen. These antibodies not only reflect infection with the hepatitis B virus but also serve as a surrogate marker for non-A, non-B hepatitis.

Recent progress in gene cloning and expression, together with the development of rapid methods for DNA sequencing and oligonucleotide synthesis, provides all the necessary tools for genome manipulations. These new technologies can, in principle, be applied to the development of live vaccines. For example, genes expressing antigens of influenza, herpes simplex, and other agents have been inserted into the genome of vaccinia, the virus of the smallpox vaccine. Genetically engineered bacteria can also be used for the production of live vaccines. An avirulent bacterial strain of *Salmonella typhi* harboring *Shigella sonnei* plasmids can colonize the gut-associated lymphoid tissue (GALT) for a limited time without systemic effect and provoke the induction of generalized, as well as local, immune mucosal response to the *Shigella* antigens. Similar results have been obtained with a strain of *S. typhimurium* transformed with a recombinant plasmid containing an antigenic protein from *Streptococcus mutans.* A mucosal immune response was manifested by the appearance of specific sIgA antibodies in the mice saliva.

Replacement therapy is the use of bacterial interference for the prevention and/or treatment of bacterial infections. The application of replacement therapy as a therapeutic approach offers considerable advantages over more traditional treatments. Ideally, one application of the effector strain to tissues at risk should lead to a persistent colonization and a lifelong protection from pathogens while requiring minimal compliance, cost, or education on the part of the patient. Moreover, such a strain may be naturally transmitted between individuals in the population. The use of bacterial interference to treat a bacterial infection was first attempted by Cantani in 1885 when he claimed to have successfully treated a case of tuberculosis by insufflating the lungs of the patient with the so-called harmless bacteria "Bact.termo." More recently, Shinefield and his collaborators noted high rates of morbidity and mortality in nurseries in the early 1960s. These deaths were caused by neonatal acquisition of the very virulent strain *Staphylococcus aureus* phage type 80/81. They implanted *S. aureus* 502A, a naturally occurring strain of low virulence, in the nasal cavity and on the umbilicus of infants before they became infected by the virulent type 80/81 strain. This replacement therapy was quite successful in blocking colonization by other *Staphylococcus* strains and preventing epidemics. Many examples of short-term uses of bacterial implantations have been reported in a wide spectrum ranging from the prevention of neonatal diarrhea in pigs to the use of attenuated (weakened) strains of *S. mutans* in the fight against dental caries. Genetic engineering offers all the necessary tools for the design of specific effector strains, which could prevent colonization or outgrowth of a pathogen before any damage is done.

The supply of natural antibiotics for direct use or chemical modification is not infinite. Genetic engineering offers the possibility for widening the range of available antibiotics. It will clearly not replace, but complement, the quest for the discovery of new antibiotics in natural isolates and the improvement of antibiotic production by mutation combined with medium and fermentation optimization. Two distinct approaches can be used to generate new types of antibiotics by altering the bacterial genotype. In the first approach, biotechnologists are investigating the differential expression of genes under the influence of specific environmental signals and by different bacterial strains. Many reports have demonstrated the production of novel compounds by recombinants generated by conjugation between Streptomycete strains. For example, the transfer of two separate DNA fragments from the actinomycin-producing *Streptomyces antibioticus* to *S. lividans* caused the production of the enzyme phenoxazinone synthase (PHS). In *S. antibioticus,* this enzyme is involved in actinomycin biosynthesis. However, neither of the two cloned DNA fragments carried a structural gene for this enzyme. In the original host, such genes are probably carefully regulated and most likely expressed under particular ecological, physiological, or developmental conditions that are different from those used during antibiotic screening. The second approach includes the production of "hybrid" antibiotics. These novel compounds can be generated by the cloning and genetic modification of some or all the genes necessary for the biosynthesis of one antibiotic.

APPLICATION OF MOLECULAR BIOTECHNOLOGY TO CLINICAL DIAGNOSIS

The application of molecular biotechnology to clinical diagnosis has given rise to a new discipline called **diagnostic molecular pathology.** This new field can be broadly defined as the use of nucleic acid probes to diagnose and study diseases. The molecular diagnostic techniques can be applied to a wide spectrum of human diseases such as infectious diseases, neoplastic diseases, and hereditary diseases. Another application is DNA fingerprinting, which can differentiate between

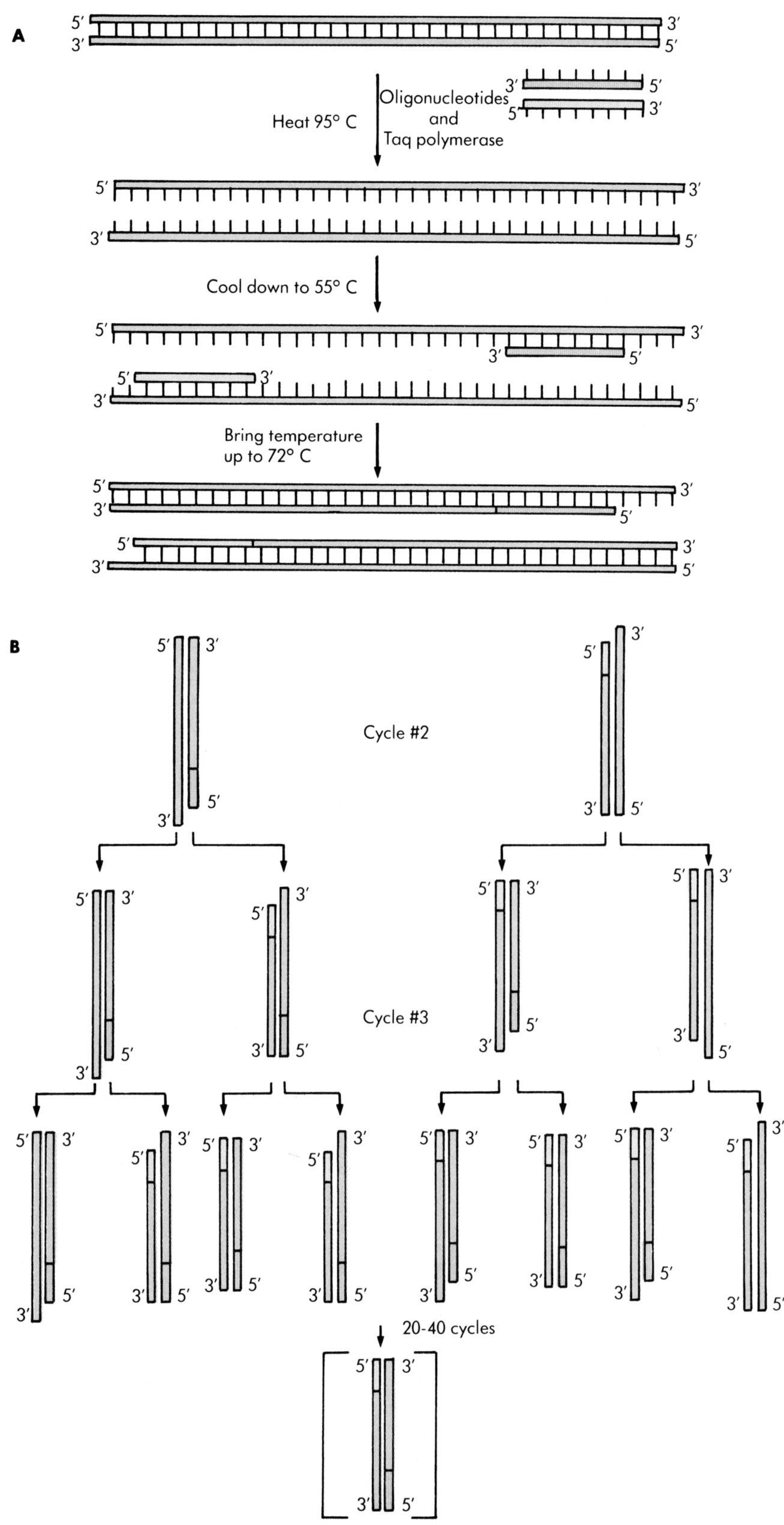

FIGURE 4-10 Polymerase chain reaction technique. **A,** First cycle of PCR. Two single-stranded primers are generated that are specific for opposite ends of the gene or sequence of interest. The samples are heated to 95° C to denature the DNA strands and cooled down to 55° C, allowing the annealing of the primers to their complementary sequences on the single-stranded DNA. These double-stranded regions act as templates for the taq polymerase when the temperature is brought back to 72° C. **B,** Following PCR cycles. The cycle in **A** is repeated 20 to 40 times, leading to an exponential accumulation of the gene of interest.

individuals using only minute tissue or blood specimens.

The common basis of all techniques of molecular pathology is the use of DNA probes in the diagnosis of diseases. To make a probe, the DNA of interest is inserted into a vector, the recombinant vector transformed into a bacterium and amplified to a high copy number in bacterial culture. The isolated recombinant vector can then be cleaved with a restriction enzyme and the pure DNA insert obtained. This DNA fragment is then labeled with some signal moiety that can be detected after hybridization. DNA labeling is achieved with the help of a polymerase, which incorporates either radioactive nucleotides or nonradioactive derivatives such as biotynilated nucleotides and digoxigenin-labeled nucleotides into newly synthesized complementary strands of DNA. By **in situ hybridization** (the direct application of DNA probes to a tissue section of intact cells on a glass slide), even the histological architecture can be retained. Many specific DNA probes used for diagnosis of bacterial diseases are now available. Those commonly used probes can detect infectious agents such as *Legionella* and *Mycobacteriae* species, *Neisseria gonorrhoeae, Chlamydia, Rickettsia,* or the toxigenic plasmids of *E. coli.*

The major concern in diagnosis by means of hybridization procedures has been the lack of sensitivity. Techniques such as in situ hybridization using nonradioactive probes are able to detect greater than 200 viral genome copies per cell. One of the most exciting developments in recombinant DNA technology is the use of a technique called **polymerase chain reaction (PCR)** (Figure 4-10). This powerful technique allows the generation of millions of exact copies of specific pieces of nucleic acid. A prerequisite for the use of PCR is that the nucleotide sequence of at least part of the target DNA be known. In approximately 2 hours, millions of copies of the specific target sequence can be obtained. Unlike the techniques described previously, the sensitivity of PCR is exquisite, with detection limits of a single bacterium. Moreover, DNA can be amplified from most clinical specimens, as well as paraffin-embedded material. The PCR technique is now commonly used in the diagnosis of many bacterial infections such as bacterial meningitis, mycobacterial diseases, *Rickettsia* species, *Treponema* and *Borrelia* strains, and for the detection of genital and congenital infections. The presence of antibiotic resistance genes can also be detected, thus allowing clinicians to prescribe earlier treatment with drugs to which the infectious organism is sensitive. Unknown organisms can also be studied by this technique using universal primers to 16S rRNA. The amplified fragment can be sequenced and the bacteria identified.

The application of molecular biotechnology to medicine represents new, exciting, and rapidly progressing research, development, and application. The cure or diagnosis of diseases, although impossible yesterday, may become routine tomorrow. See Box 4-1 for a list of the key words for this chapter.

BOX 4-1 Key Words

Apoinducer
Bacteriophage
Budding
Capsid
Codon
Competence
Complementary DNA (cDNA)
Composite transposon
Conjugation
Conservative transposition
Core antigen
Corepressor
Cosmid
Diagnostic molecular pathology
DNA-reactive chemical
Direct DNA repair
Eclipse
Electroporation
Error-prone repair
Excision repair
Frameshift mutagen
Frameshift mutation
Generalized transduction
Genomic library
Hfr cell
Incompatibility group
Inducer
Inducible
Induction
Insertion sequence (IS)
In situ hybridization
Lysogeny
Lytic cycle
Missense mutation
MobilizationMutation
Negative control
Nonsense mutation
Nucleotide base analogue
Null mutation
Operator
Operon
Plasmid
Polymerase chain reaction (PCR)
Positive control
Postreplication repair
Recombinant DNA
Recombinational repair
Replacement therapy
Replicative transposition
Replicon
Repressible
Repressor protein
Silent mutation
SOS response
Specialized transduction
Suppression
Temperate phage
TnA transposon family
Transformation
Transducing phage
Transduction
Transfer RNA (tRNA)
Transition
Translational control
Transposable phage
Transposon
Transversion
Vector
Virulent phage

QUESTIONS

1. What are the principal properties of a plasmid?
2. Give two mechanisms of regulation of bacterial gene expression using specific examples.
3. What types of mutations affect DNA, and what agents are responsible for such mutations?
4. What mechanisms may be used by a bacterial cell for the exchange of genetic material? Briefly explain each.
5. Discuss applications of molecular biotechnology to medicine, including contributions and uses in diagnosis.

Bibliography

Cohen SN: Transposable genetic elements and plasmid evolution, *Nature* 263:731-738, 1976.

Davis B, Dulbecco R, Eisen HN, and Ginsberg HS: *Microbiology,* ed 4, Philadelphia, 1990, J.B. Lippincott.

Florey HW: The use of micro-organisms for therapeutic purposes, *Yale J Biol Med* 19:101-117, 1946.

Freifelder D: *Molecular biology,* Boston, 1983, Jones & Bartlett.

Gilbert W and Villa-Komaroff L: Useful proteins from recombinant bacteria, *Scient Am* 242:74-94, 1980.

Grody WW, Gatti RA, and Naeim F: Diagnostic molecular pathology, *Mod Pathol* 2:553-568, 1989.

Hanahan D: Studies on transformation of *Escherichia coli* with plasmids, *J Mol Biol* 166:557-580, 1983.

Hardy K: *Bacterial plasmids,* Washington DC, 1981, American Society for Microbiology.

Heineman JA: Genetics of gene transfer between species, *TIG* 7:181-185, 1991.

Hillman JP and Socransky SS: The theory and application of bacterial interference to oral diseases. In Myers HM, editor: *New biotechnology in oral research,* Switzerland, 1989, Karger.

Hopwood DA: Antibiotics: opportunities for genetic manipulation, *Phil Trans R Soc Lond B* 324:549-562, 1989.

Jacob F and Monod J: Genetic regulatory mechanisms in the synthesis of proteins, *J Mol Biol* 3:318-356, 1961.

Lehninger AL: *Principles of biochemistry,* New York, 1982, Worth Publishers.

Lewin B: *Genes IV,* ed 4, New York, 1990, Oxford University Press.

Low KB and Porter DD: Modes of gene transfer and recombination in bacteria, *Ann Rev Genet* 12:249-287, 1978.

Murray K, Stahl S, and Ashton-Rickardt PG: Genetic engineering applied to the development of vaccines, *Phil Trans R Soc Lond B* 324:461-476, 1989.

Ossanna N, Peterson KR, and Mount DW: Genetics of DNA repair in bacteria, *TIG* 2:55, 1986.

Seeburg PH, Shine J, Martial JA, Ivarie RD, Morris JA, Ullrich A, Baxter JD, and Goodman HM: Synthesis of growth hormone by bacteria, *Nature* 276:795-798, 1978.

Shinefield HR, Ribble JC, Boris M, and Eichenwald HF: Bacterial interference: its effect on nursery acquired infections with *Staphylococcus aureus,* I, II, III, IV, *Am J Dis Child* 105:646-682, 1963.

Sprunt K and Leidy G: The use of bacterial interference to prevent infection, *Can J Microbiol* 34:332-338, 1988.

Watson JD, Hopkins NH, Roberts JW, Argetsinger Steitz J, and Weirner AM: *Molecular biology of the gene,* ed 4, Menlo Park, Calif, 1987, Benjamin–Cummings.

CHAPTER 5

Fungal Biology and Classification

MYCOLOGY is the branch of biology that deals with the study of fungi. The systematic study of these organisms is approximately 150 years old, yet the practical manifestations of these organisms have been known since antiquity. In addition to their disease-producing potential in humans, fungi are directly or indirectly harmful in many other ways. They contribute to food spoilage, are the major cause of plant diseases, and destroy timber, textiles, and several synthetic materials. However, as saprobes, they share with bacteria (particularly organisms such as the *Streptomyces*) a role in the decay of complex plant and animal remains in the soil, breaking them down into simpler molecules to be absorbed by future generations of plants. Without this essential decay process the growth of plants, on which life depends, would eventually cease for lack of basic materials. Fungi are also specifically beneficial to humans. They are used in the production of antibiotics, organic acids, steroids, alcoholic beverages, and products of fermentation, such as soya sauce. The carbon dioxide produced by fungi makes dough rise in bread-making, and the various ketones, aldehydes, and organic acids that result from the metabolic activities of fungi on milk curd and the juice of grapes provide the unique cheeses and wines we enjoy. Furthermore, fungi serve as scientific models to study genetics, biochemical processes, and relationships involving parasites and hosts.

Fungi are a diverse group of organisms that occupy many niches in the environment. In general they are free living and abundant in nature, with only a few in the normal flora of humans. Although tens of thousands of species have been described, fewer than 100 are routinely associated with human diseases. Unlike viruses, protozoan parasites, and some species of bacteria, fungi do not need to colonize or infect tissues of humans or animals to preserve or perpetuate the species. With only two major exceptions (candidiasis and tinea versicolor), virtually all fungal infections originate from an exogenous source, either by inhalation or by traumatic implantation.

Fungi are **eukaryotic organisms.** Most important, they possess a nucleus enclosed by a nuclear membrane. Unlike plant cells and some bacteria, fungi do not contain chlorophyll and cannot synthesize macromolecules from carbon dioxide and energy derived from light rays. Therefore all fungi lead a heterotrophic existence in nature as **saprobes** (organisms that live on dead or decaying organic matter), **symbionts** (organisms that live together in which the association is of mutual advantage), **commensals** (two organisms living in a close relationship in which one benefits by the relationship and the other neither benefits nor is harmed), or **parasites** (organisms that live on or within a host from which they derive benefits without making any useful contributions in return; in the case of pathogens the relationship is harmful to the host).

Whereas the ability of fungi to cause disease in humans or animals appears to be accidental, most disease-producing fungi have developed characteristics that enable them to adapt to hostile tissue environments and grow. Fungi that colonize the cutaneous layers of the epidermis or invade hair and nails metabolize **keratin**, the tough, fibrous, insoluble protein that forms the principal matter of these tissues. Other fungi, such as *Histoplasma capsulatum*, *Blastomyces dermatitidis*, *Paracoccidioides brasiliensis*, and *Coccidioides immitis* have developed the capacity to overcome various host cellular defense mechanisms, are able to grow at the higher temperatures of the host (37° C) and the temperatures found in natural environments (around 25° C), and can survive in a lowered oxidation-reduction state (a situation found in damaged tissues).

BIOLOGY

Morphology

Fungi can be divided into two basic morphologic forms, **yeast** and **hyphae**. Their developmental histories encompass both vegetative and reproductive phases. These phases are frequently present simultaneously in growing cultures and may not be easily separated.

Yeasts are unicellular and reproduce asexually by processes termed **blastoconidia formation** (budding; Figure 5-1, *A*) or **fission** (Figure 5-1, *B*).

Most fungi have branching, threadlike tubular fila-

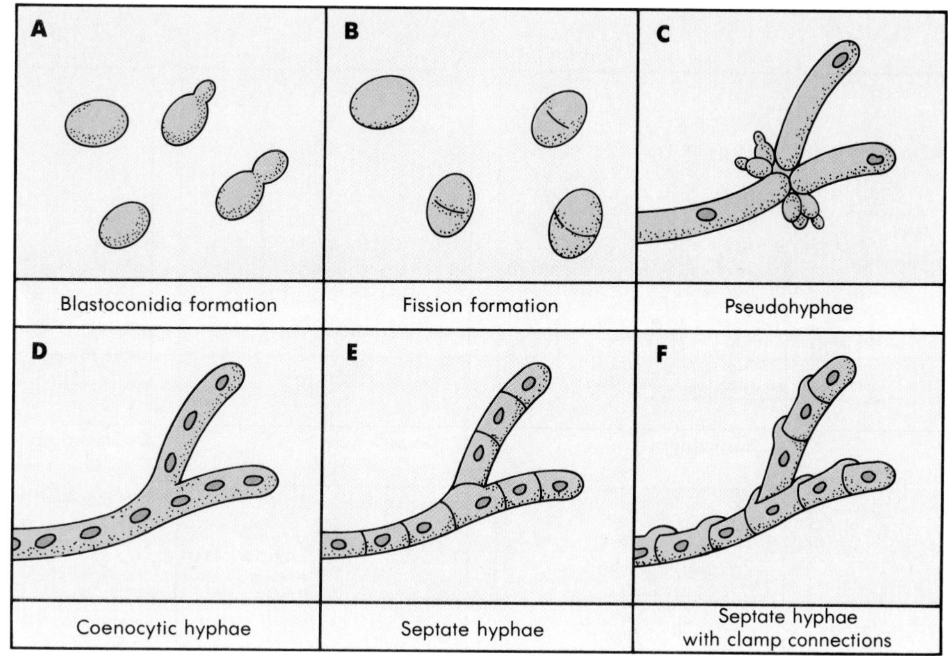

FIGURE 5-1 Fungal cell morphology. **A,** Yeast cells reproducing by blastoconidia formation; **B,** yeast cells dividing by fission; **C,** pseudohyphal development; **D,** coenocytic hyphae; **E,** septate hyphae; and **F,** septate hyphae with clamp connections.

ments called **hyphae** (Figure 5-1, *C* to *E*) that elongate at their tips by a process called **apical extension.** These filamentous structures are either **coenocytic** (hollow and multinucleate; Figure 5-1, *D*) or **septate** (divided by partitions; Figure 5-1, *E* and *F*). The collective term for a mass of hyphae is **mycelium** (synonymous with **mold**). Hyphae that grow submerged or on the surface of a culture medium are called **vegetative hyphae** because they are responsible for absorbing nutrients. Those that project above the surface of the medium are called **aerial hyphae.** Aerial hyphae often produce specialized structures called **conidia** (i.e., asexual reproductive elements also called propagules) that are easily airborne and disseminated into the environment. The shape, size, and certain developmental features of conidia are useful to the mycologist in identifying the specific species. Various examples of conidia are illustrated in Figure 5-2.

The morphology of fungi is not fixed, because some are **dimorphic** (e.g., *H. capsulatum*, *B. dermatitidis*, *C. immitis*, *P. brasiliensis*); that is, they can exist in a mycelial or yeast morphology depending on the environmental conditions of growth (in soil, on decaying vegetation, or in host tissues). The morphology of *Candida albicans*, part of the normal flora of the mouth, gastrointestinal tract, and membranes lining the mucosa of other cavities and tissues, is unique. In addition to being yeastlike or filamentous, this organism can assume a **pseudohyphal** morphology, wherein the cells are elongated and linked together like sausages (Figure 5-1, *C*). Pseudohyphal development is an exaggerated form of budding; the newly formed cells do not take on an oval shape and pinch off from the parent but rather remain attached and continue to elongate.

Cell Structure

Fungi have structures typical of eukaryotic cells. Figure 5-3 illustrates a section of a model fungal cell with its component parts. In contrast to bacterial cells, fungal cells possess a complex cytosol that contains microvesicles, microtubules, ribosomes, mitochondria, Golgi apparatus, nuclei, a double-membraned endoplasmic reticulum, and other structures. The nuclei of fungi are enclosed by a membrane and contain virtually all of the cellular DNA. They have a true nucleolus rich in RNA. An interesting and unique property of this membrane is that during the mitotic cycle it persists throughout metaphase, in contrast to the nuclear membrane of plant and animal cells, which dissolves and then re-forms after the chromosomes segregate to their centromeres.

Enclosing the complex cytosol is another membrane called the **plasmalemma** that is composed of glycoproteins, lipids, and ergosterol. The fact that fungi possess ergosterol in contrast to cholesterol, which is the major sterol found in tissues of mammals, is important because most antifungal strategies are currently based on the presence of ergosterol in fungal membranes (antifungal agents are discussed in Chapter 14).

Unlike mammalian cells, fungi possess a multilayered rigid cell wall immediately exterior to the plasmalemma. The cell wall is structurally and biochemically complex, containing **chitin,** a polymer of *N*-acetyl glucosamine, as

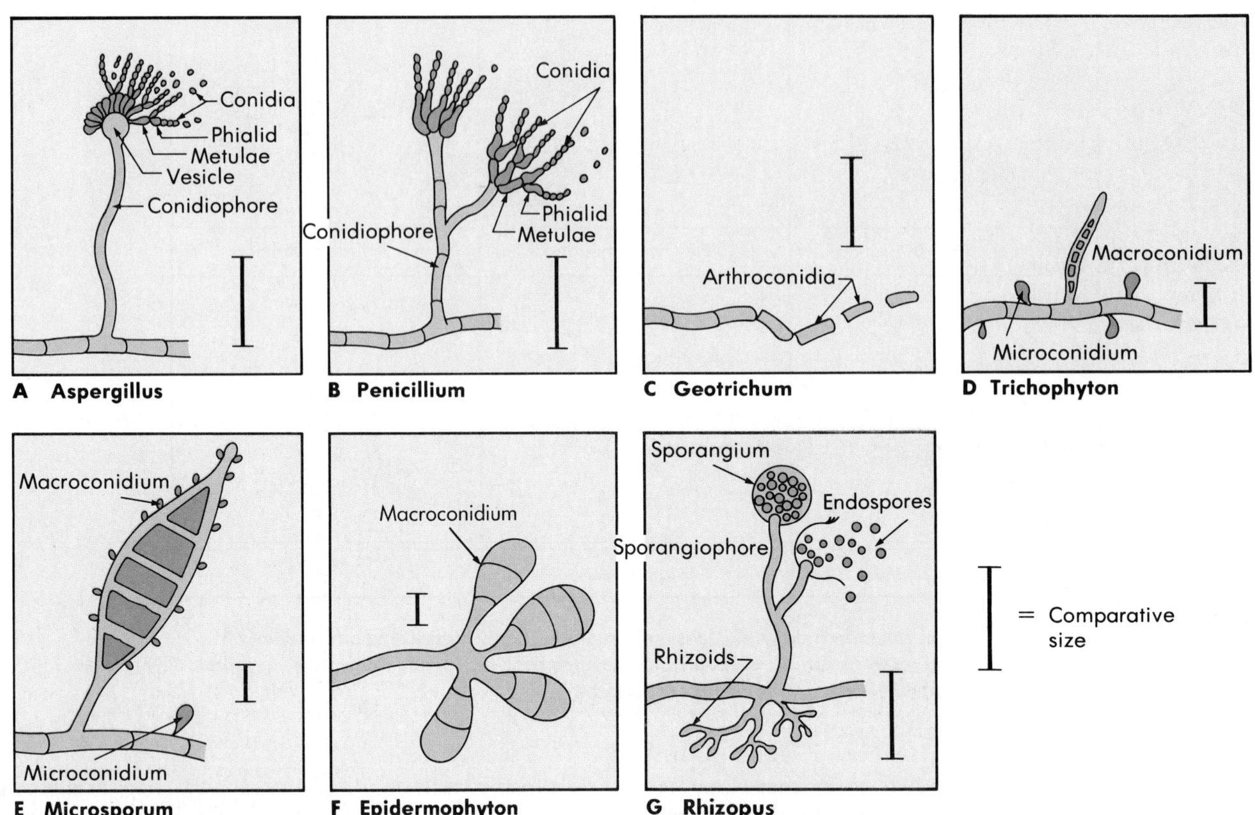

FIGURE 5-2 Conidial development in **A,** *Aspergillus;* **B,** *Penicillium;* **C,** *Geotrichum;* **D,** *Trichophyton;* **E,** *Microsporum;* **F,** *Epidermophyton;* and **G,** *Rhizopus.*

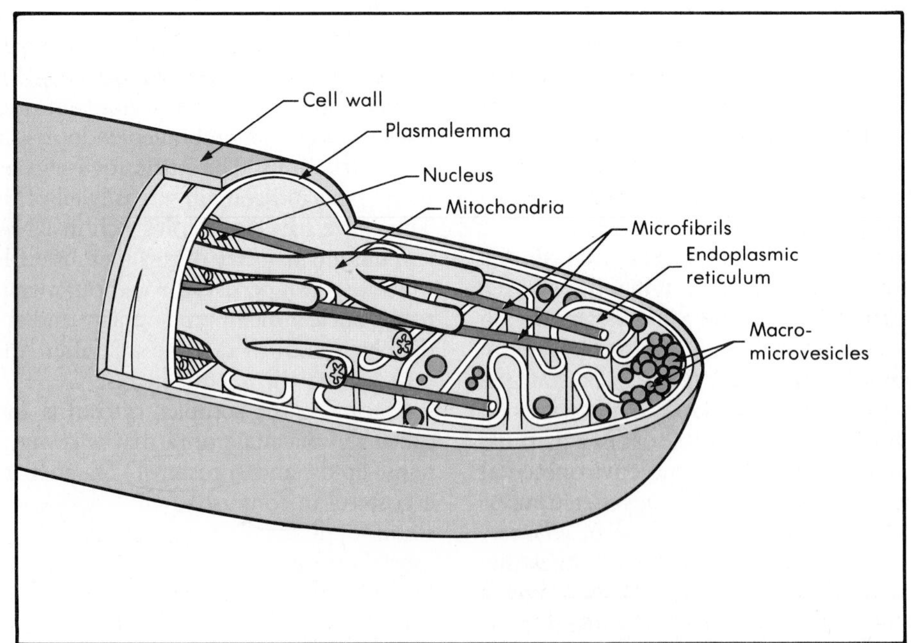

FIGURE 5-3 Diagram of the apical portion of hyphal cell illustrating its component parts.

its structural foundation. Layered on the chitin are mannans, glucans, and other complex polysaccharides in association with polypeptides. In filamentous fungi the biosynthesis of chitin occurs at the growing tip and is controlled by the activity of chitin synthase. This enzyme exists in the cytosol in discrete membrane-bound packets called chitosomes. The active form of chitin synthase is found in the plasmalemma, and polymerization of chitin microfibrils occurs outside this membrane.

In addition to the cell wall some fungi produce a capsular polysaccharide. This structure isolates the organism from its surrounding environment and at the same time serves as a communicator with that environment; in the case of pathogens this environment is host tissue. The cell wall and structures such as the capsular material determine virulence and play a role in eliciting host immune responses (see Chapter 44, the discussion of *Cryptococcus neoformans*).

Table 5-1 summarizes some of the important features of fungi.

TABLE 5-1 Summary of Important Features of Fungal Cells

Cell feature	Characteristics
Nucleus	Membrane-bound (eukaryotic); multichromosomal and can be haploid or diploid depending on whether conjugation has taken place; contains RNA-rich area (nucleolus)
Cytosol	Complex; contains several organelles such as nucleus, mitochondria, Golgi apparatus, ribosomes, a well-defined endoplasmic reticulum and other inclusions
Plasmalemma	Composed of glycoproteins, lipids, and ergosterol; differs from mammalian cell membranes, which contain cholesterol
Cell wall	Multilayered; composed of chitin, other polysaccharides such as glucans, mannans, glucomannans, galactomannans and peptides; some fungi produce an extracellular polysaccharide capsule
Shape and size	Yeasts are oval to round; 2 to 10 μm in diameter; molds are filamentous septate or coenocytic and branching; 2 to 10 μm in diameter and can be several hundred micrometers in length
Physiology	Respiration almost exclusively oxidative with limited capacity for anaerobiasis (fermentation); metabolism exclusively heterotrophic; biochemically versatile; produces various primary (e.g., citric acid, ethanol) and secondary (e.g., alpha amanitin, aflatoxin) metabolites; doubling time long (hours) compared with most bacteria (minutes)
Staining properties	Gram-positive; vegetative cells not acid-fast; in histopathological sections the fungal cell wall can be stained by special procedures (methenamine-silver or periodic acid Schiff-stain methods)

CLASSIFICATION

Organisms are classified for convenience of reference; thus the scheme of classification should reflect natural relationships between them. Biochemical, ultrastructural, molecular biological, and genetic studies support the concept that at least five kingdoms are necessary to accommodate all living things. These are the Monera (prokaryotes), Protista (protozoa), Fungi, Plantae, and Animalia. The Fungi kingdom is composed of two phyla (Table 5-2), the Zygomycota (organisms that produce a zygote during their sexual cycle) and the Dikaryomycota (organisms that have an extended dikaryotic state as a result of sexual conjugation). The phylum Dikaryomycota is divided into two subphyla, the Ascomycotina and the Basidiomycotina, which are defined according to the type of structure that forms and houses the haploid progeny. Those organisms for which a sexual phase has not been observed are classified in the form-class Deuteromycotina or Fungi imperfecti.

All fungi reproduce by asexual processes, and most can reproduce by sexual mechanisms. If a sexual phase is observed for any fungal isolate, the terms **anamorph** (asexual) and **teleomorph** (sexual) are often used to describe the taxonomic status of the organism. This is reflected mostly in the nomenclature used to refer to that organism. For example, the anamorphic designation for the organism causing histoplasmosis is *H. capsulatum*; if the specific isolate exists in the teleomorphic state, the name is changed to *Ajellomyces capsulatum*. This convention is used for all fungal organisms to maintain taxonomic consistency. However, in clinical situations it is common to refer to the organisms by their asexual designations, since the anamorphic state is isolated from clinical specimens and the sexual phase occurs only under the extremely controlled conditions of a culture.

TABLE 5-2 Taxonomic Classification of the Fungi Kingdom

Organism	Sexual characteristics	Medially important genera
Phylum Zygomycota	Sexual reproduction occurs through the fusion of two compatible gametangia to produce a zygote. Asexual reproduction is characterized by production of sporangiospores.	Agents causing zygomycosis
Phylum Dikaryomycota	Organisms whose dikaryotic life cycle includes an extended dikaryotic phase after sexual conjugation (i.e., haploid nuclei do not fuse immediately)	
Subphylum Ascomyoctina	Sexual reproduction occurs through the fusion of two compatible nuclei to form a diploid nucleus followed by meiosis to yield haploid progeny. The entire process occurs within a sac called an ascus, and the resultant spores are called ascospores.	Agents causing ringworm, histoplasmosis, and blastomycosis
Subphylum Basidiomyoctina	Sexual reproduction takes place in a sac called a basidium, where two compatible nuclei fuse to form a diploid nucleus, followed by meiosis to yield haploid progeny. These then mature on the outer surface of the basidium. The haploid progeny are called basidiospores.	Agent causing cryptococcosis
Form-class Deuteromycotina (Fungi imperfecti)	A sexual stage has not been observed in fungi classified in this category.	*Candida, Trichosporon, Torulopsis, Pityrosporum, Epidermophyton, Coccidioides, Paracoccidioides*

Conflicts often arise in considering relationships within and between certain fungi, and no universal consensus may be possible concerning the classification or even the nomenclature of a given organism. Differences of opinion occasionally arise, since one taxonomist may place greater emphasis on certain phenotypic features of an isolate than on criteria deemed more important by other individuals. Another difficulty is the conflict between those who group many organisms together and those who prefer to emphasize minor phenotype differences and split them into many groups. The result of these conflicting opinions is the controversy that frequently arises over the proper name of individual fungi.

QUESTIONS

1. How do fungi differ from bacteria?
2. What is the basic difference between the cell membrane (plasmalemma) of fungal and mammalian cells?
3. How do yeast differ from molds, and what does the term *dimorphism* mean when it is applied to fungi?
4. What do the terms *anamorph* and *teleomorph* mean, and of what importance are they?

Bibliography

Bennett JW and Laisure L, editors: *More gene manipulation in fungi*, New York, 1991, Academic Press.
Cole GT: Models of cell differentiation in conidial fungi, *Microbiol Rev* 50:95-132, 1986.
Kreger-van Rij NJW, editor: *The yeasts: A taxonomic study*, ed 3, Amsterdam, 1984, Elsevier Science Publishers.
Margulis L and Schwartz KV: *Five kingdoms*, ed 2, New York, 1988, WH Freeman & Company.
Moore-Landecker E: *Fundamentals of the fungi*, ed 3, Englewood Cliffs, N.J., 1990, Prentice-Hall Publishers.
Ruiz-Herrera J: *Fungal cell wall: Structure, synthesis, and assembly*, Boca Raton, Fla., 1991, CRC Press.

CHAPTER 6

Parasitic Classification and Physiology

THE purpose of this chapter is to provide an introduction to parasite classification and physiology. This brief review is intended to enhance the reader's comprehension of the interrelationships among parasitic organisms, their epidemiology and transmission of disease, specific disease processes involved, and possibilities for prevention and control of maladies. We have deliberately attempted to simplify the taxonomy by using it to address the major divisions involved in medical parasitology, specifically, intestinal and urogenital protozoa, blood and tissue protozoa, nematodes, trematodes, and cestodes.

THE IMPORTANCE OF PARASITES

Medical parasitology is the study of invertebrate animals capable of causing disease in humans and other animals. Although parasitic diseases are frequently considered "tropical" and thus of little importance to physicians practicing in the more temperate, developed countries of the world, it is clear that the world has become a very small place and that physician knowledge of parasitic diseases is essential. The global impact of parasitic infections and the number of parasite-associated deaths is staggering and must be of concern to all health care workers (Table 6-1). Increasingly, tourists, missionaries, Peace Corps volunteers, and others are visiting and working for extended periods of time in exotic, remote parts of the world. Thus they are at risk for parasitic and other infections that are rare in the United States and other developed countries. Another source of infected patients is the ever-increasing number of refugees from developing countries. Finally, the profound immunosuppression accompanying advances in medical therapy (e.g., organ transplantation), as well as that associated with infection with the human immunodeficiency virus (HIV), place a growing number of individuals at risk for developing infections caused by certain parasites. Given these considerations, clinicians and laboratory workers should certainly be aware of the possibility of parasitic disease and should be trained in ordering, performing, and interpreting the appropriate laboratory tests to aid in diagnosis and therapy.

CLASSIFICATION AND PHYSIOLOGY

The parasites of humans are classified within the kingdom Animalia and are separated into two subkingdoms, Protozoa and Metazoa (Table 6-2). The subkingdom Protozoa comprises animals in which all life functions occur in a single cell. The Metazoa are multicellular

TABLE 6-1 Estimated Worldwide Prevalence of Parasitic Infections

Infection	Number infected	Annual deaths*
Amebiasis	10% of world population	40,000–110,000
Malaria	400-490 million	2.2-2.5 million
African trypanosomiasis	100,000 new cases/yr	5,000
American trypanosomiasis	24 million	60,000
Leishmaniasis	1.2 million	
Schistosomiasis	>200 million	0.5-2 million
Opisthorchiasis	19 million	
Paragonimiasis	3.2 million	
Fasciolopsiasis	10 million	
Filiariasis	85-100 million	
Onchocerciasis	>30 million	
Dracunculiasis	10 million	
Ascariasis	1 billion	1550 (intestinal obstruction)
Hookworm	900 million	
Trichuriasis	500-800 million	
Strongyloidiasis	35 million	
Cestodiasis	65 million	

Modified from Sherris JC: *Medical microbiology: an introduction to infectious diseases*, ed 2, New York, 1990, Elsevier Science Publishing.
*Mortality data included where available.

TABLE 6-2 Classification of Medically Important Parasites (Kingdom Animalia)

Subkingdom	Phylum	Organisms
Protozoa	Sarcomastigophora	Ameba, flagellates
	Ciliophora	Ciliates
	Apicomplexa	Sporozoa, coccidia
	Microspora	Microsporidia
Metazoa	Nematoda	Roundworms
	Platyhelminthes	Flatworms
	Trematodes	Flukes
	Cestodes	Tapeworms
	Arthropoda	
	Chilopoda	Centipedes
	Pentastomida	Tongue worms
	Crustacea	Crabs, crayfish, shrimp, copepods
	Arachnida	Mites, ticks, spiders, scorpions
	Insecta	Mosquitoes, flies, lice, fleas, wasps, ants, beetles, moths, roaches, true bugs

animals in which life functions occur in cellular structures organized as tissue and organ systems.

Protozoa

Protozoa are simple microorganisms that range in size from 2 to 100 μm. Their protoplasm is enclosed by a cell membrane and contains numerous organelles including a membrane-bound nucleus, endoplasmic reticulum, food storage granules, and contractile and digestive vacuoles. The nucleus contains clumped or dispersed chromatin and a central karyosome. Organs of motility vary from simple cytoplasmic extrusions or pseudopods to more complex structures such as flagella or cilia. Reproduction is generally by simple binary fission **(merogony)**, although the life cycle of some protozoa includes cycles of multiple fission **(schizogony)** alternating with a period of sexual reproduction **(sporogony** or **gametogony)**.

Classification

Parasite classification takes into account the mode of reproduction and the type of locomotive organelle, as well as the morphology of intracytoplasmic structures such as the nucleus (Table 6-3). The subkingdom Protozoa comprises seven major subgroups or phyla, four of which are the concern of medical parasitology.

Sarcomastigophora. Phylum Sarcomastigophora consists of the amebae (subphylum Sarcodina) and the flagellates (subphylum Mastigophora). Locomotion of amebae is accomplished by extrusion of pseudopodia ("false feet"), whereas flagellates move by lashing of the whiplike flagella. The number and position of flagella vary a great deal in different species. In addition, specialized structures associated with the flagella may produce a characteristic morphological appearance that may be useful in species identification. Reproduction by both amebae and flagellates involves simple binary fission.

Ciliophora. Phylum Ciliophora consists of the ciliates, which include a variety of free-living and symbiotic species. Ciliate locomotion involves the coordinated movement of rows of hairlike structures or cilia. Cilia are structurally similar to flagella but are usually shorter and more numerous. Some ciliates are multinucleate. The only ciliate parasite of humans, *Balantidium coli*, contains two nuclei, a large macronucleus, and a small micronucleus. Reproduction is accomplished by binary fission or a more complex nuclear exchange called conjugation.

Apicomplexa. Phylum Apicomplexa organisms are often referred to as sporozoa or coccidia. These unicellular organisms have a system of organelles at their apical end that produce substances that help the organism penetrate host cells to become an intracellular parasite. The Apicomplexa have a complex life cycle with alternating sexual and asexual generations.

Microspora. Phylum Microspora organisms were formerly classified with the Sporozoa. The Microspora are small intracellular parasites that differ significantly in structure from the Apicomplexa. These parasites are characterized by the structure of their spores, which have a complex tubular extrusion mechanism (polar tubule) used to inject the infective material (sporoplasm) into host cells. Reproduction is accomplished by binary or multiple fission and by a process culminating in spore development (sporogony).

Physiology

The nutritional requirements of the parasitic protozoa are generally simple and require the assimilation of organic nutrients. The amebae, ameboflagellates, and certain other protozoa accomplish this assimilation by the rather primitive processes of pinocytosis or phagocytosis of soluble or particulate matter, respectively (Table 6-3). The engulfed material is enclosed in digestive vacuoles. The flagellates and ciliates generally ingest food at a definite site or structure, the peristome or cytostome. Other protozoan parasites such as the intracellular microsporidia assimilate nutrients by simple diffusion. The ingested food material may be retained in intracytoplasmic granules or vacuoles. Undigested particles and waste may be eliminated from the cell by extrusion of the material at the cell surface. Respiration in most parasitic protozoa is accomplished by facultatively anaerobic processes.

To ensure survival under harsh or unfavorable environmental conditions, many parasitic protozoa develop into a **cyst** form that is less metabolically active. This cyst is surrounded by a thick external cell wall that is capable of protecting the organism from otherwise lethal physical and chemical insults. The cyst form is an integral part of the life cycle of many protozoan parasites and facilitates the transmission of the organism from host to host in the external environment (Table 6-4). Those parasites that cannot form cysts must rely on direct transmission from host to host or require an arthropod vector to complete their life cycle (Table 6-4). In addition to cyst formation, many protozoan parasites have developed elaborate immunoevasive mechanisms that allow them to respond to attack by the host immune system by continuously changing their surface antigens, thus ensuring continued survival within the host. As mentioned previously, reproduction is usually accomplished by simple binary fission; however, the sporozoan parasites such as *Plasmo-*

TABLE 6-3 Biological, Morphological, and Physiological Characteristics of Pathogenic Parasites

Organism class	Morphology	Reproduction	Organelles of locomotion	Respiration	Nutrition
Protozoa					
Ameba	Unicellular, cyst and trophocyte forms	Binary fission	Pseudopods	Facultative anaerobe	Assimilation by pinocytosis or phagocytosis
Flagellates	Unicellular, cyst and trophozoite forms, may be intracellular	Binary fission	Flagella	Facultative anaerobe	Simple diffusion or ingestion via cytostome, pinocytosis, or phagocytosis
Ciliates	Unicellular, cysts and trophozoite	Binary fission or conjugation	Cilia	Facultative anaerobe	Ingestion via cytostome, food vacuole
Coccidia	Unicellular, frequently intracellular, multiple forms including trophozoites, sporozoi'es, cysts (oocysts), gametes	Schizogony and sporogony	None	Faculatative anaerobe	Simple diffusion
Microsporidia	Obligate intracellular forms, small simple cells, spores	Binary fission, schizogony and sporogony	None	Facultative anaerobe	Simple diffusion
Helminths					
Nematodes	Multicellular, round, smooth, spindle shaped, tubular alimentary tract, may possess teeth or plates for attachment	Separate sexes	No single organelle; active muscular motility	Adults usually anaerobic, larvae may be aerobic	Ingestion or absorption of body fluids, tissue, or digestive contents
Trematodes	Multicellular, leaf shaped with with oral and ventral suckers, blind alimentary tract	Hermaphroditic (*Schistosoma* group has separate sexes)	No single organelle, muscular, directed motility	Adults usually anaerobic	Ingestion or absorption of body fluids, tissue, or digestive contents
Cestodes	Multicellular, head with segmented body (proglottids), no alimentary tract, head equipped with hook and/or suckers for attachment	Hermaphroditic	No single organelle; usually remain attached to mucosa, proglottids may display muscular motility	Adults usually anaerobic	Absorption of nutrients from intestine
Arthropods					
Chilopoda	Elongated, many legged, possess distinct head and trunk, poison claws on first segment	Separate sexes	Legs	Aerobic	Carnivorous

Continued.

TABLE 6-3 Biological, Morphological, and Physiological Characteristics of Pathogenic Parasites—cont'd

Organism class	Morphology	Reproduction	Organelles of locomotion	Respiration	Nutrition
Pentastomida	Wormlike, cylindrical, or flattened, two distinct body regions, possess digestive and reproductive organs, lack circulatory and respiratory systems	Separate sexes	Muscular directed motility	Aerobic	Ingestion of body fluids and tissue
Crustacea	Hard external carapace, one pair maxillae, five pairs of biramous legs	Separate sexes	Legs	Aerobic	Ingestion of body fluids and tissue, carnivorous
Arachnida	Body divided into cephalothorax and abdomen, eight legs and poisonous fangs	Separate sexes	Legs	Aerobic	Carnivorous
Insecta	Body consists of head, thorax, and abdomen, one pair of antennae, three pairs of appendages, 0-2 pairs of wings	Separate sexes	Legs, wings	Aerobic	Ingestion of fluids and tissues

dium species also require cycles of multiple fission (schizogony) alternating with cycles of sexual reproduction (sporogony) to complete their life cycle.

Metazoa

The subkingdom Metazoa includes all animals that are not Protozoa. This text discusses two groups of organisms of major importance: the helminths ("worms") and the arthropods (crabs, insects, ticks, etc.).

Helminths

The helminths are complex, multicellular organisms that are elongated and bilaterally symmetrical. They are considerably larger than the protozoan parasites and generally are macroscopic, ranging in size from less than a millimeter to a meter or more. The external surface of some worms is covered with a protective cuticle, which is acellular and may be smooth or possess ridges, spines, or tubercles. The protective covering of flatworms is known as a tegument. Frequently, helminths possess elaborate attachment structures such as hooks, suckers, teeth, or plates. These structures are usually located anteriorly and may be useful in classifying and identifying the organisms (see Table 6-3). Helminths typically have primitive nervous and excretory systems. Some have alimentary tracts; however, none have a circulatory system (see Table 6-3).

Classification. The helminths are separated into two phyla.

NEMATODA. Phylum Nematoda consists of the roundworms, which have cylindrical bodies. The sexes of roundworm are separate, and these organisms have a complete digestive system. The nematodes may be intestinal parasites or may infect the blood and tissue.

PLATYHELMINTHES. Phylum Platyhelminthes consists of the flatworms, which have flattened bodies that are leaflike or resemble ribbon segments. Platyhelminthes can be further separated into trematodes and cestodes.

Trematodes, or **flukes**, have leaf-shaped bodies. Most are **hermaphroditic**, with male and female sex organs present in a single body. Their digestive systems are incomplete and have only saclike tubes. The life cycles of flukes are complex, with snails serving as first intermediate hosts and with other aquatic animals or plants as second intermediate hosts.

Cestodes, or **tapeworms**, have bodies composed of ribbons of proglottids, or segments. All are hermaphroditic, and all lack a digestive system, with nutrition being absorbed through the body wall. The life cycles of some cestodes are simple and direct, whereas those of others are complex and require one or more intermediate hosts.

Physiology. The nutritional requirements of helminthic parasites are met by active ingestion of host tissue and/or body fluids with resultant tissue destruction or by more passive absorption of nutrients from the surrounding fluids and intestinal contents (see Table 6-3). The muscular motility of many helminths expends considerable energy, and the worms rapidly metabolize carbohydrates. Nutrients are stored in the form of glycogen, the content of which is quite high in most helminths. Similar

TABLE 6-4 Transmission and Distribution of Pathogenic Parasites

Organism	Infective form	Mechanism of spread	Distribution
Intestinal Protozoa			
Entamoeba histolytica	Cyst/trophozoite	Indirect (fecal-oral) Direct (venereal)	Worldwide
Giardia lamblia	Cyst	Fecal-oral	Worldwide
Dientamoeba fragilis	Trophozoite	Fecal-oral	Worldwide
Balantidium coli	Cyst	Fecal-oral	Worldwide
Isospora belli	Oocyst	Fecal-oral	Worldwide
Cryptosporidium species	Oocyst	Fecal-oral Unknown	Worldwide
Enterocytozoon bieneusi	Spore	? Fecal-oral	North America and Europe
Urogenital Protozoa			
Trichomas vaginalis	Trophozoite	Direct (venereal)	Worldwide
Blood and Tissue Protozoa			
Naegleria and *Acanthamoeba* species	Cyst/trophozoite	Direct inoculation, inhalation	Worldwide
Plasmodium species	Sporozoite	*Anopheles* mosquito	Tropical and subtropical areas
Babesia species	Pyriform body	*Ixodes* tick	North America and Europe
Toxoplasma gondii	Oocysts and tissue cysts	Fecal-oral, carnivorism	Worldwide
Leishmania species	Promastigote	*Phlebotomus* sandfly	Tropical and subtropical areas
Trypanosoma cruzi	Trypomastigote	Reduviid bug	North, Central, and South America
Trypanosom brucei	Trypomastigote	Tsetse fly	Africa
Pneumocystis carinii	Cyst	Inhalation	Worldwide
Nematodes			
Enterobius vermicularis	Egg	Fecal-oral	Worldwide
Ascaris lumbricoides	Egg	Fecal-oral	Areas of poor sanitation
Toxocara species	Egg	Fecal-oral	Worldwide
Trichuris trichiura	Egg	Fecal-oral	Worldwide
Ancylostoma duodenale	Filariform lava	Direct skin penetration from contaminated soil	Tropical and subtropical areas
Necator americanus	Filariform larva	Direct skin penetration	Topical and subtropical areas
Strongyloides stercoralis	Filariform larva	Direct skin penetration, autoinfection	Tropical and subtropical areas
Trichinella spiralis	Encysted larva in tissue	Carnivorism	Worldwide
Wuchereria bancrofti	Third stage larva	Mosquito	Tropical and subtropical areas
Brugia malayi	Third stage larva	Mosquito	Tropical and subtropical areas
Loa loa	Filariform larva	*Chrysops* fly	Africa
Mansonella species	Third stage larva	Biting midges or black flies	Africa, Central, and South America
Onchocerca volvulus	Third stage larva	*Simulium* black fly	Africa, Central, and South America
Dracunculus medinensis	Third stage larva	Ingestion of infected cyclops	Africa and Asia
Dirofiliaria immitis	Third stage larva	Mosquito	Japan, Australia, and United States

Continued.

TABLE 6-4 Transmission and Distribution of Pathogenic Parasites—cont'd

Organism	Infective form	Mechanism of spread	Distribution
Trematodes			
Fasciolopsis buski	Metacercaria	Ingestion of metacercaria encysted on aquatic plants	China, Southeast Asia, India
Fasciola hepatica	Metacercaria	Metacercaria on water plants	Worldwide
Opisthorchis (Clonorchis) sinensis	Metacercaria	Metacercaria encysted in freshwater fish	China, Japan, Korea, Vietnam
Paragonimus westermani	Metacercaria	Metacercaria encysted in in freshwater crustacenas	Asia, Africa, India, Latin America
Schistosoma species	Cercaria	Direct penetration of skin by free swimming cercaria	Africa, Asia, India, Latin America
Cestodes			
Taenia solium	Cysticercus, embryonated egg or proglottid	Ingestion of infected pork Ingestion of egg (cysticercosis)	Pork eating countries—Africa, Southeast Asia, China, Latin America
Taenia saginata	Cysticercus	Ingestion of cysticercus in meat	Worldwide
Diphyllobothrium latum	Sparganum	Ingestion of sparganum in fish	Worldwide
Echinococcus granulosus	Embryonated egg	Ingestion of eggs from infected canines	Sheep raising countries—Europe, Asia, Africa, Australia, U.S.
Echinococcus multilocularis	Embryonated egg	Ingestion of eggs from infected animals, fecal-oral	Canada, Northern U.S., Central Europe
Hymenolepsis nana	Embryonated egg	Ingestion of eggs, fecal-oral	Worldwide
Hymenolepis diminuta	Cysticercus	Ingestion of infected beetle larvae in contaminated grain products	Worldwide
Dipylidium caninum	Cysticercoid	Ingestion of infected fleas	Worldwide

to the protozoa, respiration is primarily anaerobic, although the larval forms may require oxygen. A significant proportion of the energy requirement of helminths is dedicated to support the reproductive process. Many worms are quite prolific, producing as many as 200,000 offspring each day. In general, helminthic parasites are egg laying **(oviparous)**, although a few species may bear live young **(viviparous)**. The resulting larvae are always morphologically distinct from the adult parasites and must undergo several developmental stages or **molts** before attaining adulthood.

The major protective barrier for most helminths is the tough external layer (cuticle or tegument). Worms may also secrete enzymes that destroy host cells and neutralize immunological and cellular defense mechanisms. Similar to protozoan parasites, some helminths possess the ability to alter the antigenic properties of their external surfaces and thus evade the host immune response. This is accomplished, in part, by incorporating host antigens into their external cuticular layer. In this way the worm avoids immunological recognition and in some diseases (e.g., Schistosomiasis) it allows the parasite to survive within the host for decades.

Arthropods

Phylum Arthropoda is the largest group of animals in the kingdom Animalia. Arthropods are complex, multicellular organisms that may be involved directly in causing invasive or superficial (infestation) disease processes or indirectly as intermediate hosts and vectors of many infectious agents including protozoan and metazoan parasites (Table 6-4). In addition, envenomization by biting and stinging arthropods can result in adverse reactions in humans that range from local allergic and hypersensitivity reactions to severe anaphylactic shock and death.

Classification. There are five major classes of arthropods as follows (see Table 6-2):

CHILOPODA. Class Chilopoda consists of terrestrial forms such as centipedes. These organisms are of medical importance due to their poison claws, which may produce a painful "bite."

PENTASTOMIDA. The Pentastomids, or tongue worms, are bloodsucking endoparasites of reptiles, birds, and mammals. Adult pentastomids are white, cylindrical, or flattened parasites that possess two distinct body regions—an anterior cephalothorax and an abdomen. Humans may serve as intermediate hosts for these parasites.

CRUSTACEA. Class Crustacea consists of familiar aquatic forms such as crabs, crayfish, shrimp, and copepods. Several are involved as intermediate hosts in life cycles of various intestinal or blood and tissue helminths.

ARACHNIDA. Class Arachnida consists of familiar terrestrial forms such as mites, ticks, spiders, and scorpions. These animals have no wings or antennae, as do insects, and adults have four pairs of legs, as opposed to three pairs for insects. Of medical importance are those serving as vectors for microbial diseases (mites, ticks) or as venomous animals that bite (spiders) or sting (scorpions).

INSECTA. Class Insecta consists of familiar aquatic and terrestrial forms such as mosquitoes, flies, midges, fleas, lice, bugs, wasps, and ants. Wings and antennae are present, and adult forms have three pairs of legs. Of medical importance are the many insects that serve as vectors for various microbial diseases (mosquitoes, fleas, flies, lice, bugs) or as venomous animals that sting (bees, wasps, ants).

Physiology and Structure. Arthropods have segmented bodies, paired jointed appendages, and well-developed digestive and nervous systems. Sexes are separate. Respiration by aquatic forms is via gills and by terrestrial forms via tubular body structures. All have a hard chitin covering as an exoskeleton.

Physician awareness of parasitic diseases is undoubtedly more critical now than at any time in the history of medical practice. Physicians today must be prepared to answer questions from patients regarding protection from malaria and the risks of drinking water and eating fresh fruits and vegetables in remote areas where they may be traveling. With this knowledge of parasitic diseases, the physician can also evaluate signs, symptoms, and incubation periods in returning travelers and make a diagnosis and begin treatment for a patient with a possible parasitic disease. The risks of parasitic diseases in immunosuppressed individuals and those with AIDS must also be understood and taken into account. Proper education regarding parasitic diseases in medical curricula cannot be overemphasized as a requirement for physicians whose practice includes travelers to foreign countries and refugee populations. Many of the important parasites responsible for human diseases are transmitted by arthropod vectors or are acquired by consumption of contaminated food or water. The various modes of transmission and distribution of parasitic diseases are presented in appropriate detail in the following chapters; however, the data in Table 6-4 are provided as an outline.

QUESTIONS

1. How do protozoa adapt to harsh environmental conditions?
2. Which morphological form is important in the transmission of protozoa from host-to-host?
3. How do helminths such as Schistosomes avoid the host immune response?
4. How do arthropods cause human disease?

Bibliography

Beaver PC, Jung RC, and Cupp EW: *Clinical parasitology*, ed 9, Philadelphia, 1984, Lea & Febiger.

Brown HW and Neva FA: *Basic clinical parasitology*, ed 5, Norwalk, Conn, 1983, Appleton-Century-Crofts.

Howard BJ et al: *Clinical and pathogenic microbiology*, St Louis, 1987, Mosby.

Markell EK, Voge M, and John DT: *Medical parasitology*, ed 7, Philadelphia, 1992, WB Saunders.

Schmidt GD and Roberts LS: *Foundations of parasitology*, ed 4, St Louis, 1989, Mosby.

Washington JA II, editor: *Laboratory procedures in clinical microbiology*, ed 2, New York, 1985, Springer-Verlag.

CHAPTER 7

Viral Classification, Structure, and Replication

VIRUSES were first described as "filterable agents." Their small size allows them to pass through filters designed to retain bacteria. Unlike most bacteria, fungi, and parasites, viruses are obligate intracellular parasites that depend on the biochemical machinery of the host cell for replication. In addition, reproduction of viruses occurs by assembly of individual components rather than by binary fission (Boxes 7-1 and 7-2).

The simplest viruses consist of a genome of DNA or RNA packaged in a protective shell of protein and sometimes a membrane (Figure 7-1). Viruses lack the capacity to make energy or substrates, cannot make their own proteins, and cannot replicate their genome independent of the host cell. The virus therefore must be able to interact with the cell's biosynthetic machinery according to the biochemical rules of the cell.

The physical structure and genetics of viruses have been optimized by mutation and selection to infect human and other hosts, and to interact with the biochemical machinery of the host cell. The virus may also have to endure harsh environmental conditions, traverse the skin or other protective barriers of the host, and escape elimination by the host immune response. A knowledge of the structural (size and morphology) and genetic (type and structure of nucleic acid) features of a virus provides insight into how the virus replicates, spreads, and causes disease. The concepts presented in this chapter will be repeated in greater detail in the discussions of specific viruses in later chapters.

CLASSIFICATION

Viruses range from the structurally simple and small parvoviruses and picornaviruses to the large and complex poxviruses and herpesviruses. Their names may describe viral characteristics, the diseases they are associated with, or even the tissue or geographical locale where they were first identified. Names such as *picornavirus* (*pico*, meaning small; *rna*, ribonucleic acid [RNA]; *virus*) or *togavirus* (*toga*, Greek for mantle, referring to a membrane envelope surrounding the virus) describe the structure of the virus; whereas the name *papovavirus* describes the members of its family (*pa*pilloma, *po*lyoma, and *va*cuolating *viruses*). The name *retrovirus* (*retro*, reverse) refers to the virus-directed synthesis of deoxyribonucleic acid (DNA) from an RNA template; whereas the *poxviruses* are named for the disease smallpox, caused by one of its members. The *adenoviruses* (*adeno*ids) and the reoviruses (*r*espiratory, *e*nteric, *o*rphan) are named for the body site from which they were first isolated. *Reovirus* was discovered before it was associated with a specific disease, and thus it was designated an "orphan" virus. *Coxsackievirus* is named for Coxsackie, New York, and many of the togaviruses, arenaviruses, and bunyaviruses are named after exotic African places where they were first isolated.

BOX 7-1 Definition and Properties of a Virus

Viruses are filterable agents.
Viruses are obligate intracellular parasites.
Viruses cannot make energy or proteins independent of a host cell.
Viral components are assembled and do not replicate by "division."
Viral genomes may be RNA or DNA but not both.
Viruses have a naked capsid or envelope morphology.

BOX 7-2 Consequences of Viral Properties

Viruses are not living.
Viruses must be infectious to endure in nature.
Viruses must be able to utilize host cell processes to produce their components (viral mRNA, protein, and identical copies of the genome).
Viruses must encode any required process not provided by the cell.
Viral components must self-assemble.

Viruses can be grouped by characteristics such as their disease (e.g. hepatitis), target tissue, means of transmission (e.g. enteric, respiratory), or vector (arboviruses; *ar*thropod-*bo*rne virus) (Box 7-3). The most consistent and current means of viral classification is by physical and biochemical characteristics such as size, morphology (e.g., presence or absence of a membrane envelope), type of genome, and means of replication. The DNA viruses associated with human disease comprise six families (Tables 7-1 and 7-2). The RNA viruses may be divided into at least 13 families (Tables 7-3 and 7-4).

VIRION STRUCTURE

The units for measurement of virion size are nanometers (nm). The clinically important viruses range from 18 or 26 nm (parvoviruses) to 300 nm (poxviruses) (Figure 7-2). The latter are almost visible with a light microscope and are approximately one fourth the size of a staphylococcus. Larger virions can hold a larger genome that can code for more proteins, and they are generally more complex.

The **virion** (the virus particle) consists of a nucleic acid genome packaged into a protein coat (**capsid**) or a membrane (**envelope**) (Figure 7-3). The virion may also contain certain essential or accessory enzymes or other proteins. These proteins may associate with the genome to form a a **nucleocapsid**.

The **genome** of different viruses consists of either DNA or RNA. The DNA can be single stranded or double stranded, linear or circular. The RNA can be either positive sense (+) (like messenger RNA) or negative sense (−) (analogous to a photographic negative), double stranded (+/−) or ambisense (containing + and − regions of RNA attached end to end). The RNA genome may also be segmented into pieces, with each piece encoding an individual gene.

The outer layer of the virion is the **capsid** or **envelope.** These structures are the package, protection, and delivery vehicle during transmission of the virus from one host to another and for spread within the host to the target cell. The surface structures of the capsid and envelope mediate the interaction of the virus with the target cell. Removal or disruption of the outer package inactivates the virus. The body generates a protective antibody response against the components of these structures.

The capsid is a rigid structure able to withstand harsh environmental conditions. Viruses with naked capsids are generally resistant to drying, acid, and detergents, including the acid and bile of the enteric tract. Many of these viruses are transmitted by the fecal-oral route and can endure transmission even in sewage.

The envelope is a membrane composed of lipid, proteins, and glycoproteins. The membranous structure of the envelope can be maintained only in aqueous solutions. It is readily disrupted by drying, acidic conditions, detergents, and solvents such as ether, resulting in the inactivation of the virus. As a result, enveloped viruses must remain wet and are generally transmitted in fluids, respiratory droplets, blood, and tissue. Most cannot

BOX 7-3 Means of Classification and Naming of Viruses

Structure: size, morphology, and nucleic acid (e.g., picornavirus [small RNA]; togavirus [cloak])
Biochemical characteristics: structure and mode of replication*
Disease: (e.g., encephalitis viruses, hepatitis viruses)
Means of transmission: (e.g., arboviruses spread by insects)
Host cell (host range): animal (human, mouse, bird), plant, bacteria
Tissue or organ (tropism): (e.g., adenovirus, enterovirus)

*Current means of taxonomic classification of viruses.

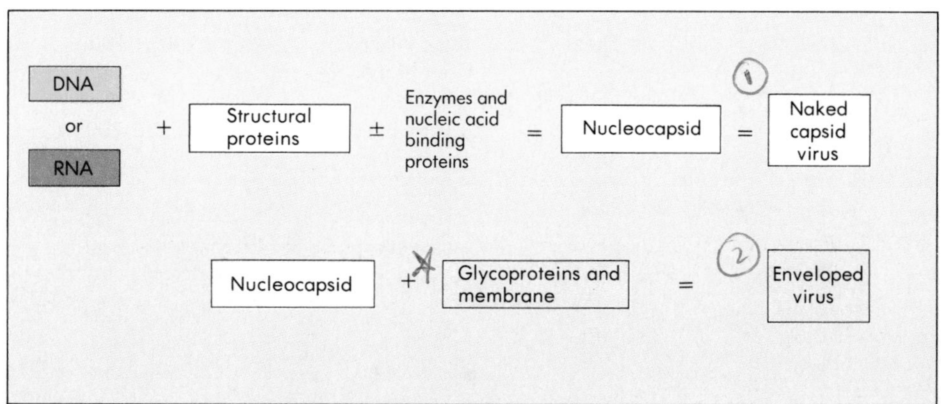

FIGURE 7-1 Schematic structure of the basic virion.

survive the harsh conditions of the gastrointestinal tract. The influence of virion structure on viral properties is summarized in Boxes 7-4 and 7-5.

Capsid Viruses

The viral capsid is assembled from individual proteins associated into progressively larger units. All of the components of the capsid have chemical features that allow them to fit together and to assemble into a larger unit. Individual structural proteins associate into subunits, then protomers, capsomers (distinguishable in electron micrographs), and finally a recognizable **procapsid** or **capsid** (Figure 7-4). A procapsid requires further processing to the final, transmissable capsid. For some viruses, the capsid forms around the genome; for others, the capsid forms as an empty shell (procapsid) to be filled by the genome.

The simplest structures that can be built stepwise are symmetrical and include **helical** and **icosahedral** structures. Helical structures appear as rods, whereas the icosahedron is an approximation of a sphere assembled from symmetrical subunits (Figure 7-5). Nonsymmetrical capsids are complex forms and are associated with certain bacterial viruses (phages).

The classic example of a virus with helical symmetry is the tobacco mosaic virus. Its capsomeres self-assemble on the RNA genome into rods extending to the length of the genome. The capsomeres cover and protect the RNA. Helical nucleocapsids are observed within the envelope of many negative-strand RNA viruses (see Figure 61-1, Chapter 61).

Simple icosahedrons are utilized by small, simple viruses such as the picornaviruses and parvoviruses. The icosahedron is made of 12 capsomers, each with five-fold symmetry (**pentamer** or **penton**). Each pentamer of the picornaviruses is made up of five protomers, each of which is composed of three subunits of four separate proteins (see Figure 7-4). X-ray crystallography and image analysis of cryoelectron microscopy have defined the structure of the picornavirus capsid to the molecular level. These studies have depicted a canyon-like cleft, which is a docking site for the receptor on the surface of the target cell (see Figure 59-2).

Larger icosahedral virions are constructed by inserting structurally distinct capsomeres between the pentons at the vertices. These capsomeres have six nearest neighbors

TABLE 7-1 DNA Viruses*

Family	Important human viruses
Poxviridae	Smallpox virus, vaccinia virus, molluscum contagiosum virus
Herpesviridae	Herpes simplex types 1 and 2, varicella-zoster virus, Epstein-Barr virus, cytomegalovirus, human herpesvirus 6 and 7
Adenoviridae	Adenovirus
Hepadnaviridae	Hepatitis B virus
Papovaviridae	Polyomaviruses (JC, BK, SV40), papillomavirus
Parvoviridae	Parvovirus B19

*Listed in order of decreasing size.

TABLE 7-2 Properties of Virions of Human DNA Viruses*

Family	Genome*: Molecular weight (× 10⁶ daltons)	Genome*: Nature	Virion: Shape	Virion: Size	Virion: DNA polymerase†
Poxviridae	85-140	ds, linear	Brick shaped, enveloped	300 × 240 × 100	+‖
Herpesviridae	100-150	ds, linear	Icosahedral, enveloped	Capsid, 100-110 Envelope, 120-200	+
Adenoviridae	20-25	ds, linear	Icosahedral	70-90	+
Hepadnaviridae	1.8	ds, circular‡	Spherical, enveloped	42	+§‖
Papovaviridae	3-5	ds, circular	Icosahedral	45-55	−
Parvoviridae	1.5-2.0	ss, linear	Icosahedral	18-26	−

ds, Double stranded; *ss*, single stranded.
*Genome invariably a single molecule.
†Polymerase encoded by virus.
‡Circular molecule is double stranded for most of its length but contains a single-stranded region.
§Reverse transcriptase.
‖Polymerase carried in the virion.

(**hexons**). This extended icosahedron is called an **icosadeltahedron**, and its size is determined by the number of hexons inserted along the edges and planes between the pentons. For example, the herpesvirus nucleocapsid has 12 pentons and 150 hexons. The herpesvirus nucleocapsid is also surrounded by an envelope. The adenovirus capsid is composed of 252 capsomeres, with 12 pentons and 240 hexons. A long fiber is attached to each penton of adenovirus to serve as the viral attachment protein to target cells and contains the type-specific antigen. The reoviruses have an icosahedral double capsid with fiber-like proteins partially extended from each vertex. The outer capsid protects the virus and promotes its uptake across the gastrointestinal tract and into target cells, whereas the inner capsid contains enzymes for the synthesis of RNA (see Figure 7-5).

TABLE 7-3 RNA Viruses*

Family	Important human viruses
Paramyxoviridae	Measles, mumps, respiratory syncytial, parainfluenza, Sendai
Orthomyxoviridae	Influenza A, B, and C
Coronaviridae	Coronavirus
Arenaviridae	Lymphocytic choriomeningitis (LCM), Lassa fever virus, Tacaribe virus complex (Junin and Machupo)
Rhabdoviridae	Rabies
Filoviridae	Marburg, Ebola
Bunyaviridae	California encephalitis, sandfly fever, Crimean Congo hemorrhagic fever, etc.
Retroviridae	Human T cell leukemia I and II; human immunodeficiency viruses I and II
Reoviridae	Rotavirus, reovirus, California tick fever
Picornaviridae	Rhinovirus, poliovirus, ECHO virus, coxsackievirus, hepatitis A virus
Togaviridae	Rubella; Western, Eastern, and Venezuelan equine encephalitis; Sindbis, Semliki Forest
Flaviviridae	Yellow fever, dengue, St. Louis encephalitis, etc.
Caliciviridae	Norwalk agent

*Listed in order of decreasing size.

TABLE 7-4 Properties of Virions of RNA Human Viruses

	Genome		Virion			
	Molecular weight ($\times 10^6$ daltons)	Nature*	Shape†	Size (nm)	RNA** polymerase	Envelope
Paramyxoviridae	5-7	ss, −	Spheric	150-300	+	+
Orthomyxoviridae	5	ss, −, seg	Spheric	80-120	+	+
Coronaviridae	6	ss, +	Spheric	80-130	−	+‡
Arenaviridae	3-5	ss, −, seg	Spheric	50-300	+	+‡
Rhabdoviridae	4	ss, −	Bullet shaped	180 × 75	+	+
Filoviridae	4	ss, −	Filamentous	800 × 80	+	+
Bunyaviridae	4-7	ss, −	Spheric	90-110	+	+‡
Retroviridae	2 × (2-3)§	ss, +	Spheric	80-110	+‖	+
Reoviridae	11-15	ds, seg	Icosahedral	60-80	+	−
Picornaviridae	2.5	ss, +	Icosahedral	25-30	−	−
Togaviridae	4	ss, +	Spheric	60-70	−	+
Flaviviridae	4	ss, +	Spheric	40-50	−	+
Caliciviridae	2.6	ss, +	Icosahedral	35-40	−	−

*ss, single stranded; ds, double stranded; seg, segmented; + or −, polarity of ss nucleic acid.
†Some enveloped viruses are very pleomorphic (sometimes filamentous).
‡No matrix protein.
§Genome has two identical ss RNA molecules.
‖Reverse transcriptase.
**Polymerase carried in the virion.

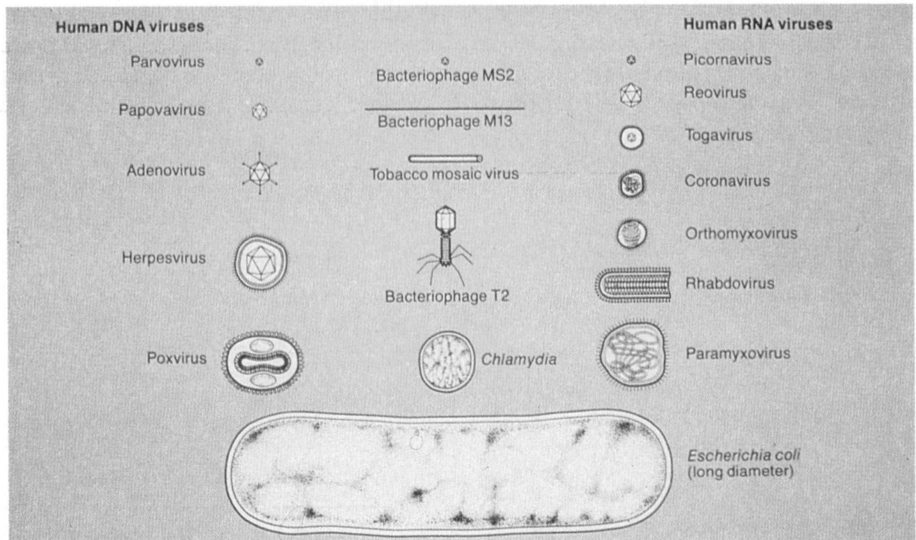

FIGURE 7-2 Relative sizes of viruses and bacteria. (Courtesy The Upjohn Company.)

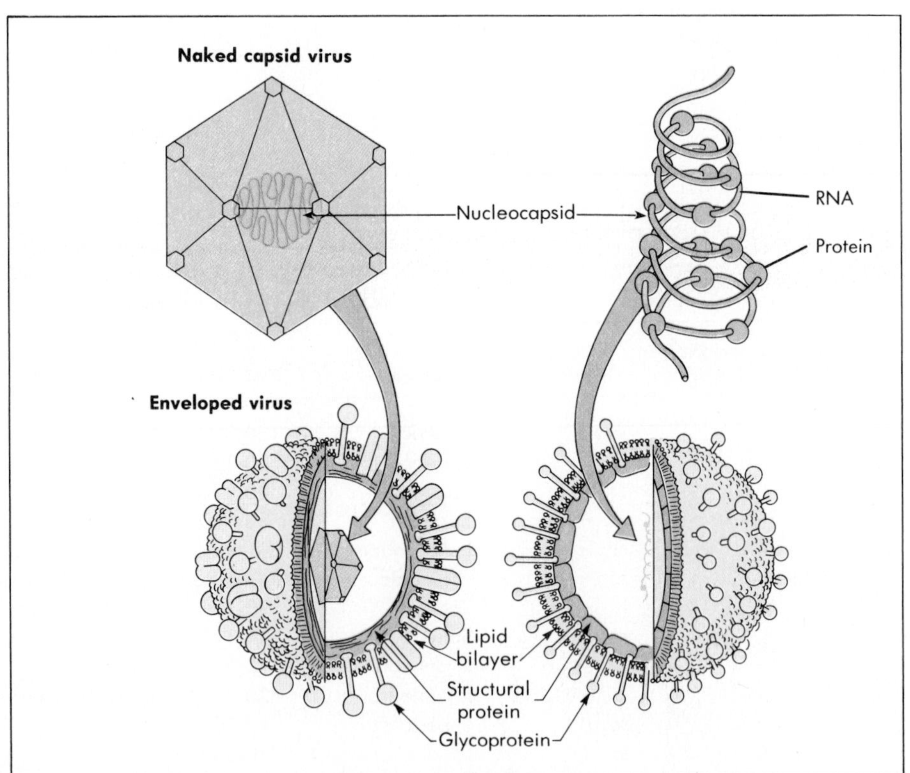

FIGURE 7-3 The structures of a naked capsid virus (*top, left*) and enveloped viruses with an icosahedral (*left*) nucleocapsid or a helical (*right*) ribonucleocapsid. The helical ribonucleocapsid is formed by viral proteins associated with an RNA genome.

Enveloped Viruses

The togaviruses, orthomyxoviruses, herpesviruses, and poxviruses are examples of enveloped viruses differing in shape, size, and complexity (See Tables 7-2 and 7-4 for complete listings of enveloped viruses). Most enveloped viruses are round or pleomorphic. Two exceptions are the poxvirus, which has a complex internal and a bricklike external structure, and the rhabdovirus, which is bullet shaped. The virion envelope has a membrane structure similar to cellular membranes and is composed of lipids, proteins, and glycoproteins (see Figure 7-3). Cellular proteins are rarely found in the viral envelope even though the envelope is obtained from cellular membranes. The viral **glycoproteins** extend through the envelope and away from the surface of the virion. For many viruses, these can be observed as **spikes** (Figure 7-6).

Most glycoproteins act as **viral attachment proteins** (VAPs; see the following) capable of binding to structures on target cells. VAPs that also bind to erythrocytes are termed **hemagglutinins** (HA). Some glycoproteins have other functions, such as the **neuraminidase** of orthomyxoviruses (e.g., influenza), the Fc receptor, and the C3b receptor associated with herpes simplex virus glycoproteins or the fusion glycoproteins of paramyxoviruses. Glycoproteins are also major antigens for protective immunity.

The envelope of the togaviruses surrounds an icosahedral nucleocapsid containing a positive-strand RNA genome. The envelope contains spikes consisting of two

BOX 7-4 Virus Structure: Naked Capsid

Components	Properties
Protein	Environmentally stable to Temperature Acid Proteases Detergents Drying Released from cell by lysis

Consequences
- Can be spread easily (on fomites, hand to hand, dust, small droplets)
- Can dry out and retain infectivity
- Can survive the adverse conditions of the gut
- Can be resistant to detergents and poor sewage treatment
- Can elicit a protective antibody response

BOX 7-5 Virus Structure: Enveloped

Components	Properties
Membrane Lipids Proteins Glycoproteins	Environmentally labile: disrupted by Acid Detergent Drying Heat Modify cell membrane during replication Released by budding and cell lysis

Consequences
- Must stay wet
- Cannot survive the G.I. tract
- Spreads in large droplets, secretions, and organ or blood transplants
- Need not kill the cell to spread
- Initiates a cell-mediated immune response
- Antibody and cell-mediated immune response may be necessary for protection and control
- Pathogenesis often due to hypersensitivity and inflammation initiated by CMI

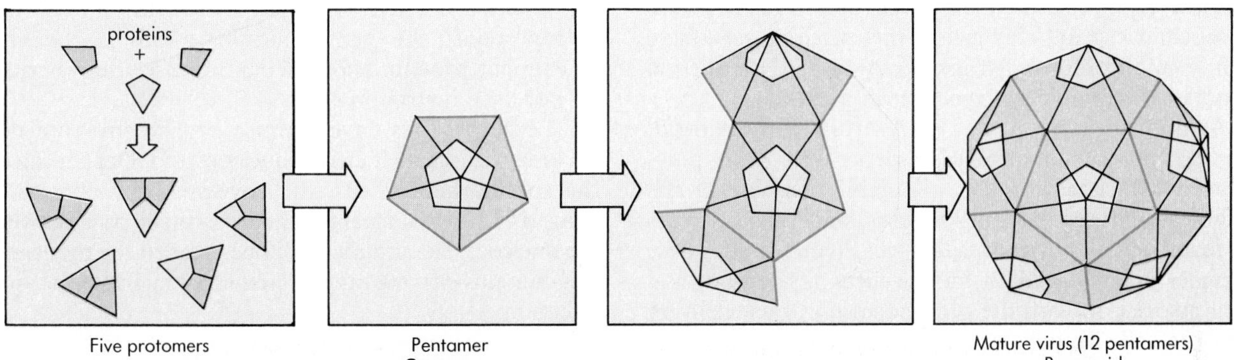

FIGURE 7-4 Capsid assembly of the icosahedral capsid of a picornavirus. Individual proteins associate into subunits, which associate into protomers, capsomeres, and an empty procapsid. Inclusion of the (+) RNA genome triggers its conversion to the final capsid form.

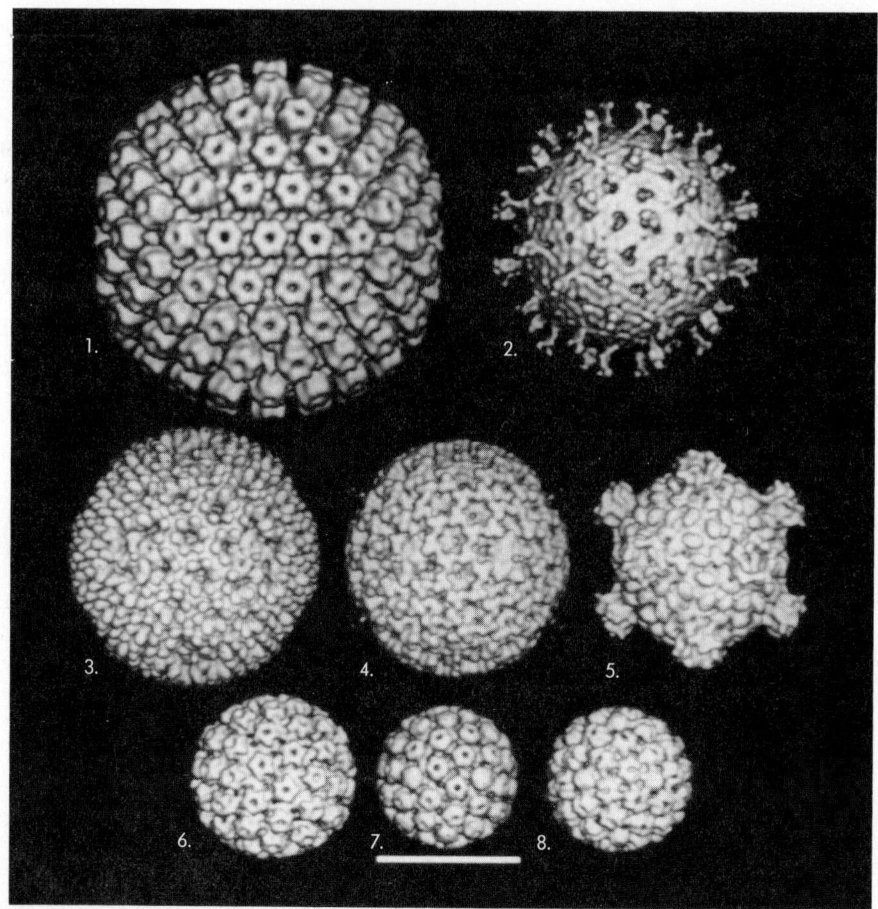

FIGURE 7-5 Cryoelectron microscopy and computer-generated three-dimensional image reconstructions of several icosahedral capsids. These images show the symmetry of the capsids and the individual capsomeres. (*1*) Equine herpesvirus nucleocapsid; (*2*) simian rotavirus; (*3*) reovirus type 1 (Lang) virion, (*4*) intermediate subviral particle (reovirus) and (*5*) core (inner capsid) particle (reovirus); (*6*) human papilloma virus type 19 (papovavirus) and (*7*) mouse polyoma virus (papovavirus); and (*8*) cauliflower mosaic virus (bar = 50 nm). During assembly, the genome may fill the capsid through the holes in the herpesvirus and papovavirus capsomeres. The structures extending from the rotavirus capsid are the sigma 1 viral attachment proteins. The different views of reovirus indicate the morphogenesis of the double capsid structure. (Courtesy Dr. Tim Baker).

or three glycoprotein subunits anchored to the virion's icosahedral capsid. This causes the envelope to adhere tightly and conform (shrink wrap) to an icosahedral structure discernible by cryoelectron microscopy.

All of the negative-strand RNA viruses are enveloped. Components of the viral RNA-dependent RNA polymerases associate with the (−) RNA genome of the orthomyxoviruses, paramyxoviruses, and rhabdoviruses to form helical nucleocapsids (see Figure 7-3). These enzymes are required to initiate virus replication, and their association with the genome ensures their delivery into the cell. **Matrix** proteins lining the inside of the envelope facilitate the assembly of the ribonucleocapsid into the virion. Influenza A (orthomyxovirus) is an example of a (−) RNA virus with a segmented genome. Its envelope is lined with matrix proteins and has two glycoproteins: the hemagglutinin, which is the viral attachment protein, and a neuraminidase. Bunyaviruses do not have matrix proteins.

The herpesvirus envelope is a baglike structure that encloses the icosadeltahedral nucleocapsid. Depending on the specific herpesvirus, the envelope may contain as many as 11 glycoproteins. The interstitial space between the nucleocapsid and the envelope is called the **tegument** and contains enzymes and proteins that facilitate the virus infection.

The poxviruses are enveloped viruses with a large, complex, bricklike shape. The envelope encloses a dumbbell-shaped, DNA-containing nucleoid structure; lateral bodies; fibrils; and many enzymes and proteins

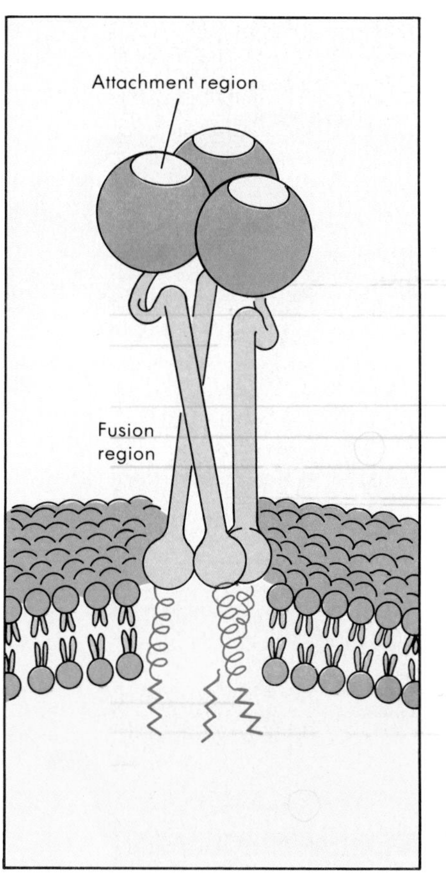

FIGURE 7-6 Diagram of the hemagglutinin glycoprotein trimer of influenza A, a representative spike protein. The region for attachment to the cellular receptor is exposed on the spike protein's surface. Under mild acidic conditions, the hemagglutinin will change conformation to expose a hydrophobic sequence at the "fusion region." (Redrawn from Schlesinger MJ and Schlesinger S: *Adv Virus Res* 33:1, 1987.)

including the enzymes and transcriptional factors required for mRNA synthesis.

VIRUS REPLICATION

The major steps in virus replication, shown in Figure 7-7 and Box 7-6, are the same for all viruses. The cell acts as a factory, providing the substrates, energy, and machinery necessary for synthesis of viral proteins and replication of the genome. Processes not provided by the cell must be encoded in the genome of the virus. The outcome of the competition between the virus and cell for the biosynthetic machinery determines the fate of the infected cell and the nature of the virus infection. The manner in which each virus accomplishes these steps and overcomes the cell's biochemical limitations is determined by the structures of both the genome and the virion that must be replicated. This is indicated in the examples in Figures 7-8 to 7-10.

The viral replication cycle can be separated into several phases. During the **early phase** of infection, the virus must recognize an appropriate target cell, attach to the cell, penetrate the plasma membrane and be taken up by the cell, release (uncoat) its genome into the cytoplasm and, if necessary, deliver the genome to the nucleus. The **late phase** begins with the start of genome replication and viral macromolecular synthesis and proceeds through viral assembly and release. Uncoating of the capsid or envelope of the virion during the early phase abolishes its infectivity and identifiable structure, which initiates the **eclipse period.** The eclipse period ends with virus assembly and the appearance of new virions. The **latent period** includes the eclipse period and ends on release of virus (Figure 7-11). Each infected cell may produce as many as 100,000 particles; however, only 1% to 10% of these particles may be infectious. The noninfectious particles (defective particles; see the following) result from mutations and errors in the manufacture and assembly of the virion. The yield of infectious virus per cell, or **burst size**, and the time required for a single cycle of virus reproduction are determined by the properties of the virus and the target cell.

Recognition of and Attachment to the Target Cell

To infect a cell, the virus must first recognize and bind to cells that permit virus replication. **Viral attachment proteins (VAP)** or structures on the surface of the virion (Table 7-5) interact with receptors on the cell (Table 7-6). The receptors on the cell may be proteins or carbohydrates. The receptor-VAP interaction is the initial determinant of which cells can be infected by a virus. Viruses that bind to receptors expressed on specific cell types may be restricted to certain species (**host range**) (e.g., human, mouse) or specific cell types. The susceptible target cell defines the tissue **tropism** (e.g., neurotropic, lymphotropic).

The viral attachment structure for a capsid virus may be part of the capsid or a protein that extends from the capsid. A canyon on the surface of rhinovirus 14, a picornavirus, serves as a keyhole for the insertion of a portion of the cellular adhesion molecule, ICAM-1. The fibers of the adenoviruses and the ς1 proteins of the reoviruses at the vertices of the capsid interact with receptors expressed on specific target cells.

The glycoproteins of enveloped viruses are the viral attachment proteins. The Epstein-Barr virus, a herpesvirus, binds to the C3d receptor (CR2), which is expressed on B lymphocytes and potentially epithelial cells of only humans and New World monkeys. The hemagglutinin of influenza A binds to sialic acid expressed on many different cells and has a broad host range and tissue tropism. Similarly, the alpha togaviruses and the flaviviruses are able to bind to receptors expressed on cells of many animal species, including arthropods, reptiles, amphibians, birds, and mammals. This allows them to

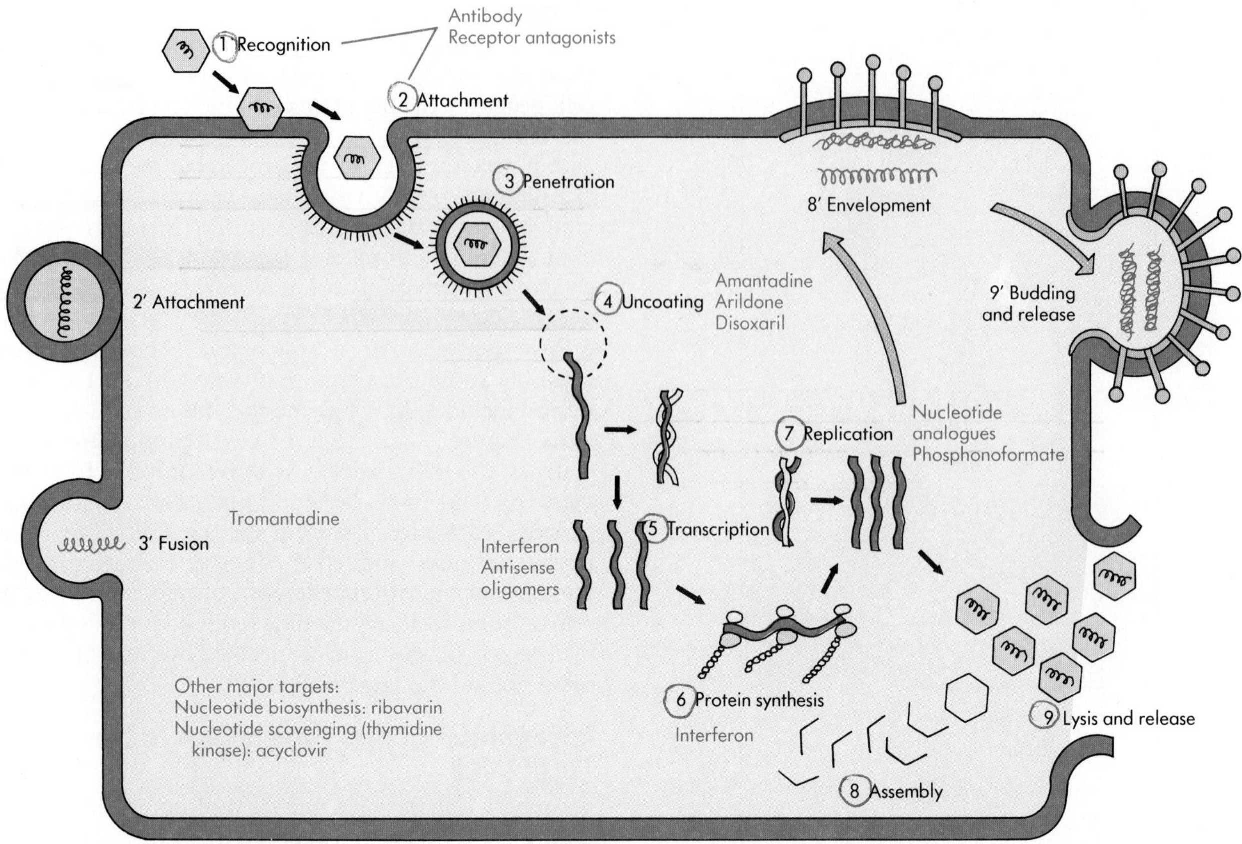

FIGURE 7-7 **A general scheme of virus replication. Enveloped viruses have alternative means of entry (step 3′), assembly, and exit from the cell (8′ and 9′). The steps in virus replication susceptible to antiviral drugs are listed in red.**

BOX 7-6 Steps in Virus Replication

1. Recognition of the target cell
2. Attachment
3. Penetration
4. Uncoating
5. Macromolecular synthesis
   a. Early mRNA and nonstructural protein synthesis: genes for enzymes and nucleic acid–binding proteins
   b. Replication of genome
   c. Late mRNA and structural protein synthesis
6. Posttranslation modification of proteins

Assembly of virus
Budding of enveloped viruses
Release of virus

infect and to be spread by animals, mosquitos, and other insects.

Penetration

Multiple interactions between the viral attachment proteins and the cellular receptors initiate the internalization of the virus into the cell. The mechanism of internalization depends on the virion structure and cell type. Most nonenveloped viruses enter the cell by receptor-mediated endocytosis, or by viropexis. **Endocytosis** is a normal process used by the cell for uptake of receptor-bound molecules such as hormones, low density lipoproteins, and transferrin. Papovaviruses may enter by **viropexis**, the direct penetration of the membrane.

Enveloped viruses can be internalized by endocytosis, or their envelope can fuse with the plasma membrane to deliver the nucleocapsid directly into the cytoplasm. The pH optimum for fusion of an enveloped virus is a major determinant for whether penetration occurs at the cell surface at neutral pH or in an endosome at acidic pH. The fusion activity may be provided by the viral attachment protein or another protein. The hemagglutinin of influenza A (see Figure 7-6) binds to sialic acid receptors on

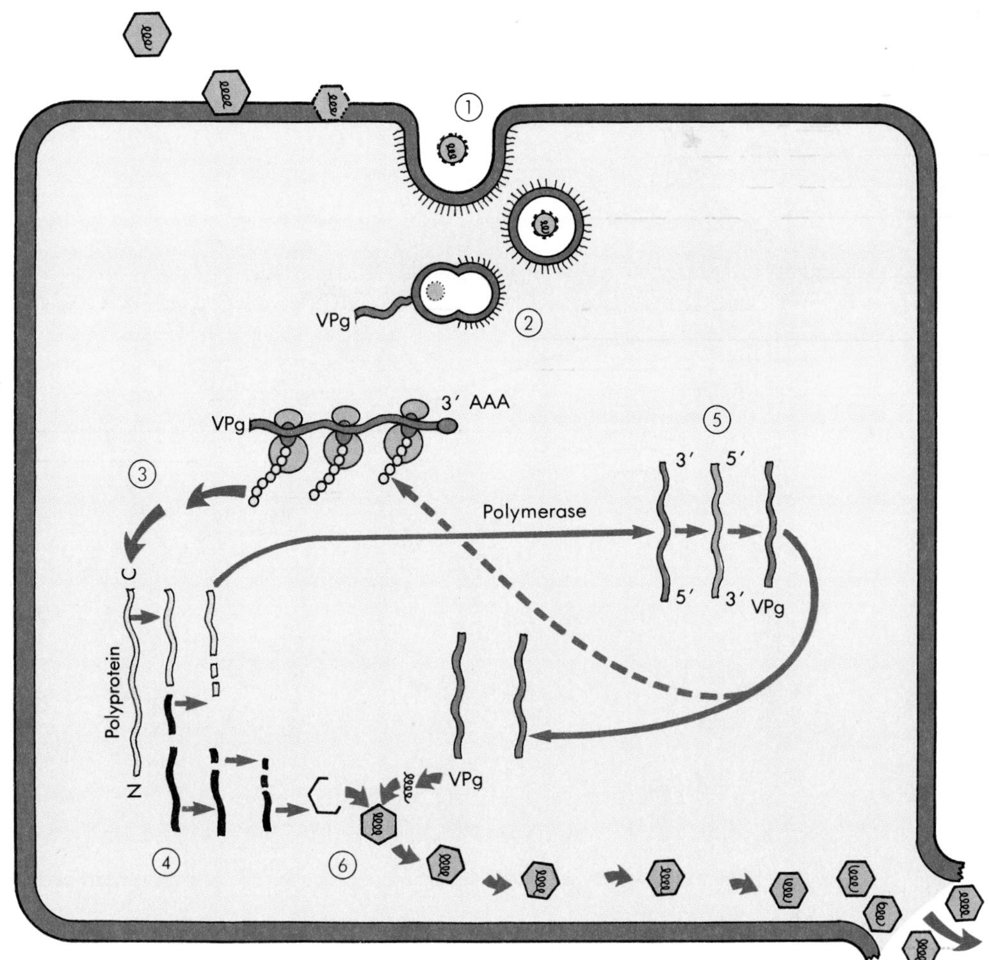

FIGURE 7-8 Replication of picornaviruses: a simple (+) RNA virus. (*1*) Interaction of the picornaviruses with receptors on the cell surface defines the target cell and weakens the capsid. (*2*) The virion is endocytosed, and the genome is released and used as a mRNA for protein synthesis. (*3*) One large polyprotein is translated from the virion genome and then (*4*) proteolytically cleaved into individual proteins, including an RNA-dependent RNA polymerase. (*5*) The polymerase makes a ([−]) strand template from the genome and replicates the genome. A protein *(VPg)* is covalently attached to the 5′ end of the viral genome. (*6*) The structural proteins associate into the capsid structure, the genome is inserted, and the virions are released upon cell lysis.

the target cell. Under the mild acidic conditions of the endosome, the hemagglutinin undergoes a dramatic conformational change to expose hydrophobic portions capable of promoting membrane fusion. Paramyxoviruses have a fusion protein that is active at neutral pH to promote virus-to-cell fusion. Paramyxoviruses can also promote cell-to-cell fusion to form multinucleated giant cells (**polykaryocytes** or **syncytia**). Some herpesviruses and retroviruses can also fuse with cells at neutral pH and induce syncytia following replication.

Uncoating

Once internalized, the nucleocapsid must be delivered to the site of replication within the cell and the capsid or envelope removed. The genome of DNA viruses, except for poxviruses, must be delivered to the nucleus, whereas most RNA viruses remain in the cytoplasm. The uncoating process may be initiated by attachment to the receptor or promoted by the acidic environment or proteases found in an endosome or lysosome. Picornavirus capsids are weakened to allow uncoating by the release of the VP4 capsid protein. VP4 is released by the insertion of the receptor into the keyhole-like canyon attachment site of the capsid. Enveloped viruses are uncoated upon fusion with cell membranes. Fusion of the herpesvirus envelope with the membrane releases its nucleocapsid, which then docks with the nuclear membrane to deliver its DNA genome directly to the site of replication.

The reovirus and poxvirus are only partially uncoated upon entry. The outer capsid of reovirus is removed, but the genome remains in an inner capsid, which contains the polymerases necessary for RNA synthesis. The initial

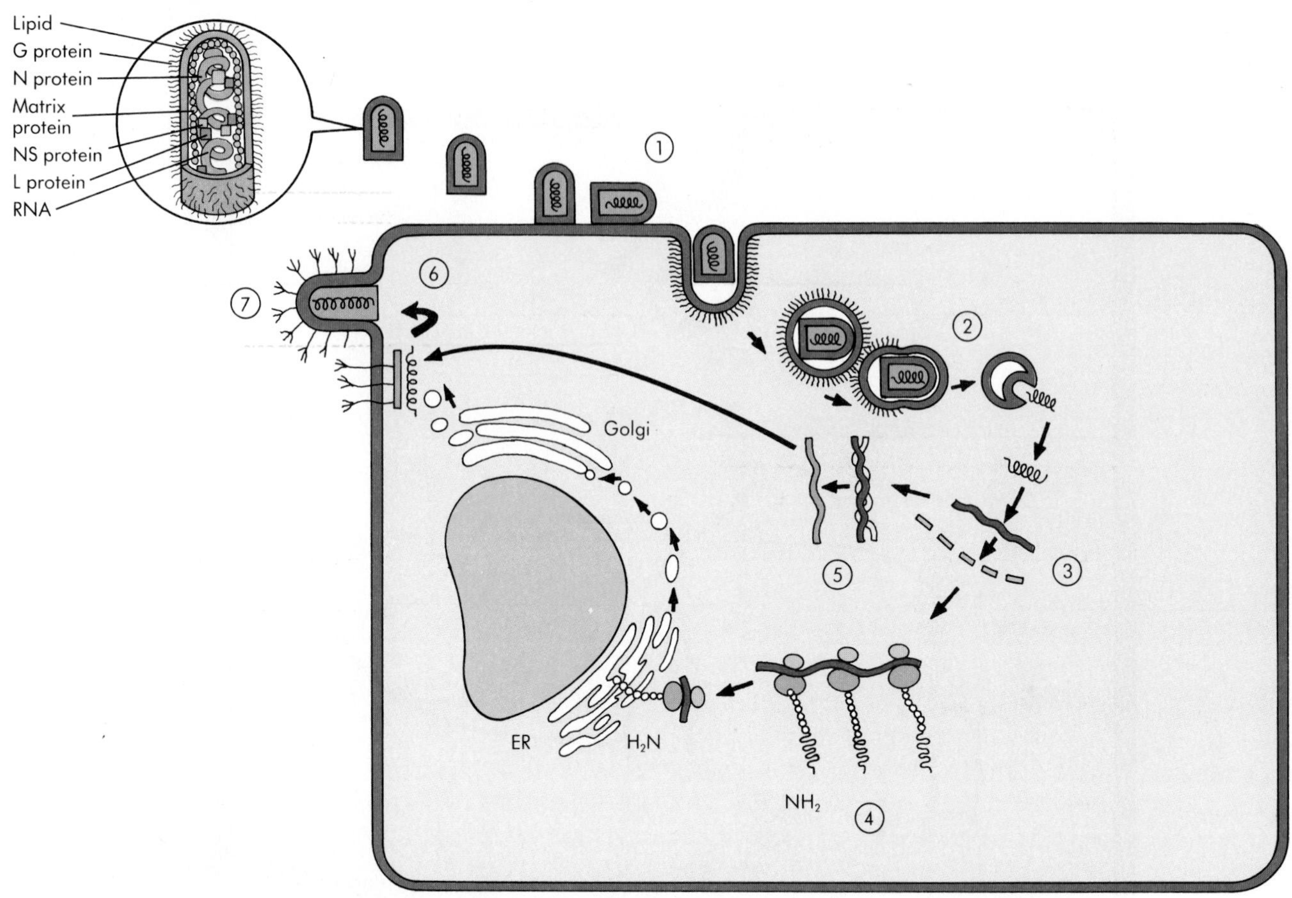

FIGURE 7-9 Replication of rhabdoviruses: a simple enveloped ([−]) RNA virus. (*1*) Rhabdoviruses bind to the cell surface and (*2*) are endocytosed. The envelope fuses with the endosome vesicle membrane to deliver the nucleocapsid to the cytoplasm. The virion must carry a polymerase and (*3*) produce five individual mRNAs and a full-length (+) RNA template. (*4*) Proteins are translated from the mRNAs, including one glycoprotein *(G),* which is co-translationally glycosylated in the endoplasmic reticulum, processed in the Golgi apparatus, and delivered to the cell membrane. (*5*) The genome is replicated from the (+) RNA template, and the N, L, and NS proteins associate with the genome to form the nucleocapsid. (*6*) The matrix protein associates with the G protein–modified membrane, which is followed by assembly of the nucleocapsid, and (*7*) the virus buds from the cell in a bullet-shaped virion.

uncoating of the poxviruses exposes a subviral particle to the cytoplasm, allowing synthesis of mRNA by virion-contained enzymes for its immediate early proteins. An uncoating enzyme can then be synthesized to release the DNA-containing core into the cytoplasm.

Macromolecular Synthesis

Each virus must make mRNA and protein and generate an identical copy of its genome. Transcription, translation, and replication of the genome are therefore probably the most important steps in virus multiplication. Once the genome has been delivered to the cell, it is useless unless it can be transcribed into functional mRNAs capable of binding to ribosomes and being translated into proteins. The means by which each virus accomplishes these steps depends on the structure of the genome (Figure 7-12) and the site of replication.

The machinery for transcription and mRNA processing is found in the nucleus. Most DNA viruses can take advantage of the cell's DNA-dependent RNA polymerase II and other enzymes used to make mRNA. For example, eukaryotic mRNAs acquire a 3′ polyadenylated (poly A) tail and a 5′ methylated cap (for binding to the ribosome) and are processed to remove introns before being exported to the cytoplasm. Viruses that replicate in the cytoplasm must provide these functions or an alternative. The poxviruses are DNA viruses, which replicate in the cytoplasm and therefore encode enzymes for all these functions. RNA viruses must encode the necessary enzymes for transcription and replication since the cell has no means of replicating RNA. The mRNAs for RNA viruses are produced in the cytoplasm and may or may not acquire a 5′ cap or poly A tail.

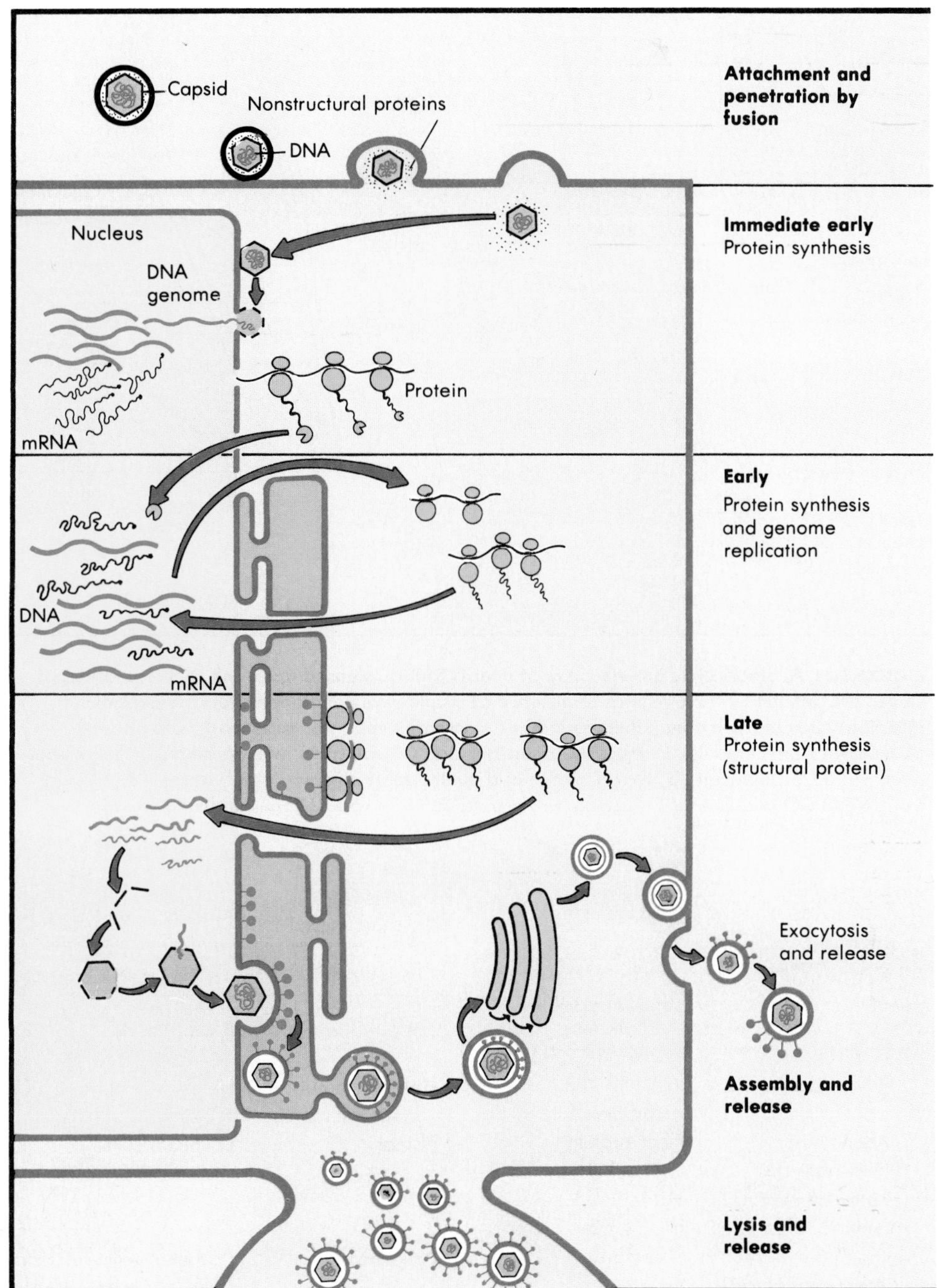

FIGURE 7-10 Replication of herpes simplex virus (HSV), a complex enveloped DNA virus. HSV binds to specific receptors and fuses with the plasma membrane. The nucleocapsid then delivers the DNA genome to the nucleus. Transcription and translation occur in three phases: immediate early, early, and late. Immediate early proteins promote the takeover of the cell; early proteins consist of enzymes, including the DNA-dependent DNA polymerase, and the late proteins are structural proteins, including the viral capsid and glycoproteins. The genome is replicated before transcription of the late genes. Capsid proteins migrate into the nucleus, assemble into icosadeltahedral capsids, and are filled with the DNA genome. The viral glycoproteins are co-translationally glycosylated in the endoplasmic reticulum and diffuse to the contiguous nuclear envelope. The capsids filled with genomes bud through these modified membranes and are transferred to the Golgi apparatus, the glycoproteins are processed, and the virus is released by exocytosis. Alternatively, the virus may be released upon cell lysis.

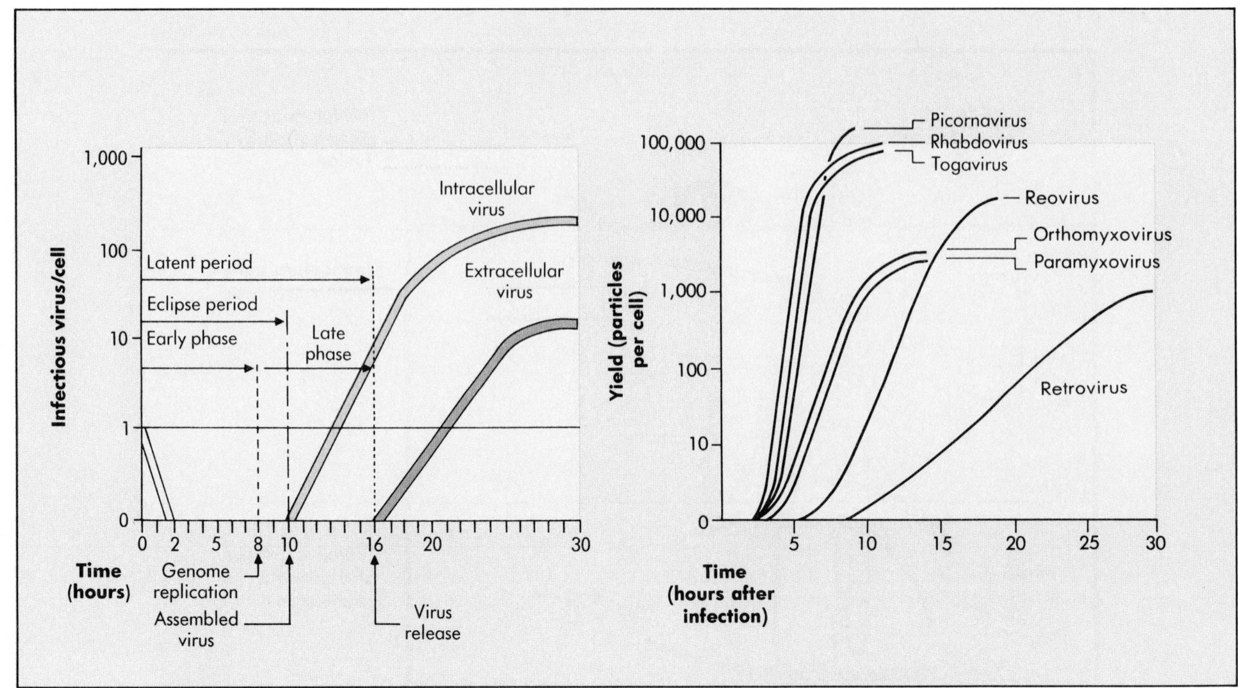

FIGURE 7-11 **A,** Single cycle growth curve of a virus that is released upon cell lysis. The different stages are defined by the presence or absence of visible viral components (eclipse period), infectious virus in the media (latent period), or macromolecular synthesis (early/late phases) (**A** redrawn from Davis BD, Dulbecco R, Eisen HN, and Ginsberg HS: *Microbiology,* ed 4, Philadelphia, 1990, JB Lippincott.) **B,** Growth curve and burst size of representative viruses. (**B** redrawn from White DO and Fenner F: *Medical virology,* ed 3, New York, 1986, Academic Press.)

TABLE 7-5 Examples of Viral Attachment Proteins

Virus family	Virus	Viral attachment protein
Picornaviridae	Rhinovirus	VP1-VP2-VP3 complex
Adenoviridae	Adenovirus	Fiber protein
Reoviridae	Reovirus	Sigma 1
	Rotavirus	VP_7
Togaviridae	Semliki Forest virus	E1, E2, E3 complex
Rhabdoviridae	Vesicular stomatitis virus	G
Orthomyxoviridae	Influenza A	Hemagglutinin
Paramyxoviridae	Measles	Hemagluttinin
Herpesviridae	Herpes simplex virus	gD and gB
	Epstein-Barr virus	gp350 and gp220
Retroviridae	Murine leukemia virus	gp70
	Human immunodeficiency virus	gp120

TABLE 7-6 Examples of Virus Receptors

Virus	Target cell	Receptor*
Epstein-Barr virus	B lymphocyte	C3 complement receptor CR2
Human immunodeficiency virus	Helper T lymphocyte	CD4 molecule
Rhinovirus	Epithelial cells	ICAM-1 (immunoglobulin superfamily adhesion protein)
Poliovirus	Epithelial cells	Immunoglobulin superfamily protein
Rabies virus	Neuron	Acetylcholine receptor
Reovirus	Neuron	Beta-adrenergic receptor
Influenza A virus	Epithelial cells	Sialyl oligosaccharides
Herpes simplex virus	Epithelial cells	Heparan sulfate

*Other receptors for these viruses may also exist.

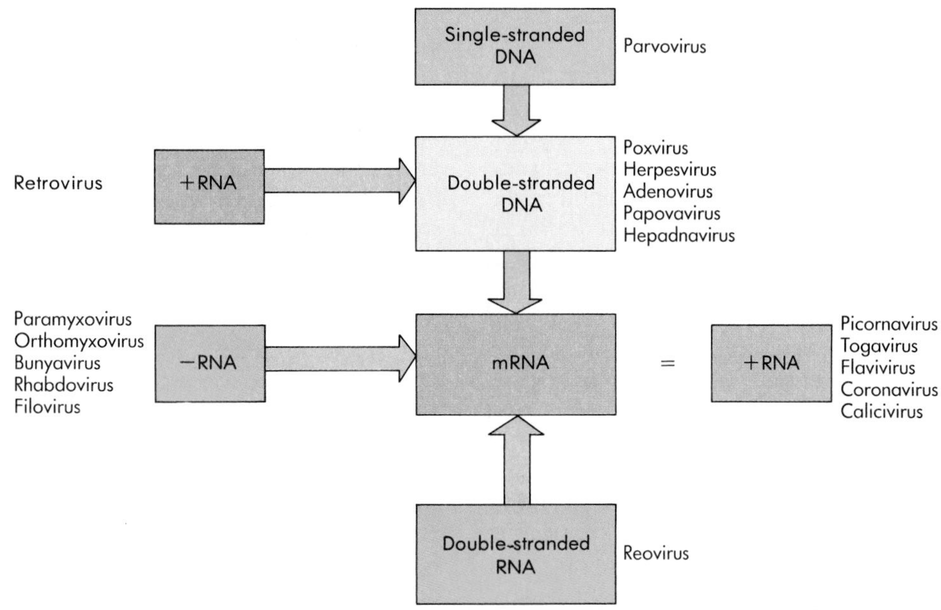

FIGURE 7-12 Strategies for production of mRNA. The arrows indicate a synthetic step. (Based on the Baltimore Schema; redrawn from Bacteriol Rev 35:235, 1971.)

DNA Viruses

Transcription of the DNA virus genome (except for poxviruses) occurs in the nucleus. These viruses utilize host cell polymerases and other enzymes for viral mRNA synthesis. The smaller the DNA virus, the more dependent the virus is on the host cell (Box 7-7). The larger DNA viruses encode a DNA polymerase and proteins to enhance and control transcription and genome replication.

Viral DNA and mRNA synthesis can be enhanced by speeding up the growth of the cell or by increasing the number of DNA templates for transcription following the replication of the genome. A growing cell provides deoxyribonucleotides, polymerases, and other materials required for DNA virus replication.

Transcription of the viral genes is regulated by the interaction of specific *DNA-binding proteins* with *promoter and enhancer elements* in the viral genome. The viral promoter and enhancer elements are similar in sequence to those of the host cell to allow binding of the cell's transcriptional activation factors and DNA-dependent RNA polymerase. Cells from different tissues or species express different DNA-binding proteins, and this is a determinant for replication of the virus in that cell.

Different DNA and RNA viruses control the duration, sequence, and quantity of viral gene and protein synthesis in different ways. The more complex viruses encode their own transcriptional activators which enhance or regulate the expression of viral genes. For example, herpes simplex virus encodes many proteins that regulate the kinetics of viral gene expression including the VMW 65/α TIF protein. VMW 65 is carried in the virion, binds to the host cell transcription activating complex (Oct-1), and

BOX 7-7 Properties of DNA Viruses

1. Viral DNA resembles host DNA for transcription and replication.
   DNA is not transient or labile.
   Viral genomes remain in the infected cell.
   Many DNA viruses establish persistent infections (e.g., latent, immortalizing).
   DNA genomes reside in the nucleus (except pox).
   Viral genes must interact with host transcriptional machinery (except pox).
   Viral gene transcription is temporarily regulated.
   Early genes encode DNA-binding proteins and enzymes.
   Late genes encode structural proteins.
   DNA polymerases require a primer to replicate the viral genome.
2. The larger DNA viruses have more control over the replication of their genome.
   Parvovirus: replicates in cells undergoing DNA synthesis.
   Papovavirus: Stimulates cell growth and DNA synthesis.
   Hepadnavirus: Stimulates cell growth (?) and encodes its own polymerase.
   Adenovirus: Stimulates cellular DNA synthesis and encodes its own polymerase.
   Herpesvirus: Stimulates cell growth, encodes its own polymerase, encodes enzymes to provide deoxyribonucleotides for DNA synthesis.
   Poxvirus: Encodes its own polymerase, enzymes to provide deoxyribonucleotides for DNA synthesis, replication machinery, and transcription machinery.

enhances its ability to stimulate transcription of the immediate early genes of the virus.

In general, mRNA for nonstructural proteins are transcribed first. **Early gene products** (nonstructural proteins) are often DNA-binding proteins and enzymes, including viral encoded polymerases. These proteins are catalytic, and only a few are required. Replication of the genome usually initiates a transition to transcription of **late gene products**. Late viral genes encode structural proteins. Many copies of these proteins are required to package the virus and are generally not required before the genome is replicated. Newly replicated genomes also provide new templates amplifying late gene mRNA synthesis. Different DNA and RNA viruses control the time and amount of viral gene and protein synthesis in different ways.

Genes may be transcribed from either DNA strand of the genome and in opposite directions. For example, the early and late genes of the papovaviruses are in opposite, nonoverlapping DNA strands. Viral genes may have introns requiring posttranscriptional processing of the mRNA by the cell's nuclear machinery **(splicing)**. The late genes of papovaviruses and adenoviruses are initially transcribed as a large RNA from a single promoter and then processed to produce several different mRNAs following removal of different intervening sequences (introns).

Replication of viral DNA follows the same biochemical rules as for cellular DNA. Replication is initiated at a unique DNA sequence of the genome, called the **origin** or **ori**. This is a site recognized by cellular or viral nuclear factors and the DNA-dependent DNA polymerase. Viral DNA synthesis is semiconservative, and viral and cellular DNA polymerases require a **primer** to initiate synthesis of the DNA chain. The parvoviruses have DNA sequences that are inverted and repeated to allow the DNA to fold back and hybridize with itself to provide a primer. Replication of the adenovirus genome is primed by a terminal protein-deoxyCMP complex. A cellular enzyme (primase) synthesizes an RNA primer to start the replication of the papovavirus genome while the herpesviruses encode a primase.

Replication of the genome of the simple DNA viruses (e.g., parvoviruses, papovaviruses) uses the host DNA-dependent DNA polymerases, whereas the larger, more complex viruses (e.g., adenoviruses, herpesviruses, poxviruses) encode their own polymerases. Viral polymerases are usually faster but less precise than host cell polymerases, causing a higher mutation rate in viruses, as well as providing a target for antiviral drugs.

Hepadnavirus replication is unique in that a circular positive-strand RNA intermediate is first synthesized by the cell's DNA-dependent RNA polymerase. An RNA-dependent DNA polymerase (reverse transcriptase) in the virion core makes a negative-strand DNA, and the RNA is degraded. Positive-strand DNA synthesis is initiated but stops when the genome and core are enveloped, yielding a partially double-stranded circular DNA genome.

Major limitations for replication of a DNA virus include availability of the DNA polymerase and deoxyribonucleotide substrates. Most cells in the resting phase of growth are not undergoing DNA synthesis, and deoxythymidine pools are limited. The parvoviruses are the smallest DNA viruses and are very dependent upon the host cell. They will replicate only in growing cells such as erythroid precursor cells or fetal tissue. The larger DNA viruses are more independent. They may provide enzymes and other proteins that stimulate cell growth, and scavenge for deoxyribonucleotides (Box 7-7). The T antigen of simian virus 40, the E7 of papillomavirus, and the E1a protein of adenovirus bind to and alter the function of a growth-inhibitory DNA-binding protein (the retinoblastoma gene product), which results in cell growth. Herpes simplex virus encodes scavenging enzymes such as DNase, ribonucleotide reductase, and thymidine kinase to generate the necessary deoxyribonucleotide substrates for replication of its genome.

RNA Viruses

Replication and transcription of RNA viruses are similar processes since the viral genomes are usually either an mRNA (positive-strand RNA) or a template for mRNA (negative-strand RNA) (Box 7-8). During replication and transcription, a **double-stranded RNA replicative intermediate** is formed, a structure not normally found in uninfected cells.

The RNA virus genome must code for **RNA-dependent RNA polymerases (replicases** and **transcriptases)** because the cell has no means of replicating RNA. Since RNA is degraded relatively quickly, the RNA-dependent RNA polymerase must be provided or synthesized soon after uncoating to generate more viral RNA, or the infection will be aborted. Replication of the genome also provides new templates for production of more mRNA, which establishes the infection and amplifies and accelerates virus replication.

The **positive-strand RNA virus** genomes of the picornaviruses, coronaviruses, flaviviruses, and togaviruses act as mRNA, bind to ribosomes, and direct protein synthesis. The naked positive-strand RNA viral genome is sufficient experimentally to initiate infection by itself. After an RNA-dependent RNA polymerase is produced, a negative-strand RNA template is synthesized. The template can then be used to generate more mRNA and to replicate the genome. The negative-sense RNA template of the togaviruses is also used to produce a smaller RNA for the structural proteins (late genes). The mRNAs for these viruses are not capped at the 5′ end, but the genome encodes a short poly A sequence. Transcription and replication of coronaviruses share many of these aspects but are more complex.

The **negative-strand RNA virus** genomes of the rhabdoviruses, orthomyxoviruses, paramyxoviruses, filovi-

BOX 7-8 Properties of RNA Viruses

RNA is labile and transient.
Most RNA viruses replicate in the cytoplasm.
Cells cannot replicate RNA. RNA viruses must encode an RNA-dependent RNA polymerase.
The genome structure determines the mechanism of transcription and replication.
RNA viruses are prone to mutation.
The genome structure and polarity determine how viral mRNA is generated and proteins are processed.
Picornaviruses, togaviruses, flaviviruses, caliciviruses, and coronaviruses
(+) RNA genome resembles mRNA, is translated into a polyprotein, which is proteolyzed. A (−) RNA template for replication.
Orthomyxoviruses, paramyxoviruses, rhabdoviruses, filoviruses, and bunyaviruses
(−) RNA genome is a template for mRNa, which may also be the (+) RNA template for replication.
Reoviruses
(+/−) segmented RNA genome is a template for mRNA, which may also be encapsulated to generate the (+/−) RNA and more mRNA.
Retroviruses
(+) retrovirus RNA genome is converted into DNA, which is integrated into the host chromatin and transcribed as a cellular gene.

ruses, and bunyaviruses are the templates for production of mRNA. The negative-strand RNA genome is not infectious by itself, and a polymerase must be carried into the cell with the genome to make mRNA and initiate viral protein synthesis. The mRNA or another positive-strand RNA species can then act as a template to generate more copies of the genome. Except for influenza, transcription and replication of negative-strand RNA viruses occurs in the cytoplasm. The influenza transcriptase requires a primer to produce mRNA. It uses the 5′ ends of cellular mRNA in the nucleus as primers for its polymerase and in the process steals the 5′ cap from the cellular mRNA. The influenza genome is also replicated in the nucleus.

The reoviruses have a **segmented, double-stranded RNA** genome and undergo a more complex means of replication and transcription. The reovirus RNA polymerase is part of the inner capsid. mRNA units are transcribed from each of the 10 or more segments of the genome while they are still in the core. The negative strands of the genome segments are used as templates for mRNA in a manner similar to the negative-strand RNA viruses. The mRNA is released into the cytoplasm where it directs protein synthesis or is sequestered into new cores. Reovirus-encoded enzymes contained in the inner capsid add the 5′ cap to viral mRNA. The mRNA does not have poly A. The positive-strand RNA in the cores acts as templates for negative-strand RNA, producing the progeny double-stranded RNA.

The arenaviruses have an **ambisense circular** genome with (+) sequences adjacent to (−) sequences. The early genes of the virus are transcribed from the negative-sense portion of the genome, and the late genes of the virus are transcribed from the full-length replicative intermediate.

Although the retroviruses have a positive-strand RNA genome, the virus provides no means for replication of the RNA in the cytoplasm. Instead, the retroviruses carry two copies of the genome, two tRNA molecules, and an RNA-dependent DNA polymerase (**reverse transcriptase**) in the virion. The tRNA is used as a primer for synthesis of a DNA copy (**cDNA**) of the genome. The cDNA is synthesized in the cytoplasm and then integrated into the host chromatin. The viral genes are then transcribed as cellular genes. Promoters in the viral genes enhance the extent of their transcription.

Viral Protein Synthesis

All viruses depend on the host cell ribosomes, transfer RNA (tRNA), and mechanisms for posttranslational modification to produce their proteins. Unlike bacterial ribosomes, which can bind to a polycistronic mRNA and translate several gene sequences into separate proteins, the eukaryotic ribosome binds to mRNA, makes a continuous protein, and then falls off the mRNA. Each virus deals with this limitation differently, depending on the structure of the genome. For example, the entire genome of a positive-strand RNA virus is read by the ribosome and translated into one giant **polyprotein**. The polyprotein is subsequently cleaved by cellular and viral proteases into functional proteins. DNA viruses, retroviruses and most negative-strand RNA viruses transcribe mRNA for smaller polyproteins or individual proteins. Most of the segments of the orthomyxovirus and reovirus genomes code for single proteins.

Viruses employ different tactics to promote preferential translation of their viral mRNA. In many cases the concentration of viral mRNA in the cell is so large that it occupies most of the ribosomes, preventing translation of cellular mRNA. Adenovirus infection blocks the egress of cellular mRNA from the nucleus. Herpes simplex virus and other viruses inhibit cellular macromolecular synthesis and induce degradation of the cell's DNA and mRNA. To promote selective translation of its mRNA, poliovirus inactivates the 200,000 d cap-binding protein of the ribosome with a viral-coded protease, preventing binding and translation of 5′ capped cellular mRNA. The pathogenic consequences of these actions are discussed further in Chapter 52.

Togaviruses and many other viruses increase the permeability of the cell's membrane, which decreases the ribosomal affinity for most cellular mRNA. All these actions also contribute to the cytopathology of the virus infection.

Some viral proteins require **posttranslational modifications** such as phosphorylation, glycosylation, acylation, or sulfation. Protein phosphorylation is accomplished by cellular protein kinases and is a means of modulating, activating, or inactivating proteins. Several herpesviruses and other viruses encode their own protein kinase. Viral glycoproteins are synthesized on membrane-bound ribosomes and have the amino acid sequences to allow insertion into the rough endoplasmic reticulum and *N*-linked glycosylation. The high mannose form of the glycoproteins is processed through the Golgi apparatus and may be expressed on the plasma and other membranes of the cell. Other modifications, such as O-glycosylation, acylation, and sulfation of the proteins, can also occur during progression through the Golgi apparatus.

Assembly

Virion assembly is analogous to a three-dimensional interlocking puzzle that puts itself together in the box. The virion is built from small, easily manufactured parts that enclose the genome into a functional package. The site and mechanism of virion assembly in the cell depend on the location of genome replication and whether the final structure is a naked capsid or enveloped virus.

Assembly of the DNA viruses, other than poxviruses, occurs in the nucleus and requires transport of the virion proteins into the nucleus. These proteins must have the appropriate peptide signals for nuclear transport in addition to structural features. RNA virus and poxvirus assembly occur in the cytoplasm.

Each part of the virion has recognition structures that allow the virus to form the appropriate protein-protein, protein-nucleic acid, and (for enveloped viruses) protein-membrane interactions needed to assemble into the final structure. The assembly process begins when the necessary pieces are synthesized and the concentration of structural proteins in the cell is sufficient to thermodynamically drive the process, much like a crystallization reaction.

Assembly may be facilitated by scaffolding proteins or other proteins that are activated or release energy upon proteolysis. For example, cleavage of the VP0 protein of poliovirus releases the VP4 peptide which solidifies the capsid. For human immunodeficiency virus and other retroviruses, polyproteins containing the protease, polymerase, and structural proteins accumulate at viral glycoprotein-modified membranes. The virion buds from the membrane and protease is activated within the virion and cleaves the polyprotein to produce the final, infectious nucleocapsid within the envelope.

Capsid viruses may be assembled as empty structures (procapsids) to be filled with the genome (e.g., picornaviruses and herpesviruses), or they may be assembled around the genome. Nucleocapsids of the retroviruses, togaviruses and the negative-strand RNA viruses assemble around the genome and are subsequently enclosed in an envelope.

Acquisition of an envelope occurs after association of the nucleocapsid with regions of host-cell membrane modified with viral glycoproteins. Matrix proteins for negative-strand RNA viruses line and promote the adhesion of nucleocapsids with the glycoprotein-modified membrane. As more interactions occur, the membrane surrounds the nucleocapsid and the virus buds from the membrane.

The site of budding is determined by the type of genome and the protein sequence of the glycoproteins. Most RNA viruses bud from the plasma membrane, and the virus is released from the cell at the same time. The flaviviruses, coronaviruses, and bunyaviruses acquire their envelope by budding into the endoplasmic reticulum and Golgi membranes and remain in these organelles. The herpes simplex virus nucleocapsid assembles in the nucleus and buds at the nuclear membrane. The enveloped herpesvirus is transported through the Golgi apparatus and released by exocytosis, or released upon cell lysis.

Assembly of a complete, functional influenza or reovirus virion requires accumulation of at least one copy of each gene segment. Although influenza has only 8 genome segments, virions can randomly package 10 to 11 segments. Statistically, this yields approximately 1 complete set of genomes and functional virus per 20 defective viruses. Reovirus genomes are likely to assemble in a similar manner.

Errors are made during virus assembly. Empty virions and virions containing defective genomes are produced. As a result, the **particle/infectious virus ratio**, also called **particle/plaque-forming unit ratio**, is high, usually greater than 10 and during rapid viral replication can even be 10^4. Defective viruses can occupy the machinery required for normal virus replication to prevent (interfere) virus production (**defective interfering particles**).

Release

Viruses can be released from cells after lysis of the cell, by exocytosis, or by budding from the plasma membrane. Naked capsid viruses are generally released after lysis of the cell. Release of some enveloped viruses occurs after budding from the plasma membrane. Lysis and plasma membrane budding are efficient means of release. Viruses that bud or acquire their membrane in the cytoplasm (e.g., flaviviruses and poxviruses) generally require cell lysis for release and are more cell associated. Viruses that bind to sialic acid receptors may also have a neuraminidase (e.g., orthomyxoviruses, certain paramyxoviruses). The neuraminidase removes potential sialic acid receptors on the glycoproteins of the virion and the host cell to prevent clumping and facilitate release.

Reinitiation of the Replication Cycle

The virus released to the extracellular medium is usually responsible for initiating new infections; however, **cell-to-cell fusion** or **vertical transmission** of the genome to daughter cells can also spread the infection. Some herpesviruses, retroviruses, and paramyxoviruses can induce cell-to-cell fusion to create multinucleated giant cells (syncytia). The retroviruses can transmit their integrated copy of the genome vertically to daughter cells on cell division.

VIRAL GENETICS

As with other genetic systems, mutations spontaneously occur in viral genomes, creating new virus strains with properties differing from the **parental,** or **wild-type, virus.** These variants can be identified by their nucleotide sequences, antigenic differences (serotypes), or differences in functional or structural properties. Most mutations have no effect or are detrimental to the virus. Mutations in essential genes inactivate the virus, but mutations in other genes can produce antiviral drug resistance or alter the antigenicity or pathogenicity of the virus.

Mutations in viral genomes can be induced chemically or by irradiation in the laboratory. In nature, mutations usually result from the poor fidelity of the viral polymerase. Errors in copying the viral genome during virus replication produce many mutations. The rates of mutation for DNA viruses are usually lower than for RNA viruses.

Mutants are identified by the changes induced by the mutation. Mutations in essential genes are termed **lethal mutations.** These mutants are difficult to isolate because the virus cannot replicate. A **deletion mutant** results from the loss or selective removal of a portion of the genome and the function that it encodes. Other mutations may produce **plaque mutants,** which differ from the wild type in the size or appearance of the plaque; **host range mutants,** which differ in the tissue type or species of target cell that can be infected; or **attenuated mutants,** which are variants that cause less serious infections in animals or humans. **Conditional mutants,** such as **temperature-sensitive** (ts) or **cold-sensitive mutants,** express a normal phenotype and grow only at certain temperatures. Ts mutants generally grow well or relatively better at 30° C to 35° C, whereas elevated temperatures of 38° C to 40° C will inactivate the mutated, essential gene product and prevent virus production.

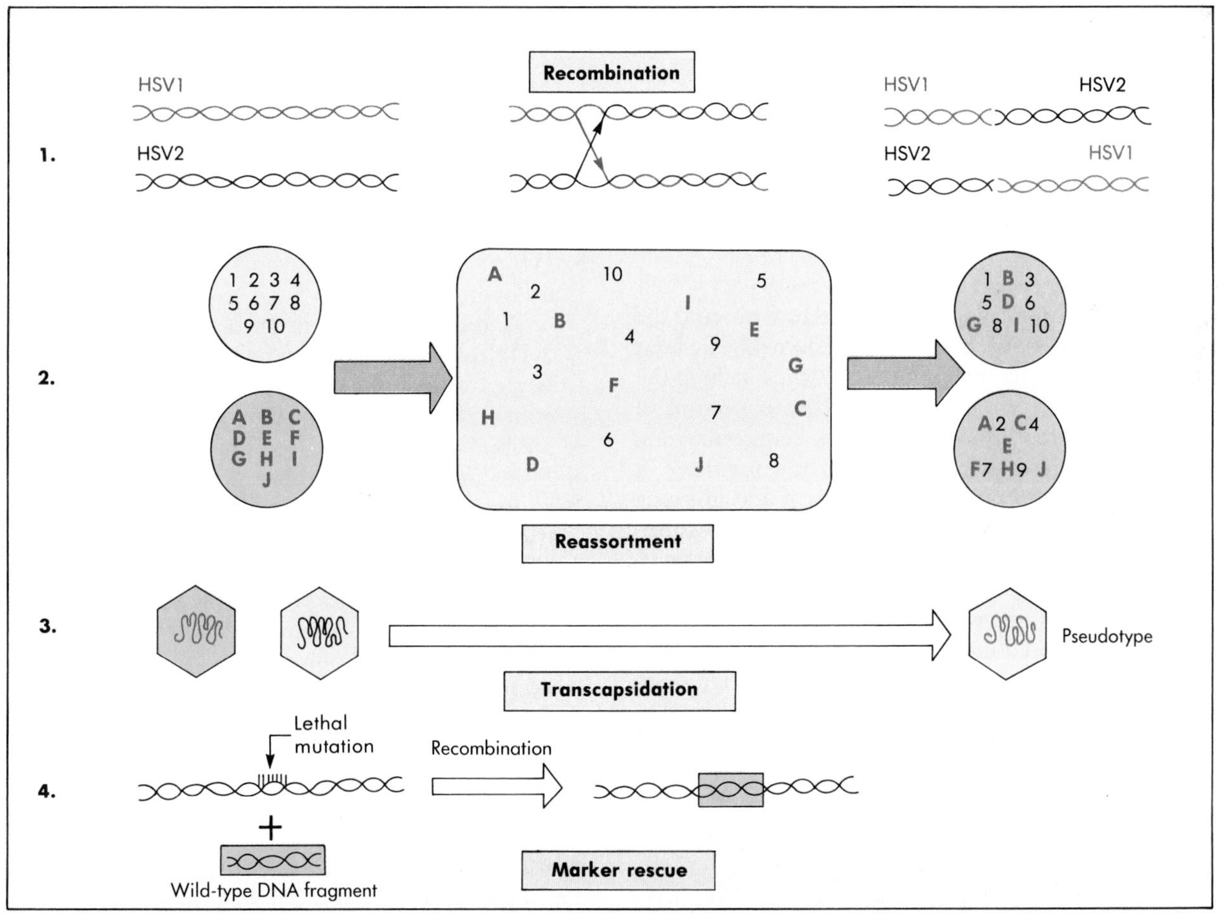

FIGURE 7-13 Genetic exchange between viral particles can give rise to new viral types, as illustrated here. Representative viruses include (*1*) intertypic recombination of herpes simplex virus types 1 and 2; (*2*) reassortment of two strains of reovirus; (3) rescue of a papovavirus defective in assembly by a complementary defective virus (transcapsidation); and (*4*) marker rescue of a lethal or conditional mutation.

New virus strains can also arise by genetic interactions between viruses or between the virus and the cell (Figure 7-13). Intramolecular genetic exchange between viruses or the virus and the host is termed **recombination.** Recombination can occur readily between two DNA viruses. For example, co-infection of a cell with the two closely related herpesviruses (herpes simplex virus types 1 and 2), will yield intertypic recombinant strains. These new hybrid strains will have genes from both types 1 and 2. Integration of retroviruses into host cell chromatin is a form of recombination.

Viruses with segmented genomes (as for influenza or reoviruses) form hybrid strains upon infection of one cell with more than one virus strain. This process, termed **reassortment**, is analogous to picking 10 marbles out of a box containing 10 black and 10 white marbles. New strains of influenza A virus are created upon co-infection with virus from different species (see Figure 60-3).

In some cases a defective viral strain can be rescued by the replication of another mutant, by the wild-type virus, or by a cell line bearing the nonfunctional viral gene. The replication of the other virus provides the missing function required by the mutant **(complementation).** Rescue of a lethal or conditional-lethal mutant with a defined genetic sequence, such as a restriction endonuclease DNA fragment, is called **marker rescue.** Marker rescue was used to map the genomes of viruses such as herpes simplex virus. Virus produced from cells infected with different virus strains may be **phenotypically mixed** and have the proteins of one strain but the genome of the other **(transcapsidation). Pseudotypes** are generated when transcapsidation occurs between different types of virus, but this is rare.

Individual virus strains or mutants are selected by their ability to use the host cell machinery and to withstand the conditions of the body and the environment. Cellular properties that can act as selection pressures include the growth rate of the cell and tissue-specific expression of certain proteins required by the virus (e.g., enzymes, glycoproteins, transcription factors). The conditions of the body, its elevated temperature, natural and immune defenses, and tissue structure are also selection pressures for viruses. The viruses that cannot endure these conditions and evade the defenses are eliminated. A small selective advantage in a mutant virus can shortly lead to its becoming the predominant viral strain.

Growth of virus under benign laboratory conditions lacks the selective pressures of the body and allows weaker strains to survive. This process is used to develop attenuated virus strains for use in vaccines.

QUESTIONS

1. What are the possible criteria for classifying each of the following pairs of viruses together?
   Poliovirus and rhinovirus
   Poliovirus and rotavirus
   Poliovirus and western equine encephalitis virus
   Yellow fever virus and dengue virus
   Epstein-Barr virus and cytomegalovirus
2. Match the characteristic(s) from column A with the appropriate viral family in column B based on your knowledge of their physical and genome structure and its implications.

   A.
   1. Resistant to detergents
   2. Resistant to drying
   3. Replication in the nucleus
   4. Replication in the cytoplasm
   5. Can be released from the cell without cell lysis
   6. Provides a good target for antiviral drug action
   7. Undergoes reassortment upon coinfection with two strains
   8. Makes DNA from an RNA template
   9. Uses a +RNA template to replicate the genome
   10. Genome translated into a polyprotein

   B.
   Picornaviruses
   Togaviruses
   Orthomyxoviruses
   Paramyxoviruses
   Rhabdoviruses
   Reoviruses
   Retroviruses
   Herpesviruses
   Papovaviruses
   Adenoviruses
   Poxviruses
   Hepadnaviruses
3. Based on structural considerations which of the virus families listed in question 2 should be able to endure fecal-oral transmission?
4. List the essential enzymes encoded by the virus families listed in question 2.
5. Which genetic mechanism(s) are occurring in the following example?
   A mutant defective in the herpes simplex virus type 1 DNA polymerase gene replicates in the presence of herpes simplex virus type 2. The progeny virus contains the HSV-1 genome but are recognized by antibodies to HSV-2.
6. How are the early and late genes of the togaviruses, papovaviruses, and herpesviruses distinguished, and how is the time of their expression regulated?
7. What are the consequences (no effect, decreased efficiency, or inhibition of replication) of a deletion mutation in the following viral enzymes?
   Epstein-Barr virus polymerase
   Herpes simplex virus thymidine kinase
   Human immunodeficiency virus reverse transcriptase
   Influenza B virus neuraminidase
   Rabies virus (rhabdovirus) G protein

Bibliography

Belshe RB, editor: *Textbook of human virology*, ed 2, St. Louis, 1991, Mosby.
Fields BN and Knipe DM: *Virology*, ed 2, New York, 1990, Raven Press.

SECTION II

HOST-PARASITE INTERACTIONS

CHAPTER 8

Microbial Flora in Health and Disease

MEDICAL microbiology is the study of the interactions between animals (primarily humans) and microorganisms such as viruses, bacteria, fungi, and parasites. Although the primary interest is in diseases precipitated by these interactions, it must also be appreciated that microorganisms play a critical role in human survival. The normal population of endogenous organisms participates in the metabolism of food products, provides essential growth factors, protects against infections with highly virulent microorganisms, and stimulates the immune response. In the absence of these organisms, life as we know it would be impossible.

The microbial flora in and on the human body is in a continual state of flux determined by such varied factors as age, diet, hormonal state, health, sanitary conditions, and personal hygiene. It is important that changes in our physical well-being can drastically disrupt the delicate balance that is maintained among the heterogeneous organisms that coexist within us. For example, hospitalization can lead to replacement of normally avirulent organisms in the oropharynx with potentially invasive gram-negative bacilli.

Two important points must be emphasized: (1) care should be taken to maintain the normal balance of microbes, and (2) an important distinction exists between colonization (also called infection) with a pathogenic organism and disease. The normal microbial flora controls the proliferation of pathogenic organisms by a variety of methods including competition for nutrients or receptors on host cells, production of **bacteriocins** (small-molecular–weight proteins that are bactericidal for other organisms), and stimulation of the immune response. Thus the pathogenic organisms residing in or on the body are controlled by the normal commensal organisms. However, if the normal flora is disrupted (e.g., by broad-spectrum antibiotics) or if the pathogenic organisms are introduced into a normally sterile environment, then disease can be produced. For example, *Streptococcus pneumoniae, Staphylococcus aureus,* and many gram-negative bacilli can be found as part of the normal oropharyngeal flora. However, when these organisms are introduced into the lower respiratory tract by aspiration of oral secretions and when local immunity is unable to contain them, bronchopulmonary disease develops.

An understanding of medical microbiology requires knowledge not only of the different classes of microbes but also of their propensity for causing disease. Some organisms (**opportunistic pathogens**) will not cause disease except in immunocompromised patients under conditions that favor the growth of the organism (e.g., *Staphylococcus epidermidis* disease at the site of an intravascular catheter). At the other end of the spectrum, some organisms (**strict pathogens**) are always associated with disease (e.g., *Mycobacterium tuberculosis, Shigella* species, *Neisseria gonorrhoeae*). Between these two extremes are the majority of organisms (**facultative pathogens**) associated with disease (e.g., *Staphylococcus aureus, Escherichia coli, Candida albicans*). The factors responsible for microbial virulence will be discussed in Chapter 11.

The microbial population that colonizes the human body is numerous and diverse. The most common organisms that form the commensal flora and their propensity to cause disease are summarized in Table 8-1 and the text that follows.

RESPIRATORY TRACT AND HEAD

Mouth, Oropharynx, and Nasopharynx

The upper respiratory tract is colonized with numerous organisms. Anaerobic bacteria are the most common, including *Peptostreptococcus, Fusobacterium, Prophyromonas, Bacteroides,* and *Actinomyces.* Aerobic organisms such as viridans group streptococci, coagulase-negative staphylococci, nonpathogenic *Neisseria,* and *Haemophilus* species (not *H. influenzae* B) are also common. These organisms are all relatively avirulent and are rarely associated with disease, unless they are introduced into normally sterile sites (e.g., sinuses, middle ear, brain). Potentially pathogenic organisms can also be found in the upper airways, including group A streptococci, *Streptococcus pneumoniae, Staphylococcus aureus, Neisseria meningitidis, Haemophilus influenzae* B, *Moraxella catarrhalis,* and Enterobacteriaceae. It must be remembered that the isolation of these organisms from an upper respiratory

TABLE 8–1 Commensal Organisms Encountered in Clinical Specimens

Site	Organism	Frequency[a]	Disease[b]
Mouth and oropharynx	Bacteria		
	Viridans *Streptococcus*	3+	L
	Group A *Streptococcus*	2+	H
	Non-group A *B-Streptococcus*	3+	L
	Streptococcus pneumoniae	2+	M
	Staphylococcus aureus	2+	M
	Coagulase-negative *Staphylococcus*	3+	L
	Neisseria	3+	L
	Haemophilus influenzae	1+	M
	Haemophilus, other species	3+	L
	Actinomyces	2+	M
	Enterobacteriaceae	1+	L
	Moraxella catarrhalis	2+	M
	Moraxella, other species	1+	L
	Capnocytophaga	2+	L
	Cardiobacteirum hominis	1+	M
	Corynebacterium	2+	L
	Eikenella corrodens	1+	L
	Kingella	1+	M
	Mycoplasma	1+	L
	Lactobacillus	1+	L
	Treponema	2+	L
	Veillonella	2+	L
	Peptostreptococcus	3+	L
	Fusobacterium	3+	M
	Porphyromonas	2+	L
	Bacteroides	2+	L
	Fungi		
	Candida	2+	L
	Parasites	2+	L
	Trichomonas tenax		
	Viruses		
	Adenovirus	1+	L
	Cytomegalovirus	1+	M
	Herpes simplex virus	1+	M
Nasopharynx	Bacteria		
	Staphylococcus aureus	1+	M
	Coagulase-negative *Staphylococcus*	3+	L
	Viridans *Streptococcus*	2+	L
	Streptococcus pneumoniae	1+	M
	Haemophilus	1+	L
	Neisseria	1+	L
Outer ear	Coagulase-negative *Staphylococcus*	3+	L
	Streptococcus pneumoniae	1+	M
	Pseudomonas	1+	M
	Enterobacteriaceae	1+	M
Eye	Coagulase-negative *Staphylococcus*	3+	L
	Haemophilus	1+	L
Stomach	*Helicobacter pylori*	1+	H
	Lactobacillus	1+	L
	Streptococcus	1+	L

TABLE 8–1 Commensal Organisms Encountered in Clinical Specimens—cont'd

Site	Organism	Frequency[(a)]	Disease[(b)]
Small intestine	Bacteria		
	Lactobacillus	3+	L
	Bacteroides	2+	M
	Prevotella	2+	L
	Porphyromonas	2+	L
	Fusobacterium	2+	L
	Clostridium	1+	M
	Peptostreptococcus	2+	L
	Staphylococcus	1+	L
	Streptococcus	2+	L
	Enterococcus	2+	M
	Enterobacteriaceae	1+	M
	Fungi		
	Candida	1+	M
	Parasites		
	Blastocystis hominis	1+	M
	Entamoeba coli	1+	L
	Endolimax nana	1+	L
	Iodamoeba butschlii	1+	L
	Trichomonas hominis	1+	L
	Chilomastix mesnili	1+	L
Large intestine	Bacteria		
	Lactobacillus	2+	L
	Clostridium	3+	M
	Bifidobacterium	3+	L
	Eubacterium	2+	L
	Bacteroides	3+	H
	Prevotella	3+	M
	Porphyromonas	3+	M
	Fusobacterium	3+	M
	Veillonella	2+	L
	Peptostreptococcus	3+	M
	Staphylococcus	1+	L
	Streptococcus	1+	L
	Enterococcus	3+	M
	Enterobacteriaceae	3+	M
	Pseudomonas	1+	M
	Aeromonas	1+	L
	Corynebacterium	1+	L
	Mycobacterium	1+	L
	Fungi		
	Candida	1+	M
	Parasites		
	Blastocystis hominis	1+	M
	Entamoeba coli	1+	L
	Endolimax nana	1+	L
	Iodamoeba butschlii	1+	L
	Trichomonas hominis	1+	L
	Chilomastix mesnili	1+	L
	Viruses		
	Adenovirus	1+	L
	Enterovirus	1+	M

TABLE 8–1 Commensal Organisms Encountered in Clinical Specimens—cont'd

Site	Organism	Frequency[a]	Disease[b]
Anterior urethra	Bacteria		
	Lactobacillus	3+	L
	Corynebacterium	3+	L
	Coagulase-negative *Staphylococcus*	2+	L
	Streptococcus	1+	L
	Enterococcus	1+	L
	Nonpathogenic *Neisseria*	1+	L
	Gardnerella vaginalis	1+	L
	Mycoplasma	1+	M
	Ureaplasma	1+	M
	Enterobacteriaceae	1+	M
	Fungi	1+	M
	Candida		
	Parasites	1+	M
	Trichomonas vaginalis		
Vagina	Bacteria		
	Lactobacillus	3+	L
	Staphylococcus	3+	L
	Enterococcus	2+	L
	Streptococcus	2+	L
	Nonpathogenic *Neisseria*	2+	L
	Mycoplasma	2+	M
	Ureaplasma	2+	M
	Gardnerella vaginalis	3+	L
	Enterobacteriaceae	2+	M
	Actinomyces	2+	M
	Bacteroides	2+	M
	Porphyromonas	2+	L
	Prevotella	2+	L
	Fusobacterium	2+	M
	Mobiluncus	2+	H
	Clostridium	1+	M
	Fungi		
	Candida	2+	M
	Torulopsis	2+	M
	Parasites		
	Trichomonas vaginalis	1+	M
Skin	Bacteria		
	Staphylococcus aureus	1+	H
	Coagulase-negative *Staphylococcus*	3+	M
	Corynebacterium	3+	L
	Propionibacterium	3+	L
	Clostridium	1+	L
	Fungi		
	Candida	1+	M
	Malassezia furfur	1+	M

[a]Frequency of recovery from healthy individuals: *1+*, rare; *2+*, frequently isolated; *3+*, commonly present.
[b]Cause of disease: *H*, high; *M* moderate; *L*, low.

tract specimen does not define their pathogenicity. Their involvement with a disease process must be demonstrated to the exclusion of other pathogens. For example, with the exception of group A streptococci, these organisms are rarely responsible for pharyngitis even though they can be isolated from patients with this disease.

Ear

The most common organism found to colonize the outer ear is coagulase-negative *Staphylococcus.* Other organisms colonizing the skin have been isolated from this site, as well as potential pathogens such as *Streptococcus pneumoniae, Pseudomonas aeruginosa,* and the Enterobacteriaceae.

This latter group of organisms has also been associated with disease at this site.

Eye

The surface of the eye is colonized with coagulase-negative staphylococci, as well as rare numbers of organisms found in the nasopharynx (e.g., *Haemophilus* spp., *Neisseria* spp., viridans streptococci).

Lower Respiratory Tract

The larynx, trachea, bronchioles, and lower airways are generally sterile, although transient colonization with upper respiratory secretions may occur following aspiration. Acute lower airway disease is usually caused by the more virulent bacteria present in the mouth (e.g., *S. pneumoniae, S. aureus, H. influenzae,* and members of the Enterobacteriaceae such as *Klebsiella*). Chronic aspiration may lead to a polymicrobial disease with anaerobes as the predominant pathogens, particularly peptostreptococci and anaerobic gram-negative bacilli. Fungi such as *Candida* can cause lower airway disease, but organisms must be demonstrated in tissue to exclude simple colonization. In contrast, the presence of the dimorphic fungi (e.g., *Histoplasma, Coccidioides, Blastomyces*) is diagnostic because colonization with these organisms does not occur.

GASTROINTESTINAL TRACT

The gastrointestinal tract is colonized with microbes at birth and remains the home for a diverse collection of organisms throughout the life of the host. Although the opportunity for colonization with new organisms occurs daily with ingestion of food and water, the population remains relatively constant unless exogenous factors such as antibiotic treatment disrupt the balanced flora.

Stomach

This area is generally colonized with small numbers of acid-tolerant organisms such as the lactic acid–producing bacteria, lactobacilli and streptococci. *Helicobacter pylori,* a cause of gastritis and ulcerative disease, is also commonly found in this area. The microbial population can dramatically change in numbers and diversity in patients receiving drugs that neutralize or reduce the production of gastric acids.

Small Intestine

In contrast with the anterior portion of the digestive tract, the small intestine is colonized with many different bacteria, fungi, and parasites. Most of these organisms are anaerobes. Common causes of gastroenteritis (e.g., *Salmonella, Campylobacter*) can be present in small numbers as asymptomatic residents; however, their detection in the clinical laboratory is generally indicative of disease production. If obstruction of the small intestine occurs, such as following abdominal surgery, then a condition called "blind loop syndrome" can occur. In this case stasis of the intestinal contents leads to colonization and proliferation of organisms typically present in the large intestine, with a subsequent malabsorption syndrome.

Large Intestine

More microbes are present in this site than anywhere else in the human body. It has been estimated that more than 10^{11} bacteria per gram of feces can be found, with anaerobic bacteria in excess by a thousandfold. Many of these anaerobes are the relatively avirulent bifidobacteria and eubacteria. However, the peptostreptococci and the anaerobic gram-negative bacilli (particularly *Bacteroides fragilis* group) are common. Members of the family Enterobacteriaceae and the enterococci are the most common facultative anaerobes present in the large intestine. Antibiotic treatment can rapidly alter this population, with the proliferation of antibiotic-resistant organisms such as enterococci, *Pseudomonas,* and fungi. *Clostridium difficile* can also grow rapidly in this situation, leading to disease ranging from diarrhea to pseudomembranous colitis. Exposure to other enteric pathogens, such as *Shigella,* enterohemorrhagic *Escherichia coli,* and *Entamoeba histolytica* can also rapidly disrupt the colonic flora and produce significant intestinal disease.

GENITOURINARY SYSTEM

In general, the anterior urethra and vagina are the only anatomical areas of the genitourinary system that are colonized with microbes. Although the urinary bladder can be transiently colonized with bacteria migrating upstream from the urethra, these should be rapidly cleared by the bactericidal activity of the uroepithelial cells and the flushing action of voided urine. The other structures of the urinary system should be sterile except when disease or an anatomical abnormality is present. Likewise, the uterus should also remain free of organisms.

Anterior Urethra

The indigenous population of the urethra consists of a variety of organisms, with lactobacilli, corynebacteria, and coagulase-negative staphylococci the most numerous. These organisms are relatively avirulent and are rarely associated with human disease. In contrast, the urethra can be colonized with enterococci, Enterobacteriaceae, and *Candida*—all of which can invade the urinary tract and lead to significant disease. Organisms such as *Neisseria gonorrhoeae* and *Chlamydia trachomatis* are common causes of urethritis and can persist as asymptomatic colonizers of the urethra. The isolation of these organisms in clinical specimens should always be considered significant, irrespective of the presence or absence of clinical symptoms.

Vagina

The microbial population of the vagina is dramatically influenced by hormonal factors. Newborn girls are colonized with lactobacilli at the time of birth, and these bacteria predominate for approximately 6 weeks. After that time, the levels of maternal estrogen have declined and the vaginal flora changes to include staphylococci, streptococci, and Enterobacteriaceae. When estrogen production is initiated at puberty, the microbial flora again changes. Lactobacilli reemerge as the predominant organisms, and many other organisms are also isolated, including staphylococci (*S. aureus* less commonly than the coagulase-negative species), streptococci including group B *Streptococcus,* enterococci, *Gardnerella vaginalis, Mycoplasma* and the related *Ureaplasma,* Enterobacteriaceae, and a variety of anaerobic bacteria. Although *Neisseria gonorrhoeae* and *Chlamydia trachomatis* are common causes of genital disease, a significant proportion of disease develops when the balance of vaginal bacteria is disrupted, resulting in decreases in lactobacilli and increases in *Mobiluncus* and *Gardnerella. Mycoplasma hominis* may also be involved in this process, and *Trichomonas vaginalis, Candida albicans,* and *Torulopsis glabrata* are certainly important causes of vaginitis. Although herpes simplex virus and papillomavirus would not be considered normal flora of the genitourinary tract, these viruses can establish persistent infections.

SKIN

Although many organisms come into contact with the skin surface, this relatively hostile environment does not support the survival of most organisms. Coagulase-negative staphylococci and less commonly *Staphylococcus aureus,* corynebacteria, and propionibacteria are the most common organisms found on the skin surface. *Clostridium perfringens* is isolated on the skin of approximately 20% of healthy individuals, and the fungi *Candida* and *Malassezia* are also found on skin surfaces, particularly in moist sites. Streptococci can transiently colonize the skin, but the volatile fatty acids produced by the anaerobe propionibacteria are toxic for these organisms. Gram-negative bacilli do not permanently colonize the skin surface (with the exception of *Acinetobacter* and a few other less common genera), because the skin is too dry.

QUESTIONS

1. What is the distinction between infection and disease?
2. Give examples of opportunistic pathogens, facultative pathogens, and strict pathogens.
3. What factors regulate the microbial population that colonize humans?

Bibliography

Isenberg H and D'Amato R: Indigenous and pathogenic microorganisms of humans. In Balows A, Hausler W, Herrmann K, Isenberg H, Shadomy HJ, editors: *Manual of clinical microbiology*, ed 5, Washington DC, 1991 ASM Publications.

CHAPTER 9

Natural Immunity and Physiological Defense Mechanisms

ENTRY of a pathogenic microorganism into a susceptible host can be followed by invasion and colonization of tissues, circumvention of the host immune response, and injury to the host tissues. The skill with which pathogenic microorganisms resist the host's immune defenses governs their survival and pathogenicity. Paradoxically, the host response to a pathogenic microorganism, rather than the microbe itself, may induce injury to host tissues. This chapter will examine the role of the host's natural immune response in infection (Figure 9-1); acquired immunity will be discussed in Chapter 10.

MICROBIAL COMPETITION

As discussed in Chapter 8, the human body is inhabited by microorganisms that provide a number of important physiological functions, including protection from colonization and subsequent infection with exogenous pathogenic organisms. This normal commensal population of organisms is commonly present on the skin, as well as mucous membranes of the conjunctiva, nose, mouth, intestinal tract, and lower urogenital tract. These organisms can inhibit colonization of pathogenic organisms by a number of methods, including competition for cell surface receptors (e.g., fibronectin on epithelial cells), production of bacteriocins that inhibit the growth of other organisms, competitive depletion of essential nutrients, production of toxic by-products (e.g., vaginal colonization is regulated by lactobacilli, which convert glycogen to lactic acid yielding a pH of 4 to 5), and stimulation of natural antibodies that cross-react with pathogenic organisms. This protective mechanism can be disrupted by disease or the use of broad spectrum antibiotics. The resultant changes in the commensal flora may lead to colonization with enterococci, gram-negative bacilli, *Clostridium difficile,* or yeast.

MECHANICAL BARRIERS

The skin and mucous membranes serve as barriers to the microorganisms (Box 9-1). With the exception of a few organisms (e.g., papilloma virus, dermatophytes ["skin loving" fungi]), most microorganisms cannot establish infections without penetrating the skin or mucous membranes. Free fatty acids produced in sebaceous glands and by organisms on the skin surface, lactic acid in perspiration, and the low pH and relatively dry environment of the skin are all unfavorable for the survival of most organisms. Lysozyme and lactoferrin are antimicrobial substances found in secretions at mucosal surfaces. Lysozyme induces lysis of bacteria through disruption of the linkage connecting *N*-acetylmuraminic acid and *N*-acetylglucosamine in the walls of gram-positive bacteria. Lactoferrin, an iron binding protein, competes with microorganisms for this substance. By chelating iron, lactoferrin deprives microbes of the free iron they need for growth. Secretory IgA is also present on mucosal surfaces. These immunoglobulins can interfere with the attach-

BOX 9-1 Mechanical Barriers Against Infection

- Intact skin
- Mucus
  - Motion of cilia
  - Coughing/sneezing
- Cell shedding
- Flushing of microbes by tears, saliva, urine, perspiration, other body fluids
- Emesis and diarrhea aid microbial elimination

ment of bacteria to host cells, inhibit microbial motility, agglutinate the organisms, and neutralize their exotoxins. The acidic environment of the stomach and intestinal peristalsis also regulate the organisms that can colonize the intestinal tract.

Inhaled microorganisms in dust or droplets greater than 5 μm adhere to the mucosa lining the upper respiratory tract and are swept upward by cilia to the posterior pharynx and then expectorated or swallowed. Particles less than 5 μm are able to reach the lower airways but should be rapidly phagocytized by alveolar macrophages. However, cigarette smoke or other pollutants, as well as some bacteria and viruses (e.g., *Bordetella pertussis,* influenza virus), can interfere with this clearance mechanism by damaging the ciliated epithelial cells, thus rendering the patient susceptible to secondary bacterial pneumonia. Intubation or tracheostomy also decreases the normal defense mechanisms.

Even though urine can support bacterial growth in the bladder, the acidic pH of urine and voiding serve as effective defensive mechanisms against most uropathogens. Urinary tract infections are also generally less common in males than females because of the longer urethra in males. Urinary stasis caused by reflux, prostatic hypertrophy, or calculi facilitates growth of organisms in the retained urine and subsequent infections.

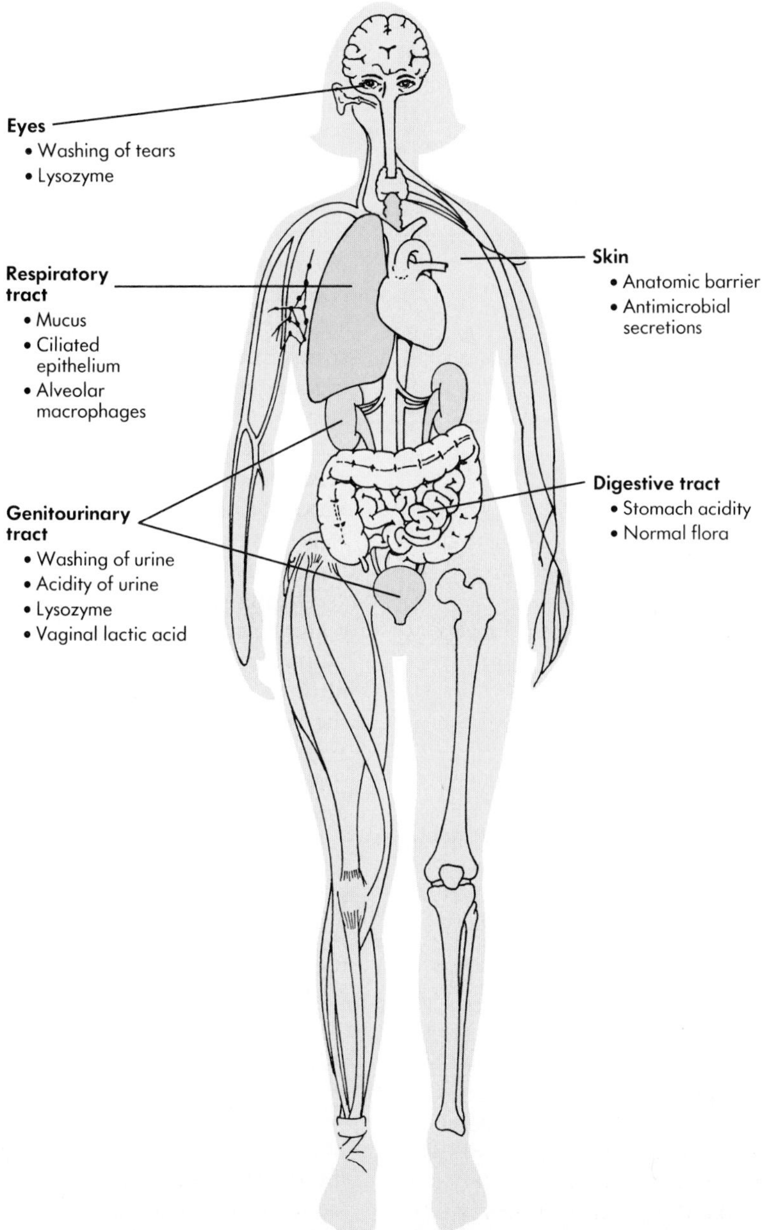

FIGURE 9-1 External defense barriers of the human body.

NONSPECIFIC HUMORAL DEFENSE MECHANISMS

Numerous enzymes, proteins, and other factors contribute to a host's nonspecific immunity. Some are humoral defenses (Table 9-1) and others, to be discussed later, are cellular defenses.

Inflammatory Response

Acute inflammation represents an early defense mechanism to contain an infection and prevent its spread from the initial focus (Figure 9-2). When microbes multiply in host tissues, two principal defensive mechanisms mounted against them are antibodies and leukocytes. The three major events in acute inflammation are (1) dilatation of capillaries to increase blood flow, (2) changes in the microvasculature structure leading to escape of plasma proteins and leukocytes from the circulation, and (3) leukocyte emigration from the capillaries and accumulation at the site of injury. Widening of interendothelial cell junctions of venules or injury of endothelial cells facilitates escape of plasma proteins from the vessels. Neutrophils, attached to the endothelium through adhesion molecules, escape the microvasculature and are attracted to sites of injury by chemotactic agents. This is followed by phagocytosis of the microorganisms that may lead to their intracellular destruction. Activated leukocytes may produce toxic metabolites and proteases that injure endothelium and tissues when they are released. Activation of the third component of complement (C3) is also a critical step in inflammation.

Multiple chemical mediators of inflammation derived from either plasma or cells have been described. Mediators in plasma, such as complement, are present as precursors that require activation for them to become biologically active. Mediators derived from cells are present as precursors in intracellular granules, such as histamine in mast cells. Following activation, these substances are secreted. Other mediators such as prostaglandins may be synthesized following stimulation. These mediators are quickly activated by enzymes or other substances such as antioxidants. A chemical mediator may also cause a target cell to release a secondary mediator with a similar or opposing action.

Besides histamine, other preformed chemical mediators in cells include serotonin and lysosomal enzymes. Those that are newly synthesized include prostaglandins, leukotrienes, platelet-activating factors, cytokines, and nitric oxide. Chemical mediators in plasma include complement fragments C3a and C5a and the C5b-9 sequence. Three plasma-derived factors, including kinins, complement, and clotting factors, are involved in inflammation. Bradykinin is produced by activation of the kinin system. It induces arteriolar dilatation and increased venule permeability through contraction of endothelial cells and extravascular smooth muscle contraction. Activation of bradykinin precursors involves activated factor XII (Hageman factor) generated by its contact with injured tissues.

During clotting, fibrinopeptides produced during the conversion of fibrinogen to fibrin increase vascular permeability and are chemotactic for leukocytes. The fibrinolytic system participates in inflammation through the kinin system. Products produced during arachidonic acid metabolism also affect inflammation. These include prostaglandins and leukotrienes, which can mediate essentially every aspect of acute inflammation.

TABLE 9-1 Nonspecific Humoral Defense Mechanisms

Factor	Function	Source
Lysozyme	Catalyses hydrolysis of cell wall mucopeptide layer	Tears, saliva, nasal secretions, body fluids, lysosomal granules
Lactoferrin, transferrin	Binds iron and competes with microorganisms for it	Specific granules of PMNs
Lactoperoxidase	May be inhibitory to many microorganisms	Milk and saliva
Beta-lysin	Effective mainly against gram-positive bacteria	Thrombocytes, normal serum
Chemotactic factors	Induce reorientation and directed migration of PMNs, monocytes and other cells	Bacterial substances and products of cell injury and denatured proteins
Properdin	Activates complement in the absence of antibody-antigen complex	Normal plasma
Interferons	Act as immunomodulators to increase the activities of macrophages	Leukocytes, fibroblasts, natural killer cells, T cells
Defensins	Block cell transport activities	Polymorphonuclear granules

PMNs, Polymorphonuclear leukocytes.

Cytokines

Cells responding to invading microorganisms may produce a variety of peptides called **cytokines** that are able to modulate the immune system. Cytokines produced by macrophages and monocytes are known as **monokines,** and those produced by lymphocytes are known as **lymphokines.** Cytokines are not antigen specific but play an important function in modifying the immune response. Examples of cytokines are interleukin 1 (IL-1) and tumor necrosis factor (TNF) produced by macrophages, and interleukin 2 (IL-2), interferons, and colony-stimulating factors synthesized by T lymphocytes (Box 9-2).

Cytokines with the greatest role in inflammation are IL-1, TNF, and IL-8. IL-1 and TNF both are produced by activated macrophages, although other types of cells

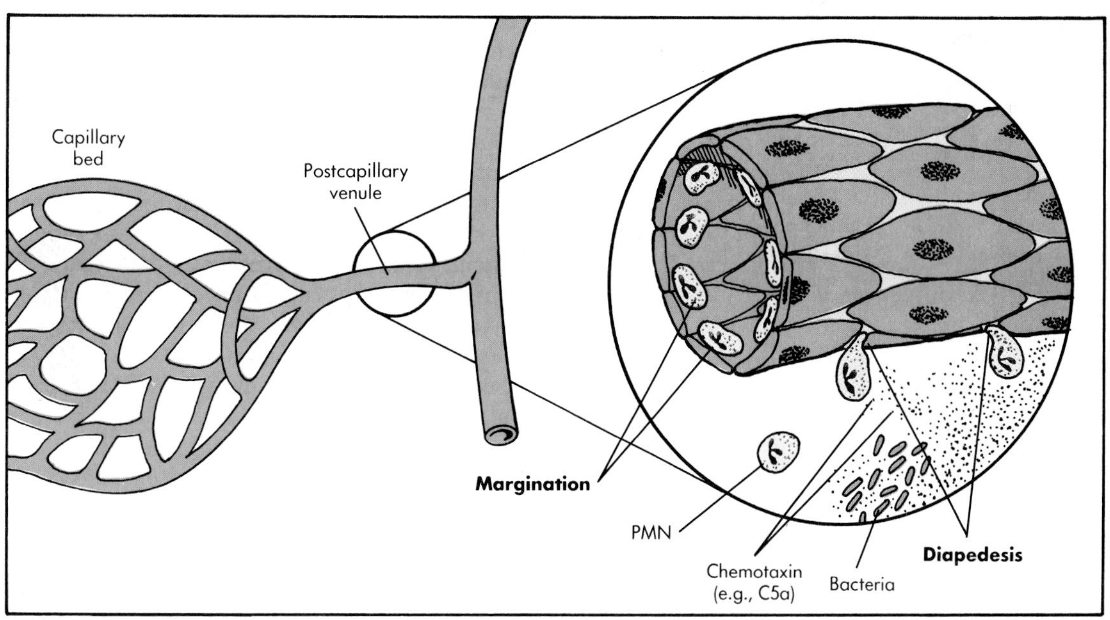

FIGURE 9-2 A schematic illustration showing margination of polymorphonuclear leukocytes *(PMNs)* along the lumen of a postcapillary venule and migration through the wall into the surrounding tissue by diapedesis. The PMNs then move by chemotaxis toward a chemotactic agent.

may also produce IL-1. Cytokine secretion is promoted by endotoxin, immune complexes, toxins, physical injury, and inflammation. Cytokines that act on the cells producing them are said to have an **autocrine action,** whereas those that affect neighboring cells are said to have a **paracrine effect.** When they act like any other hormone (i.e., on cells distant from their site of synthesis), they have an **endocrine effect.** In inflammation, they act locally on the endothelium, participate in systemic acute phase reactions, and affect fibroblasts. They promote the synthesis and surface expression of adhesion molecules on the endothelial surface, which leads to increased adherence of leukocytes and increased thrombogenicity of the endothelium. They are pyrogenic (induce fever) during acute inflammation. TNF promotes neutrophil aggregation and activation and the escape of proteolytic enzymes from mesenchymal cells, thereby promoting tissue injury. IL-8 has powerful chemoattractant qualities and activates neutrophils.

Oxygen-derived metabolites from leukocytes may contribute to inflammation. They may injure endothelial cells, causing increased vascular permeability, inactivation of antiproteases, and injury to other cells. The effect of oxygen-derived free radicals in inflammation depends on their synthesis and inactivation by host cells.

Acute Phase Response

The acute phase response is a nonspecific reaction by an individual stimulated by infection, inflammation, tissue injury, and infrequently neoplasm; it is mediated by IL-1, IL-6, tumor necrosis factor, prostaglandin (PGE_1), and interferons. Serum proteins elevated in the circulation during the acute phase response include complement, coagulation proteins, transport proteins, protease inhibitors, and adherence proteins that activate complement, promote phagocytosis, and stimulate migration of leukocytes (Box 9-3).

C-reactive protein (CRP) is produced by IL-1 stimulation of the liver. Within 24 to 48 hours of the onset of acute inflammation, the CRP concentration increases a thousandfold (thus elevated levels are a nonspecific indicator of inflammation). CRP complexes with polysaccharides of numerous bacteria and fungi; it activates the alternate complement pathway, which facilitates removal of these organisms from the body through increased phagocytosis.

Interleukin-1, tumor necrosis factor α, and α-interferon released during the acute phase response act on the hypothalamus to induce fever (Table 9-2).

BOX 9-2 Cytokines

Monokines
- α-interferon
- Interleukin-1
- Tumor necrosis factor–α
- Colony-stimulating factors

Lymphokines
- Tumor necrosis factor–β
- τ-interferon
- Interleukins (e.g., IL-2)
- Granulocyte-macrophage colony-stimulating factor
- Lymphotoxin

BOX 9-3 Acute Phase Reactants

alpha-1 antitrypsin	Ceruloplasmin
alpha-1 glycoprotein	Fibrinogen
Amyloid A and P	Haptoglobin
Antithrombin III	Orosomucoid
C-reactive protein	Plasminogen
C1 esterase inhibitor	Transferrin
C3 complement	

Complement

Multiple plasma proteins may be activated during inflammation. Immune complexes activate the classic pathway of complement, whereas bacterial products activate the alternative pathway without participation by specific antibody. Many antimicrobial effects are mediated by complement. For example, C5a, C5b67, and C3a induce chemotaxis of leukocytes, and C3b has opsonic properties.

Classical Pathway

The first complement component, designated C1, consists of a complex of three separate proteins designated C1q, C1r, and C1s (Figure 9-3). One molecule each of C1q and C1s with two molecules of C1r compose the C1 complex or **recognition unit.** C1q facilitates binding of the recognition unit to cell surface antigen-antibody complexes. Activation of the classical complement cascade requires linkage of C1q to two IgG antibodies through their Fc regions. In contrast, one pentameric IgM molecule attached to a cell surface may interact with C1q to initiate the classical pathway. Binding of C1q activates C1r (referred to now as C1r*) and in turn C1s (C1s*). C1s* then splits C4 (to C4a and C4b) and C2 (to C2a and C2b). The ability of a single recognition unit to split numerous C2 and C4 molecules represents an amplification mechanism in the complement cascade. The union of C4b and C2a produces C4b2a, which is known as **C3 convertase.** This complex binds to the cell membrane and splits C3 into C3a and C3b fragments. The ability to split multiple C3 molecules is another amplification mechanism. The interaction of C3b with C4b2a bound to the cell membrane produces a complete activation unit, C4b3b2a, which is termed **C5 convertase.** This **activation unit** splits C5 into C5a and C5b fragments and represents yet another amplification step.

The terminal stage of the classical pathway involves creation of the **membrane attack complex,** which is also called the **lytic unit.** C5b binds to the cell membrane, followed by the successive interaction of single molecules of C6, C7, C8, and C9 with the membrane-bound C5b. Formation of a membrane attack complex leads to a cell membrane lesion that permits loss of potassium and ingress of sodium and water, leading to hypotonic lysis of cells.

Not all C3b produced in the classical complement activation unites with C4b2a to produce C5 convertase. Some of it binds directly to the cell membrane and makes it more attractive for phagocytic cells such as neutrophils and macrophages, which have receptors for C3b. Complement fragments C3a and C5a also serve as powerful **anaphylatoxins** that stimulate mast cells to release histamine, which enhances vascular permeability and smooth muscle contraction. C5a also acts as an attractant for neutrophils and macrophages that release hydrolytic enzymes and stimulate platelet aggregation, leading to microthrombosis, blood stasis, edema, and local tissue injury and destruction.

Selected microorganisms such as *Escherichia coli,* low virulence strains of *Salmonella,* and certain viruses (e.g., parainfluenzae) can react directly with C1q in the absence of antibody, leading to C1 activation. Various other substances such as myelin basic protein, denatured bacterial endotoxin, heparin, and urate crystal surfaces may also directly activate the classical complement pathway.

Alternate Pathway

Endotoxin, human IgA, microbial polysaccharides, and other factors may activate complement by an alternative pathway (see Figure 9-3). This pathway does not depend on antibody activation and does not involve the early complement components (C1, C2, and C4). The initial activation of the alternate pathway is mediated by **properdin factor B** binding to C3b and then with properdin factor D, which splits factor B in the complex to yield the Bb active fragment that remains linked to C3b (activation unit). Inactive Ba is split off from this complex, which leads to C3 activation and then continuation of the complement cascade in a manner analogous to the classical pathway. Activation of the late components results in opsonic activity, chemotaxis of leukocytes, enhanced permeability of organisms, and cytolysis.

Membrane Attack Complex

Five terminal complement proteins (C5-C9) associate into a membrane attack complex (MAC) on target cell membranes to mediate injury. Initiation of MAC assembly begins with C5 cleavage into C5a and C5b fragments. A $(C5b,6,7,8)_1(C9)_n$ complex then either forms on natural membranes or, in their absence, combines with plasma inhibitors such as lipoproteins, antithrombin III, and S protein.

Mechanisms proposed for complement-mediated cytolysis include incorporation of extrinsic protein channels into the plasma membrane or membrane deformation and destruction. Only scant data are available concerning the domains or segments that link the MAC or its precursors to the membrane. The central regions of C5, C7, C8 alpha, C8 beta, and C9 have been postulated to contain amphilic structures that may be membrane anchors. Binding of a single C9 molecule to the C5b-C8 complex is sufficient to lead to erythrocyte lysis. Gram-negative bacilli are able to resist complement cytolysis by lengthening the surface carbohydrate content and interfering with MAC binding.

TABLE 9-2 Nonspecific Cellular Defense Mechanisms

Factor	Function	Source
Monokines α-Interferon	Inhibits cell proliferation and tumor growth, enhances natural killer cell activity and phagocytosis	Leukocytes
Interleukin-1	Induces lymphokine production, enhances B cell proliferation and antibody production, increases phagocytosis, acts as chemoattractant, increases T cell activation and IL-2 receptor expression	Macrophages, dendritic cells, B lymphocytes, PMNs, endothelial and smooth muscle cells, and others
Tumor necrosis factor α	Many functions shared with IL-1	Activated macrophages, others
Colony-stimulating factors	Specific factors stimulate the growth of specific cell lines such as neutrophils, monocytes, eosinophils, erythrocytes, megakaryocytes and basophils	Monocytes, fibroblasts, T cells, B cells, endothelial and epithelial cells, kidney cells
Lymphokines	T cell, B cell and hematopoietic growth factors; multiple effector functions	Lymphocytes
τ-Interferon	Activates macrophages, maintains MHC class II expression on cell surfaces, inhibits cell proliferation, enhances accessory cell function of macrophages	Stimulated T lymphocytes, natural killer cells
Lymphotoxin (tumor necrosis factor β)	Target cell destruction	Lymphocytes
Interleukin-2	Induces proliferation of activated T cells, B cells, and natural killer cells, stimulates lymphokine and immunoglobulin production	Activated CD4+ T cells
Interleukin-3	Acts on pluripotent stem cells to stimulate growth of neutrophils, monocytes, erythrocytes, basophils, eosinophils, and megakaryocytes	Activated T lymphocytes
Interleukin-4	Stimulates B cells, promotes immunoglobulin subtype switching, stimulates mast cells and hemopoiesis, activates macrophages	T helper cells, mast cells
Interleukin-5	Helps stimulate B cell proliferation and growth, stimulates eosinophils, promotes immunoglobulin subtype switching, enhances expression of IL-2 receptor	T helper cells
Interleukin-6	Increases immunoglobulin secretion, stimulates production of acute phase proteins, stimulates T cells and thymocytes, enhances differentiation of myelomonocytic cell lines	T and B cells, monocytes, fibroblasts, epithelial and endothelial cells
Interleukin-7	Stimulates pre-B cells and thymocytes, stimulates mature T cells, stimulates megakaryotes and myeloid precursors	Bone marrow stromal cells
Interleukin-8	Stimulates migration of monocytes and neutrophils, stimulates release of superoxide anions and lysosomal enzymes, chemotactic for basophils and T lymphocytes, stimulates release of histamine from basophils	Monocytes, fibroblasts, epithelial and endothelial cells, synovial cells
Interleukin-9	Enhances mast cell growth and CD4+ T cell	T cells, spleen cells
Interleukin-10	Regulates the class of immune response, modulates accessory cell (APC) function	T cells
Interleukin-11	Acts as a megakaryocyte potentiator, stimulates IgG production	Fibroblasts, stromal cells

PMNs, Polymorphonuclear neutrophilic leukocytes; *APC*, antigen presenting cells.

Hereditary Complement Deficiencies and Microbial Infection

Inherited deficiencies of C1q, C1r, C1s, C4, or C2 components are associated with defects in activation of the classical pathway that lead to increased susceptibility to **pyogenic** (pus-producing) infections. A deficiency of C3 leads to a defect in activation of both the classical and alternative pathways, which also results in an increased incidence of pyogenic infections. As would be expected, such individuals also have defective opsonization and phagocytosis (see the following). Defects of the properdin factors impair activation of the alternative pathway,

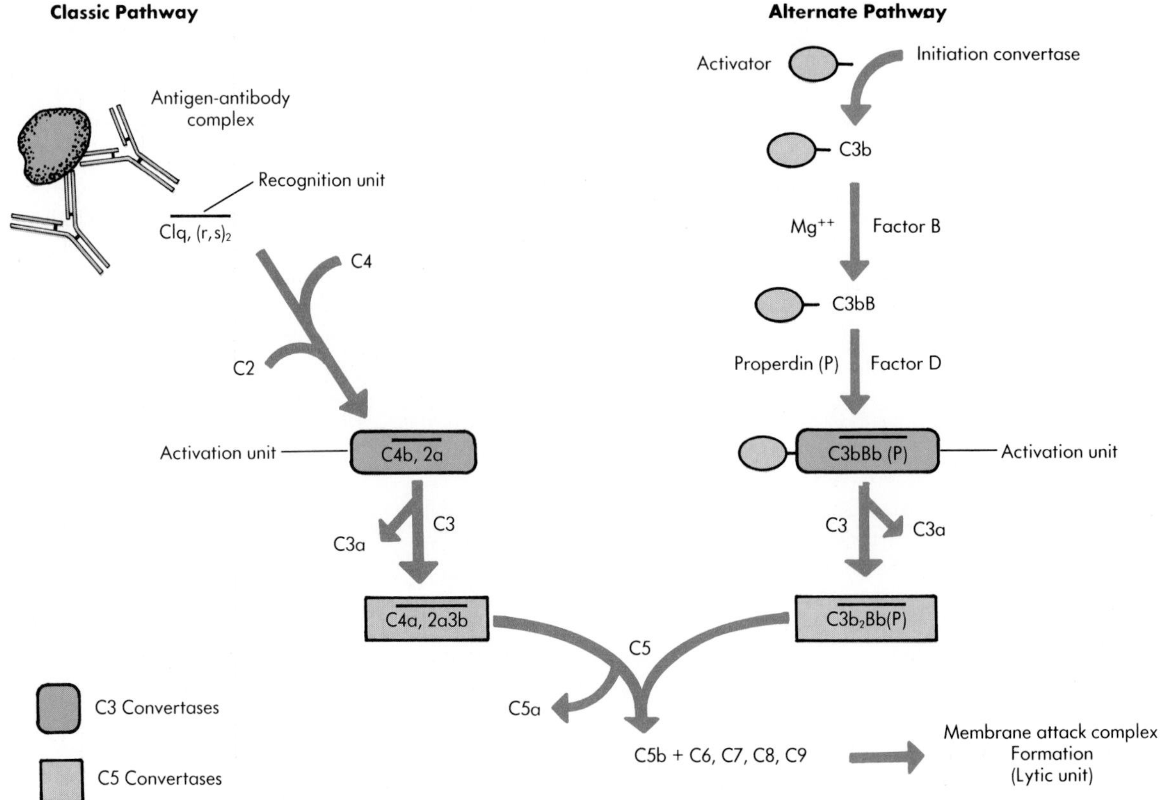

FIGURE 9-3 The classical and alternate pathways of complement activation.

which also results in an increased susceptibility to pyogenic infections. Finally, deficiencies of C5 through C9 are associated with defective MAC activity. This action increases the susceptibility to disseminated *Neisseria* infections.

Opsonins and Opsonization

An **opsonin** is a substance that adheres to the surface of a microorganism and makes it more attractive to a phagocytic cell. Opsonins enhance phagocytosis of microbes, constituting a cornerstone of defense against infection. Both nonimmune and immune substances may serve as opsonins. C3b, produced during complement activation, covalently binds to microbes. This complex can then bind to the C3b/C4b glycoprotein receptor (also known as CR1) present on the membrane of human erythrocytes, monocytes, polymorphonuclear cells, B cells, T cell subsets, and mast cells. Complement receptor-1 (CR1) facilitates attachment of the opsonized microbe to the phagocytic cell and phagocytosis. Proteolytic cleavage of bound C3b yields C3d, g, and C3bi molecules that interact with specific receptors. The C3dg complex binds with CR2, a membrane glycoprotein present only on B lymphocytes and selected tumor cell lines. C3dg can also bind to CR4, a glycoprotein membrane receptor on polymorphonuclear neutrophils and monocytes. C3bi binds to CR3, which is found on polymorphonuclear leukocytes, natural killer (NK) cells, monocytes, and some cytotoxic T lymphocytes.

Fibronectin

This is a glycoprotein of relatively high molecular weight found on cells and in plasma. It may serve as an opsonin, as well as function as an adhesion molecule in cellular interactions. Fibronectin may also react with complement components.

Interferons

These low molecular weight glycoproteins are characterized as alpha, beta, and gamma. Alpha and beta interferon are activated by viral infections and induce antiviral proteins that prevent viral mRNA translation. The activity of interferon is cell specific and not virus specific (e.g., chicken interferon will not protect humans). Interferon-γ modulates the immune response. Interferons act at the cell surface through specific receptors with a common receptor for alpha and beta interferon. Interferon can also activate NK cells and macrophages.

NONSPECIFIC CELLULAR DEFENSE MECHANISMS

Phagocytic Cells

Phagocytosis is an important clearance mechanism for the removal and disposition of microbes or damaged cells. Macrophages, monocytes, eosinophils, and polymorpho-

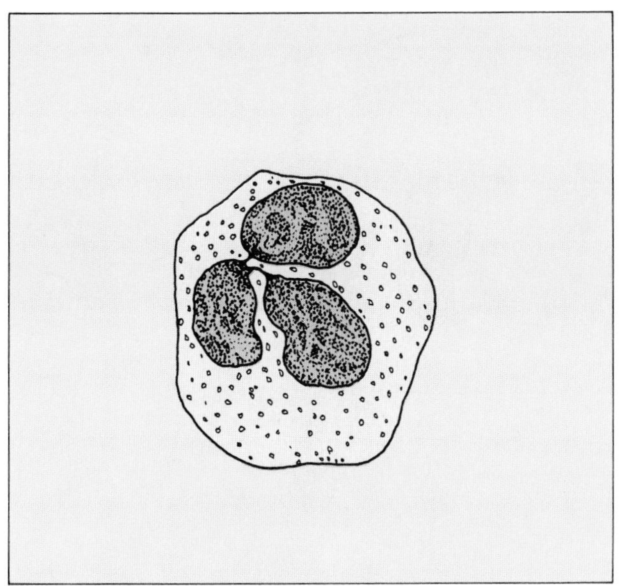

FIGURE 9-4 Distinguishing characteristics of a neutrophil *(PMN).*

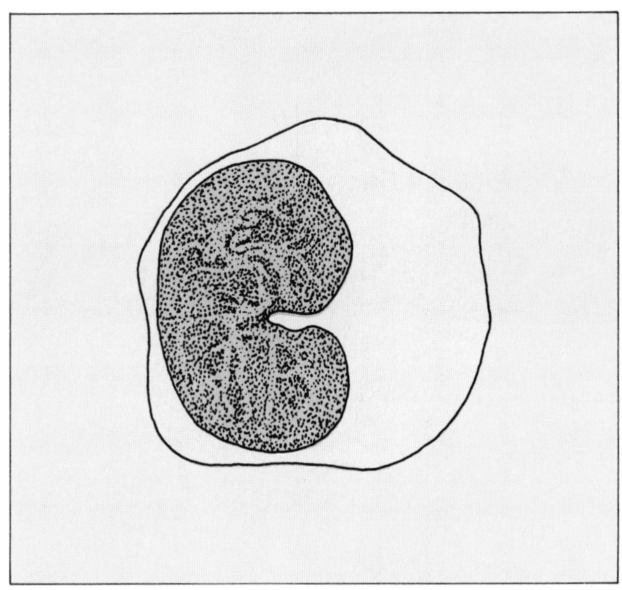

FIGURE 9-5 Distinguishing characteristics of a circulating monocyte.

nuclear (PMN) leukocytes are phagocytic cells. In special circumstances other cells such as fibroblasts may show phagocytic properties; these cells are called **facultative phagocytes.** PMNs are the first cells to arrive at the infected focus (Figure 9-4). The cells contain both primary or azurophilic granules and secondary or specific granules. **Azurophilic granules** serve as reservoirs for myeloperoxidase and also for other lysosomal hydrolases such as β-glucuronidase, elastase, and cathepsin G. **Specific granules** serve as reservoirs for lysozyme and lactoferrin. These digestive and hydrolytic enzymes are delivered to phagosomes to aid in the breakdown of ingested material. Frequently, the PMNs die after ingesting and destroying the invading microorganisms—a property commonly observed with pyogenic bacteria (e.g., *Staphylococcus, Streptococcus, Neisseria*).

Mononuclear Phagocytes

These include monocytes (Figure 9-5) in the blood and macrophages in the tissues (Figure 9-6). These cells have cell surface receptors for Fc gamma and C3b. They are also able to phagocytize microorganisms coated with opsonins and kill many but not all of them. Some microorganisms (including but not limited to mycobacteria, *Listeria, Brucella, Cryptococcus, Toxoplasma*) survive and multiply within macrophages. In this case the cell may serve as a protective reservoir or transport system to help spread the organisms throughout the body. However, in the presence of cell-mediated immunity, the macrophages are activated and can kill the intracellular pathogens.

Phagocytosis

PMNs, eosinophils, and macrophages have an important role in defending the host against microbial infection.

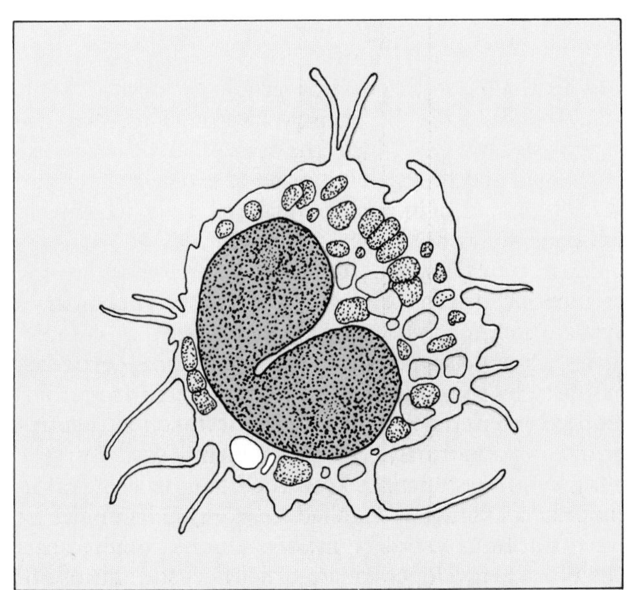

FIGURE 9-6 Distinguishing characteristics of an activated macrophage.

PMNs and occasionally eosinophils appear first in response to acute inflammation, followed later by macrophages. Chemotactic factors (e.g., formyl-methionyl-leucyl-phenylalanine [f-met-leu-phe]) are released by actively multiplying microbes. These chemotactic factors are powerful attractants for phagocytic cells, which have specific membrane receptors for the factors.

Phagocytosis of microbes involves several steps: attachment, internalization, and digestion. After attachment, the particle is engulfed within a membrane

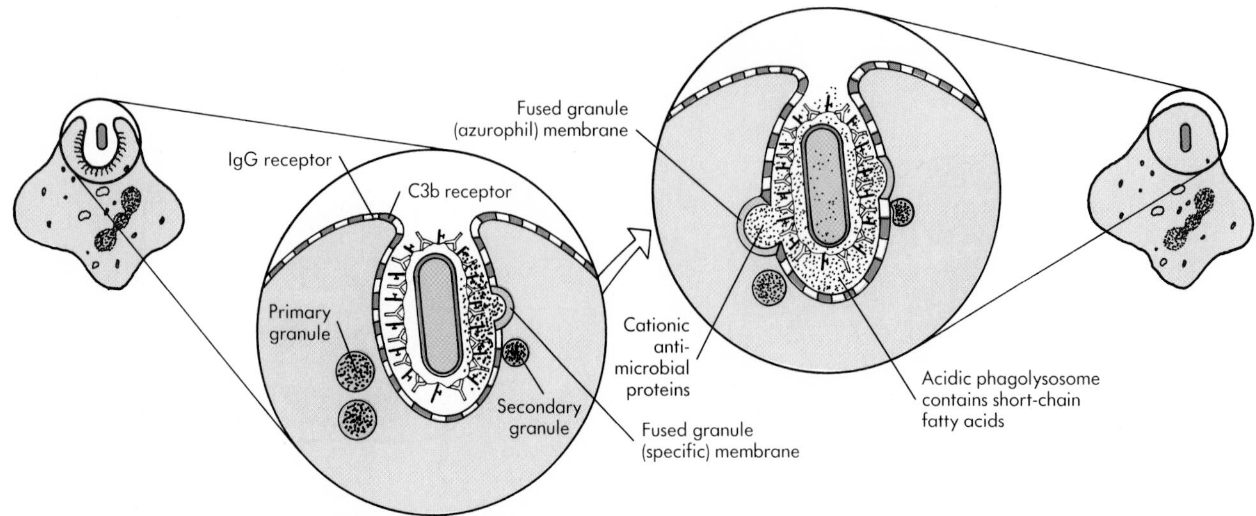

FIGURE 9-7 Schematic representation of the progressive steps of phagocytic endocytosis. Fusion with the specific granule membranes releases lactoferrin, lysozyme, collagenase, and vitamin B_{12}-binding protein, whereas fusion with azurophil granule membranes releases cationic antimicrobial proteins CAP57 and CAP37, defensins, lysozyme, cathepsin G, elastase, and myeloperoxidase.

fragment and a phagocytic vacuole is formed. This vacuole fuses with the primary lysosomes to form the phagolysosome, in which the lysosomal enzymes are discharged and the enclosed material is digested (Figure 9-7). Remnants of indigestible material can be recognized subsequently as residual bodies.

Phagocytic dysfunction may be due to either extrinsic or intrinsic defects. The extrinsic variety encompasses opsonin deficiencies secondary to antibody or complement factor deficiencies, suppression of phagocytic cell numbers by immunosuppressive agents, corticosteroid-induced interference with phagocytic function, neutropenia, or abnormal neutrophil chemotaxis. Intrinsic phagocytic dysfunction is related to deficiencies in enzymatic killing of engulfed organisms. Examples of these intrinsic disorders include chronic granulomatous disease, myeloperoxidase deficiency, and glucose-6-phosphate dehydrogenase deficiency. Consequences of phagocytic dysfunction include increased susceptibility to bacterial infections but not to viral or protozoal infections. Selected phagocytic function disorders may be associated with severe fungal infections. The severity of bacterial infections associated with phagocytic dysfunction may range from mild skin infections to fatal systemic infections.

Chemotaxis

The locomotion of cells may be stimulated by the presence of certain substances in their environment. This locomotion may be random in direction (not oriented with respect to the stimulus) or directed with respect to the inducing stimulus. The latter form of cell movement is called **chemotaxis** and may be direct toward the stimulant (attractant), or repulsed by the stimulant (repellent).

Substances that may stimulate the random cell locomotion are called **cytotoxigens,** and those that stimulate directed migration are called **cytotoxins** or **chemotactic factors.** The main element in the effect of chemotactic factors is the presence of a concentration gradient that determines the direction of cell migration. In the absence of a gradient, chemotactic factors enhance random migration.

Oxygen-Dependent Killing

Phagocytic killing of microbes is either oxygen dependent or oxygen independent. Oxygen-dependent killing is activated by a powerful oxidative burst that culminates in the formation of hydrogen peroxide and other antimicrobial substances. In oxygen-dependent killing, the membranes of specific lysosomal granules and phagosomes fuse (Figure 9-8). This permits the interaction of NADPH oxidase with cytochrome b. With the aid of quinone, this combination reduces oxygen to superoxide anion (O_2^-), which in the presence of a catalyst (e.g., superoxide dismutase) is converted to hydrogen peroxide. Hydrogen peroxide with myeloperoxidase (released by azurophil granules during fusion to the phagolysosome) transforms chloride ions into hypochlorous ions that kill the microorganisms. The clinical relevance of oxygen-dependent killing is illustrated by chronic granulomatous disease (CGD) in children who have diminished cytochrome b and fail to form superoxide anions. Even though phagocytosis is normal, they have impaired ability

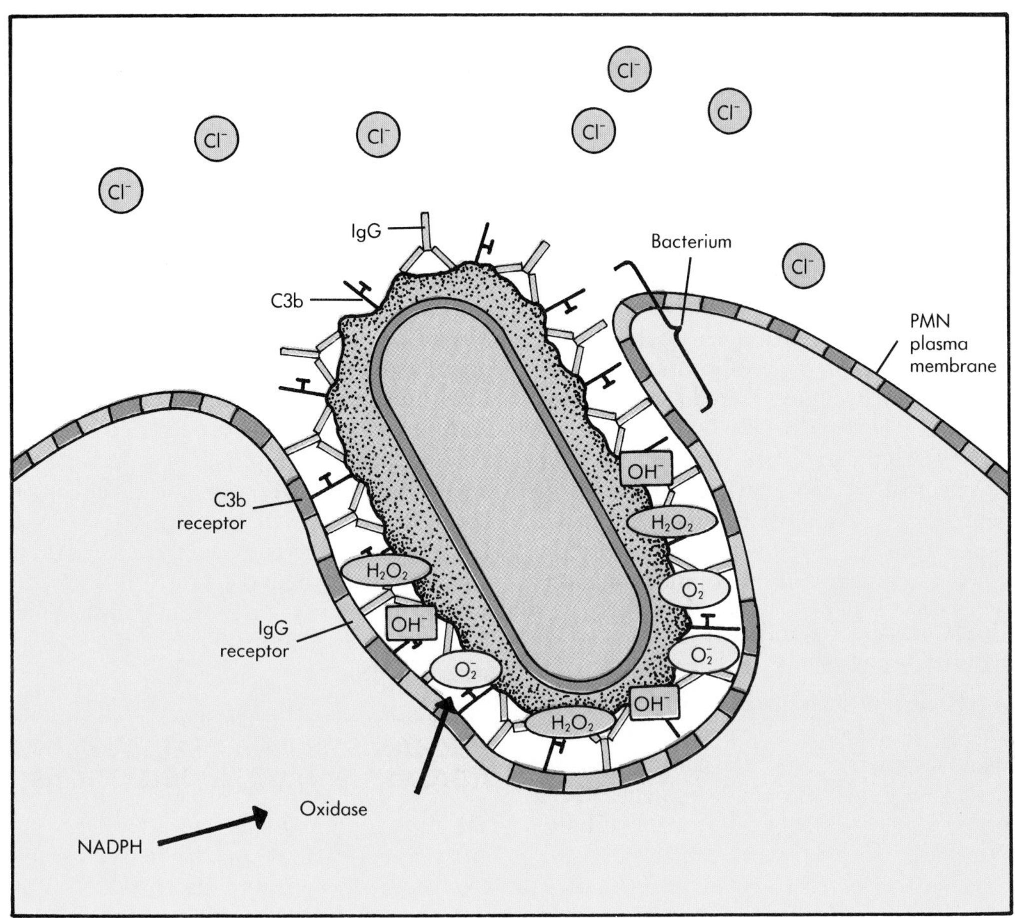

FIGURE 9-8 Formation of bactericide and hydrogen peroxide catalyzed by NADPH oxidase.

to oxidize NADPH and destroy bacteria through the oxidative pathway.

Oxygen-Independent Killing

Following adherence of opsonized microbes to the neutrophil plasma membrane and engulfment, cationic proteins (e.g., cathepsin G) from azurophil granules and lysozyme and lactoferrin from specific granules are discharged into the phagosomes. These proteins kill gram-negative bacteria by interrupting their cell membrane integrity but are far less effective against gram-positive bacteria (which are killed principally through the oxygen-dependent mechanism).

Cationic protein deficiency may be associated with chronic skin infections or abscesses. In patients with Chédiak-Higashi syndrome, the neutrophil granules fuse when the cells are immature in the bone marrow. Thus neutrophils from these patients can phagocytize bacteria but have greatly diminished ability to kill them.

Leukocyte Activation

Hydrogen peroxide production by PMNs exposed to macrophages and lymphocytes may be associated with a large prolonged respiratory burst by surface adherent leukocytes. Recombinant tumor necrosis factor α (TNF α) delays hydrogen peroxide release, demonstrating that soluble factors from macrophages and lymphocytes can affect the cytotoxic potential of adherent PMNs. Studies on regulation of neutrophil activation by platelets reveal that platelet-derived growth factor (PDGF) does not alter the resting level of superoxide generation but inhibits the rate and extent of the f-met-leu-phe–induced oxidative burst. Intracellular Ca^{++} increases up-regulation of the cell surface expression of f-met-leu-phe receptors in neutrophils, whereas phorbol myristate acetate (PMA) activates down-regulation of these receptors. A pertussis toxin–sensitive GTP-binding protein regulates monocyte phagocytic function.

Complement receptor 3 (CR3) facilitates the ability of phagocytes to bind and ingest opsonized particles. A relatively large family of adhesion-promoting receptor proteins, including leukocyte proteins, identifies the sequence arg-gly-asp in these opsonized particles and bacterial or tissue cells. Molecules found to be powerful stimulators of leukocyte activity include recombinant γ-interferon, granulocyte-macrophage colony-stimulating factor, tumor necrosis factor, and lymphotoxin. Investigation of storage sites for the several protein receptors has revealed a mobile intracellular storage compartment in human neutrophils. Chemotactic stimuli, such as f-met-leu-phe, may cause translocation of granules acting as storage sites to the cell surface, which could be requisite for neutrophil adhesion and chemotaxis.

Dephosphorylation pathways for inositol triphosphate isomers culminate in the elevation of intracellular Ca^{++} and activation of protein kinase C. NADPH oxidase, which utilizes NADPH generated by the hexose monophosphate shunt, catalyzes the respiratory burst. Both Ca^{++} and protein kinase C play a key role in the activated pathway. Activated human neutrophils manifest an elevated expression of complement decay-accelerating factor, which protects erythrocytes from injury by autologous complement. Transduction of decay-accelerating factors to the cell surface following stimulation by chemoattractants may be significant in protecting neutrophils from complement-mediated injury. This type of process would permit neutrophils to manifest unreserved function in sites of inflammation.

Natural Killer Cells and Antibody-Dependent Cytotoxic Cells

Although natural killer (NK) cells are not phagocytic, they can attack and destroy certain virus-infected cells. They constitute an important part of the natural immune system, do not require prior contact with antigen, and are not MHC restricted by the major histocompatibility complex (MHC) antigens (described in Chapter 10). On contact with the virus-infected cell, NK cells produce perforin that leads to the formation of pores in the infected cell membrane and subsequent osmotic lysis. Interferon enhances NK cell activity.

The natural immune system, in which the NK cells are key participants, does not involve memory, require sensitization, and cannot be enhanced by specific immunization. Other nonmemory cells include polymorphonuclear leukocytes and macrophages. NK cells are also able to lyse selected tumor target cells without prior sensitization and in the absence of antibody or complement. NK and cytotoxic T cells share similar lytic mechanisms. Both cell types have granules that contain perforin or C9-related protein, which lyses target cells without antibody or complement.

Both NK cells and killer (K) cells or antibody-dependent cell-mediated cytotoxicity (ADCC) cells can induce lysis through the action of antibody. With the demonstration of Fc receptors that bind IgG antibody on their surface, NK cells may actually be responsible for the antibody-dependent cell-mediated cytotoxicity previously ascribed to K cells. The ADCC cells mediate their classic effects through cell surface receptors for target cell antigens.

Circulating monocytes or macrophages also mediate cell lysis through antibody molecules. **Cytotoxic T cells (CTLs)** apparently recognize specific target cells through interaction with MHC antigens on the cell surface. Whereas either helper or killer T cells are directed to MHC proteins, NK cells apparently do not recognize MHC determinants. NK cell activity is located in the low density population of lymphocytes, which have large granules in their cytoplasm (i.e., large granular lymphocytes [LGLs]). NK cells are also believed to play a regulatory role in the immune system, encompassing down-regulation of antibody responses.

Lymphokine Activated Killer (LAK) Cells

LAK cells are IL-2 activated effectors that are able to bind and kill many types of tumor and virally infected cells. Most LAK activity is derived from NK cells. The large granular lymphocyte (LGL) compartment contains all LAK precursor activity and all active NK cells. In accord with the phenotype of precursor cells, LAK effector cells are also granular lymphocytes expressing markers associated with human NK cells. The asialo Gm_1 + population, known to be expressed by murine NK cells, contains most LAK precursor activity. Analysis of LAK precursor and effector phenotype has revealed that essentially all LAK activity resides in the LGL population, which contains all NK cell activity and manifests surface markers associated with NK cells.

MECHANISMS OF INNATE IMMUNITY AGAINST INVADING ORGANISMS

The capacity of pathogenic microorganisms to resist the rapid microbicidal action of phagocytosis by neutrophils, monocytes, and tissue macrophages is an important feature of their virulence. Complement activation represents a significant mechanism for the infected host to eliminate invading microorganisms. The peptidoglycan layer in bacterial cell walls (particularly in gram-positive bacteria) and lipopolysaccharide (LPS) in gram-negative

BOX 9-4 Secreted Products of Macrophages That Have a Protective Effect on the Body

Cell differentiation factors
CSF
Cytotoxic factors
TNF α
Cachectin
Hydrolytic enzymes
- Collagenase
- Lipase
- Phosphatase

Endogenous pyrogen
- IL-1

Complement components
- C1 to C5
- Properdin
- Factors B, D, I, H

α-interferon
Plasma proteins
Coagulation factors
Oxygen metabolites
- H_2O_2
- Superoxide anion

Arachidonic acid metabolites
- Prostaglandins
- Thromboxanes
- Leukotrienes

bacterial cell walls can activate the alternative complement pathway (in the absence of antibody). LPS (endotoxin) induces macrophages and selected other cells (e.g., endothelial cells) to synthesize cytokines such as interleukin-1, interleukin-6, interleukin-8, and tumor necrosis factor that participate in the inflammatory process (Box 9-4).

The natural immune mechanism of phagocytosis is of little use in controlling infection by intracellular microorganisms. Indeed, the intracellular residence of these organisms protects them from extracellular defense mechanisms of the host, which may lead to chronic infections. Virus-infected cells synthesize type I interferon, which can block virus replication and accentuate natural killer cell action.

Both complement and phagocytosis play significant roles in removal of extracellular viruses. Protozoa and helminths are adept at survival within the host through successful resistance to the host's innate immune mechanisms, such as complement lysis. In helminth infections, eosinophils and IgE levels are increased in the blood. Eosinophils localize near parasites, where they degranulate by fusing their intracellular granules with the plasma membrane. The contents are released against the target parasite, which is too large to be phagocytized, facilitating its elimination. Reducing surface antigenicity by molecule masking, shedding, or sequestration of antigen represents a successful mechanism for parasites to escape the immune system. Whereas macrophages may ingest protozoa, numerous pathogenic parasites may resist intracellular killing or even replicate within the phagocyte.

QUESTIONS

1. Describe the inflammatory response.
2. Compare and contrast the classical versus alternative complement pathway.
3. List and describe nonspecific cellular defense mechanisms.
4. What is innate immunity?
5. List and describe nonspecific humoral defense mechanisms.

Bibliography

Abbas AK, Lichtman AH, Pober JS: *Cellular and molecular immunology,* Philadelphia, 1991, WB Saunders.

Benjamini E, Leskowitz S: *Immunology, a short course,* ed 2, New York, 1991, Wiley-Liss.

Bona C, Francisco AB: *Immunology for medical students,* New York, 1990, Harwood Academic Publishers.

Cruse JM, Lewis RE Jr: *Complement today,* vol 1, Basel and New York, 1993, S. Karger Publishers.

Eisen HN: *General immunology,* ed 2, Philadelphia, 1990, JB Lippincott.

Gorbach SL, Bartlett JG, Blacklow NR: *Infectious diseases,* Philadelphia, 1992, WB Saunders.

Mandell GL, Douglas RG Jr, Bennett JE: *Principles and practices of infectious diseases,* ed 3, New York, 1990, Churchill Livingstone.

Oppenheim JJ, Shevach EM: *Immunophysiology,* Oxford, 1990, Oxford University Press.

Roitt IM: *Essential immunology,* ed 7, Oxford, 1991, Blackwell Scientific Publications.

Roitt IM, Brostoff J, Male DK, editors: *Immunology,* ed 2, London, 1989, Gower Medical Publishing.

Ruby J: *Immunology,* New York, 1992, WH Freeman.

Samter M, Talmadge DW, Frank MM, et al.: *Immunological diseases,* vol I and II, ed 4, Boston, 1988, Little, Brown.

Sell S: *Immunology, immunopathology and immunity,* ed 4, New York, 1987, Elsevier.

Stites DP, Abba TF: *Basic and clinical immunology,* ed 7, Norwalk, Conn, 1991, Appleton-Lange.

CHAPTER 10

Acquired Immunity

HUMANS are confronted with a host of microorganisms that have the potential to induce serious or fatal infections. Yet nature has provided appropriate molecules, cells, and receptors that can protect against these microbes. As discussed in the preceding chapter, many of these defenses are general or nonspecific and do not require previous exposure to the offending pathogen (or closely related organism). These important mechanisms constitute the **innate** or **constitutive** defense system. Another important defense system is acquired immunity, which can develop after previous contact with the organism through infection (overt or subclinical) or by deliberate immunization with a vaccine prepared from the etiological agent. Acquired immunity is the subject of this chapter. The brief treatment of the fundamentals of immunology in this chapter is in no way a substitute for a course on immunology. The purpose of this section is to provide a minimum number of concepts requisite for a proper understanding of the host immune response to the infecting agents.

Naturally acquired immunity describes the protection provided by previous exposure to a pathogenic microorganism or antigenically related organism. In contrast, **artificially acquired immunity** develops as a result of immunization with vaccines—either with attenuated organisms or with killed organisms or subunit components. Toxoids provide excellent immunity against the effects of microorganisms such as *Corynebacterium diphtheriae* and *Clostridium tetani* that produce powerful exotoxins. Active immunization with appropriate booster injections leads to the development of IgG, which provides immunity of long duration. Acquired immunity depends on antibodies and T cells.

Passive immunity involves the transfer of resistance against an infectious disease agent from an immune individual to a previously susceptible recipient. **Natural passive immunity** describes the transfer of IgG antibodies across the placenta from mother to child. IgA secretory antibodies may also be passively transferred from mother to child in breast milk. **Artificially acquired passive immunity** describes the transfer of immunoglobulins from an immune individual to a nonimmune, susceptible recipient. Passive immunity of this type is more often used for prophylaxis than for therapy. It provides immediate protection of the recipient for relatively short periods (few weeks). Human sera are preferred for passive immunization to avoid serum sickness induced by foreign serum proteins. **Adoptive immunization** refers to the transfer of specifically immune lymphoid cells from one individual to another, such as occurs in bone marrow transplantation.

ANTIGEN

An infectious agent, whether a bacterium, fungus, virus, or parasite, contains a plethora of substances called **antigens** or **immunogens** that are capable of inducing an immune response. After exposure to an antigen, immunological tolerance or antibody synthesis and/or cell-mediated immunity may result. To stimulate an immunogenic response, a substance usually needs to be foreign, although some autoantigens are exceptions. Antigens usually have a molecular weight of at least 10,000 d and are either proteins or polysaccharides. Nevertheless, immunogenicity depends on the genetic capacity of the host to respond and on the immunogenic properties of the antigen.

A **complete** antigen is one that both induces an immune response (antibodies or T lymphocytes) and also reacts with the products. An incomplete antigen or **hapten** is unable to induce an immune response alone but will react with the products. Haptens can be rendered **immunogenic** (capable of stimulating an immune response) by covalently linking them to a carrier molecule such as a foreign protein. In addition, haptens often have highly reactive chemical groupings that permit them to couple with a substance such as a tissue protein. This type of reaction occurs in individuals who develop contact hypersensitivity to poison ivy or poison oak.

The specific parts of antigen molecules that elicit immune reactivity are known as **antigenic determinants** or **epitopes.** The epitope reacts with the specific antigen binding site in the variable region of an antibody molecule known as a **paratope** (Figure 10-1). The excellent fit between epitope and paratope is based on their three-dimensional interaction and noncovalent union. An epitope may also react with a T cell receptor for which it is specific. A single antigen molecule may have several different epitopes. Whereas an epitope interacts with the antigen binding region of an antibody molecule or with

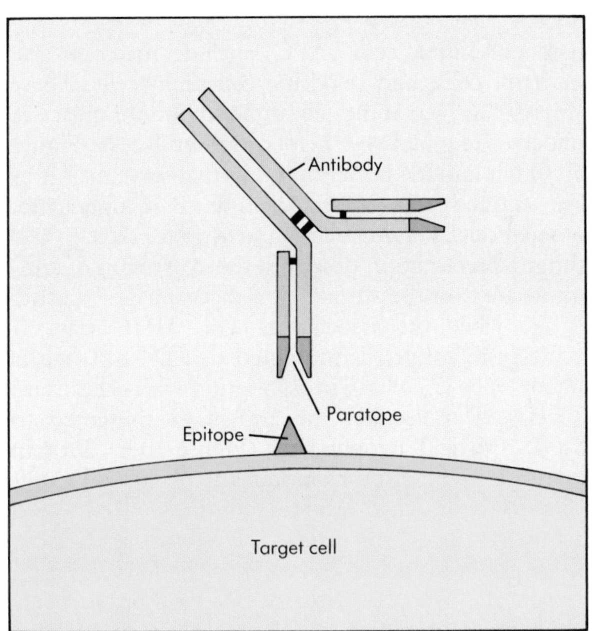

FIGURE 10-1 Antigen binding site (paratope) on an antibody molecule combines with an antigenic determinant of an antigen molecule (epitope).

TABLE 10-1 Comparison of T-cell Dependent with T-cell Independent Antigens

	T-cell dependent antigen	T-cell independent antigen
Structural properties	Complex	Simple
Chemistry	Proteins; protein-nucleoprotein conjugates; glycoproteins; lipoproteins	Polysaccharide of pneumococcus; dextran polyvinyl pyrolidone; bacterial lipo-polysaccharide
Antibody class induced	IgG, IgM, IgA (+IgD and IgE)	IgM
Immunological memory response	Yes	No
Present in most pathogenic microbes	Yes	No

the T cell receptor, a separate region of the antigen that combines with class II major histocompatibility (MHC) molecules is known as an **agretope.**

Antigenic determinants may be either conformational or linear. A **conformational determinant** is produced by spatial juxtaposition during folding of amino acid residues from different segments of the linear amino acid sequence. Conformational determinants are usually associated with natural rather than denatured proteins. A **linear determinant** is one produced by adjacent amino acid residues in the proteins. They usually interact with antibody only after denaturation and are not customarily in the native configuration. Antigens derived exclusively by laboratory synthesis are termed **synthetic antigens.**

An antigen has two or more epitopes per molecule. Epitopes consist of approximately six amino acids or six monosaccharides. Epitopes that stimulate a greater antibody response than others are referred to as **immunodominant epitopes.** Antigens must be degradable by phagocytes to be able to stimulate an immune response. Antigen processing includes enzymatic digestion to prepare soluble macromolecules. Substances that cannot be digested (e.g., D-amino acid polypeptides) cannot function as antigens.

Foreignness is another characteristic that is critical for **antigenicity** (i.e., immunogenicity). During development, the body becomes tolerant to self-antigens, as well as any foreign antigens that may be introduced before the development of the immune system. The latter situation describes the induction of actively acquired **immunological tolerance.** Tolerance is a type of antigen-induced specific immunosuppression, and antigen must remain in contact with immunocompetent cells for the tolerant state to be maintained. An antigen that induces tolerance is often referred to as a **tolerogen.**

Immunoresponsiveness to antigens requires the presence of appropriate **immune response (Ir) genes.** Lymphocyte proteins in humans encoded by Ir genes include the class II MHC molecules designated DP, DQ, and DR that are found on human B cells, and macrophages. Antigens may be classified as either T-cell dependent (TD) or T-cell independent (TI). As shown in Table 10-1, the TD antigens are much more complex than the TI antigens, are usually proteins, stimulate all five classes of immunoglobulins, elicit an anamnestic or memory response, and are present in most pathogenic microorganisms. These properties ensure that an effective immune response can be generated in a host infected with these pathogens. By contrast, the simpler TI antigens are often polysaccharides or lipopolysaccharides, elicit an IgM response only, and fail to stimulate an anamnestic response.

A **superantigen** is a substance such as a bacterial toxin that is capable of stimulating multiple T lymphocytes, leading to the release of relatively large quantities of cytokines. Superantigens are TD antigens that do not require phagocytic processing. Instead of fitting into the T-cell receptor (TCR) internal groove where a typical processed peptide antigen fits, superantigens bind to the external region of the TCR and simultaneously link to DP, DQ, or DR molecules on antigen presenting cells. Superantigens react with multiple TCR molecules whose peripheral structure is similar (Figure 10-2). Thus they stimulate multiple T cells that augment a protective T and

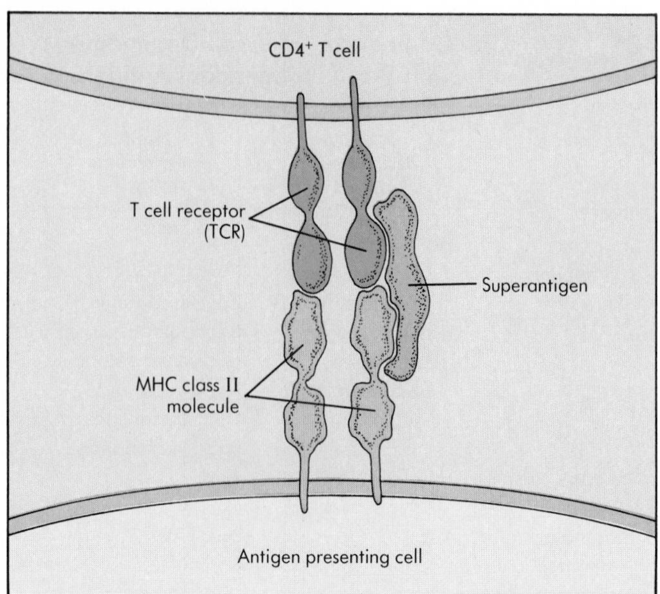

FIGURE 10-2 Superantigen binding to external regions of the T-cell receptor and of the MHC class II molecules.

B cell antibody response. This enhanced responsiveness to antigens such as toxins produced by staphylococci and streptococci is an important protective mechanism in the infected individual.

CELLS OF IMMUNITY

To properly understand the process of antigen presentation, it is necessary to understand the types of lymphocytes and MHC molecules with which an antigen must interact. All lymphocytes develop from hematopoietic stem cells in the bone marrow (Figure 10-3). Precursor cells destined to follow the T-lymphocyte lineage migrate from the bone marrow to the thymus, whereas the B-lymphocyte precursors remain in the bone marrow. The immune response consists of two limbs: a T-cell limb responsible for cell-mediated immunity and a B-cell or humoral limb concerned with antibody production. A successful immune response against many microorganisms often involves stimulation of both T and B cells and involves a cooperative interaction between these two cell populations.

T and B lymphocytes do not function in isolation. They actively communicate through specialized surface molecules, including the class I and class II MHC molecules. The class I molecules consist of one three-domain MHC polypeptide chain and a B_2 microglobulin component, are important for presenting endogenous antigens to T lymphocytes, and are present on all nucleated cells. Class II MHC molecules consist of an alpha and a beta MHC polypeptide chain, are primarily responsible for presentation of exogenous antigens, and are present only on macrophages, B lymphocytes, and a few other cell types.

Antigen Presenting Cells

Antigen presenting cells (APC) include macrophages, Langerhans' cells, and dendritic reticulum cells. These cells present antigen at the cell surface to immunoreactive lymphocytes (e.g., CD4+ helper/inducer T cells; Figure 10-4). Other antigen presenting cells that serve mainly as passive antigen transporters include B lymphocytes, endothelial cells, keratinocytes, and Kupffer cells.

Antigen presentation describes the expression of antigen molecules on the surface of a macrophage or other APC (1) when, in association with MHC class II molecules, the antigen is presented to CD4+ T-helper lymphocytes or (2) when, in association with cell surface MHC class I molecules, the antigen is presented to CD8+ cytotoxic T lymphocytes (Figure 10-5). Protein antigens are ingested by mononuclear phagocytes, split into 8 to 10 amino acid residues, and then linked to cell surface MHC class II molecules. For appropriate presentation, peptides must bind securely to the MHC class II molecules. Those peptides that do not bind or bind only weakly are not presented and fail to elicit an immune response. Following interaction of the peptide and CD4 helper T-lymphocyte receptor, the CD4 cell is activated, interleukin-2 (IL-2) is released, and IL-2 receptors are expressed on the CD4 lymphocyte surface. The IL-2 produced by the activated cell stimulates its own receptors, as well as those of mononuclear phagocytes, increasing their killing activity. IL-2 also stimulates B cells to synthesize antibody. Whereas B cells may recognize a protein antigen in its native state, T lymphocytes recognize the oligopeptides that result from antigen processing.

Lymphocytes

Lymphocytes are classified as B cells, T cells, or null cells (i.e., natural killer [NK] cells, large granular lymphocytes [LGL]). B cells release immunoglobulins into the circulation following antigenic stimulation of the cells. In contrast, the T cells have specific receptors that are retained on the cell surface and facilitate participation of the lymphocyte in cell-mediated immunity. When the T cell is stimulated, it produces powerful immunoregulatory chemicals (lymphokines) that affect B cell function. The function of null or NK cells has been discussed in Chapter 9.

In general, lymphocytes constitute approximately 30% of human leukocytes, with the NK cells and LGLs responsible for only about 5% of the lymphocyte population. In contrast with B cells that mature in the bone marrow, the T-cell populations migrate to the thymus where during maturation some surface markers are lost and others gained. These markers can be used to classify the T cells by immunophenotyping with monoclonal antibodies and flow cytometry techniques. Functionally, the CD4+ cell population is predominantly helper/inducer T cells, while the CD8+ population is suppressor/cytotoxic T cells. After maturation of T and B cells, they will migrate to the peripheral lymphoid tissues such as lymph nodes and spleen.

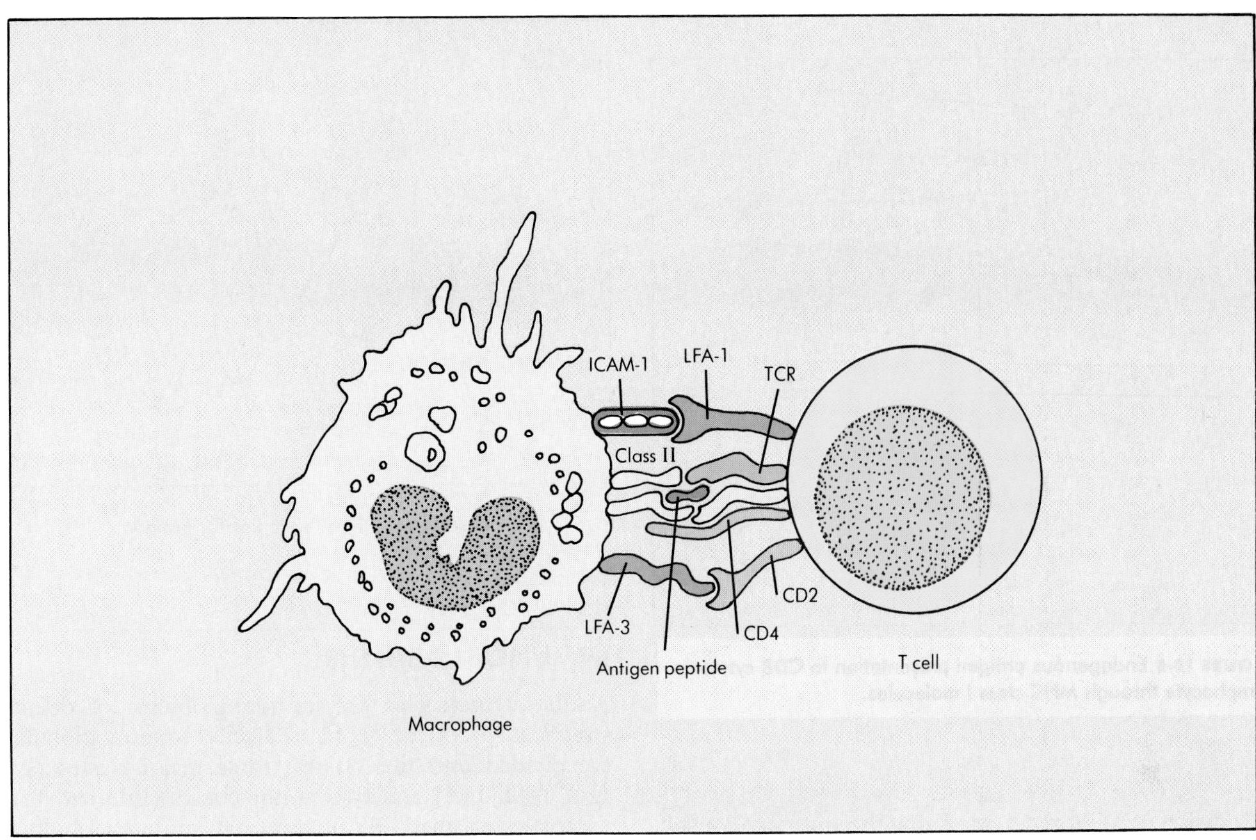

FIGURE 10-3 Distribution of the central and peripheral lymphoid tissues in human.

T Lymphocytes

T-lymphocyte precursors are detectable in the human fetus at 7 weeks of gestation. Between 7 and 14 weeks of gestation, thymic changes begin to imprint thymic lymphocytes as T cells. The maturation (mediated by hormones such as thymosin, thymulin, thymopoietin II) can be followed by identification of surface (cluster of differentiation [CD]) markers detectable by immunophenotyping methods. CD3, a widespread T-cell marker, serves as a signal transducer from the antigen receptor to the cell interior. Thus the CD3 molecule is intimately associated with the T-cell antigen receptor (Figure 10-6).

T lymphocytes in the medulla initially express both CD4+ and CD8+ markers; however, these cells will later differentiate into either CD4+ helper cells or CD8+ suppressor cells. The CD4+ cells, characterized by a 55,000 d surface marker, communicate with macrophages and B cells bearing MHC class II molecules during antigen presentation. The CD8+ suppressor/cytotoxic cells interact with antigen presenting cells with MHC class I molecules.

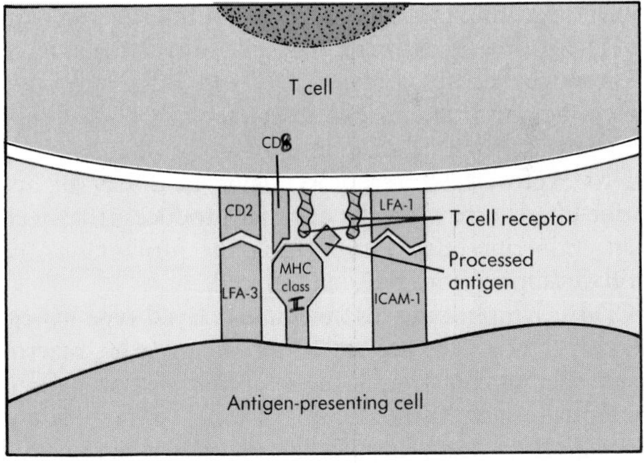

FIGURE 10-4 Antigen nonspecific CD2 and LFA-1 on the T cell bind with LFA-3 and ICAM-1 on the antigen presenting macrophage to assist the linkage of these two cells. TCR and CD4 on the T cell have the more specific role of binding the epitope and the class II MHC protein.

T-Cell Receptor

There are two types of T-cell antigen receptors: TCR1, which appears first in ontogeny, and TCR2. TCR2 is a heterodimer of two polypeptides (alpha and beta); TCR1 consists of gamma and delta polypeptides. Each of the two polypeptides comprising each receptor has a constant and a variable region (similar to immunoglobulins). Reminiscent of the diversity in antibody molecules, T-cell antigen receptors can likewise identify a tremendous number of antigenic specificities (estimated to be able to recognize 10^{15} separate epitopes). For a more detailed

FIGURE 10-4 Antigen nonspecific CD2 and LFA-1 on the T cell bind with LFA-3 and ICAM-1 on the antigen presenting macrophage to assist the linkage of these two cells. TCR and CD4 on the T cell have the more specific role of binding the epitope and the class II MHC protein.

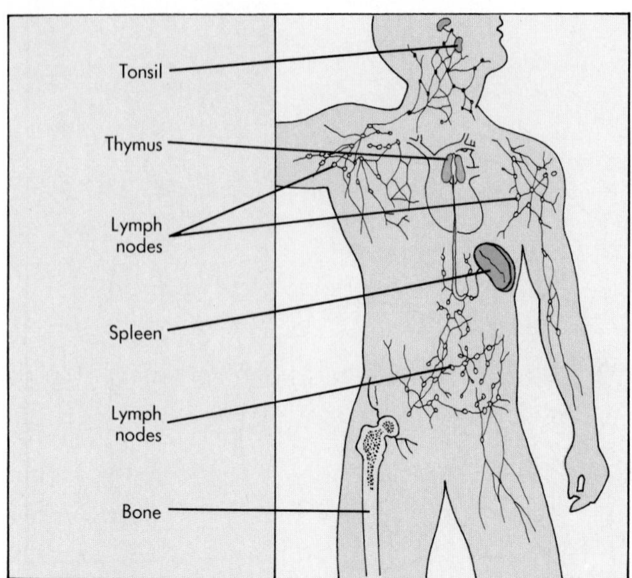

FIGURE 10-3 Distribution of the central and peripheral lymphoid tissues in human.

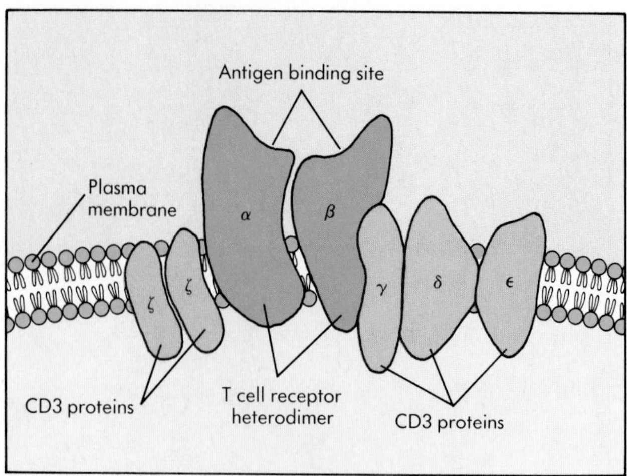

FIGURE 10-6 T-cell receptor for antigen.

discussion of TCR genes regulating this diversity, consult one of the textbooks on immunology listed in the Bibliography.

T cells may be activated by the interaction of antigen, in the context of MHC, with the T-cell receptor. This involves transmission of a signal to the interior through the CD3 protein to activate the cell. Among the surface receptors on T cells are the IL-1 and IL-2 receptors. The monokine interleukin-1 interacts with IL-1 receptors, causing the T cells to synthesize interleukin-2 and to express IL-2 receptors. Thus IL-2 has an autocrine effect, acting on the cell that produces it, as well as an endocrine effect, stimulating the proliferation of cytotoxic/suppressor, NK, and B cells.

CD4+ lymphocytes also mediate delayed-type hypersensitivity. The cells secrete lymphokines (e.g., macrophage chemotaxin, migration inhibitory factor [MIF], macrophage activating factor [MAF]) that produce histological changes in the tissues (described in the section on hypersensitivity disorders).

Suppressor T Lymphocytes

Some CD8+ T lymphocytes are responsible for suppressor cell activity. The inability to confirm the presence of receptor molecules on suppressor cells has cast a cloud over the suppressor cell; however, functional suppressor cell effects are indisputable. Some suppressor T lymphocytes are antigen specific and are important in the regulation of T-helper cell function. Like cytotoxic T cells, T-suppressor cells are MHC class I restricted.

IMMUNOGLOBULINS

Antibody molecules are immunoglobulins of defined specificity produced by plasma cells. Immunoglobulins are divided into five classes: three major classes (i.e., IgG, IgM, IgA) and two minor classes (IgD and IgE; comprise less than 1% of the total immunoglobulins). Secretory IgA is found in body secretions such as saliva, milk, and intestinal and bronchial secretions. IgD and IgM are present as membrane-bound immunoglobulins on B cells, where they interact with antigen to activate B cells (Table 10-2).

The immunoglobulin molecule consists of heavy (H) and light (L) chains fastened together by disulfide bonds. The molecules are subdivided into classes and subclasses based on the antigenic specificity of their heavy chains. Heavy chains are designated by lower case Greek letters (μ, γ, α, δ, and ϵ), and the immunoglobulins are designated IgM, IgG, IgA, IgD, and IgE, respectively. The two types of light chains (termed kappa and lambda) are present in all five immunoglobulin classes, although only one type is present in an individual molecule.

IgG, IgD, and IgE have two H and two L polypeptide chains, whereas IgM and IgA consist of multimers of this basic chain structure. Disulfide bridges and noncovalent forces stabilize the immunoglobulin structure. The basic monomeric unit is Y-shaped, with a hinge region rich in proline and susceptible to cleavage by proteolytic enzymes. Both H and L chains have a constant region at the carboxyl terminus and a variable region at the amino terminus. The two heavy chains are alike, as are the two light chains in any individual immunoglobulin molecule. Approximately 60% of human immunoglobulin molecules have kappa light chains, and 40% have lambda light chains.

The five immunoglobulin classes are termed **isotypes** based on the heavy chain specificity of each immunoglob-

TABLE 10-2 The Immunoglobulins

Ig	IgG	IgM	IgA	IgD	IgE
Serum concentration (mg/dl)	800-1700	50-190	140-420	0.3-0.40	<0.001
Total Ig (%)	85	5-10	5-15	<1	<1
Complement fixation	+	++++	–	–	–
Principal biological effect	Resistance—opsonin; secondary response	Resistance—precipitin; primary response	Resistance—prevents movement across mucous membranes	?	Anaphylaxis
Principal site of action	Serum	Serum	Secretions	?; Receptor for B cells	Mast cells
Molecular weight (kd)	154	900	160 (+ dimer)	185	190
Serum half-life (days)	23	5	6	2-3	2-3
Antibacterial lysis	+	+++	+	?	?
Antiviral lysis	+	+	+++	?	?
H-chain class	γ	μ	α	δ	ϵ
Subclass	$\gamma_1\gamma_2\gamma_3\gamma_4$	$\mu_1\mu_2$	$\alpha_1\alpha_2$		

ulin class. Two immunoglobulin classes, IgA and IgG, may be further subdivided into subclasses based on H-chain differences. There are four IgG subclasses designated as IgG1 through IgG4, and two IgA subclasses (IgA1 and IgA2). These various molecules are depicted in Figure 10-7.

Digestion of IgG molecules with papain yields two Fab and one Fc fragments (Figure 10-8, *A*). Each Fab fragment has one antigen binding site. By contrast, the Fc fragment has no antigen binding site but is responsible for fixation of complement and attachment of the molecule to a cell surface. Pepsin cleaves the molecule to the right of the central disulfide bond, yielding an $F(ab')_2$ fragment and a pFc′ fragment. $F(ab')_2$ fragments have two antigen binding sites (Figure 10-8, *B*). Immunoglobulin domains have a variable and a constant sequence: L chains have a single variable and constant domain, whereas H chains possess one variable and three to four constant domains.

Immunoglobulin Supergene Family

Several molecules that participate in the immune response show similarities in structure that have caused them to be grouped into the immunoglobulin supergene family. Included are CD2, CD3, CD4, CD7, CD8, CD28, T-cell receptor (TCR), MHC class I and MHC class II molecules, leukocyte function associated antigen 3 (LFA3), the IgG receptor, and a dozen other proteins.

Antibody Response

Within 5 days to 2 weeks after exposure to a novel immunogen, antibodies will appear in the blood. The first antibodies produced react with residual antigen and therefore are rapidly cleared. However, after the initial lag phase, the antibody titer increases logarithmically to reach a plateau. This primary antibody response is characterized by the production of IgM immunoglobulins initially and then, as these antibodies decline, IgG antibodies rapidly increase in concentration.

Reexposure to an immunogen induces a heightened antibody response (also termed **anamnestic response**). The antibodies develop more rapidly, last longer, and reach a higher titer. The secondary antibodies are principally of the IgG class, although IgM antibodies can also be detected in response to some infections.

Antibodies against epitopes of microorganisms are polyclonal (i.e., they are the products of multiple antibody producing cell clones). Kohler and Millstein in 1975 developed a remarkable technique for producing monoclonal antibodies from B-cell hybridomas. This method involves fusion of a myeloma cell line with an antibody producing cell. This process forms a hybridoma that is immortal and produces a single (monoclonal) antibody. This technique has been extensively employed by investigators in essentially every branch of immunology to prepare monoclonal antibodies against hundreds of antigens. Indeed, these antibodies have been commercially produced for both diagnostic reagents and therapeutic purposes.

Immunoglobulin G

IgG comprises approximately 85% of the immunoglobulins in adults. It has a molecular weight of 154 kd based on two L chains of 22,000 d each and two H chains of 55,000 d each. It has the longest half-life (23 days) of the five immunoglobulin classes, crosses the placenta, and is the principal antibody in the anamnestic or booster

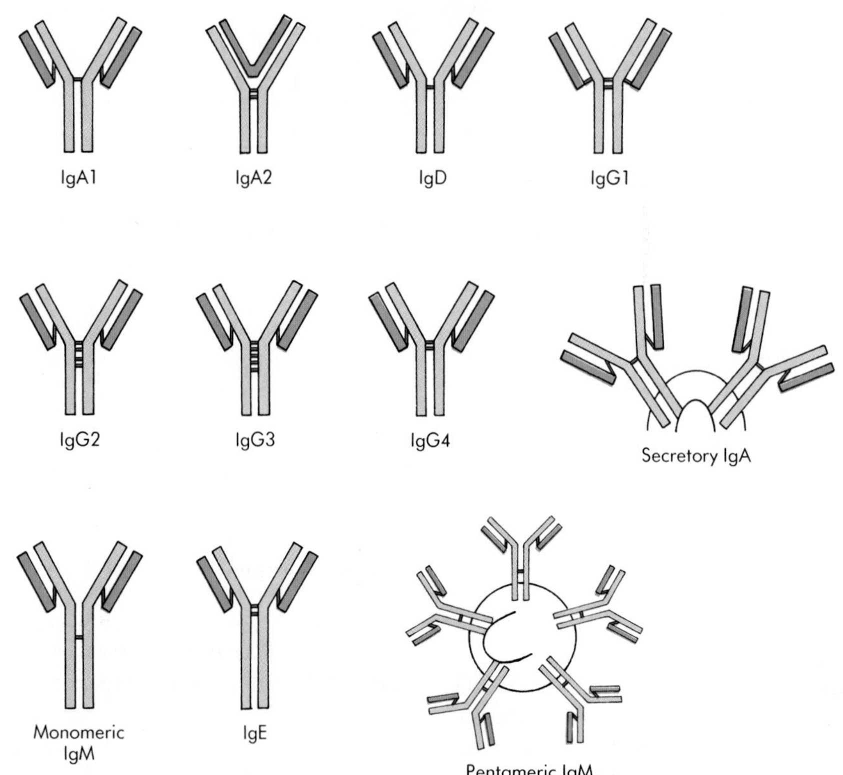

FIGURE 10-7 Comparative structures of the immunoglobulin classes and subclasses in humans.

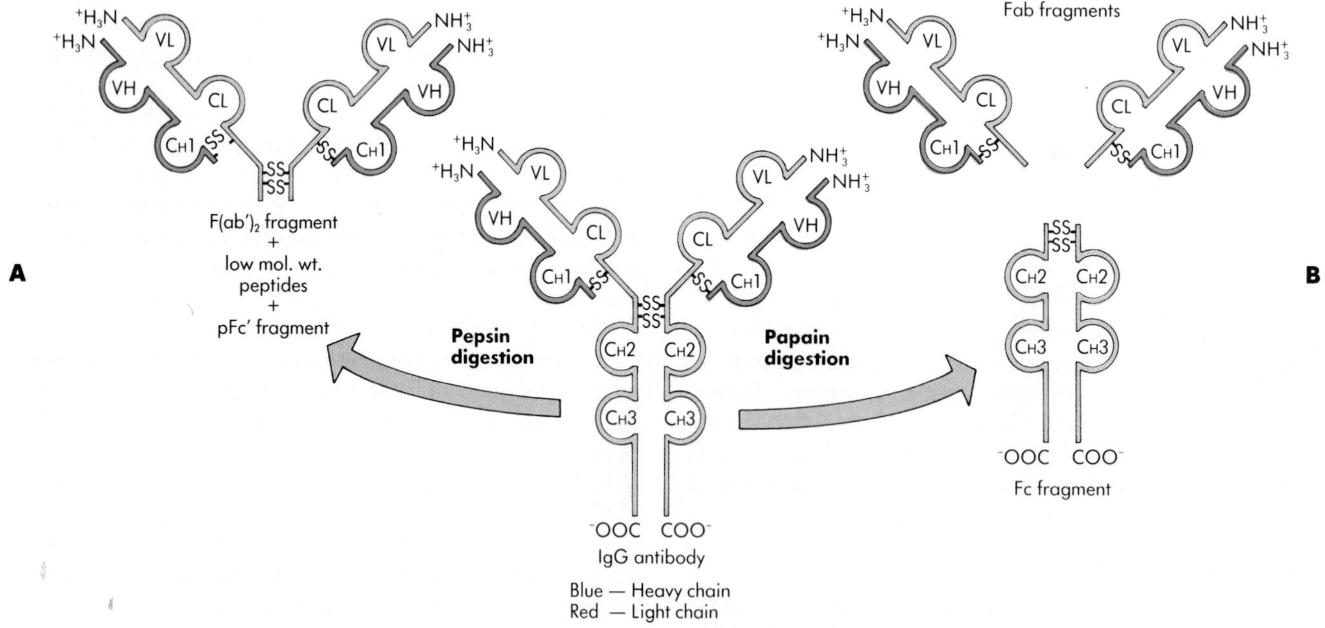

FIGURE 10-8 A, Pepsin digestion of IgG. **B,** Papain digestion of IgG.

response. IgG shows high avidity or binding capacity for antigens, fixes complement, stimulates chemotaxis, and acts as an opsonin to facilitate phagocytosis.

Immunoglobulin M

IgM comprises 5% to 10% of the total immunoglobulins in adults and has a half-life of 5 days. It is a pentameric molecule with five four-chain monomers joined by disulfide bonds and the J chain, with a total molecular weight of 900 kd. Theoretically this immunoglobulin has 10 antigen binding sites. IgM is the most efficient immunoglobulin in fixing complement. A single IgM pentamer can activate the classic pathway. Monomeric IgM is found with IgD on the B-lymphocyte cell surface, where it serves as the receptor for antigen. Because IgM is relatively large, it is confined to intravascular locations. IgM is particularly important for immunity against polysaccharide antigens on the exterior of pathogenic microorganisms. It also promotes phagocytosis and promotes bacteriolysis through its complement activation activity.

Immunoglobulin A

IgA comprises 5% to 15% of the serum immunoglobulins and has a half-life of 6 days. It has a molecular weight of 160 kd and a basic four-chain monomeric structure. However, it can occur as monomers, dimers, trimers, and multimers. It contains alpha heavy chains and kappa or lambda light chains. IgA2 does not have disulfide bonds linking H to L chains. In addition to serum IgA, a secretory or exocrine variety appears in body secretions and provides localized immunity. For example, the Sabin oral polio vaccine stimulates secretory IgA antibodies in the gut, which provide effective immunity against poliomyelitis. IgA deficient individuals have increased incidence of respiratory infections associated with a lack of secretory IgA in the respiratory system. Secretory or exocrine IgA appears in colostrum, intestinal and respiratory secretions, saliva, tears, and other secretions.

Immunoglobulin D

IgD, which has a molecular weight of 185 kd, comprises less than 1% of serum immunoglobulins. It has the basic four-chain monomeric structure with two delta heavy chains (molecular weight 63,000 d each) and either two kappa or two lambda light chains (molecular weight 22,000 d each). The half-life of IgD is only 2 to 3 days, and the role of IgD in immunity remains elusive. As indicated previously, membrane IgD serves with IgM as an antigen receptor on B-cell membranes.

Immunoglobulin E

IgE constitutes less than 1% of the total immunoglobulins and has a half-life of approximately 2.5 days. This antibody has a four-chain unit structure with two epsilon heavy chains (molecular weight 75,000 d each) and either two kappa or two lambda light chains per molecule (total molecular weight 190 kd). IgE does not precipitate with antigen in vitro and is heat labile. IgE is responsible for anaphylactic hypersensitivity, discussed later.

Immunoglobulin Genetics

Human chromosomes 2, 22, and 14 contain immunoglobulin genes for kappa, lambda, and H chains, respectively. There are multiple V genes. Once a cell starts to synthesize antibody, it chooses a V gene and translocates it proximal to the constant or C gene. The formation of multiple antigen specificities of light chains requires numerous V or J genes to connect with the C gene. Thus V, J, and C genes dictate L chain structure. In heavy chain genes, a diversity (D) gene is positioned between the V and J genes. Thus V, D, J, and C genes govern the structure of H chains. Class switching, or the ability to change to a fixed class of antibody synthesis, is driven by antigen and is governed by switch sequences. For a discussion of immunoglobulin genetics, see the immunology texts cited in the Bibliography.

COMPLEMENT

The complement system has been discussed in Chapter 9. For a more detailed discussion of its significance in resistance to infectious diseases, see the reference entitled *Complement Today*.

AUTOIMMUNITY

Immune reactivity involving either antibody-mediated (humoral) or cell-mediated limbs of the immune response against the body's own (self) constituents is termed **autoimmunity.** When autoantibodies or autoreactive T lymphocytes interact with self-epitopes, tissue injury may occur (e.g., in rheumatic fever the autoimmune reactivity against heart muscle sarcolemmal membranes occurs as a result of cross-reactivity with antibodies against streptococcal antigens [molecular mimicry]). Thus the immune response can be a two-edged sword, producing both beneficial, protective effects while also leading to severe injury to host tissues. Reactions of this deleterious nature are referred to as **hypersensitivity reactions,** which have been subgrouped into four types (I-IV).

Type I Anaphylactic Hypersensitivity

Type I hypersensitivity is mediated by IgE antibodies reactive with specific allergens (antigens that induce allergy) attached to basophil or mast cell Fc receptors (Figure 10-9). Cross-linking of the cell-bound IgE antibodies by antigen is followed by mast cell or basophil degranulation, with release of pharmacological mediators. These mediators include vasoactive amines such as histamine, which causes increased vascular permeability, vasodilation, bronchospasm, and mucus secretion. Secondary mediators of type I hypersensitivity include leukotrienes, prostaglandin D_2, platelet-activating factor, and various cytokines. Systemic anaphylaxis is a serious clinical problem and can follow the injection of such protein antigens as antitoxin or drugs such as penicillin.

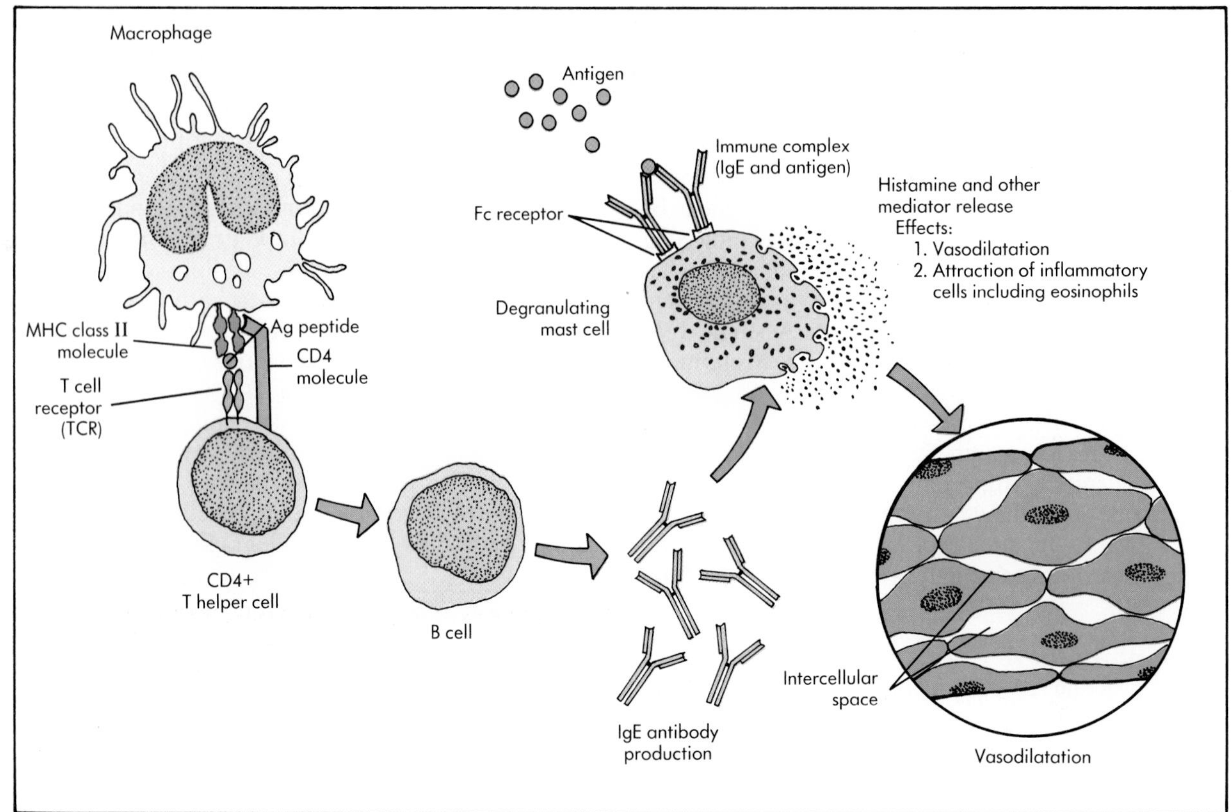

FIGURE 10-9 Type I (IgE-mediated) hypersensitivity.

Type II Antibody-Mediated Hypersensitivity

These antibodies are directed against antigens intrinsic to specific target tissues. The classic type of hypersensitivity involves the interaction of antibody with cell membrane antigens followed by complement lysis. Antibody-coated cells also have increased susceptibility to phagocytosis. Examples of type II hypersensitivity include the antiglomerular basement membrane antibody that develops in Goodpasture's syndrome and antibodies that develop against erythrocytes in Rh incompatibility leading to erythroblastosis fetalis or autoimmune hemolytic anemia (Figure 10-10, *A*).

A second variety of type II hypersensitivity is antibody-dependent cell-mediated cytotoxicity (ADCC). Killer (K) cells or NK cells, which have Fc receptors on their surfaces, may bind to the Fc region of IgG molecules. They may react with surface antigens on target cells to produce lysis of the antibody-coated cell. Complement fixation is not required. Complement does not participate in this reaction. In addition to K and NK cells, neutrophils, eosinophils, and macrophages may participate in ADCC (Figure 10-10, *B*).

A third form of type II hypersensitivity is antibody against cell surface receptors that interfere with function, as in the case of antibodies against acetylcholine receptors in motor endplates of skeletal muscle in myasthenia gravis. This interference with neuromuscular transmission results in muscular weakness, ultimately affecting the muscles of respiration to produce death. By contrast, stimulatory antibodies develop in hyperthyroidism (Graves' disease). They react with thyroid stimulating hormone receptors on thyroid epithelial cells to produce hyperthyroidism (Figure 10-10, *C*).

Type III Immune Complex-Mediated Hypersensitivity

Antigen-antibody complexes can stimulate an acute inflammatory response that leads to complement activation and PMN leukocyte infiltration (Figure 10-11). The immune complexes are formed either by exogenous antigens such as those from microbes or by endogenous antigens such as DNA, a target for antibodies produced in systemic lupus erythematosus. Immune complex–mediated injury may be either systemic or localized. In the systemic variety, antigen-antibody complexes are produced in the circulation, deposited in the tissues, and initiate inflammation. Acute serum sickness occurred in children treated with diphtheria antitoxin earlier in this century as a consequence of antibodies produced against the horse serum protein. When immune complexes are deposited in tissues, complement is fixed, and PMNs are attracted to the site, where lysosomal enzymes are

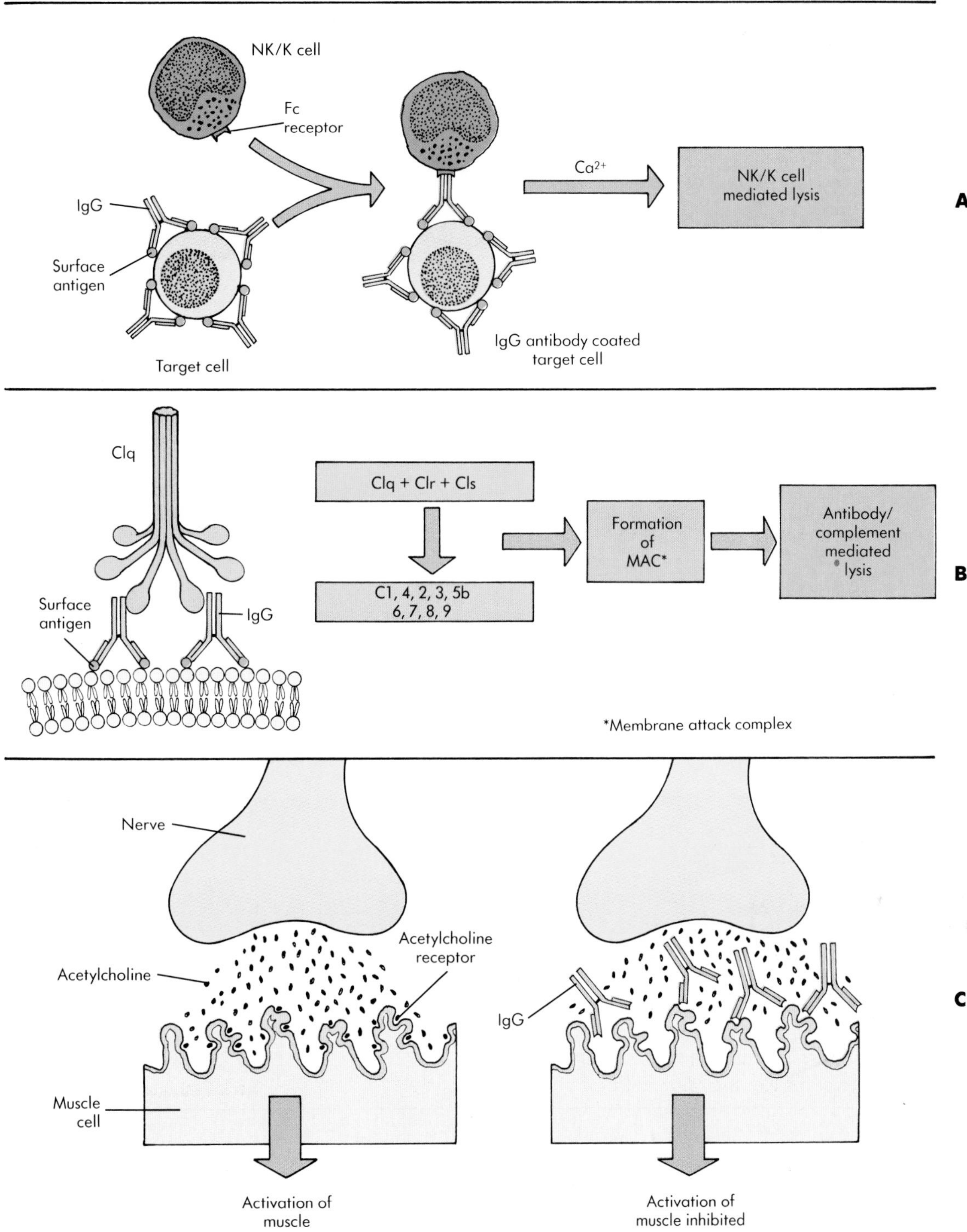

FIGURE 10-10 Type II hypersensitivity. **A,** Antibody-complement–mediated lysis of membranes. **B,** Antibody-dependent cell–mediated cytotoxicity (ADCC). **C,** Antibody against cell surface receptors.

released resulting in tissue injury. Localized immune complex disease, sometimes called the **Arthus reaction,** is characterized by an acute immune complex vasculitis with acute fibrinoid necrosis occurring in the walls of small vessels.

Type IV Cell-Mediated Hypersensitivity

Whereas antibodies participate in type I, II, and III reactions, T lymphocytes mediate type IV hypersensitivity (Figure 10-12). Two types of reactions, mediated by separate T-cell subsets, are observed. Delayed type

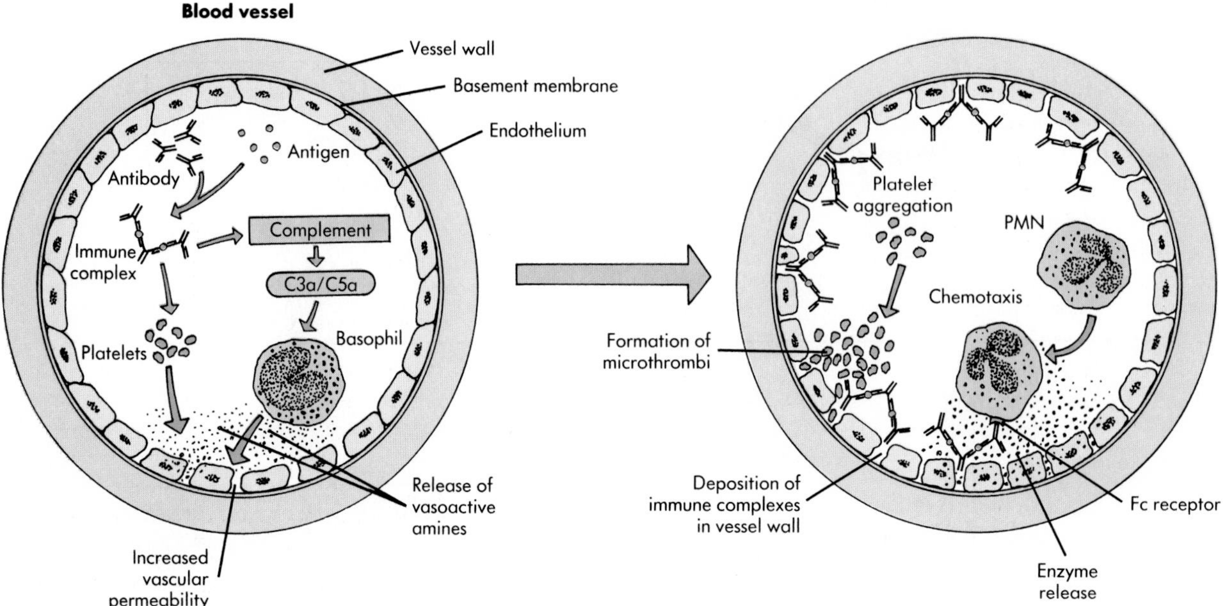

FIGURE 10-11 Type III hypersensitivity resulting from immune complex formation and deposition in vessel walls followed by inflammation initiated by complement fragments C3a and C5a.

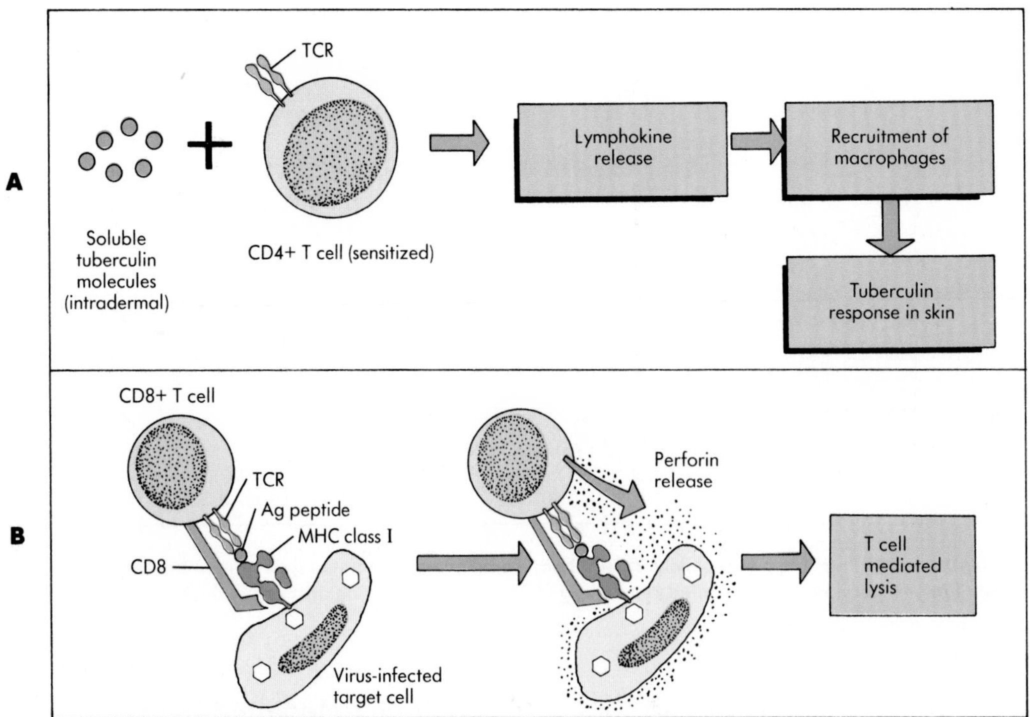

FIGURE 10-12 Type IV hypersensitivity. **A,** Tuberculin hypersensitivity mediated by CD4+ T lymphocytes. **B,** CD8+ T lymphocyte–mediated cytotoxicity of cells presenting endogenous antigen (e.g., virus-infected cell).

hypersensitivity (DTH) is mediated by CD4+ T cells, and cellular cytotoxicity is mediated principally by CD8+ T cells.

A classic delayed hypersensitivity reaction is the tuberculin or Mantoux reaction. Following exposure to *Mycobacterium tuberculosis,* CD4+ lymphocytes recognize the microbe's antigens complexed with class II MHC molecules on the surface of the antigen presenting cell that processed the mycobacterial antigens. Memory T cells develop and remain in the circulation for prolonged periods. When tuberculin antigen is injected intradermally, sensitized T cells react with the antigen on the antigen presenting cell surface, undergo transformation, and secrete lymphokines that lead to the manifestations of delayed hypersensitivity. Unlike in antibody-mediated hypersensitivity, lymphokines are not antigen specific.

In T-cell–mediated cytotoxicity, CD8+ T lymphocytes kill antigen bearing target cells. The cytotoxic T lymphocytes play a significant role in resistance to viral infections. Class I MHC molecules present viral antigens to CD8+ T lymphocytes as a viral peptide class I molecular complex, which is transported to the infected cell's surface. Cytotoxic CD8+ cells recognize this and lyse the target before the virus can replicate, thereby stopping the infection.

IMMUNODEFICIENCY DISEASES

Immunodeficiencies are classified as either primary diseases with a genetic origin or those that are secondary to an underlying disorder. X-linked (congenital) agammaglobulinemia (e.g., Bruton's disease) results from a failure of pre-B cells to differentiate into mature B cells. The defect in Bruton's disease is in rearrangement of immunoglobulin heavy chain genes. It occurs almost entirely in males and is apparent after 6 months of age following disappearance of the passively transferred maternal immunoglobulins. Patients have recurrent sinopulmonary infections caused by *Haemophilus influenzae, Streptococcus pyogenes, Staphylococcus aureus,* and *Streptococcus pneumoniae.* These patients have absent or decreased B cells and decreased serum levels of all immunoglobulin classes. The T-cell system and cell-mediated immunity appear normal.

Thymic hypoplasia (DiGeorge's syndrome) occurs when the immune system in infants is deprived of thymic influence. T cells are absent or deficient in the blood and thymus-dependent areas of lymph nodes and spleen. Infants with this condition are highly susceptible to infection by viruses, fungi, protozoa, or intracellular bacteria due to defective intracellular microbial killing by phagocytic cells with interferon (IFN-τ). By contrast, B cells and immunoglobulins are not affected.

Severe combined immunodeficiency (Swiss-typeagammaglobulinemia) comprises a group of conditions manifesting variable defects in both B and T cell immunity. In general, there is a lymphopenia with deficiency of T and B cell numbers and function. The thymus is hypoplastic or absent. Lymph nodes and other peripheral lymphoid tissues reveal depleted B- and T-cell regions. Infants with severe combined immunodeficiency show increased susceptibility to infections by viruses, fungi, and bacteria, and often succumb during the first year.

Secondary immunodeficiencies are more common than the primary forms. The best known is acquired immunodeficiency disease (e.g., AIDS), which results from destruction of the helper/inducer (CD4+) lymphocyte. Most of these individuals develop opportunistic infections caused by viruses, fungi, protozoa, and bacteria that are not commonly pathogenic.

SPECIFIC IMMUNE DEFENSE MECHANISMS

Specific Immune Responses to Extracellular Bacteria

Antibodies are the primary agents that protect the body against extracellular bacteria (Box 10-1). Microbial cell wall polysaccharides serve as thymus-independent antigens that stimulate specific IgM antibody responses. Cytokine production may even permit switching from IgM to IgG production. Protein antigens of extracellular bacteria primarily stimulate CD4+ T cells. Toxins of extracellular bacteria may activate multiple CD4+ T lymphocytes. Immune stimulation of this type may lead to the production of abundant quantities of cytokines that lead to pathological sequelae.

The resistance mechanisms against extracellular bacteria regrettably may include two reactions that produce tissue injury: acute inflammation and endotoxin shock. In addition, late in the course of a bacterial infection, pathogenic antibodies may appear (e.g., antibodies produced in poststreptococcal glomerulonephritis and rheumatic fever). The multiple lymphocyte clones stimulated by either bacterial endotoxins or superantigens may lead to the production of autoimmunity through overriding specific T-cell bypass mechanisms. Autoreactive lymphocytes may also be activated during this process.

BOX 10-1 Antimicrobial Action of Antibodies

Opsonic—promote ingestion and killing by phagocytic cells (IgG)
Block attachment (IgA)
Neutralize toxins
Agglutinate bacteria—may aid in clearing
Render motile organisms nonmotile
Abs only rarely affect metabolism or growth of bacteria (Mycoplasma)
Abs, combining with antigens of the bacterial surface, activate the complement cascade, thus inducing an inflammatory response and bringing fresh phagocytes and serum Abs into the site
Abs, combining with antigens of the bacterial surface, activate the complement cascade, and through the final sequences the (MAC) membrane attack complex is formed involving C5b-C9

Evasion of Immune Mechanisms by Extracellular Bacteria

The ability of extracellular bacteria to adhere to tissues through their surface proteins, to inhibit or inactivate complement, and to discourage phagocytosis all represent virulence mechanisms that facilitate invasion and colonization of tissues. Sialic acid–containing capsules can interfere with the alternate complement pathway. Bacterial capsules are also known to circumvent phagocytosis. Antigenic variation is another mechanism whereby bacteria may escape the development of an immune response specific for their surface antigens.

Specific Immune Responses to Intracellular Bacteria and Fungi

Some bacteria reproduce inside cells of the host. For example, mycobacteria and *Listeria monocytogenes* are organisms of high pathogenicity that survive in phagocytic cells such as macrophages. Within the macrophage, they are not exposed to specific antibody. A number of fungi are also intracellular pathogens.

Cell-mediated immunity attributable to T lymphocytes is the principal mechanism whereby intracellular bacteria are eliminated by macrophages activated by γ-interferon derived from T cells. Intracellular bacterial protein antigens activate powerful T-lymphocyte responsiveness, and their cell wall components stimulate macrophages. CD4+ helper/inducer and CD8+ suppressor/cytotoxic T-lymphocyte subsets protect against intracellular bacteria. Both CD4+ and CD8+ T-lymphocyte subsets produce γ-interferon, which activates both phagocytosis and functional degradation of ingested microorganisms by macrophages.

Some intracellular microorganisms within macrophages remain resistant even in the presence of specific cell-mediated immunity. They activate macrophages, which encircle the bacteria and inhibit their distribution. Infections by both mycobacteria and fungi may produce granulomatous inflammation, which leads to necrosis of tissues, fibrosis, and interference with function. This represents a pathogenic immune response by the host reacting against selected intracellular bacteria.

Evasion of Immune Mechanisms by Intracellular Bacteria and Fungi

The principal evasion mechanism of intracellular bacteria is their ability to circumvent killing by phagocytes. Two such microorganisms, *Mycobacterium tuberculosis* and *Legionella pneumophila,* survive by preventing fusion of phagolysosomes. *Listeria monocytogenes* synthesizes a hemolysin that facilitates survival within host cells by the formation of pores within phagolysosomes, permitting bacteria to escape back into the cytoplasm.

Specific Immune Responses to Viruses

Viruses are obligate intracellular parasites that multiply within host cells whose nucleic acids and protein synthesis capability are subverted and appropriated for virus propagation. Viruses may interfere with the cell's protein synthesis and normal functioning, leading to host cell death. This constitutes a cytopathic effect. Viruses that are not cytopathic may induce a latent infection in which they remain inside host cells and induce synthesis of proteins that provoke a specific immune response. This consists of cytolytic T lymphocytes that are specific for the virus and destroy the virus-infected cell. Viral proteins may induce delayed-type hypersensitivity that leads to cellular injury. Both antibodies from B cells and specifically sensitized T cells confer immunity against viruses. Before host cell invasion, specific antibodies may neutralize virions. However, following penetration of host cells, T-cell–mediated immunity is requisite for destruction of the virus-infected host cells.

Antibodies specific for viral antigenic determinants may offer early protection following viral infection. They interact with viral capsid or envelope antigens, thereby inhibiting adherence and invasion of host cells. Antibodies may also act as opsonins that increase the attractiveness of viral particles to phagocytic cells. Secretory IgA antibody is important in neutralizing viruses on mucosal surfaces. Complement also facilitates phagocytosis and may be significant in viral lysis.

Immunization or vaccination against viruses often involves the use of an attenuated or killed virus vaccine. The antibody induced is specific for the particular serologic type of the virus. Protection is restricted to that serotype, leaving the individual susceptible to the virus's remaining serotypes. Humoral immunity is of value only early during the course of virus infection and provides no immunity once host cells have been invaded. Antiviral immunity based on antibody alone is insufficient to protect an individual against a viral infection. Virus neutralization does not necessarily reflect the protective action of a particular antibody.

Antiviral immunity depends primarily on cytotoxic T cells. These cells are virus-specific CD8+ lymphocytes that can identify viral antigens presented in the context of class I MHC molecules on any virus-infected host cell with which they come into contact. The cytotoxic T lymphocytes lyse virus-infected host cells, activate intracellular enzymes that disassemble viral genomes, and secrete lymphokines such as interferon.

Viruses that induce chronic infection persist for an extended period, complex with antibodies in the blood, and are deposited in the vessels, leading to vasculitis. Viruses may also produce disease through "molecular mimicry" in which an immune response is produced against selected amino acid sequences of the virus that are shared in common with host "self"-antigens. Therefore products of the immune reaction (antibodies or T cells) cross-react with host tissues bearing the shared antigenic determinants, leading to injury.

Evasion of Immune Mechanisms by Viruses

Besides the sanctuary viruses enjoy once they have entered host cells, these disease agents have additional means to escape host immune mechanisms. Viruses are especially adept at antigenic variation whereby they may alter their surface antigenic structure once antibodies are formed against their original epitopes. This process may be repeated many times, leading to the production of numerous strains of a particular virus that are antigenically and therefore serologically distinct. The influenza and AIDS viruses are especially versatile in this regard.

Viruses may also induce immunosuppression in the host they infect. The AIDS virus (HIV-1) is well known to target CD4+ helper/inducer lymphocytes that are central to mounting any type of immune response. Selected viruses such as the Epstein-Barr virus may induce immunosuppression by mechanisms that are yet to be determined but possibly attributable to genes that encode substances that dampen antiviral immune responsiveness.

Specific Immune Responses to Parasites

Parasites such as protozoa and helminths elicit a variety of immune responses. Helminthic infections including *Nippostrongylus,* schistosomes, and filaria evoke titers of IgE that exceed those induced by other infectious agents. Helminths specifically stimulate CD4+ helper T lymphocytes that form IL-4 and IL-5. ADCC involving eosinophils and IgE antibody is believed to be effective in immunity against helminths since the major basic protein in eosinophil granules is toxic to helminths. Coating helminths with IgE specific antibody followed by eosinophil attachment through the Fc regions leads to ADCC by eosinophils.

Parasites such as *Schistosoma mansoni* produce eggs that induce granuloma formation in such organs as the liver. Stimulated CD4+ T lymphocytes activate macrophages, which leads to granuloma formation and isolation of the eggs. The development of fibrosis interrupts the venous blood supply to the liver, leading to hypertension and cirrhosis.

Intracellular protozoa often activate specific cytotoxic T cells. They represent a critical mechanism to prevent dissemination of intracellular malarial parasites. Parasite antigen-antibody (immune) complexes may be trapped in the renal microvasculature, leading to immune complex glomerulonephritis.

Evasion of Immune Mechanisms by Parasites

Animal parasites have developed remarkable mechanisms to establish chronic infections in the vertebrate host. Natural immunity to them is weak, and the parasites have devised novel and ingenious mechanisms to circumvent specific immunity. Parasites either camouflage their own antigens or interfere with host immunity. Some parasites mask their antigens by coating themselves with host proteins, which prevents their detection by host immune mechanisms. Some develop resistance by biochemical alterations of their surface coat. They are also adept at changing their surface antigens by antigenic variation, which may frustrate attempts for prophylactic immunization. Other parasites, such as *Entamoeba histolytica,* may shed their antigenic coats.

QUESTIONS

1. List and describe the function of the cells of immunity.
2. Describe the structure of all major and minor immunoglobulin molecules.
3. Describe the four types of hypersensitivity, and give examples of each.
4. Describe specific immune responses to parasites, viruses, fungi, and bacteria.
5. Describe an antigen, and tell what makes it antigenic.

Bibliography

Abbas AK, Lichtman AH, Pober JS: *Cellular and molecular immunology,* Philadelphia, 1991, WB Saunders.

Barrett JT: *Medical immunology,* Philadelphia, 1991, FA Davis.

Benjamin E, Leskowitz S: *Immunology, a short course,* ed 2, New York, 1991, Wiley-Liss.

Bona CA, Francisco AB: *Immunology for medical students,* New York, 1990, Harwood Academic Publishers.

Brostoff J, Scadding GK, Male D, Roitt IM: *Clinical immunology,* London, 1991, Gower Medical Publishing.

Cruse JM, Lewis RE Jr, editors: *Complement today,* vol 1, Complement Profiles, Basel and New York, 1993, S. Karger Publishers.

Eisen HN: *General immunology,* ed 2, Philadelphia, 1990, JB Lippincott.

Golub ES, Green DR: *Immunology, a synthesis,* ed 2, Suderland, Mass., 1991, Sinauer Associates.

Gorbach SL, Bartlett JG, Blacklow NR: *Infectious diseases,* Philadelphia, 1992, WB Saunders.

Haynes BF, Eisenbath GS: *Monoclonal antibodies,* Orlando, Fla., 1983, Academic Press.

Hudson L, Hay FC: *Practical immunology,* ed 3, Oxford, 1989, Blackwell Scientific Publications.

Kumar V, Cotran RS, Robbins SL: *Basic pathology,* ed 5, Philadelphia, 1992, WB Saunders.

McMichael AJ, Fabre JW: *Monoclonal antibodies in clinical medicine,* London, 1983, Academic Press.

Mandrell GL, Douglas RG Jr, Bennett JE: *Principles and practices of infectious diseases,* ed 3, New York, 1990, Churchill Livingstone.

Oppenheim JJ, Shevach EM: *Immunophysiology,* Oxford, 1990, Oxford University Press.

Paul WE, editor: *Fundamental immunology,* ed 2, New York, 1989, Raven Press.

Paul WE, Fathman CG, Metzger H: *Annual review of immunology,* vols 1-10, Palo Alto, CA, 1983-1992, Annual Reviews.

Roitt IM: *Essential immunology,* ed 7, Oxford, 1991, Blackwell Scientific Publications.

Roitt IM, Brostoff J, Male DK, editors: *Immunology,* ed 2, London, 1989, Gower Medical Publishing.

Ruby J: *Immunology,* New York, 1992, WH Freeman.

Samter M, Talmage DW, Frank MM, et al.: *Immunological diseases,* vols 1 and 2, ed 4, Boston, Mass, 1988, Little, Brown.

Sell S: *Immunology, immunopathology and immunity,* ed 4, New York, 1987, Elsevier.

Stites DP, Terr AI: *Basic and clinical immunology,* ed 7, Norwalk, Conn., 1991, Appleton-Lange.

CHAPTER 11

Microbial Virulence Factors

Of the numerous microorganisms to which humans are exposed, very few produce disease. The ability to initiate disease is determined by an organism's virulence, as well as by specific host factors. As would be expected, exposure of a nonimmune individual to organisms with a high virulence potential usually results in disease. Likewise, patients with compromised natural or acquired immunity are more susceptible to diseases caused by less virulent organisms. Host defense mechanisms were discussed in Chapters 9 and 10, and microbial virulence factors are examined in this chapter.

Disease can be initiated by exposure to a microbial toxin such as *Clostridium botulinum* toxin in food-borne botulism, *Staphylococcus aureus* enterotoxin in staphylococcal food poisoning, or mushroom intoxication. In each example, the etiological organism does not need to be present for initiation of disease. However, this process is atypical. Production of most infectious diseases requires exposure to the pathogen, colonization of the host, microbial penetration into host tissues, and production of toxic products.

EXPOSURE

As was discussed in Chapter 8, the human body is colonized with large numbers of microbes, of which many provide important functions for their hosts, such as digestion of food, transport of metabolites, and protection from colonization with pathogenic microbes. Disease with these **endogenous** organisms can be established if the normal balance of organisms is disrupted (e.g., during antibiotic therapy) or if the organisms are introduced into normally sterile sites (e.g., aspiration of oral bacteria into the lower airways, traumatic introduction of organisms on the mucosal surface into deep tissues, spillage of intestinal organisms into the intra-abdominal cavity after intestinal perforation). Another source of pathogenic organisms is from **exogenous** sites. These organisms normally enter the body through one of three routes: ingestion, inhalation, or direct penetration. Examples of bacteria, fungi, viruses, and parasites that can

TABLE 11-1 Microbial Port of Entry

Route	Examples
Ingestion	
Bacteria:	*Salmonella, Shigella, Yersinia enterocolitica,* enterotoxigenic *Escherichia coli, Vibrio, Campylobacter, Clostridium botulinum, Bacillus cereus, Listeria, Brucella*
Parasites:	*Giardia, Entamoeba histolytica, Cryptosporidium,* cestodes
Viruses:	*Enterovirus,* poliovirus, hepatitis A virus
Inhalation	
Bacteria:	*Mycobacterium, Nocardia, Mycoplasma pneumoniae, Legionella, Bordetella, Chlamydia psittaci, Chlamydia pneumoniae*
Fungi:	*Histoplasma, Blastomyces, Coccidioides, Cryptococcus*
Viruses:	Respiratory syncytical virus, Orthomyxovirus, Paramyxovirus, Varicella-zoster
Direct Penetration	
Trauma:	*Clostridium tetani, Erysipelothrix, Sporothrix,* rabies virus
Needle stick:	*Staphylococcus aureus, Pseudomonas,* hepatitis B, human immunodeficiency virus (HIV)
Arthropod bite:	*Rickettsia, Ehrlichia, Coxiella, Francisella, Borrelia, Yersinia pestis,* malaria, *Babesia*
Sexual transmission:	*Neisseria gonorrhoeae, Chlamydia trachomatis, Treponema pallidum,* papillomavirus, herpes simplex viruses, HIV
Transplacental:	*Treponema pallidum, Toxoplasma,* rubella virus, cytomegalovirus
Organism directed:	Hookworm, *Strongyloides, Schistosoma*

produce exogenous infections are listed in Table 11-1. By no means should this compilation be considered exhaustive; rather, the listing illustrates the diversity of organisms that confront the human body.

Additional factors that determine the consequences of the interaction between pathogen and host are the **route of exposure** and **inoculum size.** Many pathogenic organisms have a limited range of organs or host cells in which they are able to replicate. For example, simple skin contact with Varicella-zoster virus does not result in disease; rather, the virus must be inhaled for the disease process to be initiated. Likewise, a minimum number of organisms is required to establish infection. This may be relatively small (e.g., fewer than 200 *Shigella* needed for shigellosis) or quite large (e.g., 10^8 *Vibrio cholerae* or *Campylobacter* to produce their respective gastrointestinal infections). It is important to recognize that the inoculum required to establish disease can vary enormously depending on host factors. For example, although a million or more *Salmonella* are required to establish gastroenteritis in a healthy individual, only a few hundred or thousand organisms are required if the gastric pH is neutral. Likewise, the presence of a foreign body (e.g., prosthesis, catheter, suture material) can dramatically reduce the number of staphylococci required to produce a wound infection.

COLONIZATION

Most infections are initiated by the attachment of the microbe to host tissues, followed by microbial replication to establish colonization. The attachment can be relatively nonspecific, mediated by production of polysaccharide capsules or slime, or require the interaction between structures on the bacterial surface known as **adhesins** and specific glycoprotein or glycolipid receptors on the host cells. Specific microbial surface structures that facilitate adhesion include lipoteichoic acids, outer membrane proteins, hemagglutinin, flagella, and fimbriae or pili. Examples of some of the many adhesins that have been identified in microbes are listed in Table 11-2.

Escherichia coli is a good model of the importance of adhesins in virulence. A large variety of fimbriae have been identified in *E. coli* strains and demonstrated to mediate specific adherence to receptors in host cells. The enteropathogenic strains of *E. coli* that induce diarrhea adhere to specific receptors on epithelial cells in the small gut of susceptible hosts. This adherence facilitates the multiplication of the microbes and release of bacterial enterotoxins that induce hypersecretion of fluids. The adhesin molecules are situated at the fimbrial tips, permitting attachment to a target receptor.

Various adhesin molecules have been associated with specific infections. For example, the majority of *E. coli* strains producing pyelonephritis manifest a fimbrial adhesin termed *P fimbriae.* This adhesin is able to bind to receptors for alpha-D-galactosyl-beta-D-galactoside (Gal-Gal), which is part of the P blood group antigen structure on human erythrocytes and uroepithelial cells. *Neisseria gonorrhoeae* pili are also important in site-specific disease. Gonococcal pili bind to oligosaccharide receptors on epithelial cells, which overcome the repulsive force generated by the negatively charged bacteria and eukaryotic cells.

MICROBIAL PENETRATION AND GROWTH

Although some organisms such as *Corynebacterium diphtheriae* and *Bordetella pertussis* can establish disease by

TABLE 11-2 Examples of Microbial Adherence Mechanisms

Microbe	Adhesin	Receptor
Bacteria		
Staphylococcus aureus	Lipoteichoic acid	Unknown
Staphylococcus spp.	Slime	Unknown
Streptococcus, group A	LTA-M protein complex	Unknown
Streptococcus, group B	Protein	*N*-acetyl-D-glucosamine
Escherichia coli	Type 1 fimbriae	D-mannose
	CFA/1 fimbriae	GM ganglioside
	P fimbriae	P blood group glycolipid
Other Enterobacteriaceae	Type 1 fimbriae	D-mannose
Neisseria gonorrhoeae	Fimbriae	GD_1 ganglioside
Treponema pallidum	P_1, P_2, P_3	Fibronectin
Chlamydia	Cell surface lectin	*N*-acetyl-D-glucosamine
Mycoplasma pneumoniae	Protein P1	Sialic acid
Fungi		
Candida albicans	Mannan	Unknown
Parasites		
Plasmodium vivax	Apical complex	Duffy blood group antigen
P. falciparum	Apical coplex	*N*-acetyl-D-glucosamine
Entamoeba histolytica	Cell surface lectin	*N*-acetylglucosamine
Giardia lamblia	Gripping disk	Mechanical
Viruses		
Orthomyxovirus	Hemagglutinin	Sialic acid
Picornavirus	Capsid protein	Four receptor "families"
Adenovirus	Fiber protein	Unknown
HIV	gp120	CD4 on T cells

Modified from Mandell G, Douglas G, Bennett J: *Principles and practice of infectious diseases*, ed 3, New York, 1990, Churchill Livingstone.

localized multiplication at the site of attachment, most organisms initiate the disease process by invading into normally sterile tissues and replicating. For example, *Shigella* invade the epithelial cells of the colonic mucosa, are nourished by blood nutrients, and multiply. Ultimately, the epithelium is destroyed and mucosal inflammation or ulceration occurs as the organisms spread to the lamina propria.

The predilection of a microbe for a certain tissue of the body may reflect the presence of a specific receptor, a plentiful supply of growth factors, or other substances that favor the survival and proliferation of that particular microorganism. For example, some bacteria have perfected ingenious methods to acquire and utilize host iron not readily available to them but required for growth. Essentially all iron in the human body is sequestered in heme-binding proteins (hemoglobin, myoglobin, transferrin, lactoferrin). Confronted with this paucity of available iron, bacteria have evolved high-affinity iron-capturing systems called *siderophores* to acquire iron from the environment. In addition, bacteria that produce hemolysins are able to lyse erythrocytes and release heme-containing iron proteins.

The spread of organisms through tissues is mediated by release of degradative enzymes (e.g., hyaluronidase, nucleases, collagenase, elastase). This process of tissue destruction is frequently sufficient to initiate clinical disease. However, for the disease process to be maintained, the organisms must be able to avoid the host's immunological defense mechanisms (e.g., phagocytic killing). This is accomplished by a variety of approaches (Box 11-1).

Many bacteria are encapsulated (Box 11-2). The hydrophilic nature of capsules inhibits phagocytosis. In addition, capsules can mask surface components such as lipopolysaccharide (LPS), which can activate the alternate complement pathway. Free soluble capsular material can interact with opsonic antibodies and prevent phagocytic removal of the organisms. Capsules can also mimic host antigens; for example the capsule of *Streptococcus pyogenes* consists of hyaluronic acid present in human connective tissue. Thus the host fails to recognize the encapsulated bacteria as a foreign antigen.

Organisms can shift antigenic expression, such as is observed with influenza A virus or with the pilin proteins in *Neisseria gonorrhoeae.* Rapid variation of expression of different pilin proteins is an effective means for the gonococci to avoid immune clearance (and unfortunately renders vaccines directed against pili ineffective). Microbial antigens can be masked when the organism assumes an intracellular location in the host cells. In addition, antibody activity can be destroyed by production of proteases specific for IgA antibodies (e.g., *N. gonorrhoeae*) or rendered ineffective by interference with complement activation.

Phagocytic killing can be circumvented in a variety of ways. The microbe can produce enzymes capable of lysing phagocytic cells (e.g., streptolysin produced by *Streptococcus pyogenes* or alpha toxin by *Clostridium perfringens*). Chemotaxis can be inhibited by microbial products such as *Staphylococcus aureus* protein A. Phagocytosis can be inhibited (e.g., effect of capsule and M protein in *S. pyogenes*), or intracellular killing obviated. Mechanisms developed to avoid intracellular killing have included prevention of phagolysosome fusion, resistance to killing following exposure to the lysosomal enzymes, or release of phagocytosed cells into the host cytoplasm before exposure to lysosomal enzymes (Table 11-3).

MICROBIAL TOXINS

Even though organisms may attach and colonize mucosal surfaces and then invade into the deeper tissues, disease is frequently determined by the production of microbial

BOX 11-1 Microbial Defenses Against Host Immunological Clearance

Encapsulation
Antigenic mimicry
Antigenic masking
Antigenic shift
Production of anti-immunoglobulin proteases
Phagocytic destruction
Inhibition of chemotaxis
Inhibition of phagocytosis
Inhibition of phagolysosome fusion
Resistance to lysosomal enzymes
Adaptation to cytoplasmic replication

BOX 11-2 Examples of Encapsulated Microorganisms

Staphylococcus aureus
Streptococcus pneumoniae
Streptococcus pyogenes (group A)
Streptococcus agalactiae (group B)
Bacillus anthracis
Bacillus subtilis
Neisseria gonorrhoeae
Neisseria meningitidis
Haemophilus influenzae
Escherichia coli
Klebsiella pneumoniae
Salmonella
Yersinia pestis
Campylobacter fetus
Pseudomonas aeruginosa
Bacteroides fragilis
Cryptococcus neoformans

TABLE 11-3 Methods Developed to Circumvent Phagocytic Killing

Method	Example
Inhibition of phagolysome fusion	*Legionella, Mycobacterium tuberculosis, Chlamydia*
Resistance to lysosomal enzymes	*Salmonella typhimurium, Coxiella, Ehrlichia, Mycobacterium leprae, Leishmania*
Adaptation to cytoplasmic replication	*Listeria, Francisella, Rickettsia*

toxins. They have been classified as either endotoxin or exotoxins.

Endotoxin (discussed in Chapter 2) is a lipopolysaccharide that forms an integral component of gram-negative cell walls. The active component of endotoxin is lipid A, which has multiple biological properties including the ability to induce fever, initiate the complement and blood coagulation cascades, activate B lymphocytes, and stimulate production of tumor necrosis factor, interleukin-1, and prostaglandins. The effects of endotoxin are dose related with exposure to large quantities such as during gram-negative bloodstream infections leading to fever, hypotension, shock, and possibly death.

The effects of exotoxins have been known for more than a century. The early bacteriologists including von

TABLE 11-4 Properties of A-B Type Bacterial Toxins

Toxin	Organism	Genetic Control	Subunit Structure	Target Cell Receptor	Biological Effects
Anthrax toxins	*B. anthracis*	Plasmid	Three separate proteins (EF, LF, PA)	Unknown, probably glycoprotein	EF + PA: increase in target cell cAMP level, localized edema; LF + PA: death of target cells and experimental animals
Bordetella adenylate cyclase toxin	*Bordetella* species	Chromosomal	A-B	Unknown, probably glycolipid	Increase in target cell cAMP level; modified cell function or cell death
Botulinum toxin	*C. botulinum*	Phage	A-B	Possibly ganglioside (GD_{1b})	Decrease in peripheral, presynaptic acetylcholine release; flaccid paralysis
Cholera toxin	*V. cholera*	Chromosomal	A-5B	Ganglioside (GM_1)	Activation of adenylate cyclase, increase in cAMP level; secretory diarrhea
Diphtheria toxin	*C. diphtheriae*	Phage	A-B	Probably glycoprotein	Inhibition of protein synthesis; cell death
Heat-labile enterotoxins	*E. coli*	Plasmid	Similar or identical to cholera toxin		
Pertussis toxin	*B. pertussis*	Chromosomal	A-5B	Unknown, probably glycoprotein	Block of signal transduction mediated by target G proteins
Pseudomonas exotoxin A	*P. aeruginosa*	Chromosomal	A-B	Unknown, but different from diphtheria toxin	Similar or identical to diphtheria toxin
Shiga toxin	*S. dysenteriae*	Chromosomal	A-5B	Glycoprotein or glycolipid	Inhibition of protein synthesis, cell death
Shiga-like toxins	*Shigella* species, *E. coli*	Phage	Similar or identical to shiga toxin		
Tetanus toxin	*C. tetani*	Plasmid	A-B	Ganglioside (GT_1) and/or GD_{1b}	Decrease in neurotransmitter release from inhibitory neurons; spastic paralysis

Modified from Mandell G, Douglas G, and Bennett J: *Pricniples and practice of infectious disease*, ed 3, New York, 1990, Churchill Livingstone.

Behring, Kitasato, and Ehrlich raised antibodies against the exotoxins of *Corynebacterium diphtheriae, Clostridium tetani,* and *Clostridium botulinum.* By treating these toxins chemically to render them immunogenic but no longer toxic, protective immunity was induced in susceptible hosts. Even though multiple exotoxins have been discovered since that time, few have been as amenable to the development of effective immunogenic toxoids as were the earliest ones discovered. Some bacterial exotoxins are among the most poisonous substances known. The consumption of a single bean in home-canned vegetables contaminated with *Clostridium botulinum* toxin, unheated before serving, may produce death. Likewise, the lethal dose of tetanus toxin is less than the immunizing dose.

Bacterial exotoxins are either **cytolytic** or **bipartite.** The effect of cytolytic toxins on susceptible cells is dose dependent. Whereas relatively large amounts of a cytolytic toxin may interrupt the structural integrity of cell membrane leading to cell death, lesser quantities may only interfere with specific functions. An example of a cytolytic toxin is the alpha toxin (phospholipase C) of *Clostridium perfringens,* which enzymatically attacks sphingomyelin and other membrane phospholipids, resulting in cell lysis. Bipartite exotoxins consist of A and B subunits. The toxins bind to the cell surface through the B subunit, and then the A subunit is transferred into the interior of the cell where cell injury is produced. Examples of common bipartite exotoxins and their biological effects are summarized in Table 11-4. The functional properties of cytolytic and bipartite exotoxins are discussed in greater detail in the chapters dealing with their specific diseases.

QUESTIONS

1. What is the distinction between endogenous and exogenous infections?
2. Name three routes by which exogenous pathogens can infect an individual. List five examples of organisms that use each route.
3. Give at least one example of an adhesin for each major group of organisms (bacteria, fungi, parasites, viruses).
4. How are microbes able to resist immunological clearance? Give at least one specific example of each mechanism.
5. What are the two general types of exotoxins? List examples of each type.

Bibliography

Gorbach S, Bartlett J, Blacklow NR: *Infectious diseases,* Philadelphia, 1992, WB Saunders.

McGee J, Isaacson P, Wright N: *Oxford textbook of pathology,* vol 1, Oxford, 1992, Oxford University Press.

Mandell G, Douglas G, Bennett J: *Principles and practice of infectious diseases,* ed 3, New York, 1990, Churchill Livingstone.

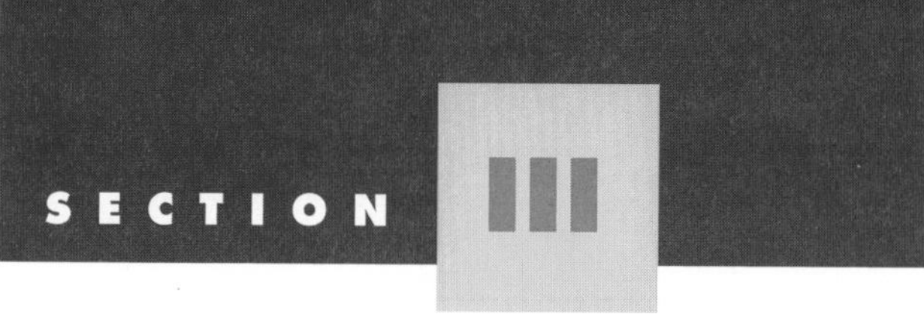

STERILIZATION, DISINFECTION, CHEMOTHERAPY, AND VACCINATION

CHAPTER 12

Sterilization, Disinfection, and Antisepsis

MEDICAL microbiology is logically concerned with understanding the pathogenesis and chemotherapy of infectious diseases. However, it is just as important to know how diseases are prevented. An important component of infection control is an understanding of the principles of sterilization, disinfection, and antisepsis (Box 12-1), which are the subject of this chapter. The subsequent chapters in this section (Chapters 13 through 17) will examine chemotherapeutic and immunotherapeutic control of infections.

STERILIZATION

Sterilization is the total destruction of all microbes including the more resilient forms such as bacterial spores, mycobacteria, nonlipid viruses, and fungi (Figure 12-1). This can be accomplished by physical means (e.g., use of steam under pressure, dry heat, ultraviolet or gamma radiation) or by chemical germicides (e.g., ethylene oxide gas or various liquids; Table 12-1). Obviously sterilization procedures cannot be used on living tissues; however, these procedures are important for eliminating all microbes on surfaces where any microbial contamination will have serious consequences (e.g., on surgical instruments).

BOX 12-1 Definitions

Sterilization	Use of physical procedures or chemical agents to destroy all microbial forms, including bacterial spores
Disinfection	Use of physical procedures or chemical agents to destroy most microbial forms; bacterial spores and other relatively resistant organisms (e.g., mycobacteria, nonlipid viruses, fungi) may remain viable; disinfectants are subdivided into high-level, intermediate-level, and low-level agents
Antisepsis	Use of chemical agents on skin or living tissue to inhibit or eliminate microbes
Germicide	Chemical agent capable of killing microbes
Sporicide	Germicide capable of killing bacterial spores

DISINFECTION

Disinfection also refers to elimination of microbes, although the more resilient ones can survive. Unfortunately, the terms *disinfection* and *sterilization* are casually intermingled, which can result in some confusion. This

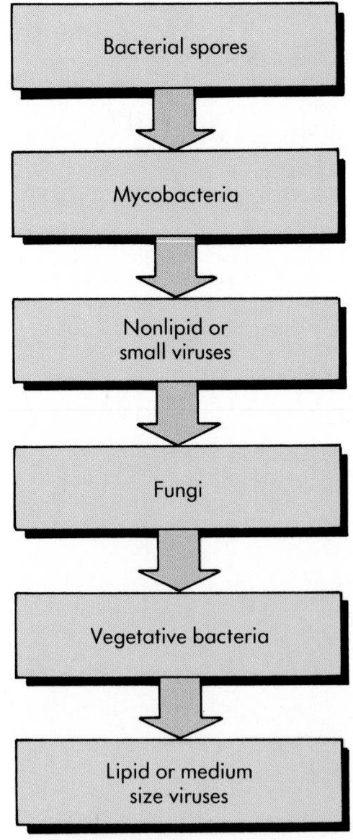

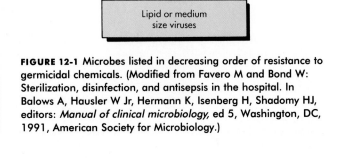

FIGURE 12-1 Microbes listed in decreasing order of resistance to germicidal chemicals. (Modified from Favero M and Bond W: Sterilization, disinfection, and antisepsis in the hospital. In Balows A, Hausler W Jr, Hermann K, Isenberg H, Shadomy HJ, editors: *Manual of clinical microbiology,* ed 5, Washington, DC, 1991, American Society for Microbiology.)

occurs because disinfection processes have been categorized as high level, intermediate level, and low level. High-level disinfection can generally approach sterilization in effectiveness, whereas spore forms can survive intermediate-level disinfection and many microbes can remain viable when exposed to low-level disinfection.

Even the classification of disinfectants by their level of activity is misleading. The effectiveness of these procedures is influenced by the nature of the item to be disinfected, number and resilience of the contaminating organism(s), amount of organic material present (which can inactivate the disinfectant), type and concentration of disinfectant, and duration and temperature of exposure.

High-level disinfectants are used for items involved with invasive procedures that cannot withstand sterilization procedures (e.g., certain types of endoscopes, surgical instruments with plastic or other components that cannot be autoclaved). Disinfection of these and other items is most effective if treatment is preceded by cleaning of the surface to remove organic matter. Examples of high-level disinfectants, as well as all other disinfectants, are listed in Table 12-1.

Intermediate-level disinfection is used to clean surfaces

TABLE 12-1 Methods of Sterilization or Disinfection; Activity Levels of Selected Liquid Germicides

Method	Concentration or level	Disinfectant activity
Sterilization		
Heat		
Moist heat (steam under pressure)	250° F (121° C) or 271° F (132° C) for various time intervals	
Dry heat	171° C for 1 hr; 160° C for 2 hr; 121° C for 16 hr	
Gas		
Ethylene oxide	450-500 mg/liter at 55-60° C	
Liquid		
Glutaraldehyde	Variable	
Hydrogen peroxide	6%-30%	
Formaldehyde	6%-8%	
Chlorine dioxide	Variable	
Peracetic acid	Variable	
Disinfection		
Heat		
Moist heat (includes hot water pasteurization)	75° C-100° C	High
Liquid		
Glutaraldehyde	Variable	High to intermediate
Hydrogen peroxide	3%-6%	High to intermediate
Formaldehyde	1%-8%	High to low
Chlorine dioxide	Variable	High
Peracetic acid	Variable	High
Chlorine compounds	500-5000 mg of free or available chlorine/liter	Intermediate
Alcohols (ethyl, isopropyl)	70%	Intermediate
Phenolic compounds	0.5%-3%	Intermediate to low
Iodophor compounds	30-50 mg of free iodine/liter; up to 10,000 mg of available iodine/liter	Intermediate to low
Quaternary ammonium compounds	0.1%-0.2%	Low
Antisepsis		
Alcohols (ethyl, isopropyl)	70%	
Iodophors	1-2 mg of free iodine/liter; 1%-2% available iodine	
Chlorhexidine	0.75%-4%	
Hexachlorophene	1%-3%	
Parachlorometaxylenol	0.5%-4%	

From Favero M, Bond W.: Sterilization, disinfection, and antisepsis in the hospital. In Balows A, Hausler WJ Jr, Herrmann KL et al., editors: *Manual of clinical microbiology*, ed 5, Washington, DC, 1991, American Society for Microbiology.

or instruments in which contamination with bacterial spores and other highly resilient organisms is unlikely. These have been referred to as semicritical instruments and devices and include flexible fiberoptic endoscopes, laryngoscopes, vaginal specula, anesthesia breathing circuits, and so forth. Low-level disinfectants are used to treat noncritical instruments and devices such as blood culture cuffs, electrocardiogram electrodes, and stethoscopes. Although these items come into contact with patients, they do not penetrate through mucosal surfaces or into sterile tissues.

The level of disinfectants that are used for environmental surfaces is determined by the relative risk these surfaces pose as a reservoir for pathogenic organisms. For example, a higher level of disinfectant should be used to clean the surface of instruments contaminated with blood than those surfaces that are "dirty," such as floors, sinks, and countertops. The exception to this rule is if a particular surface has been implicated in a nosocomial infection, such as a bathroom contaminated with *Clostridium difficile* (spore-forming anaerobic bacterium) or a sink contaminated with *Pseudomonas aeruginosa.* In these cases a disinfectant with appropriate activity against the implicated pathogen should be selected.

MECHANISMS OF ACTION

The following section will briefly review the mechanism(s) by which the most common sterilants, disinfectants, and antiseptics work.

Moist Heat

Attempts to sterilize items using boiling water are inefficient because only a relatively low temperature (100° C) can be maintained. Indeed, spore formation by a bacterium is commonly demonstrated by boiling a solution of organisms and then subculturing the solution. Vegetative organisms are killed by boiling, but the spores remain viable. If organisms grow on the subculture plate, then the bacteria were capable of sporulating. In contrast with boiling, steam under pressure in an autoclave is a very effective form of sterilization; the higher temperature causes denaturation of microbial proteins. The rate of killing organisms during the autoclave process is rapid but will be influenced by the temperature and duration of autoclaving, size of the autoclave and flow rate of the steam, density and size of the load, and placement of the load in the chamber. Care must be used to avoid creating air pockets, which will inhibit penetration of the steam into the load. In general most autoclaves are operated at 121° C to 132° C for 15 minutes or longer. The effectiveness of sterilization can be monitored by including commercial preparations of *Bacillus stearothemophilus* spores. An ampule of these spores is placed in the center of the load, removed at the end of the autoclave process, and incubated at 37° C. If the sterilization process was successful, the organisms will fail to sporulate and will not grow.

Dry Heat

Hot air can also be used to sterilize items such as glassware. This is not as efficient as with moist air because diffusion and penetration of heat is slow, long sterilization periods and high temperatures are required, materials can be damaged by the oxidation process of this prolonged heating, and dry heat tends to stratify in the processing chamber. Sterilization requires processing for 1 hour at 171° C, 2 hours at 160° C, or 16 hours at 121° C. Effectiveness is monitored with spore tests using *Bacillus subtilis,* which is relatively resistant to killing by dry air (in contrast with *Bacillus stearothermophilus*).

Ethylene Oxide

Ethylene oxide is a colorless gas, soluble in water and common organic solvents, that is used to sterilize items that are heat sensitive. The sterilization process is relatively slow and influenced by concentration of gas, relative humidity and moisture content of the item to be sterilized, exposure time, and temperature. The exposure time is reduced by 50% for each doubling of ethylene oxide concentration. Likewise, the activity of ethylene oxide approximately doubles with each 10° C temperature increase. Sterilization with ethylene oxide is optimum in a relative humidity of approximately 30%, with decreased activity at higher or lower humidity. This is particularly problematic if the contaminated organisms are dried onto a surface or lyophilized. Ethylene oxide exerts its sporicidal activity through the alkylation of terminal hydroxyl, carboxyl, amino, and sulfhydryl groups. This process blocks the reactive groups required for many essential metabolic processes. Examples of other strong alkylating gases used as sterilants are formaldehyde and beta-propiolactone. Because ethylene oxide can damage viable tissues, the gas must be dissipated before the item can be used. This aeration period is generally 24 hours or longer. The effectiveness of sterilization is monitored with the *Bacillus subtilis* spore test.

Aldehydes

As with ethylene oxide, the aldehydes exert their effect through alkylation. The two best known aldehydes are formaldehyde and glutaraldehyde, both of which can be used as sterilants or high-level disinfectants. **Formaldehyde** gas can be dissolved in water (called formalin) at a final concentration of 37%. Stabilizers such as methanol are added to formalin. Low concentrations of formalin are bacteriostatic (inhibit but don't kill organisms), whereas higher concentrations (e.g., 20%) can kill all organisms. This microbicidal activity can be enhanced by combining formaldehyde with alcohol (e.g., 20% formalin in 70% alcohol). Exposure of skin or mucous membranes to formaldehyde can be toxic. **Glutaraldehyde** is less toxic for viable tissues, but it can still cause burns on the skin or mucous membranes. Glutaraldehyde is more active at alkaline pHs ("activated" by sodium hydroxide) but less stable. Glutaraldehyde is also inactivated by organic material so items to be treated must first be cleaned.

Oxidizing Agents

Examples of oxidants include ozone, peracetic acid, and hydrogen peroxide, with the latter used most commonly. **Hydrogen peroxide** effectively kills most bacteria at a concentration of 3% to 6% and kills all organisms including spores at higher concentrations (10% to 25%). The active oxidant form is not hydrogen peroxide but rather the free hydroxyl radical formed by the decomposition of hydrogen peroxide. Hydrogen peroxide is used to disinfect plastic implants, contact lenses, and surgical prostheses.

Halogens

Halogens, such as compounds containing iodine or chlorine, are extensively used as disinfectants.

Iodine compounds are the most effective halogens available for disinfection. Iodine is a highly reactive element that precipitates proteins and oxidizes essential enzymes. It is microbicidal against virtually all organisms including spore-forming bacteria and mycobacteria. Neither the concentration of iodine nor the pH of the iodine solution affect the microbicidal activity, although the efficiency of iodine solutions is increased in acid solutions because more free iodine is liberated. Iodine acts more rapidly than other halogen compounds or quaternary ammonium compounds. However, the activity of iodine can be reduced in the presence of some organic and inorganic compounds, including serum, feces, ascitic fluid, sputum, urine, sodium thiosulfate, and ammonia. Thus skin surfaces must be cleaned before iodine compounds are used as a disinfectant. Elemental iodine can be dissolved in aqueous potassium iodide or alcohol, or complexed with a carrier. The latter compound is referred to as an **iodophor** (iodo-iodine and phor-carrier). Povidone iodine (iodine complexed with polyvinylpyrrolidone) is used most commonly, relatively stable and nontoxic to tissues and metal surfaces, but expensive compared with other iodine solutions.

Chlorine compounds are also used extensively as disinfectants. Aqueous solutions of chlorine are rapidly bactericidal, although their mechanism(s) of action are not defined. Three forms of chlorine may be present in water: elemental chlorine (Cl_2), which is a very strong oxidizing agent, hypochlorous acid (HOCl), and hypochlorite ion (OCl^-). Chlorine will also combine with ammonia and other nitrogenous compounds to form chloramines or *N*-chloro compounds. Chlorine can exert its effect by the irreversible oxidation of SH groups of essential enzymes. Hypochlorites are believed to interact with cytoplasmic components to form toxic *N*-chloro compounds, which interfere with cellular metabolism. The efficacy of chlorine is inversely proportional to the pH, with greater activity observed at acid pHs. This is consistent with greater activity associated with hypochlorous acid rather than hypochlorite ion concentration. The activity of chlorine compounds also increases with concentration (e.g., a twofold increase in concentration results in a 30% decrease in time required for killing) and temperature (e.g., a 50% to 65% reduction in killing time with a 10° C increase in temperature). Organic matter and alkaline detergents can reduce the effectiveness of chlorine compounds. These compounds demonstrate good germicidal activity, although spore-forming organisms are tenfold to a thousandfold more resistant to chlorine than vegetative bacteria.

Phenolic Compounds

These germicides are rarely used now as a disinfectant. However, they are of historical interest because they were used as a comparative standard for assessing the activity of other germicidal compounds. The ratio of germicidal activity by a test compound to that by a specified concentration of phenol yielded the **phenol coefficient.** A value of 1 indicated equivalent activity, greater than 1 indicated activity less than phenol, and less than 1 indicated activity greater than phenol. These tests are limited by the fact that phenol is not sporicidal at room temperature (but is at temperatures approaching 100° C) and has poor activity against nonlipid-containing viruses. This is understandable because phenol is believed to act by disrupting lipid-containing membranes, resulting in leakage of cellular contents. Phenolic compounds are active against the normally resilient mycobacteria because the cell wall of these organisms has a very high concentration of lipids. Exposure of phenolics to alkaline compounds significantly reduces their activity, whereas halogenation of the phenolics enhances their activity. Introduction of aliphatic or aromatic groups into the nucleus of halogen phenols also increases their activity. **Bis-phenols** are two phenol compounds linked together. The activity of these compounds can also be potentiated by halogenation. One example of a halogenated bisphenol is hexachlorophene, an antiseptic with activity against gram-positive bacteria.

Quaternary Ammonium Compounds

These compounds consist of four organic groups covalently linked to nitrogen. Germicidal activity of these cationic compounds is determined by the nature of the organic groups, with the greatest activity observed with compounds with 8 to 18 carbon long groups. Examples of quaternary ammonium compounds include benzalkonium chloride and cetylpyridinium chloride. These compounds act by denaturing cell membranes to release the intracellular components. Quaternary ammonium compounds are bacteriostatic at low concentration, bactericidal at high concentrations. However, organisms such as *Pseudomonas, Mycobacterium,* and the fungus *Trichophyton* among others are resistant to these compounds. Indeed, some *Pseudomonas* strains can grow readily in quaternary ammonium solutions. Many viruses and all bacterial spores are also resistant. Quaternary ammonium compounds are neutralized by ionic detergents, organic matter, and dilution.

Alcohols

The germicidal activity of alcohols increases with increasing chain length (maximum of 5 to 8 carbons). The two most commonly used alcohols are ethanol and isopropanol. These are rapidly bactericidal against vegetative bacteria, mycobacteria, some fungi, and lipid-containing viruses. Unfortunately, alcohols have no activity against bacterial spores, and poor activity against some fungi and non–lipid-containing viruses. Activity is greater in the presence of water. Thus 70% alcohol is more active than 95% alcohol. Alcohol is a common disinfectant used for skin surfaces and, when followed by treatment with an iodophor, is extremely effective for this purpose. Alcohols are also used to disinfect items such as thermometers.

QUESTIONS

1. Define the following terms and give examples of each: sterilization, disinfection, antisepsis, germicide, sporicide.
2. Define the three levels of disinfection and give examples of each. When world each type of disinfectant be used?
3. What factors influence the effectiveness of sterilization with moist heat, dry heat, and with ethylene oxide?
4. Give examples of each of the following disinfectants and their mode of action: iodine compounds, chlorine compounds, phenolic compounds, and quarternary ammonium compounds.

Bibliography

Block SS: *Disinfection, sterilization, and preservation,* ed 2, Philadelphia, 1977, Lea & Febiger.

Favero M and Bond W: Sterilization, disinfection, and antisepsis in the hospital, 1991. In Balows A, Hausler W Jr, Herrmann K, Isenberg H, and Shadomy HJ, editors: *Manual of clinical microbiology,* ed 5, Washington, DC, American Society for Microbiology.

Wingard L, Brody T, Larner J, and Schwartz A, editors: *Human pharmacology: molecular to clinical,* St. Louis, 1991, Mosby.

CHAPTER 13

Chemotherapy of Bacterial Infections

THIS chapter will provide an overview of the mechanisms of action and antibacterial spectrum of the most commonly used antibiotics, as well as common mechanisms of bacterial resistance. Terminology appropriate for this discussion is summarized in Box 13-1. For additional information about specific antibiotics, consult the textbooks by Lorian and by Wingard et al. listed in the Bibliography.

An important year in chemotherapy of systemic bacterial infections was 1935. Although antiseptics had been applied topically to prevent growth of microorganisms, systemic bacterial infections did not respond to any existing agents. In 1935 the red azo dye *protosil* was shown to protect mice against systemic streptococcal infection and was curative in patients suffering from such infections. It was soon demonstrated that protosil was cleaved in the body to release *p*-aminobenzenesulfonamide, or sulfanilamide, which was subsequently shown to have antibacterial activity. These observations with the first sulfa drug initiated a new era in medicine. Compounds (antibiotics) produced by microorganisms were eventually discovered to inhibit the growth of other microorganisms. Fleming first noted that the mold *Penicillium* prevented the multiplication of staphylococci. A concentrate from a culture of this mold was prepared, and the remarkable activity and lack of toxicity of the first antibiotic, penicillin, was demonstrated. Later, in the 1940s and 1950s, streptomycin and the tetracyclines were developed and were followed rapidly by additional aminoglycosides, semisynthetic penicillins, cephalosporins, quinolones and other antimicrobials. All greatly increased the range and effectiveness of antibacterial agents.

Despite the rapidity with which new chemotherapeutic agents are introduced, bacteria have shown a remarkable ability to develop resistance to these agents. Thus antibiotic therapy will not be the predicted magic bullet against infections but rather one weapon, albeit an important one, against infectious diseases. It is also important to recognize that because resistance to antibiotics is frequently not predictable, the physician must rely

BOX 13-1 Terminology

Antibacterial spectrum	Range of activity of a compound against microorganisms. A **broad-spectrum** antibacterial drug can inhibit a wide variety of both gram-positive and gram-negative bacteria, whereas a **narrow spectrum** drug is active only against selected organisms.
Antimicrobial (bacteriostatic) activity	Activity of a chemotherapeutic agent tested in the laboratory and expressed as the lowest concentration at which the drug inhibits multiplication of the microorganism (minimum inhibitory concentration, or **MIC**).
Bactericidal activity	Ability of a chemotherapeutic agent to kill a microorganism; expressed as the minimum bactericidal concentration (**MBC**).
Antibiotic combinations	Combinations of antibiotics may be used (1) to broaden the antibacterial spectrum in presumed mixed infections pending culture results, (2) to prevent emergence of resistant organisms during therapy, and (3) for a synergistic killing effect.
Antibiotic synergism	Combination of two antibiotics (e.g., penicillin and streptomycin) that have enhanced bactericidal activity when tested together compared with each alone.
Antibiotic antagonism	Situation in which one antibiotic interferes with the killing action of another antibiotic.
β-lactamase	An enzyme that breaks β-lactam ring in penicillins (**penicillinase**) or cephalosporins (**cephalosporinase**). Hydrolysis of the ring protects the bacteria from the antimicrobial activity of the antibiotic.

on clinical experience for the initial selection of empirical therapy. Guidelines for the management of infections caused by specific organisms will be discussed in the relevant chapters of this text.

The results of in vitro antimicrobial susceptibility testing are valuable for selecting chemotherapeutic agents active against the infecting organism. Please refer to the Bibliography for additional information regarding methods for performing these laboratory tests. Extensive work has been performed to standardize the testing methods and improve the clinical predictive value of the results. Despite these efforts, the in vitro tests are simply a measurement of the effect of the antibiotic against the organism. Selection of an antibiotic and the patient's outcome are influenced by a variety of interrelated factors, including the pharmacokinetic properties of the antibiotic, drug toxicity, and the patient's general medical status.

The five basic sites of antibiotic activity are summarized in Box 13-2.

INHIBITION OF CELL WALL SYNTHESIS

By far the most common site of antibiotic activity is interference with bacterial cell wall synthesis. The majority of the cell wall active antibiotics are classified as β-lactam antibiotics (e.g., penicillins, cephalosporins, cephamycins, carbapenems, monobactams, and β-lactamase inhibitors), so named because they share a common β-lactam ring structure (Figure 13-1). Other antibiotics that interfere with construction of the bacterial cell wall include vancomycin, bacitracin, and the antimycobacterial agents isoniazid, cycloserine, and ethionamide.

BOX 13-2 Basic Mechanisms of Antibiotic Action

Inhibition of cell wall synthesis
- Penicillins
- Cephalosporins
- Cephamycins
- Carbapenems
- Monobactams
- β-lactamase inhibitors
- Vancomycin
- Bacitracin
- Isoniazid
- Cycloserine
- Ethionamide

Alteration of cell membranes
- Polymyxins

Inhibition of protein synthesis
- Aminoglycosides
- Tetracyclines
- Chloramphenicol
- Macrolides
- Clindamycin

Inhibition of nucleic acid synthesis
- Rifampin
- Quinolones
- Metronidazole

Antimetabolites
- Sulfonamides
- Trimethoprim
- Dapsone

β-Lactam Antibiotics

Mode of Action

Synthesis of the bacterial cell wall is catalyzed by specific enzymes (e.g., transpeptidases, carboxypeptidases, and endopeptidases). These regulatory proteins are also called penicillin binding proteins (PBPs) because they can be bound by β-lactam antibiotics (Figure 13-2). When growing bacteria are exposed to these antibiotics, the antibiotic binds to the PBPs in the cell membrane, synthesis of the cell wall peptidoglycan layer is inhibited, and autolytic enzymes are released that degrade the preformed cell wall, resulting in bacterial cell death (Figure 13-3). Thus the β-lactam antibiotics generally act as bactericidal agents.

Spectrum of Activity

Penicillins. Penicillin compounds are highly effective antibiotics with extremely low toxicity. The base compound is an organic acid with a β-lactam ring (see Figure 13-1) obtained from culture of the mold *Penicillium chrysogenum*. If the mold is grown by a fermentation process, large amounts of a key intermediate, 6-aminopenicillanic acid, are produced. Biochemical substitution of this intermediate yields derivatives (Box 13-3) that have decreased acid lability and thus increased gastrointestinal absorption, resistance to destruction by penicillinase, or a widening of the spectrum so that gram-negative organisms are susceptible to the compound.

Penicillin G is incompletely absorbed because it is inactivated by gastric acid. Thus it is used mainly as an intravenous drug for serious infections with penicillin-sensitive organisms (e.g., streptococci, gonococcus). Penicillin V is more resistant to acid and is the preferred oral form for treatment of susceptible streptococci. Penicillinase-resistant penicillins such as nafcillin and cloxacillin are used to treat infections caused by penicillinase-producing staphylococci. Ampicillin was the first penicillin active against gram-negative bacilli, although the spectrum was limited. However, parenteral penicillins (e.g., carbenicillin, ticarcillin, piperacillin) have been now been developed that can be effective against a broad spectrum of gram-negative bacteria including *Klebsiella*, *Enterobacter*, and *Pseudomonas*.

Cephalosporins and Cephamycins. The cephalosporins (see Figure 13-1) are β-lactam antibiotics derived from 7-aminocephalosporanic acid, which was originally isolated for a *Cephalosporium* mold. The cephamycins are closely related to the cephalosporins, except that cephamycins contain oxygen in place of sulfur in the dihydrothiazine ring, rendering the antibiotics more stable to β-lactamase hydrolysis. The cephalosporins and cephamycins have the same mechanism of action as the penicillins but have a wider antibacterial spectrum, are resistant to many β-lactamases, and have improved pharmacokinetic properties.

Biochemical modification of the basic antibiotic molecules results in significant improvements in antibiotic activity and pharmacokinetic properties. The activity of the first-generation antibiotics is similar to that of ampicillin (Table 13-1). Many of the second-generation antibiotics (e.g., cefaclor) have expanded activity to include *Haemophilus influenzae,* an important pediatric pathogen, and cefoxitin and cefotetan are active against *Bacteroides fragilis*, an important anaerobic pathogen. The third-generation antibiotics further extend the antibacterial spectrum to include virtually all Enterobacteriaceae and *Pseudomonas aeruginosa*.

Unfortunately, with these refinements the second- and third-generation antibiotics were frequently less active against gram-positive cocci. Furthermore, all cephalosporin-type antibiotics are ineffective against penicillin-resistant *Streptococcus pneumoniae,* methicillin-resistant *Staphylococcus*, as well as *Enterococcus*, and *Listeria*. In addition, organisms such as *Enterobacter, Serratia,* and *Pseudomonas* can develop resistance during therapy with the cephalosporins and then display cross-resistance to all β-lactam antibiotics.

Other β-Lactam Antibiotics. Several β-lactam antibiotics have slightly different biochemical structures from the penicillins and cephalosporins but have similar potent antibacterial activity. Imipenem is a **carbapenem** with excellent in vitro and in vivo activity against aerobic and anaerobic gram-positive and gram-negative bacteria. Aztreonam, a **monobactam**, is a narrow-spectrum antibiotic with activity specific for gram-negative bacilli (e.g., Enterobacteriaceae, *Pseudomonas*). Finally, **β-lactamase inhibitors** (e.g., clavulanic acid, sulbactam) are relatively inactive by themselves but have been combined with some penicillins (e.g., ampicillin, amoxicillin, ticarcillin) to treat infections caused by β-lactamase producing bacteria. This latter group of antibiotics will irreversibly bind and inactivate bacterial β-lactamases, permitting the companion drug to enter the cell and disrupt bacterial cell wall synthesis.

Mechanisms of Resistance

Three general mechanisms of resistance occur (Figure 13-4): failure of the antibiotic to penetrate through the outer membrane, failure to bind to the target site (penicillin binding proteins), and hydrolysis of the antibiotic by β-lactamases. Examples of all three mecha-

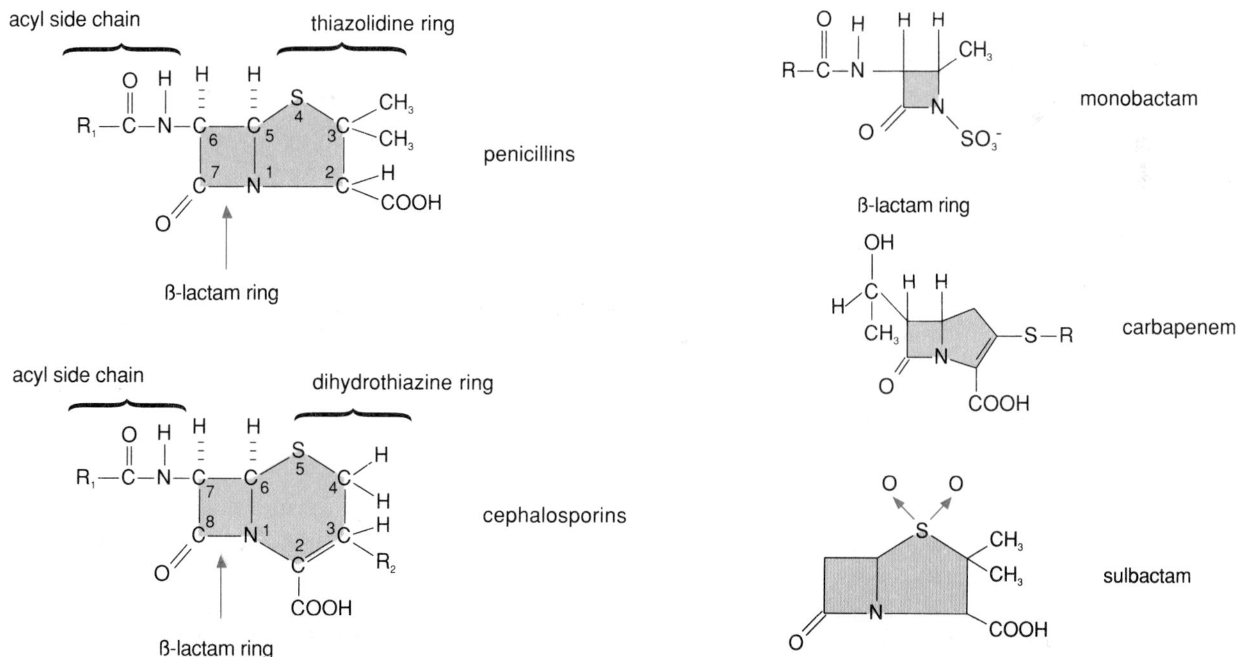

FIGURE 13-1 General structures of the main classes of β-lactam antibiotics. Additional variations are possible at some of the non-R group positions. For example, the cephamycins and cephalosporins differ by replacing the sulfur molecule at the 5 position with oxygen. The arrow points to the bond that is broken during β-lactamase catalyzed hydrolysis. (Modified from Wingard LB, Brody TM, Larner J, et al., editors: *Human pharmacology: molecular to clinical*, St. Louis, 1991, Mosby.)

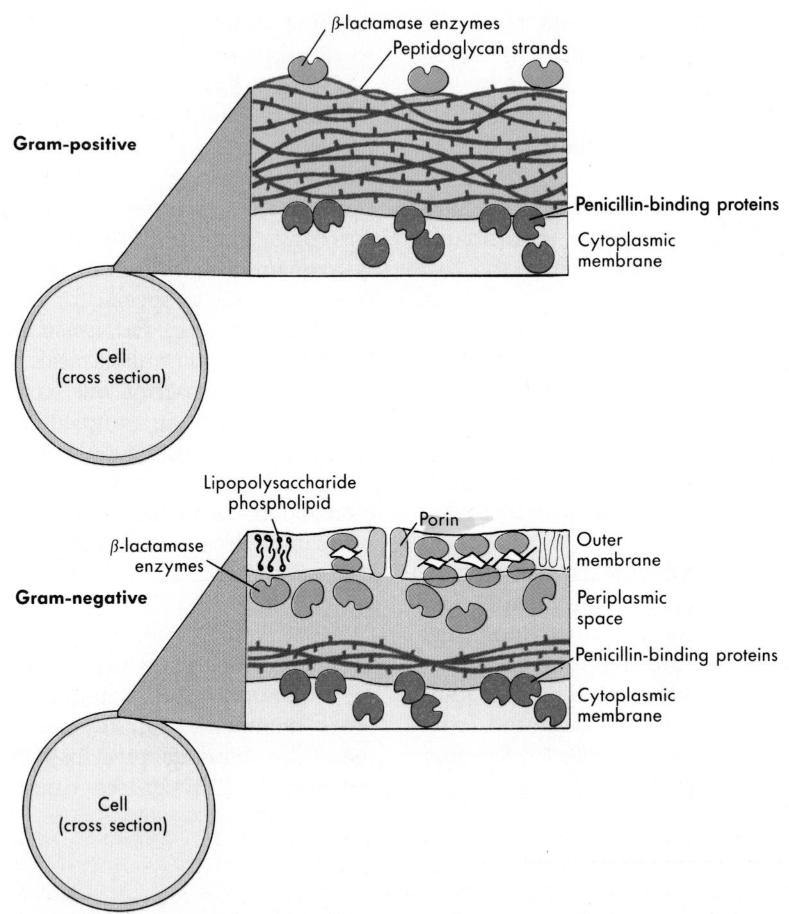

FIGURE 13-2 Cell wall structure of gram-positive and gram-negative bacteria. The β-lactam antibiotics act by inhibiting the synthesis of the rigid peptidoglycan part of the cell wall. The bacteria can protect themselves from some of these antibiotics by production of β-lactamase, enzymes which can hydrolyze the β-lactam ring. (Modified from Wingard LB, Brody TM, Larner J, et al., *Human pharmacology: molecular to clinical*, St. Louis, 1991, Mosby.)

nisms are well recognized. Penetration of β-lactams into gram-negative bacilli requires transit through the porin channels in the outer membrane. Mutation of the porin proteins can render the organism resistant to the β-lactam antibiotic (e.g., resistance of *Pseudomonas aeruginosa* to imipenem). Likewise, mutation in the penicillin binding proteins can lead to antibiotic resistance. This mechanism is responsible for oxacillin resistance in staphylococci and penicillin resistance in *Streptococcus pneumoniae*. Despite the initial success of penicillin G against staphylococci, resistance mediated by β-lactamase hydrolysis developed rapidly. Unfortunately this resistance was not restricted to the early β-lactam antibiotics. Simple point mutations in the genes for the initial β-lactamases (enzymes with a narrow spectrum of activity and present in many bacteria) have now rendered these enzymes active against most penicillins and cephalosporins, including the broad spectrum agents. Because these potent β-lactamases are present on plasmids and can be exchanged among bacterial species, the utility of β-lactam antibiotics may be severely limited in the future.

Vancomycin: Mode of Action, Spectrum of Activity, and Mechanisms of Resistance

Vancomycin, obtained from an actinomycete, is a complex glycopeptide that interferes with cell wall synthesis in growing gram-positive bacteria. Vancomycin acts by sterically interfering with elongation of the peptidoglycan chain by interacting with the terminal D-alanyl-D-alanine present on the pentapeptide side chains of the peptidoglycan precursors. Vancomycin is inactive against gram-negative bacteria because the molecule is too large to pass through the outer membrane and reach the peptidoglycan target site.

Vancomycin is used for the management of infections with oxacillin-resistant staphylococci, *Clostridium difficile*, and other gram-positive bacteria that are resistant to β-lactam antibiotics. Resistance among gram-positive bacteria is uncommon but has been reported for *Leuconostoc, Lactobacillus, Pediococcus, Erysipelothrix,* and for rare isolates of *Enterococcus* and *Staphylococcus*. Vancomycin resistance occurs in bacteria with alterations of the terminal side chain (presence of L-alanine rather than

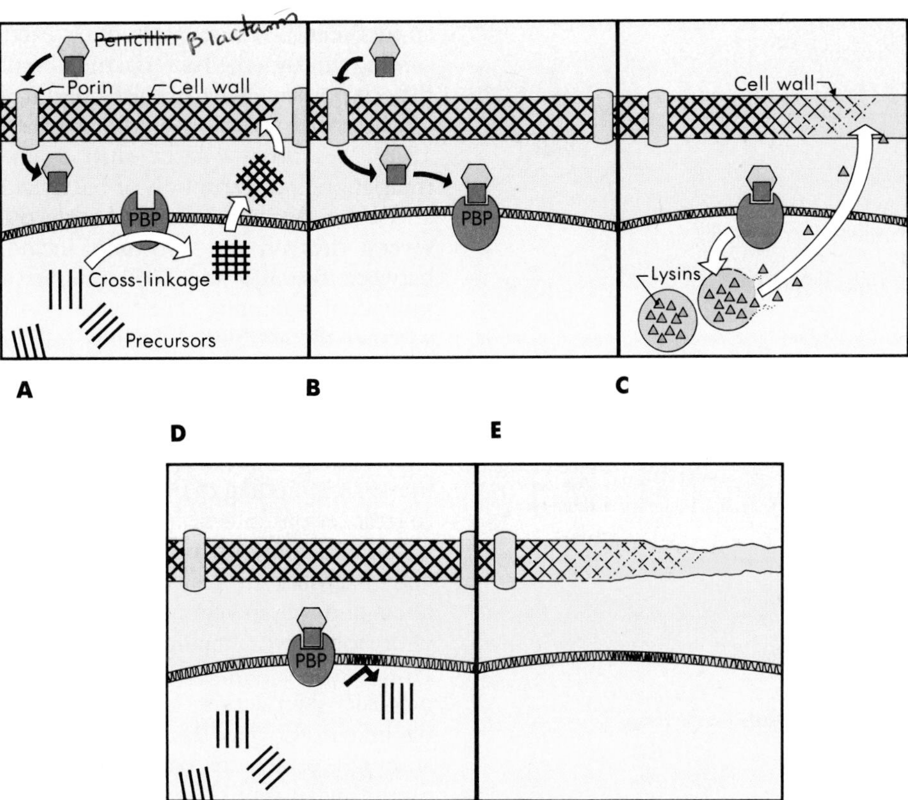

FIGURE 13-3 Inhibition of cell wall synthesis. **A,** Precursors are cross-linked by the enzymatic action of penicillin binding proteins (PBP) and then added to the cell wall. **B,** The β-lactam enters the cell and binds to PBP. **C,** Binding leads to release of autolysins, which break down preformed cell wall. **D,** After β-lactams bind to PBP, PBP can no longer catalyze cell wall synthesis. **E,** Cell wall loses integrity and can no longer preserve osmotic pressure.

L-alanine) or in strains producing a protein that interferes with vancomycin binding to its target site.

Bacitracin: Mode of Action, Spectrum of Activity, and Mechanism of Resistance

Bacitracin, another cell wall–active antibiotic, is a mixture of polypeptides used topically for skin infections caused by gram-positive bacteria. It inhibits cell wall synthesis by interfering with dephosphorylation of the lipid carrier responsible for moving the peptidoglycan precursors through the cytoplasmic membrane to the cell wall. It may also damage the bacterial cytoplasmic membrane and inhibit RNA transcription. Resistance is most likely due to failure of the antibiotic to penetrate into the bacterial cell.

Cycloserine, Ethionamide, and Isoniazid: Modes of Action, Spectrum of Activity, and Mechanisms of Resistance

Cycloserine, ethionamide, and isoniazid are antibiotics useful for the management of some mycobacterial infections. Cycloserine inhibits two enzymes that catalyze cell wall synthesis, D-alanyl-D-alanine synthetase and alanine racemase. Ethionamide and isoniazid interfere with mycobacterial replication at multiple levels. Although these drugs inhibit synthesis of cell wall components, the exact mode of action has not been defined. Resistance is mediated by either reduced drug uptake into the bacterial cell or alteration of the target sites.

BOX 13-3 Penicillins With Improved Pharmacokinetic Properties or Enhanced Antimicrobial Spectrum

Acid-Stable Pencillins
Penicillin V, ampicillin, amoxicillin
Pencillinase-Resistant Penicillins
Nafcillin, oxacillin, methicillin, dicloxacillin, cloxacillin
Enhanced Spectrum of Activity
Carbenicillin, ticarcillin, mezlocillin, piperacillin

ALTERATION OF CELL MEMBRANES

Another mechanism of antibiotic action is alteration of the bacterial cell membranes. The polymyxin class of

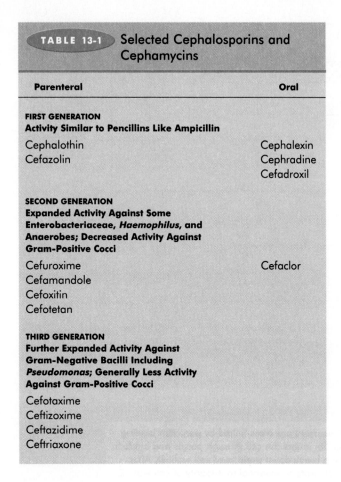

TABLE 13-1 Selected Cephalosporins and Cephamycins

Parenteral	Oral
FIRST GENERATION	
Activity Similar to Pencillins Like Ampicillin	
Cephalothin	Cephalexin
Cefazolin	Cephradine
	Cefadroxil
SECOND GENERATION	
Expanded Activity Against Some Enterobacteriaceae, *Haemophilus*, and Anaerobes; Decreased Activity Against Gram-Positive Cocci	
Cefuroxime	Cefaclor
Cefamandole	
Cefoxitin	
Cefotetan	
THIRD GENERATION	
Further Expanded Activity Against Gram-Negative Bacilli Including *Pseudomonas*; Generally Less Activity Against Gram-Positive Cocci	
Cefotaxime	
Ceftizoxime	
Ceftazidime	
Ceftriaxone	

antibiotics is an important example of this activity. These antibiotics consist of cationic branched cyclic decapeptides that destroy the cytoplasmic membranes of susceptible bacteria (Figure 13-5). Members of this class of antibiotics include polymyxin B and colistin. These antibiotics are active against gram-negative bacteria; however, serious nephrotoxicity has limited their use chiefly to the external treatment of localized infections such as external otitis, eye infections, and skin infections with sensitive organisms. The detergent-like activity of the polymyxins is prevented when the antibiotic is unable to penetrate through the outer cell wall to the inner cytoplasmic membrane. Other antibiotics acting on the cell membrane include the antifungal polyene antibiotics (e.g., amphotericin B, nystatin), which are discussed in Chapter 14.

INHIBITION OF PROTEIN SYNTHESIS

The second largest class of antibiotics consists of those whose primary action is to inhibit protein synthesis (see Box 13-2 for examples).

Aminoglycosides: Modes of Action

The aminoglycoside antibiotics (Box 13-4) consist of aminosugars linked through glycosidic bonds to an aminocyclitol. These antibiotics exert their effect by passing through the bacterial membranes and cell wall to the cytoplasm, where they inhibit bacterial protein synthesis by irreversibly binding to the ribosomes (Figure 13-6). Secondary effects, such as induction of faulty translation and disruption of bacterial membranes, have also been documented. Aminoglycosides can bind to several sites on the ribosome, including the interface between the 30S and 50S subunits as well as to the individual subunits. The binding site will influence whether the antibiotic prevents polysome formation or misreading of the mRNA.

Aminoglycosides: Spectrum of Activity

The aminoglycosides are bactericidal antibiotics due to irreversible binding to ribosomes and are commonly used to treat serious infections caused by many gram-negative bacilli and some gram-positive organisms. Streptococci and anaerobes are resistant to aminoglycosides. Gentamicin and tobramycin have a broad spectrum of activity, with tobramycin being slightly more active against *Pseudomonas aeruginosa*. Netilmicin is reported to be less ototoxic than either gentamicin or tobramycin, but netilmicin also has less antibacterial activity. All three aminoglycosides are used to treat systemic infections caused by susceptible gram-negative bacteria, including the Enterobacteriaceae and *Pseudomonas*. Because enzymatic modification of amikacin is rare, this aminoglycoside is used to treat infections caused by gram-negative bacteria that are resistant to other aminoglycosides. Streptomycin has been used for the treatment of tuberculosis, tularemia, and streptococcal endocarditis (when combined with a penicillin). Although kanamycin was one of the first aminoglycosides with broad activity against gram-negative bacteria, it is now rarely used because it is inactive against *Pseudomonas*.

Mechanisms of Resistance

Resistance to the antibacterial action of aminoglycosides can develop in one of three ways: mutation of the ribosome binding site, decreased antibiotic uptake into the bacterial cell, and enzymatic modification (e.g., acetylation, phosphorylation) of the antibiotic. Resistance caused by alteration of the bacterial ribosome is relatively uncommon, except in members of the genus *Enterococcus*. Because the synergistic combination of an aminoglycoside with a cell wall–active antibiotic is required for the killing of these important gram-positive cocci, this resistance is clinically significant. Resistance caused by inhibition of transport into the bacterial cell is occasionally observed with *Pseudomonas* but more commonly seen with anaerobic bacteria. This is because aminoglycoside uptake by the cell is oxygen dependent. Enzymatic phosphorylation, adenylation, or acetylation of the amino and hydroxyl groups of the aminoglycoside are the most common mechanisms of resistance. The differences in antibacterial activity among the aminoglycosides are due to their relative susceptibility to these enzymes.

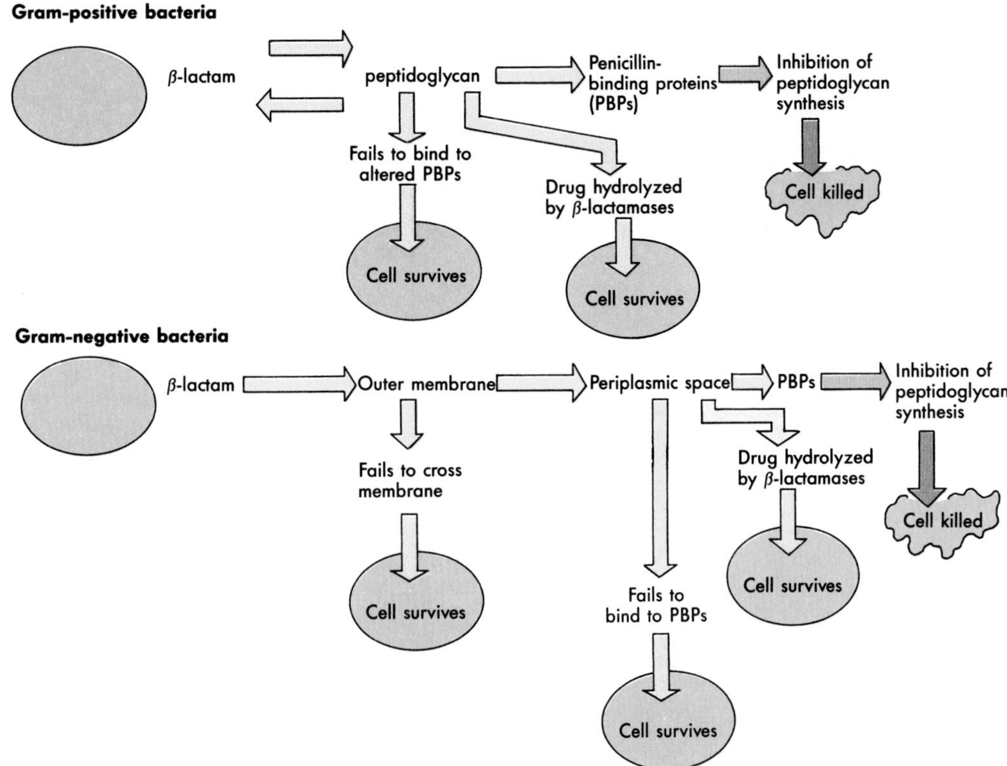

FIGURE 13-4 Mechanisms of resistance to β-lactam antibiotics. (Modified from Wingard LB, Brody TM, Larner J, et al., editors: *Human pharmacology: molecular to clinical*, St. Louis, 1991, Mosby.)

Tetracyclines: Mode of Action, Spectrum of Activity, and Mechanisms of Resistance

The tetracycline antibiotics (e.g., tetracycline, minocycline, doxycycline) are broad-spectrum, bacteriostatic antibiotics that inhibit protein synthesis in bacteria by blocking the binding of tRNA to the 30S ribosomal subunit (Figure 13-6). Because the interaction between antibiotic and ribosome is weak, tetracycline antibiotics are bacteriostatic. Tetracyclines are effective in treatment of *Mycoplasma pneumoniae* infections, cholera, rickettsial disease, brucellosis, chlamydial urethritis, as well as gonorrhea, uncomplicated urinary tract infections, and acne.

Resistance to the tetracyclines is primarily due to increased efflux of the antibiotic from the cell. The gene encoding for this mechanism is on a transferable plasmid. Less commonly, resistance can also be the result of chromosomally mediated alteration of the cell surface proteins.

Chloramphenicol: Mode of Action, Spectrum of Activity, and Mechanisms of Resistance

Chloramphenicol has a broad antibacterial spectrum similar to that of tetracycline but is considered the drug of choice only for treatment of typhoid fever. The reason is that, in addition to interfering with bacterial protein synthesis, chloramphenicol disrupts protein synthesis in human bone marrow cells and can produce blood dyscrasias such as aplastic anemia (1 case per 24,000 treated patients). Chloramphenicol exerts its effect on bacterial protein synthesis by binding to the 50S subunit and blocking peptide bond formation (see Figure 13-6). Resistance to chloramphenicol is observed in bacteria producing chloramphenicol acetyltransferase, which catalyzes acetylation of the 3-hydroxy group of chloramphenicol. Less commonly resistant strains have altered permeability or ribosomal proteins.

Macrolides: Mode of Action, Spectrum of Activity, and Mechanism of Resistance

Erythromycin, a macrolide antibiotic, is a bacteriostatic organic base used mainly to treat pulmonary infections caused by *Mycoplasma*, *Legionella*, *Chlamydia*, *Campylobacter*, and gram-positive organisms in patients allergic to penicillin. The antibiotic disrupts protein synthesis by binding to the 50S ribosomal subunit. Bacterial resistance to erythromycin develops by modification of ribosomal 23S RNA, which in turn prevents binding by the antibiotic. Modification of the macrolide structure has led to the development of newer agents including azithromycin and clarithromycin. These macrolides are notewor-

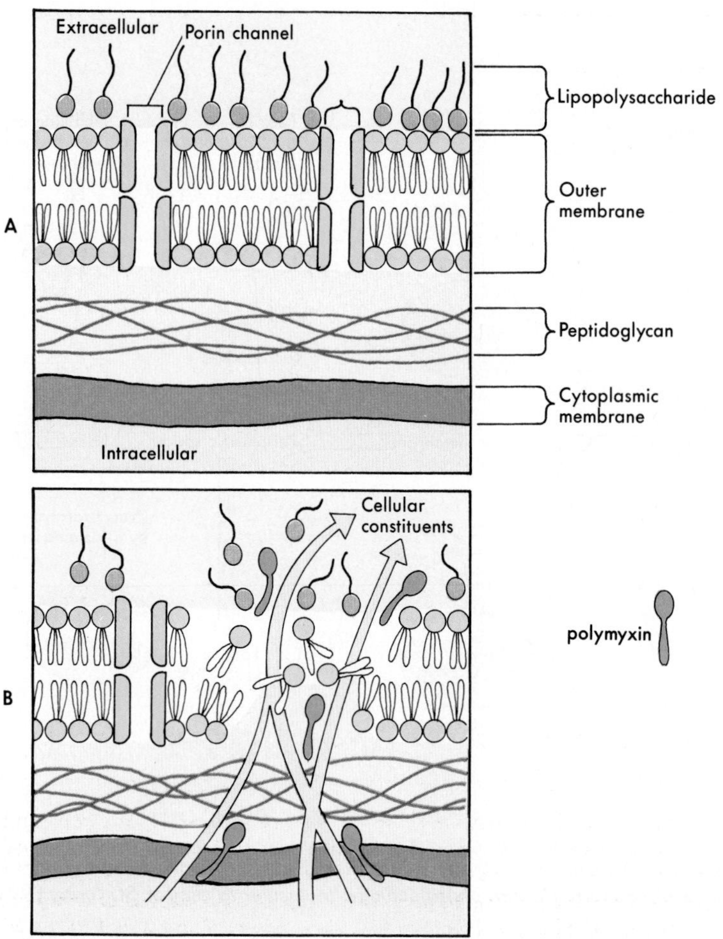

FIGURE 13-5 Mechanism of action of polymyxin. **A** illustrates the normal structure of the cell wall of gram-negative bacteria. **B** illustrates the disruption of the cytoplasmic membrane after exposure to polymyxin. (From Wingard LB, Brody TM, Larner J, et al., editors: *Human pharmacology: molecular to clinical*, St. Louis, 1991, Mosby).

BOX 13-4 Aminoglycosides

Streptomycin	Tobramycin
Kanamycin	Amikacin
Gentamicin	Netilmicin

thy because they have better pharmacological properties, as well as improved antibacterial activity.

Clindamycin: Mode of Action, Spectrum of Activity, and Mechanisms of Resistance

Clindamycin, like chloramphenicol and the macrolides, blocks protein synthesis by binding to the 50S ribosome. It inhibits peptidyl transferase by interfering with binding of the amino acid-acyl-tRNA complex. Clindamycin is active against staphylococci and anaerobic gram-negative bacilli but generally inactive against aerobic gram-negative bacteria. Bacterial resistance is mediated by induction of an enzyme that methylates the 50S ribosomal RNA. Because both erythromycin and clindamycin can induce this enzymatic resistance (also plasmid-mediated), cross-resistance between these two classes of antibiotics is observed.

INHIBITION OF NUCLEIC ACID SYNTHESIS

Another mechanism of antibacterial activity involves inhibition of synthesis of bacterial DNA and RNA (Figure 13-7).

Rifampin: Mode of Action, Spectrum of Activity, and Mechanisms of Resistance

Rifampin, a semisynthetic derivative of rifamycin B produced by *Streptomyces mediterranei*, binds to DNA-dependent RNA polymerase and inhibits initiation of RNA synthesis (Figure 13-8). Rifampin is bactericidal for *Mycobacterium tuberculosis* and is very active against aerobic gram-positive cocci, including staphylococci (in-

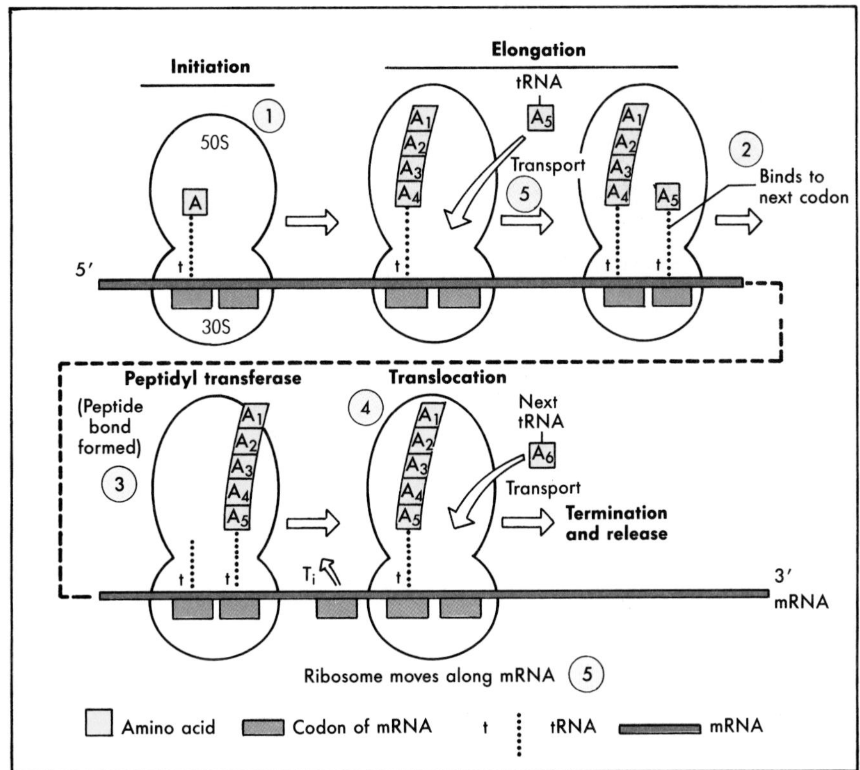

FIGURE 13-6 Bacterial protein synthesis and sites of antibiotic activity. (*1*) Streptomycin and other aminoglycosides freeze initiation so the ribosome does not progress along the mRNA. (*2*) Tetracycline and chloramphenicol prevent tRNA from binding to mRNA codon. (*3*) Chloramphenicol and the macrolides (e.g., erythromycin) block peptide bond formation. (*4*) The macrolides and clindamycin block translocation. (*5*) Streptomycin and other aminoglycosides cause misreading of mRNA so the wrong amino acid is added. (From Wingard LB, Brody TM, Larner J, et al., editors: *Human pharmacology: molecular to clinical*, St. Louis, 1991, Mosby.)

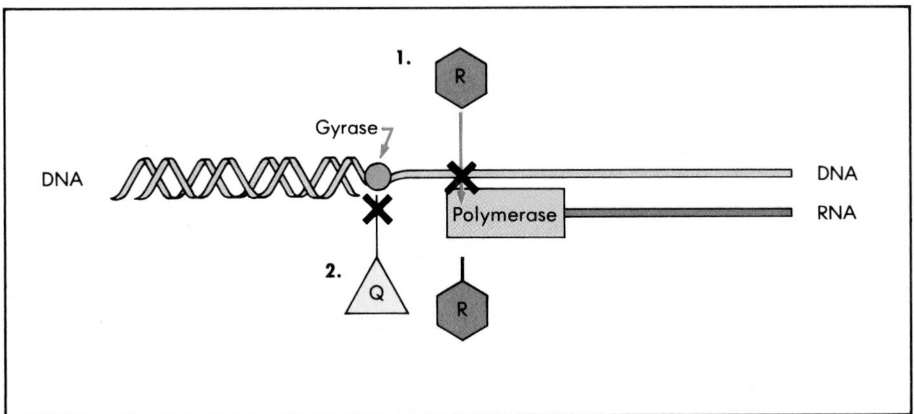

FIGURE 13-7 Inhibition of nucleic acid synthesis. *1*, Rifampin (*R*) binds to DNA-dependent RNA polymerase and inhibits RNA synthesis. *2*, Quinolones (*Q*) inhibit DNA gyrase and prevent supercoiling of DNA.

cluding oxacillin-resistant strains) and streptococci. Because resistance can develop rapidly, rifampin is usually combined with one or more other effective antibiotics. Alteration of the polymerase leads to rifampin resistance.

Quinolones: Mode of Action, Spectrum of Activity, and Mechanisms of Resistance

The quinolones (Box 13-5) are synthetic chemotherapeutic agents that inhibit bacterial DNA gyrases or topoisomerases, which are required to supercoil strands of

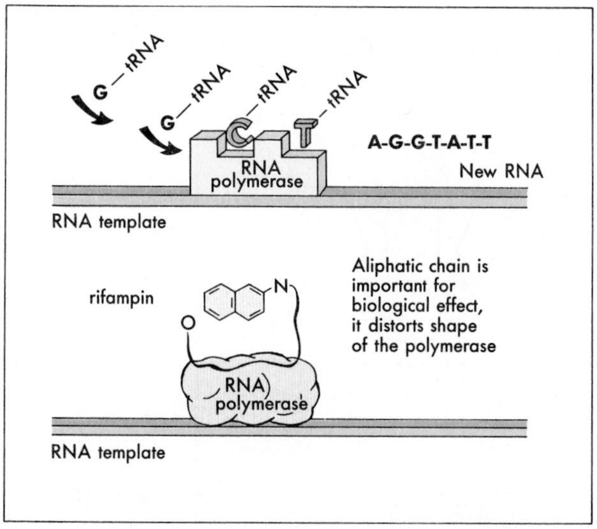

FIGURE 13-8. Mechanism of rifampin action. The antibiotic binds to the beta subunit of DNA-dependent RNA polymerase and inhibits initiation (but not ongoing) RNA synthesis. **A**, Drug absent. **B**, The drug binds to the polymerase molecule, distorts its conformation, and prevents the binding of the enzyme to new DNA molecules. (From Wingard LB, Brody TM, Larner J, Schwartz A, editors: *Human pharmacology: molecular to clinical*, St. Louis, 1991, Mosby.)

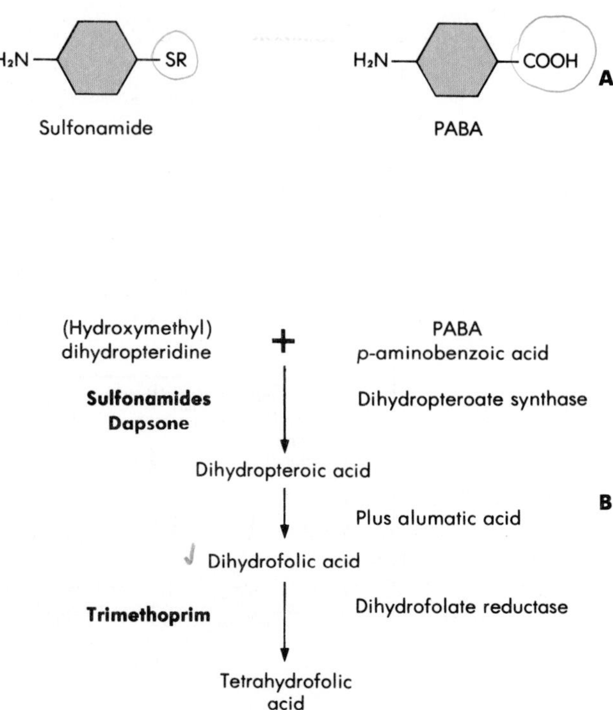

FIGURE 13-9 Antimetabolic activity or competitive antagonism. **A**, Sulfonamides, which resemble PABA, and dapsone competitively inhibit dihydropteroate synthase. **B**, Trimethoprim inhibits enzymatic action of dihydrofolate reductase. Both steps interfere with synthesis of folic acid, which is required by bacteria.

BOX 13-5 Quinolones

Nalidixic acid	Cinoxacin
Norfloxacin	Ofloxacin
Ciprofloxacin	

bacterial DNA into the bacterial cell. Nalidixic acid was used to treat urinary tract infections caused by a variety of gram-negative bacteria, but resistance to the drug developed rapidly. This drug has now been replaced by newer, more active quinolones such as norfloxacin, ciprofloxacin, and ofloxacin.

DNA gyrase consists of alpha and beta subunits, with binding of the quinolones to the alpha subunit. Alteration of this subunit is the principal mechanism of bacterial resistance, although decreased drug uptake has also been observed. Decreased uptake is mediated by changes in porin proteins on the bacterial surface. Both resistance mechanisms are chromosomally mediated.

Metronidazole: Mode of Action, Spectrum of Activity, and Mechanisms of Resistance

Metronidazole was originally introduced as an oral agent for treatment of *Trichomonas* vaginitis. It is also effective in treatment of amebiasis, giardiasis, and serious anaerobic bacterial infections (including *Bacteriodes fragilis*) but has no significant activity against aerobic or facultatively anaerobic bacteria. The antimicrobial properties of metronidazole appear to be mediated by a partially reduced intermediate, which results in DNA breakage. A decreased rate of reduction of metronidazole to its active form has been observed in resistant strains of bacteria (e.g., *Bacteroides fragilis*).

ANTIMETABOLITES

The final mechanism of antibiotic activity is illustrated by the sulfonamides, trimethoprim, and the antileprosy drug, dapsone (Figure 13-9). The sulfonamides compete with *p*-aminobenzoic acid, preventing synthesis of folic acid that is required by certain microorganisms. Because mammalian organisms do not synthesize folic acid (required as a vitamin), sulfonamides do not interfere with mammalian cell metabolism. Dapsone's activity is at the same site as the sulfonamides. Trimethoprim has a high affinity for dihydrofolate reductase, and competitively prevents conversion of dihydrofolate to tetrahydrofolate. This blocks the formation of thymidine, some purines, methionine, and glycine. Trimethoprim is commonly combined with sulfamethoxazole to produce a synergistic combination active at two steps in the synthesis of folic acid.

Sulfonamides are effective against a broad range of gram-positive and gram-negative organisms, such as *Nocardia, Chlamydia,* and some protozoa. Short-acting sulfonamides such as sulfisoxazole are among the drugs of choice for treatment of acute urinary tract infections caused by susceptible bacteria such as *Escherichia coli*. Trimethoprim-sulfamethoxazole is effective against a large variety of gram-positive and gram-negative microorganisms and is the drug of choice for acute and chronic urinary tract infections. The combination is active in infections caused by *Pneumocystis carinii,* bacterial infections of the lower respiratory tract, otitis media, and uncomplicated gonorrhea.

QUESTIONS

1. Describe the mode of action of the following antibiotics: penicillin, imipenem, vancomycin, polymyxin, gentamicin, tetracycline, erythromycin, ciprofloxicin, sulfamethoxazole.
2. What three mechanisms of resistance are observed with β-lactam antibiotics? What is the mechanism responsible for oxacillin resistance in *Staphylococcus*? *Pseudomonas* to imipenem? *Staphylococcus* to penicillin?
3. By what three mechanisms have organisms developed resistance to aminoglycosides?

Bibliography

Balows A, Hausler WJ, Herrmann KL, Isenberg HD, Shadomy HJ: *Manual of clinical microbiology*, ed 5, Washington, DC, 1991, American Society for Microbiology.

Kucers A, Bennett NM: *The use of antibiotics: a comprehensive review with clinical emphasis*, ed 4, Philadelphia, 1989.

Lorian V: *Antibiotics in Laboratory Medicine*, ed 3, Baltimore, 1991, Williams & Wilkins.

Mandell GL, Douglas RG, Bennett JE: *Principles and practice of infectious diseases*, ed 3, New York, 1991, Churchill Livingstone.

Pratt WB and Fekety R: *The antimicrobial drugs*, New York, 1986, Oxford University Press.

Wingard LB, Brody TM, Larner J, Schwartz A. *Human Pharmacology: molecular to clinical*, St. Louis, 1991, Mosby.

CHAPTER 14

Chemotherapy of Fungal Infections

IN general, healthy immunologically competent individuals have a high degree of innate resistance against fungi. In most cases infections are asymptomatic and subclinical. However, this is dependent on exposure and inoculum of organisms. In considering the therapeutic strategy to be used in the management of infections caused by fungi, one must take into account the etiological agent and the tissues involved. The fungal pathogens that colonize humans and cause disease possess features that allow categorization into groups according to primarily colonized tissues (Box 14-1). Considering these facts serves to dictate the best clinical approach that can be used to manage the infection.

The agents causing **superficial infections** tend to grow only on the outermost layers of the skin or cuticle of the hair shaft, rarely inducing an immune reaction. These infections cause minimal destructive disease, are cosmetic in nature, and are readily diagnosed. In general, excellent clinical responses result from using topical antifungals combined with good personal hygiene. The agents causing **cutaneous infections (tineas or dermatophytes)** are limited to keratinized tissues of the epidermis, hairs, and nails. However, they do have greater invasive properties and, depending on the species involved, may evoke a highly inflammatory reaction from the host. Although these infections respond well to topical agents, systemic therapy may be required, particularly with widespread involvement of the skin, scalp, or nails (see description of griseofulvin). The **subcutaneous** agents of disease generally have a low degree of infectivity, and infections caused by these organisms are usually associated with some form of traumatic injury. Depending on the organism and the degree of tissue involvement, specific strategies are used to treat the infection. As examples, the drug of choice in treating lymphocutaneous sporotrichosis is a saturated solution of potassium iodide (SSKI) and, depending on the etiological agent, some forms of chromoblastomycosis respond to high doses of orally administered 5-fluorocytosine (see the following). Other infections in this group are refractory to antifungal therapy and may require amputation or surgical excision of the involved area. The **systemic** agents of disease all involve the respiratory tract, and they possess unique morphological features that appear to contribute to the organism's ability to survive within the host. Depending on the immune status of the patient and other underlying host factors, these diseases can be life threatening; they require rapid diagnosis and aggressive therapy with systemic antifungal compounds.

BOX 14-1 Categories of Fungal Infections	
Superficial	Systemic
Cutaneous	Opportunistic
Subcutaneous	

Whereas a large number of antibiotics are available to treat bacterial infections, a similar situation does not exist for therapy of systemic fungal infections. Several reasons can be given for this difference. For example, there has not been a great impetus for development of antifungal agents because systemic fungal infections are less common than bacterial infections. Furthermore, fungal cells, like mammalian cells, are eukaryotic and it has been difficult to develop compounds with a high degree of specificity for fungal cells that are not toxic to the host cells that are parasitized.

The antifungals presently used in treating systemic fungal infections fall into three major classes of compounds: polyenes, azoles, and nucleotides (Table 14-1). The polyenes affect cytosolic membranes; the azole derivatives inhibit ergosterol biosynthesis; and the fluorinated pyrimidine analog, 5-fluorocytosine, interferes with DNA and RNA synthesis. The increasing incidence of life-threatening fungal infections has created a need to develop newer antifungals that are safer and more effective. This is particularly important in patients with AIDS or in those who are otherwise immunosuppressed because they are receiving radiation or chemotherapy for various cancers or who are candidates for organ transplants. Even with these efforts, it must be emphasized that in most cases the immune defect must be corrected to achieve successful antifungal results.

ANTIFUNGALS USED IN TREATING SYSTEMIC FUNGAL INFECTIONS

Polyenes

The polyenes are secondary metabolites produced by various species of *Streptomyces*. More than 150 have been isolated and chemically characterized; they are cyclic macrolide lactones containing a variable number of hydroxyls and between two to seven conjugated double bonds (Figure 14-1). These compounds are classified according to the degree of unsaturation of the ring structure (i.e., diene, triene, tetraene, pentaene, hexaene, and heptaene). Although the mechanism of their action is complex, it is based primarily on the ability of these compounds to bind to sterols in cytosolic membranes of susceptible cells. Because fungal membranes contain ergosterol, mammals cholesterol, plants sitosterol, and certain protozoa ergosterol, all are susceptible to the action of polyenes. This fact serves as the basis for the toxicity of these compounds when used to treat patients with systemic fungal infections.

Amphotericin B, a heptaene macrolide, is the only clinically useful polyene because it possesses a greater potency in damaging fungal than mammalian cells (Figure 14-1, *A*). The generally accepted reason for this selectivity is the preferential binding of amphotericin B to ergosterol-containing membranes compared with cholesterol-containing membranes. Although the structural aspects of the polyene:sterol binding are unclear, experimental evidence indicates that the amphotericin B molecule inserts into the cytoplasmic membrane of susceptible cells. Several molecules of the drug orient themselves parallel to the acyl side chains of the membrane phospholipids to form a cylindrical channel (Figure 14-2). The pores that are formed by amphotericin B increase permeability of the membrane in a dose-dependent manner, leading to leakage of essential ions from the cytosol at low concentrations and destruction of the cell at high doses. In addition to its direct effects on membranes, amphotericin B has immunomodulatory properties that may play a role in its biological activity in vivo. Amphotericin B is insoluble in water at pH 6 to 7. It is used clinically as a mixture of amphotericin B, deoxycholate, and phosphate buffer. In aqueous solutions amphotericin B dissociates from deoxycholate and, depending on its concentration, forms self-associated or monomeric species. When injected intravenously, amphotericin B interacts with plasma proteins and binds to cholesterol in lipoproteins, whereupon it is delivered mainly to tissues of the liver, spleen, lung, and kidney.

Nystatin (formerly called fungicidin) is a structural analogue of amphotericin B. The only difference between the two polyenes is the stretch of conjugated double bonds. In the nystatin ring it is interrupted to yield a diene-tetraene chromophore. Nystatin resembles amphotericin B in its permeabilizing and lethal effects on eukaryotic cells; however, little research has been done on its potential use as a systemic agent. At present, it is available only in topical, cream, suspension, or suppository form, primarily for the treatment of mucocutaneous, oropharyngeal, and vaginal candidiasis.

TABLE 14-1 Antifungal Agents and Primary Sites of Activity

Antifungal agents	Target
Polyenes (e.g., amphotericin B, nystatin)	Membrane sterols (binds to ergosterol)
Azole derivatives (e.g., miconazole, ketoconazole, fluconazole, itraconazole)	Ergosterol biosynthesis (inhibits cytochrome-P450–dependent enzymes)
Nucleotide (e.g., 5-fluorocytosine)	Inhibits DNA and RNA synthesis
Grisans (e.g., griseofulvin)	Microtubules (inhibits microtubular function)
Allylamines (e.g., naftifine, terbinafine)	Squalene epoxidase
Thiocarbamates (e.g., tolnaftate, tolciclate)	Squalene epoxidase
Morpholines (e.g., amorolfine)	Ergosterol biosynthesis (inhibits Δ_{14}-reductase and Δ_7-Δ_8-isomerase)
Potassium iodide (e.g., SSKI)	Unknown (possibly activates lysomal enzymes and breaks down granulomas)

Azole Derivatives

The development of antifungal azole derivatives has progressed at a rapid rate over the past 20 years with the discovery that benzimidazole and the antiparasitic compound thiobendizole had activity against fungi. The azole derivatives constitute the largest group of antifungals that are commercially available. They have a broad spectrum of activity against fungi and, to some extent, against gram-positive bacteria. These compounds are fungistatic and act by inhibiting the 14α-demethylation of 24-methylenedihydrolanosterol, a precursor of ergosterol. The 14α-demethylation step in ergosterol biosynthesis is a cytochrome-P450–dependent process. The azoles are highly selective and act by binding to the heme moiety of cytochrome-P450, resulting in an interference with certain mixed oxidase reactions. As a result, synthesis of ergosterol is blocked and 14α-methyl sterols accumulate.

These compounds are divided into two major groups both characterized by five-membered azole rings with a

A. Amphotericin B (polyene)

B. Ketoconazole (imidazole)

C. Fluconazole (triazole)

D. 5-fluorocytosine (nucleotide)

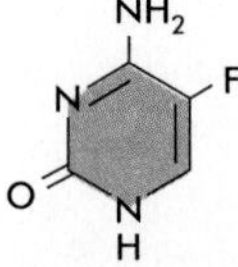

FIGURE 14-1 Chemical structures of systemic antifungal agents: **A,** Amphotericin B; **B,** ketoconazole (imidazole); **C,** fluconazole (triazole); **D,** 5-fluorocytosine.

N-linked methyl group, which is derivatized by the addition of various halogenated phenyl or other complex chemical groups. The **imidazoles** such as chlotrimazole, miconazole, econazole, ketoconazole (Figure 14-1, *B*) are those derivatives that have two nitrogens in the ring, and the **triazoles** such as fluconazole, itraconazole, terconazole (Figure 14-1, *C*) are those with three nitrogens in the ring.

Nucleotide Analogues

5-fluorocytosine (Figure 14-1, *D*) is a polar fluorinated pyrimidine that has a narrow spectrum of activity. It is used orally for the treatment of systemic infections caused by specific fungi mainly in the genera *Candida*, *Cryptococcus*, *Aspergillus*, and certain fungi that cause chromoblastomycosis. This drug is well absorbed from the gastrointestinal tract, has low protein binding, is met-

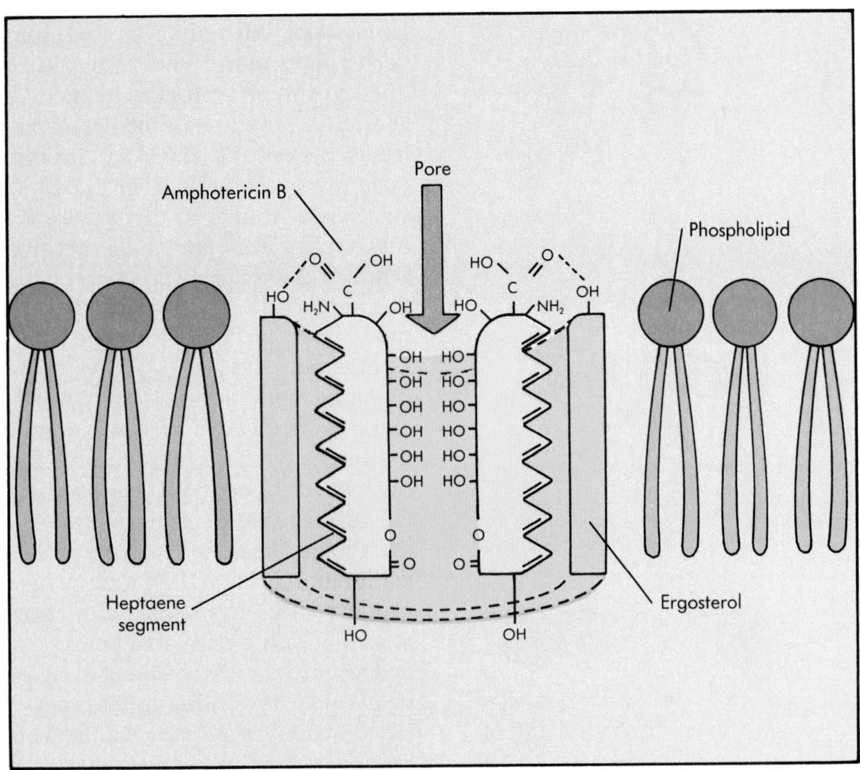

FIGURE 14-2 Mechanism of action of amphotericin B.

abolically stable, and exhibits high bioavailability in human subjects. Unfortunately, it has a narrow spectrum of antifungal activity and rapidly induces resistance in susceptible organisms. In susceptible fungi, 5-fluorocytosine is taken up by a cytosine permease and is rapidly deaminated to 5-fluoruracil. This compound is then converted either to 5-fluorouridylic acid monophosphate and inhibits RNA function or to 5-fluorodeoxyuridine monophosphate, a potent inhibitor of DNA synthesis.

ANTIFUNGALS USED IN TREATING DERMATOPHYTE INFECTIONS

Griseofulvin, an orally administered antifungal agent used in the management of dermatophyte infections, is a grisan derivative produced by *Penicillium griseofulvum* (Figure 14-3, *A*). Griseofulvin interacts specifically with tubulin and acts as a mitotic poison in susceptible fungi. The exact mechanism of action is unknown, but it appears to alter function of tubulin rather than disaggregation or assembly of its subunits. Griseofulvin is active against dermatophytes but inactive against *C. albicans* and the agents causing systemic mycoses. The mechanism of resistance appears to be lack of uptake since griseofulvin reacts in vitro with tubulins isolated from a variety of sources including mammalian, dermatophyte, and amphibian cells.

The **allylamines** include the topical agent, **naftifine**, and the orally active antifungal agent, **terbinafine**. The allylamines inhibit squalene epoxidase, a complex membrane-bound system that requires phospholipids and oxygen as a source of reducing equivalents (Figure 14-3, *B*). These compounds are very active in vitro against dermatophytes, have good effects against filamentous and dimorphic fungi but have very poor activity against yeasts.

Tolnaftate and **tolciclate** are thiocarbamates whose mechanism of action is similar to the allylamines (Figure 14-3, *C*). They inhibit ergosterol biosynthesis in dermatophytes at the level of squalene epoxidase but are less active against yeasts. These antifungals are used topically in the management of dermatophyte infections.

Amorolfine is a morpholine derivative that is highly active against dermatophytes and exhibits moderate activity against yeasts, but the response in filamentous fungi is variable (Figure 14-3, *D*). Amorolfine has no effect on DNA, RNA, protein, or carbohydrate synthesis but appears to inhibit Δ_{14}-reductase and Δ_7-Δ_8-isomerase in the pathway of ergosterol biosynthesis.

Other preparations, such as those containing 10-undecenoic (undecylenic acid), caprylic, or propionic acid as active ingredients, have also been used in the management of ringworm infections. These compounds do not possess fungicidal properties, and the role they play in eradicating the fungus from the skin has not been established. Good hygienic practices in addition to use of preparations containing these compounds no doubt play an important role in the clinical responses that result.

A. Griseofulvin (grisan)

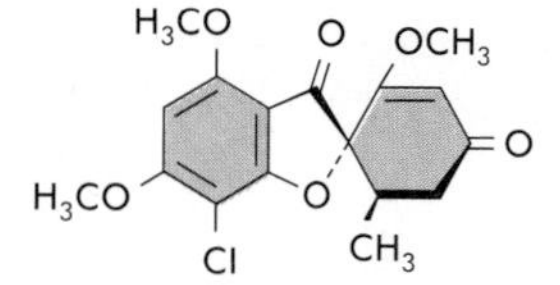

B. Naftifine (allylamine)

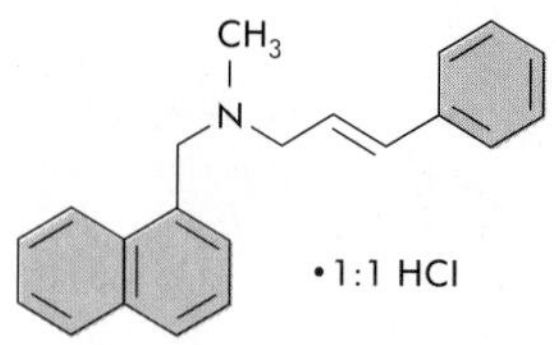

C. Tolnaftate (thiocarbamate)

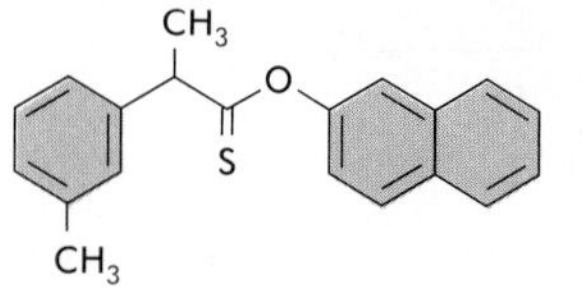

D. Amorolfine (morpholine)

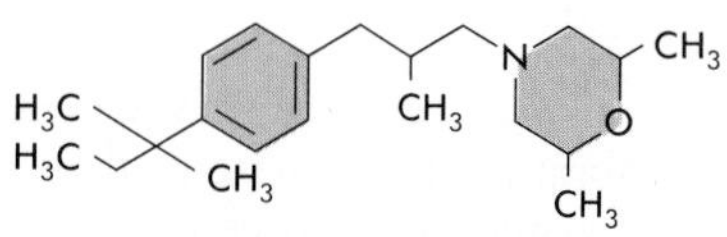

FIGURE 14-3 Chemical structures of agents used primarily for dermatophyte infections.

FUTURE CONSIDERATIONS

Identifying Novel Targets for Development of Agents

The cytosolic membrane has been the main focus for development of antifungals. Unfortunately those currently in use are toxic to host cells or are fungistatic and have a limited spectrum of activity. There is clearly a need to look for other targets. In addition to the cytosolic membrane, the cell wall is a major constituent of the fungal envelope. It determines the shape of the cell, serves as a protective permeability barrier to large molecules, and is essential for survival of the fungus. The fungal wall structure is multilayered and composed mainly of glucan, mannoproteins and chitin. Chitin and β-glucans are absent in host cells and unique to fungi. Thus the cell wall is an attractive target for antifungal drug development, and several efforts have been made to design compounds that interfere with its synthesis. Polyoxins are analogues of *UDP-N*-acetylglucosamine, a class of compounds that are specific competitive inhibitors of chitin synthase. Antifungal activity has been demonstrated in vitro against *C. albicans*, but only a limited number of studies have been conducted in vivo. There is some question about uptake of these analogues by medically important fungi; as a result, progress in the development of the polyoxins has not been made. More promising have been the nikkomycins, a related group of compounds that are structurally similar to the polyoxins. Like the polyoxins, nikkomycin Z is also a competitive inhibitor of chitin synthase. It has been shown to be highly effective against murine coccidioidomycosis, blastomycosis, and histoplasmosis and prolongs the life of mice infected with *C. albicans*.

Along with the development of agents that inhibit chitin synthase have been efforts to find compounds that inhibit the synthesis of β-glucan. One compound that was discovered about 20 years ago and found to be very effective against yeast is echinocandin B, a cyclic lipopeptide metabolite produced by *Aspergillus nidulans*. Recently, cilofungin (LY121019), a derivative of echinocandin B produced by enzymatic deacylation using *Actinoplanes utahensis* with *p*-octyl-oxo-benzoic acid, was synthesized and found to be less toxic and more potent than the parent compound. Promising in vitro and in vivo results led to clinical trials for invasive candidiasis and esophageal disease. Unfortunately, development of this compound has been abandoned for the present time because the vehicle in which it is delivered is toxic.

In Vitro Susceptibility Testing

Paralleling the development and discovery of newer antifungal compounds has been the increasing use of these agents to treat the growing number of common and exotic fungal infections that occur. This situation has brought about demands for in vitro antifungal testing methods that will accurately predict in vivo activity. Unfortunately, in vitro susceptibility testing with fungi is not yet standardized, and results of the presently used tests are not always predictive of clinical responses. This is particularly true of the azole derivatives and, to some extent, 5-fluorocytosine. Efforts are being expended to develop standardized methods for in vitro susceptibility testing and to develop animal models of infection to evaluate these agents.

Need to Monitor Patients Who Are Receiving Therapy

Although therapy for life-threatening fungal infections is far from ideal, it is obvious that progress has been made. Despite these advances, significant problems still exist in the treatment of fungal infections, particularly in patients with AIDS and in those who are otherwise severely immunosuppressed. None of the agents currently in use appears to be curative in these patient populations, and lifelong suppressive therapy is often necessary to prevent recurrence of disease. This is a significant problem because these patients are taking a variety of medications to suppress the AIDS virus, as well as other opportunistic organisms. It is known that some of the available antifungals potentially have clinically important drug interactions. In patients who are being treated with combinations of drugs, monitoring plasma levels and relevant pharmacological parameters may be necessary so that adverse drug effects can be minimized. To complicate therapy, drug resistance in fungi exists and may explain the emergence of recurrent disease.

QUESTIONS

1. What is the current thought on the mechanism of action of amphotericin B?
2. How do the azoles work?
3. How does 5-fluorocytosine work, and what major problem is encountered with its use?
4. If you were to design an antifungal agent that was targeted specifically for fungi, what strategy would you use?

Bibliography

Riley JF, editor: *Chemotherapy of fungal diseases*, New York, 1990, Springer-Verlag.

Sutcliffe JA and Georgopapadakou NH, editors: *Emerging targets in antibacterial and antifungal chemotherapy*, New York, 1992, Chapman & Hall.

Yamaguchi H, Kobayashi GS, and Takahashi H, editors: *Recent advances in antifungal chemotherapy*, New York, 1992, Marcel Dekker.

CHAPTER 15

Chemotherapy of Parasitic Infections

THE chemotherapeutic approach to the management of infectious diseases has clearly changed the face of medicine. Unfortunately, very few of the antiinfective agents that have proved so successful against bacterial pathogens have been effective against parasites. In many instances we must continue to rely on antiparasitic agents from the pre-antibiotic era. These and some newer agents remain limited in number and relatively toxic. Many antiparasitic agents require prolonged or parenteral administration and may be effective only in certain disease states. Fortunately, in the last 5 to 10 years several new agents have appeared that constitute significant advances in the treatment of parasitic diseases. In each case the previously available drugs were toxic and often ineffective.

In large part the difficulties in treatment of parasitic diseases stem from the fact that parasites are eukaryotic organisms and thus are more similar to the human host than the more successfully treated prokaryotic bacterial pathogens. Furthermore, the more chronic and prolonged course of infection and the complex life cycles and multiple developmental stages of many parasites add to the difficulties of effective chemotherapeutic intervention. Additional complicating factors in the developing world, where the majority of parasitic diseases occurs, include (1) the presence of multiple infections and the high probability of reinfection, (2) the large number of persons immunocompromised by malnutrition and HIV infection, and (3) the overwhelming influence of poverty and poor sanitation, which facilitates the transmission of many parasitic infections. Although chemotherapeutic approaches may be used effectively to treat and prevent many parasitic infections, some agents have adverse effects or are eventually met with resistance (microbial and social) and most antiparasitic agents are too expensive for widespread use in developing countries. Thus the global approach to the prevention and treatment of parasitic diseases must involve several strategies including improved hygiene and sanitation, control of the disease vector, use of vaccinations if available (largely unavailable for parasitic diseases), and prophylactic and therapeutic administration of safe and effective chemotherapy. These strategies now must also include efforts to decrease the transmission of HIV infection.

TARGETS FOR ANTIPARASITE DRUG ACTION

As mentioned previously, parasites are eukaryotic organisms and thus have more similarities than differences with the human host. Consequently, many antiparasitic agents act on pathways (nucleic acid synthesis, carbohydrate metabolism) or targets (neuromuscular function) shared by both the parasite and the host. For this reason developing safe and effective antiparasitic drugs based on biochemical differences between the parasite and host has been difficult. Differential toxicity is commonly achieved by preferential uptake, metabolic alteration of the drug by the parasite, or differences in the susceptibility of functionally equivalent sites in parasite and host. Fortunately, as our understanding of the basic biology and biochemistry of parasites and the mechanism of action of antimicrobial agents has improved, so has our recognition of potential parasite-specific targets for chemotherapeutic attack. Examples of the current chemotherapeutic strategies to exploit differences between parasite and host are provided in Table 15-1. These will be discussed in greater detail as we deal with the specific agents later in the chapter.

DRUG RESISTANCE

Resistance to antimicrobial agents is an important consideration in the treatment of infections due to bacteria and fungal pathogens and certainly plays a role in the chemotherapy of parasitic diseases. Unfortunately, our understanding of the molecular and genetic basis for resistance to most antiparasitic agents is quite limited. Most of the information regarding the molecular mechanisms of drug resistance in parasites has come from studies in plasmodia. Resistance to chloroquine, a major antimalarial agent, is most likely due to the presence of an active chloroquine efflux mechanism similar to that producing the rapid efflux of anticancer drugs observed in multidrug-resistant mammalian cancer cells. In addition,

TABLE 15-1 Chemotherapeutic Strategies to Exploit Differences Between the Parasite and Host

Unique site of attack	Drug	Organism
Drug-concentrating mechanism unique to parasite	Chloroquine	*Plasmodium*
Folic acid pathway-parasite unable to use exogenous folate	Pyrimethamine or trimethoprim plus sulfa	*Plasmodium* *Toxoplasma* *Pneumocystis*
Inhibitor of trypanothion-dependent mechanism for reducing oxidized thiol groups	Arsenicals Difluoromethyl-ornithine	Trypanosomes
Interfere with neuro-mediators unique to parasites	Pyrantel pamoate Piperazine	*Ascaris*
Inhibitors of GABA-mediated conduction in the peripheral nervous system of parasites	Ivermectin	Filaria
Interaction with tubulin unique to parasites	Benzimidazoles	Many helminths

the development of plasmodial resistance to antifolate compounds such as pyrimethamine has been shown to be due to a series of mutations in the parasite's combined dihydrofolate reductase–thymidylate synthetase enzyme. Further insights into the mechanisms of action and resistance to antiparasitic agents will be necessary to optimize the effectiveness of antiparasite chemotherapy.

ANTIPARASITIC AGENTS

Although the number of effective antiparasitic agents is small relative to the vast array of antibacterial agents, the list is expanding (Table 15-2). Certainly in many cases the goal of antiparasitic therapy is similar to that of antibacterial therapy: to eradicate the organism rapidly and completely. In many cases, however, the agents and treatment regimens used for parasitic diseases are designed simply to decrease the parasite burden and/or prevent the systemic complications of chronic infection. Thus the goals of antiparasitic therapy, particularly as applied in endemic areas, may be quite different from those usually considered for therapy of microbial infection in the United States or other developed countries. Given the significant toxicity of many of these agents, in every case the need for treatment must be weighed against the toxicity of the drug. A decision to withhold therapy may often be correct, particularly when the drug can cause severe adverse effects.

Immunocompromised individuals pose a particular problem with respect to antiparasitic chemotherapy. On the one hand, prophylaxis, such as that administered for *Pneumocystis carinii*, is essential and effective in preventing infection. However, once infection is established, radical cure may not be possible and long-term suppressive therapy may be indicated. In some diseases, such as cryptosporidiosis and microsporidiosis, effective therapy is not available and care must be taken to avoid unnecessary toxicity while providing supportive care for the patient.

The remainder of this chapter will provide an overview of the major classes of antiprotozoal and antihelminthic agents. These and additional antiparasitic agents, their mechanisms of action, and clinical indications are listed in Table 15-2. Treatment of specific infections is discussed in the chapters dealing with the individual parasites. Refer to several excellent reviews listed in the Bibliography for more complete listings and discussions of the available antiparasitic agents.

Antiprotozoal Agents

Similar to antibacterial and antifungal agents, the antiprotozoal agents are generally targeted at relatively rapidly proliferating, young, growing cells. Most commonly these agents target nucleic acid synthesis, protein synthesis, or specific metabolical pathways (e.g., folate metabolism) unique to the protozoan parasites.

Heavy Metals

The heavy metals used for treatment of parasitic infections include arsenical (melarsoprol) and antimonial compounds (sodium stibogluconate, meglumine antimonate). These agents are thought to oxidize sulfhydryl groups of enzymes, which are essential catalysts in carbohydrate metabolism. Melarsoprol inhibits parasite pyruvate kinase, causing decreased concentrations of ATP, pyruvate, and phosphoenolpyruvate. Arsenicals also inhibit *sn*-glycerol 3-phosphate oxidase, needed for regeneration of NAD in trypanosomes but not found in mammalian cells. The antimonials, sodium stibogluconate and meglumine antimonate, inhibit the glycolytic enzyme phosphofructokinase and certain Krebs cycle enzymes in *Leishmania* organisms. In each instance the inhibition of parasite metabolism is parasiticidal. Unfortunately, the heavy metal compounds are toxic to the host, as well as the parasite. The toxicity is greatest on cells that are most metabolically active, such as neuronal, renal tubular, intestinal and bone marrow stem cells. Their differential toxicity and therapeutic value are largely due to enhanced uptake by the parasite and its intense metabolic activity.

Melarsoprol is the drug of choice for trypanosomiasis involving the central nervous system. It is capable of penetrating the blood-brain barrier and is effective in all stages of trypanosomiasis. The antimonial compounds are restricted to the management of leishmaniasis. Meglumine antimonate and sodium stibogluconate are the

TABLE 15-2 Mechanisms of Action and Clinical Indications for the Major Antiparasitic Agents

Drug class	Mechanism of action	Examples	Clinical indication
ANTIPROTOZOAL AGENTS			
Heavy metals arsenicals and antimonials	Inactivate SH groups	Melarsoprol Sodium stibogluconate Meglumine antimonate	Trypanosomiasis Leishmaniasis
Aminoquinoline analogues	Accumulate in parasitized cells; interfere with DNA replication; bind to ferriprotoporphyrin IX; raise intravesicular pH; interfere with hemoglobin digestion	Chloroquine Mefloquine Quinine Primaquine	Malaria prophylaxis and therapy Radical cure (exoerythrocytic-primaquine only)
Folic acid antagonists	Inhibit dihydropteroate synthetase and dihydrofolate reductase	Sulfonamides Pyrimethamine Trimethoprim	Toxoplasmosis Pneumocystosis Malaria
Inhibitors of protein synthesis	Block peptide synthesis at the level of the ribosome	Clindamycin Spiramycin Tetracycline Doxycycline	Malaria Babesiosis Amebiasis Cryptosporidiosis
Diamidines	Bind DNA Interfere with uptake and function of polyamines	Pentamidine	Pneumocystosis Leishmaniasis Trypanosomiasis
Nitroimidazoles	Unclear Interaction with DNA Inhibit metabolism of glucose and interfere with mitochondrial function	Metronidazole Benzimidazole Tinidazole	Amebiasis Giardiasis Trichomoniasis
Quinolones	Inhibit DNA gyrase	Ciprofloxacin	Malaria
Oxidants	Overwhelm or inhibit antioxidant defenses of parasite	Quinghaosu	Malaria
Ornithine analogue	Inhibits ornithine decarboxylase Interferes with polyamine metabolism	Difluoromethylornithine (DFMO)	African trypanosomiasis
Inhibitors of nucleic acid synthesis	Inhibition of enzymes in purine salvage pathway	Allopurinol	Leishmaniasis
Acetanilide	Unknown	Diloxanide furoate	Intestinal amebiasis
Sulfated naphthylamine	Inhibits *sn*-glycerol phosphate oxidase and glycerol 3-phosphate dehydrogenase, causing decreased ATP synthesis	Suramin	African trypanosomiasis
ANTIHELMINTHIC AGENTS			
Benzimidazoles	Inhibition of fumarate reductase Inhibition of glucose transport Disruption of microtubular function	Mebendazole Thiabendazole Albendazole	Broad-spectrum antihelminthics Nematodes Cestodes
Tetrahydropyrimidine	Neuromuscular blockage Inhibits fumarate reductase	Pyrantel pamoate	Ascariasis Pinworm Hookworm
Piperazines	GABA agonist Neuromuscular paralysis Stimulation of phagocytic cells	Piperazine Diethylcarbamazine	*Ascaris* and pinworm infections filarial infections

TABLE 15-2 Mechanisms of Action and Clinical Indications for the Major Antiparasitic Agents—cont'd

Drug class	Mechanism of action	Examples	Clinical indication
Avermectins	Neuromuscular blockade GABA antagonist Inhibits filarial reproduction	Ivermectin	Filarial infections
Pyrazinoisoquinoline	Calcium agonist; tetanic muscular contractions; tegumental disruption; synergy with host defenses	Praziquantel	Broad-spectrum anti-helminthics Cestodes Trematodes
Phenol	Uncouples oxidative phosphorylation	Niclosamide Bithionol	Intestinal tapeworm Paragonimiasis
Quinolone	Alkylates DNA; inhibits DNA, RNA, and protein synthesis	Oxamniquine	Schistosomiasis
Organophosphate	Anticholinesterase; neuro-muscular blockade	Metrifonate	Schistosomiasis
Sulfated naphthylamidine	Inhibits glycerophosphate oxidase and dehydrogenase	Suramin	Onchocerciasis

drugs of first choice for leishmaniasis and are active against all forms of the disease. Prolonged therapy is usually required for disseminated leishmaniasis, and relapses are common.

Aminoquinoline Analogues

The aminoquinoline analogues include the 4-aminoquinolines (chloroquine), the 8-aminoquinolines (primaquine), and the 4-quinolinemethanols (mefloquine). Additional quinoline analogues include quinine, quinidine, quinacrine, and amodiaquine. These compounds all have antimalarial activity and accumulate preferentially in parasitized red blood cells. Several potential mechanisms of action have been proposed, including (1) binding to DNA and interfering with DNA replication, (2) binding to ferriprotoporphyrin IX, released from hemoglobin in infected erythrocytes, producing a toxic complex, and (3) raising the pH of the parasite's intracellular acid vesicles, thus interfering with its ability to degrade hemoglobin. Quinine, the 4-aminoquinolines, and 4-quinolinemethanols all rapidly destroy the erythrocytic stage of malaria and thus may be used prophylactically to suppress clinical illness or therapeutically to terminate an acute attack. The 8-aminoquinolines (e.g., primaquine) accumulate in tissue cells and destroy the extra erythrocytic (hepatic) stages of malaria, resulting in a radical cure of the infection.

Chloroquine remains the drug of choice for prophylaxis and treatment of susceptible malaria strains. Chloroquine is active against all four *Plasmodium* species (*P. falciparum*, *P. vivax*, *P. ovale*, and *P. malariae*) and is well tolerated, inexpensive, and effective orally. Unfortunately, resistance of *P. falciparum* to chloroquine is widespread in Asia, Africa, and South America, greatly limiting the use of this agent. Recently, *P. vivax* resistant to chloroquine has been reported from Papua New Guinea, the Solomon Islands, and Indonesia.

Quinine is currently used primarily to treat chloroquine-resistant *P. falciparum* infection. Presumably, it is active against the rare chloroquine-resistant strains of *P. vivax* as well. Quinine is used orally only to treat mild attacks and by the IV route to treat acute attacks of multidrug-resistant *P. falciparum*. Quinine is quite toxic and not rapidly parasiticidal; thus it is never used alone but is often combined with a sulfonamide or tetracycline antibiotic with antimalarial activity.

Mefloquine is a new 4-quinolinemethanol antimalarial agent that is used for the prophylaxis and treatment of falciparum malaria. Presently it displays a high level of activity against most chloroquine-resistant parasites. Unfortunately, mefloquine-resistant strains of falciparum malaria have recently been reported from Southeast Asia.

Folic Acid Antagonists

Similar to other organisms, protozoan parasites require folic acid for the synthesis of nucleic acids and ultimately DNA. Protozoa are unable to absorb exogenous folate and thus are susceptible to drugs that inhibit folate synthesis. The folic acid antagonists that are useful in treating protozoan infections include the diaminopyrimidines (pyrimethamine and trimethoprim) and the sulfonamides. These compounds block separate steps in the folic acid pathway. The sulfonamides inhibit the conversion of aminobenzoic acid to dihydropteroic acid. The diaminopyrimidines inhibit dihydrofolate reductase, which effectively blocks the synthesis of tetrahydrofolate, a precursor necessary for the formation of purines, pyrimidines, and certain amino acids. These agents are effective at concentrations far below those needed to inhibit the mammalian enzyme, so selectivity can be attained. When a diaminopyrimidine is used with a sulfonamide, a synergistic effect is achieved by blockade of two steps in the same metabolic pathway, resulting in very effective inhibition of protozoan growth.

The diaminopyrimidine, trimethoprim, is used in combination with sulfamethoxazole to treat *Pneumocystis carinii* pneumonia and toxoplasmosis. Another diaminopyrimidine, pyrimethamine, has a high affinity for sporozoan dihydrofolate reductase and has been quite effective when combined with a sulfonamide in the treatment of malaria and toxoplasmosis. Resistance to antifolates has been shown to be due to specific point mutations at the active site of the parasites dihydrofolate reductase and has been largely confined to species of plasmodia.

Inhibitors of Protein Synthesis

Several antibiotics that inhibit protein synthesis in bacteria also exhibit antiparasitic activity in vitro and in vivo. These agents include clindamycin, spiramycin, tetracycline, and doxycycline.

Clindamycin and the tetracyclines are active against plasmodia, *Babesia,* and amebae. Doxycycline is used for the chemoprophylaxis of chloroquine-resistant *P. falciparum* malaria, and tetracycline may be used in combination with quinine for the treatment of chloroquine-resistant *P. falciparum* infection. Clindamycin may be useful in the treatment of central nervous system toxoplasmosis. Spiramycin is recommended as an alternative to the antifolates in the treatment of toxoplasmosis. Although spiramycin appears active against *Cryptosporidium* in vitro, neither spiramycin nor any other agent has been shown to be effective clinically for human cryptosporidiosis.

Diamidines

Pentamidine, a diamidine, is a relatively toxic agent that has become extremely important as an alternative to the antifolates for the prevention and treatment of *Pneumocystis carinii* pneumonia in AIDS patients and other immunocompromised hosts. Although its mechanism of action is unknown, pentamidine is a polycation and may interact with DNA, or it may interfere with the uptake and function of polyamines.

In addition to its role in the prevention and therapy of *Pneumocystis* pneumonia, pentamidine is effective in treating the tissue forms of leishmania and the early (pre-CNS) forms of African trypanosomiasis. Pentamidine does not penetrate the CNS and therefore is not useful in the late CNS stages of infection with *Trypanosoma brucei gambiense* or *T. b. rhodesiense.*

Nitroimidazoles

The nitroimidazoles include the well-known antibacterial agent metronidazole, as well as benzimidazole and tinidazole. The mechanism of action of these compounds is unclear. It has been suggested that they inhibit DNA and RNA synthesis and also inhibit the metabolism of glucose and interfere with mitochondrial function. Metronidazole binds to parasite guanine and cytosine residues, causing loss of helical structure and breakage of DNA strands.

The nitroimidazoles have excellent penetration into tissues and thus are particularly effective for the treatment of disseminated amebiasis. Metronidazole is the drug of choice for trichomoniasis and is effective in the treatment of giardiasis. Tinidazole appears to be more effective and less mutagenic than metronidazole; however, it is not yet available for use in the United States.

Other Antiprotozoal Agents

A number of additional agents used in therapy, their mechanism of action (if known), and clinical use are listed in Table 15-2.

Antihelminthic Agents

The strategy for the use of antihelminthic drugs is quite different from that employed in the treatment of most protozoal infections. Most antihelminthic drugs are targeted at nonproliferating adult organisms, whereas with protozoa the targets are generally younger, more rapidly proliferating cells. The helminthic life cycle is frequently quite complex, and the adaptation to survival in the human host is strongly dependent on the following factors: (1) neuromuscular coordination for worm feeding movements and for maintaining a favorable location of the worm within the host; (2) carbohydrate metabolism as the major source of energy, with glucose the primary substrate; and (3) microtubular integrity, since egg laying and hatching, larval development, glucose transport, and enzyme activity and secretion are impaired when the microtubules are modified. Most antihelminthic agents are targeted at one of these three biochemical functions in the adult organism.

The mechanisms of action and clinical indications for the commonly employed antihelminthic agents are listed in Table 15-2.

Benzimidazoles

The benzimidazoles are broad-spectrum antihelminthic agents and include mebendazole, thiabendazole, and albendazole (not available in the United States). The basic structure of these agents consists of linked imidazole and benzene rings. Three mechanisms of action have been proposed for the benzimidazoles: (1) inhibition of fumarate reductase; (2) inhibition of glucose transport, resulting in glycogen depletion, cessation of ATP formation, and paralysis or death; and (3) disruption of microtubular function. Benzimidazoles block the assembly of tubulin dimers into tubulin polymers in a process mimicked by colchicine, a powerful antimitotic and embryotoxic drug. Because tubulin is important for parasite motility, drugs such as the benzimidazoles, which bind to parasite tubulin, are thought to act against nematode parasites by reducing or eliminating their motility.

The benzimidazoles have a wide spectrum of activity including intestinal nematodes (*Ascaris*, *Trichuris*, *Necator*, *Ancylostoma*, *Enterobius vermicularis*), as well as a number of cestodes (*Taenia*, *Hymenolepis*, and *Echinococcus*). Thiabendazole acts against both larval and adult nematodes and is useful in the management of cutaneous larval migrans, trichinosis, and most intestinal nematode infections. Mebendazole is active against the intestinal nematodes and also is effective against the cestodes listed previously. Albendazole has a spectrum similar to mebendazole and may have greater activity against *Echinococcus*.

Tetrahydropyrimidines

Pyrantel pamoate, a tetrahydropyrimidine, is a cholinergic agonist that produces a powerful effect on nematode muscle cells by binding to cholinergic receptors, which results in cell depolarization and muscle contraction. This paralytic action on intestinal nematodes leads to expulsion of the worm from the host intestinal tract.

Pyrantel pamoate is not readily absorbed from the intestine and is active against *Ascaris*, pinworm, and hookworm. An analogue of pyrantel, oxantel, may be used in combination with pyrantel to provide effective therapy for the three major soil-transmitted nematodes: *Ascaris*, hookworm, and *Trichuris* species.

Piperazines

The piperazine antihelminthics include piperazine and diethylcarbamazine. Piperazine is thought to act by hyperpolarization of the muscle membrane, producing a flaccid paralysis. The current hypothesis is that piperazine acts against nematodes as a low-potency GABA (gamma amino benzoic acid) agonist. Diethylcarbamazine may act by stimulating cholinergic receptors and depolarizing muscle cells, with subsequent paralysis of the worms. However, additional evidence suggests that it enhances the adherence of leukocytes to microfilariae and thus may act by altering the parasite surface membrane or by directly stimulating phagocytic cells.

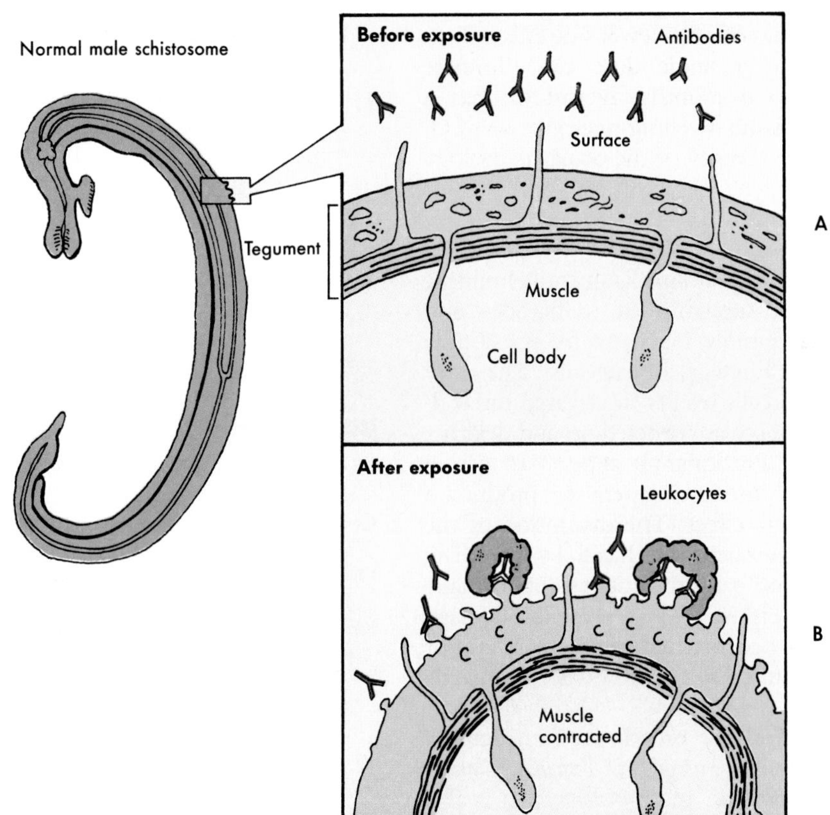

FIGURE 15-1 Before exposure to praziquantel, the schistosome is capable of avoiding the numerous antibodies directed toward surface and internally located antigens. **A**, Cross section of the dorsal surface of a normal male schistosome. Within 1 to 2 seconds after exposure to praziquantel, the muscles of the schistosome contract because of drug-induced influx of calcium ions into the schistosome tegument. **B**, The change in permeability of the schistosome surface toward external ions initiates the appearance of small holes and balloon-like structures, making the parasite vulnerable to antibody-mediated adherence of host leukocytes that kill the helminth. (From Wingard LB Jr, Brody TM, Larner J, Schwartz A, editors: *Human pharmacology: molecular to clinical,* St. Louis, 1991, Mosby.)

The piperazines are active against *Ascaris* and pinworm (*Enterobius vermicularis*). In addition, diethylcarbamazine is active against the filariae that produce river blindness (*Onchocerca volvulus*) and lymphatic filariasis (*Wuchereria bancrofti* and *Brugia malayi*). Unfortunately, destruction of the microfilariae in the tissues may actually increase the pathology because of the host inflammatory response to the parasite antigens released upon exposure to diethylcarbamazine.

Avermectins

Ivermectin, an avermectin, acts by interacting with the chloride channel on the helminth GABA receptor complex, thus inhibiting GABA-ergic synapses in the peripheral nervous system of nematode parasites. As a result, the parasites become paralyzed and may be eliminated by the host. The drug also inhibits the reproductive function of the adult female *Onchocerca volvulus* and alters the ability of the *O. volvulus* microfilariae to evade the host immune system.

Although ivermectin is used extensively to control gut-dwelling nematode infections in domestic and farm animals, its use in humans is limited to treating ocular and lymphatic filariasis. Ivermectin has fewer side effects than diethylcarbamazine, and a single dose can eliminate microfilariae for up to 6 months. Ivermectin has a dramatic effect on the tissue-dwelling microfilariae of *O. volvulus* and reduces the severity of the ocular pathology seen in onchocerciasis.

Pyrazinoisoquinolines

Praziquantel, a pyrazinoisoquinoline, is an antihelminthic active against a broad spectrum of trematodes and cestodes. The drug is rapidly taken up by susceptible helminths in which it acts as a calcium agonist. The entry of calcium into various cells results in elevated intracellular calcium, tetanic muscular contraction, and destruction of the tegument. Praziquantel appears to act in concert with the host immune system to produce a synergistic antihelminthic effect. The disruption of the parasite surface and tegument produced by the drug allows antibodies to attack parasite antigens not normally exposed on the surface (Figure 15-1). Irreversible damage to the parasite probably occurs when complement and/or host leukocytes are recruited to the sites where antibody is bound.

Praziquantel has extremely broad-spectrum activity against trematodes including *Fasciolopsis*, *Fasciola*, *Clonorchis*, *Opisthorchis*, *Paragonimus*, and *Schistosoma*. It is also active against cestodes including *Echinococcus*, *Taenia*, and *Dipylidium*. Praziquantel is currently the drug of choice for the treatment of schistosomiasis, clonorchiasis, opisthorchiasis, and neurocysticercosis. Importantly, there is now good evidence that praziquantel reduces hepatosplenomegaly and portal hypertension in schistosomiasis. Good activity has also been demonstrated against other common trematode and cestode infections.

Phenols

Niclosamide, a phenol, is a nonabsorbable antihelminthic with selective activity against intestinal tapeworms. The drug is absorbed by gut-dwelling cestodes but not by nematodes. It acts by uncoupling oxidative phosphorylation in mitochondria, resulting in a loss of helminth ATP that ultimately immobilizes the parasite so that it is expelled with the feces. Niclosamide is effective in the treatment of intestinal tapeworms in both humans and animals.

Other Antihelminthic Agents

Additional antihelminthic agents including oxamniquine, metrifonate, and suramin are described in Table 15-2. These agents are generally considered secondary agents for the treatment of trematode (oxamniquine and metrifonate) and filarial (suramin) infections.

QUESTIONS

1. What are the obstacles to effective treatment and prophylaxis of parasitic diseases in developing countries?
2. What are the goals of antiparasitic therapy, and how are they different from antibacterial therapy?
3. What is the importance of aminoquinoline analogues?
4. How does the strategy for use of antihelminthic agents differ from that employed in the treatment of protozoal infections?

Bibliography

Campbell WC and Rew RS, editors: *Chemotherapy of parasitic diseases*, New York, 1986, Plenum Publishing.

Cook GC: Antihelminthic agents: some recent developments and their clinical application, *Postgrad Med* J 67:16-22, 1991.

Drugs for parasitic infections, *Med Lett Drugs Ther* 32:23-32, 1990.

Krogstad DJ: Antiparasitic drugs: mechanisms of action and resistance, pharmacokinetics, pharmacodynamics, and in vitro and in vivo assays of drug activity. In Lorian V, editor: *Antibiotics in laboratory medicine*, ed 3, Baltimore, 1991, Williams & Wilkins.

Rosenblatt JE: Antiparasitic agents, *Mayo Clin Proc* 67: 276-287, 1992.

Schwartz IK: Prevention of malaria, *Infect Dis Clin North Am* 6: 313-331, 1992.

Wingard LB Jr, Brody TM, Larner J, Schwartz A, editors: *Human pharmacology: molecular to clinical*, St. Louis, 1991, Mosby.

CHAPTER 16

Chemotherapy of Viral Infections

THE development of antiviral chemotherapy has lagged significantly behind the development of antibacterial drugs. Antibacterial drugs, such as the β-lactam and aminoglycoside antibiotics, are targeted at enzymes and structures that are unique and essential to the viability of almost all prokaryotes. Viruses, unlike most bacteria, are obligate intracellular parasites and utilize the host cell's biosynthetic machinery and enzymes for replication (see Chapter 7). Hence inhibition of viral replication without toxicity to the host is more difficult.

Early antiviral drugs were selective poisons targeted at cells with extensive DNA and RNA synthesis similar to cancer chemotherapies. Newer antiviral drugs are targeted toward viral encoded enzymes or structures of the virus that are important to the replication of the virus. Many of these compounds are classical biochemical inhibitors of viral encoded enzymes (Box 16-1). Newer approaches to antiviral therapy are being directed at blocking the expression of the viral genome (e.g., with antisense RNA) and promoting immune resolution of the viral infection (e.g. with interferon). Unfortunately, most targets for antiviral drugs are unique to a viral family, which limit the drug's spectrum of antiviral activity. Antiviral drugs have been developed against those viruses that cause significant morbidity and mortality and also provide reasonable targets for drug action (Box 16-2). As with antibacterial drugs, antiviral drug resistance is becoming more of a problem with the increased long-term treatment of immunocompromised individuals (e.g., AIDS patients).

BOX 16-1 Antiviral Drug Targets

Cellular activity important for the virus but not for cell viability (*good*)
Activity important for viral replication (facilitates, speeds, or extends the host range of the virus; *better*)
Viral activity or structure essential for replication (*best*)

TARGETS FOR ANTIVIRAL DRUGS

An analysis of the steps of the viral replication cycle identifies potential targets for antiviral drug development, such as structures, enzymes, or processes that are important or essential for virus production. These targets are described in this chapter with examples of antiviral drugs and are listed in Table 16-1.

Attachment is the first step in virus replication. Attachment is mediated by the interaction of a viral attachment protein and its cell surface receptor. This interaction can be blocked by **neutralizing antibodies**, which bind and coat the virion, or by **receptor antagonists**. Administration of specific antibodies (**passive immunization**) is the oldest form of antiviral therapy. Receptor antagonists include peptide or sugar analogues of the cell receptor or the viral attachment protein, which competitively block the interaction of the virus with the cell. Specific peptides of the human immunodeficiency virus (HIV) glycoprotein gp120 or its receptor, the CD4 molecule of T cells, block infection and are being investigated for their clinical potential. Acidic polysaccharides, such as heparan and dextran sulfate, interfere with viral binding and have been suggested for use against herpes simplex, HIV, and other viruses.

BOX 16-2 Viruses Treatable With Antiviral Drugs

Herpes simplex virus
Varicella zoster virus
Cytomegalovirus
Human immunodeficiency virus
Influenza A virus
Respiratory syncytial virus
Hepatitis A, B, C viruses*
Papillomavirus*

*Experimental protocols are available.

TABLE 16-1 Examples of Targets for Antiviral Drugs

Replication step or target	Agent	Targeted virus
Attachment	Peptide analogues of receptor viral attachment protein	Human immunodeficiency virus gp120/CD4 receptor
	Neutralizing antibodies	Most viruses
	Dextran sulfate, heparin	Human immunodeficiency virus, herpes simplex virus
Penetration and uncoating	Amantadine, rimantadine	Influenza A virus
	Tromantadine	Herpes simplex virus
	Arildone, disoxaril	Picornaviruses
Transcription	Interferon	Hepatitis A, hepatitis B, hepatitis C, papillomavirus
	Antisense oligonucleotides	Papillomavirus
Protein synthesis	Interferon	Hepatitis B, hepatitis C, papillomavirus
DNA replication (polymerase)	Nucleotide analogues	Herpesviruses, human immunodeficiency virus
	Phosphonoformate, phosphonacetic acid	Herpesviruses
Nucleoside biosynthesis	Ribavirin	Respiratory syncitial virus
Nucleotide scavenging (thymidine kinase)	Nucleoside analogues	Herpes simplex and varicella zoster viruses
Glycoprotein processing		Human immunodeficiency virus
Assembly (protease)		Human immunodeficiency virus
Virion integrity	Nonoxynol-9	Human immunodeficiency virus, herpes simplex virus

Penetration and uncoating of the virus are required to deliver the viral genome into the cytoplasm of the host cell. Uptake of many viruses utilizes the acidic environment of the endocytic vesicle to initiate uncoating. Amantadine, rimantadine and other hydrophobic amines (weak organic bases) can neutralize these compartments and inhibit virion uncoating. Amantadine, however, is clinically effective only for influenza A. Tromantadine, a derivative of amantadine, inhibits penetration of herpes simplex virus. Arildone, disoxaril and other methylisoxazole compounds fit into a cleft in the receptor binding canyon of the picornavirus capsid and block uncoating.

Although mRNA synthesis is essential for production of virus, it is difficult to inhibit viral mRNA synthesis without affecting cellular mRNA synthesis. DNA viruses use the host cell's transcriptases for mRNA synthesis, making this a poor target for antiviral drugs. The RNA polymerases encoded by RNA viruses may not be sufficiently different from host transcriptases to allow antiviral drug development. Alternatively, the high rate of mutation for RNA viruses may generate many drug-resistant strains. However, rifampin, an antibacterial drug targeted toward RNA polymerase, will inhibit the poxvirus and adenovirus polymerase. Guanidine and 2-hydroxybenzylbenzimidine will block picornavirus RNA synthesis by binding to the 2C picornavirus protein, which is essential for RNA synthesis.

Viral mRNA expression and utilization are targets for antiviral action. Virus infection of an interferon-treated cell triggers a cascade of biochemical events, which blocks viral replication. Viral and cellular mRNA degradation is enhanced, and mRNA binding to the ribosome is blocked, preventing protein synthesis and viral replication. Interferon will be described further in Chapter 52. Interferon and artificial interferon inducers (Ampligen: poly rI:rC) are in clinical trials for viruses such as hepatitis A, B, and C, papilloma viruses, and herpesviruses.

A new approach to block specifically the function of viral mRNA is the use of **antisense oligonucleotides**. Antisense drugs are short, oligomeric sequences (20 nucleotides), which are complementary to specific sequences of the viral genome. These oligomers are chemically synthesized from nucleotide analogues and are resistant to nuclease digestion. Antisense oligonucleotide binding to newly transcribed viral RNA blocks its utilization by preventing processing to mRNA in the nucleus, delivery to the cytoplasm, and binding to the ribosome. An antisense oligonucleotide is in trials for treatment of human papilloma virus infection.

RO 24-7429, an inhibitor of the tat gene-product of HIV, uses another approach to blocking expression of mRNA. The tat protein regulates the processing and delivery of HIV mRNA to the cytoplasm. Inhibition of tat function inhibits HIV replication. Another alternative mechanism is used by isatin-β-thiosemicarbazone. This drug induces mRNA degradation in poxvirus-infected cells and was used as a treatment for smallpox.

Most antiviral drugs are nucleoside analogues, which inhibit viral polymerases. The nucleosides are sequentially phosphorylated to the triphosphate by viral (e.g., thymidine kinase) and cellular enzymes in the infected cells. Viral polymerases are essential for virus replication and are the prime target for most antiviral drugs. Many viral polymerases are less specific for substrate than are host enzymes. The viral polymerase will bind a nucleotide analogue with modifications of the base and/or sugar several hundredfold better than the host enzyme. These drugs prevent chain elongation or proper recognition and base pairing, respectively (Figure 16-1). Antiviral drugs that cause termination of the DNA chain because of modified nucleoside sugar residues include acyclovir, ganciclovir, adenosine arabinoside (Vidarabine), zidovudine, dideoxycytidine (DDC), and dideoxyinosine (DDI). Antiviral drugs that become incorporated into the viral genome and cause errors in replication (mutation) and transcription (inactive mRNA and proteins) because of modified nucleoside bases include 5′iododeoxyuridine (Idoxuridine) and trifluorothymidine (Trifluridine). The rapid rate and large extent of nucleotide incorporation during virus replication makes DNA virus replication especially susceptible to these drugs. Pyrophosphate analogues resembling the byproduct of the polymerase reaction, such as phosphonoformic acid (Foscarnet or PFA), or phosphonoacetate (PAA) are classical inhibitors of the herpesvirus polymerases. A variety of other nucleoside analogues are also being developed as antiviral drugs.

Deoxyribonucleotide scavenging enzymes (e.g., thymidine kinase [TK] and ribonucleotide reductase of the herpesviruses) are also enzyme targets of antiviral drugs. These enzymes provide nucleotide substrates to facilitate the replication of the DNA viral genome. The thymidine kinase also phosphorylates both purine and pyrimidine nucleoside analogues, including acyclovir. HSV mutants lacking thymidine kinase activity are resistant to acyclovir since the drug cannot be activated.

Cellular enzymes or pathways important to viral replication but not cell viability are also targets for antiviral drugs. Ribavirin resembles guanosine monophosphate (GMP) and inhibits nucleoside biosynthesis, mRNA capping, and other processes important to the replication of many viruses.

Although bacterial protein synthesis is the target for several antibacterial compounds, viral protein synthesis is a poor target for antiviral drugs because the virus utilizes host ribosomes and synthetic mechanisms. However, inhibition of posttranslational modification of proteins, such as proteolysis of a viral polyprotein, glycoprotein processing (castanospermine, deoxynojirimycin) or phosphorylation (D609:xanthate) will inhibit virus replication. For example, the HIV protease is unique and essential to virion assembly and release. X-ray crystallographic and molecular biological studies have allowed computer-assisted molecular modeling of site-directed inhibitors and the development of potential antiviral drugs for the HIV protease and other enzyme targets of antiviral drugs. Inhibitors of glycoprotein processing of HIV or HSV block virus release and inhibit glycoprotein functions such as attachment and fusion, preventing both the production and spread of the virus.

In addition to inhibiting the production of virus, other targets for antiviral therapy include preventing the acquisition of the virus, preventing the spread of the virus, and promoting the antiviral immune response of the host. Enveloped viruses are susceptible to certain lipid and detergent-like molecules, which disperse or disrupt the envelope membrane. Nonoxynol-9, a detergent-like component in birth control jellies, will inactivate herpes simplex and human immunodeficiency virus and prevent sexual acquisition of the virus. Antibodies, acquired naturally or by passive immunization (see Chapter 17), prevent both the acquisition and spread of the virus. Interferon, interferon inducers, and other immunomodulatory biological response modifiers stimulate resolution of the infection by the host. Biological response modifiers under investigation include adjuvants consisting of bacterial components (e.g., OK432:killed streptococcal vaccine), mismatched polynucleotides (e.g., ampligen: poly rI:rC), and immunomodulatory chemicals. These agents stimulate the production and release of interferon and other lymphokines, which have antiviral activity and also activate natural killer and killer cell immune responses. These antiviral activities are not specific to one virus and usually work best prophylactically or when administered early in the course of disease.

ANTIVIRAL DRUGS AVAILABLE FOR CLINICAL USE

Most of the antiviral drugs approved by the Food and Drug Administration in the United States (Table 16-2) are nucleoside analogues, which inhibit viral polymerases. These drugs are generally activated by phosphorylation by cellular or viral kinases. Selective inhibition of virus replication is due to either enhanced nucleoside phosphorylation, preferential binding to viral rather than cellular DNA polymerases, or the increased rate of DNA synthesis in infected cells.

Acyclovir

Acyclovir (acycloguanosine; ACV) differs from the nucleoside guanosine by having an acyclic (hydroxyethoxymethyl) side chain instead of a ribose or deoxyribose sugar. ACV has selective action against those herpesviruses that encode a thymidine kinase (TK) (Figure 16-2). The viral thymidine kinase activates the drug by phosphorylation, and host cell enzymes complete the progression to the diphosphate and finally the triphosphate. No initial phosphorylation occurs in uninfected cells, and thus there is no active drug to inhibit cellular DNA synthesis or to cause toxicity. ACV triphosphate competes with guanosine triphosphate and causes termination of the growing viral DNA chain because there is no 3′-hydroxyl group on the ACV molecule to allow chain elongation. The selectivity and minimal toxicity of ACV is also due to its hundredfold or

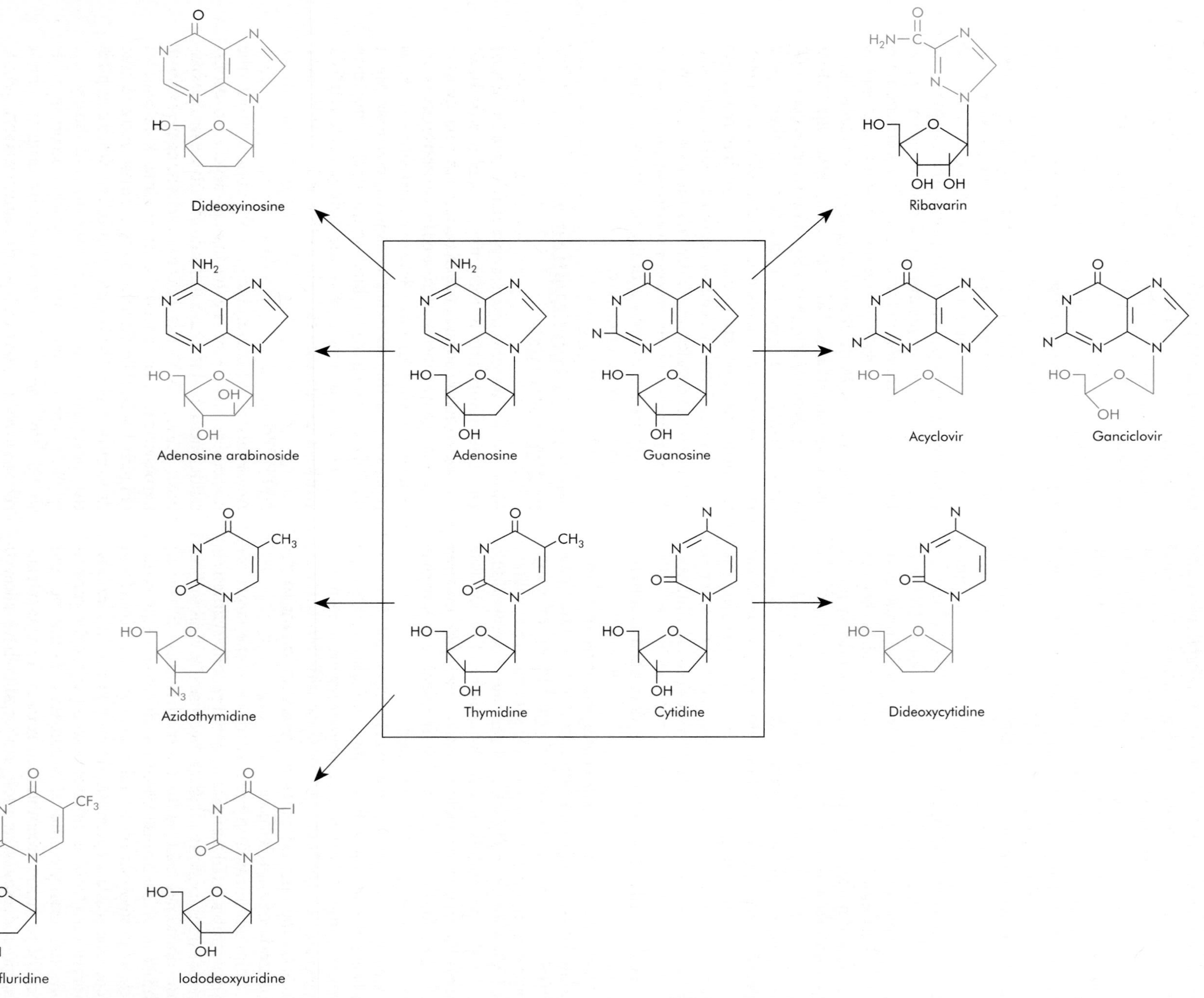

FIGURE 16-1. Structure of nucleoside analogues that are antiviral drugs. The chemical distinctions between the natural deoxynucleoside and the antiviral drug analogues are highlighted.

TABLE 16-2 Antiviral Drug Therapies Approved by the U.S. Food and Drug Administration

Virus	Antiviral drug	Trade names
Herpes simplex virus	Acyclovir	Zovirax
	Adenosine arabinoside (Ara A)	Vidarabine, Vira A
	Iododeoxyuridine*	Stoxil, Idoxuridine
	Trifluorothymidine*	Viroptic, Trifluridine
Cytomegalovirus	Ganciclovir	Cytovene
	Phosphonoformate	Foscarnet, Foscavir
Human immunodeficiency virus	Azidothymidine	Retrovir, Zidovudine
	Dideoxyinosine (DDI)	Didanosine
	Dideoxycytidine	
Influenza A virus	Amantadine	Symmetrel
Hepatitis C	Interferon-α	IFN-α-2a: Roferon A; IFN-α-2b: Intron A
Papillomavirus	Interferon-α	
Respiratory syncytial virus, Lassa fever	Ribavirin	Virazole

*Topical use only.

greater utilization by the viral DNA polymerase than by cellular DNA polymerases. Mutations in either the thymidine kinase or the polymerase can generate acyclovir-resistant strains. These resistant strains are less virulent but can still cause disease in immunocompromised patients, especially patients with AIDS.

Activity of ACV against herpesviruses directly correlates with the capacity of the virus to produce a TK. The order of TK induction and ACV sensitivity is HSV-1 and HSV-2 > Epstein-Barr virus = varicella zoster virus > > cytomegalovirus.

Acyclovir is most effective against herpes simplex viral infections such as encephalitis, disseminated herpes and other serious herpes presentations. ACV can also be used as a prophylactic treatment to prevent recurrent outbreaks, especially in immunosuppressed individuals. A recurrent episode may be prevented if treated within 48 hours of the stimulus of recurrence, before the onset of inflammatory responses. ACV inhibits the replication of HSV but cannot resolve the latent HSV infection. The virus can recur upon cessation of treatment.

ACV can also be used for varicella zoster virus infection, especially if the eye is affected and for Epstein-Barr virus–induced hairy cell leukoplakia. These viruses are much less sensitive to ACV, and intravenous treatment is necessary to deliver higher blood levels of drug.

Ganciclovir

Ganciclovir (dihydroxypropoxymethyl guanine, DHPG), differs from ACV by the addition of a single hydroxymethyl group in the acyclic side chain (see Figure 16-1). The remarkable result of this single addition to the side chain is that it confers considerable activity against cytomegalovirus (CMV). Although CMV does not encode a thymidine kinase, DHPG is phosphorylated to a greater degree in CMV-infected cells than in uninfected cells. Once activated by phosphorylation, DHPG inhibits all herpesvirus DNA polymerases. The viral DNA polymerases have nearly 30 times greater affinity for the drug than does the cellular DNA polymerase. Strains of CMV resistant to DHPG have been described.

DHPG is effective in the treatment of CMV retinitis in patients with AIDS. Studies are in progress to determine its efficacy for CMV esophagitis, colitis, and pneumonia. DHPG is currently available only for intravenous administration. The drug's bone marrow toxicity limits its use to CMV infections in AIDS patients.

Adenine Arabinoside

Adenine arabinoside, (Vidarabine; Ara A) is a purine nucleoside analogue identical in structure to adenosine, except arabinose is substituted for ribose as the sugar moiety (see Figure 16-1). It is phosphorylated by cellular enzymes (especially adenosine kinase) even in uninfected cells and thus has a greater potential for toxicity than acyclovir. Both cellular and viral DNA polymerases are inhibited by Ara A triphosphate, but the viral enzyme is 6 to 12 times more sensitive. This is the basis for a somewhat favorable therapeutic/toxic ratio. Ara A is also incorporated into viral DNA, as well as cellular DNA.

Ara A exhibits activity against HSV and varicella zoster but not Epstein-Barr virus and cytomegalovirus. Resistance can develop by mutation of the viral DNA polymerase.

Ara A was the principal antiviral drug used in the treatment of herpesvirus infections until the introduction of acyclovir. The drug is rapidly deactivated by host enzymes to produce an inactive metabolite and is relatively insoluble in physiological solutions. These properties make it difficult to deliver an effective inhibitory dose.

Azidothymidine

Azidothymidine (Zovirax [AZT]), a nucleoside analogue of thymidine, inhibits the reverse transcriptase of HIV (see Figure 16-1). As with other nucleosides, AZT must be phosphorylated, in this case by host cell enzymes. AZT lacks the 3′ hydroxyl necessary for DNA chain elongation. The basis for the relatively selective therapeutic effect of

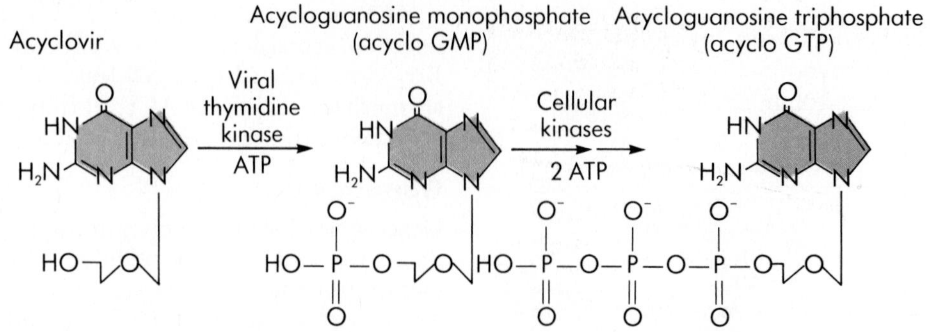

FIGURE 16-2 Activation of acyclovir (acycloguanosine) in herpes simplex viral infected cells. Acyclovir is converted to acycloguanosine monophosphate (acyclo GMP) by the herpes-specific viral thymidine kinase and then to acyclo GTP by cellular kinases.

AZT is that the host cell DNA polymerase is more than 100 times less sensitive to AZT triphosphate than is the HIV reverse transcriptase.

First developed as an anticancer drug, AZT was the first useful therapy for HIV infection. Continuous oral AZT treatment is administered to HIV-infected individuals with depleted CD4 T-cell counts (less than 500 cells per ml) to prevent progression of disease. Toxicity to AZT ranges from nausea to life-threatening bone marrow toxicity.

Dideoxyinosine and Dideoxycytidine

Dideoxyinosine (Didanosine [ddI]) is a nucleoside analogue that is converted to dideoxyadenosine triphosphate (ddA-TP) to inhibit the HIV reverse transcriptase (see Figure 16-1). Dideoxyinosine lacks a 3′hydroxyl group, like AZT, and inhibits the HIV reverse transcriptase by preventing DNA chain elongation. ddI is available for treatment of AIDS patients unresponsive to AZT therapy. *Dideoxycytidine* also inhibits HIV replication and has been approved for treatment of advanced cases of AIDS in conjunction with AZT therapy.

Ribavirin

Ribavirin is an analog of the nucleoside guanosine (see Figure 16-1), but ribavirin differs from guanosine in that the base ring is incomplete and open. As with other nucleoside analogs, ribavirin must be phosphorylated. The drug is active against a broad range of viruses in vitro.

Ribavirin monophosphate resembles guanosine monophosphate (GMP) and inhibits nucleoside biosynthesis, mRNA capping, and other processes important to the replication of many viruses. Ribavirin depletes cellular stores of guanine by inhibiting inosine monophosphate dehydrogenase, an enzyme important in the synthetic pathway of guanosine. It also prevents the synthesis of the mRNA 5′ cap by interference with both guanylation and methylation of the nucleic acid base. In addition, ribavarin triphosphate inhibits RNA polymerases. The multiple sites of action may explain the lack of ribavirin-resistant mutants of respiratory syncytial virus or influenza A virus.

Ribavirin is administered in an aerosol for treatment of children with severe respiratory syncytial virus bronchopneumonia and potentially adults with severe influenza or measles. Oral and IV administration of the drug may be effective for treatment of Lassa fever, and Korean and Argentine hemorrhagic fevers.

Other Nucleoside Analogues

Iododeoxyuridine ([IUDR] Idoxuridine), *trifluorothymidine (trifluridine)* (see Figure 16-1), and *fluorouracil* are analogues of thymidine. These drugs can inhibit the biosynthesis of thymidine, an essential nucleotide for DNA synthesis, or replace thymidine and become incorporated into the viral DNA. This action inhibits further synthesis or causes extensive misreading of the genome, leading to mutation and inactivation of virus. These drugs target cells with extensive DNA replication as occurs in cells infected with herpes simplex virus.

IUDR was the first anti-HSV drug approved for human use. IUDR was indicated for topical treatment of herpes keratitis but has been replaced by trifluridine and other more effective and less toxic treatments. Fluorouracil is an antineoplastic drug that kills rapidly growing cells but has also been used for topical treatment of warts caused by human papillomaviruses.

Many other nucleoside analogues have antiviral activity and are being investigated for clinical use against the herpesviruses and HIV. These compounds include modified pyrimidines such as *bromovinyldeoxyuridine* (BVdU) with a modified base, *fluoroiodoaracytosine* (FIAC) with a modified base and a 2-fluoro arabinose sugar instead of ribose, and *2-fluoromethylarauridine* (FMAU) with the same modified sugar as FIAC. Purine analogues have also been developed that lack or have alternate sugar residues attached to the nucleoside base, similar in concept to acyclovir.

Foscarnet

Foscarnet (phosphonoformate [PFA]) (Figure 16-3) and the related phosphonoacetic acid (PAA) are simple compounds that resemble pyrophosphate. These drugs

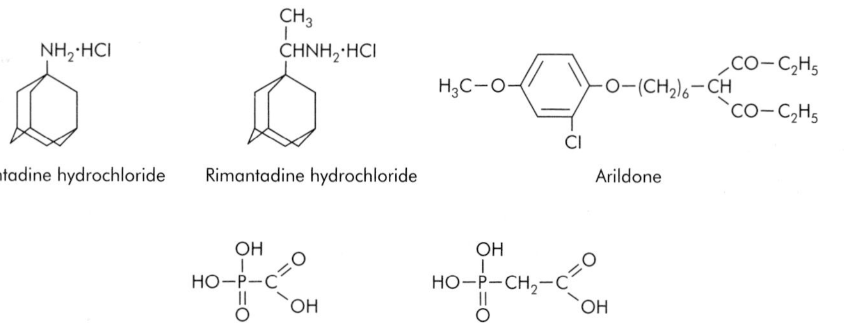

FIGURE 16-3 Structures of some non-nucleoside antiviral drugs.

inhibit viral replication by binding to the pyrophosphate binding site of the DNA polymerase to block nucleotide binding. PFA and PAA do not inhibit cellular polymerases at pharmacological concentrations, but they can cause renal and other problems because of their ability to chelate divalent metal ions (e.g., calcium) and become incorporated into bone. PFA inhibits the DNA polymerase of all herpesviruses and the HIV reverse transcriptase without requiring phosphorylation by nucleotide kinases (e.g., thymidine kinase). PFA has been approved for treatment of cytomegalovirus retinitis in AIDS patients.

Amantadine and Rimantadine

Amantadine and rimantadine (see Figure 16-3) are amphipathic amine compounds with clinical efficacy against influenza A virus but not influenza B or other viruses. Amantadine has two activities on influenza A replication. These two compounds are acidotrophic and concentrate in and buffer the contents of the cytoplasmic vesicles involved in entry of many viruses and glycoprotein processing and transport. Amantadine inhibits the uncoating of influenza A virus by preventing viral envelope fusion with cell membranes following endosomal uptake. At lower concentrations, amantadine binds to and blocks a membrane channel formed by the influenza A virus M2 matrix protein. The M2 protein channel prevents the normal acidification of Golgi and other cytoplasmic vesicles. In the presence of amantadine, newly synthesized hemagglutinins traverse an acidic compartment on their way to the plasma membrane and undergo a mild acid-induced conformation change that can inactivate the progeny virus. Influenza A strains with an altered M2 matrix or hemagglutinin protein may be resistant to these drugs.

Amantadine is effective in preventing influenza A and may be useful in treating this viral infection if taken within 48 hours of exposure. Amantadine is a useful prophylactic treatment in lieu of vaccination. The principal toxic effect is upon the central nervous system and consists of nervousness, irritability, and insomnia.

Interferon

Genetically engineered forms of interferon-α have been approved for human use. Interferon-α is normally produced by leukocytes in response to viral challenge. Interferons bind to cell surface receptors and initiate a cellular antiviral response. In addition, interferons stimulate the immune response and promote immune clearance of viral infection. Interferon-α is active toward many viral infections, including hepatitis A and B, herpes simplex virus, papillomavirus, and rhinovirus. It has been approved for treatment of condyloma acuminatum (genital warts; a presentation of papillomavirus) and hepatitis C. Interferon causes the flu-like symptoms observed during many viremic and respiratory infections and causes similar side effects during treatment. Further discussion of interferon may be found in Chapter 52.

QUESTIONS

1. List the steps in viral replication that are poor targets of antiviral drug development. Why?
2. List the viruses that can be treated with an antiviral drug. Distinguish those viruses treatable with an antiviral nucleoside analog.
3. A mutation in the gene for which enzymes or proteins would confer resistance to the following antiviral drugs: acyclovir, adenosine arabinoside, phosphonoformate, amantadine, azidothymidine?
4. A patient was exposed to influenza A virus and was in his third day of symptoms. He had heard that an antiinfluenza drug was available and requested therapy. You indicate that therapy is not appropriate. What therapeutic agent was the patient referring to, and why did you decline to use the treatment?
5. After treating an AIDS patient for 6 months of prophylactic treatment with acyclovir, viral disease becomes evident. The acyclovir treatment was stopped for 2 weeks and then resumed. No virus was observed upon resumption of therapy.

Which virus is being treated by the acyclovir? Why did the treatment become ineffective? Why did the disease disappear after cessation and resumption of therapy?

Bibliography

Baron S. et al: The interferons. Mechanisms of action and clinical applications, *JAMA* 266:1375-1383, 1991.

Bartlett JG: *1991-1992 pocketbook of infectious disease therapy*, Baltimore, 1991, Williams & Wilkins.

DeClerq E: *Design of anti-AIDS drugs*, Amsterdam, 1990, Elsevier.

Diasio RB, Sommadossi JP. *Advances in chemotherapy of AIDS*, New York, 1990, Pergamon Press.

Fischl MA et al.: The efficacy of azidothymidine (AZT) in the treatment of patients with AIDS and AIDS-related complex: a double-blind, placebo-controlled trial, *N Eng J Med* 317:185-191, 1987.

Havlichek DH, Neu HC. Antiviral drugs. In Wingard LB Jr, Brody TM, Larner J, Schwarz A, editors: *Human pharmacology: molecular to clinical*, St. Louis, 1991, Mosby.

Hirsch M.S. Chemotherapy of human immunodeficiency virus infections: current practice and future prospects, *J Infect Dis* 161:845-857, 1990.

Minor JR, Hay AJ, Belshe RB. In Belshe RB, editor: *Textbook of human virology*, ed 2, St. Louis, 1991, Mosby.

Myers MW: New antiretroviral agents in the clinic, *Rev Infect Dis* 12:944-950, 1990.

Pharmaceutical Manufacturer's Association. *1991 survey report on AIDS medicines in development. AIDS patient care.* April 1992, The Association.

Richman DD: Antiviral therapy of HIV infection, *Ann Rev Med* 42:69-90, 1991.

Yarchoan R and Broder S: Anti-retroviral therapy of AIDS and related disorders: general principles and specific development of dideoxynucleosides, *Pharmacol Ther* 40:329-348, 1989.

CHAPTER 17

Antibacterial and Antiviral Vaccines

ANTIBODIES produced in response to immunization or provided as therapy can prevent or lessen the serious symptoms of disease by blocking the spread of a bacterium, bacterial toxin, or virus to its target organ. Preventing infection is better and cheaper than treating an infectious disease. Immunization of a population, like personal immunity, stops the spread of the infectious agent by reducing the number of susceptible hosts (**herd immunity**). National and international immunization programs have succeeded in protecting the populace from the symptoms of pertussis, diphtheria, tetanus, and rabies; in controlling the spread of measles, mumps, rubella, and poliomyelitis; and led to the elimination of smallpox. In conjunction with immunization of the individual and the populace, diseases can be prevented by limiting exposure to infected individuals (**quarantine**) and by eliminating the source (e.g., water purification) or means of spread (e.g., mosquito eradication). Vaccine-preventable diseases still occur where immunization programs are unavailable or too expensive (Third World countries) or neglected (United States, etc.). For example, measles causes 2 million deaths annually worldwide, and outbreaks are becoming more frequent in the United States. Smallpox was eliminated as of 1977 through a successful World Health Organization program combining vaccination and quarantine.

TYPES OF IMMUNIZATION

Injection of purified antibody or antibody-containing serum for rapid, temporary protection or treatment of an individual is termed **passive immunization.** Newborns receive natural passive immunity from maternal immunoglobulin that has crossed the placenta or is present in the mother's milk.

Stimulation of an immune response and immunological memory by challenge with an immunogen is termed **active immunization.** Active immunization occurs after each exposure to an infectious agent (**natural immunization**) and through exposure to microbes or their antigens in **vaccines**. The term *vaccine* is derived from vaccinia virus, a less virulent member of the poxvirus family, which was used to immunize against smallpox. Vaccines can be subdivided into two groups based on whether they infect the individual (**live vaccines** like vaccinia) or not (**inactivated [killed] vaccines**) (Figure 17-1).

Passive Immunization

Passive immunity may be administered in the following cases: to prevent disease following a known exposure (e.g., needlestick with hepatitis B virus–contaminated blood), to ameliorate the symptoms of an ongoing disease, to protect immunosuppressed patients, or as a therapy to block the action and diseases caused by bacterial toxins. Immune serum globulin preparations derived from seropositive humans or animals (e.g., horses) are available for several bacterial and viral diseases (Table 17-1). Human serum globulin is prepared from pooled plasma and contains the normal repertoire of antibodies for an adult. Special high-titered immunoglobulin preparations are available for hepatitis B virus (HBIG), varicella zoster virus (VZIG), rabies (RIG) and tetanus (TIG). Human immunoglobulin is preferable to animal immunoglobulin because there is less risk of a hypersensitivity reaction (serum sickness).

Monoclonal antibody preparations are being developed for protection against various agents and diseases. Monoclonal antibodies are also being developed to block the pathogenic mechanisms associated with infection, such as neutrophil adherence or lipopolysaccharide action.

Active Immunization

Inactivated Vaccines

Inactivated vaccines, rather than live vaccines, are used for most bacteria and for those viruses that may be too virulent or have the potential for recurrence or oncogenicity. Inactivated vaccines can be produced by chemical (e.g., formalin) or heat inactivation of bacteria, bacterial toxins, or viruses, or by purification of the components or subunits of the infectious agents. These vaccines are usually administered with an adjuvant, such as alum, which functions to boost their immunogenicity. Inacti-

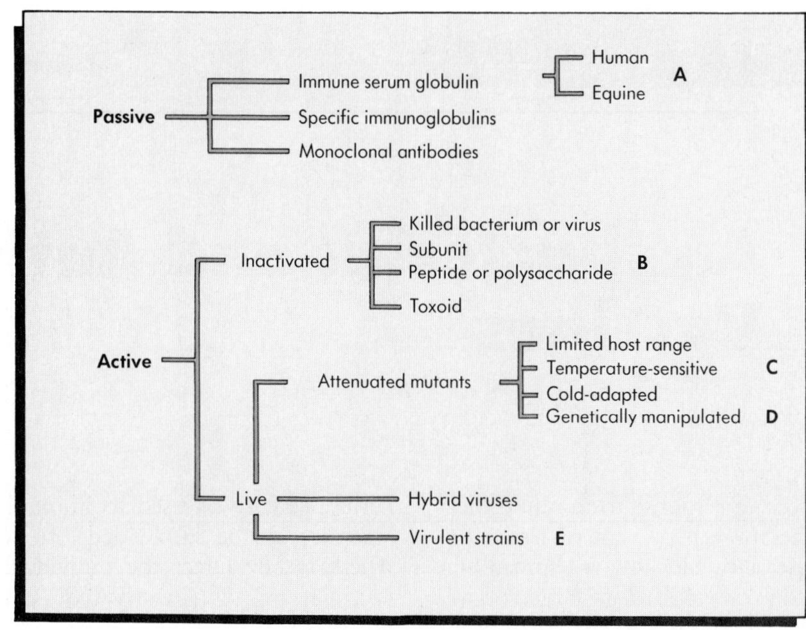

FIGURE 17-1 *Types of immunizations.* Antibodies (passive immunization) can be provided to block the action of an infectious agent or an immune response can be elicited (active immunization) by natural infection or vaccination. The different forms of passive and active immunization are indicated in the figure. **A,** Equine antibodies can be used if human antibody is not available. **B,** Vaccine consisting of components purified from the infectious agent or developed through genetic engineering. **C,** Vaccine selected by passage in animals, embryonated eggs, or tissue culture cells. **D,** Includes deletion, insertion, reassortment, and other laboratory–derived mutants. **E,** Vaccine composed of a virus from a different species, which has a common antigen with the human virus.

TABLE 17-1 Immune Globulins Available for Postexposure Prophylaxis

Disease	Source
Hepatitis A	Human
Hepatitis B	Human*
Measles	Human
Rabies	Human*
Chickenpox, zoster	Human*
Tetanus	Human*, equine
Botulism	Equine
Diphtheria	Equine

*Specific, high-titer antibody is available and the preferred therapy.

vated vaccines are generally safe, except for allergic reactions to vaccine components. The immunity is usually not lifelong, may be limited to humoral and not to cell-mediated immunity, does not elicit a local IgA response, requires booster shots, and demands a larger dose of vaccine than a live vaccine (Table 17-2).

There are three major types of inactivated bacterial vaccines: **toxoid** (inactivated toxins), **inactivated (killed)** bacteria, and **capsule or protein subunits** of the bacteria. Currently available bacterial vaccines are listed in Table 17-3. Most antibacterial vaccines elicit protection against the pathogenic action of toxins.

Inactivated viral vaccines are available for polio, influenza, rabies, and other viruses. The Salk polio (IPV) and the influenza vaccines are prepared by formaldehyde inactivation of virions. In the past, rabies vaccine was prepared by formalin inactivation of infected rabbit neurons or duck embryos, but it is now prepared by chemical inactivation of virions grown in human diploid tissue culture cells. The slow course of rabies disease allows this vaccine to be administered immediately after exposure and still elicit a protective antibody response.

Identification of the bacterial or viral components that elicit a protective immune response allows development of a **subunit vaccine**. Subunit vaccines are prepared by biochemical isolation of the immunogenic component from the bacterium, virus, or viral-infected cells, or by expression of cloned viral genes in bacteria or eukaryotic cells. The hepatitis B virus subunit vaccine was initially prepared from surface antigen obtained from human sera of chronic carriers of the virus (no longer used in the United States), but this vaccine is now purified from yeast bearing the gene for the antigen. The antigen is purified, chemically treated, and absorbed onto alum for immunization. Vaccines against *Haemophilus influenzae B*, *Neisseria meningitidis*, and *Streptococcus pneumoniae* are

monkey kidney tissue culture cells. At least 57 mutations are accumulated in the polio type 1 vaccine strain. Oral administration of this vaccine elicits both secretory IgA in the gut and IgG in the serum. This provides protection along the normal route of infection by the wild virus.

Measles, mumps, and rubella are live vaccines that are often administered together. The initial measles vaccine consisted of the Edmonston B strain developed by Enders and colleagues. This virus was extensively passaged at 35° C–36° C through primary human kidney cells, human amnion cells, and chicken embryo cells. The currently used Moraten (United States) and Schwarz (other nations) vaccine strains of measles were obtained by further passage of the Edmonston B strain in chick embryos at 32° C. The mumps vaccine (Jerryl-Lynn strain) and rubella vaccine (RA 27/3) viruses were also attenuated by extensive passage in cell culture.

FUTURE DIRECTIONS FOR VACCINATION

New vaccines are being developed using molecular biological techniques. New live vaccines can be created by genetically engineering mutations that inactivate or delete a virulence gene instead of random attenuation through tissue culture passage. Genes from infectious agents that cannot be properly attenuated can be inserted into safe viruses (e.g., vaccinia) to form **hybrid virus vaccines**. This promising approach allows development of a polyvalent vaccine to many agents in a single, safe, inexpensive, and relatively stable vector. Upon infection, the hybrid virus vaccine expresses and initiates an immune response to itself and the inserted antigens. The vaccinia virus vector system has been used in several experimental hybrid vaccines. A human immunodeficiency virus (HIV)/ vaccinia hybrid vaccine is currently under evaluation. Other vectors that have been considered include retroviruses, adenovirus, and herpes simplex virus.

Genetically engineered **subunit vaccines** are being developed by cloning genes encoding immunogenic proteins into bacterial and eukaryotic vectors. The most difficult phase in development of subunit vaccines is identification of the appropriate subunit or peptide immunogen. Once identified, its gene can be isolated, cloned, and expressed in bacteria or yeast cells. Large quantities of these proteins can then be produced. Genes for protective immunogens such as the surface antigen of hepatitis B, the gp120 of HIV, the hemagglutinin of influenza, the G antigen of rabies, the gD antigen of herpes simplex virus have been cloned and grown in bacteria or eukaryotic cells for use or potential use as subunit vaccines.

Peptide subunit vaccines consist of specific epitopes of microbial proteins that elicit neutralizing antibody responses. To generate a response, the peptide must contain sequences that allow it to be processed by an antigen presenting cell, bind to an MHC antigen for presentation to T cells, and be recognized by helper T cells to facilitate antibody production. The immunogenicity of the peptide can be enhanced by covalent attachment to a carrier protein. Further understanding of the mechanisms of antigen presentation and T-cell receptor-specific antigens will allow construction of better vaccines.

Antiidiotype antibodies are also being investigated as potential vaccines. Antiidiotype antibodies recognize the variable region of a monoclonal antiviral antibody. The monoclonal antibody is like a cast of the viral epitope. The antiidiotype resembles the original viral epitope, as if molded in the cast. Immunization with an antiidiotype antibody or the viral peptide would elicit similar antibodies.

New technology should allow development of vaccines against infectious agents such as *Streptococcus mutans* (to prevent tooth decay), the herpesviruses, HIV, and parasites such as *Plasmodium falciparum* (malaria) and *Leishmania*. Identification of the appropriate protective immunogen and isolation of its gene should allow production of a vaccine to almost any infectious agent.

IMMUNIZATION PROGRAMS

Immunization may be the best means of protection against infection, but vaccines cannot and should not be developed for all infectious agents. An effective vaccine program can save millions of dollars in health care costs. Effective vaccination of the public protects the individual against infection and disease and reduces the number of susceptible individuals, preventing the spread of the

BOX 17-1 Properties of a Good Candidate for Vaccine Development

Organism causes significant illness
Organism exists as only one serotype
Antibody will block infection or systemic spread
Organism does not have oncogenic potential
Vaccine should be heat stable to allow transport to endemic areas

BOX 17-2 Problems With Vaccine Use

Live vaccines can occasionally revert to virulent forms
Interference by other organisms may prevent infection by the virus (e.g., rubella will prevent polio virus replication)
Vaccination of an immunocompromised person with a live vaccine can be life threatening
Side effects to vaccination can occur, such as hypersensitivity or allergic reactions to the antigen, to nonmicrobial material in the vaccine, or to contaminants
Vaccine development and liability insurance for the manufacturer are very expensive
Organisms with many serotypes are difficult to control by vaccination

TABLE 17-5 Recommended Schedule of Vaccinations for All Children

2 months	4 months	6 months	12 months	15 months	4-6 years (before beginning school)
DPT	DPT	DPT		DPT*	DPT
Polio	Polio			Polio*	Polio
				MMR†	MMR‡
HbCV:					
HbCV§	HbCV	HbCV		HbCV	
HbCV§	HbCV		HbCV		
	At birth (before hospital discharge)		**1-2 months**	**4 months**	**6-18 months**
HBv:					
Option 1	HBv		HBv‖		HBv‖
Option 2			HBv‖	HBv‖	HBv‖

From *MMWR* 40:RR-12, 1991.
DPT, Diphtheria, Pertussis and Tetanus Vaccine. *Polio,* Live oral polio vaccine drops (OPV) or killed (inactivated) polio vaccine shots (IPV). *MMR,* Measles, mumps, and rubella vaccine. *HbCV, Haemophilus influenzae* type b conjugate vaccine. *HBv,* Hepatitis B vaccine.
*Many experts recommend these vaccines at 18 months.
†In some areas this dose of MMR vaccine may be administered at 12 months.
‡Many experts recommend this dose of MMR vaccine be administered at entry into middle school or junior high school.
§HbCV vaccine is administered in either a 4-dose schedule (1) or a 3-dose schedule (2), depending on the type of vaccine used.
‖HBv can be administered at the same time as DPT and/or HbCV.

infectious agent within the population. However, vaccine development and testing are time-consuming and very costly. Considerations for choosing a candidate for a vaccine program are listed in Box 17-1.

Smallpox was eliminated by an effective vaccine program because the virus existed in only one serotype, symptoms were always present, and the vaccine was relatively benign and stable. Elimination of smallpox required a concerted, cooperative effort of the WHO and local health agencies worldwide. Rhinovirus is an example of a poor candidate for vaccine development, because the viral disease is not serious and there are too many serotypes for successful vaccination. Practical aspects and problems with vaccine development are indicated in Box 17-2.

On an individual basis, the ideal vaccine should elicit dependable, lifelong immunity to infection without serious side effects. Factors that influence the success of an immunization include not only the composition of the vaccine, but also the time, site, concentration, and conditions of administration.

The recommended schedule of vaccinations for children is presented in Table 17-5. Infants are immunized with the diphtheria, tetanus, pertussis, and *Haemophilus influenzae* B conjugate inactivated vaccines, and the live, oral polio vaccine. The live measles, mumps, and rubella vaccines are administered at 15 months after the baby's immune response has matured and maternal antibodies have dissipated. Booster immunizations are required for inactivated vaccines later in life. Adults should be immunized with vaccines for *S. pneumoniae* (pneumococcus), influenza, hepatitis B virus and other vaccines, depending on job, travel, or other risk factors that make the individual susceptible to specific infectious agents.

QUESTIONS

1. Why is an inactivated rather than a live vaccine used for the following immunizations? Rabies, influenza, tetanus, hepatitis B virus, *Haemophilus influenzae* B, diphtheria, and pertussis.
2. Tetanus is treated with passive immunization and prevented by active immunization. Compare the nature and function of each of these therapies.
3. The inactivated polio vaccine is administered intramuscularly, whereas the live polio vaccine is administered as an oral vaccine. How does the course of the immune response and the immunoglobulins produced in response to each vaccine differ? What step in polio virus infection is blocked in an individual vaccinated by each vaccine?
4. Why have large-scale vaccine programs not been developed for rhinovirus, herpes simplex virus, or respiratory syncytial virus?
5. Describe the public or personal health benefits that justify the development of the following major vaccine programs: measles, mumps, rubella, polio, smallpox, tetanus, and pertussis.

Bibliography

Centers for Disease Control. Update on Adult Immunization: Recommendations of the Immunization Practices Advisory Committee, *MMWR* 40:RR-12, 1991.

Hill DR: Immunizations, *Infect Dis Clin North Am* 6:291, 1992.

Plotkin SA and Mortimer EA: *Vaccines*, Philadelphia, 1988, WB Saunders.

SECTION IV

BACTERIOLOGY

CHAPTER 18

Laboratory Diagnosis of Bacterial Diseases

MICROBIOLOGY differs from all other specialties in clinical pathology in that the objective of most tests is to isolate viable organisms. This means that the proper specimen must be collected, delivered expeditiously to the laboratory in the appropriate transport system, and inoculated onto media that will support the growth of the most likely pathogens. Collection of the proper specimen and rapid delivery to the clinical laboratory are primarily the responsibility of the patient's physician, whereas selection of the appropriate transport system and culture methods are determined by the clinical microbiologist. However, these responsibilities are not mutually exclusive: the microbiologist should be prepared to instruct the physician about the most appropriate specimen that should be collected for a specific diagnosis, and the physician must provide the microbiologist with information about the clinical diagnosis so the right culture media and growth conditions can be selected. For information about selection of culture media for specific pathogens, see the texts by Balows et al. and Baron and Finegold listed in the Bibliography. The primary focus of this chapter is to provide guidelines for the proper collection and transport of different specimens (summarized in Table 18-1), as well as general information about the laboratory processing of specimens. Whenever an unusual or fastidious pathogen is suspected (e.g., *Bordetella pertussis, Francisella tularensis*, etc.), the laboratory should be notified so the appropriate transport system and culture media can be obtained.

BLOOD

The culture of blood is one of the most important procedures performed in the clinical microbiology laboratory. The success of this test is directly related to the methods used to collect the blood sample. Bacteremia and fungemia are defined as the presence of bacteria or fungi, respectively, in the bloodstream, and these infections are referred to collectively as **septicemia**. Clinical studies have demonstrated that septicemia can be either continuous or intermittent. **Continuous septicemia** is observed primarily in intravascular infections (e.g., endocarditis, septic thrombophlebitis, intravascular catheter infections) or in overwhelming sepsis (e.g., septic shock). **Intermittent septicemia** is observed in most other infections where the focus is at a distal site (e.g., lungs, urinary tract, soft tissue infections). The timing of blood collection is not important for patients with continuous septicemias, whereas it is critical for patients with intermittent septicemias. In addition, because clinical signs of sepsis (e.g., fever, chills, hypotension) are a response to the release of endotoxins or exotoxins from the organisms, these signs may occur as long as 1 hour after clearance of the organisms from the bloodstream. Thus collection of blood samples during a febrile episode may be the worst time for isolation of organisms. Two to three blood samples should be collected at random times during a 24-hour period. For the reasons stated previously, the number of samples collected is more important if an intermittent septicemia is suspected. Collecting more than three samples per 24 hours has been found unnecessary even in patients receiving antibiotics.

A large volume of blood should be collected because more than one half of all septic patients have fewer than one organism per ml of blood. Approximately 20 ml of blood should be collected from an adult for each blood culture and proportionally smaller volumes for children and neonates. The volume of cultured blood is critically important because a 40% increase in significant positive cultures occurs when the cultured volume of blood increases from 10 ml to 20 ml. Because many hospitalized patients are susceptible to infections with organisms colonizing their skin, careful disinfection of the skin with alcohol followed by 2% iodine is important.

Most blood samples are inoculated into bottles filled with enriched nutrient broths. This should be done when the sample is collected. To ensure the maximum recovery of important organisms, two bottles of media are inoculated for each culture. When these inoculated bottles of broth are received in the laboratory, they will be incubated at 37° C and inspected at regular intervals for evidence of microbial growth. When growth is detected, the broths are subcultured to isolate the organism for identification and antimicrobial susceptibility testing.

TABLE 18-1 Specimen Collection for Bacterial Pathogens

Specimen	Transport system	Specimen volume	Other considerations
Blood—routine bacterial culture	Blood culture bottle with nutrient medium	Adults: 20 ml/culture Children: 5-10 ml/culture Neontes: 1-2 ml/culture	Disinfect skin with 70% alcohol followed by 2% iodine or iodophor; collect 2-3 cultures/24 hr period unless patient is in septic shock or antibiotics will be started immediately; blood collections should be separated by 30-60 minutes; blood divided equally into two bottles of nutrient media
Blood—intracellular bacteria (e.g., *Brucella, Francisella, Neisseria*)	As with routine blood cultures; lysis-centrifugation system	As with routine blood cultures	As with routine blood cultures; release of intracellular bacteria may improve their recovery; *Neisseria* inhibited by some anticoagulants (sodium polyanetholsulfonate)
Blood—*Leptospira*	Sterile, heparinized tube	1-5 ml	Useful only during the first week of illness; afterward, urine should be cultured
Cerebrospinal fluid	Sterile, screw-capped tube	Bacterial culture: 1-5 ml Mycobacterial culture: as large a volume as possible	Specimen must be collected aseptically; deliver immediately to lab; do not expose to heat or refrigeration
Other normally sterile fluids (e.g., abdominal, chest, synovial, pericardial)	Small volume: sterile, screw-capped tube; large volume: blood culture bottle with nutrient medium	As large a volume as possible; pathogens can be diluted to small numbers per ml of fluid	Collect specimens with a needle and syringe; do not use a swab because the quantity of collected specimen is inadequate; do not inject an "air bubble" into the culture bottle—this will inhibit the growth of anaerobes
Catheter (venous, arterial)	Sterile screw-capped tube or specimen cup	N/A	Disinfect the entry site with alcohol; aseptically remove the catheter; upon receipt of the specimen in the laboratory, the catheter is rolled across a blood agar plate and then discarded; a semiquantitative culture is performed
Respiratory—throat	Swab immersed in transport medium	N/A	Swab area of inflammation; collect exudate if present; avoid contact with saliva because this can inhibit the recovery of group A streptococci
Respiratory—epiglottis	Collect blood for culture	See above for blood culture	Swabbing the epiglottis can precipitate complete airway closure; collect blood cultures for specific diagnosis
Respiratory—sinuses	Sterile, anaerobic tube or vial	1-5 ml	Specimens must be collected with needle and syringe; culture of nasopharynx or oropharynx has no predictive value; culture specimen for aerobic and anaerobic bacteria
Respiratory—lower airways	Sterile, screw-capped bottle; anaerobic tube or vial only for specimens collected by avoiding upper tract flora	1-2 ml	Expectorated sputum: if possible have the patient rinse his/her mouth with water before collection of the specimen; cough deeply and ask patient to expectorate lower airway secretions directly into sterile cup; avoid contamination with saliva. Bronchoscopy specimen: anesthetics can inhibit the growth of bacteria so specimens should be processed immediately; if a "protected" bronchoscope is used, anaerobic cultures can be performed. Transtracheal aspirate or direct lung aspirate: specimens can be processed for aerobic and anaerobic bacteria
Ear	Capped, needle-less syringe; sterile, screw-capped tube	Whatever volume is collected	Aspirate specimen with a needle and syringe; culture of external ear has no predictive value for otitis media

Continued

TABLE 18-1 Specimen Collection for Bacterial Pathogens—cont'd

Specimen	Transport system	Specimen volume	Other considerations
Eye	Inoculate plates at bedside, seal, and transport to lab immediately	Whatever volume can be collected	For infections on the surface of the eye, specimens are collected with a swab or by corneal scrapings; for deep-seated infections, aspiration of aqueous or vitreous fluid is performed; all specimens should be inoculated onto appropriate media at collection; delays will result in significant loss of organisms
Exudates (transudates, drainage, ulcers)	Swab immersed in transport medium; aspirate in sterile screw-capped tube	Bacteria: 1-5 ml Mycobacteria: 3-5 ml	Avoid contamination with surface material; specimens are generally unsuitable for anaerobic culture
Wounds (abscess, pus)	Aspirate in sterile screw-capped tube or sterile anaerobic tube or vial	1-5 ml of pus	Specimens should be collected with a sterile needle and syringe; use curette to collect specimen at base of wound; swabbed specimens should be avoided
Tissues	Sterile screw-capped tube; sterile anaerobic tube or vial	Representative sample for center and border of lesion	Place aseptically into appropriate sterile container; an adequate quantity of specimen must be collected to recover small numbers of organisms
Urine—midstream	Sterile urine container	Bacteria: 1-10 ml Mycobacteria: ≥10 ml	Avoid contamination of the specimen with bacteria in the urethra or vagina so discard the first portion of the voided specimen; organisms can grow rapidly in urine so the specimens must be transported immediately to the laboratory, held in a bacteriostatic preservative, or refrigerated
Urine—catheterized	Sterile urine container	Bacteria: 1-10 ml Mycobacteria: ≥10 ml	Catheterization is not recommended for routine cultures (risk of inducing an infection); first portion of collected specimen is contaminated with urethral bacteria so it should be discarded (similar to midstream voided specimen); transport rapidly to the laboratory
Urine—suprapubic aspirate	Sterile anaerobic tube or vial	Bacteria: 1-10 ml Mycobacteria: ≥10 ml	Invasive specimen so urethral bacteria are avoided; only valid method available for collecting specimens for anaerobic culture; useful also for collection of specimens from children or adults unable to void an uncontaminated specimen
Genitals	Swab immersed in transport medium; anaerobic transport system if endocervical specimen is collected by aspiration; directly inoculate media for isolation of *Neisseria gonorrhoeae*; specialized transport system for *Chlamydia*	N/A	Some genital pathogens are extremely labile (e.g., *N. gonorrhoeae*, *Chlamydia*); the area of inflammation or exudate should be sampled; avoid collection of normal flora because they may inhibit or overgrow the pathogens
Feces (stool)	Sterile screw-capped container	N/A	Rapid transport to laboratory required to prevent production of acid (bactericidal for some enteric pathogens) by normal fecal bacteria; unsuitable for anaerobic culture; because a large number of different media will be inoculated, a swab should not be used for specimen collection

Most clinically significant isolates will be detected within the first 2 days of incubation; however, all cultures should be incubated for a minimum of 5 to 7 days.

CEREBROSPINAL FLUID

Bacterial meningitis is a serious disease with high morbidity and mortality if the etiological diagnosis is delayed. Because some common pathogens are labile (e.g., *Neisseria meningiditis*, *Streptococcus pneumoniae*), cerebrospinal fluid (CSF) should be processed immediately. CSF is collected aseptically after skin disinfection with alcohol and iodine. The specimen is collected into sterile, screw-capped tubes, which should be transported immediately to the laboratory. Under no circumstance should the specimen be subjected to refrigeration or heating. Upon receipt in the laboratory, the specimen is concentrated by centrifugation, and the pellet is used to inoculate bacteriological media, prepare a Gram stain (and other stains if fungal or mycobacterial infections are suspected), and perform tests for the direct detection of bacterial antigens (e.g., for *Haemophilus influenzae, Neisseria meningiditis, Streptococcus pneumoniae*, and group B *Streptococcus*). The antigen tests have very limited value but may be useful for patients with partially treated infections. The laboratory should contact the physician immediately if any test (stain, antigen test, culture) is positive.

OTHER NORMALLY STERILE FLUID

A variety of other normally sterile fluids may be collected for bacteriological culture, including abdominal (peritoneal), chest (pleural), synovial, and pericardial fluids. If a large volume of fluid can be collected by percutaneous aspiration (e.g., abdominal or chest fluids), it should be inoculated into blood culture bottles with nutrient media. A small portion should also be sent to the laboratory in a sterile tube so appropriate smears (e.g., Gram, KOH, acid-fast) can be prepared. For smaller quantities of fluid, the specimen can be inoculated directly onto agar media or into a sterile container and transported to the laboratory. Transport of specimens in syringes should be discouraged. Because relatively few organisms may be present in the sample (due to dilution of organisms or microbial elimination by the host immune response), it is important to culture as large a volume of fluid as possible. Anaerobes may be present in the sample (particularly for intraabdominal and pulmonary infections); therefore exposure of the specimen to oxygen should be avoided.

UPPER RESPIRATORY SPECIMENS

Group A streptococci are the most important bacteria responsible for bacterial pharyngitis. Other potentially pathogenic bacteria, such as *Staphylococcus aureus, Streptococcus pneumoniae, Haemophilus influenzae, Moraxella catarrhalis,* Enterobacteriaceae, and *Pseudomonas* may be present in the oropharynx, but they are rarely responsible for significant upper respiratory tract disease. Although *Corynebacterium diphtheriae* and *Bordetella pertussis* are relatively uncommon in the United States, these organisms can cause significant disease. *Neisseria gonorrhoeae, Chlamydia* species, and *Mycoplasma pneumoniae* are also upper respiratory tract pathogens.

The specimen should be collected with a Dacron or calcium alginate swab. The tonsillar areas, posterior pharynx, and any exudate or ulcerative area should be sampled. Contamination of the specimen with saliva should be avoided because bacteria in saliva can either overgrow or inhibit the growth of the important pathogen. If a pseudomembrane is present (e.g., as with *C. diphtheriae* infections), a portion should be dislodged and submitted for culture. Group A streptococci and *C. diphtheriae* are very resistant to drying so special precautions are not required for transport to the laboratory. In contrast, specimens collected for the recovery of *B. pertussis* and *N. gonorrhoeae* should be inoculated onto culture media immediately after collection and before sending the specimen to the laboratory. Transport of specimens for the isolation of *Chlamydia* and *M. pneumoniae* requires the use of special transport medium.

Group A streptococci can be detected directly in the clinical specimen by use of immunoassays specific for the group-specific antigen. Although these tests are very specific, they are currently insensitive and cannot reliably exclude the diagnosis of group A streptococcal pharyngitis.

Other upper respiratory tract infections can involve the epiglottis and sinuses. Complete airway obstruction can be precipitated by attempts to culture the epiglottis in infected patients (particularly children). For this reason, these cultures should be avoided. The specific diagnosis of a sinus infection requires direct aspiration of the sinus, appropriate anaerobic transport to the laboratory (using a system that avoids exposing anaerobes to oxygen and drying), and prompt processing. *S. pneumoniae, H. influenzae, M. catarrhalis, S. aureus*, and anaerobes are the most common pathogens responsible for sinusitis.

LOWER RESPIRATORY SPECIMENS

A variety of techniques can be used to collect lower respiratory specimens, including expectoration, induction with saline, bronchoscopy and bronchial alveolar lavage, transtracheal aspiration (rarely used today), and direct aspiration through the chest wall. Expectorated and induced sputa, as well as most types of bronchoscopy specimens, can potentially be contaminated with upper airway bacteria. For this reason the specimen should be microscopically inspected to assess the magnitude of oral contamination and value of processing the specimen. Specimens with large numbers of squamous epithelial cells (greater than or equal to 25 cells per low power microscopic field) and no predominant bacteria associated with leukocytes should not be submitted for culture.

Upper airway contamination of the specimen can be avoided by using a protected bronchoscope, transtracheal aspiration, or direct lung aspiration. Use of these invasive procedures to collect an uncontaminated specimen is required for anaerobic pleuropulmonary infections. Most lower respiratory pathogens grow within 2 to 3 days, although additional time may be required for isolation and identification of the bacterium.

EAR AND EYE

Tympanocentesis (aspiration of fluid in the middle ear) is required to make the specific diagnosis of a middle ear infection. However, this is unnecessary for most infections because the most common pathogens (*S. pneumoniae, H. influenzae, M. catarrhalis*) can be treated empirically. Culture of the nasopharynx or pharynx is not useful and should not be performed.

Collection of specimens for ocular infections is difficult because the sample obtained is generally very small and relatively few organisms may be present. Samples should be collected by swab before the topical anesthetics are used, followed by corneal scrapings whenever necessary. The culture media should be inoculated at the time the specimen is collected and then sent to the laboratory. All media should be incubated for a minimum of 5 days. Although most common ocular pathogens grow rapidly (e.g., *S. aureus, S. pneumoniae, H. influenzae, P. aeruginosa*), some may require prolonged incubation before detection (e.g., coagulase-negative staphylococci, *N. gonorrhoeae*). Specialized cultures must be performed if *C. trachomatis* ocular infection is suspected.

WOUNDS, ABSCESSES, AND TISSUES

Open, draining wounds can frequently be colonized with potentially pathogenic organisms that are unrelated to the specific infectious process. For this reason it is important to collect samples from deep in the wound after the surface has been cleaned. Use of swabs should be avoided whenever possible because it is difficult to obtain a representative sample without contamination with organisms colonizing the surface. Likewise, aspirates from a closed abscess should be collected from both the center of the abscess and the abscess wall. Drainage from soft tissue infections can be collected by aspiration and, if fluctuance is not obtained, a small quantity of saline can be infused into the tissue and then withdrawn for culture. Do not use saline containing a bactericidal preservative.

Tissues should be obtained from representative portions, with multiple samples collected whenever possible. The tissue specimen should be transported in a sterile, screw-capped container, and sterile saline should be added to prevent drying if a small sample (e.g., punch biopsy) is collected. A sample of tissue should also be submitted for histological examination. The outer surface of the tissue should be sterilized, and then the specimen is homogenized and inoculated onto bacteriological media. Because collection of tissue specimens requires invasive procedures, every effort should be made to collect the proper specimen and ensure it is cultured for all clinically significant organisms that may be responsible for the infection. This process requires close communication between the physician and microbiologist.

URINE

Urine is one of the most frequently submitted specimens for culture. Because potentially pathogenic bacteria colonize the urethra, the first portion of urine voided or collected by catheterization should be discarded. Urinary tract pathogens can also grow in urine, so delays in transport to the laboratory should be avoided. If the specimen cannot be cultured immediately, it should be refrigerated or placed in a bacteriostatic urine preservative. Upon receipt of the specimen in the laboratory, 1 μl to 10 μl of urine is inoculated onto each culture medium (generally one nonselective agar medium and one selective medium). In this manner the number of organisms in the urine can be quantitated. This process is useful for assessing the significance of an isolate, although small numbers of organisms in the presence of pyuria can be clinically significant. A number of urine screening procedures have been developed and are used widely; however, these procedures are invariably insensitive for clinically significant, low grade bacteriuria.

GENITALS

Despite the variety of bacteria that have been associated with sexually transmitted diseases, most laboratories concentrate on isolating *Neisseria gonorrhoeae* and *Chlamydia trachomatis*. Both organisms are labile so proper handling of the specimen is required. Urethral discharge or endocervical exudate should be inoculated immediately onto appropriate selective media for the recovery of *N. gonorrhoeae* (e.g., Thayer-Martin medium). The media contain antibiotics to suppress the growth of other organisms that may be present in the specimen. However, a nonselective medium should also be inoculated because some strains of *N. gonorrhoeae* are inhibited by the antibiotics. *N. gonorrhoeae* is sensitive to cold and requires carbon dioxide for growth; therefore the media must be warmed before inoculation and then should be placed into a CO_2-enriched atmosphere. A number of innovative transport-culture systems have been developed to provide this atmosphere. A portion of the exudate should also be smeared on a glass slide, Gram stained, and examined microscopically. For many male patients, this procedure is all that is necessary to make the diagnosis.

The most common cause of sexually transmitted disease in the United States is *Chlamydia trachomatis*. Specimens collected for the recovery of this organism must be rapidly transported to the laboratory in special transport media (2-SP). Upon receipt in the laboratory, cell cultures are inoculated and then monitored for the growth of this intracellular pathogen. Cytoplasmic inclusions indicative of the chlamydia are usually observed after 1 to 2 days of incubation.

As can be imagined, numerous problems can be encountered recovering *N. gonorrhoeae* and *C. trachomatis*. For this reason, nonculture methods have been developed, including use of commercial molecular probes for both organisms and direct immunofluorescent staining and antigen-directed immunoassays for chlamydia. The direct stains and immunoassays have proved to be relatively insensitive, particularly for asymptomatic carriers. However, the probes are both sensitive and specific and are rapidly replacing the use of culture for these organisms.

The other major bacterium responsible for sexually transmitted diseases is *Treponema pallidum*, the etiological agent of syphilis. This organism cannot be cultured in the clinical laboratory so the diagnosis is made by either microscopy or serology. Material from lesions must be examined by darkfield microscopy because the organism is too thin to be detected by brightfield microscopy. In addition, the organisms die rapidly when exposed to air and drying so the microscopic examination must be performed at the time the specimen is collected. The serologic diagnosis of syphilis will be discussed in Chapter 36.

FECES

A large variety of bacteria can cause gastrointestinal infections. Their recovery in culture requires collection of an adequate stool sample (generally not a problem), transport to the laboratory in a manner to ensure their viability, and inoculation onto the appropriate selective media. Because a variety of selective media must be inoculated for the recovery of the various pathogens, rectal swabs should not be submitted. The quantity of feces collected on the swab would be inadequate unless enrichment culture for a specific pathogen is performed (e.g., screening for carriage of *Salmonella*).

Stool specimens should be passed into a clean pan and then transferred into a tightly sealed, waterproof container. The specimens should be transported promptly to the laboratory to prevent acidic changes in the stool (caused by bacterial metabolism), which are toxic for organisms such as *Shigella*. If a delay is anticipated, the feces should be mixed with a preservative such as phosphate buffer mixed with glycerol or, if campylobacter infection is suspected, Cary-Blair transport medium. In general, however, rapid transport to the laboratory is always superior to the use of any transport medium.

It is important to notify the laboratory if a particular enteric pathogen is suspected because this will help the laboratory select the appropriate culture medium. For example, although *Vibrio* species will grow on the common selective media used for stool specimens, specific media selected for *Vibrio* will facilitate the rapid isolation and detection of this organism. In addition, some organisms are not routinely isolated by the laboratory procedures (e.g., enterotoxigenic *Escherichia coli*), whereas others would not be expected to be present in the stool sample because their disease is caused by toxin production in the food and not by growth in the gastrointestinal tract (e.g., *Staphylococcus aureus*). *C. difficile* is a significant cause of antibiotic-associated gastrointestinal disease. Although the organism can be cultured from stool specimens if they are promptly delivered to the laboratory, the most specific diagnostic test is detection in fetal extracts of the *C. difficile* toxin responsible for the disease.

Because a large number of different organisms are present in fecal specimens (pathogenic and nonpathogenic bacteria), the isolation and identification of the enteric pathogen frequently takes 3 days or more. For this reason, stool cultures are frequently used to confirm the clinical diagnosis, and therapy, if indicated, should not be delayed while waiting for the culture results. Indeed, antimicrobial susceptibility testing is usually not performed with most enteric pathogens.

QUESTIONS

1. Name four factors that influence recovery of microorganisms in blood collected from septic patients. Which factor is the most important?
2. When are antigen tests useful for the diagnosis of bacterial meningitis?
3. How can the clinical diagnosis of epiglottitis be confirmed?
4. What criteria should be used to assess the quality of a lower respiratory tract specimen?
5. What technical problems are associated with the recovery of *Neisseria gonorrhoeae* and *Chlamydia trachomatis* from genital specimens?

Bibliography

Balows A, Hausler WJ, Lennette EH: *Laboratory diagnosis of infectious diseases—principles and practice*, vol 1, New York, 1988, Springer-Verlag.

Balows A, Hausler WJ, Herrmann KL, Isenberg HD, Shadomy HJ: *Manual of clinical microbiology*, ed 5, Washington, DC, 1991, American Society for Microbiology.

Baron EJ, Finegold SM: *Bailey and Scott's diagnostic microbiology*, ed 8, St. Louis, 1991, Mosby.

CHAPTER 19

Staphylococcus

THE family Micrococcaceae consists of four genera: *Planococcus, Stomatococcus, Micrococcus,* and *Staphylococcus. Planococcus,* a genus of motile, gram-positive cocci, has not been found in humans, and *Micrococcus* is usually recovered as a laboratory contaminant. Infections caused by *Stomatococcus mucilaginosus*, part of the normal flora of the human mouth, are relatively uncommon but have been reported with increasing frequency in immunocompromised patients. The most common clinical manifestations are endocarditis, septicemia, and catheter-related infections. Infections with this opportunistic pathogen are facilitated by its ability to form adherent mucoid colonies. *Staphylococcus* is a significant human pathogen, causing a wide spectrum of diseases ranging from superficial cutaneous infections to life-threatening systemic maladies. The remainder of this chapter will concentrate on *Staphylococcus* and its role in human disease.

The name *Staphylococcus* is derived from the Greek term for grapelike cocci. This name is appropriate because the cellular arrangement of these gram-positive cocci resembles a cluster of grapes, although this is most characteristic for staphylococci grown on agar media. Organisms in clinical material are seen as single cells, pairs, or short chains.

Staphylococci are gram-positive cocci, 0.5 to 1.5 μm in diameter, nonmotile, facultatively anaerobic, catalase positive, and able to grow in a medium containing 10% sodium chloride and in a temperature range from 18° C to 40° C. The organisms normally grow on the skin and mucous membranes of humans, as well as that of other mammals and birds. A total of 27 species and seven subspecies are currently recognized in the genus, with 14 species and 2 subspecies found on humans (Table 19-1). The species most commonly associated with human infections are *S. aureus* (the most virulent and best-known member of the genus), *S. epidermidis, S. haemolyticus, S. lugdunensis, S. saprophyticus, and S. schleiferi*. *S. aureus* is the only species found in humans that produces the enzyme coagulase; thus all other species are commonly referred to as **"coagulase-negative staphylococci."**

PHYSIOLOGY AND STRUCTURE

Staphylococcal structure and function are outlined in Table 19-2 and Figure 19-1.

Capsule

A loose-fitting, polysaccharide layer is only occasionally found on staphylococci cultured in vitro but is believed to be more commonly present in vivo. This capsule protects the bacteria by inhibiting chemotaxis and phagocytosis by polymorphonuclear leukocytes and proliferation of mononuclear cells following mitogen exposure. It also facilitates adherence of bacteria to catheters and other synthetic material (e.g., graft, prosthetic valves and joints, and shunts) (Figure 19-2). This property is particularly

TABLE 19-1 *Staphylococcus* Species Found on Humans

Species	Cause of human disease
S. aureus	Common
S. epidermidis	Common
S. saprophyticus	Common
S. haemolyticus	Uncommon
S. lugdunensis	Uncommon
S. schleiferi	Uncommon
S. saccharolyticus	Rare
S. warneri	Rare
S. hominis	Rare
S. auricularis	Rare
S. xylosus	Rare
S. simulans	Rare
S. capitis	Rare
S. capitis ssp. *ureolyticus*	Rare
S. cohnii	Rare
S. cohnii ssp. *urealyticum*	Rare

important for the relatively avirulent coagulase-negative staphylococci.

Peptidoglycan

The peptidoglycan layer, composed of peptide cross-linked glycan chains, is the major structural component of the staphylococcal cell wall (Figure 19-3). The glycan chains are built with approximately 10 to 12 alternating subunits of *N*-acetylmuramic acid and *N*-acetylglucosamine. Tetrapeptide side chains are attached to the *N*-acetylmuramic acid subunits, and the glycan chains are then cross-linked with peptide bridges between the side chains. This layer has endotoxin-like activity, can attract polymorphonuclear leukocytes (abscess formation), and can activate complement. Lysozyme (muramidase) present in tears, saliva, and human leukocytes, monocytes, and macrophages can hydrolyze the linkage between the glycan subunits and thus form a natural barrier to staphylococcal infections.

Protein A

The surface of most *S. aureus* strains (but not the coagulase-negative staphylococci) is uniformly coated with protein A. This protein is covalently linked to the peptidoglycan layer and has the unique affinity for binding the Fc receptor of immunoglobulins IgG1, IgG2, and IgG4, thus effectively preventing the antibody-mediated immune clearance of the organism. Extracellular protein A can also bind antibodies, forming immune complexes with the subsequent consumption of complement.

The presence of protein A has been exploited in some serological tests in which protein-A–coated *S. aureus* is used as a nonspecific carrier of antibodies directed against other antigens.

TABLE 19-2 Staphylococcal Structure and Function

Structure	Function
Capsule	Inhibits opsonization and phagocytosis Protects from C′-mediated leukocyte destruction
Peptidoglycan	Osmotic stability Stimulates production of endogenous pyrogen Leukocyte chemoattractant Inhibits phagocytosis and chemotaxis
Protein A	Binds IgG1, IgG2, IgG4 Fc receptors Inhibits opsonization and phagocytosis Leukocyte chemoattractant Anticomplementary
Teichoic acid	Regulates cationic concentration at cell membrane Receptor for bacteriophages Attachment site for mucosal surface receptors
Cytoplasmic membrane	Osmotic barrier Regulates transport into and out of cell Site of biosynthetic and respiratory enzymes

Teichoic Acid

Teichoic acids are complex, phosphate-containing polysaccharides bound to both the peptidoglycan layer and cytoplasmic membrane. These polysaccharides are species specific. For example, ribitol teichoic acid with *N*-acetylglucosamine residues (polysaccharide A) are present in *S. aureus,* and glycerol teichoic acid with glucosyl residues (polysaccharide B) are present in *S. epidermidis*. Attachment of staphylococci to mucosal surfaces is mediated by the cell wall teichoic acids through their specific binding to fibronectin. Although the teichoic acids are poor immunogens, a specific antibody response is stimulated when they are bound to peptidoglycan. The monitoring of this antibody response has been used to detect systemic staphylococcal disease.

Clumping Factor

The outer surface of most strains of *S. aureus* contains clumping factor or **bound coagulase**. This protein binds fibrinogen and can cause the staphylococci to clump or aggregate.

Cytoplasmic Membrane

The cytoplasmic membrane is a complex of protein, lipids, and a small amount of carbohydrates that forms an osmotic barrier for the cell and provides an anchor site for the cellular biosynthetic and respiratory enzymes.

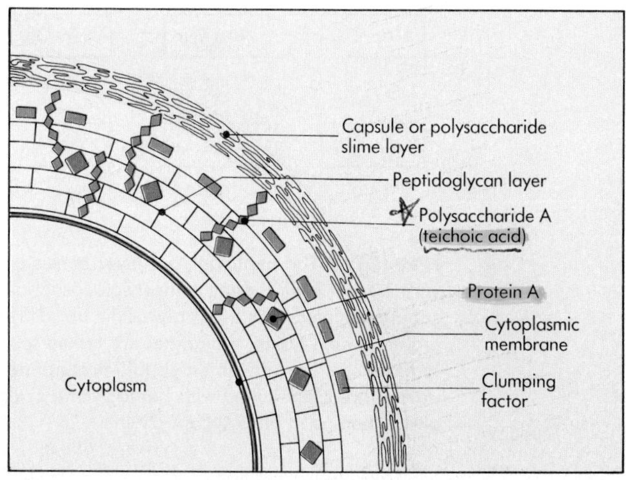

FIGURE 19-1 Staphylococcal cell wall structure.

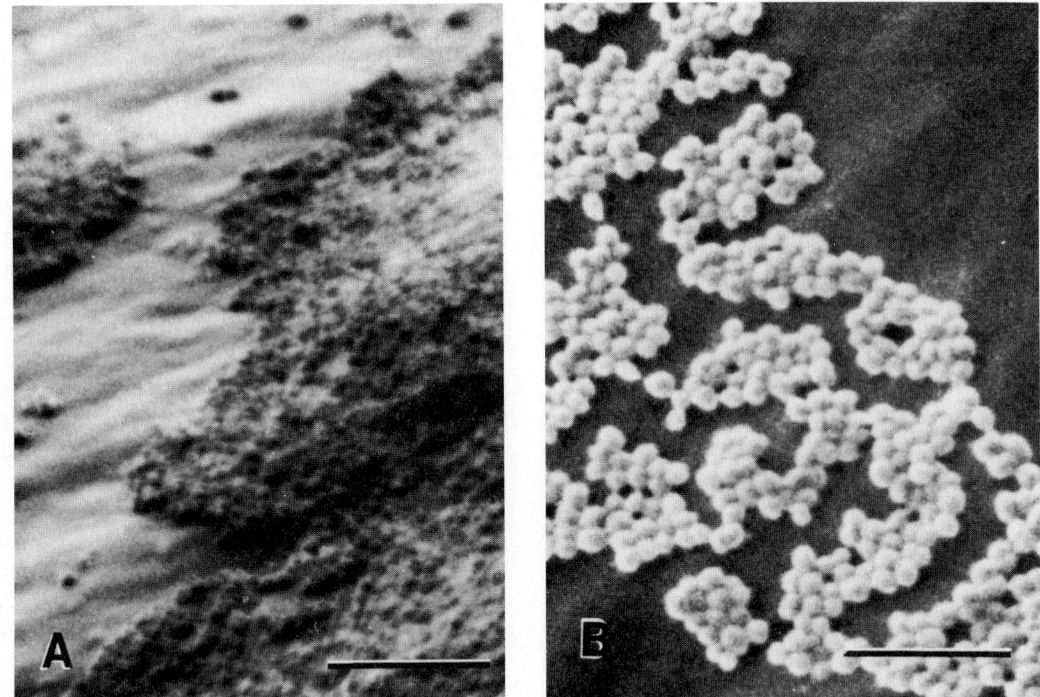

FIGURE 19-2 *S. epidermidis* and other coagulase-negative staphylococci are commonly associated with infections of prosthetic devices, shunts, and catheters. The ability of these organisms to form slime facilitates their colonization of plastic surfaces. Following attachment to the plastic, the organisms are able to erode the surface. This interaction with the surface and production of polysaccharide slime renders the organisms relatively resistant to natural immune mechanisms and antibiotic activity. In many patients the foreign body must be removed for an effective cure. **A,** Slime-producing strain forming an indistinct mat encased in the polysaccharide matrix. **B,** Non–slime-producing strain present as a mat of clearly defined cells without the adherent matrix. (From Christensen GD et al: *Inf Immun* 37:324, 1982.)

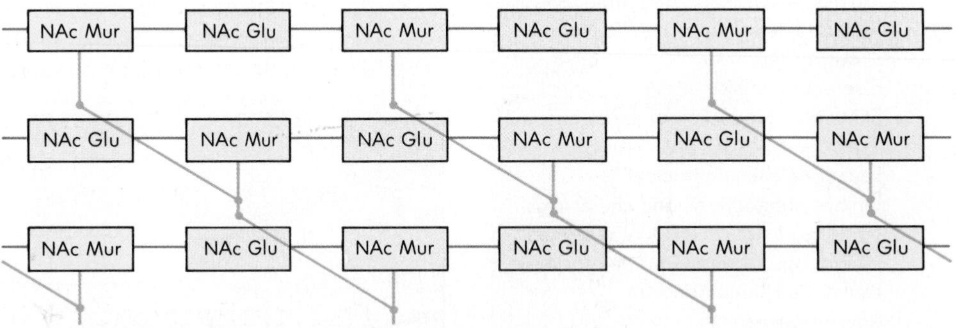

FIGURE 19-3 The peptidoglycan layer consists of three integral parts. The glycan chains are built with 10 to 12 alternating *N*-acetylglucosamine (NAc Glu) and *N*-acetylmuramic acid (NAc Mur) subunits jointed with b-1,4 glycosidic bonds. Vertical tetrapeptide side chains (L-alanine, D-glutamine, L-lysine, D-alanine) are linked to the muramic acid subunits, and the side chains are in turn cross-linked with diagonal intrapeptide bridges. For example, the glycan chains in *S. aureus* are cross-linked with pentaglycine bridges attached to L-lysine in one tetrapeptide chain and D-alanine in an adjacent chain.

PATHOGENESIS AND IMMUNITY

Staphylococcal Toxins

S. aureus produces a large number of virulence factors (Figure 19-4) including at least five **cytolytic**, or membrane-damaging toxins (alpha, beta, delta, gamma, and leukocidin), as well as exfoliative toxin, toxic shock syndrome toxin-1, and five enterotoxins. The cytolytic toxins have also been described as hemolysins, but the activities of the first four toxins are not restricted to red blood cells and leukocidin is unable to lyse erythrocytes. The cytotoxins are capable of lysing neutrophils, with the release of the lysosomal enzymes that subsequently damage the surrounding tissues.

Alpha Toxin

This toxin is cytotoxic for a number of cells, including erythrocytes, leukocytes, hepatocytes, platelets, human diploid fibroblasts, HeLa cells, and Ehrlich ascites carcinoma cells. The toxin also disrupts the smooth muscle in blood vessels. Species variation in erythrocyte susceptibility to alpha toxin is observed (e.g., rabbit erythrocytes are 100 times more sensitive to alpha toxin than are human erythrocytes). Alpha toxin is a protein that is genetically encoded on both the bacterial chromosome and a plasmid. Although the precise mechanism of toxin action is not known, the toxin appears to insert into hydrophobic regions of the cell membrane, with the subsequent disruption of membrane integrity. The alpha toxin is believed to be an important mediator of tissue damage in staphylococcal disease and causes necrosis when injected subcutaneously.

Beta Toxin

This toxin, also called **sphingomyelinase C**, is a heat-labile protein that is toxic for a variety of cells, including erythrocytes, leukocytes, macrophages, and fibroblasts. This enzyme catalyzes the hydrolysis of membrane phospholipids in susceptible cells, with the amount of lysis proportional to the concentration of sphingomyelin exposed on the cell surface. Beta toxin, together with alpha toxin, is believed to be responsible for the tissue destruction and abscess formation characteristic of staphylococcal diseases and the ability of *S. aureus* to proliferate in the presence of a vigorous inflammatory response.

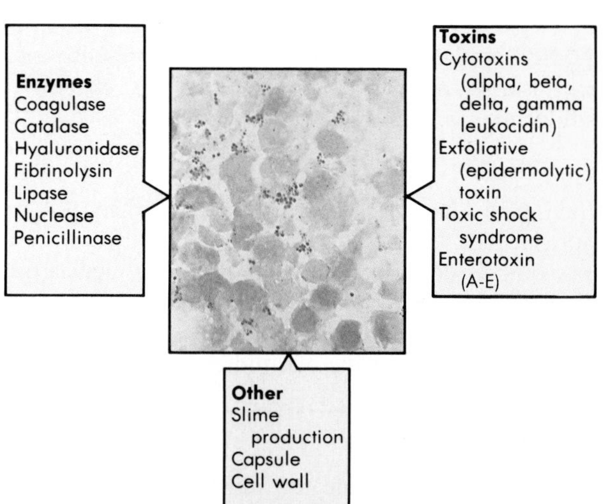

FIGURE 19-4 Staphylococcal virulence factors.

Delta Toxin

This is a thermostable, large, heterogeneous protein. The toxin has a wide spectrum of cytolytic activity, which is consistent with the belief that delta toxin disrupts cellular membranes by a detergent-like action.

Gamma Toxin

This toxin is able to lyse a variety of species of erythrocytes, including human, sheep, and rabbit, as well as human lymphoblastic cells. Although two separate proteins are required for toxin activity, the mode of action is not defined.

Leukocidin

This toxin has an F component and an S component. Neither component alone has appreciable activity against the leukocyte membrane. However, the combination of the two molecules facilitates structural changes in the cell membrane, pore formation, and increased permeability. Bacteria producing leukocidin have increased resistance to phagocytosis.

Exfoliative Toxin

Staphylococcal scalded skin syndrome (SSSS), a spectrum of diseases characterized by exfoliative dermatitis, is mediated by the action of **exfoliative toxin**, also known as **exfoliatin** or **epidermolytic toxin**. The majority of stains associated with SSSS belong to phage group II, although disease has been reported with isolates of groups I and III. Two distinct forms of exfoliative toxin (A and B) have been identified (Table 19-3), but no clear relationship between specific phage groups and toxin types has been established.

Ultrastructural studies have demonstrated that exposure to the toxin is followed by the splitting of the intercellular bridges (desmosomes) in the stratum gran-

TABLE 19-3 Characteristics of Exfoliative Toxins

Properties	Exfoliative toxin A	Exfoliative toxin B
Size	24,000 daltons	24,000 daltons
Temperature tolerance	Stable (100° C, 20 min)	Labile (60° C, 30 min)
EDTA treatment	Inactivated	No effect
DNA	Chromosomal	Plasmid

ulosum layer of the outer epidermis. The toxins are not associated with cytolysis or inflammation. Following exposure to the toxin, protective neutralizing antibodies develop, leading to resolution of the toxic process. SSSS is seen only in young children and only rarely develops in older children or adults, which may be due to the presence of protective antibodies or an insensitivity of the adult epidermis to the toxin.

Toxic Shock Syndrome Toxin-1

Toxic shock syndrome, characterized by fever, hypotension, rash followed by desquamation, and involvement of multiple organ systems, is toxin mediated. **Toxic shock syndrome toxin-1 (TSST-1)**, formerly called pyrogenic exotoxin C and enterotoxin F, is an exotoxin secreted during growth of some strains of *S. aureus* and can reproduce most of the clinical manifestations of toxic shock syndrome in an experimental rabbit model (rash and desquamation are not seen). TSST-1 has not been found in staphylococcal isolates from all patients with toxic shock syndrome; however, most of these non-TSST-1–producing isolates are reported to produce enterotoxin B. The role of this second toxin in toxic shock syndrome has not been adequately defined. The presence of TSST-1 toxin in species other than *S. aureus* remains controversial. However, it is now clear that coagulase-negative staphylococci and group A streptococci can cause toxic shock syndrome.

Enterotoxins

Five serologically distinct staphylococcal enterotoxins (A through E) have been described. The enterotoxins are resistant to hydrolysis by gastric and jejunal enzymes and are stable to heating at 100° C for 30 minutes. Thus once enterotoxin-producing staphylococci have contaminated a food product and produced their toxins, reheating the food will not be protective.

These toxins are found in both *S. aureus* and *S. epidermidis,* with 30% to 50% of all *S. aureus* strains producing an enterotoxin. Although primarily associated with phage group III, other phage groups also produce the enterotoxins. Enterotoxin A is most commonly associated with disease. Enterotoxins C and D are associated with contaminated milk products, and enterotoxin B is associated with staphylococcal pseudomembranous enterocolitis. The mechanism of toxin activity is not understood because a satisfactory animal model is not available. However, the enterotoxins and TSST-1 are strong inducers of interleukin-1. The enterotoxins also stimulate intestinal peristalsis and have a central nervous system effect, as manifested by the intense vomiting associated with this gastrointestinal disease.

Staphylococcal Enzymes

Coagulase

S. aureus strains possess two forms of coagulase: bound (also called clumping factor) and free. Coagulase bound to the staphylococcal cell wall can directly convert fibrinogen to insoluble fibrin and cause the staphylococci to clump together. The cell-free coagulase accomplishes the same result by reacting with a globulin plasma factor (coagulase-reacting factor [CRF]) to form a thrombin-like factor, staphylothrombin. This factor catalyzes the conversion of fibrinogen to insoluble fibrin. Coagulase is used as a marker for virulence for *S. aureus*. The role of coagulase in the pathogenesis of disease is speculative, but coagulase may cause the formation of a fibrin layer around a staphylococcal abscess, thus localizing the infection and protecting the organisms from phagocytosis.

Catalase

All staphylococci produce catalase, a protective enzyme that catalyzes the conversion of toxic hydrogen peroxide, which accumulates during bacterial metabolism or is released following phagocytosis, to water and oxygen.

Hyaluronidase

This enzyme hydrolyzes hyaluronic acids, the acidic mucopolysaccharides present in the acellular matrix of connective tissue. Hyaluronidase facilitates the spread of *S. aureus* in tissues. More than 90% of *S. aureus* strains produce this enzyme.

Fibrinolysin

This enzyme, also called **staphylokinase**, is produced by virtually all *S. aureus* strains and can dissolve fibrin clots. Staphylokinase is distinct from the fibrinolytic enzymes produced by streptococci.

Lipases

All *S. aureus* and more than 30% of coagulase-negative staphylococci produce several different lipases. As their name implies, these enzymes hydrolyze lipids, which is essential for the survival of staphylococci in the sebaceous areas of the body. It is believed that these enzymes are required for invasion of staphylococci into cutaneous and subcutaneous tissues and the formation of superficial skin infections (e.g., furuncles [boils], carbuncles).

Nuclease

Another marker for *S. aureus* is the presence of a thermostable nuclease. The role of this enzyme in pathogenesis is unknown.

Penicillinase

When penicillin was introduced, more than 90% of staphylococcal isolates were susceptible. However, resistance quickly developed and was primarily mediated by the production of penicillinase **(β-lactamase)**. The widespread distribution of this enzyme is ensured by its presence on transmissible plasmids.

EPIDEMIOLOGY

Staphylococci are ubiquitous. Virtually all persons have coagulase-negative staphylococci on their skin surface, and transient colonization of moist skin folds is common with *S. aureus* (Boxes 19-1 and 19-2). *S. aureus* and

BOX 19-1 Epidemiology of *Staphylococcus aureus* Infection

DISEASE/BACTERIAL FACTORS

Staphylococcal scalded skin syndrome (SSSS), cutaneous infections (impetigo, furuncle, carbuncle), toxic shock syndrome, endocarditis, pneumonia, food poisoning, septic arthritis

Common on skin, orophayrnx, gastrointestinal and urogenital tracts

Numerous virulence factors (see Table 19-2 and Figure 19-4): capsule, peptidoglycan, protein A, teichoic acid, toxins, enzymes

Lysozyme in tears, saliva, and human leukocytes, monocytes, and macrophages form a natural barrier to *S. aureus* infection

Organisms can survive on dry surfaces for long periods

TRANSMISSION

Person to person via direct contact or by fomites (contaminated clothing, bed linens)

Food poisoning: ingestion of food or dairy products contaminated with organisms producing heat-stable toxin

Pneumonia: aspiration of oral secretions

WHO IS AT RISK?

Hospitalized patients with trauma or after surgery and a foreign body focus of infection (e.g., stitches)

Persons taking antibiotics that suppress the normal flora

SSSS: infants and young children

Toxic shock syndrome: menstruating women and adults with localized staphylococcal infection

Impetigo: young children

Bacteremia, endocarditis: hospitalized patients with a contaminated intravascular catheter; use of intravenous needles

Pneumonia: children, hospitalized patients, elderly, patients with compromised pulmonary function or antecedent viral respiratory infection

Joint disease: hematogenous spread or secondary infection resulting from trauma or overlying staphylococcal infection

GEOGRAPHY/SEASON

Ubiquitous and worldwide

Food poisoning more common in summer and late-year holidays

MODES OF CONTROL

Most strains resistant to penicillins; use β-lactamase–resistant penicillins

Vancomycin is drug of choice for strains resistant to β-lactam antibiotics

Bacteremia and endocarditis: prompt treatment is essential

Food poisoning: treatment is symptomatic
avoid food preparation by persons with staphylococcal skin infection

Proper cleansing of wound and disinfectant use

Medical personnel: thorough handwashing and covering of exposed skin surfaces

BOX 19-2 Epidemiology of Coagulase-Negative Staphylococci

DISEASE/BACTERIAL FACTORS

Endocarditis, catheter and shunt infections, prosthetic joint infections, urinary tract infections

Common on skin, oropharynx, gastrointestinal and urogenital tracts

Numerous virulence factors (see Table 19-2 and Figure 19-4): capsule, peptidoglycan, teichoic acid, cytoplasmic membrane, toxins, enzymes

Organisms can survive on dry surfaces for long periods

TRANSMISSION

Endocarditis: inoculation of organisms onto a damaged or artificial heart valve

Inoculation via prosthetic device, catheters, shunts, prosthetic joints

WHO IS AT RISK?

Hospitalized patients with catheters, shunts, prosthetic joint or heart valve implants

GEOGRAPHY/SEASON

Ubiquitous and worldwide

No seasonal incidence

MODES OF CONTROL

Most strains resistant to penicillins

Vancomycin is drug of choice for strains resistant to β-lactam antibiotics

Endocarditis: prompt treatment is essential

Maintenance of sterile intravascular lines

coagulase-negative staphylococci are also found in the oropharynx, gastrointestinal tract, and urogenital tract. Colonization of neonates with *S. aureus* is common on the umbilical stump, skin surface, and perineal area. Short-term or persistent carriage in older children and adults is more common in the anterior nasopharynx. Adherence to the mucosal epithelium is regulated by receptors for staphylococcal teichoic acids. Approximately 15% of normal healthy adults are persistent nasopharyngeal carriers of *S. aureus*, with a higher incidence of carriage reported in hospitalized patients, medical personnel, individuals with eczematous skin diseases, and in individuals who regularly use needles illicitly (drug abusers) or for medical reasons (e.g., insulin-dependent diabetics, patients receiving allergy injections, or those undergoing hemodialysis).

Because staphylococci are carried on the skin surface and in the nasopharynx, shedding of the bacteria is common and is responsible for many hospital-acquired infections. Staphylococci are susceptible to high temperature, as well as to disinfectants and antiseptic solutions. However, the organisms are capable of survival on dry surfaces for long periods. Transfer of the organisms to a susceptible individual can be either by direct contact or by means of fomites (e.g., contaminated clothing or bed linens). Therefore medical personnel must use proper handwashing techniques to prevent transfer of staphylococci from themselves to patients or between patients.

CLINICAL SYNDROMES

Staphylococcus aureus

S. aureus causes disease by either production of toxin or direct invasion and destruction of tissue. The clinical manifestations of some staphylococcal diseases are almost exclusively due to toxin activity (e.g., staphylococcal

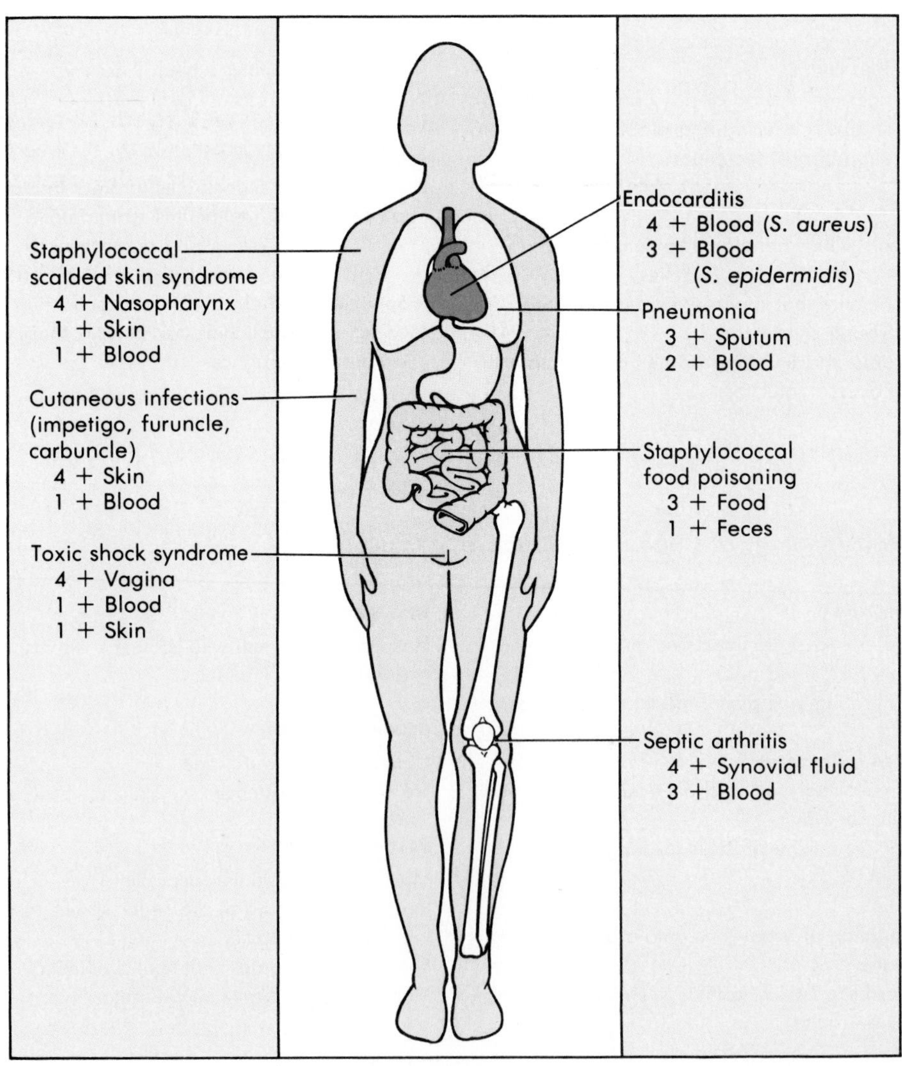

FIGURE 19-5 Staphylococcal diseases. Isolation of staphylococci from sites of infection. *1+*, <10% positive cultures; *2+*, 10% to 50% positive cultures; *3+*, 50% to 90% positive cultures; *4+*, >90% positive cultures.

scalded skin syndrome, toxic shock syndrome, and staphylococcal food poisoning), whereas other diseases involve proliferation of the organisms with abscess formation and tissue destruction (Figure 19-5).

Staphylococcal Scalded Skin Syndrome

In 1878 Gottfried Ritter von Rittershain described 297 infants younger than 1 month of age who had bullous exfoliative dermatitis. The disease, now called Ritter's disease or staphylococcal scalded skin syndrome (SSSS), was characterized by an abrupt onset with localized perioral erythema (redness and inflammation around the mouth) that spread to cover the entire body within 2 days. Under slight pressure the skin can be displaced (a positive Nikolsky sign). Soon afterward large bullae or cutaneous blisters formed, followed by desquamation of the epithelium (Figure 19-6). The blisters contained clear fluid with no organisms or leukocytes present consistent with the fact the pathogenesis is due to the bacterial toxin rather than enzymatic activity of growing bacteria. Recovery of intact epithelium occurred within 7 to 10 days when protective antibodies appear. Scarring is absent because only the top layer of epidermis is sloughed. Mortality is low and when observed is due to secondary bacterial infection of the denuded skin areas.

A localized form of SSSS is **bullous impetigo**. Specific strains of toxin-producing *S. aureus* (e.g., phage type 71) are associated with superficial skin blisters (Figure 19-7). In contrast with the disseminated manifestations of SSSS, bullous impetigo is seen with localized blisters that are culture positive. Erythema does not extend beyond the borders of the blister, and the Nikolsky sign is not present. The disease is primarily restricted to infants and young children and is highly communicable.

Toxic Shock Syndrome (TSS)

TSS was initially described in children in 1978, although it is now primarily a disease in menstruating women and other adults with localized staphylococcal infections. When the pathogenesis of this disease was first recognized, 80% to 90% of patients with TSS were menstruating women. However, this proportion has gradually decreased with the recognition that use of hyperabsorbent tampons represented a significant risk factor.

The disease starts with an abrupt onset of fever, hypotension, and a diffuse macular erythematous rash, as well as involvement of multiple organ systems (gastrointestinal, musculature, renal, hepatic, hematologic, central nervous system). The rash is followed by desquamation involving the entire skin surface including the palms and soles. The initial fatality rate of 5% to 10% has been decreased with a better understanding of the etiology and epidemiology of this disease.

Specific strains of *S. aureus,* those producing toxic shock syndrome toxin-1 (TSST-1) or a related toxin, are responsible for TSS. Vaginal carriage of toxin-producing strains has been reported in virtually all women with TSS but in less than 10% of healthy women. In the presence of hyperabsorbent tampons these organisms can multiply rapidly and release toxin for systemic distribution. Toxin production has also been associated with staphylococcal strains isolated in wounds in patients with TSS.

TSST-1 enhances by more than 1000 times the

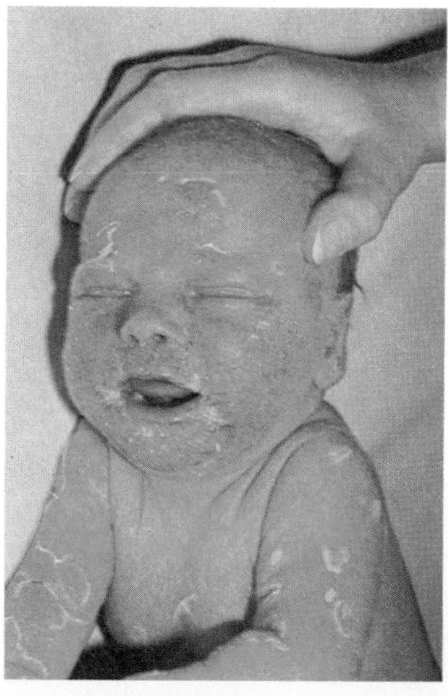

FIGURE 19-6 Ritter's disease or staphylococcal scalded skin syndrome. (From Emond R and Rowland H: *A colour atlas of infectious diseases,* London, 1987, Wolfe Medical Publications).

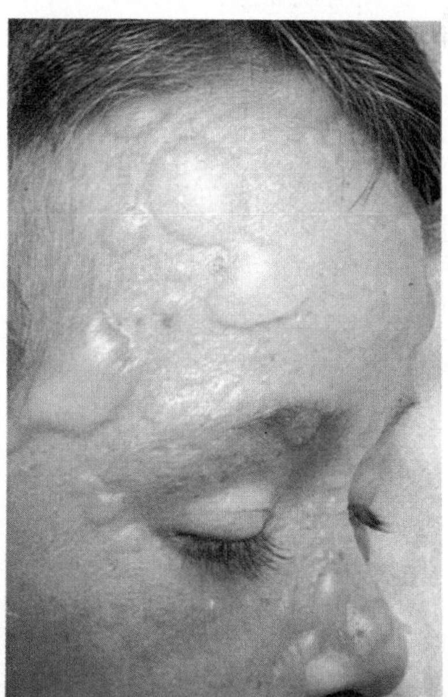

FIGURE 19-7 Bullous impetigo, a localized form of staphylococcal scalded skin syndrome. (From Emond R and Rowland H: *A colour atlas of infectious diseases,* London, 1987, Wolfe Medical Publications).

susceptibility of rabbits to the lethal effect of endotoxin. This may explain the observed shock in TSS. Furthermore, the toxin can induce fever and dilation of peripheral blood vessels, with subsequent rash formation. The role of other staphylococcal toxins in this disease has not been defined. Unless the patient is specifically treated with an effective antibiotic, the risk for recurrent disease is as great as 65%.

Staphylococcal Food Poisoning

Staphylococcal food poisoning, one of the most common food-borne illnesses, is an intoxication rather than infection. Disease is due to ingestion of toxin-contaminated food rather than the organisms. The foods most commonly implicated are processed meats such as ham and salted pork, custard-filled pastries, potato salad, and ice cream (Table 19-4). Growth of *S. aureus* in salted meats is consistent with the ability of this organism to replicate selectively in nutrient media supplemented with as much as 15% sodium chloride. In contrast with many other forms of food poisoning in which an animal reservoir is important, staphylococcal food poisoning is the result of contamination of the food by a human carrier. Although contamination can be avoided by excluding individuals with an obvious staphylococcal skin infection from preparing food, approximately half of the carriers are asymptomatic, with colonization most commonly occurring in the nasopharynx. After the staphylococci have been introduced into the food, the food must remain at room temperature or warmer to permit the growth of the organisms and release of the toxin. Subsequent heating of the food will kill the bacteria but not inactivate the heat-stable toxin. Furthermore, the contaminated food will not appear or taste tainted. Figure 19-8 illustrates the proportion of outbreaks of staphylococcal food poisoning during a 12-month period.

Following ingestion of the food, the onset of disease is abrupt and rapid with a mean incubation period of 4 hours, consistent with a disease mediated by preformed toxin. Further production of toxin by ingested staphylococci does not occur, so the course of disease is rapid, with symptoms lasting generally less than 24 hours. Staphylococcal food poisoning is characterized by severe vomiting, diarrhea, and abdominal pain or nausea. Sweating and headache may occur, but an elevated fever is not seen. Diarrhea is watery and nonbloody, and dehydration may result from significant fluid loss.

The toxin-producing organisms can be cultured from the contaminated food if the organisms are not killed during the food preparation. Because the enterotoxins are heat stable, the food can be submitted to a public health facility for toxin testing (these tests are not performed in most hospital laboratories).

Treatment is symptomatic for relief of the abdominal cramping and diarrhea and replacement of fluids. Antibiotic therapy is not indicated because disease is not mediated by in situ production of toxin. Neutralizing antibodies to the toxin can develop and can be protective. However, a second episode of staphylococcal food poisoning can occur with a serologically distinct enterotoxin.

Certain strains of *S. aureus* can also cause enterocolitis, manifested clinically by profuse watery diarrhea, fever, and dehydration. This is primarily observed in patients who have received broad-spectrum antibiotics, which suppress the normal colonic flora and permit the growth of *S. aureus*. The diagnosis of staphylococcal enterocolitis can be confirmed only after other infectious causes have been excluded (e.g., *Clostridium difficile* colitis). Abundant staphylococci are present, and the normal gram-negative flora are absent by Gram stain and culture of stool specimens. Fecal leukocytes are observed, and white plaques on the colonic mucosa with ulceration will be seen.

TABLE 19-4 Food Incriminated in 131 Staphylococcal Food Poisoning Outbreaks Reported to the Centers for Disease Control During a 5-Year Period

Food product	Number of outbreaks	Percentage of total
Meat (ham, pork, beef)	50	38
Salad (potato, egg, other)	20	15
Baked foods	13	10
Poultry	13	10
Dairy (milk, cheese, butter)	4	3
Shellfish	2	2
Vegetables, fruits	2	2
Multiple sources or unknown	27	20

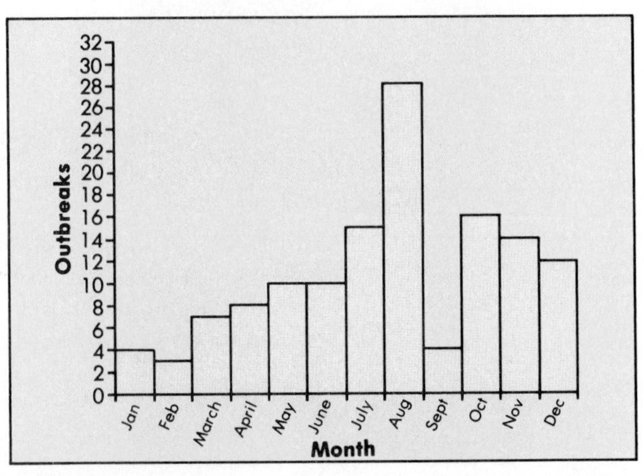

FIGURE 19-8 Staphylococcal food poisoning can be seen year-round but is most common during the summer and late-year holidays (Thanksgiving and Christmas).

Cutaneous Infections

Localized pyogenic staphylococcal infections include impetigo, folliculitis, furuncles, and carbuncles. **Impetigo** is a superficial infection affecting mostly young children and is manifested primarily on the face and limbs. The initial presentation is a small macule (flattened red spot) that develops into a pus-filled vesicle (pustule) on an erythematous base. After the pustule ruptures, crusting will occur. Multiple vesicles at different stages of development are common. Impetigo is usually caused by group A *Streptococcus*, alone or in combination with *S. aureus*, with group A *Streptococcus* responsible for 20% of the cases.

Folliculitis is a pyogenic infection localized to the hair follicle. The base of the follicle is raised and reddened, with a small collection of pus beneath the epidermal surface. If this occurs at the base of the eyelid, it is called a **stye**. **Furuncles**, or boils, are an extension of folliculitis. Large, painful, raised nodules with an underlying collection of dead and necrotic tissue are characteristic. These can drain spontaneously or with a surgical incision.

Carbuncles result from the coalescence of furuncles and extend to the deeper subcutaneous tissue. Multiple sinus tracts are usually present. In contrast with folliculitis and furuncles, chills and fevers are associated with carbuncles and indicate systemic spread of the staphylococci. Bacteremia with secondary spread to other tissues is common with carbuncles.

Staphylococcal wound infections can also occur following surgery or a traumatic injury, with the introduction into the wound of organisms colonizing the skin. In an immunocompetent individual the staphylococci are not able to establish an infection unless a foreign body is present in the wound (e.g., stitches, splinter, dirt). Infections are characterized by edema, erythema, pain, and an accumulation of purulent material. If the wound is reopened and the foreign matter removed with drainage of the purulence, the infection can be easily managed. If signs such as fever and malaise are observed, or if the wound does not clear with localized management, then antibiotic therapy directed against *S. aureus* is indicated.

Bacteremia and Endocarditis

S. aureus is a common cause of bacteremia. Whereas bacteremias with most other organisms originate from an identifiable focus such as an infection of the lungs, urinary tract, or gastrointestinal tract, the initial focus of infection in approximately one third of *S. aureus* bacteremias is not known. Most likely the infection spreads to the bloodstream from an innocuous-appearing skin infection. More than half of *S. aureus* bacteremias are acquired in the hospital following a surgical procedure or result from continued use of a contaminated intravascular catheter. *S. aureus* bacteremias, particularly long-dwelling episodes, are associated with dissemination to other body sites, including the heart.

Acute endocarditis caused by *S. aureus* is a serious disease, with a mortality rate approaching 50%. *S. aureus* endocarditis may initially be seen with nonspecific flu-like symptoms; however, the patient's condition deteriorates rapidly with disruption of cardiac output and peripheral evidence of septic embolization. Unless appropriate medical and surgical intervention is immediate, the patient's prognosis is poor. An exception to this rule is *S. aureus* endocarditis in parenteral drug abusers, whose disease normally involves the right side of the heart (tricuspid valve) rather than the left side. The initial symptoms may be mild, although fever, chills, and pleuritic chest pain caused by pulmonary emboli are generally present. Clinical cure of the endocarditis is the rule, although complications from secondary spread to other organs are common.

Pneumonia and Empyema

S. aureus respiratory disease can develop following aspiration of oral secretions or hematogenous spread of the organism from a distant site. Aspiration pneumonia is primarily seen in the very young and the aged and in patients with cystic fibrosis, influenza, chronic obstructive pulmonary disease (COPD), or bronchiectasis. The clinical and radiologic presentations are not unique for this organism. Radiographic examination will reveal patchy infiltrates with consolidation or abscess formation, consistent with the ability of the organism to form localized abscesses. Hematogenous pneumonias are common in patients with endocarditis and in patients with bacteremias from contamination of either intravascular catheters or access sites for hemodialysis.

Empyema will occur in 10% of patients with pneumonia, and *S. aureus* is responsible for one third of all cases of empyema. Because the organism is able to form walled-off areas of consolidation (loculation), drainage of the purulent material is sometimes difficult.

Osteomyelitis and Septic Arthritis

S. aureus osteomyelitis can be a result of hematogenous infection or secondary infection resulting from trauma or an overlying staphylococcal infection. Hematogenous spread in children, generally from a cutaneous staphylococcal infection, usually involves the metaphyseal area of long bones, a highly vascularized area of bony growth. Hematogenous osteomyelitis in children is characterized by sudden onset of localized pain over the involved bone and high fever. Positive blood cultures are documented in about half of all infections. Hematogenous osteomyelitis in adults commonly occurs as vertebral osteomyelitis but rarely as an infection of the long bones. Intense back pain with fever is the initial symptom. Radiographic evidence of osteomyelitis is not seen until 2 to 3 weeks after initial signs (in both children and adults). **Brodie's abscess** is a sequestered focus of staphylococcal osteomyelitis of the metaphyseal area of a long bone in adults. Staphylococcal osteomyelitis following trauma or surgery is generally accompanied with evidence of inflammation and purulent drainage from the wound or sinus tract overlying the infected bone. With appropriate antibiotic therapy, and surgery when indicated, the cure rate for staphylococcal osteomyelitis is excellent.

S. aureus is the primary cause of septic arthritis in young children and in adults receiving intraarticular injections or with mechanically abnormal joints. *S. aureus* is replaced by *Neisseria gonorrhoeae* as the most common cause of septic arthritis in sexually active persons. Staphylococcal arthritis is characterized by a painful, erythematous joint with purulence on aspiration. Infection is usually demonstrated in the large joints (e.g., shoulder, knee, hip, elbow). The prognosis is excellent in children, although in adults it is influenced by the underlying disease and the occurrence of secondary infectious complications.

Staphylococcus epidermidis and Other Coagulase-Negative Staphylococci

Endocarditis

S. epidermidis and the related coagulase-negative staphylococci can infect native and prosthetic heart valves (Figure 19-9). Infections of native valves are believed to be due to the inoculation of organisms onto a damaged heart valve (e.g., congenital malformation, secondary to rheumatic heart disease). This form of staphylococcal endocarditis is relatively rare and more commonly associated with streptococci. In contrast, staphylococci are a major cause of artificial valve endocarditis. The organisms are introduced at the time of heart surgery, and the infection characteristically has an indolent course with clinical signs and symptoms not developing for as long as 1 year after surgery. Although infection can involve the heart valve, the more common occurrence is infection at the site where the valve is sewn to the heart tissue. Thus infection with abscess formation can lead to separation of the valve at the suture line, with mechanical heart failure. Septic embolization and persistent bacteremia are less common with staphylococcal prosthetic valve endocarditis than with other forms of endocarditis because of the nature and site of infection. Prognosis is guarded for this infection, and prompt medical and surgical management is critical.

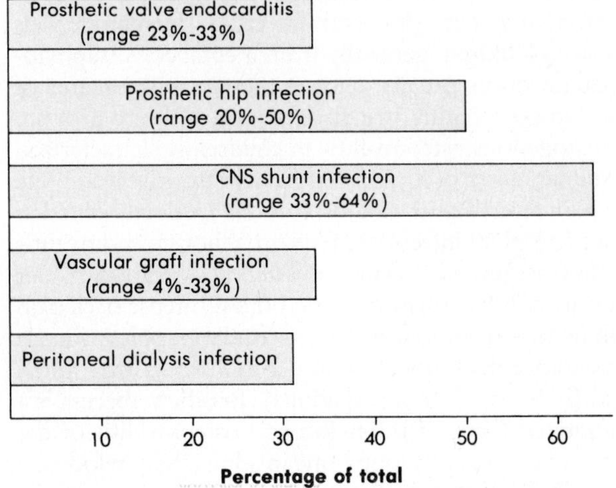

FIGURE 19-9. Role of *S. epidermidis* in infections associated with prosthetic devices.

Catheter and Shunt Infections

From 20% to 65% of all infections of prosthetic devices, catheters, and shunts are caused by coagulase-negative staphylococci. This has become a major medical problem with the introduction of long-dwelling catheters for feeding and medical management of critically ill patients. The coagulase-negative staphylococci are particularly well suited for these infections by their ability to produce a polysaccharide slime that can bond them to catheters and shunts and protect them from antibiotics and inflammatory cells. Infections of cerebrospinal fluid shunts can lead to meningitis. Persistent bacteremia is generally observed because the organisms have continual access to the bloodstream. Immune complex–mediated glomerulonephritis occurs in patients with long-standing disease.

Prosthetic Joint Infections

Infections of artificial joints, particularly the hip, can be caused by coagulase-negative staphylococci. Clinical manifestations are usually limited to localized pain and mechanical failure of the joint. Systemic signs such as fever and leukocytosis are not prominent, and blood cultures are usually noncontributory. Surgical replacement of the joint, together with antimicrobial therapy, is required. The risk of reinfection of the new joint is significantly increased.

Staphylococcus saprophyticus

S. saprophyticus has a predilection for causing urinary tract infections in young, sexually active women. The organism appears to be restricted to this population and is only infrequently found as an asymptomatic colonizer of the urinary tract. Infected women usually have dysuria (pain on urination), pyuria (pus in urine), and large numbers of organisms in their urine. Rapid response to appropriate antibiotics and the absence of reinfections are common.

LABORATORY DIAGNOSIS

Microscopy

Staphylococcus is a gram-positive coccus that will form clusters of cocci when grown on agar media, but it is commonly seen as single cells or small groups of organisms when clinical material is examined by microscopy. The success of detecting the organism in a clinical specimen depends on the type of the infection (e.g., abscess, bacteremia, impetigo) and the quality of the material submitted for analysis. If abscess material is examined, the base of the abscess should be scraped with a swab or curette; large numbers of organisms should be observed by Gram stain and isolated in culture. Aspirated pus consists primarily of necrotic material with relatively few organisms, so this specimen should not be processed. Small numbers of organisms are generally present in the blood of bacteremic patients (an average of less than 1 organism/ml of blood), so Gram stains of blood are unrewarding. Staphylococci are seen in the nasopharynx of patients with staphylococcal scalded skin syndrome or in the vagina of patients with toxic shock syndrome, but these organisms cannot be differentiated from the staphylococci that normally colonize these sites. Large numbers of staphylococci are seen in food implicated in staphylococcal food poisoning in more than 50% of documented outbreaks, but organisms are generally not seen in fecal specimens collected from ill patients.

Culture

Clinical specimens should be inoculated onto nutritionally enriched agar media supplemented with sheep blood. If a mixture of organisms is present in the specimen, *S. aureus* can be isolated on agar media supplemented with 7.5% sodium chloride (inhibitory for most other organisms) and mannitol (fermented by *S. aureus*). Staphylococci will grow rapidly on nonselective media both aerobically and anaerobically, with large, smooth colonies seen within 24 hours. Yellow pigmentation caused by carotenoids is common with *S. aureus* (hence the name aureus for gold), particularly when the cultures are incubated at room temperature. On sheep blood agar hemolysis caused by cytotoxins is seen with almost all isolates of *S. aureus* and relatively few strains of coagulase-negative staphylococci.

Serology

Attempts to detect staphylococcal structural antigens in blood or clinical specimens have been generally unsuccessful. However, antibodies to cell wall teichoic acids are present in many patients with long-standing *S. aureus* infections (e.g., endocarditis, osteomyelitis). Antibodies develop within 2 weeks of the onset of disease and are positive in most patients with staphylococcal endocarditis. This test is less reliable for staphylococcal osteomyelitis because the focus of infection is sequestered and organisms do not stimulate a humoral immune response. The presence of elevated antibody titers in a bacteremic patient is considered consistent with the need for a prolonged course of antimicrobial therapy. However, the significance of negative serology must be carefully evaluated because the test is relatively insensitive. Antibody titers are measured by either counterimmunoelectrophoresis (CIE) or immunodiffusion. CIE is more sensitive but less specific, and at present the immunodiffusion assay is the preferred method for measuring teichoic acid antibodies.

Identification

Staphylococci can be separated from other gram-positive cocci by their microscopic and colonial morphology and biochemical properties (Table 19-5). *S. aureus* can be differentiated from the other staphylococci by relatively simple biochemical tests. However, separation of the coagulase-negative staphylococci is more complex and is not undertaken in many clinical laboratories.

TABLE 19-5 Key Tests for Identification of the Most Clinically Significant Species

	Test*																			
													Acid (aerobically) from:							
Species	Colony pigment†	Staphylocoagulase	Clumping factor	Heat-stable nuclease	Alkaline phosphatase	Pyrrolidonyl arylamidase	Ornithine decarboxylase	Urease	β-Galactosidase	Acetoin production	Novobiocin resistance	Polymyxin B resistance	D-Trehalose	D-Mannitol	D-Mannose	D-Turanose	D-Xylose	D-Cellbiose	Maltose	Sucrose
S. aureus	+	+	+	+	+	−	−	d	−	+	−	+	+	+	+	+	−	−	+	+
S. epidermidis	−	−	−	−	+	−	(d)	+	−	+	−	+	−	−	(+)	(d)	−	−	+	+
S. haemolyticus	d	−	−	−	−	+	−	−	−	+	−	−	+	d	−	(d)	−	−	+	+
S. lugdunensis	d	−	(+)	−	−	+	+	d	−	+	−	d	+	−	+	(d)	−	−	+	+
S. schleiferi	−	−	+	+	+	+	−	−	(+)	+	−	−	d	−	+	−	−	−	−	−
S. saprophyticus	d	−	−	−	−	−	−	+	+	+	+	−	+	d	−	+	−	−	+	+

From Balows A, Hausler WJ, Herrman KL et al: *Manual of clinical microbiology*, ed 5, Washington, DC, 1991, American Society of Microbiology.

*+, 90% or more strains positive; ±, 90% or more strains weakly positive; −, 90% or more strains negative; d, 11% to 89% of strains positive; ( ), delayed reaction.

†Presence of carotenoid pigments.

Intraspecies characterization of isolates for epidemiological purposes can be performed by analysis of antibiotic susceptibility patterns (antibiograms), biochemical profiles (biotyping), susceptibility to bacteriophages (phage typing), or nucleic acid analysis. Whereas the first two procedures can be performed in most laboratories and are reproducible if the tests are carefully performed, phage typing and nucleic acid analysis are performed more selectively. Phage typing distinguishes staphylococcal strains by their pattern of susceptibility to lysis by an international collection of specific bacteriophages. Currently, five lytic groups are recognized (groups I through V). Particular strains are identified by their susceptibility to specific bacteriophages (e.g., phage type 80/81 is lysed by bacteriophages 80 and 81). Nucleic acid analysis has rapidly evolved to be the most sensitive procedure for characterizing isolates. Refinement of this molecular technology is developing rapidly so that many laboratories will soon be able to exploit this epidemiological approach.

TREATMENT, PREVENTION, AND CONTROL

Resistance quickly developed in staphylococci after penicillin was introduced, and today fewer than 10% of the strains are susceptible to this antibiotic. Resistance is mediated by production of penicillinase (β-lactamase), which hydrolyzes the β-lactam ring of penicillin. The genetic information encoding production of this enzyme is carried on transmissible plasmids, which facilitate the rapid dissemination of resistance among staphylococci.

With the problems with penicillin-resistant staphylococci, semisynthetic penicillins resistant to β-lactamase hydrolysis (e.g., methicillin, naficillin, oxacillin, dicloxacillin) were developed. Unfortunately, resistance to these antibiotics also followed, first in Europe, Scandinavia, and Japan and then more recently in the United States. Although the majority of patients with serious staphylococcal infections can be treated with these penicillins, approximately 10% to 25% of *S. aureus* strains and as many as 40% of coagulase-negative staphylococci are resistant to these penicillins. This is a particularly serious problem in large academic medical centers where resistant *S. aureus* have become well established. The mechanism of this resistance is due to alterations in the antibiotic target sites (i.e., penicillin-binding proteins [PBPs]) in the cell wall, which prevents binding of the antibiotics to the bacteria. This phenomenon appears to be chromosomally mediated. Some strains of staphylococci also produce large quantities of β-lactamases that, when present in sufficient amounts, can hydrolyze these antibiotics. Resistance to these semisynthetic penicillins is also frequently associated with resistance to other classes of antibiotics, including clindamycin, erythromycin, and the aminoglycosides. The detection of resistance to the semisynthetic penicillins is sometimes difficult because resistance is preferentially expressed in vitro at low temperatures (30° C).

Despite the propensity for staphylococci to develop resistance to antibiotics, virtually all strains are uniformly susceptible to vancomycin. This is the antibiotic of choice in treatment of disease caused by staphylococci resistant to β-lactam antibiotics.

Staphylococci are ubiquitous organisms present on the skin and mucous membranes. Introduction through breaks in the skin is frequently unavoidable. However, the number of organisms required to establish an infection (infectious dose) is generally large unless a foreign body is present in the wound (e.g., dirt, splinter, stitch). Proper cleansing of the wound and application of an appropriate disinfectant (e.g., germicidal soap, iodine solution, hexachlorophene) will prevent most infections in healthy individuals.

The spread of staphylococci from person to person is more difficult to manage. Surgical infections with organisms contaminating the operative site can be established by relatively few organisms because foreign bodies and devitalized tissue are present. Although it is unrealistic to sterilize the operating room personnel and environment, proper handwashing and the covering of exposed skin surfaces should minimize the risk of contamination during the operative procedure. The spread of methicillin-resistant organisms can also be difficult to control because asymptomatic nasopharyngeal carriage is the most frequent source of these organisms. Some success has been seen with chemoprophylaxis with the combination of vancomycin and rifampin.

CASE STUDY AND QUESTIONS

An 18-year-old boy fell on his knee while playing basketball. The knee was painful, but the overlying skin was unbroken. The next day, the knee was swollen and remained painful, so the boy was taken to the local emergency room. Clear fluid was aspirated from the knee, and the physician prescribed symptomatic treatment. Two days later, the swelling returned, pain increased, and erythema developed over the knee. Because the patient also felt systemically ill and had an oral temperature of 102° F, he returned to the emergency room. Aspiration of the knee yielded cloudy fluid, and cultures of the fluid and blood were positive with *Staphylococcus aureus.*

1. Name two possible sources of this organism.
2. Staphylococci cause a variety of diseases including scalded skin syndrome, toxic shock syndrome, food poisoning, cutaneous infections, and endocarditis. How do the clinical symptoms of these diseases differ from the infection in this case? Which of these diseases are intoxications?
3. What toxins have been implicated in staphylococcal diseases? Which staphylococcal enzymes have been proposed as virulence factors?
4. Which structures in the staphylococcal cell and which toxins protect the bacterium from phagocytosis?

5. What is the role of *S. epidermidis* in infections associated with prosthetic devices? What virulence property helps establish these infections? What infection is caused by *S. saprophyticus*? What population is most susceptible to this infection?

Bibliography

Balows A, Hausler WJ, Herrman KL, Isenberg HD, and Shadomy HJ: *Manual of clinical microbiology*, ed 5, Washington, DC, 1991, American Society of Microbiology.

Christensen GD, Simpson WA, Bisno AL, and Beachey EH: Adherence of slime-producing strains of *Staphylococcus epidermidis* to smooth surfaces, *Inf Immun* 37:318-326, 1982.

Committee on Toxic Shock Syndrome. Report of toxic shock syndrome conference. I and II, *Ann Intern Med* 96: 1982.

Fidalgo S, Vazquez F, Mendoza M et al: Bacteremia due to *Staphylococcus epidermidis*: microbiologic, epidemiologic, clinical, and prognostic features, *Rev Infect Dis* 12:520-528, 1990.

Holmberg SD and Blake PA: Staphylococcal food poisoning in the United States: new facts and old misconceptions, *JAMA* 251:487-489, 1984.

Hovelius B and Mardh PA: *Staphylococcus saprophyticus* as a common cause of urinary tract infections, *Rev Infect Dis* 6:328-337, 1984.

Kaplan MH and Tenenbaum MJ: *Staphylococcus aureus:* cellular biology and clinical application, *Am J Med* 72:248-258, 1982.

McWhinney PHM, Kibbler CC, Gillespie SH et al: *Stomatococcus mucilaginosus*: an emerging pathogen in neutropenic patients, *Clin Infect Dis* 14:641-646, 1992.

Mandell GL, Douglas RG, and Bennett JE: *Principles and practice of infectious diseases*, ed 3, New York, 1991, John Wiley & Sons.

Pfaller M and Herwaldt L: Laboratory, clinical, and epidemiological aspects of coagulase-negative staphylococci, *Clin Microbiol Rev* 1:281-299, 1988.

Rogolsky M: Nonenteric toxins of *Staphylococcus aureus, Microbiol Rev* 43:320-360, 1979.

Sheagren JN: *Staphylococcus aureus:* the persistent pathogen, *N Engl J Med* 310:1368-1373, 1437-1442, 1984.

CHAPTER 20

Streptococcus and Related Gram-Positive Bacteria

In recent years the classification of gram-positive cocci has become increasingly complex. Currently, seven genera of catalase-negative, gram-positive cocci are recognized as human pathogens. Although *Streptococcus* and *Enterococcus* are the best known and most frequently isolated genera, *Aerococcus*, *Gemella*, *Lactococcus*, *Leuconostoc*, and *Pediococcus* cause significant albeit rare human disease. Differentiation of these bacteria is important for the therapeutic management of infected patients and understanding the epidemiology and pathogenesis of their infections (Table 20-1).

STREPTOCOCCUS

The genus *Streptococcus* encompasses a diverse collection of species of gram-positive cocci that are commonly arranged in pairs or chains. Most species are facultative anaerobes, although atmospheric requirements may range from strictly anaerobic to **capnophilic** (growth dependent on carbon dioxide). The nutritional requirements are complex, necessitating the use of blood or serum-enriched medium for their isolation. Carbohydrates are fermented with the production of lactic acid and, unlike *Staphylococcus* species, the organisms are catalase negative.

The role of streptococci in human disease was appreciated very early (Box 20-1). However, the differentiation of species within the genus is complicated because at least four different schemes for classifying these organisms are used: clinical presentation (pyogenic, oral, enteric streptococci); serological properties (Lancefield groupings A through H, K through V); hemolytic patterns (complete [β] hemolysis, incomplete [α] hemolysis, and no [γ] hemolysis); and biochemical (physiological) properties. The serological classification scheme was developed by Lancefield in 1933 for differentiating pathogenic β-hemolytic strains. Most β-hemolytic strains and some α- and nonhemolytic strains possess group-specific antigens, which are either cell wall carbohydrates or teichoic acids. These antigens can be readily detected by immunological probes and have been useful for rapid identification of the most common streptococcal pathogens. Not all streptococci possess these group-specific cell wall antigens. Thus organisms such as *S. pneumoniae* and the

TABLE 20-1 Differentiation of Catalase-Negative, Gram-Positive Cocci

		Test*						
Genus	Gram stain morphology	Vanco	Gas from glucose	PYR	LAP	NaCl broth	45° C	10° C
Streptococcus	Chains, pairs	S	−	−†	+	−	V	−
Enterococcus	Short chains, pairs	S	−	+	+	+	+	+
Aerococcus	Pairs, tetrads, clusters	S	−	−	−	V	−	+
Gemella	Chains, pairs, tetrads, clusters	S	−	+	V	−	−	−
Lactococcus	Chains, pairs	S	−	−†	+	V	−	+
Leuconostoc	Chains, pairs	R	+	−	−	V	−	+
Pediococcus	Pairs, tetrads, clusters	R	−	−	+	V	+	−

Modified from Lennette EH, Balows A, Hausler WJ Jr, et al.: *Manual of clinical microbiology*, ed 5, Washington, DC, 1991, American Society of Microbiology.
**Vanco*, vancomycin (*S*, susceptible; *R*, resistance); *PYR*, pyrrolidonyl arylamidase; *LAP*, leucine aminopeptidase; *NaCl*, growth in 6.5% broth; growth at 45° C or 10° C; +, positive reaction; −, negative reaction; *V*, variable reaction.
†*S. pyogenes* (group A Streptococcus) and *Lactococcus garviae* are positive for PYR.

BOX 20-1 Common Streptococci and Their Diseases

S. pneumoniae	Pneumonia, sinusitis, otitis media, meningitis, bacteremia
S. pyogenes (group A)	Pharyngitis, scarlet fever, streptococcal toxic shock syndrome, erysipelas, pyoderma, rheumatic fever, glomerulonephritis
S. agalactiae (group B)	Neonatal infections (meningitis, pneumonia, bacteremia), postpartum sepsis
S. intermedius-anginosus group ("*S. milleri*" group)	Bacteremia, abscess formation
Viridans group	Bacteremia, endocarditis, dental caries

TABLE 20-2 Classification of Common Streptococcal Pathogens in Humans

Serological classification	Biochemical classification	Hemolytic patterns
A	*S. pyogenes*	β
B	*S. agalactiae*	β; occasionally alpha or nonhemolytic
C	*S. anginosus*, *S. equisimilis*	β; occasionally alpha or nonhemolytic
D	*S. bovis*, *Enterococcus* spp.	α, nonhemolytic; occasionally beta
F	*S. anginosus*	β
G	*S. anginosus*	β
—	*S. pneumoniae*	α
(Viridans group)	*S. adjacens*, *S. anginosus*, *S. bovis*, *S. defectivus*, *S. mitis*, *S. mutans*, *S. salivarius*, *S. sanguis*, *S. vestibularis*	α, nonhemolytic

numerous species of α- and nonhemolytic streptococci (collectively termed the viridans group of streptococci) must be identified by their physiological properties. Unfortunately the classification schemes are not mutually exclusive (Table 20-2). For example, *S. anginosus* strains may be nontypeable (viridans group) or react with the antisera for groups C, F, and G. Likewise, *S. agalactiae* (group B) is usually β-hemolytic but may also be α-hemolytic or nonhemolytic.

Group A *Streptococcus*

Group A *Streptococcus*, also called *Streptococcus pyogenes*, is an important cause of pharyngitis, scarlet fever, streptococcal toxic shock syndrome, erysipelas, and pyoderma. In addition, the organism is responsible for nonsuppurative sequelae—acute rheumatic fever and glomerulonephritis.

Physiology and Structure

Group A streptococci are 0.5 to 1.0 μm spherical cocci that form short chains in clinical specimens and longer chains when grown in liquid media (Figure 20-1). Growth is optimal on enriched blood agar media but is inhibited if the medium contains a high concentration of glucose. After 24 hours of incubation, 1 to 2 mm white colonies with a large zone of β-hemolysis are observed. Encapsulated strains will appear mucoid on freshly prepared media, but on dry media they appear wrinkled (matt appearance). Nonencapsulated colonies are smaller and glossy.

The antigenic structure of group A streptococci is well defined (Figure 20-2). The outermost layer of the cell is the capsule, which is composed of hyaluronic acid, identical to that found in connective tissue. For this reason the capsule is nonimmunogenic. Although the capsule is present in actively growing cells, it rapidly diffuses into the extracellular space in nondividing cells.

The basic structural framework of the cell wall is the peptidoglycan layer, similar in composition to that found in other gram-positive bacteria. Within the cell wall are the group- and type-specific antigens of group A streptococci. The **group-specific carbohydrate** of group A streptococci, which is approximately 10% of the dry weight of the cell, is a dimer of *N*-acetylglucosamine and rhamnose. Three type-specific protein antigens have also been identified. The **M protein** is a major antigen associated with virulent streptococci. In the absence of the M protein the strains are not infectious. This protein is located on the end of the hairlike fimbriae that are anchored in the cell wall and extend through the capsule. Thus the M protein is exposed in encapsulated strains. The M protein and a second type-specific protein, **T or trypsin-resistant protein**, are important epidemiological markers of group A strains. The third type-specific protein in the cell wall is the **R protein**. Finally, two other cell surface antigens have been described: the **F protein** or fibronectin-binding protein and **lipoteichoic acid**, which is associated with fimbriae.

Pathogenesis and Immunity

The virulence of group A streptococci is determined by a variety of structural molecules and elaborated toxins and enzymes (Table 20-3). Although the precise role each

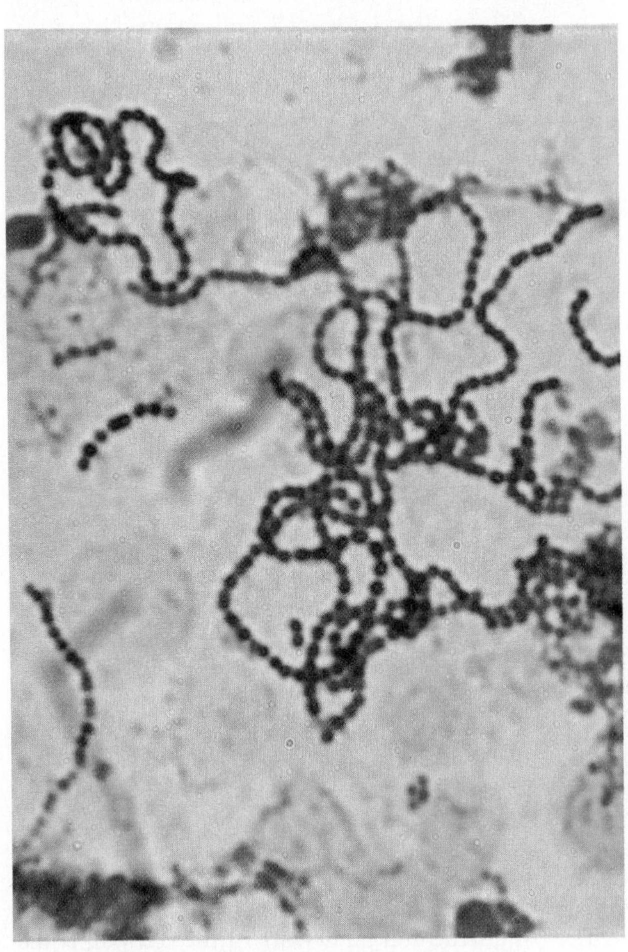

FIGURE 20-1 Gram stain of group A *Streptococcus*.

plays in pathogenesis is often not well defined, it is likely that M protein, F protein, and possibly lipoteichoic acid are important in the establishment of infection, and that the observed clinical manifestations can be directly attributed to molecules such as the pyrogenic exotoxins and streptolysins.

Capsule. The hyaluronic acid capsule of group A streptococci is nonimmunogenic and protects the cells against phagocytosis. However, the major antiphagocytic structural component is the M protein.

M Protein. In the absence of specific antibodies against the M protein, the cells are protected against phagocytosis. The M protein also prevents interaction with complement. Recent studies in the United States have demonstrated that M serotypes 1, 3, and 18 are associated with serious, invasive streptococcal disease and serotypes M3 and M18 with rheumatic fever.

F Protein. This protein has a receptor for fibronectin, a matrix protein on eukaryotic cells, and may be the major adhesin for bacterial attachment to the epithelial cells of the pharynx and skin.

Lipoteichoic acid. The lipid moiety of lipoteichoic acid has been implicated in binding to fibronectin. However, because this molecule is normally imbedded in the streptococcal cell membrane, what role this plays in binding to epithelial cells is unclear.

Pyrogenic exotoxins. These toxins, also called **erythrogenic toxins**, are produced by lysogenic strains of streptococci, similar to the toxin produced in *Corynebacterium diphtheriae*. Three immunologically distinct, heat-labile toxins (A, B, and C) have been described in group A streptococci and in rare strains of groups C and G streptococci. These toxins have a variety of important effects, including enhancement of delayed hypersensitiv-

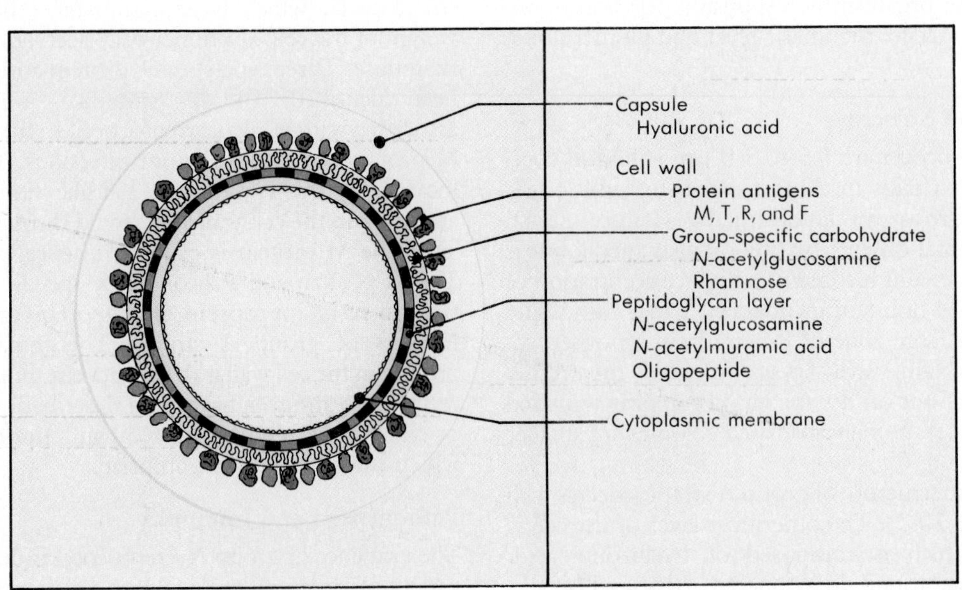

FIGURE 20-2 Schematic diagram of group A *Streptococcus*.

TABLE 20-3 Group A Streptococcus Virulence Factors

Virulence factor	Action
Capsule	Nonimmunogenic; antiphagocytic
M protein	Antiphagocytic; anticomplementary
F protein	Mediates adherence to epithelial cells
Lipoteichoic acid	Possibly mediates adherence to epithelial cells
Exotoxins (erythrogenic toxins)	Mediates pyrogenicity, enhancement of delayed hypersensitivity and susceptibility to endotoxin, cytotoxicity, nonspecific mitogenicity for T lymphocytes, immunosuppression of B lymphocyte function, and production of scarlatiniform rash
Streptolysin S	Lyses leukocytes, platelets, and erythrocytes; stimulates release of lysosomal enzymes; nonimmunogenic
Streptolysin O	Lyses leukocytes, platelets, and erythrocytes; stimulates release of lysosomal enzymes; immunogenic
Streptokinases	Lyses blood clots; facilitates spread of bacteria in tissues
DNase	Depolymerizes cell-free DNA in purulent material

ity and susceptibility to endotoxin, cytotoxicity, nonspecific mitogenicity for T lymphocytes, and immunosuppression of B-lymphocyte function. The toxins are also responsible for the rash observed in scarlet fever, although it is unclear whether this is due to the direct effect of the toxin on the capillary bed or (more likely) is secondary to a hypersensitivity reaction. Toxin injected intradermally will produce localized erythema at 24 hours in a susceptible individual **(Dick test)**. Antitoxin injected intradermally in a patient with scarlet fever will produce localized blanching, indicating neutralization of the toxin **(Schultz-Charlton reaction)**. Neither test is currently used for diagnostic purposes. Exotoxin A has been found in more than half of the group A streptococcal strains responsible for severe streptococcal toxic shock disease. Although this toxin may be important in this disease, other factors are certainly also significant.

Streptolysins S and O. Streptolysin S is an oxygen-stable, nonimmunogenic cell-bound hemolysin capable of lysing erythrocytes, as well as leukocytes and platelets, following direct cell contact. Streptolysin S can also stimulate release of lysosomal contents after engulfment, with subsequent death of the phagocytic cell. Streptolysin O is inactivated reversibly by oxygen and irreversibly by cholesterol. Unlike streptolysin S, antibodies are readily formed against streptolysin O and are useful for documenting a recent infection **(ASO test)**. This hemolysin will cross-react with similar oxygen-labile toxins produced by *S. pneumoniae* and *Clostridium* species. Streptolysin O is also capable of killing leukocytes by lysis of their cytoplasmic granules with release of hydrolytic enzymes.

Streptokinases. At least two forms (A and B) have been described. These enzymes are capable of lysing blood clots and may be responsible for the rapid spread of group A streptococci in infected tissues.

DNase. Four immunologically distinct deoxyribonucleases (A through D) have been identified. These enzymes are not cytolytic but are capable of depolymerizing free DNA present in pus. This reduces the viscosity of the abscess material and facilitates spread of the organisms. Antibodies developed against DNase B are an important marker of cutaneous group A streptococcal infections.

Other enzymes. Other enzymes have been described, including hyaluronidase ("spreading factor") and diphosphopyridine nucleotidase (DPNase). Their role in pathogenesis is unknown.

Epidemiology

Group A streptococci commonly colonize the oropharynx of healthy children and young adults (Box 20-2). Although the incidence of carriage is reported to be 15% to 20%, these figures are misleading. Highly selective culture techniques are required to detect small numbers of organisms in oropharyngeal secretions. Colonization with group A streptococci is transient, regulated by the individual's ability to mount specific immunity to the M protein of the colonizing strain and the presence of competitive organisms in the oropharynx. Bacteria such as the α- and nonhemolytic streptococci are able to produce antibiotic-like substances called **bacteriocins,** which suppress the growth of group A streptococci. In general, group A streptococcal disease is caused by recently acquired strains that are able to establish an infection of the pharynx or skin before specific antibodies are produced or competitive organisms are able to proliferate.

Clinical Syndromes

Suppurative Streptococcal Disease

PHARYNGITIS. Group A *Streptococcus* is the major cause of bacterial pharyngitis, with group C and G occasionally involved. This is primarily a disease of children between the ages of 5 to 15 years, but infants and adults are also susceptible. The pathogen is spread by person-to-person contact via respiratory droplets. Crowding, such as in classrooms and with play activities for children, increases the opportunity for spread of the organism.

Infection generally develops 2 to 4 days after exposure, with an abrupt onset of sore throat, fever, malaise, and headache. The posterior pharynx can appear erythema-

BOX 20-2 Epidemiology of Group A Streptococcal Infections

DISEASE/BACTERIAL FACTORS

Pharyngitis, scarlet fever, streptococcal toxic shock syndrome, erysipelas, pyoderma, acute rheumatic fever, glomerulonephritis

Numerous virulence factors (see Table 20-3): capsule, M and F proteins, lipoteichoic acid, pyrogenic exotoxins, streptolysins S and O, streptokinase, DNase, other enzymes

Transient colonization of oropharynx is common; disease occurs when strains establish an infection of pharynx or skin before specific antibodies develop or competitive organisms proliferate

TRANSMISSION

Person to person via respiratory droplets (pharyngitis) or through break in skin via direct contact with infected person, fomite, or arthropod vector (pyoderma)

Rheumatic fever: nonsuppurative complication of upper respiratory infections with group A streptococci

Acute glomerulonephritis: nonsuppurative complication of upper respiratory or cutaneous infection with group A streptococci

WHO IS AT RISK?

Pharyngitis: children 5 to 15 years old at greatest risk

Streptococcal toxic shock syndrome: immunocompetent persons with bacteremia and extensive soft tissue infections

Erysipelas: young children and older adults with preceding respiratory or skin infections with group A streptococci

Pyoderma: children 2-5 years old with poor personal hygiene

Rheumatic fever: children with severe streptococcal disease

Pharyngitis-associated glomerulonephritis: school-age children

Pyoderma-associated glomerulonephritis: preschool-age children

GEOGRAPHY/SEASON

Pharyngitis, rheumatic fever: more common in winter and fall

Pyoderma: most common in warm, moist environments and during summer

Pharyngitis-associated glomerulonephritis: more common in temperate and cold climates and during winter and spring

Pyoderma-associated glomerulonephritis: more common in hot or tropical climates and during late summer and early fall

MODES OF CONTROL

Penicillin drug of choice; erythromycin for patients allergic to penicillin

Oropharyngeal carriage after treatment can be treated with additional antibiotic course; however, retreatment is *not* indicated with prolonged asymptomatic carriage because antibiotics will disrupt normal flora

Starting antibiotic therapy within 10 days for patients with pharyngitis will prevent rheumatic fever

Rheumatic fever: antibiotic prophylaxis prevents recurrence with subsequent streptococcal infections;antibiotic prophylaxis required before procedures (e.g., dental) that can induce bacteremias leading to endocarditis

Glomerulonephritis: no specific antibiotic treatment or prophylaxis is indicated

tous with an exudate, and cervical lymphadenopathy can be prominent. Despite these clinical signs and symptoms, differentiating streptococcal pharyngitis from viral pharyngitis is difficult. For example, only about 50% of patients with "strep throat" will have pharyngeal or tonsillar exudates. Likewise, most young children with exudative pharyngitis will have viral disease. The specific diagnosis can be made only by bacteriological or serological tests.

Scarlet fever is a complication of streptococcal pharyngitis (Figure 20-3) seen when the infecting strain is lysogenized by a temperate bacteriophage that stimulates production of a pyrogenic exotoxin. Within 1 to 2 days after the initial clinical symptoms of pharyngitis, a diffuse erythematous rash will initially appear on the upper chest and then spread to the extremities. The area around the mouth is generally spared (circumoral pallor), as are the palms and soles. The tongue will initially be covered with a yellowish-white coating that later will be shed, revealing a red, raw surface ("strawberry tongue"). The rash, which blanches upon pressure, is best seen on the abdomen and in skin folds (Pastia's lines). The rash will disappear over the next 5 to 7 days and is followed by desquamation.

Suppurative complications of streptococcal pharyngitis rarely occur with the advent of antimicrobial therapy. However, abscesses of the peritonsillar and retropharyngeal areas can be observed, as well as disseminated infections to the brain, heart, bones, and joints.

STREPTOCOCCAL TOXIC SHOCK SYNDROME (also called toxic shock-like syndrome). Although severe group A streptococcal disease had steadily declined with the introduction of antibiotics, this trend was dramatically altered in the late 1980s when severe streptococcal soft tissue infections (e.g., cellulitis, necrotizing fasciitis) associated with multisystem toxicity were reported. Most affected patients had hypotension, diffuse erythroderma, hypoalbuminemia, hypocalcemia, and multiorgan failure (e.g., kidney, lungs, liver, heart)—features similar to

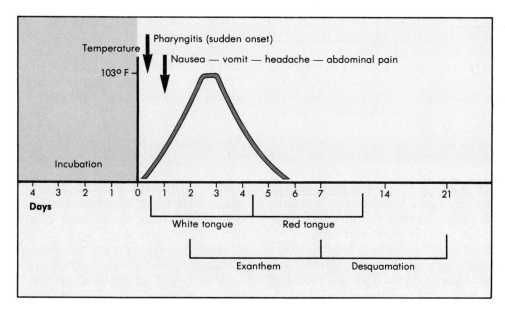

FIGURE 20-3 Evolution of signs and symptoms of scarlet fever. (Modified from Habif TP: *Clinical dermatology: a color guide to diagnosis and therapy,* St. Louis, 1985, Mosby.)

staphylococcal toxic shock syndrome. These patients were bacteremic and had extensive soft tissue infections, in contrast with those with staphylococcal infections. Most patients were younger than 50 years of age and were not immunocompromised. The group A streptococci responsible for this syndrome differ from the strains causing pharyngitis in that most are serotypes M1, M3, or M18, and some have prominent hyaluronic acid capsules (mucoid strains). Production of pyrogenic exotoxins, particularly exotoxin A, is also a prominent feature of these organisms, which may explain the severe systemic toxicity (see Table 20-3).

ERYSIPELAS. This is an acute superficial cellulitis of the skin with prominent lymphatic involvement. Erysipelas occurs most commonly in young children or older adults, involves the face and less frequently the trunk or extremities, and usually is preceded by either respiratory or skin infections with group A *Streptococcus* (less frequently with groups C or G streptococci). The cutaneous manifestations (Figure 20-4) are accompanied by chills, fever, and systemic toxicity.

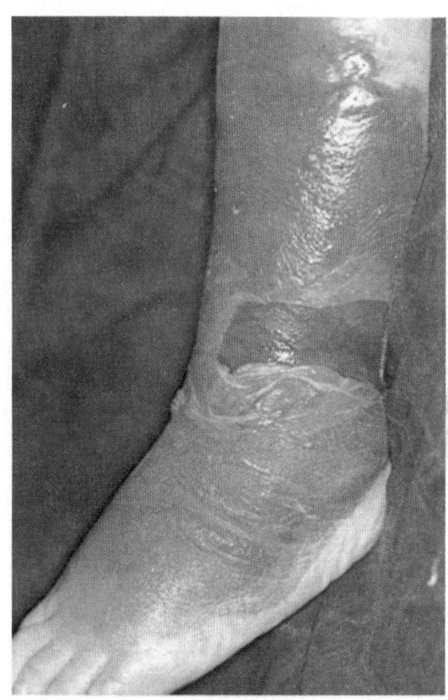

FIGURE 20-4 Acute stage of erysipelas of leg. Note erythema in involved area and bullae formation. (From Emond RTD and Rowland HAK: *A colour atlas of infectious diseases,* ed 2, London, 1989, Wolfe Medical Publications.)

PYODERMA. Streptococcal skin infections most commonly occur in warm, moist environments during the summer months. Pyoderma is seen primarily in young children (2 to 5 years of age) with poor personal hygiene. Clinical disease is preceded by initial colonization of the skin with group A streptococci via direct contact with another infected child or fomite, or transfer by an arthropod vector. Introduction into the subcutaneous tissues is by minor break in the skin integrity (e.g., scratch or insect bite). Group A streptococci are responsible for the majority of streptococcal skin infections, although groups C and G have also been implicated. The strains of streptococci that cause skin infections are different from those that cause pharyngitis, although pyoderma serotypes can colonize the pharynx and establish a persistent carriage state.

OTHER SUPPURATIVE DISEASES. Group A streptococci have been associated with a variety of other suppurative infections, including puerperal sepsis, lymphangitis, pneumonia, and others. Although these infections can be seen occasionally, they have become exceedingly rare with the introduction of antibiotic therapy.

Nonsuppurative Streptococcal Disease

RHEUMATIC FEVER. Rheumatic fever is a nonsuppurative complication of group A streptococcal disease. It is characterized by inflammatory changes of the heart, joints, blood vessels, and subcutaneous tissues. Chronic, progressive damage to the heart valves may occur, although the specific mechanisms of tissue damage are unknown. A number of theories have been proposed, including (1) direct destruction of the tissue by the organism or a streptococcal enzyme (e.g., streptolysin), (2) serum sickness–like reaction mediated by complexes of antibodies and antigens, and (3) an autoimmune reaction. This latter explanation is currently favored because antibodies directed against heart tissue have been identified in patients with uncomplicated streptococcal disease and rheumatic heart disease. These antibodies can bind to cardiac and skeletal muscles, as well as to the smooth muscles in blood vessels.

Rheumatic fever had steadily decreased over the last 30 years from a peak incidence of more than 10,000 reported cases to fewer than 150 cases. However, the disease is still observed (127 cases reported in 1991), and some recent evidence indicates that it may be increasing in frequency. Disease is associated with specific serotypes of group A *Streptococcus* (e.g., M18 and M3, and to a lesser extent M5). As discussed previously, disease caused by serotype M18 has become more prevalent in recent years. Rheumatic fever is also associated only with upper respiratory infections. Cutaneous streptococcal infections do not initiate rheumatic fever. The epidemiology of the disease mimics streptococcal pharyngitis: it most commonly occurs in young school-age children, with no male or female predilection, and it occurs during the fall or winter months (Table 20-4). Rheumatic fever usually follows severe streptococcal disease, although as many as one third of the patients will have had an asymptomatic infection with group A *Streptococcus*. Recurrence will occur with subsequent streptococcal infection if antibiotic prophylaxis is not used. The risk for recurrence will decrease with time.

Because no specific diagnostic test is available to identify patients with rheumatic fever, diagnosis is made by clinical parameters. The revised criteria of Jones are currently used (Box 20-3). Critical to the diagnosis is documentation of recent group A streptococcal disease by either culture, antigen detection, or serologic testing.

ACUTE GLOMERULONEPHRITIS. The other nonsuppurative complication of streptococcal disease is acute glomerulonephritis, which is characterized by acute inflammation of the renal glomeruli with edema, hypertension, hematuria, and proteinuria. Specific nephritogenic strains of group A streptococci are associated with this disease. The pharyngeal strains and pyodermal strains differ. The epidemiology of the disease is similar to the initial streptococcal infection (Table 20-4). The clinical diagnosis is based on the clinical presentation and evidence of a recent group A streptococcal infection. Young patients generally have an uneventful recovery, whereas the long-term prognosis for adult patients is unclear. Progressive, irreversible loss of renal function has been reported in adults.

Laboratory Diagnosis

Microscopy. A rapid, preliminary diagnosis of group A streptococcal soft tissue infections or pyoderma can be made with a Gram stain. Streptococci do not normally colonize the skin surface; thus the presence of gram-positive cocci in pairs and chains associated with leukocytes is significant. In contrast, streptococci are part of the normal oropharyngeal flora, so their presence in a respiratory specimen collected from a patient with pharyngitis has poor predictive value.

Antigen detection. Group A streptococci can be detected directly in clinical specimens by a variety of immunological tests that react with the group-specific

TABLE 20-4 Epidemiological Features of Streptococcal Glomerulonephritis

Feature	Pharyngitis-associated acute glomerulonephritis	Pyoderma-associated acute glomerulonephritis
Seasonal occurrence	Winter and spring	Late summer and early fall
Geographic distribution	Common in temperate and cold climates	Common in hot or tropical climates
Age	School-age children	Preschool-age children
Familial occurrence	Common	Common
Attack rate after infection with nephritogenic strain	10% to 15%	10% to 15%
Carrier state	Pharynx (common)	Skin (rare)
Serologic types	Limited in pharynx	Limited to skin
Antistreptolysin O response	Common	Uncommon
Anti-DNase B response	Common	Common

Modified from Wannamaker LW: Differences between streptococcal infections of the throat and of the skin, *N Engl J Med* 282:23, 1970.

carbohydrate in the bacterial cell wall. The antigen is extracted by treating the clinical specimen (e.g., throat swab) with nitrous acid or less commonly by enzymatic methods. The extract is then mixed with specific antibodies, either bound to latex particles or immobilized on a filter membrane (EIA procedure). Agglutination of the latex particles or development of a positive indicator in the EIA procedure represents a positive test. These assays have been shown to be very specific. However, the test sensitivity is low (probably no better than 75% to 80%), so all negative tests must be confirmed by culture.

Culture. The proper specimen must be collected for the isolation of group A streptococci. Specimens collected from posterior oropharyngeal sites from infected patients (e.g., tonsils, posterior pharynx, posterior tongue) yield quantitatively more group A streptococci than do specimens from the anterior areas of the mouth. This is logical because there is a greater chance of isolating the pathogen when the site of infection is sampled. However, it should also be appreciated that the mouth, particularly saliva, is colonized with bacteria that inhibit the growth of group A streptococci. Contamination of even a well-collected specimen may obscure or suppress the growth of group A streptococci. The recovery of group A streptococci from skin infections is less of a problem. The crusted top of the lesion is raised, and the purulent material and base of the lesion cultured. Group A streptococci should be recovered in large numbers. Open, draining skin pustules should be avoided because these might be superinfected with staphylococci.

As discussed previously, streptococci have fastidious growth requirements. To suppress the oral bacterial flora, antibiotics (e.g., trimethoprim-sulfamethoxazole) have been added to blood agar plates. Although these selective plates have proved very useful, a delay in the growth of group A streptococci has been observed and necessitates prolonged incubation (2 to 3 days) of the cultures. It is also unclear what atmosphere of incubation should be used. Although both streptolysin O and S are expressed in an anaerobic atmosphere, group A streptococci will be confused under these conditions with other β-hemolytic streptococci present in the oropharynx. Because virtually all group A streptococci produce streptolysin S, cultures can be incubated in air.

Identification. Group A streptococci historically were identified by their susceptibility to bacitracin (Table 20-5). A disk saturated with bacitracin is placed onto a plate seeded with group A streptococci and, after overnight incubation, a zone of inhibited growth is considered positive for group A streptococci. Some α-hemolytic strains are inhibited by bacitracin. If errors in interpretation of the hemolytic patterns are made, then these organisms would be misidentified. This is particularly a problem in small laboratories with limited technical experience, such as in a physician's office. A bacitracin disk can be placed directly onto the primarily seeded culture (direct test). This procedure will identify approximately 50% of the positive cultures, so negative tests must be confirmed. Group A streptococci are definitively identified by demonstrating the group-specific carbohydrate. This was not routinely practical until the introduction of direct antigen detection tests.

Antibody detection. Patients with group A streptococcal disease produce antibodies to a number of specific enzymes. Although antibodies against the M protein are produced and are important for immunity to develop, these antibodies are not measured because they appear late in the clinical course of disease and are type-specific. Antibodies against streptolysin O (ASO test) are measured most commonly. The antibodies appear 3 to 4 weeks after the initial exposure to the organism and persist. Measurement of these antibodies is particularly useful for documenting recent streptococcal pharyngitis in a patient with rheumatic fever or acute glomerulonephritis. An elevated ASO titer is not observed in patients with streptococcal pyoderma. It is thought that the streptolysin is inactivated by the lipids present on the skin. Other antibodies produced against streptococcal enzymes, particularly DNase B, have been documented in patients with streptococcal pyoderma and pharyngitis. This test should be performed to confirm the role of streptococci in the development of glomerulonephritis.

BOX 20-3 1992 Revised Jones Criteria for the Diagnosis of Rheumatic Fever

The diagnosis of rheumatic fever is highly likely if supported by evidence of a preceding group A streptococcal infection and the presence of two major manifestations or one major and two minor manifestations.

SUPPORTING EVIDENCE OF ANTECEDENT GROUP A STREPTOCOCCAL INFECTION

Positive throat culture
Positive streptococcal antigen test
Elevated or rising streptococcal antibody titer

MAJOR MANIFESTATIONS

Carditis
Polyarthritis
Chorea
Erythema marginatum
Subcutaneous nodules

MINOR MANIFESTATIONS

Clinical findings: arthralgia, fever
Laboratory findings
- Elevated acute phase reactants (erythrocyte sedimentation rate, C-reactive protein)
- Prolonged PR interval on electrocardiography

From *JAMA* 268: 2069-2073, 1992.

TABLE 20-5 Presumptive Identification of Streptococci

Organism	Susceptibility to: Bacitracin	Optochin	CAMP	Hydrolysis of: Hippurate	Esculin	Growth in: Bile	6.5% NaCl	Lysis by bile
β-hemolytic streptococci								
Group A	S	R	−	−	−	−	−	−
Group B	R*	R	+	+	−	−	+*	−
Groups C, F, G	R	R	−	−	−	−	−	−
Viridans group	R*	R	−	−	−*	−*	−	−
S. pneumoniae	R	S	−	−	−	−	−	+

*Test variations can be seen.

Treatment, Prevention, and Control

Group A streptococci are very sensitive to penicillin. For patients with a history of penicillin allergy, erythromycin can be used. Persistent oropharyngeal carriage of group A streptococci after a complete course of therapy can occur. This may represent poor compliance with the prescribed course of therapy, reinfection with a new strain, or persistent carriage in a sequestered focus. Antibiotic resistance has not been reported; thus an additional course of treatment can be initiated. If carriage persists, retreatment is not indicated because prolonged antibiotic therapy can disrupt the normal protective bacterial flora. Carriers have not been shown to be at increased risk for relapse infections or transmission of their organism to susceptible individuals. Antibiotic therapy in patients with pharyngitis will speed the relief of symptoms and, if initiated within 10 days of initial clinical disease, prevent rheumatic fever. Antibiotic therapy does not appear to influence the progression to acute glomerulonephritis.

Patients with a history of rheumatic fever require long-term use of antibiotic prophylaxis to prevent recurrent disease. In addition, damage to the heart valve predisposes the patient to subsequent endocarditis. Antibiotic prophylaxis is required before the use of procedures that induce transient bacteremias (e.g., dental procedures). Specific antibiotic therapy will not alter the course of acute glomerulonephritis and is not indicated for prophylaxis because recurrent disease is not observed.

Group B *Streptococcus*

Group B *Streptococcus*, or *Streptococcus agalactiae*, was initially recognized as a cause of puerperal sepsis. Although the organism is still associated with this disease, it has gained more notoriety as a significant cause of septicemia, pneumonia, and meningitis in newborn children.

Physiology and Structure

Group B streptococci are gram-positive cocci (0.6 to 1.2 μm) that form short chains in clinical specimens and longer chains in culture. The organism grows well on nutritionally enriched medium as buttery colonies, larger than seen with group A streptococci, and surrounded by a narrow zone of β-hemolysis. Rare strains will be nonhemolytic or α-hemolytic.

The group-specific cell wall polysaccharide antigen is composed of rhamnose, *N*-acetylglucosamine, and galactose (Figure 20-5). Serologic cross-reactions have been observed between some group B and group G streptococci. Six immunologically distinct serotypes have been described based on the type-specific capsular polysaccharide antigen and surface protein antigen: Ia, Ib/c, Ia/c, II, III, and IV. These serotypes are important epidemiological markers.

Pathogenesis and Immunity

Antibodies developed against the type-specific capsular antigens in group B streptococci are protective. This in part explains the predilection of this organism for neonates. In the absence of type-specific maternal antibodies the infant is at increased risk for infection. Bactericidal activity for group B streptococci also requires complement. If the level of complement is low in the neonate, then there is a greater likelihood of systemic spread of the organism in colonized infants.

Group B streptococci produce a number of enzymes, including deoxyribonucleases, hyaluronidase, neuraminidase, proteases, hippurase, and hemolysins. Although these enzymes are useful for identification of the organism, their role in the pathogenesis of infection is unknown.

Epidemiology

Group B streptococci colonize the upper respiratory tract, lower gastrointestinal tract, and vagina (Box 20-4). Transient vaginal carriage has been reported in as many as 40% of pregnant women, although this is influenced by the time of sampling during the gestation period and culture techniques employed. The serotype distribution for asymptomatic colonization is evenly divided among types I, II, and III.

Infection, with subsequent development of disease in the neonate, can occur in utero, at the time of birth, or

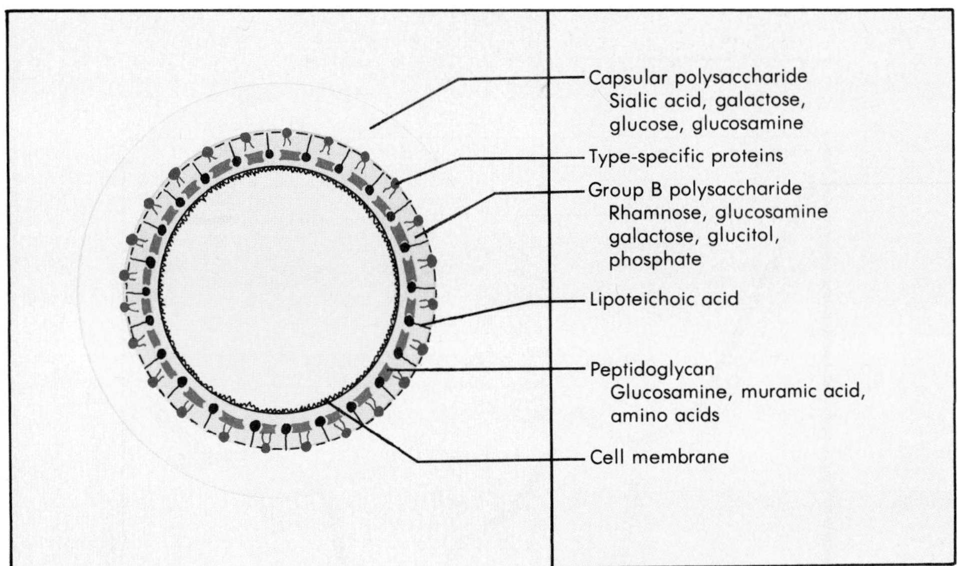

FIGURE 20-5 Schematic representation of group B *Streptococcus.* (Redrawn from Christensen KK, Christensen P, and Ferrieri P: *Neonatal group B streptococcal infections*, vol 35, Basel, Switzerland, 1985, Karger.)

during the first few months of life (Figure 20-6). Infections at or before birth are called early-onset disease (Table 20-6). Premature rupture of membranes, prolonged labor, preterm delivery, or maternal disease increases the risk of fetal infection in colonized women. Approximately 60% of infants born of colonized mothers will become colonized with their mother's serotype organism. The likelihood of colonization at the time of birth is increased if the mother is heavily colonized, although neonatal disease is not more common in these infants (emphasizing the maternal immune status is more important than exposure to the bacteria). The incidence of neonatal disease is approximately 3 per 1000 live births, with early-onset disease about twice as frequent as late-onset disease. Late-onset disease generally occurs in infants from 1 week to 3 months of life.

Early-onset disease is associated with all serotypes of group B *Streptococcus* in a proportion similar to maternal colonization. One exception would be infants with early-onset meningitis – 80% of these infants are infected with serotype III. Serotype III is also responsible for more than 70% of late-onset infections.

Clinical Syndromes

Early-onset neonatal disease. Clinical symptoms of group B streptococcal disease acquired in utero or at the time of delivery generally will develop during the first 5 days of life. Early-onset disease, characterized by bacteremia, pneumonia, or meningitis, will appear indistinguishable from sepsis caused by other organisms. Mortality has been decreased with rapid diagnosis and better supportive care. However, 60% of infected, low birth weight, premature infants will die, and a significant proportion of survivors will have neurological sequelae

BOX 20-4 Epidemiology of Group B Streptococcal Infection

DISEASE/BACTERIAL FACTORS

Neonatal meningitis, pneumonia, bacteremia; postpartum sepsis

Disease can occur in utero, at birth, or during first few months of life

TRANSMISSION

Early-onset neonatal disease: inoculation from mother via colonized birth canal, premature rupture of membranes, prolonged labor, preterm delivery, or disseminated maternal group B streptococcal disease

Late-onset neonatal disease: person to person via contact with infected infant or mother

Postpartum sepsis: spread of organisms colonizing vagina to surgical incision site or uterus

WHO IS AT RISK?

Neonates, particularly those without type-specific maternal antibodies and with low complement levels

GEOGRAPHY

Ubiquitous

No seasonal incidence

MODES OF CONTROL

Penicillin G drug of choice; combination of penicillin and aminoglycoside used in serious infections

High-risk babies: antibiotic therapy and passive immunization by transfusion with blood containing type-specific antibodies

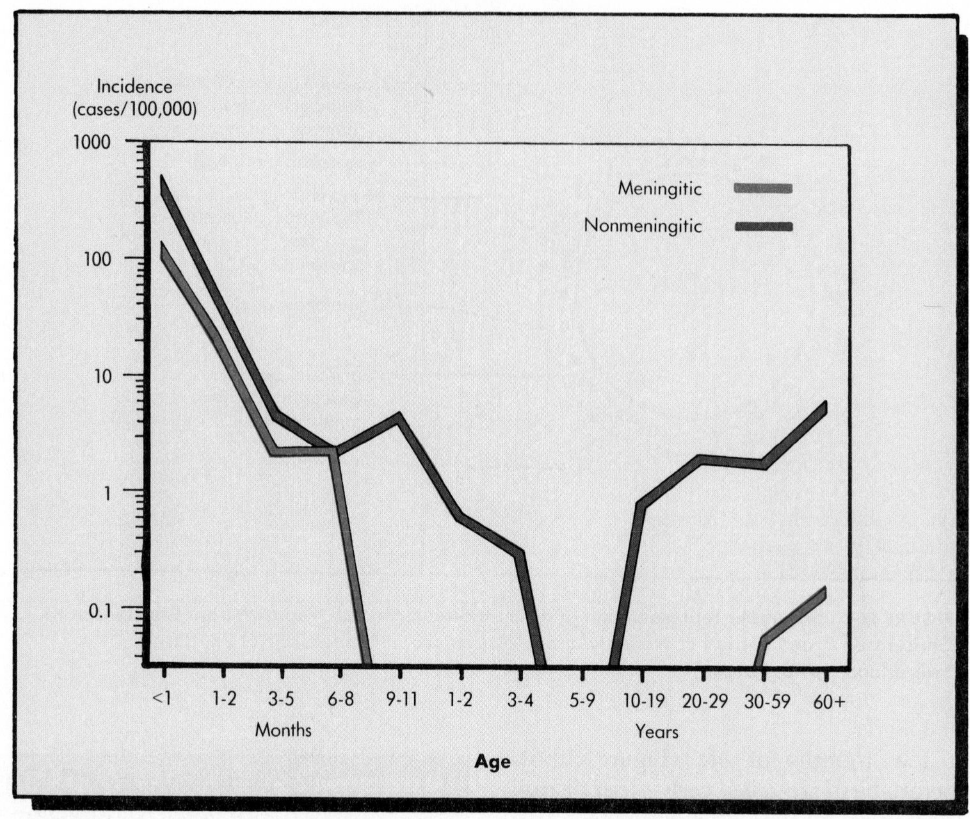

FIGURE 20-6 Age-specific attack rates of group B streptococcal disease. (Modified from Wenger JD et al., J Infect Dis *162:1316, 1990.)*

TABLE 20-6 Epidemiology of Neonatal Group B Streptococcal Disease

Features	Early-onset disease	Late-onset disease
Age of onset	<7 days	1 week to 3 months
Obstetrical complications	Yes	Infrequent
Time of acquisition	In utero or at delivery	Postpartum
Clinical disease	Bacteremia, pneumonia, meninigitis	Bacteremia, meningitis, osteomyelitis
Mortality rate	High	Low (<20%)
Streptococcal serotype	I, II, or III	III most common

including blindness, deafness, and severe mental retardation.

Late-onset neonatal disease. Disease in older infants is acquired from an exogenous source (e.g., mother, another infant). The predominant manifestation is bacteremia with meningitis, which again resembles disease caused by other bacterial pathogens. Although survival (greater than 80%) is significantly better than with early-onset disease, neurological complications in children with meningitis are common.

Postpartum sepsis. Postpartum group B streptococcal disease generally is seen as endometritis or a wound infection, with bacteremia frequently documented. Because child-bearing women are generally in good health, the prognosis is excellent when appropriate therapy is initiated. Secondary complications following bacteremia, such as endocarditis, meningitis, or osteomyelitis, have been rarely reported.

Laboratory Diagnosis

Antigen detection. Direct detection of the organism with antibodies prepared against the group-specific carbohydrate is useful for the rapid detection of group B streptococcal disease in neonates. A variety of methods have been used, including counterimmunoelectrophoresis, staphylococcal coagglutination, and latex agglutination. In the latter two methods, antibodies developed against the group-specific antigen are attached to killed staphylococci or latex particles. These assay methods are sensitive, specific, and can be used with cerebrospinal fluid, urine, or serum. Unfortunately, the direct antigen

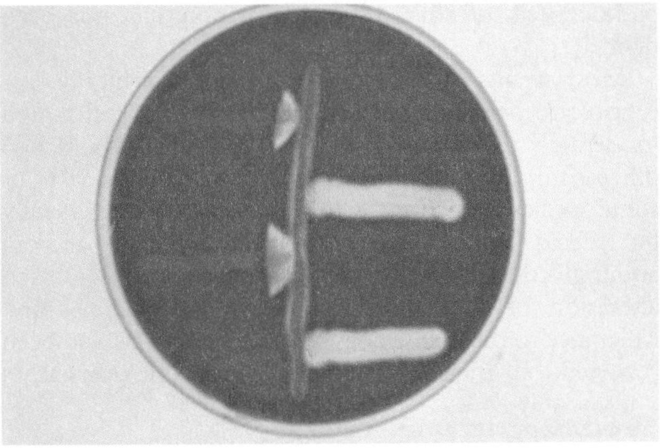

FIGURE 20-7 CAMP reaction with group B *Streptococcus.* Group B streptococci produce a diffusible, heat-stable protein (CAMP factor) that enhances β-hemolysis of *S. aureus. S. aureus* produces sphingomyelinase C, which can bind to erythrocyte membranes. When exposed to the group B CAMP factor, the cells undergo hemolysis. Although most group B streptococci produce CAMP factor and stimulate enhanced hemolysis, it has also been found in some group C, F, and G streptococci. (From Howard BJ: *Clinical and pathogenic microbiology,* St Louis, 1987, Mosby.)

test has not proven reliable for screening mothers to predict which newborns will be at increased risk for developing neonatal disease.

Culture. Group B streptococci readily grow on a nutritionally enriched medium, producing large colonies after 24 hours of incubation. β-hemolysis may be either difficult to detect or absent, which will present a problem in the detection of the organism in mixed cultures. A selective medium, with antibiotics used to suppress the growth of other organisms, has been used with some success. Carriage of small numbers of organisms can be detected by inoculating specimens into an enrichment broth.

Identification. A preliminary identification of an isolate can be made by demonstration of a positive CAMP test (Figure 20-7) or hydrolysis of hippurate. Group B streptococci are definitively identified by demonstrating the group-specific carbohydrate (similar to group A streptococci).

Treatment, Prevention, and Control

Group B streptococci are generally susceptible to penicillin G, which is the drug of choice. However, the minimum inhibitory concentration (MIC) is approximately 10 times greater than with group A streptococci. In addition, **tolerance** to penicillin (ability to inhibit but not kill the organism) has been reported. For these reasons, a combination of penicillin plus an aminoglycoside is frequently used in serious infections. Resistance to erythromycin and tetracycline has also been observed. Thus specific antimicrobial susceptibility tests will have to be performed for isolates from patients allergic to penicillin.

Attempts to prevent neonatal disease have met with limited success. Although early-onset disease occurs in infants of colonized women, the incidence of colonization is high. Only a small proportion of these women will deliver infants who will become colonized and subsequently develop disease, and infants at greatest risk for disease cannot be identified unless maternal antibodies are measured (a procedure rarely done). Intrapartum antibiotic therapy reduces the incidence of neonatal disease, but the routine treatment of all colonized women is not currently recommended.

Passive immunization of high-risk babies by transfusion with blood containing type-specific antibodies has reduced morbidity and mortality associated with group B streptococcal disease. However, most whole blood has inadequate levels of protective antibodies. Future efforts to eliminate this disease will be directed toward the detection and immunization of women of childbearing age without protective antibodies.

Other β-Hemolytic Streptococci

Although a large variety of other groupable β-hemolytic streptococci have been described, the most commonly isolated strains belong to groups C, F, and G. These groups can be subdivided into large colony or "*S. pyogenes*-like" strains and small colony strains. Most small colony strains are *S. anginosus* (also referred to as *S. milleri* group) and can be distinguished from other β-hemolytic streptococci by a positive Voges-Proskauer reaction (production of acetylmethylcarbinol).

The taxonomic classification of group C streptococci has undergone recent changes. The two species most commonly associated with human disease, *S. equisimilis* and *S. anginosus*, can be part of the normal microbial flora of the pharynx, gastrointestinal tract, and genitourinary tract. Other species (e.g., *S. equi* and *S. zooepidemicus*) are primarily isolated only in zoonotic infections. Group C streptococci have been implicated in a variety of infections including pharyngitis (sometimes complicated by acute glomerulonephritis but never rheumatic fever), epiglottitis, sinusitis, meningitis, soft tissue and bone infections, intraabdominal abscesses, pericarditis, and endocarditis.

All group F streptococci are considered to be *S. anginosus*. These organisms colonize the same body sites as group C streptococci and have been associated with a wide distribution of infections. Abscess formation is a prominent feature of these infections.

Group G streptococci are a heterogeneous collection of organisms sharing reactivity with antibodies directed against the group G carbohydrate. The "small colony" variants have been classified as *S. anginosus* and are associated with the same diseases attributed to the other serogroups of this species. These include respiratory infections (possibly complicated by acute glomerulonephritis), cutaneous infections, bacteremia, endocarditis, meningitis, arthritis, and puerperal sepsis.

Viridans Streptococci

The viridans group of streptococci are a heterogeneous collection of α- and nonhemolytic streptococci. Taxonomic nomenclature for these species is confusing because a consensus between European and American microbiologists has not been reached. Thus different species names are often used interchangeably in the literature. Although most isolates of viridans streptococci do not possess a group-specific carbohydrate, reactivity with some groups has been reported (e.g., A, C, E, F, H, K, M, and O).

Like most other streptococci, these species are nutritionally fastidious, requiring complex media supplemented with blood products and an incubation atmosphere frequently augmented with 5% to 10% carbon dioxide. Some strains are "nutritionally deficient streptococci" because they can grow only in the presence of exogenously supplied pyridoxal, the active form of vitamin B_6. These organisms will usually grow initially in blood cultures but will fail to grow when subcultured unless pyridoxal-supplemented media are used. These strains have been recently organized within two new species: *S. defectivus* and *S. adjacens*.

The viridans streptococci are the most common group of organisms in the oropharynx and can also be isolated from the gastrointestinal and urogenital tracts. Although these organisms can cause a variety of infections, they are most commonly associated with dental caries, subacute endocarditis, and suppurative intraabdominal infections. Adherence to tooth enamel or previously damaged heart valves is believed to be due to the production of insoluble dextran from glucose. This is most commonly observed with *S. mutans* and *S. sanguis*. *S. anginosus* is the species most commonly associated with pyogenic infections. The pathogenesis of this abscess formation has not been defined.

Most strains of viridans streptococci are highly susceptible to penicillin with MICs ≤0.1 μg/ml, although moderately resistant streptococci (penicillin MIC 0.2 to 0.5 μg/ml) have been observed in as many as 10% of some species. Infections with these isolates can generally be treated with a combination of penicillin and an aminoglycoside. High-level resistance, because of an alteration of the penicillin-binding proteins, is rare. Tolerance to the killing activity of penicillin has also been reported, but the clinical significance is controversial.

Streptococcus pneumoniae

Streptococcus pneumoniae was initially isolated independently by Pasteur and Steinberg more than 100 years ago. Since that time research with this organism has increased our understanding of molecular genetics (Figure 20-8), antibiotic resistance, and vaccine-related immunoprophylaxis. Unfortunately, pneumococcal disease is still a leading cause of morbidity and mortality.

Physiology and Structure

The pneumococcus is an encapsulated gram-positive coccus. The cells are 0.5 to 1.2 μm in diameter, oval or lancet-shaped, and arranged in pairs or short chains. Older cultures will decolorize readily and appear gram-negative. Colonial morphology will vary. Encapsulated strains are generally large (1 to 3 mm on blood agar; smaller on chocolatized or heated blood agar), round, mucoid, and unpigmented; nonencapsulated strains are smaller and appear flat. All colonies will undergo autolysis with aging (the central portion of the colony will dissolve, leaving a dimpled colony). Colonies will be α-hemolytic

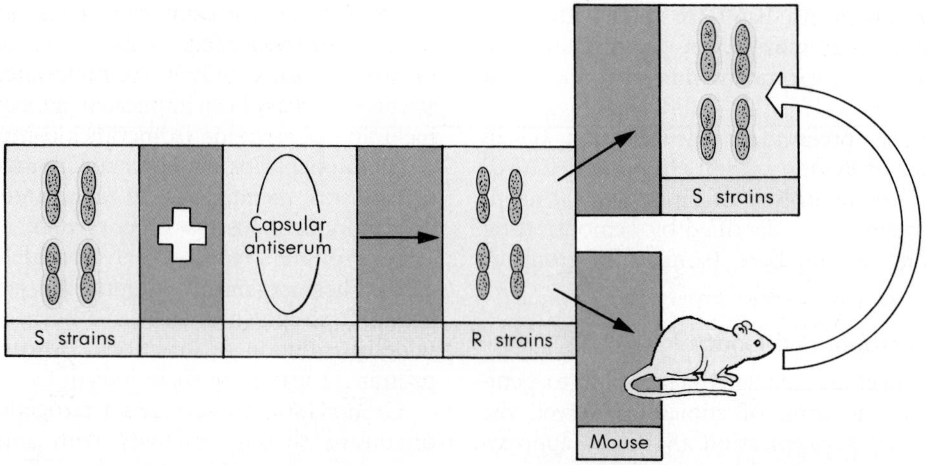

FIGURE 20-8 Genetic variation. Under the selective pressure of type-specific antiserum, rough variants of encapsulated strains of *S. pneumoniae* are selected. These R strains can revert to encapsulated S strains by spontaneous back mutations. S strains can also be selected by passage through a mouse, where the virulent S strains will rapidly overgrow the avirulent R strains. Passage of pneumococci in mice is a means to maintain virulent strains in the laboratory. Avery, MacLeod, and McCarty demonstrated the DNA from a smooth strain could transform a different strain from rough to smooth. This observation formed the beginning of molecular genetics.

on blood agar when incubated aerobically and may be β-hemolytic when grown anaerobically.

The organism has fastidious nutritional requirements and is capable of growth only on enriched media (e.g., tryptic soy agar or brain heart infusion agar) supplemented with blood products. *S. pneumoniae* is able to ferment a number of carbohydrates, with lactic acid as the primary metabolic by-product. In media with high glucose concentrations, *S. pneumoniae* grow poorly because lactic acid rapidly reaches toxic levels. Like all streptococci the organism lacks catalase. Unless an exogenous source of catalase is provided (e.g., from blood), the accumulation of hydrogen peroxide will inhibit growth of *S. pneumoniae*. The poor growth of isolates on chocolatized blood agar is the result of the heat-denaturation of catalase present in the blood.

Virulent strains of *S. pneumoniae* are covered with a complex polysaccharide capsule. The capsular polysaccharides are antigenically distinct and have been used for serologic classification of strains. At present, 84 serotypes are recognized. Purified capsular material from the most commonly isolated serotypes are used in a polyvalent vaccine. Antibodies directed against the capsules have also been used for diagnostic purposes.

The cell wall peptidoglycan layer of the pneumococcus is typical of gram-positive cocci, with alternating subunits of *N*-acetylglucosamine and *N*-acetylmuramic acid cross-linked by peptide bridges. The other major component of the cell wall is teichoic acid rich in galactosamine, phosphate, and choline. The presence of choline is unique to the cell wall of *S. pneumoniae* and plays an important regulatory role in cell wall hydrolysis. In the absence of choline the pneumococcal autolytic enzyme is unable to function and cell division ceases. Two forms of teichoic acid exist in the pneumococcal cell wall: one exposed on the cell surface and a similar form covalently bound to the plasma membrane lipids. The exposed teichoic acid (also called **C-substance**) is species-specific and unrelated to the group-specific carbohydrates described by Lancefield in β-hemolytic streptococci. The C-substance will precipitate a serum globulin fraction **(C-reactive protein [CRP])** in the presence of calcium. CRP is present in low concentrations in healthy individuals but is elevated in patients with acute inflammatory diseases. The membrane lipoteichoic acid can cross-react with the Forssman surface antigens on mammalian cells. Other somatic antigens include the poorly characterized species-specific R protein and the type-specific M protein. Neither antigen protects against phagocytosis.

Pathogenesis and Immunity

Capsule. The virulence of *S. pneumoniae* is directly associated with the capsule, which inhibits phagocytosis in the absence of specific antibodies (Table 20-7). Encapsulated (smooth) strains are able to cause disease in humans and experimental animals, whereas nonencapsulated (rough) strains are avirulent. Antibodies directed against the capsular polysaccharides protect against disease caused by immunologically related strains. The capsular polysaccharides are soluble and have been referred to as **specific soluble substance (SSS)**. Free polysaccharides can protect viable organisms from phagocytosis by binding with opsonic antibodies.

The role of toxins in the pathogenesis of pneumococcal disease has not been demonstrated. However, an undefined or presently unrecognized factor is very likely responsible for the rapid onset of pneumococcal disease and the fulminant course observed in some groups of patients (e.g., patients with splenectomy). The following toxins and enzymes have been described.

Pneumolysin. This is a temperature- and oxygen-labile hemolysin immunologically related to streptolysin O. Pneumolysin is responsible for the β-hemolysis observed when *S. pneumoniae* is grown anaerobically. The protein is dermatoxic and causes hemolytic anemia in experimental rabbit infections.

Purpura-Producing Principle. This substance is released during cell autolysis and can cause dermal hemorrhage in experimental animals. A role in human disease has not been identified.

Neuraminidase. This enzyme is active against cell glycoproteins and glycolipids and may play a role in the spread of pneumococci through infected tissues.

Autolysins. The pneumococcal autolysin, amidase, hydrolyzes the peptidoglycan layer at the bond between

TABLE 20-7 *Streptococcus pneumoniae* Virulence Factors

Virulence factor	Action
Capsule	Inhibits phagocytosis in absence of antibodies
Pneumolysin	Hemolysin, dermotoxic
Purpura-producing principle	Causes dermal hemorrhage
Neuraminidase	Spreading factor
Amidase	Autolysin important for cell division

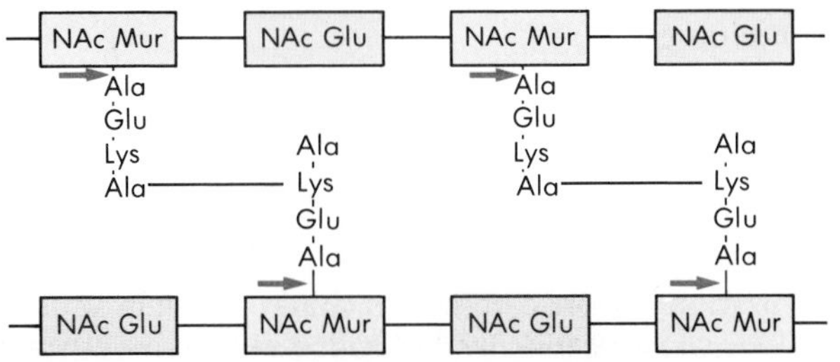

FIGURE 20-9 Pneumococcal cell wall. The peptidoglycan layer consists of alternating *N*-acetylglucosamine and *N*-acetylmuramic acid residues cross-linked with tetrapeptide bridges. The site of amidase activity is indicated by the arrows.

BOX 20-5 Epidemiology of *Streptococcus pneumoniae* Infection

DISEASE/BACTERIAL FACTORS

Pneumonia, sinusitis, otitis media, meningitis, bacteremia
Numerous virulence factors (see Table 20-7): capsule, pneumolysin, purpura-producing principle, neuraminidase, autolysins

TRANSMISSION

Endogenous spread from colonized nasopharynx or oropharynx to distal site: lungs, sinuses, ears, meninges, blood
Person to person via infectious droplets (rare)

WHO IS AT RISK?

Persons with antecedent viral respiratory disease or other conditions that interfere with bacterial clearance from respiratory tract
Children and the elderly
Persons with hematological disorder (malignancy, sickle cell disease)
Persons with asplenia
Renal transplant recipients

GEOGRAPHY/SEASON

Ubiquitous
Disease more common in winter and spring

MODES OF CONTROL

Penicillin drug of choice; cephalosporins, erythromycin, chloramphenicol (for meningitis) for patients allergic to penicillin
Penicillin resistance increasingly common
Vaccine less satisfactory for patients at risk for pneumococcal disease

N-acetylmuramic acid and the alanine residue on the peptide cross-bridge (Figure 20-9). If choline is absent from the cell wall teichoic acid, the amidase is inactive. Although its role in cell division is well defined, the importance of the amidase in pathogenesis is not known.

Epidemiology

S. pneumoniae is a common inhabitant of the throat and nasopharynx of healthy individuals (Box 20-5). Carriage has been reported to range from 5% to 75%, but these percentages are significantly affected by the methods used to detect the organism and the population studied. Colonization is more common in children than in adults, with *S. pneumoniae* initially detected at about 6 months of age (Figure 20-10). Subsequently, the child is transiently colonized with other serotypes of the organism. The duration of carriage decreases with each successive serotype carried, in part related to the development of serotype-specific immunity. Acquisition of new serotypes occurs throughout the year, although carriage and associated disease is highest during the winter and spring months. The strains of pneumococci that cause disease are the same ones associated with carriage. When infection occurs, it is generally with a newly acquired serotype rather than one associated with prolonged carriage.

Pneumococcal disease originates from spread of organisms colonizing the nasopharynx and oropharynx to distal loci: lungs (pneumonia), paranasal sinuses (sinusitis), ears (otitis media), and meninges (meningitis). Bacteremia, with subsequent spread to other body sites, can occur with all of these infections.

S. pneumoniae is the most common cause of bacterial pneumonia (estimated 500,000 cases per year in the United States), as well as bacterial meningitis. In addition, the organism is a common cause of otitis and sinusitis. The incidence of disease is highest in children and the elderly (Figure 20-11) (i.e., populations with low levels of protective antibodies directed against the pneumococcal capsular polysaccharides).

Clinical Syndromes

Pneumonia. Infections are caused by aspiration of the endogenous oral organisms. Although strains can be transferred from one person to another by droplets in a closed population, epidemics are rare.

Disease occurs when the natural defense mechanisms (epiglottal reflex, trapping of bacteria by the mucus-producing cells lining the bronchus, removal of organisms by the ciliated respiratory epithelium and cough reflex) are circumvented, permitting organisms colonizing the oropharynx to gain access into the lower airways. Pneumococcal disease is most commonly associated with an antecedent viral respiratory disease such as influenza or measles, or with other conditions that interfere with bacterial clearance, such as chronic pulmonary disease, alcoholism, congestive heart failure, diabetes mellitus, and chronic renal disease.

The pathogenesis of pneumococcal pneumonia is due to bacterial multiplication in the alveolar spaces. Following aspiration, the bacteria undergo rapid growth in nutrient-rich edema fluid. Erythrocytes, leaking from congested capillaries, accumulate in the alveoli, followed by the migration first of neutrophils and then alveolar macrophages, with the subsequent phagocytosis and destruction of the organisms. The clinical manifestations of pneumococcal pneumonia are abrupt in onset, with a severe shaking chill and sustained fever of 102° F to 105° F. The patient commonly has symptoms of a viral respiratory infection 1 to 3 days before the initial onset. A productive cough with blood-tinged sputum is seen in most patients, and chest pain (pleurisy) is common. Because the disease is associated with aspiration, disease is generally localized in the lower lobes of the lungs (hence the name **lobar pneumonia**). However, a more generalized bronchopneumonia can be seen in children or the elderly. Recovery is usually rapid after the initiation of

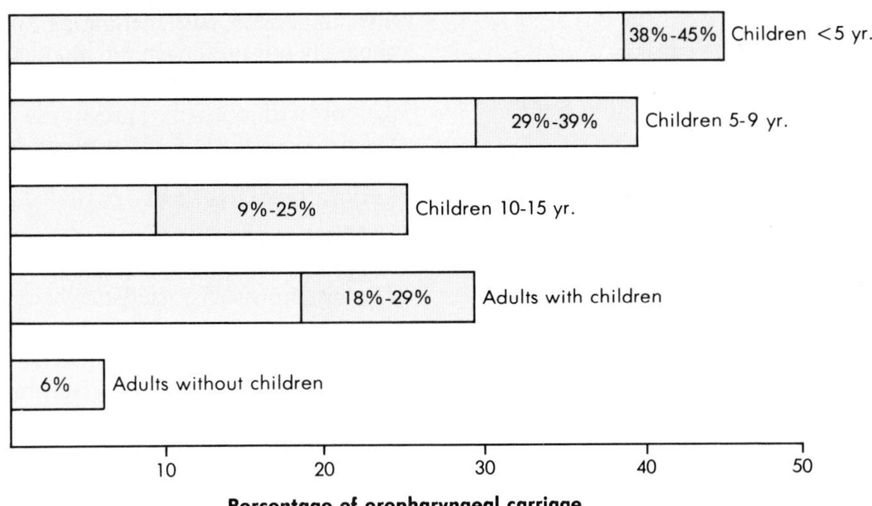

FIGURE 20-10 Carriage of *S. pneumoniae* is age related. The highest incidence is observed in young children and adults with young children present in the home.

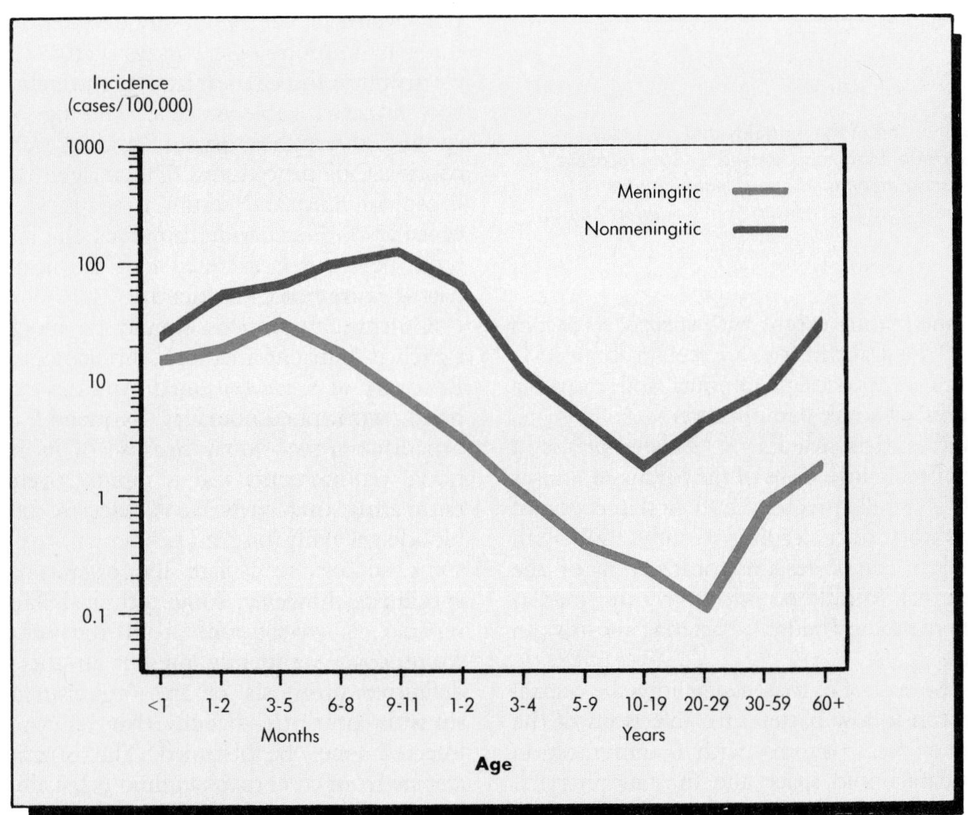

FIGURE 20-11 Age-specific attack rates of *S. pneumoniae* disease. *(From Wenger JD et al.:* J Infect Dis *162:1316, 1990).*

appropriate antimicrobial therapy, with complete radiological resolution in 2 to 3 weeks. The overall mortality is 5%, although this is influenced by the serotype of the organism and the age and underlying disease of the patient. Mortality is significantly increased in disease caused by *S. pneumoniae* type 3, as well as in elderly patients or in patients for whom bacteremia is documented. Severe pneumococcal disease is also observed in patients with splenic dysfunction or splenectomy caused by decreased bacterial clearance from the bloodstream and defective production of early antibodies.

Abscess formation is not commonly associated with

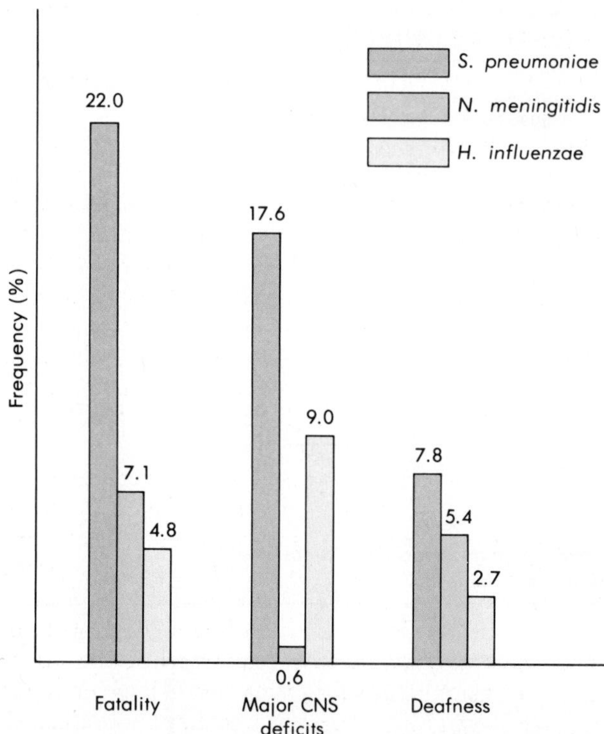

FIGURE 20-12 Comparison of the mortality and morbidity associated with bacterial meningitis caused by *Streptococcus pneumoniae, Neisseria meningitidis,* and *Haemophilus influenzae.* (Redrawn from Christensen G et al.: *Infect Immun* 37:318, 1982.)

pneumococcal pneumonia except with specific serotypes (e.g., serotype 3). Pleural effusions are seen in about 25% of patients with pneumococcal pneumonia, and empyema (purulent effusion) is a rare complication.

Sinusitis and Otitis Media. *S. pneumoniae* is a common cause of acute infections of the paranasal sinuses and ear. Disease is usually preceded by a viral infection of the upper respiratory tract, leading to infiltration with polymorphonuclear leukocytes and obstruction of the sinuses and ear canal. Middle ear infection (otitis media) is primarily seen in young children; bacterial sinusitis can occur at all ages.

Meningitis. Spread of *S. pneumoniae* into the central nervous system can follow bacteremia, infections of the ear or sinuses, or head trauma with communication between the subarachnoid space and the nasopharynx. Bacterial meningitis can occur at all ages, although it is primarily a pediatric disease. Pneumococcal meningitis is relatively uncommon in neonates; however, about 15% of meningitis in children and 30% to 50% of adult disease is caused by *S. pneumoniae.* Mortality and severe neurological deficits are from four times to 20 times more common with disease caused by *S. pneumoniae* compared with the other common causes of bacterial meningitis (Figure 20-12).

Bacteremia. Bacteremia will occur in 25% to 30% of patients with pneumococcal pneumonia and more than 80% of patients with meningitis. In contrast, bacteria are generally not present in the bloodstream of patients with sinusitis or otitis media. Endocarditis can occur in patients with normal or previously damaged heart valves. Destruction of the valve tissue is common.

Laboratory Diagnosis

Microscopy. Examination of sputum by Gram stain is a rapid method for diagnosing pneumococcal disease. The organisms characteristically appear as lancet-shaped diplococci surrounded by an unstained capsule; however, they may appear gram-negative because they tend not to stain well (particularly older cultures) and their morphology may be distorted by concomitant antibiotic therapy. If the Gram stain is consistent with *S. pneumoniae,* this can be confirmed with the quellung reaction. In this test anticapsular antibodies are mixed with the bacteria and then the mixture is examined microscopically. A positive reaction for *S. pneumoniae* is seen by an increased refractiveness around the bacteria.

Antigen detection. Soluble pneumococcal capsular polysaccharide can be rapidly detected in infected body fluids by immunological assays such as counterimmunoelectrophoresis (CIE) or latex agglutination. The tests are very sensitive (able to detect 50 ng of antigen) and specific, although serotypes 7 and 14 are not detected by routine CIE procedures. The antigen detected in cerebrospinal fluid and serum is identical to the purified capsular polysaccharide; however, the antigen is hydrolyzed before it is excreted into the urine and has only partial immunological identity.

Culture. Specimens should be inoculated onto an enriched nutrient medium supplemented with blood. Recovery of *S. pneumoniae* in sputum cultures from patients with pneumonia is frequently difficult as the organism grows slowly because of its fastidious nutritional requirements and is rapidly overgrown by contaminating oral bacteria. A selective medium such as blood agar with 5 μg/ml gentamicin has been used with some success to isolate the organism from sputum specimens; however, some technical skill is required to separate *S. pneumoniae* from the other α-hemolytic streptococci frequently present in the specimen. The definitive diagnosis of the organism responsible for sinusitis or otitis dictates that an aspirate from the infected focus be obtained. The isolation of *S. pneumoniae* from cerebrospinal fluid is usually without problems, unless antibiotic therapy is initiated before the specimen is collected. In the presence of even a single dose of antibiotics as many as half of the infected patients will have negative cultures.

Identification. Isolates of *S. pneumoniae* undergo rapid lysis when the autolysins are activated following exposure to bile. A presumptive identification can be made by placing a drop of bile on an isolated colony. Colonies of *S. pneumoniae* will be solubilized within a few minutes, whereas other α-hemolytic streptococci will be unchanged. This test can also be performed by adding bile to a broth culture of *S. pneumoniae* with the rapid lysis of the organisms and clearing of the broth. *S. pneumoniae* can also be identified by its susceptibility to optochin (ethylhydrocupreine dihydrochloride). The isolate is streaked onto a blood agar plate, and a disk saturated with optochin is placed in the middle of the inoculum. After overnight incubation a zone of inhibited bacterial growth will be seen around the disk. Additional biochemical and serologic tests can be performed for a definitive identification.

Treatment, Prevention, and Control

Before the availability of antibiotics, specific treatment was guided by the passive infusion of type-specific capsular antibodies. These opsonizing antibodies enhanced polymorphonuclear leukocyte–mediated phagocytosis and killing of the bacteria. However, this immunotherapy was discontinued with the advent of antimicrobial therapy. Penicillin rapidly became the treatment of choice for pneumococcal disease. For patients allergic to penicillin, alternative effective agents have included the cephalosporins, erythromycin, and chloramphenicol (for meningitis). Resistance to tetracycline is well documented. In 1977 isolates of *S. pneumoniae* resistant to multiple antibiotics, including penicillin, were reported in South Africa. Until recently high-level resistance to penicillin (MIC ≥ 2 μg/ml) was relatively uncommon, and only 5% of all strains of *S. pneumoniae* isolated in the United States were considered to be moderately resistant (MIC between 0.1 and 1.0 μg/ml). However, this has changed dramatically in recent years; resistance to penicillin has been reported for as many as one third of U.S. isolates and a higher proportion in other countries. The overall mortality rate is higher with the moderately and highly resistant strains. Increased resistance to penicillins is associated with a decreased affinity of the antibiotic for the penicillin-binding proteins present in the bacterial cell wall.

Because the pneumococcal capsule is the primary virulence factor associated with this organism, efforts to prevent or control the disease have focused on the development of an effective vaccine. The first vaccine was used in 1914 in South African gold miners, a population at high risk for pneumococcal disease. Over the following years the vaccines have been refined and improved. The current vaccine contains 23 different capsular polysaccharides. Approximately 94% of all strains isolated from infected patients are either included in the vaccine or are serologically related to the vaccine serotypes. Longitudinal studies have documented that the introduction of the vaccine has not influenced the serotypes of *S. pneumoniae* that are associated with disease. The vaccine is immunogenic in normal adults, and the immunity is long lived. However, the effectiveness of the vaccine in patients at risk for pneumococcal disease (e.g., patients with asplenia, sickle cell disease, hematological malignancy, renal transplant, or young children and the elderly) is less satisfactory.

ENTEROCOCCUS

The enterococci were previously classified as group D streptococci because they possess the group D cell wall antigen (glycerol teichoic acid associated with the cytoplasmic membrane). Despite this observation, it was recognized that these organisms were distinct from other group D streptococci (referred to as nonenterococcal group D streptococci, e.g., *S. bovis*). The enterococcal and nonenterococcal groups were originally differentiated by their physiological properties and more recently by DNA-DNA hybridization studies. At present, 12 species of enterococci are recognized, although the species most commonly responsible for human infections are *E. faecalis* and *E. faecium*.

The enterococci are gram-positive cocci typically arranged in pairs and short chains. The microscopic morphology of these isolates frequently cannot be differentiated from *S. pneumoniae* when grown in broth culture. They grow readily on blood agar media, producing large white colonies after 24 hours of incubation.

E. faecalis is found in small numbers in the upper respiratory tract and small intestine and in large numbers (e.g., 10^7 org/gm of feces) in the large intestine. *E. faecium* has a similar distribution, although it is found less frequently. The enterococci are uniquely suited for survival. They are able to grow in the presence of a high concentration of bile and sodium chloride, which is necessary for survival in the bowel and gall bladder.

Enterococci are a common cause of urinary tract infections in hospitalized patients, particularly those patients with an indwelling catheter and receiving broad-spectrum antibiotics with limited activity against these organisms. The etiological role of enterococci in intraabdominal abscesses and wound infections is less clear because the infections are generally polymicrobic. Enterococci are also able to cause bacterial endocarditis.

Antimicrobial therapy for enterococcal infections is complicated because most antibiotics are not bactericidal at clinically relevant concentrations. Therapy has traditionally consisted of the synergistic combination of an aminoglycoside and a cell-wall active antibiotic (e.g., penicillin, ampicillin, vancomycin). However, resistance to aminoglycosides, ampicillin, penicillin, and vancomycin has been reported. These strains are particularly troublesome because this resistance is plasmid mediated and can be transferred to other bacteria. At present, no combination of antibiotics has proven bactericidal activity against these organisms.

OTHER CATALASE-NEGATIVE GRAM-POSITIVE COCCI

Other catalase-negative, gram-positive cocci or coccobacilli that have been associated with human disease include *Aerococcus*, *Gemella*, *Lactococcus*, *Leuconostoc*, and *Pediococcus*. All are relatively avirulent, opportunistic pathogens that are rarely isolated in clinical specimens. Precise identification of most isolates is difficult and generally performed only in reference laboratories. *Leuconostoc* and *Pediococcus* are important because these organisms are typically resistant to vancomycin, an antibiotic commonly used to treat infections with gram-positive cocci.

CASE STUDY AND QUESTIONS

A 62-year-old man with a history of chronic obstructive pulmonary disease (COPD) entered the emergency room with a fever of 102° F, chills, nausea, vomiting, and hypotension. The patient also produced tenacious, yellowish sputum, increasing in productivity over the preceding 3 days. The patient had a respiration rate of 18 per min and blood pressure of 94/52 mm Hg. Chest x-ray examination demonstrated extensive infiltrates in the left lower lung involving both the lower lobe and the lingula. Multiple blood cultures and culture of the sputum yielded *Streptococcus pneumoniae*. The isolate was susceptible to cefazolin, vancomycin, and erythromycin but resistant to penicillin.

1. What predisposing condition made this patient more susceptible to pneumonia and bacteremia caused by *S. pneumoniae*? What other populations of patients are susceptible to these infections? What other infections are caused by this organism, and what populations are most susceptible?
2. What is the mechanism most likely responsible for this isolate's resistance to penicillin?
3. What are the major virulence factors of *S. pneumoniae*, group A Streptococcus, and group B Streptococcus? What infections are caused by groups A and B streptococci and in what patient populations?
4. Group A streptococci can produce streptococcal toxic shock syndrome. Compare the pathogenesis of this disease with that produced by staphylococci.
5. What two nonsuppurative diseases can develop after localized group A streptococcal disease? What is the most likely site of infection for the initial disease? Which serologic tests can be used to confirm the clinical diagnosis of each nonsuppurative disease?

Bibliography

Breese BB: A simple scorecard for the tentative diagnosis of streptococcal pharyngitis, *Am J Dis Child* 131:514-517, 1977.

Bruyn GAW, Zegers BJM, and van Furth R: Mechanisms of host defense against infection with *Streptococcus pneumoniae*, *Clin Infect Dis* 14:251-262, 1992.

Crowe CC, Sanders WE, and Longley S: Bacterial interference. II. Role of the normal throat flora in prevention of colonization by group A streptococcus, *J Infect Dis* 128:527-532, 1973.

Handwerger S, Horowitz H, Coburn K et al: Infection due to *Leuconostoc* species: six cases and review, *Rev Infect Dis* 12:602-610, 1990.

Hendley JO, Sande MA, Stewart PM, and Gwaltney JM Jr: Spread of *Streptococcus pneumoniae* in families. I. Carriage rates and distribution of types, *J Infect Dis* 132:55-61, 1975.

Johnson DR, Stevens DL, and Kaplan EL: Epidemiologic analysis of group A streptococcal serotypes associated with severe systemic infections, rheumatic fever, or uncomplicated pharyngitis, *J Infect Dis* 166:374-382, 1992.

Katz AR and Morens DM: Severe streptococcal infections in historical perspective, *Clin Infect Dis* 14:298-307, 1992.

Klugman KP: Pneumococcal resistance to antibiotics, *Clin Microbiol Rev* 3:171-196, 1990.

Mandell GL, Douglas RG Jr, and Bennett JE: *Principles and practice of infectious diseases*, ed 3, New York, 1990, John Wiley & Sons.

Moellering RC: Emergence of *Enterococcus* as a significant pathogen, *Clin Infect Dis* 14:1173-1178, 1992.

Murray BE: The life and times of the *Enterococcus*, *Clin Microbiol Rev* 3:46-65, 1990.

Musher DM: Infections caused by *Streptococcus pneumoniae*: clinical spectrum, pathogenesis, immunity, and treatment, *Clin Infect Dis* 14:801-809, 1992.

Peter G and Smith AL: Group A streptococcal infections of the skin and pharynx, *N Engl J Med* 297:311-317, 365-370, 1977.

Quie PG, Giebink GS, and Winkelstein JA: Symposium: the pneumococcus, *Rev Infect Dis* 3:183-395, 1981.

Ruoff KL: *Streptococcus anginosus* ("Streptococcus milleri"): the unrecognized pathogen, *Clin Microbiol Rev* 1:102-108, 1988.

Stevens DL, Tanner MH, Winship J et al: Severe group A streptococcal infections associated with a toxic shock-like syndrome and scarlet fever toxin A, *N Engl J Med* 321:1-7, 1989.

Wannamaker LW: Differences between streptococcal infections of the throat and of the skin, *N Engl J Med* 282:23, 1970.

Wenger JD, Hightower AW, Facklam RR et al: Bacterial meningitis in the United States, 1986: report of a multistate surveillance study, *J Infect Dis* 162:1316-1323, 1990.

CHAPTER 21

Bacillus

THE medically important, aerobic and facultatively anaerobic, gram-positive bacilli that form spores are classified in the genus *Bacillus*. *Bergey's Manual of Systematic Bacteriology* lists 34 *Bacillus* species; however, only *Bacillus anthracis* is always considered a pathogen. *Bacillus cereus* can cause disease or be isolated as an insignificant contaminant. Other *Bacillus* species, such as *Bacillus subtilis*, are opportunistic pathogens, causing disease in the presence of a foreign body (e.g., catheter, shunt, prosthesis) when introduced by surgery or trauma into normally sterile tissues, or in intravenous drug abusers (Table 21-1).

BACILLUS ANTHRACIS

Physiology and Structure

Bacillus anthracis is a large (1 × 3 to 5 μm) organism that is arranged as single or paired bacilli in clinical specimens (Figure 21-1) and in long serpentine chains and clumps in culture. Although spores are readily observed in 2- or 3-day-old cultures, they are not seen in clinical specimens. A prominent polypeptide capsule (consisting of glutamic acid) is observed in clinical specimens, but it is not produced in vitro unless special growth conditions are used. In addition to the capsular antigen, a polysaccharide cell wall somatic antigen and a toxin are associated with *B. anthracis*. **Anthrax toxin** consists of three antigenically distinct, heat-labile components: protective antigen, lethal factor, and edema factor. Although none of the components is active alone, the combination of protective antigen with either of the other two components has toxic properties.

Pathogenesis

The two major factors responsible for *B. anthracis* virulence are presence of the capsule and toxin production. The capsule is antiphagocytic, and antibodies directed against the capsule are not protective. Only one capsular type has been identified, presumably because the capsule is composed of only glutamic acid. The anthrax toxin protective antigen produces edema in experimental animals when combined with the edema factor and death when combined with the lethal factor. This toxin can be detected in edematous fluid collected from patients with anthrax.

TABLE 21-1 *Bacillus* Species and Their Diseases

Organism	Disease
Bacillus anthracis	Anthrax
Bacillus cereus	Gastroenteritis
	Emetic form
	Diarrheal form
	Panophthalmitis
	Opportunistic infections
Bacillus subtilis	Opportunistic infections
Other *Bacillus* species	Opportunistic infections

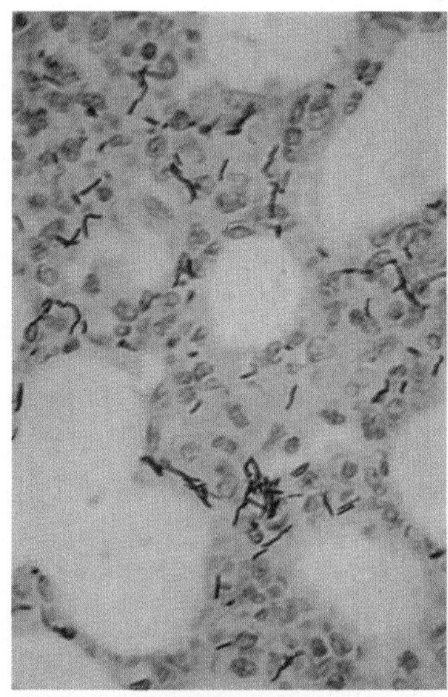

FIGURE 21-1 Gram stain of anthrax bacilli in pulmonary capillaries. The large bacilli will typically form long chains when grown in culture. (From Emond RTD and Rowland HAK: *A colour atlas of infectious diseases,* ed 2, London, 1987, Wolfe Medical Publications.)

Epidemiology

B. anthracis is an organism found in soil and on vegetation (Figure 21-2 and Box 21-1). The ability to form spores allows the organism to survive under adverse conditions for years without the need to replicate. Anthrax is a disease primarily of herbivores; humans may be accidentally infected by exposure to contaminated animals or animal products. Anthrax is rarely seen in the United States (only four cases reported between 1981 and 1990), and most infections are reported in Iran, Turkey, Pakistan, and Sudan.

Human disease is acquired by one of three routes: inoculation, inhalation, or ingestion. Approximately 95% of anthrax infections are due to the inoculation of *Bacillus* spores through exposed skin surfaces, either from contaminated soil or infected animal products such as hides, goat hair, or wool. Inhalation anthrax, also called **Woolsorter's disease,** results from inhalation of *B. anthracis* spores during the processing of goat hair. Ingestion anthrax is very rare in humans but is a common route of infection in herbivores. Person-to-person transmission does not occur.

Clinical Syndromes

Cutaneous anthrax is characterized by the development of a painless papule at the site of inoculation that rapidly progresses to an ulcer surrounded by vesicles and then to a necrotic eschar. Massive edema due to the anthrax toxin and systemic signs can develop. Mortality in patients with untreated cutaneous anthrax is 20%.

Inhalation anthrax may initially mimic a viral respiratory illness and then rapidly progress to diffuse pulmonary involvement leading to respiratory failure. Mortality is high even in appropriately treated patients because the disease is usually not suspected until the course is irreversible.

Gastrointestinal anthrax is a very rare human disease with varied clinical presentations. Mesenteric adenopathy, hemorrhage, and ascites production are all reported and associated with high mortality.

Laboratory Diagnosis

B. anthracis can be readily detected by the microscopic examination and culture of cutaneous papules or ulcers. Large gram-positive bacilli, without spores, are seen in

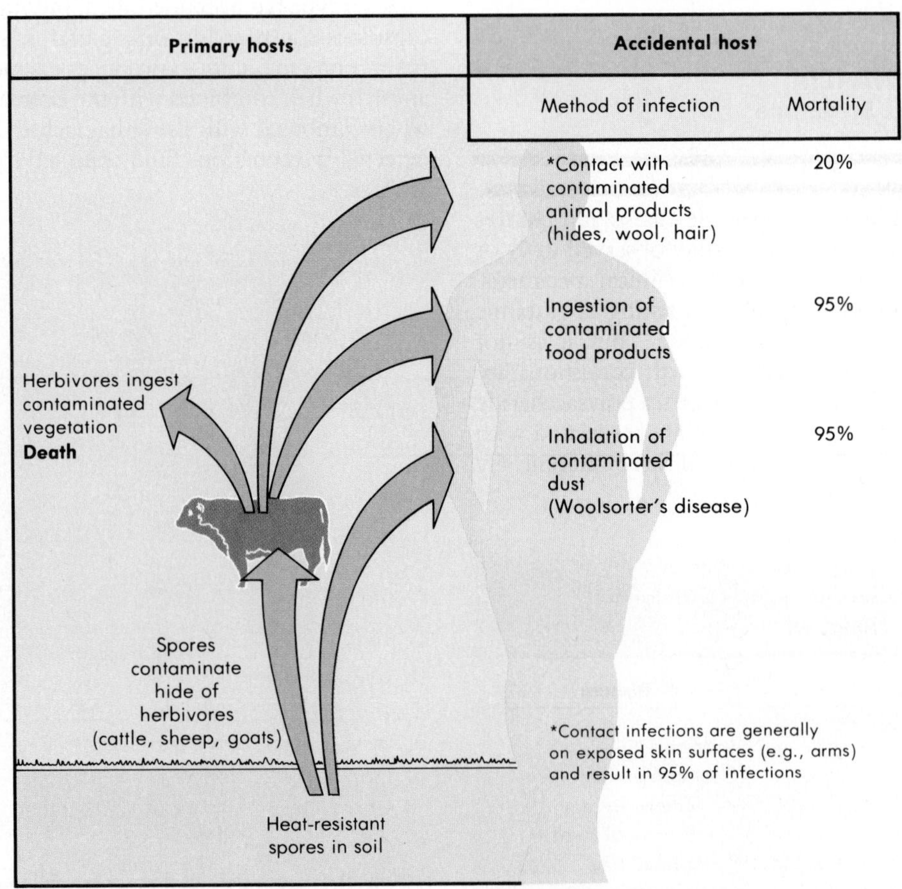

FIGURE 21-2 Epidemiology of anthrax in animal and human hosts.

the tissue. Staining with specific fluorescein-labeled antibodies can confirm the clinical suspicion, although these reagents are available only in special reference laboratories. *B. anthracis* will grow on nonselective laboratory media, with the appearance of nonhemolytic, rapidly growing, adherent colonies. The absence of hemolysis, the sticky consistency of the colonies, and the microscopic appearance of serpentine chains of bacilli ("medusa head") are useful characteristics for distinguishing *B. anthracis* from other *Bacillus* species. Definitive identification of *B. anthracis* requires the use of selected biochemical tests and demonstration that *B. anthracis* is nonmotile.

Treatment, Prevention, and Control

Penicillin is the antibiotic of choice for treating anthrax, with tetracycline or chloramphenicol used as alternative agents for penicillin-allergic patients. Control of human disease requires control of animal anthrax. This involves vaccination of animal herds in endemic regions and burning or burial of animals who die of anthrax. Vaccination is an effective control measure in animal herds. It has also been used to protect humans in areas with endemic disease or humans who work with animal hides, furs, bone meal, wool, and animal hair imported from countries with endemic anthrax. Complete eradication of anthrax is unlikely because the spores of the organism can exist for many years in soil.

BOX 21-1 Epidemiology of Anthrax

DISEASE/BACTERIAL FACTORS

Prominent polypeptide capsule
Polysaccharide somatic antigen present in cell wall
Anthrax toxin has three components: alone none are active, but the protective antigen with either the lethal factor or the edema factor is toxic
Spores can survive in soil for years

TRANSMISSION

Inoculation (most common)
Inhalation (rare in humans)
Ingestion (rare in humans)

WHO IS AT RISK?

People in endemic areas
People who work with animal material (hides, fur, wool, hair) imported from endemic areas

GEOGRAPHY/SEASON

Most common in Iran, Turkey, Pakistan, Sudan
No seasonal incidence

MODES OF CONTROL

Penicillin; tetracycline or chloramphenicol for patients allergic to penicillin
Vaccination of people and herds in endemic areas
Disposal of animals that die of anthrax

BACILLUS CEREUS AND OTHER *BACILLUS* SPECIES

Pathogenesis

Gastroenteritis caused by *Bacillus cereus* is mediated by one of two enterotoxins. The heat-stable enterotoxin is responsible for disease characterized by vomiting **(emetic form)**, and the heat-labile enterotoxin causes the **diarrheal form** of *B. cereus* disease. The heat-labile enterotoxin is similar to the enterotoxin produced by *Escherichia coli* and *Vibrio cholera;* each stimulates the adenylate cyclase—cyclic AMP system in intestinal epithelial cells and can be assayed by measuring fluid accumulation in rabbit ileal loops inoculated with the toxin. The mechanism of action of the heat-stable enterotoxin is unknown.

The pathogenesis of *B. cereus* panophthalmitis is also incompletely defined. At least three toxins have been implicated: **necrotic toxin** (a heat-labile enterotoxin), **cereolysin** (a potent hemolysin named after the species), and **phospholipase C** (a potent lecithinase). It is likely that the rapid destruction of the eye that is characteristic of *B. cereus* infections is the result of the interaction of these toxins and other unidentified factors.

Epidemiology

B. cereus, *B. subtilis*, and other *Bacillus* species are ubiquitous organisms, present in virtually all environmental sites (Box 21-2). The isolation of the bacteria from clinical specimens, in the absence of characteristic disease, usually represents insignificant contamination.

Clinical Syndromes

As mentioned previously, *B. cereus* is responsible for two forms of food poisoning (Table 21-2): vomiting disease (emetic form) and diarrheal disease (diarrheal form). The emetic form is associated with consumption of contaminated rice. During the initial cooking of the rice, the vegetative bacilli are killed but the heat-resistant spores survive. If the rice is not refrigerated, the spores germinate and the bacilli can multiply rapidly. The heat-stable enterotoxin that is released is not destroyed when the rice is reheated. After ingestion of the enterotoxin and a 1- to 6-hour incubation period, the patient develops a disease of short duration (less than 24 hrs), characterized by vomiting, nausea, and abdominal cramps. Fever and diarrhea are generally absent. In contrast, the diarrheal form of *B. cereus* food poisoning is associated with consumption of contaminated meat or vegetables. There is a longer incubation period during which the organism multiplies in situ and produces a heat-labile toxin, and then the diarrhea,

BOX 21-2 Epidemiology of *Bacillus cereus* Infection

DISEASE/BACTERIAL FACTORS

Heat-stable enterotoxin causes vomiting
Heat-labile enterotoxin causes diarrhea
Cereolysin (a hemolysin) and phospholipase C (a lecithinase) are involved in panophthalmitis
Organisms are ubiquitous

TRANSMISSION

Ingestion causes gastroenteritis (food poisoning)
Contaminated soil in direct contact with eye or direct inoculation through eye surface causes panophthalmitis
IV catheters and CNS shunt infections are possible

WHO IS AT RISK?

Individuals eating contaminated foods (e.g., rice, meat)
Patients with eye trauma
Patients with IV catheters or CNS shunts

GEOGRAPHY/SEASON

Organisms are ubiquitous
No seasonal incidence

MODES OF CONTROL

Clindamycin, vancomycin, and aminoglycosides can be used if susceptible
Refrigeration of foods after cooking

TABLE 21-2 *Bacillus cereus* Food Poisoning

	Emetic form	Diarrheal form
Implicated food	Rice	Meat, vegetables
Incubation period	<6 hours (mean, 2 hours)	>6 hours (mean, 9 hours)
Symptoms	Vomiting, nausea, abdominal cramps	Diarrhea, nausea, abdominal cramps
Duration	8-10 hours (mean, 9 hours)	20-36 hours (mean, 24 hours)
Enterotoxin	Heat stable	Heat labile

nausea, and abdominal cramps develop. This form of disease generally lasts 1 day or longer.

B. cereus is the most common cause of traumatic eye infections. The source of the organisms can be either soil contamination of the object penetrating the eye or direct inoculation of organisms colonizing the eye surface. Bacillus panophthalmitis is a rapidly progressive disease that almost universally ends in complete loss of light perception within 48 hours of the injury. Massive destruction of the vitreal and retinal tissue is observed.

Other infections seen with *B. cereus*, *B. subtilis*, and other *Bacillus* species include intraveneous catheter and central nervous system shunt infections, endocarditis (most commonly in drug abusers), as well as pneumonitis, bacteremia, and meningitis in severely immunosuppressed patients. Most isolates of *Bacillus* in blood cultures represent insignificant contaminants from the patient's skin surface or in the blood culturing system.

Laboratory Diagnosis

As with *B. anthracis,* the other *Bacillus* species can be readily grown in the laboratory. For confirmation of food-borne disease, the implicated food (e.g., rice, meat, vegetables) should be cultured. Isolation of the organism from the patient should not be attempted because fecal colonization is commonplace. The heat-labile enterotoxin can be detected using an animal model (e.g., rabbit ileal loop); however, the heat-stable emeric toxin is detected only when grown on media prepared from rice (consistent with the fact that rice is the food most commonly contaminated with this organism). *Bacillus* grows rapidly and is readily detected in specimens collected from infected eyes, intravenous culture sites, and other locations.

Treatment, Prevention, and Control

Because of the short and uncomplicated course of *B. cereus* gastroenteritis, symptomatic treatment is adequate. Treatment of other *Bacillus* infections is complicated by the rapid, progressive course of the infections and the high incidence of multidrug resistance that is observed with these organisms (most isolates are resistant to penicillins and cephalosporins, as well as other antibiotics). Clindamycin, vancomycin, and the aminoglycosides can be used, although susceptibility must be confirmed by in vitro testing. Food poisoning can be prevented by the proper refrigeration of food products after cooking and before serving.

CASE STUDY AND QUESTIONS

A family of three ate dinner at a local restaurant. Two hours after eating, all three developed severe abdominal cramps, nausea, and vomiting. They went to a local emergency room where they were found to have normal blood pressure, no temperature elevation, and a normal WBC count and differential. They were treated symptomatically for food poisoning and sent home. Within 24 hours the symptoms subsided for all three.

1. Describe the two forms of Bacillus food poisoning. Which form do these patients have?
2. What is the most likely food responsible for this disease? Why was the onset of symptoms so rapid and the duration so short?

3. This organism can also cause eye infections. What risk factors are associated with these infections?
4. *Bacillus anthracis* is responsible for three clinical forms of anthrax. Name them, the method of acquisition, and the prognosis.
5. What are the two major virulence factors of *B. anthracis*?

Bibliography

Davey RT Jr and Tauber WB: Posttraumatic endophthalmitis: the emerging role of *Bacillus cereus* infection, *Rev Infect Dis* 9:110-123, 1987.

Ihde DC and Armstrong D: Clinical spectrum of infection due to *Bacillus* species, *Am J Med* 55:839-845, 1973.

Shamsuddin D, Tuazon CU, Levy C, and Curtin J: *Bacillus cereus* panophthalmitis: source of the organisms, *Rev Infect Dis* 4:97-103, 1982.

Terranova W and Blake PA: *Bacillus cereus* food poisoning, *N Engl J Med* 298:143-144, 1978.

Tuazon CU, Murray HW, Levy C, et al: Serious infections from *Bacillus* sp, *JAMA* 241:1137-1140, 1979.

Van Ness GB: Ecology of anthrax, *Science* 172:103-109, 1971.

CHAPTER 22

Miscellaneous Gram-Positive Bacilli

THE aerobic, non–spore-forming, gram-positive bacilli are a heterogeneous group of organisms, many of which are poorly characterized. The most common isolates are collectively called **coryneform** bacteria or **diphtheroids** (named after the most prominent member, *Corynebacterium diphtheriae*). However, despite the fact that most of these organisms are morphologically similar (i.e., small, pleomorphic gram-positive bacilli that stain irregularly), many isolates that were originally classified in the genus *Corynebacterium* are now known to belong to other genera (Table 22-1). The coryneform bacilli that are discussed in this chapter are *Corynebacterium* and *Arcanobacterium*. *Actinomyces* and *Rhodococcus* are discussed in Chapters 31 and 34, respectively. Three other genera of aerobic gram-positive bacilli are also discussed in this chapter: *Listeria*, *Erysipelothrix*, and *Gardnerella*. The isolation of *Listeria* and *Erysipelothrix* in clinical specimens is virtually always significant. *Gardnerella* strains, which are commonly isolated in genital specimens, play a poorly defined role in the pathogenesis of bacterial vaginosis (vaginitis) (see Table 22-1).

CORYNEBACTERIUM

Physiology and Structure

The corynebacteria are small, usually pleomorphic, gram-positive bacilli that appear in short chains (V or Y configurations) or in clumps resembling "Chinese letters." Metachromatic granules within the cells may be seen with special stains. The genus *Corynebacterium* is restricted to bacteria with cell walls containing meso-diaminopimelic acid, arabino-galactan polymers, and short-chain mycolic acids. These characteristics place these bacilli in a taxonomic position closely related to nocardia, mycobacteria, and *Rhodococcus*. Corynebacteria are aerobic or facultatively anaerobic and generally grow slowly on enriched media. The organisms are nonmotile, catalase-positive, and ferment carbohydrates, producing lactic acid. Corynebacteria are ubiquitous in plants and animals, and they normally colonize the skin, upper respiratory tract, gastrointestinal tract, and urogenital tract of humans.

Pathogenesis and Immunity

Although most of these organisms are opportunistic pathogens, specific virulence factors have been identified in the more pathogenic species (Table 22-2).

Diphtheria Exotoxin

The mechanism of action of diphtheria exotoxin is well known. The **"tox" gene** that codes for the exotoxin is

TABLE 22-1 Aerobic Gram-Positive Bacilli Associated With Human Diseases

Organism	Diseases
Corynebacterium diphtheriae	Diphtheria
C. jeikeium (CDC group JK)	Opportunistic infections
C. urealyticum (Coryneform group D-2)	Urinary tract infections
C. pseudodiphtheriticum	Endocarditis; lower respiratory tract infections
C. minutissimum	Skin infections (erythrasma); systemic infections
C. ulcerans	Pharyngitis (mild to diphtheria-like)
C. xerosis	Opportunistic infections
Arcanobacterium (Corynebacterium) haemolyticum	Pharyngitis
Actinomyces (Corynebacterium) pyogenes	Granulomatous ulcerative infections
Rhodococcus (Corynebacterium) equi	Suppurative pneumonia; opportunistic infections
Listeria monocytogenes	Meningitis; septicemia; granulomatosis infantiseptica; endocarditis
Erysipelothrix rhusiopathiae	Erysipeloid; septicemia; endocarditis
Gardnerella vaginalis	Bacterial vaginosis

introduced into strains of *Corynebacterium diphtheriae*, *Corynebacterium pseudotuberculosis*, and *Corynebacterum ulcerans* by a lysogenic bacteriophage **(B-corynephage).** Diphtheria exotoxin is a 63,000 d protein that consists of two fragments (A-B toxin). The B fragment mediates binding to the cell surface, permitting the enzymatically active A fragment to enter the cell. In the presence of limiting amounts of iron, the A fragment blocks protein synthesis in a manner similar to *Pseudomonas aeruginosa* exotoxin A (see Chapter 27). The A fragment catalyzes the irreversible inactivation of elongation factor 2 (EF-2), which is required for movement of nascent peptide chains on ribosomes. Because the turnover of EF-2 is very slow and only about one molecule per ribosome is present in a cell, it has been estimated that one exotoxin molecule can inactivate the entire content of EF-2 in a cell. The concentration of diphtheria exotoxin found in strains of *C. ulcerans* and *C. pseudotuberculosis* that have the "tox" B-corynephage is generally lower than in *C. diphtheriae*.

Phospholipase D

Phospholipase D (also called **dermonecrotic toxin**) is produced by strains of *C. pseudotuberculosis* and *C. ulcerans*. This toxin promotes the spread of the organisms by increasing vascular permeability through hydrolysis of sphingomyelin in endothelial cell membranes.

Urease Production

The concentration of urease produced by *C. urealyticum* is sufficient to cause alkalinization of urine with subsequent formation of struvite calculi or stones. The association between high urease production and renal stone formation is also seen with some other urinary tract pathogens, such as *Staphylococcus saprophyticus, Klebsiella pneumoniae,* and *Proteus mirabilis*.

Antibiotic Resistance

Although a number of different species of corynebacteria colonize the skin and mucosal surfaces, *C. jeikeium* is a common cause of hospital-acquired infections in immunocompromised patients. This is largely due to the selection of these antibiotic-resistant coryneforms during antibiotic therapy. Likewise, *C. urealyticum* is resistant to most antibiotics commonly used to manage urinary tract infections.

TABLE 22-2 Virulence Factors in Corynebacterium Species

Organism	Virulence factors
C. diphtheriae	Diphtheria exotoxin
C. jeikeium	Antibiotic resistance
C. urealyticum	Antibiotic resistance; urease production
C. pseudotuberculosis	Diphtheria exotoxin; phospholipase D
C. ulcerans	Diphtheria exotoxin; phospholipase D

Epidemiology

Diphtheria is a disease with worldwide distribution among poor urban areas where crowding exists and a protective level of vaccine-induced immunity is low (Box 22-1). *Corynebacterium diphtheriae* is maintained in the population by asymptomatic carriage in the oropharynx or on the skin of immune individuals (after either exposure to *C. diphtheriae* or immunization). It is transmitted person to person by respiratory droplets or skin contact.

An active immunization program has made diphtheria uncommon in the United States. Whereas more than 200,000 cases were reported in 1921, only 28 cases of respiratory diphtheria were reported from 1980 to 1990 (Figure 22-1). Although primarily a pediatric disease, the incidence of disease has shifted toward older age-groups in populations where active immunization programs for children exist. Skin infection with toxigenic *C. diphtheriae* (cutaneous or wound diphtheria) also occurs but is not a reportable disease in the United States, so the actual incidence is unknown.

BOX 22-1 Epidemiology of Diphtheria

DISEASE/BACTERIAL FACTORS

Diphtheria exotoxin disrupts peptide formation in ribosomes

Phospholipase D increases vascular permeability and promotes spread of organism

TRANSMISSION

Person to person by inhalation or skin contact

Asymptomatic carriage maintains bacteria in population

WHO IS AT RISK?

Unvaccinated people

People in crowded, poor urban areas

Children

GEOGRAPHY/SEASON

Worldwide, where vaccination programs are not in place

No seasonal incidence

MODES OF CONTROL

Early use of diphtheria antitoxin to neutralize exotoxin

Penicillin or erythromycin effective for infected patients and asymptomatic carriers

Active immunization with diphtheria toxoid during childhood (DPT vaccine), then booster shots every 10 years for life

Antimicrobial prophylaxis for close contacts of patients with diphtheria

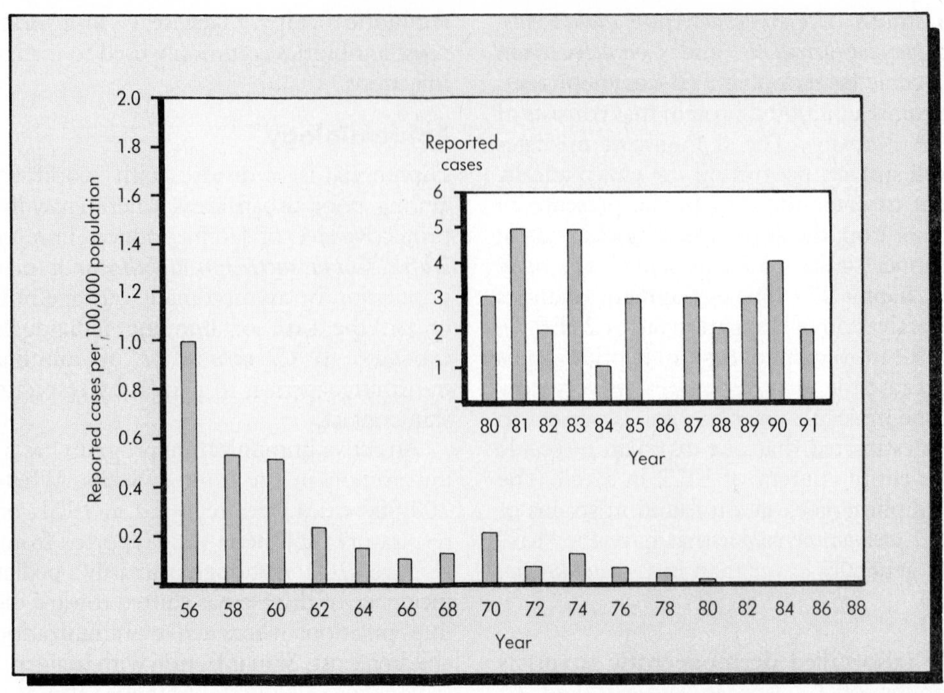

FIGURE 22-1 Incidence of diphtheria in the United States, 1955-1990. (Redrawn from *MMWR* 39:22, 1992.)

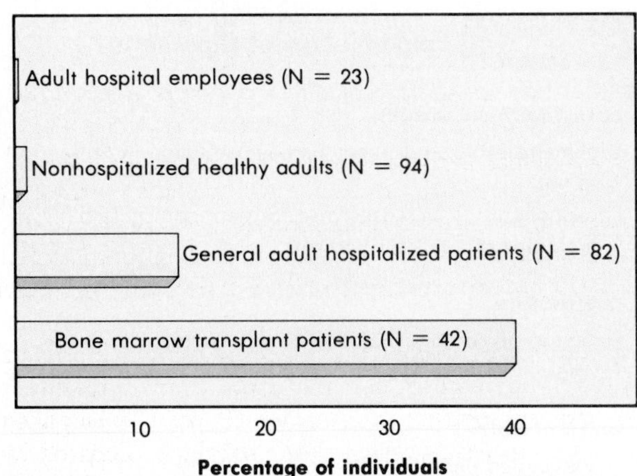

FIGURE 22-2 *C. jeikeium* colonization in four adult populations. Although *C. jeikeium* does not commonly colonize healthy individuals or hospital employees, there is an increased incidence of colonization in hospitalized patients, particularly highly immunocompromised patients who have received broad-spectrum antibiotics during a prolonged hospitalization. (Redrawn from Stamm WE et al: *Ann Intern Med* 91:167, 1979.)

Human infection with some strains of corynebacteria (e.g., *C. ulcerans* and *C. pseudotuberculosis*) requires exposure to an animal reservoir (e.g., cattle, sheep, horses, goats, deer). Other corynebacteria are part of the indigenous human oropharyngeal or skin flora (e.g., *C. jeikeium, C. urealyticum, C. pseudodiphtheriticum, C. xerosis*). With only a few exceptions the incidence of disease caused by these organisms is relatively rare. *C. jeikeium* is a well-recognized opportunistic pathogen in immunocompromised patients, particularly those with hematologic disorders, and patients with intravascular catheters. Carriage of this organism is uncommon in healthy persons, but as many as 40% of hospitalized patients can be colonized (Figure 22-2). Predisposing conditions for disease include prolonged hospitalization, granulocytopenia, prior or concurrent antimicrobial therapy or chemotherapy, and a mucocutaneous portal of entry. The highest incidence of disease is seen in elderly men.

Risk factors associated with *C. urealyticum* infections include immunosuppression, underlying genitourinary disorders, an antecedent urologic procedure, and prior antibiotic therapy. Since as many as one fourth to one third of all hospitalized patients are colonized with *C. urealyticum*, prior antibiotic therapy may select for the organism. A urologic procedure may introduce organisms on the skin surface into previously damaged tissue.

Clinical Syndromes

Diphtheria

The clinical presentation of diphtheria is determined by the site of infection, immune status of the patient, and virulence of the organism. Exposure to *Corynebacterium diphtheriae* can result in asymptomatic colonization in fully immune individuals, mild respiratory disease in partially immune patients, or a fulminant, sometimes fatal disease in nonimmune patients. The Centers for Disease Control has defined respiratory diphtheria as an upper respiratory tract illness characterized by sore throat, low-grade fever, and an adherent membrane of the tonsil, pharynx, and/or nose without other apparent cause.

Patients with diphtheria involving the respiratory tract will develop symptoms after a 2- to 6-day incubation period. Organisms will multiply locally on epithelial cells in the pharynx or adjacent surfaces and initially produce localized damage by exotoxin activity. The onset is sudden, with malaise, sore throat, exudative pharyngitis, and a low-grade temperature. The exudate evolves into a thick **pseudomembrane,** composed of bacteria, lymphocytes, plasma cells, fibrin, and dead cells, that can cover the tonsils, uvula, and palate and extend up into the nasopharynx or down into the larynx. The pseudomembrane firmly adheres to the respiratory tissue and is difficult to dislodge without causing bleeding of the underlying tissue. As the patient recovers after the approximately 1-week course of the disease, the membrane dislodges and is expectorated. Complications in patients with severe disease include breathing obstruction and myocarditis.

Cutaneous diphtheria is acquired by skin contact with other infected persons. The organism colonizes the skin surface and gains entry into the subcutaneous tissue through breaks in the skin (e.g., following an insect bite). A papule will develop and evolve into a chronic nonhealing ulcer, sometimes covered with a grayish membrane. Systemic signs of disease due to the exotoxin can be seen.

Other Clinical Syndromes

A variety of diseases have been associated with other species of *Corynebacterium* (see Table 22-1). The most important include mild to severe pharyngitis or a diphtheria-like illness produced by toxigenic *C. ulcerans*, opportunistic infections by *C. jeikeium*, and urinary tract infections by *C. urealyticum*. The development of catheter-related infections with bacteremia, as well as pneumonitis, wound infections, and other diseases by *C. jeikeium*, is particularly troublesome because successful treatment is frequently difficult with these antibiotic-resistant bacteria. A similar problem is observed with *C. urealyticum* infections. In addition, therapeutic concentrations of effective antibiotics may be difficult to maintain in the presence of renal stones.

Laboratory Diagnosis

Diagnosis of diphtheria depends on clinical parameters because definitive laboratory tests can take 1 week or more.

Microscopy

Microscopic examination of clinical material is unreliable. Metachromatic granules in *C. diphtheriae* stained with methylene blue have been described. However, this appearance is not specific for this organism, and interpretation of the smear requires technical expertise.

Culture

Corynebacteria grow on common laboratory media, although some species may require prolonged incubation. Specimens for the recovery of *C. diphtheriae* should be collected from both the nasopharynx and throat and then inoculated onto nonselective media, as well as media developed specifically for this organism (e. g., cysteine-tellurite agar, serum tellurite agar, Löffler medium). *C. diphtheriae* has a characteristic gray-to-black color on tellurite agar, and the microscopic morphology is best seen on Löffler medium. Three colonial morphologies of *C. diphtheriae* have been described on cysteine-tellurite agar: **gravis, intermedius,** and **mitis**. Gravis-type colonies are large, irregular, gray colonies; intermedius colonies are small, flat, and gray; and mitis-type colonies are small, round, convex, black colonies. Although these morphologies were initially related to the severity of illness, the distinctions are not valid now. However, the colonial morphologies are useful for epidemiologic classification of isolates. Precise identification of *C. diphtheriae* and the other corynebacteria is based on specific biochemical tests. Resistance to all antibiotics except vancomycin is a helpful property for recognizing *C. jeikeium* and *C. urealyticum*.

Toxigenicity Testing

All isolates of *C. diphtheriae* should be tested for production of exotoxin. This can be done by either an in vitro immunodiffusion assay (Elek test), tissue culture neutralization assay using specific antitoxin, or an in vivo animal assay (Figure 22-3).

Treatment, Prevention, and Control

The most important factor for treatment of diphtheria is early use of diphtheria antitoxin for the specific neutralization of exotoxin. Antibiotic therapy with penicillin or erythromycin has proved effective in eliminating *C. diphtheriae* from patients who have the disease and also from those who are asymptomatic carriers. Bed rest, isolation to prevent secondary spread, and maintenance of an open airway in patients with respiratory diphtheria are all appropriate.

Symptomatic diphtheria can be prevented by active immunization with diphtheria toxoid during childhood and booster immunizations every 10 years throughout life. The nontoxic, immunogenic toxoid is prepared by formalin treatment of toxin. Immunization with this preparation, in conjunction with pertussis and tetanus **(DPT vaccine),** is initially performed in three monthly injections followed by regular booster injections (normally combined with tetanus only).

Immunity to diphtheria can be determined by measuring for the presence of neutralizing antibodies in an individual's circulatory system (**Schick test**). This is done by injecting diphtheria toxin intradermally. No skin reaction will be observed if neutralizing antibodies are present, but localized edema with necrosis indicates neutralizing antibodies are absent and the individual is susceptible to diphtheria.

Close contacts of patients with documented diphtheria are at risk for developing disease. Nasopharyngeal cultures should be collected from all close contacts and antimicrobial prophylaxis with either penicillin or erythromycin should be start^d immediately. Contacts who

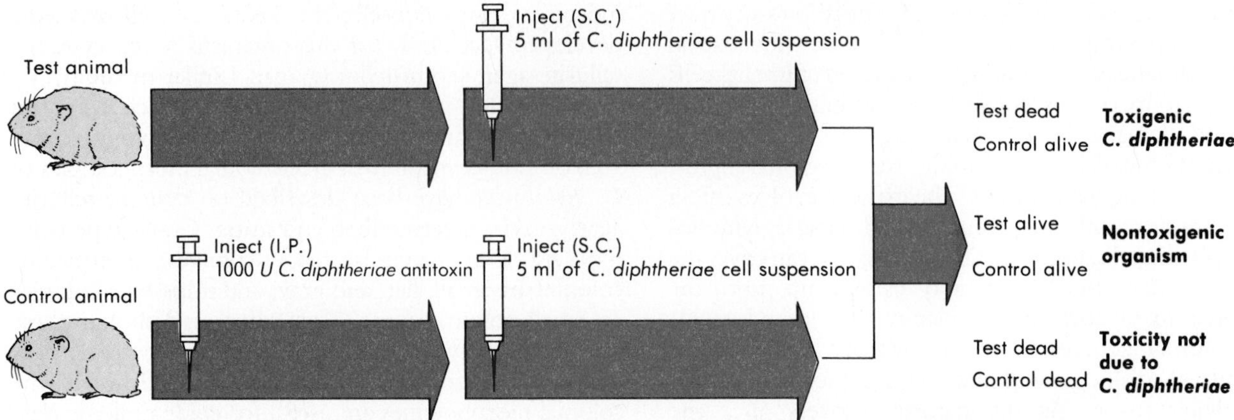

FIGURE 22-3 In vivo detection of *Corynebacterium diphtheriae* exotoxin. The clinical presentation of diphtheria is caused by production of exotoxin by "tox" positive strains of *C. diphtheriae.* The most sensitive way to detect toxin production is by injecting a guinea pig subcutaneously with a suspension of *C. diphtheriae* grown in broth culture. After 1 to 4 days the test animal will show signs of localized tissue necrosis and systemic signs of disease, including death. To ensure this is due to toxin, a control guinea pig is preimmunized with an intraperitoneal injection of diphtheria antitoxin. When this control is injected with the toxic cell suspension, the antitoxin will neutralize the exotoxin and protect the animal.

have not completed the series of diphtheria immunizations or who have not received a booster dose within the previous 5 years should receive a booster dose of toxoid. Exposure to cutaneous diphtheria should be managed in the same manner as respiratory diphtheria. If the respiratory or cutaneous infection is known to be caused by a nontoxigenic strain, then prophylaxis of contacts is unnecessary.

ARCANOBACTERIUM

Arcanobacterium haemolyticum is a small, pleomorphic gram-positive bacillus that was formerly classified in the genus *Corynebacterium*. Arcanobacteria colonize humans and are responsible for pharyngitis, with or without a scarlet fever–like rash, as well as cutaneous infections, endocarditis, and meningitis. The frequency of pharyngitis caused by this bacterium is unknown but has been estimated to be between 5% and 13% of that caused by *Streptococcus pyogenes*. *Arcanobacterium* infections occur in older patients, but pharyngitis caused by this organism and *S. pyogenes* cannot be distinguished clinically. A prominent erythematous, maculopapular rash is observed in more than half of the patients.

The pathogenesis of these infections is not completely understood. Arcanobacteria produce at least two toxins, phospholipase D and hemolysin, and the enzyme neuraminidase. The phospholipase D is similar to that found in the *C. pseudotuberculosis* and *C. ulcerans*, although it is antigenically distinct.

Detection of the organism in culture is problematic. Despite its name, *A. haemolyticum* grows slowly and is only weakly hemolytic on sheep blood agar. Growth and hemolysis are much better on agar medium supplemented with human or rabbit blood, but these media are rarely used in clinical laboratories.

LISTERIA

The genus *Listeria* consists of seven species, with human disease caused by *Listeria monocytogenes* and rarely by the animal pathogen, *Listeria ivanovii*. *L. monocytogenes* is a gram-positive, non–spore-forming, facultatively anaerobic bacillus capable of causing meningoencephalitis, bacteremia, and endocarditis, as well as a variety of other diseases. These small coccobacilli (0.4 × 0.5 to 2 μm) can microscopically resemble corynebacteria or gram-positive diplococci (e.g., *Streptococcus pneumoniae, Enterococcus*). The organisms are motile, with a characteristic tumbling motility in liquids incubated at room temperature. This differential characteristic is useful for their preliminary identification. Although listeria have a widespread distribution in nature, human disease is uncommon and restricted to several well-defined populations: neonates and the elderly, pregnant women, and immunocompromised patients, particularly those with defective cell-mediated immunity.

Pathogenesis and Immunity

L. monocytogenes is a facultative intracellular pathogen, capable of growth in macrophages, epithelial cells, and cultured fibroblasts. All virulent strains produce a β-hemolysin, **listeriolysin O**, that is related to streptolysin O (as the name implies). This hemolysin is required for release of the bacterium after phagocytosis and intracellular growth (Figure 22-4). Phagocytosis of the bacteria by activated macrophages leads to bacterial death, most likely because the oxygen-labile hemolysin is

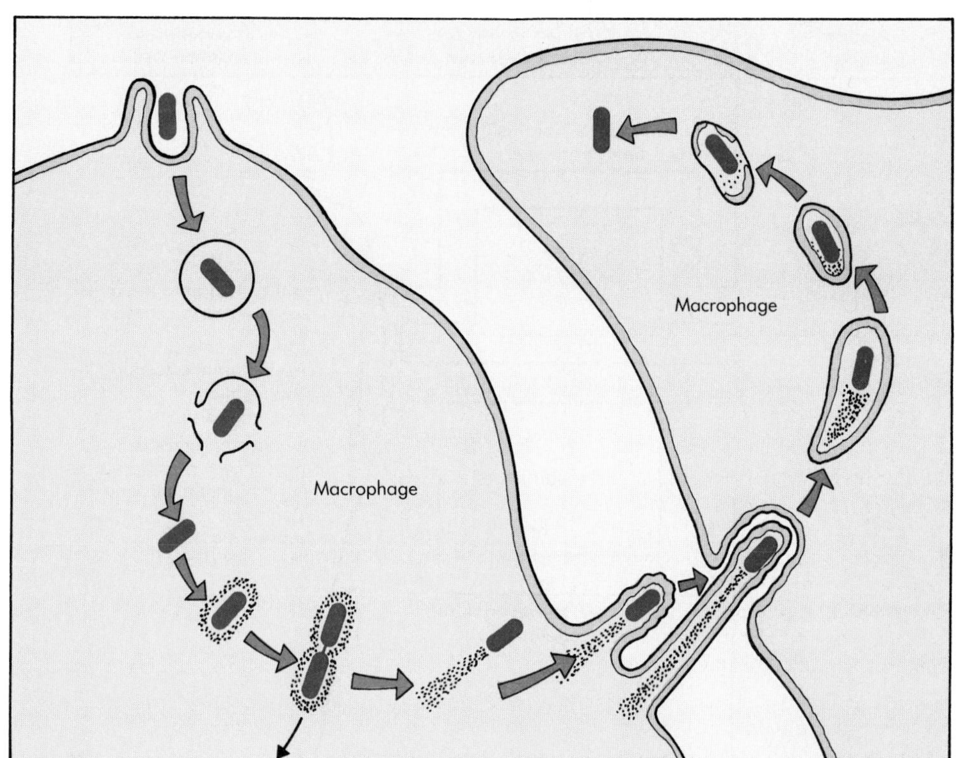

FIGURE 22-4 *Listeria* is an intracellular pathogen. After phagocytosis, the bacillus moves into the cell in an endosome that fuses with lysosomes. Before the bacterium is damaged by the lysosomal enzymes, the phagolysosome membrane is dissolved, presumably by listeriolysin O. A halo of actin filaments then surrounds the organism that, following bacteria replication, will orient into a tail and push the bacteria to the macrophage surface. A pseudopod extension then forms and facilitates transfer into another phagocyte. This process protects listeria from exposure to antibodies and other extracellular bactericidal factors. (Redrawn from Tilney LG and Portnoy DA: *J Cell Biol* 109:1597-1608, 1989).

inactivated by the oxidative metabolites of the macrophages. Intracellular survival and spread of the bacilli is critically important because no other virulence factors have been identified.

Epidemiology

L. monocytogenes is isolated from soil, water, vegetation, and a variety of mammals, birds, fish, insects, and other animals (Figure 22-5 and Box 22-2). Asymptomatic carriage, as well as disease, is well-documented in both mammals and humans. Although the incidence of human carriage is unknown, fecal carriage in healthy individuals is estimated to be 1% to 5%. Recent studies have documented that the annual incidence of invasive human disease is 12.7 cases per 100,000 live births and 7.4 cases per million population. Approximately 1700 cases occur annually in the United States, with 450 adult deaths and 100 fetal and postnatal deaths. Listeria are the most common cause of meningitis in renal transplant patients and in adult patients with cancer and the fifth most common cause of meningitis overall.

Human listeriosis is a sporadic disease seen throughout the year, with a peak in the warmer months. Focal epidemics have been associated with consumption of contaminated milk, soft cheese, undercooked meat (e.g., turkey franks, cold cuts), unwashed raw vegetables, and cabbage. Recent studies have demonstrated that most cases of sporadic listeriosis are also foodborne. Listeria are able to grow in a wide pH range, as well as in cold temperatures—a fact that has been exploited for the selective isolation of this organism **("cold enrichment").** Thus refrigeration of contaminated food products permits the slow multiplication of the organism to an infectious dose.

Clinical Syndromes

Neonatal Disease

Two forms of neonatal disease have been described: **early-onset disease** acquired transplacentally in utero and **late-onset disease** acquired at or soon after birth. Early-onset disease, also called **granulomatosis infantiseptica,** is a devastating disease with a high mortality unless promptly treated. The disease is characterized by disseminated abscesses and granulomas in multiple organs. Late-onset disease occurs 2 to 3 weeks after birth as meningitis or meningoencephalitis with septicemia. The

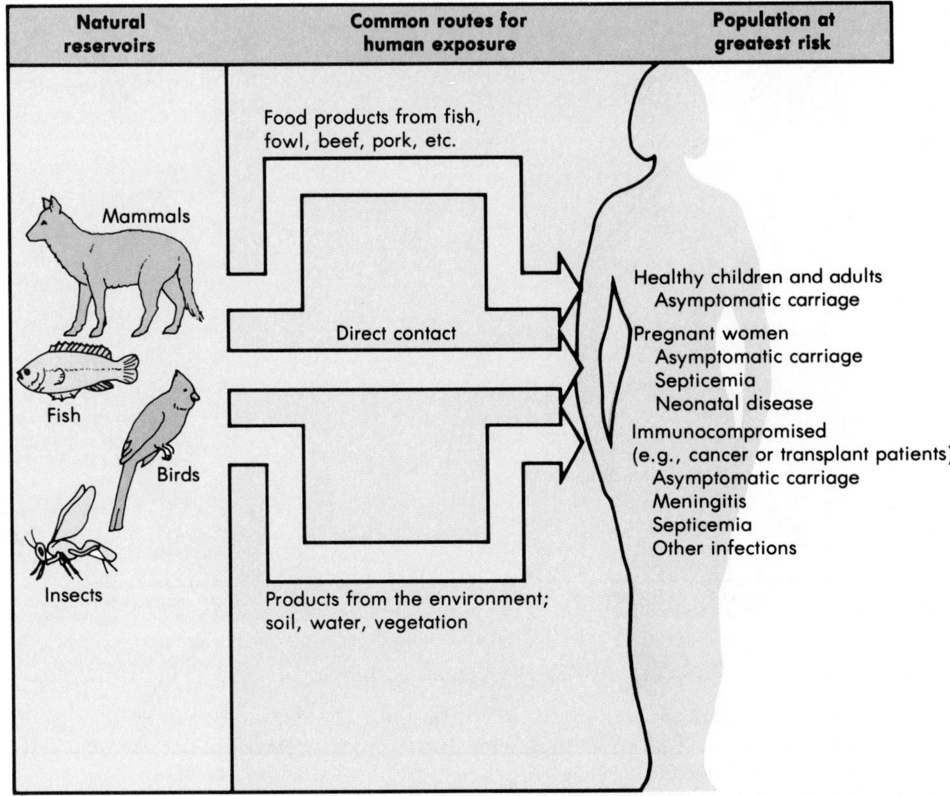

FIGURE 22-5 Epidemiology of *Listeria* infections.

BOX 22-2 Epidemiology of *Listeria* Infection

DISEASE/BACTERIAL FACTORS

Organism can grow in macrophages and epithelial cells
Asymptomatic carriage is possible
Virulent strains produce listeriolysin O
Can grow in cold temperatures (refrigerators)

TRANSMISSION

Ingestion of contaminated food products
Transplacental

WHO IS AT RISK?

Neonates
Elderly
Pregnant women
Immunocompromised patients

GEOGRAPHY/SEASON

Ubiquitous and worldwide
Sporadic, with peak occurrence in the warmer months

MODES OF CONTROL

Penicillin or ampicillin, alone or in combination with an aminoglycoside
People at high risk should avoid eating raw or partially cooked food of animal origin, soft cheeses, and unwashed raw vegetables

clinical signs and symptoms are not unique; thus other causes of neonatal central nervous system disease, such as group B streptococcal disease, must be excluded.

Meningitis in Adults

Meningitis is the most common form of listeria infections in adults, with most infections in patients with depressed cell-mediated immunity (Figure 22-6). Although the presentation is not specific for this organism, listeria should always be suspected in organ transplant patients or patients with a malignancy who develop meningitis.

Primary Bacteremia

Bacteremic patients may have an unremarkable history of chills and fever (commonly observed in pregnant women) or have a more acute presentation with high-grade fever and hypotension. Mortality appears to be restricted to severely immunocompromised patients and the infants of septic pregnant women.

Endocarditis and Other Infections

One complication of listeria bacteremia is endocarditis. A variety of other inflammatory and purulent infections have also been reported.

Laboratory Diagnosis

Microscopy

Gram stain preparations of cerebrospinal fluid are usually negative because listeria are generally present in concen-

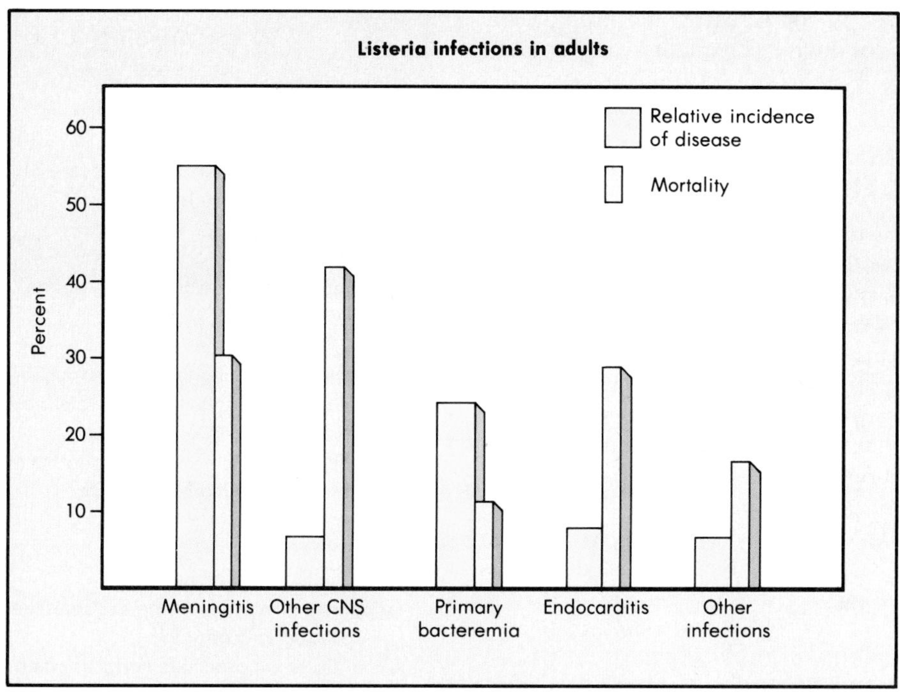

FIGURE 22-6 *Listeria* infections in adults. The most common manifestation of *Listeria* disease in adults is meningitis or meningoencephalitis. Less commonly seen diseases include septicemia, endocarditis, endophthalmitis, peritonitis, amnionitis, osteomyelitis, lymphadenitis, and cholecystitis. (Data from Nieman RE and Lorber B: *Rev Infect Dis* 2:207-227, 1980.)

trations 100 to 1000 times less than observed with other causes of bacterial meningitis. In a positive stain, intracellular and extracellular gram-positive coccobacilli are seen. Care must be used in interpreting the Gram stain because the organism can resemble corynebacteria, *Streptococcus pneumoniae,* or (if the preparation is overdecolorized) *Haemophilus.*

Culture

Listeria grow on most conventional laboratory media, with small, round colonies observed on agar media after incubation for 1 to 2 days. The use of selective media and cold enrichment may be required to detect listeria in specimens contaminated with rapidly growing bacteria. Useful differential tests for the preliminary identification of listeria are listed in Table 22-3. β-hemolysis on sheep blood agar media can separate listeria from morphologically similar bacteria; however, the hemolysis is generally weak and may not be observed initially. Motility in liquid medium or semisolid agar is also helpful for the preliminary identification of listeria. All gram-positive bacilli isolated from blood and cerebrospinal fluid should be identified to distinguish between *Corynebacterium* (presumably contaminants) and *Listeria.*

Identification

Definitive identification is achieved with selected biochemical and serologic tests. Eleven serotypes have been described, with 1/2a, 1/2b, and 4b responsible for most human infections. Because relatively few serotypes are isolated from human disease, serotyping is generally not useful in epidemiologic investigations and molecular characterization of isolates is required.

TABLE 22-3 Differential Features of *Listeria monocytogenes, Erysielothrix rhusiopathiae* , and *Corynebacterium* Species

Test reactions	*Listeria*	*Erysipelothrix*	*Corynebacterium*
Hemolysis on blood agar	beta	alpha	variable
Motility	+	−	−
Catalase	+	−	+
H_2S on triple sugar agar	−	+	−

Treatment, Prevention, and Control

Penicillin or ampicillin, either alone or in combination with an aminoglycoside, is the treatment of choice for infections with *L. monocytogenes.* Because listeria are ubiquitous and most infections are sporadic, prevention and control are difficult. However, high-risk individuals (e.g., pregnant women, immunocompromised persons, the elderly) should avoid eating raw or partially cooked foods of animal origin, soft cheeses, and unwashed raw vegetables. A vaccine is not available, and prophylactic antibiotic therapy for high-risk patients has not been evaluated.

ERYSIPELOTHRIX

Physiology and Structure

Erysipelothrix rhusiopathiae, the sole member of the genus, is a gram-positive, non–spore-forming, facultative anaerobic bacillus that has worldwide distribution in wild and domestic animals. The bacilli are small, slender (0.2 to 0.4 × 0.8 to 2.5 μm), and sometimes pleomorphic with a tendency to form long filaments. They may decolorize readily and appear gram negative. The organisms are microaerophilic, preferring growth in a reduced oxygen atmosphere and supplemented carbon dioxide. Small, grayish, α-hemolytic colonies are observed after 2 to 3 days of incubation. Animal disease—particularly in swine—is widely recognized, but human disease is uncommon.

Pathogenesis

Little is known about specific virulence factors in *Erysipelothrix.* Disease in swine has been associated with hyaluronidase and neuraminidase production. However, because this organism is an uncommon human pathogen, similar studies in humans have not been performed.

BOX 22-3 Epidemiology of *Erysipelothrix* Infection

DISEASE/BACTERIAL FACTORS

Disease is common in swine but rare in humans
Organism is ubiquitous

TRANSMISSION

Inoculation through abrasion or wound

WHO IS AT RISK?

Those who occupationally handle meat (butchers), poultry, fish, or animals (farmers, veterinarians)

GEOGRAPHY/SEASON

Worldwide distribution in animals

MODES OF CONTROL

Penicillin is very effective
Organism is resistant to the sulfonamides, aminoglycosides, and vancomycin
Covering of exposed skin surfaces when exposed occupationally to animals
No vaccine available

Epidemiology

Erysipelothrix is a ubiquitous organism with worldwide distribution in many wild and domestic animals, including mammals, birds, and fish (Box 22-3). Swine and fish are the most important animals associated with human disease. **Erysipeloid** is an occupational disease in humans, with greatest risk for butchers, meat processors, farmers, poultry workers, fish handlers, and veterinarians. Infections follow subcutaneous inoculation of the organism through an abrasion or puncture wound while handling contaminated animal products or soil.

Clinical Syndromes

Three forms of human disease with *Erysipelothrix rhusiopathiae* have been described: (1) a localized skin infection, erysipeloid; (2) a generalized cutaneous form; and (3) a septicemic form, often associated with endocarditis. Erysipeloid is an inflammatory skin lesion that develops at the site of trauma after a 1- to 4-day incubation period. The lesion, most commonly present on the fingers or hands, is characterized by an erythematous, raised edge that slowly spreads peripherally as the discoloration in the central area fades. The painful lesion is pruritic with a burning or throbbing sensation, and suppuration is uncommon. Spontaneous resolution can occur but can be hastened with appropriate antibiotic therapy. The diffuse cutaneous infection is rare and is often associated with systemic manifestions, but blood cultures are negative. The septicemic form of *Erysipelothrix* infections is also uncommon, but when present it is frequently associated with endocarditis. *Erysipelothrix* endocarditis may have an acute onset but is usually subacute. Involvement of previously undamaged heart valves (particularly the aortic valve) is common. Valvular destruction and metastatic pyogenic complications are reported with this rare disease.

Laboratory Diagnosis

Bacilli are located only in the deep tissue of the lesion. Thus full thickness biopsies or deep aspirates must be collected. Specimens collected from the surface will invariably be negative by microscopy and culture.

E. rhusiopathiae is not fastidious and will grow on most conventional laboratory media. Initial classification of the organism can be performed as detailed in Table 22-3, with definitive identification by biochemical testing.

Treatment, Prevention, and Control

Erysipelothrix is highly susceptible to penicillin, the antibiotic treatment of choice. Cephalosporins, erythromycin, and clindamycin are also active in vitro, but the organism is resistant to the sulfonamides, aminoglycosides, and vancomycin. Although erysipeloid is generally a nonfatal disease, approximately one third of the patients with endocarditis die despite appropriate antibiotic therapy.

Infections in individuals with an increased occupational risk are prevented by use of gloves and appropriate covering of exposed skin surfaces. Vaccination is not available.

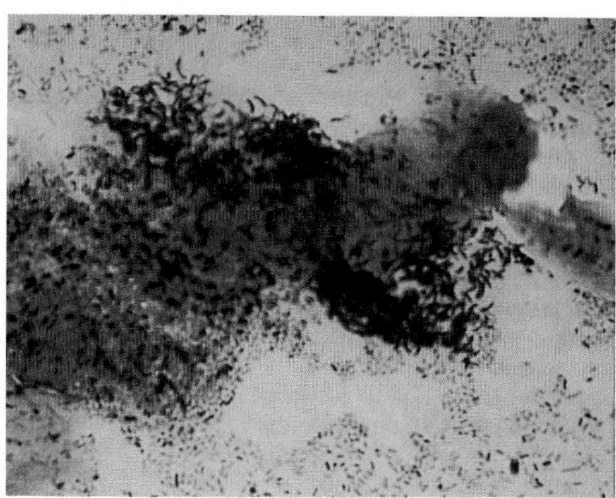

FIGURE 22-7 Vaginal epithelial cell covered with organisms resembling *G. vaginalis* and *Mobiluncus*. The abundance of these small gram-negative and gram-variable bacilli and the absence of larger gram-positive bacilli (lactobacilli) is consistent with bacterial vaginosis. (From Nugent et al: *J Clin Microbiol* 29:297-301, 1991.)

GARDNERELLA

Gardnerella vaginalis, an organism formerly classified in the genera *Haemophilus* and *Corynebacterium,* morphologically resembles a gram-negative bacilli but has the cell wall structure of a gram-positive organism. *G. vaginalis* is pleomorphic, averaging 0.5 × 1.5 μm, nonmotile, and does not form spores or possess a capsule. The organism is facultatively anaerobic and grows slowly in a carbon dioxide enriched atmosphere.

G. vaginalis is part of the normal vaginal flora in 20% to 40% of healthy women. In women with bacterial vaginosis (nonspecific vaginitis), the number of *Gardnerella* and various obligate anaerobes (primarily *Bacteroides* species, *Mobiluncus*, and *Peptostreptococcus* species) significantly increases. However, the pathogenic role of *G. vaginalis* in this disease is incompletely defined. This organism has also been associated with postpartum bacteremia, endometritis, and vaginal abscesses.

The simple isolation of *Gardnerella* from vaginal secretions has little diagnostic significance because the organism is frequently recovered in healthy women. The diagnostic test for bacterial vaginosis is microscopic examination of vaginal secretions. The clinical diagnosis is supported by the observation of **"clue cells"** (Figure 22-7), epithelial cells covered with gram-positive or gram-variable bacilli (resembling *G. vaginalis*) and small curved gram-negative bacilli (resembling the anaerobe *Mobiluncus*; see Chapter 33).

G. vaginalis is inhibited by ampicillin and metronidazole, both of which have been used to treat bacterial vaginosis.

CASE STUDY AND QUESTIONS

A 35-year-old man was hospitalized for headache, fever, and confusion. Seven months previously he had received a transplanted kidney. Physical examination of the patient revealed a temperature of 39° C and obtundation. Analysis of CSF disclosed a WBC count of 36 cells/mm^3 (96% polymorphonuclear leukocytes), glucose concentration of 40 mg/dl, and protein concentration of 172 mg/dl. Gram stain of CSF was negative, but culture of blood and urine revealed gram-positive coccobacilli.

1. What is the most likely cause of this patient's meningitis? What is the significance of his immunosuppression?
2. What are potential sources of this organism? What other individuals would be at increased risk for infection?
3. What is the significance of the negative Gram stain? What growth and biochemical characteristics would be useful for identifying this organism?
4. List the most important gram-positive bacilli discussed in this chapter and the diseases they cause.
5. What is the epidemiology of infections cause by *Corynebacterium diphtheriae, C. jeikeium, C. urealyticum, Archanobacterium haemolyticum,* and *Erysipelothrix rhusiopathiae*?

Bibliography

Catlin BW: *Gardnerella vaginalis*: characteristics, clinical considerations, and controversies, *Clin Microbiol Rev* 5:213-237, 1992.

Coyle MB and Lipsky BA: Coryneform bacteria in infectious diseases: clinical and laboratory aspects, *Clin Microbiol Rev* 3:227-246, 1990.

Gorby GL and Peacock JE Jr: *Erysipelothrix rhusiopathiae* endocarditis: microbiologic, epidemiologic, and clinical features of an occupational disease, *Rev Infect Dis* 10:317-325, 1988.

Hodges HL: Diphtheria, *Pediatr Clin North Am* 26:445-459, 1979.

Lipsky BA, Goldberger AC, Tompkins LS, and Plorde JJ: Infections caused by nondiphtheria corynebacteria, *Rev Infect Dis* 4:1220-1235, 1982.

Miller RA, Brancato F, and Holmes KK: *Corynebacterium haemolyticum* as a cause of pharyngitis and scarlatiniform rash in young adults, *Ann Intern Med* 105:867-872, 1986.

Nieman RE and Lorber B: Listeriosis in adults: a changing pattern. Report of eight cases and review of the literature, 1968-1978, *Rev Infect Dis* 2:207-227, 1980.

Papenheimer AM, Jr and Gill DM: Diphtheria, *Science* 182:353-358, 1973.

Pinner RW, Schuchat A, Swaminathan B et al: Role of foods in sporadic listeriosis. II. Microbiologic and epidemiologic investigation, *JAMA* 267:2046-2050, 1992.

Reboli AC and Farrar WE: *Erysipelothrix rhusiopathiae*: an occupational pathogen, *Clin Microbiol Rev* 2:354-359, 1989.

Schuchat A, Deaver KA, Jenger JD et al: Role of foods in sporadic listeriosis. I. Case-control study of dietary risk factors, *JAMA* 267:2041-2045, 1992.

Schuchat A, Swaminathan B, and Broome CV: Epidemiology of human listeriosis, *Clin Microbiol Rev* 4:169-183, 1991.

Soriano F, Aguado JM, Ponte C et al: Urinary tract infection caused by *Corynebacterium* group D2: report of 82 cases and review, *Rev Infect Dis* 12:1019-1034, 1990.

Stamm AM, Dismukes WE, Simmons BP et al: Listeriosis in renal transplant recipients: report of an outbreak and review of 102 cases, *Rev Infect Dis* 4:665-682, 1982.

Stamm WE, Tompkins LS, Wagner KF et al: Infection due to *Corynebacterium* species in marrow transplant patients, *Ann Intern Med* 91:167-173, 1979.

Tilney LG and Portnoy DA: Actin filaments and the growth, movement, and spread of the intracellular bacterial parasite, *Listeria monocytogenes*, *J Cell Biol* 109:1597-1608, 1989.

CHAPTER 23

Neisseria

RECENT studies of the family Neisseriaceae using DNA-rRNA hybridization and 16S rRNA sequence analysis have led to the taxonomic reorganization of the family. Members of the genera *Branhamella*, *Moraxella*, and *Acinetobacter* have been transferred into a new family, Moraxellaceae (see Chapter 27 for further discussion of these organisms). Members of the genera *Neisseria* can be easily differentiated from the other genera by morphological and biochemical parameters (Table 23-1). The best known *Neisseria* species are *Neisseria meningitidis* and *Neisseria gonorrhoeae*. *N. meningitidis* can either colonize the upper respiratory tract or cause significant human disease. In contrast, *N. gonorrhoeae* is always considered pathogenic, even in individuals with asymptomatic colonization. The other *Neisseria* species normally colonize mucous membranes and the skin surface and are rare causes of disease.

NEISSERIA MENINGITIDIS

The meningococci are encapsulated, gram-negative diplococci that can asymptomatically colonize the nasopharynx of healthy individuals or cause fulminant meningitis, pneumonia, or overwhelming sepsis (**meningococcemia**) (Box 23-1).

TABLE 23-1 Differentiation of *Neisseria* From *Moraxella* and *Acinetobacter*

Characteristics	*Neisseria*	*Moraxella*	*Acinetobacter*
Cell morphology			
Cocci	+	+	−
Coccobacilli	−	+	+
Oxidase	+	+	−
Catalase	+	+	+
Acid from glucose	+	−	±
Nitrate reduction	+	±	−
Mol% G + C of DNA	46-54	40-48	38-47

Physiology and Structure

The meningococci form transparent, nonpigmented, nonhemolytic colonies on chocolate blood agar, with enhanced growth in a moist atmosphere with 5% carbon dioxide. Isolates with large capsules appear as mucoid colonies. Meningococci are oxidase positive and are differentiated from other neisseria by acid production from glucose and maltose but not sucrose or lactose (Table 23-2).

N. meningitidis is subdivided into serogroups and immunotypes (Table 23-3). Serogroups A, B, C, Y, and W135 are most commonly associated with meningococcal disease. All group A meningococci have the same outer membrane proteins and belong to a single serotype, whereas multiple serotypes have been described for groups B and C. Membrane proteins and serotype classification are shared between the two groups.

Pathogenesis and Immunity

Three major factors are responsible for meningococcal disease: the ability of *N. meningitidis* to colonize the nasopharynx (mediated by pili), systemic spread without

BOX 23-1 Infections Associated With *Neisseria meningitidis* and *Neisseria gonorrhoeae*

N. meningitidis	Meningitis Septicemia Pneumonia Urethritis Arthritis
N. gonorrhoeae	Urethritis Cervicitis Salpingitis Proctitis Septicemia Arthritis Conjunctivitis Pharyngitis Pelvic inflammatory disease

TABLE 23-2 Differential Characteristics of Commonly Isolated *Neisseria* Species

Characteristics	*N. gonorrhoeae*	*N. meningitidis*	*N. lactamica*	*N. sicca*	*N. flavescens*	*N. mucosa*	*N. subflava*
Growth on:							
MTM, ML*	+	+	+	−	−	+	−
Blood agar	−	−	+	+	+	+	+
Nutrient agar	−	−	+	+	+	+	+
Acid from:							
Glucose	+	+	+	+	−	+	+
Maltose	−	+	+	+	−	+	+
Lactose	−	−	+	−	−	−	−
Sucrose	−	−	−	+	−	+	+
Nitrate reduction	−	−	−	−	−	+	−

**MTM*, Modified Thayer-Martin agar; *ML*, Martin-Lewis agar.

TABLE 23-3 Antigenic Determinants of *Neisseria meningitidis*

Epidemiologic classification	Antigenic determinant	Number described
Serogroup	Polysaccharide capsule	13
Serotype	Outer membrane protein	>20
Immunotype	Lipopolysaccharide	8

antibody-mediated phagocytosis (protection afforded by polysaccharide capsule), and expression of toxic effects (mediated by the lipooligosaccharide endotoxin). Experiments with nasopharyngeal tissue organ cultures have demonstrated that meningococci attach selectively to specific receptors for meningococcal pili on nonciliated columnar cells of the nasopharynx (Figure 23-1). Meningococci without pili have decreased binding to these cells. The organisms are then internalized in phagocytic vacuoles, and after 18 to 24 hours the meningococci are found in the subepithelial space. The antiphagocytic properties of the polysaccharide capsule protect *N. meningitidis* from phagocytic destruction. The diffuse vascular damage associated with meningococcal infections (e.g., endothelial damage, inflammation of vessel walls, thrombosis, disseminated intravascular coagulation [DIC]) is in large part attributed to the action of the lipooligosaccharide endotoxin. The endotoxin is present in the outer membrane. *N. meningitidis* produces excess membrane fragments that are released into the extracellular space (Figure 23-2). This continuous hyperproduction of endotoxin is most likely responsible for the severe endotoxic reaction associated with meningococcal disease.

Serum bactericidal antibodies are important for preventing systemic meningococcal disease. Thus infants younger than 1 year of age are more susceptible to disease related to the decline in maternal antibodies. Bactericidal activity also requires complement activity. Individuals with deficiencies in C5, C6, C7, or C8 in the complement system are at increased risk (6000-fold) for meningococcal disease. Although immunity is primarily mediated by the humoral immune response, lymphocyte responsiveness to meningococcal antigens is markedly depressed in patients with acute disease.

Epidemiology

Endemic meningococcal disease occurs worldwide, and epidemics are common in developing countries (Box 23-2). Pandemic outbreaks of disease have been uncommon in developed countries since one swept Europe and North America following World War II (Figure 23-3). Approximately 90% of meningococcal disease is caused by serogroups A, B, and C, with B responsible for most endemic disease in the United States and serogroup A the major pathogen in Africa and Asia. Transmission of *N. meningitidis* is by respiratory droplets among persons who have prolonged close contact, such as family members living in the same household, and within crowded communities such as the military. Classmates and hospital employees are not considered close contacts and are not at significantly increased risk unless they are in direct contact with respiratory secretions.

Humans are the only natural carriers for *N. meningitidis*, so the bacterium is spread from person to person by aerosolization of respiratory secretions. Tremendous variation in prevalence (e.g., less than 1% to greater than 30%) has been reported in studies of asymptomatic carriage of *N. meningitidis*. The oral and nasopharyngeal carriage rates are highest in school-age children and young adults, higher in lower socioeconomic populations (possibly caused by crowding), and do not vary with seasons of the year (even though disease is most common during the dry season). Endemic disease is most common in children younger than 5 years of age, with the highest attack rates in infants from 3 months to 1 year of age

A

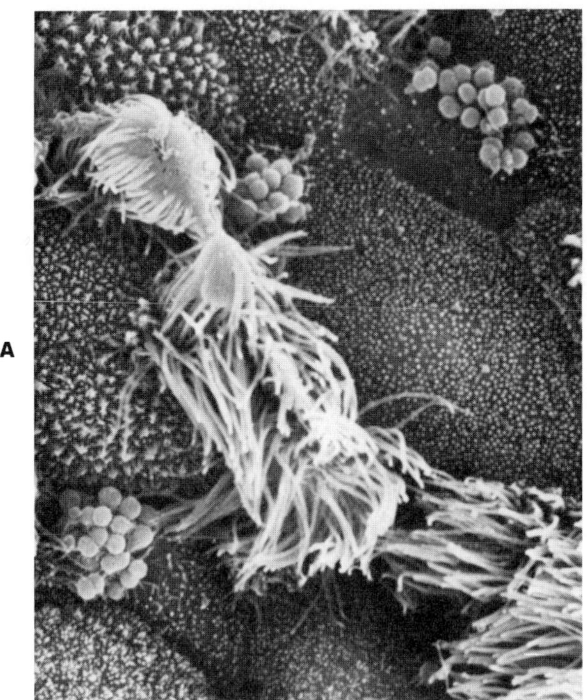

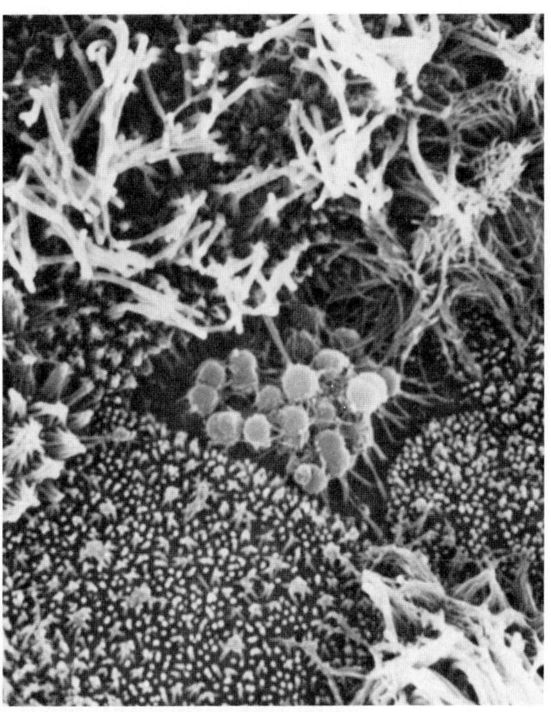

B

FIGURE 23-1 Scanning electron micrographs showing interaction of *Neisseria meningitidis* with human nasopharyngeal mucosa. **A,** The meningococci attach by pili to the microvilli of nonciliated cells but not to ciliated cells. **B,** Attachment stimulates folding of the epithelial cell membrane around the bacteria and subsequent internalization. (From Stephens DS, Hoffman LH, and McGee ZA: *J Infect Dis* 148:369, 1983.)

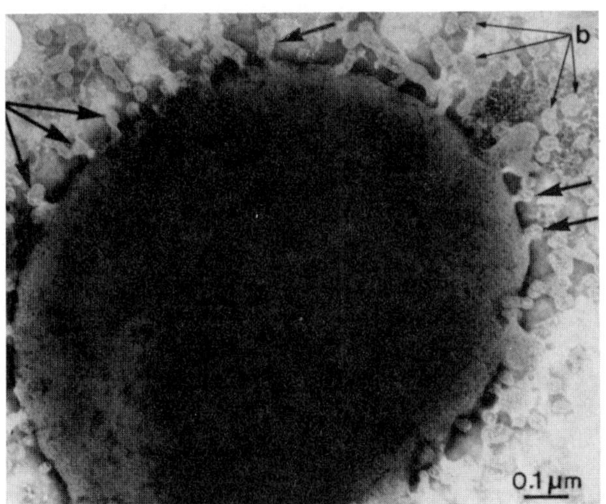

FIGURE 23-2 Negative-stained electron micrograph of *Neisseria* meningitidis. Excess outer membrane fragments containing endotoxin are released into the extracellular space in actively growing cells. (From *J Exp Med* 138:1156, 1973.)

(Figure 23-4). Older individuals, particularly those living in closed populations (e.g., military, prisons) are infected during epidemics.

During the first months of life, maternal bactericidal antibodies are protective. However, as passive immunity wanes and before acquired immunity develops, children are susceptible to infection. Acquired immunity develops in asymptomatically colonized persons, with bactericidal antibodies detectable within 2 weeks of colonization. Cross-reacting antibodies providing immunity to *N. meningitidis* can occur with antigenically related strains of meningococci or with bacteria of other genera (e.g., *Escherichia coli* serotype K1 cross-reacts with group B *N. meningitidis*). The majority of meningococcal strains acquired during carriage are typable.

Clinical Syndromes

Meningitis

Between 2500 and 3000 cases of meningococcal meningitis occur in the United States each year. Disease usually begins abruptly with headache, meningeal signs, and fever. However, very young children may have only nonspecific signs such as fever and vomiting. Mortality approaches 100% in untreated patients but is less than 15% when appropriate antibiotics are promptly instituted. The incidence of neurologic sequelae is low, with hearing deficits and arthritis most commonly reported.

Meningococcemia

Septicemia (meningococcemia) with or without meningitis is a life-threatening disease with a mortality rate of 25%, even in patients who are promptly treated. Thrombosis of small blood vessels and multiorgan involvement

BOX 23-2 Epidemiology of Meningococcal Disease

DISEASE/BACTERIAL FACTORS

Humans are the only natural carriers of *N. meningitidis*
Specific receptors for meningococcal pili allow colonization of nasopharynx
Polysaccharide capsule protects bacteria from antibody-mediated phagocytosis

TRANSMISSION

Person to person by aerosolization of respiratory secretions

WHO IS AT RISK?

Children less than 5 years old, particularly those less than 1 year old without protective maternal antibodies
Patients with late complement deficiencies
Close contacts of infected individuals (family members, military personnel)

GEOGRAPHY/SEASON

Worldwide distribution; epidemics more common in developing countries
Disease more common in dry months

MODES OF CONTROL

Infants: breast-feeding (first 6 months)
Penicillin (drug of choice), chloramphenicol, broad-spectrum cephalosporins
Prophylaxis with: sulfonamide for patients with sulfonamide-susceptible strains; rifampin for patients with sulfonamide-resistant strains
Polyvalent vaccine against capsular polysaccharide groups A, C, Y, and W135 available for children older than 2 years
Vaccination useful during outbreaks of groups A, C, Y, or W135, for travelers to hyperendemic areas, and for patients at increased risk

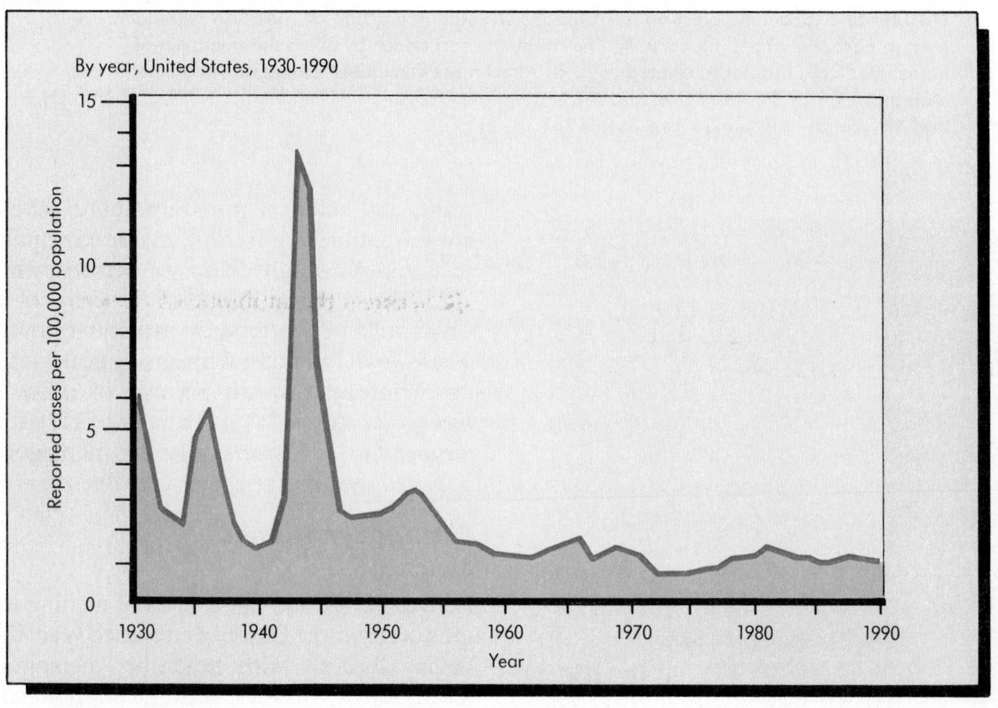

FIGURE 23-3 Meningococcal disease in the United States from 1930 to 1990. (Redrawn from *MMWR* 39:32, 1991).

are characteristic. Small petechial skin lesions on the trunk and lower extremities are common and may coalesce to form larger hemorrhagic lesions. The disease may progress to overwhelming disseminated intravascular coagulation with shock and includes bilateral destruction of the adrenal glands **(Waterhouse-Friderichsen syndrome).**

A milder, chronic septicemia has also been described. Bacteremia can persist for days or weeks in these patients, with the only signs of infection being low-grade fever, arthritis, and petechial skin lesions. Response to antibiotic therapy is generally excellent.

Other Syndromes

Additional infections associated with *N. meningitidis* include pneumonia, arthritis, and urethritis. Meningo-

FIGURE 23-4 Attack rate of meningococcal disease in the United States from 1975 to 1980. The highest incidence of disease is in children less than 1 year of age. (Redrawn from Band JD et al: *J Infect Dis* 148:754, 1983.)

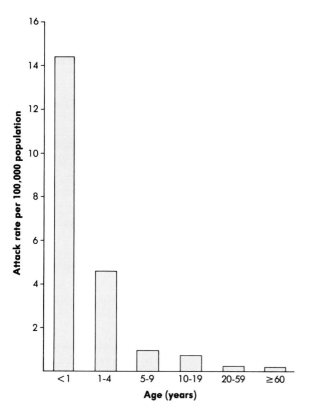

coccal pneumonia is usually preceded by a respiratory infection. Symptoms include cough, chest pain, rales, fever, and chills. Evidence of pharyngitis is observed in the majority of patients. The prognosis for this infection is good.

Laboratory Diagnosis

Definitive identification of *N. meningitidis* is important for the initiation of specific therapy and prophylaxis for contacts when indicated. The most useful specimens for detection of meningococci are blood and cerebrospinal fluid (CSF). Although most patients with systemic disease have positive blood cultures, additives present in the blood culture broths can be toxic for *Neisseria* and inhibit or delay bacterial growth. The laboratory should be notified that meningococcal disease is suspected, so that alternative blood-culturing methods can be selected. Detection and growth of the organism from CSF are relatively easy in untreated patients because more than 10^7 org/ml of fluid are normally found. However, the viability of organisms can be adversely affected in patients previously treated with antibiotics.

Because the bacterial count in CSF is high, the gram-negative diplococci are readily seen with polymorphonuclear leukocytes in Gram-stained specimens (Figure 23-5). Soluble polysaccharide antigen can also be detected in CSF by counterimmunoelectrophoresis or

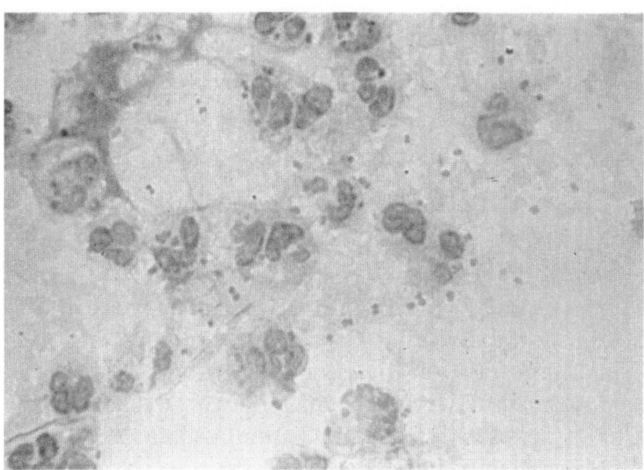

FIGURE 23-5 Gram stain of *Neisseria meningitidis* in cerebrospinal fluid.

agglutination of latex particles coated with specific antibodies. However, these tests have limited usefulness because serogroup B *N. meningitidis*, the most common group responsible for disease in developed countries, is relatively nonimmunogenic and does not react with the test reagents.

Treatment, Prevention, and Control

Antibiotic therapy and supportive management of the complications of meningococcal disease have significantly reduced the associated mortality. Although sulfonamides were the basis for the initial therapeutic successes, widespread resistance has negated their effectiveness. Penicillin is the antibiotic of choice; however, resistance to penicillin is becoming more common. High-level resistance (MIC greater than or equal to 2 ug/ml) mediated by the production of β-lactamase is very rare. However, moderate resistance (MIC 0.1 to 1.0 μg/ml) caused by the genetic alteration of penicillin-binding proteins (specifically, PBP 2) has been reported with increasing frequency in Spain, the United Kingdom, and South Africa. Alternative antibiotics include chloramphenicol and the broad-spectrum cephalosporins that remain active in vitro.

Eradication of the pool of healthy carriers is unlikely. Efforts have concentrated instead on the prophylactic treatment of persons who have significant exposure to diseased patients and the enhancement of immunity to serogroups most commonly associated with disease. Although sulfonamides were used for prophylaxis, this practice is no longer considered reliable because of the increased resistance. In addition, penicillin is ineffective in eliminating the carrier state. Minocycline and rifampin have both been used effectively for antibiotic-mediated chemoprophylaxis; however, toxic effects have been associated with minocycline, and rifampin-resistant *N. meningitidis* can arise during rifampin treatment. At present, prophylaxis with a sulfonamide is recommended for persons exposed to sulfonamide-susceptible strains, with rifampin used for sulfonamide-resistant strains.

Vaccines directed against the group-specific capsular polysaccharides have been developed for antibody-mediated immunoprophylaxis. An effective polyvalent vaccine, which can be administered to children older than 2 years of age, has been developed against groups A, C, Y, and W135. However, the vaccine cannot be administered to high-risk children in a younger age-group. Moreover, the group B polysaccharide is a weak immunogen and cannot induce a protective antibody response. Thus immunity to *N. meningitidis* group B, the most common cause of significant meningococcal disease in the United States, must develop naturally after exposure to cross-reacting antigens. Vaccination can be used to control an outbreak of disease with a serogroup present in the vaccine, for travelers to hyperendemic areas, or for individuals at increased risk for disease (e.g., patients with complement deficiency).

NEISSERIA GONORRHOEAE

Infection with *Neisseria gonorrhoeae* is the most common sexually transmitted disease in the United States. Clinical manifestations include urethritis, cervicitis, arthritis, conjunctivitis, and a number of local and systemic complications (see Box 23-1).

Physiology and Structure

Gonococci, like meningococci, are small, gram-negative diplococci. Five morphologically distinct colony types (T1 through T5) have been described, based on such features as color, size, and opacity, with virulence associated with T1 and T2. In vitro transfer of isolates results in a phase transition from T1 and T2 to T3 through T5, with reversion accomplished by in vitro inoculation onto human tissue culture cells. Identification of isolates is based on typical morphology, the presence of cytochrome oxidase, and strict oxidative metabolism of glucose but not other carbohydrates (see Table 23-2).

The structure of the gonococcus is similar to *N. meningitidis* (Figure 23-6). The outer surface is covered with a loosely associated capsule of unknown composition. Protruding through the surface of the bacteria are filamentous, protein pili, which are present only in the virulent T1 and T2 colony types. Considerable heterogeneity exists in the pilin protein, with antigenic variation exhibited during infection and only limited relatedness observed in pili from different strains. The major protein in the outer membrane is Protein I, which is arranged in trimers forming hydrophilic surface pores. Sixteen serotypes of Protein I have been described and are useful for the epidemiologic classification of isolates. Protein II is a minor membrane protein found in avirulent, opaque colonies. The presence of this protein is associated with intercellular adhesiveness, as well as increased adherence of gonococci to cultured mammalian cells. Protein III is a highly conserved surface protein closely associated with Protein I. A 37,000 d protein common to all gonococci is responsible for the removal of iron from host iron-binding proteins (e.g., lactoferrin, transferrin). Iron is essential for the growth and metabolism of gonococci. The endotoxin lipooligosaccharide of *N. gonorrhoeae* resembles that found in *N. meningitidis.* The endotoxin contains lipid A and a core polysaccharide, although the strain-specific O side chains that are present in many gram-negative bacilli are absent. The lipooligosaccharide is present on the outermost portion of the cell membrane and is released in an active form into the extracellular space much like with *N. meningitidis.* Other proteins associated with the gonococci are a protease capable of cleaving immunoglobulin A and β-lactamase that hydrolytically destroys penicillin.

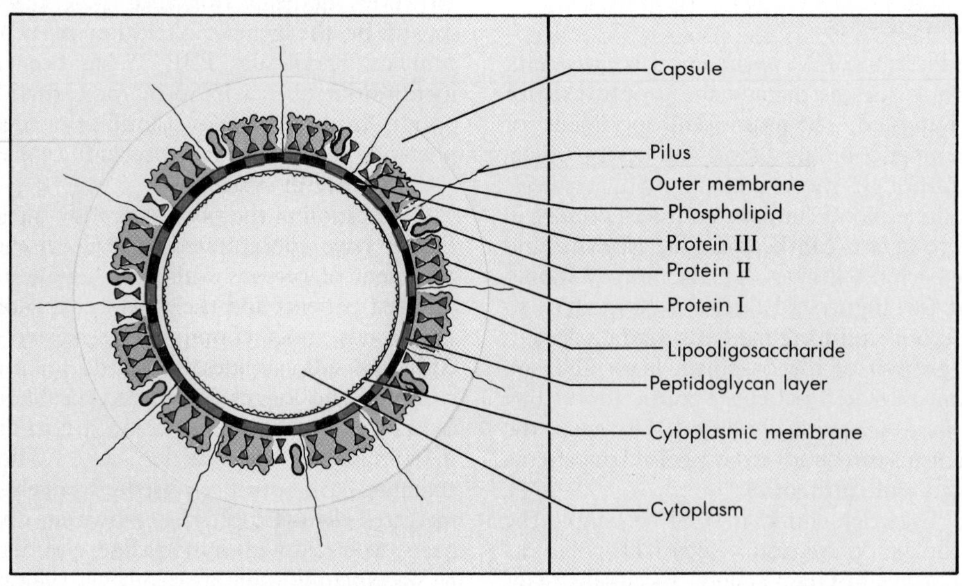

FIGURE 23-6 Surface structure of *Neisseria gonorrhoeae.*

TABLE 23-4 *Neisseria gonorrhoeae* Virulence Factors

Virulence factors	Biological effects
Capsule	Antiphagocytic actions
Pili	Attachment to human cells, including epithelium of vagina, fallopian tube, and buccal cavity; antiphagocytic; facilitates genetic transformation
Protein I	Major surface antigen; forms surface pores; specific serotypes associated with virulence
Protein II	Presence associated with avirulent, opaque colonies; responsible for intracellular adherence
Protein III	May protect other surface antigens from bactericidal interaction with antibodies
Lipooligosaccharide	Endotoxin activity
Iron-binding protein	Binds iron required for gonococcal metabolism
IgA protease	Destroys IgA1
β-lactamase	Hydrolyzes β-lactam ring in penicillin

BOX 23-3 Epidemiology of Gonococcal Disease

DISEASE/BACTERIAL FACTORS (SEE ALSO TABLE 23-4)

Humans are the only natural carriers of *N. gonorrhoeae*
Pili facilitate attachment to cells
Protein I interferes with neutrophil degranulation
Capsule protects against phagocytosis
Endotoxin causes tissue destruction

TRANSMISSION

Primarily by sexual contact
Asymptomatic carriage is largest reservoir

WHO IS AT RISK?

Patients with inherited complement deficiencies
Patients with multiple sexual encounters

GEOGRAPHY/SEASON

Worldwide
Disease corresponds to sexual activity

MODES OF CONTROL

Ceftriaxone in uncomplicated cases
Ceftriaxone and tetracycline in cases complicated by *Chlamydia* infection
Neonates: chemoprophylaxis with 1% silver nitrate, 1% tetracycline, or 0.5% erythromycin eye drops to protect against ophthalmia neonatorum
Patient education, aggressive documentation of frequency of disease, and follow-up with sexual contacts will help control disease

Pathogenesis and Immunity

Similar to infections with *N. meningitidis,* gonococci attach to mucosal cells, penetrate into the cells and multiply, and then pass through the cells into the subepithelial space where infection is established. The presence of pili is important for the initial attachment (Table 23-4). Nonpiliated cells such as those present in colony types T3 to T5 are avirulent. In the absence of specific opsonic antibodies and complement, the capsule protects against phagocytosis by polymorphonuclear leukocytes. Piliated strains are also more resistant to phagocytosis than are strains without pili.

Protein I can interfere with neutrophil degranulation. Whether this blocks intracellular killing of phagocytosed bacteria is unclear. The biologic roles of Protein II and Protein III are unknown. The gonococcal endotoxin is responsible for tissue destruction in cell culture and is believed to be the major virulence factor in vivo. In persistent infection, chronic inflammation and fibrosis occur, which can lead to sterility, arthritis with joint destruction, or blindness.

IgG_3 is the predominant IgG antibody response to gonococcal infection. Whereas the antibody response to Protein I is minimal, serum antibodies to pilin protein, Protein II, and lipooligosaccharide are readily detected. Antibodies to lipooligosaccharide can activate complement, releasing C5a, which is chemotaxic to neutrophils. However, IgG and secretory IgA antibodies directed against Protein III can block this bactericidal antibody response. As observed with *N. meningitidis*, individuals with inherited complement deficiencies are at significantly increased risk for systemic disease.

Epidemiology

Gonorrhea is a disease found only in humans; it has no other known reservoir (Box 23-3). Although the incidence of disease has decreased since 1975 (Figure 23-7), almost 700,000 cases are reported annually in the United States. Even this large number is an underestimation of the true incidence of disease because diagnosis and reporting of gonococcal infections are incomplete. Studies have documented that private physicians report fewer than 20% of the patients treated for gonorrhea. The peak incidence of disease is in the 20- to 24-year age-group, with significant increases since 1970 in the incidence of disease in teenage patients.

Transmission of *N. gonorrhoeae* is primarily by sexual contact. The risk of infection for women after a single exposure to an infected man is 50%; the risk for men after exposure to an infected woman is approximately 20%. The incidence of infection increases with multiple sexual

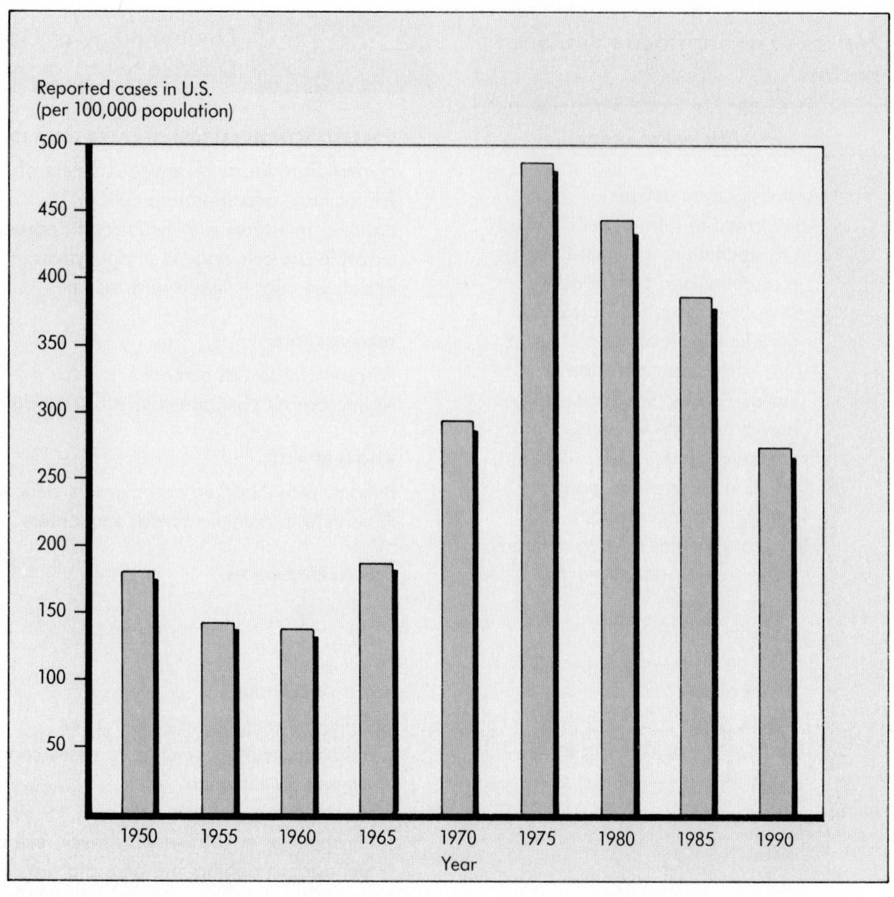

FIGURE 23-7 Gonorrhea in the United States from 1950 to 1990. (Data from *MMWR* 39:55-59, 1991).

encounters. Gonorrhea is more common in homosexual and bisexual men than in heterosexual men.

The major reservoir for the gonococcus is the asymptomatically infected individual. Determining a true incidence of asymptomatic infection is difficult. Although disease is more commonly diagnosed in men than in women (Figure 23-8), asymptomatic carriage is more common in women than in men. As many as half of all infected women have mild or asymptomatic infections, whereas most men are initially symptomatic. In untreated disease, however, the symptoms generally clear within a few weeks and asymptomatic carriage may become established. These carriers can transmit disease. Carriage is also influenced by the site of infection; rectal and pharyngeal infections are more commonly asymptomatic than are genital infections.

Clinical Syndromes

Genital infection in men is primarily restricted to the urethra. Purulent urethral discharge and dysuria develop after a 2- to 7-day incubation period. Approximately 95% of all infected men have acute symptoms. Although complications are rare, epididymitis, prostatitis, and periurethral abscesses can occur.

The primary site of infection in women is the cervix, although gonococci can be isolated in the vagina, urethra, and rectum. Vaginal discharge, dysuria, and abdominal pain are commonly reported in symptomatic patients. Ascending genital infection, including salpingitis, tubo-ovarian abscesses, and pelvic inflammatory disease (PID) are reported in 10% to 20% of women. Disseminated infections with septicemia and infection of skin and joints occurs in 1% to 3% of infections in women and in a much lower percentage of infected men. The increased proportion of disseminated infections in women is caused by the large number of untreated asymptomatic infections in this population (Box 23-4). Clinical manifestation of disseminated disease includes fever, migratory arthralgias, suppurative arthritis in the wrists, knees, and ankles, and a pustular rash on an erythematous base over the extremities but sparing the head and trunk. *N. gonorrhoeae* is a leading cause of purulent arthritis in adults.

Other diseases associated with *N. gonorrhoeae* include perihepatitis **(Fitz-Hugh-Curtis syndrome)**, purulent conjunctivitis (particularly in newborns infected during vaginal delivery **[ophthalmia neonatorum]**), anorectal gonorrhea in homosexual males, and pharyngitis.

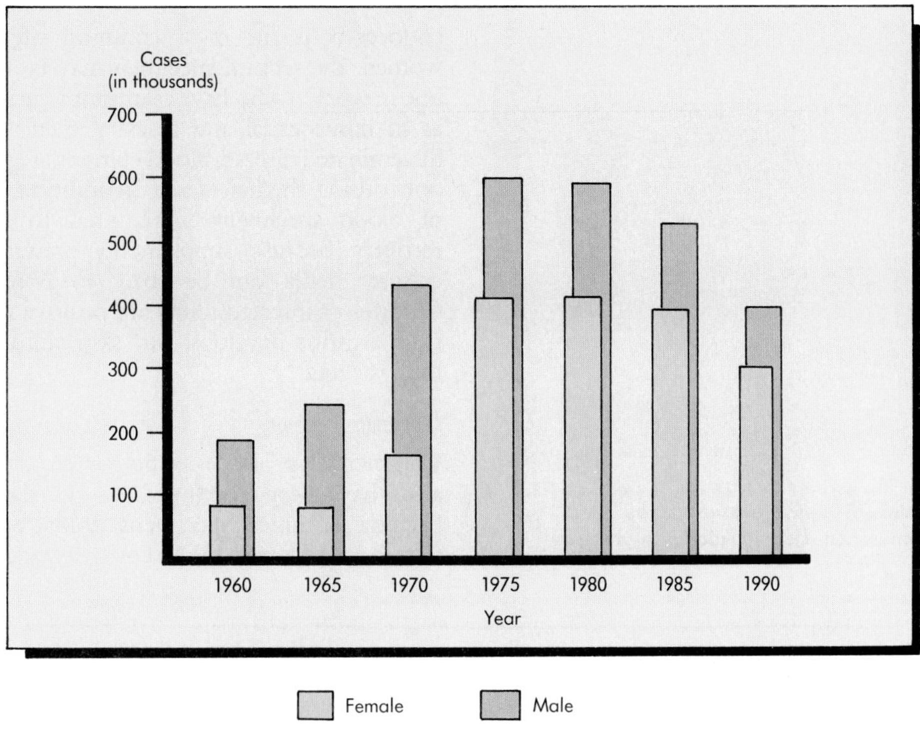

FIGURE 23-8 Incidence of gonorrhea by sex in the United States from 1960 to 1990. (Redrawn from *MMWR* 39:22, 1991).

Laboratory Diagnosis

Microscopy

The Gram stain is a very sensitive (greater than 90%) and specific (98%) test for the detection of gonococcal infection in men with purulent urethritis (Figure 23-9). However, the test sensitivity is 60% or less for asymptomatic men. The test is also relatively insensitive for detection of gonococcal cervicitis in both symptomatic and asymptomatic women, although a positive result is reliable when an experienced microscopist sees gram-negative diplococci within polymorphonuclear leukocytes. Thus the Gram stain can be reliably used to diagnose infections in men with purulent urethritis, but all negative results in women and asymptomatic men must be confirmed by culture. The Gram stain is useful early in the course of purulent arthritis but is insensitive for detection of *N. gonorrhoeae* in skin lesions, anorectal infections, and pharyngitis. The presence of commensal *Neisseria* in the oropharynx and morphologically similar bacteria in the gastrointestinal tract compromises the specificity of the stain for these specimens.

Culture

N. gonorrhoeae can be readily isolated from clinical specimens if appropriate precautions are followed (Figure 23-10). Because other commensal organisms normally colonize mucosal surfaces, all genital, rectal, and pharyngeal specimens must be inoculated onto both selective media (e.g., modified Thayer-Martin medium) and nonselective media (e.g., chocolate blood agar). The use of selective media suppresses the growth of contaminating organisms. However, a nonselective medium should also be inoculated because some gonococcal strains are inhibited by vancomycin present in most selective media. The organisms are also inhibited by the fatty acids and trace metals present in the peptone hydrolysates and agar in other common laboratory media (e.g., blood agar, nutrient agar). The gonococci are susceptible to desiccation and generally require an atmosphere of 5% carbon dioxide and incubation temperature of 35° C to 37° C for initial growth in culture. Drying and cold temperatures should be avoided by inoculating the specimen directly onto prewarmed media at the time of collection.

The endocervix must be properly exposed to ensure that an adequate specimen is collected. Although the

BOX 23-4 Characteristics of Disseminated *Neisseria gonorrhoeae* Infection

Patient	Primarily women
Initial infection	Usually asymptomatic genital infection
Site of dissemination	Blood, skin, joints
Strain characteristics	Resistant to serum killing; very susceptible to penicillin*; auxotrophic growth requirements for arginine, hypoxanthine, and uracil*

*Penicillin susceptibility and growth requirements may vary depending on the prevalent strain in the community.

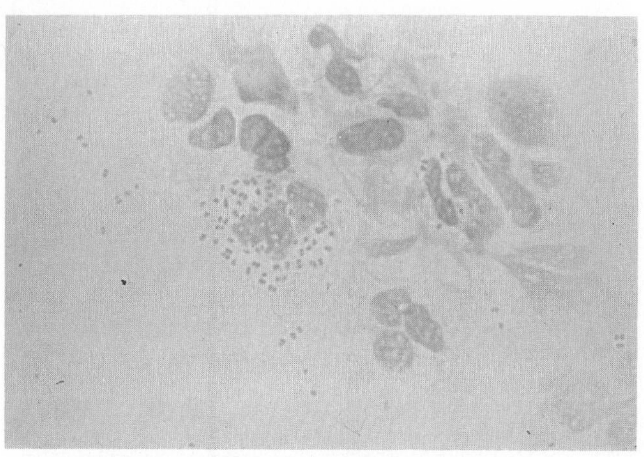

FIGURE 23-9 Gram stain of *Neisseria gonorrhoeae* associated with polymorphonuclear leukocytes in urethral discharge.

endocervix is the most common site of infection in women, the rectum specimen may be the only positive one in women who have asymptomatic infections, as well as in homosexual and bisexual men. In patients with disseminated disease, blood cultures are generally positive only during the first week. In addition, special handling of blood specimens is required to ensure adequate recovery because supplements present in the blood culture media can be toxic to *Neisseria* organisms. Cultures of infected joints are positive if collected at the time arthritis develops, but skin cultures are generally unrewarding.

Genetic Probes

Commercial probes specific for *N. gonorrhoeae* nucleic acids have been developed for the direct detection of bacteria in clinical specimens. Initial evaluations of the tests have reported high sensitivity and specificity. The

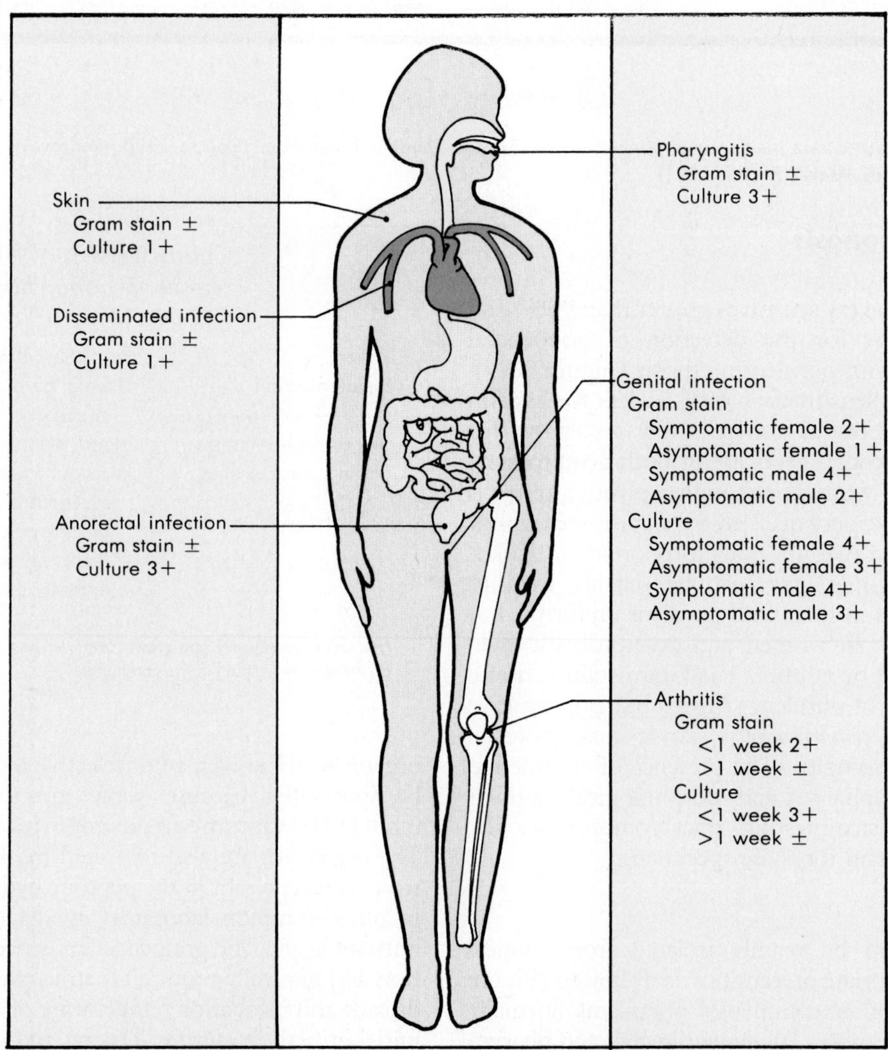

FIGURE 23-10 Laboratory detection of *Neisseria gonorrhoeae*. The reliability of the Gram stain is compromised when specimens are collected from sites such as the cervix, pharynx, or rectum that are contaminated with commensal *Neisseria* and morphologically similar organisms. Rapidly growing commensal organisms can also overgrow and obscure *N. gonorrhoeae*, unless selective media are used.

tests are rapid (2 hours or less) and particularly useful for initially treated patients or when delays in transport of specimens may compromise bacterial viability. These tests will likely become the test procedure of choice.

Serology

Although serologic tests have been developed to detect both gonococcal antigens and antibodies directed against the organism, these tests are neither sensitive nor specific and cannot be recommended.

Treatment, Prevention, and Control

Penicillin historically has been the treatment of choice. However, three changes have been observed. First, the concentration of penicillin required to inhibit growth of *N. gonorrhoeae* has steadily increased, necessitating significantly higher doses for clinical cures. The recommended therapeutic dose of penicillin G for uncomplicated gonorrhea has risen from 200,000 units in 1945 to 4.8 million units currently. Second, penicillin resistance mediated by enzymatic hydrolysis of the β-lactam ring was initially reported in Southeast Asia and now has worldwide distribution. The first β-lactamase producing *N. gonorrhoeae* in the United States was reported in March 1976. During the next 4 years relatively few new cases were detected and most were related to imported cases. However, since 1980 the number of resistant strains has risen rapidly (Figure 23-11), and the increase is not related to foreign travel. The genetic information for this resistance is encoded on a transmissible plasmid. Thus this increase in resistance should continue. Finally, strains of penicillin-resistant *N. gonorrhoeae* that do not produce β-lactamase have been isolated. This chromosomally mediated resistance is not limited to the penicillin antibiotics but also includes resistance to tetracyclines, erythromycin, and aminoglycosides. This resistance appears to be the result of changes on the cell surface that prevent antibiotic penetration into the gonococcal cell. Because the incidence of penicillin resistance is now relatively high, the Centers for Disease Control recommends ceftriaxone should be used as initial therapy for uncomplicated gonorrhea, combined with tetracycline to manage dual infections with *Chlamydia*.

Immunity to infections with *N. gonorrhoeae* is poorly understood. Antibodies can be detected to pili antigens, as well as to Protein I and the lipooligosaccharide. However, multiple infections in sexually promiscuous individuals are common. This lack of protective immunity is explained in part by the antigenic diversity of gonococcal strains. The variable region at the carboxy terminus of the pilin protein is the immunodominant portion of the molecule. Antibodies developed against this region protect against reinfection with a homologous strain, but cross-protection against heterologous strains is incomplete. This also explains the ineffectiveness of vaccines developed against pilin proteins.

Chemoprophylaxis is also ineffective, except in protection against gonococcal eye infections in newborns (ophthalmia neonatorum) in which 1% silver nitrate, 1% tetracycline, or 0.5% erythromycin eye ointments are

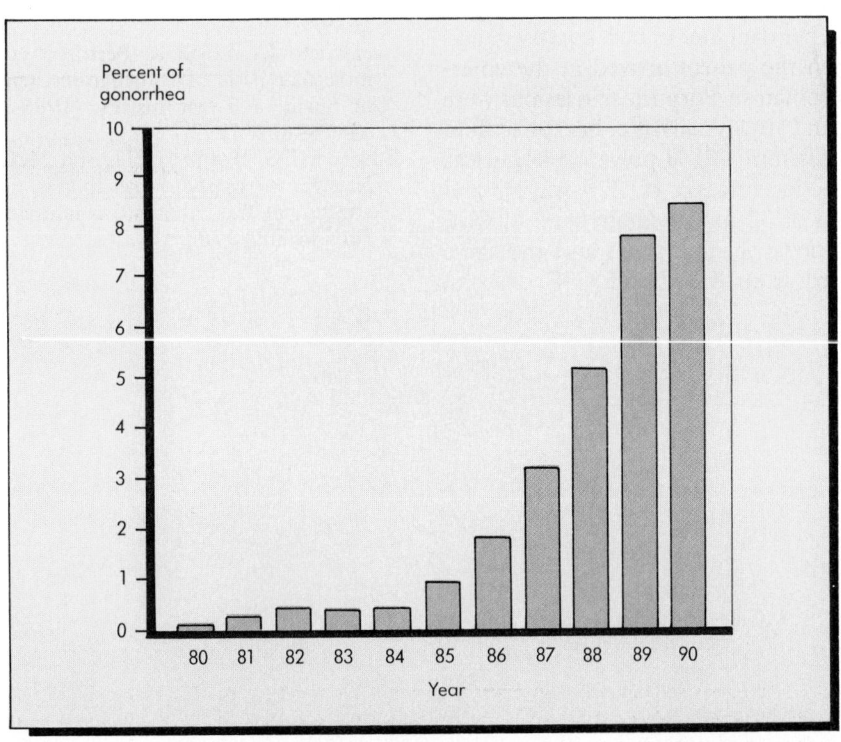

FIGURE 23-11 Cases of β-lactamase producing *Neisseria* gonorrhoeae isolated in the United States from 1980 to 1990. (Redrawn from *MMWR* 39:24, 1991).

routinely used. Prophylactic use of penicillin to prevent genital disease has been demonstrated to be ineffective and may select for resistant strains.

The major efforts to stem the epidemic of gonorrhea encompass education, aggressive documentation of disease by culture, and follow-up screening of sexual contacts. It is important to realize that gonorrhea is not an insignificant disease. Chronic infections can lead to sterility, and asymptomatic infections perpetuate the reservoir of disease and lead to a higher incidence of disseminated infections.

OTHER *NEISSERIA* SPECIES

Neisseria species such as *N. sicca* and *N. mucosa* are commensal organisms in the oropharynx and genital tract. These organisms are associated with isolated reports of meningitis, osteomyelitis, and endocarditis, as well as bronchopulmonary infections, acute otitis media, and acute sinusitis. The true incidence of respiratory infections caused by these organisms is not known because most specimens are contaminated with oral secretions. Most isolates of *N. sicca* and *N. mucosa* are susceptible to penicillin, although low-level resistance caused by altered penicillin binding protein (PBP 2) has been observed.

CASE STUDY AND QUESTIONS

A 22-year-old female school teacher entered the emergency room with a 2-day history of headache and fever. On the day of admission the woman failed to come to school. When the woman's mother went to her apartment, she found her daughter in bed, confused, and highly agitated. When the patient arrived in the emergency room, she was comatose. Purpuric skin lesions were present on her trunk and arms. Analysis of her spinal fluid demonstrated 380 cells/mm^3 (93% polymorphonuclear leukocytes), protein concentration of 220 mg/dl, and glucose concentration of 32 mg/dl. Gram stain of CSF showed many gram-negative diplococci, and the same organism was isolated from blood and CSF. Despite prompt initiation of therapy with penicillin, the patient expired.

1. What is the most likely organism responsible for this fulminant disease? What virulence factors could be responsible for this disease?
2. What is the most likely source of this organism? What should be done for the students in contact with this teacher?
3. What other diseases are caused by this organism?
4. What virulence factors have been associated with *Neisseria gonorrhoeae*? What is their mode of action?
5. What measures should be used to control infections with *Neisseria gonorrhoeae*?

Bibilography

Band JD, Chamberland ME, Platt T, Weaver RE, Thornsberry C, and Fraser DW: Trends in meningococcal disease in the United States, 1975-1980, *J Infect Dis* 148:754, 1983.

Campos J, Fuste MC, Trujillo G et al: Genetic diversity of penicillin-resistant *Neisseria meningitidis*, *J Infect Dis* 166:173-177, 1992.

DeVoe IW: The meningococcus and mechanisms of pathogenicity, *Microbiol Rev* 46:162, 1982.

Ellison RT, Kohler PF, Curd JG, Judson FN, and Reller LB: Prevalence of congenital or acquired complement deficiency in patients with sporadic meningococcal disease, *N Engl J Med* 308:913, 1983.

Feldman HA: The meningococcus: a twenty year perspective, *Rev Infect Dis* 8:288, 1986.

Hook EW and Holmes KK: Gonococcal infections, *Ann Intern Med* 102:229, 1985.

Morris SA, Broome CV, Cannon J et al: Perspectives on pathogenic Neisseriae, *Clin Microbiol Rev* 2(suppl):1-149, 1989.

Saez-Nieto JA, Lujan R, Berron S et al: Epidemiology and molecular basis of penicillin-resistant *Neisseria meningitidis* in Spain: a 5-year history (1985-1989), *Clin Infect Dis* 14:394-402, 1992.

Stephens DS, Hoffman LH, and McGee ZA: Interaction of *Neisseria meningitidis* with human nasopharyngeal mucosa: attachment and entry into columnar epithelial cells, *J Infect Dis* 148:369, 1983.

CHAPTER 24

Enterobacteriaceae

THE family Enterobacteriaceae is the largest, most heterogeneous collection of medically important gram-negative bacilli. At present, at least 27 genera and 102 species, as well as eight enteric groups (isolates with undefined genus affiliation), have been described (Table 24-1). These genera have been classified on the basis of DNA homology, biochemical properties, serologic reactions, susceptibility to genus-specific and species-specific bacteriophages, and antibiotic susceptibility patterns. The genetic relationship among the more common genera is illustrated in Figure 24-1. Despite the complexity of this family, more than 95% of medically important isolates belong to fewer than 25 species.

Enterobacteriaceae are ubiquitous organisms that are found worldwide in soil, water, vegetation and are part of the normal intestinal flora of most animals, including humans. Some members of the family (e.g., *Shigella, Salmonella, Yersinia pestis*) are always associated with disease when isolated from humans, whereas others (e.g., *Escherichia coli, Klebsiella pneumoniae, Proteus mirabilis*) are members of the normal commensal flora that can cause opportunistic infections. Infections can originate from an animal reservoir (e.g., most *Salmonella* infections), from a human carrier (e.g., *Shigella* and *Salmonella typhi*), or by endogenous spread of organisms in a susceptible patient (e.g., *Escherichia*), involving virtually all body sites (Figure 24-2). The Enterobacteriaceae are responsible for 30% to 35% of all septicemias, more than 70% of urinary tract infections, and many intestinal infections.

TABLE 24-1 Family Enterobacteriaceae

Genus	No. of species
Citrobacter	4
Edwardsiella	4
Enterobacter	13
Escherichia	5
Shigella	4
Ewingella	1
Hafnia	2
Klebsiella	7
Kluyvera	2
Morganella	2
Proteus	4
Providencia	5
Salmonella	7 subgroups
Serratia	10
Yersinia	11

Other genera included in the family Enterobacteriaceae are *Budvicia, Buttiauxella, Cedecea, Koserella, Leclercia, Leminorella, Moellerella, Obesumbacterium, Pragia, Rahnella, Tatumella, Xenorhabdus*, and eight enteric groups.

PHYSIOLOGY AND STRUCTURE

Members of this family are moderate-size (0.3-1.0 × 1.0-6.0 μm) gram-negative bacilli, usually motile with peritrichous flagella or nonmotile, and do not form spores. All members grow aerobically and anaerobically (facultative anaerobes), with growth observed generally after 18 to 24 hours of incubation on a variety of nonselective media (e.g., blood agar) and selective media (e.g., MacConkey agar). The Enterobacteriaceae have simple nutritional requirements, ferment glucose, reduce nitrate, and are catalase-positive and oxidase-negative. The absence of cytochrome oxidase activity is an important characteristic because it can be rapidly measured and used to distinguish the Enterobacteriaceae from many other fermentative and nonfermentative gram-negative bacilli.

Morphological characteristics on differential selective media have been used to identify members of the family Enterobacteriaceae. For example, the ability to ferment lactose has been exploited as a differential characteristic for separating lactose-fermenting strains (e.g., *Escherichia, Klebsiella, Enterobacter, Citrobacter, Serratia*) from strains that do not ferment lactose (e.g., *Salmonella, Shigella, Yersinia*). The red-colored colonies of lactose-fermenting organisms are readily differentiated on MacConkey agar (a selective medium commonly used for isolation of gram-negative bacilli) from the colorless non-lactose fermenting colonies. Resistance to bile salts present in some selective media has also been used to separate the enteric pathogens *Shigella* and *Salmonella* from commensal Enterobacteriaceae and other organisms present in the gastrointestinal tract. Some members of the family have prominent capsules (e.g., *Klebsiella*), whereas other strains are surrounded by a loose-fitting, diffusible slime layer.

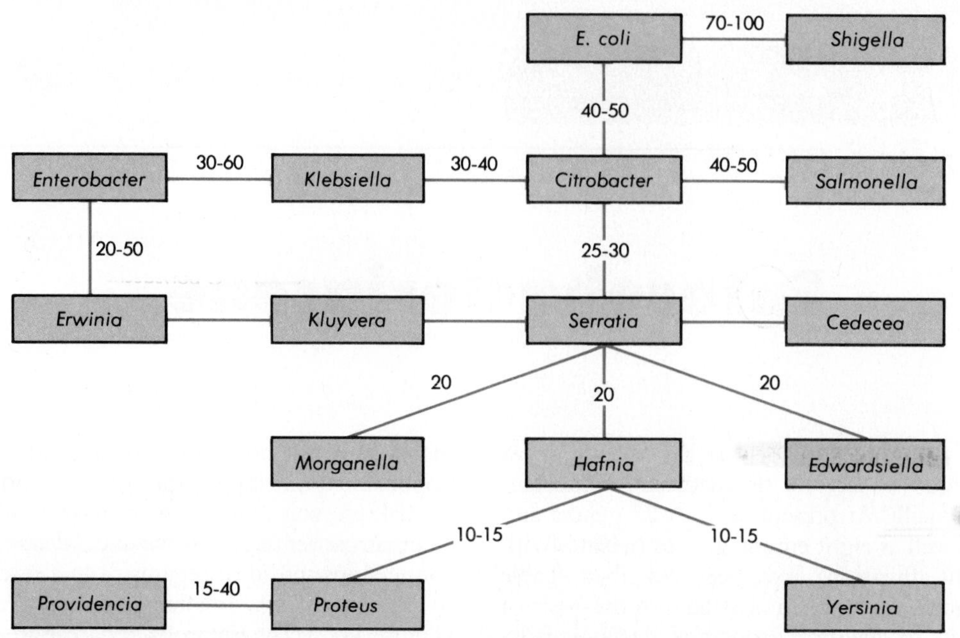

FIGURE 24-1 DNA relatedness among common Enterobacteriaceae. The numbers represent the approximate percentage of relatedness. (Redrawn from Krieg NR and Holt JG, editors: *Bergey's manual of systematic bacteriology*, vol 1, Baltimore, 1984, Williams & Wilkins.)

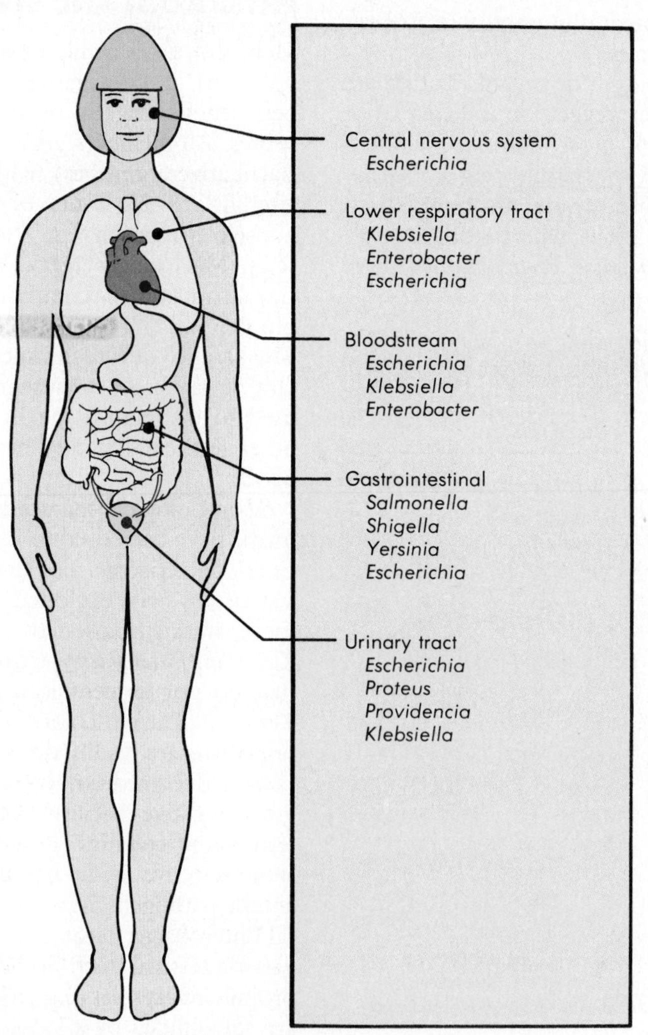

FIGURE 24-2 Sites of infections with members of the Enterobacteriaceae.

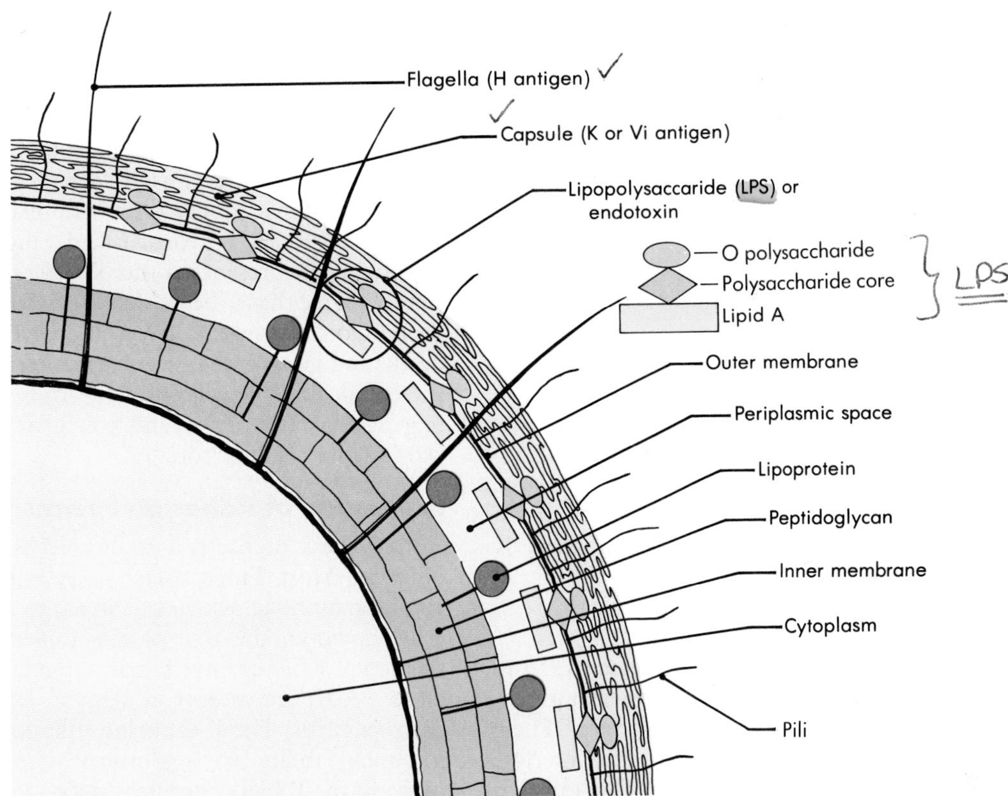

FIGURE 24-3 Antigenic structure of Enterobacteriaceae.

The serologic classification of Enterobacteriaceae is based on three major groups of antigens: somatic O lipopolysaccharides, capsular K antigens, and the flagellar H proteins (Figure 24-3). The heat-stable lipopolysaccharide (LPS) is the major cell wall antigen and consists of three components: the antigenically variable O polysaccharide, a core polysaccharide common to all Enterobacteriaceae (common antigen), and lipid A. Endotoxin activity is associated with the lipid A component of LPS. Specific O antigens are present in each genus, although cross-reactions between closely related genera are common (e.g., *Salmonella* with *Citrobacter; Escherichia* with *Shigella*). The antigens are detected by agglutination with specific antisera. The capsular K antigens are either protein or polysaccharides. The heat-labile K antigens may interfere with detection of the O antigens, necessitating the removal of the capsular antigen by boiling the suspension of organisms. The capsular antigen of *Salmonella typhi* is referred to as the Vi antigen. K antigens are shared by different genera both within and outside the family Enterobacteriaceae (e.g., *Escherichia coli* K1 cross-reacts with *Neisseria meningitidis* and *Haemophilus influenzae; Klebsiella pneumoniae* cross-reacts with *Streptococcus pneumoniae*). The H antigens are heat-labile, flagellar proteins. These can be absent from a cell or undergo antigenic variation and be present in two phases.

BOX 24-1 Virulence Factors Associated With Enterobacteriaceae

Endotoxin
Capsule
Antigenic phase variation
Exotoxin production
Expression of adhesion factors
Intracellular survival and multiplication
Sequestration of growth factors
Resistance to serum killing
Antimicrobial resistance

PATHOGENESIS AND IMMUNITY

Consistent with the large and diverse composition of the family Enterobacteriaceae is the observation of many virulence factors in the pathogenic strains (Box 24-1). The following is a summary of the more important factors.

Endotoxin

Endotoxin is a virulence factor shared among all aerobic and some anaerobic gram-negative bacteria. This toxicity

BOX 24-2 Endotoxin-Mediated Toxicity

Fever
Leukopenia followed by leukocytosis
Activation of complement
Thrombocytopenia
Disseminated intravascular coagulation
Decreased peripheral circulation and perfusion to major organs
Shock
Death

resides in the lipid A component of LPS, which is released upon cell death and lysis. Many of the systemic manifestations of gram-negative infections are initiated by endotoxin (Box 24-2).

Capsule

Encapsulated Enterobacteriaceae are protected from phagocytosis because the hydrophilic capsular antigens repel the hydrophobic phagocytic cell surface. These antigens also obscure cell wall antigens and thus interfere with antibody binding to the bacteria. The capsular antigens are also poor immunogens or activators of complement. However, when specific anticapsular antibodies develop, the protected role of the capsule is diminished.

Antigenic Phase Variation

Expression of capsular (K) and flagellar (H) antigens is under genetic control of the organism. Each of these antigens can be alternately expressed or not **(phase variation),** which can serve to protect bacteria from antibody mediated cell death.

Exotoxin Production

A number of important toxins have been identified in the Enterobacteriaceae, including **heat-stable** and **heat-labile enterotoxins**, **Shiga** and **Shiga-like** toxins, and **hemolysins**. The heat-labile enterotoxins, as well as Shiga and Shiga-like toxins, are A-B type toxins (i.e., they consist of an A subunit and one or more B subunits). The A subunit is responsible for the enzymatic, intracellular activity of the toxin, while the B subunit(s) mediates cell binding to facilitate intracellular transfer of the A subunit.

Heat-labile enterotoxin is virtually identical to cholera toxin (see Chapter 25). This toxin, produced primarily by *E. coli* and occasional isolates of *Klebsiella* and *Salmonella*, catalyzes the ADP ribosylation of the adenylate-cyclase regulatory protein, G_5. This leads to elevated levels of cyclic AMP and subsequent altered electrolyte transport with a resultant secretory diarrhea. The heat-stable toxin, present in *E. coli* and occasional *Yersinia enterocolitica* and *Citrobacter freundii*, is a small molecular weight protein extensively cross-linked with disulfide bonds that impart heat stability. This toxin also stimulates a secretory diarrhea by increasing cyclic activation of guanylate cyclase. *Shigella dysenteriae* produces Shiga toxin, which in animal models has been demonstrated to be neurotoxic, enterotoxic, and cytotoxic. The role this toxin plays in human disease, however, is ill defined. The toxin inhibits protein synthesis by the enzymatic inactivation of 60S ribosomes. Related toxins, called Shiga-like toxins or verotoxins, are present in other *Shigella* species and *E. coli*. These toxins have been demonstrated to produce a pronounced cytopathic effect in tissue culture, mouse death, and gastrointestinal toxicity. Hemolysins are also present in many species and can cause cell destruction (e.g., lysis of erythrocytes and leukocytes) and increase the extracellular pool of iron.

Expression of Adhesion Factors

Adhesiveness of bacteria to host cells is mediated by fimbriae. Most Enterobacteriaceae express the Type I common fimbriae, which can attach to a number of host cells; however, the role of this molecule in disease is unknown. Colonization factor antigen fimbriae (CFA/I and CFA/II) are present in many *E. coli* responsible for gastroenteritis. The **P fimbriae** adhesion factors, named for their ability to agglutinate human erythrocytes carrying the P blood group antigen, are associated with uropathogenic *E. coli*. Finally, the **S fimbriae** (bind to sialyl galactosides on human erythrocytes) are commonly associated with *E. coli* responsible for neonatal sepsis and meningitis. Phase variation of all fimbrial antigens protects the bacteria from immune-mediated clearance.

Intracellular Survival and Multiplication

Intracellular survival has the obvious benefit of protecting the bacteria from many antibiotics and the patient's immune reaction. *Shigella*, *Salmonella*, enteroinvasive *E. coli*, and *Yersinia* are facultative intracellular parasites (i.e., these organisms can invade and multiply inside cells but do not require intracellular host factors for survival). *Shigella* enters the colonic epithelium through bacterial-directed endocytosis. The genetic controls for this process are encoded in the *Shigella* chromosome, as well as a 220-kb virulence plasmid. Similar to the phagocytic process of *Listeria*, actin filaments in the host cell are mobilized to facilitate the phagocytosis of *Shigella*. After internalization, the bacteria rapidly escape from the phagocytic vacuole and initiate replication, leading to the eventual lysis of the host cell and spread to adjoining cells. Polymerization of actin filaments at the late stages of this replicative cycle coordinates the migration of bacteria from one cell to another.

Enteroinvasive pathogenic *E. coli* are very closely related to *Shigella* on the taxonomic scale. Likewise, the process of invasion, replication, and spread in colonic epithelium is believed to be similar. *Salmonella* has adopted a different mechanism of intracellular survival. *Salmonella* initiates uptake by binding to apical microvilli of epithelial cells. This induces rearrangement of host cell actin filaments, which form at the site of uptake. Regulation of this uptake process is genetically complicated, involving at least six bacterial genes. On entry into the host cell, the bacteria remain in the phagocytic vacuole and replicate; this process is possible because phagosome-lysosome fusion is blocked by the bacteria. *Yersinia* species can also resist phagosome-lysosome fusion and multiply inside the phagocytic vacuole.

Sequestration of Growth Factors

In contrast with in vitro growth of organisms in enriched media, in vivo growth forces the bacteria to be nutritional scavengers. Iron is an important growth factor required by bacteria, but it is bound in heme-proteins (e.g., hemoglobin, myoglobin) or in iron-chelating proteins (e.g., transferrin, lactoferrin). The bacteria counter this by producing their own competitive iron-chelating compounds—the siderophores enterobactin and aerobactin. Iron can also be released from host cells by production of hemolysins.

Resistance to Serum Killing

Whereas many bacteria can be rapidly cleared from the bloodstream, virulent organisms capable of producing systemic infections are frequently resistant to serum killing. Although this can be mediated by capsule formation, other poorly defined factors prevent binding of complement components to the bacteria and complement-mediated immune clearance.

Antimicrobial Resistance

As rapidly as new antibiotics are introduced, organisms are able to develop resistance. This process can be dramatically illustrated by examining the speed with which resistant strains of bacteria can develop following exposure to an antibiotic. The spread of this resistance is also a significant problem because resistance can be encoded on transferable plasmids and exchanged among species, genera, and even families of bacteria.

ESCHERICHIA COLI

Epidemiology

The genus *Escherichia* consists of five species, with *Escherichia coli* the most frequently isolated (Box 24-3). Large numbers of *E. coli* are present in the gastrointestinal tract and are the Enterobacteriaceae most frequently associated with bacterial sepsis, neonatal meningitis, infections of the urinary tract, and gastroenteritis in travelers to countries with poor hygiene. Most infections (with the exception of neonatal meningitis and gastroenteritis) are endogenous (i.e., the individual's normal microbial flora is able to establish infection under conditions in which the host defenses are compromised).

The antigenic composition of *E. coli* is complex, with a very large number of O, H, and K antigens described. The serologic classification of *E. coli* isolates is useful for epidemiologic purposes, and specific serotypes are associated with increased virulence.

BOX 24-3 Epidemiology of *E. coli* Infection

DISEASE/BACTERIAL FACTORS

Septicemia, urinary tract infections, neonatal meningitis, gastroenteritis
Present in soil, water, vegetation, and part of normal GI flora
Numerous virulence factors (see Box 24-1)

TRANSMISSION

Endogenous spread in susceptible patients
Ingestion of contaminated food or water
Nosocomial infection

WHO IS AT RISK?

Individuals at risk for developing urinary tract infections (in community or hospital)
Individuals with intestinal perforation
Hospitalized patients at increased risk for nosocomial infections
Travelers to countries with poor hygiene standards

GEOGRAPHY/SEASON

Worldwide
No seasonal incidence

MODES OF CONTROL

Treatment with antibiotics demonstrating in vitro activity
Appropriate hospital control of nosocomial infections
Improved hygiene

Clinical Syndromes

Septicemia

E. coli is the most common gram-negative bacillus isolated from septic patients (Figure 24-4). The focus of infection from which the organisms spread into the bloodstream is commonly either the urinary tract or the gastrointestinal tract. The mortality associated with *E. coli* septicemia is influenced by the source of infection and the underlying disease of the patient, with a significantly higher incidence of death in immunocompromised patients or with infections originating from intestinal perforation.

Urinary Tract Infections

E. coli is responsible for more than 80% of all community-acquired urinary tract infections and the majority of hospital-acquired infections. Infecting strains originate from the gastrointestinal tract, with disease associated with specific serotypes, primarily O4, O6, and O75. The ability of these bacteria to resist killing in serum, produce hemolysins, and bind to uroepithelial cells is associated with increased virulence.

Neonatal Meningitis

E. coli, together with group B streptococci, is the most common cause of neonatal meningitis; 75% of these strains possess the K1 capsular antigen. Although colonization of infants with *E. coli* at the time of delivery is common, disease is relatively infrequent.

Gastroenteritis

Strains of *E. coli* that cause gastroenteritis are subdivided into five groups: enterotoxigenic, enteroinvasive, enteropathogenic, enterohemorrhagic, and enteroaggregative (Table 24-2).

Gastroenteritis produced by **enterotoxigenic *E. coli* (ETEC)** is mediated by heat-labile and heat-stable enterotoxins described previously. The production of both toxins is plasmid mediated, and maximum virulence is associated with specific adhesive pili: K88 in piglets, K99 in calves, and **colonization factors CFA/I and CFA/II** in humans. Secretory diarrhea caused by ETEC follows a 1- to 2-day incubation period and persists for an average of 3 to 4 days. Symptoms are characteristically mild, with cramps, nausea, vomiting, and watery diarrhea. Disease mediated by either toxin is indistinguishable. Toxin production is not associated with specific serotypes, so detection of toxigenic strains requires tissue culture or animal model assays for toxin activity. Nucleic acid probes have also been used to detect the toxin genes. Disease caused by these pathogenic *E. coli* is rarely observed in the United States.

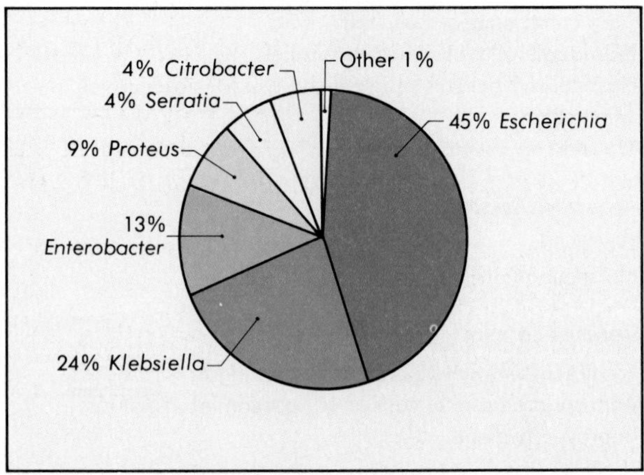

FIGURE 24-4 Enterobacteriaceae associated with bacteremia. (Data courtesy Barnes Hospital, St. Louis.)

Enteroinvasive *E. coli* (EIEC) are able to invade and destroy the colonic epithelium, producing a disease characterized by fever and cramps, with blood and leukocytes in stool specimens. Disease has been associated with specific O serotypes of *E. coli*; however, serologic classification of isolates cannot reliably identify invasive strains. Invasiveness must be confirmed by the **Sereny test**, in which EIEC inoculated into the eye of a guinea pig causes keratoconjunctivitis.

Enteropathogenic *E. coli* (EPEC) are historically important agents of childhood diarrhea, particularly in impoverished countries. Although specific O serotypes have been associated with nursery outbreaks of EPEC diarrhea, serotyping *E. coli* isolated in random or endemic disease is discouraged except in epidemiologic investigations. Disease is caused by the ability of the organism to adhere to the enterocyte plasma membrane and cause destruction of the adjacent microvilli. Thus these strains

TABLE 24-2 Gastroenteritis Caused by *Escherichia coli*

Organism	Site of action	Disease	Pathogenesis
Enterotoxigenic *E. coli* (ETEC)	Small intestine	Traveler's diarrhea; infant diarrhea in underdeveloped countries; watery diarrhea, cramps, nausea, low-grade fever	Heat-stable and/or heat-labile enterotoxins; stimulate guanylate or adenylate cyclase activity with fluid and electrolyte loss
Enteroinvasive *E. coli* (EIEC)	Large intestine	Fever, cramping, watery diarrhea followed by development of dysentery with scant, bloody stools	Plasmid-mediated invasion and destruction of epithelial cells lining colon
Enteropathogenic *E. coli* (EPEC)	Small intestine	Infant diarrhea with fever, nausea, vomiting, nonbloody stools	Plasmid-mediated adherence and destruction of epithelial cells
Enterohemorrhagic *E. coli* (EHEC)	Large intestine	Hemorrhagic colitis with severe abdominal cramps, watery diarrhea initially, followed by grossly bloody diarrhea, little or no fever; hemolytic uremic syndrome (HUS)	Mediated by cytotoxic "verotoxin"
Enteroaggregative *E. coli* (EAggEC)	Small intestine	Persistent infant diarrhea, sometimes with gross blood, low-grade fever	Aggregative adherence mediated by 60 MDa plasmid

have also been called **enteroadherent E. coli**. Two adhesion molecules have been characterized: one encoded on the bacterial chromosome and the other plasmid-mediated. Some strains also produce a Shiga-like toxin.

Enterohemorrhagic *E. coli* (EHEC) produce a Shiga-like toxin also called **verotoxin**, which was so named because the toxin causes a cytopathic effect in the Vero cell line of tissue culture cells. Two verotoxins have been described in EHEC: one homologous to *Shigella dysenteriae* toxin except for a single amino acid substitution in the A subunit; the other toxin with 60% homology to the *Shigella* toxin. The range of disease caused by EHEC varies from mild uncomplicated diarrhea to hemorrhagic colitis with severe abdominal pain, bloody diarrhea, and little or no fever. **Hemolytic uremic syndrome** (acute renal failure, thrombocytopenia, and microangiopathic hemolytic anemia) is also associated with this organism. Serologic classification of isolates has limited usefulness; however, approximately half of EHEC strains are serotype O157:H7. Disease is most prevalent in the warm months of the year, with the greatest incidence in children younger than 5 years of age. Most cases of epidemic and endemic disease have been attributed to consumption of undercooked ground beef or other beef products, as well as unpasteurized milk.

Enteroaggregative *E. coli* (EAggEC), originally called enteroadherent *E. coli*, have been implicated as a cause of persistent diarrhea in infants in developing countries. The bacteria are characterized by their D-mannose resistant aggregative adherence pattern to HEp-2 tissue culture cells. Expression of the aggregative pattern is mediated by a 60 MDa plasmid.

SALMONELLA

The taxonomic classification of the genus *Salmonella* has been fraught with problems, with more than 1500 unique serotypes of *Salmonella* described. Careful analysis of DNA homology reveals that the genus consists of a single species subdivided into seven subgroups. Although the single species designation (*Salmonella enterica*) has been recommended, this taxonomically correct approach has not been widely adopted. Most authorities continue to use the conventional approach of designating the serotype epithet as the species name.

Epidemiology

Salmonella are found in virtually all animals, including poultry, reptiles, livestock, rodents, domestic animals, birds, and humans (Box 24-4). An animal reservoir is maintained by animal-to-animal spread and the use of *Salmonella*-contaminated animal feeds. Serotypes such as *Salmonella typhi* and *Salmonella paratyphi* are highly adapted to man and do not cause disease in nonhuman hosts. Other *Salmonella* strains are adapted to animals and, when they infect humans, can cause severe human disease (e.g., *Salmonella choleraesuis*). Finally, many strains have no host specificity and cause disease in both human and nonhuman hosts.

The source of most infections is ingestion of contaminated water or food products or direct fecal-oral spread in children. The peak incidence of disease is in young children infected during the warm months of the year when consumption of contaminated food such as egg salad can occur at outdoor social gatherings. The most common sources of human infections are poultry, eggs, and dairy products. Interestingly, the outside surface of eggs, as well as the yolk, can be contaminated with the bacteria. Thus consumption of foods with undercooked or raw eggs substantially increases the risk of infection. Approximately 50,000 cases of *Salmonella* infections are reported annually, although this probably represents only 10% of all human infections (Figure 24-5). The most common incidence of salmonellosis is in children, particularly those younger than 1 year of age, and infections are most severe in the very young and the elderly.

Salmonella typhi is spread by ingestion of food or water contaminated by infected food handlers. In contrast with other *Salmonella* infections, approximately 500 *S. typhi*

BOX 24-4 Epidemiology of *Salmonella* Infection

DISEASE/BACTERIAL FACTORS

Enteritis, septicemia, enteric fever, asymptomatic carriage
Animals are main reservoir of human disease except for bacteria responsible for typhoid and paratyphoid fevers
Numerous virulence factors (see Box 24-1)

TRANSMISSION

Ingestion of contaminated food products (especially poultry, eggs, dairy products)
Direct fecal-oral spread in children

WHO IS AT RISK?

Anyone consuming foods contaminated with large numbers of *Salmonella*, particularly children younger than 1 year old, elderly, patients with reduced gastric acids, and patients with AIDS
S. typhi: foreign travelers or individuals exposed to carriers

GEOGRAPHY/SEASON

Worldwide
More common in warm months

MODES OF CONTROL

Symptomatic treatment rather than antibiotics
Proper preparation and refrigeration of foods
Improved hygiene

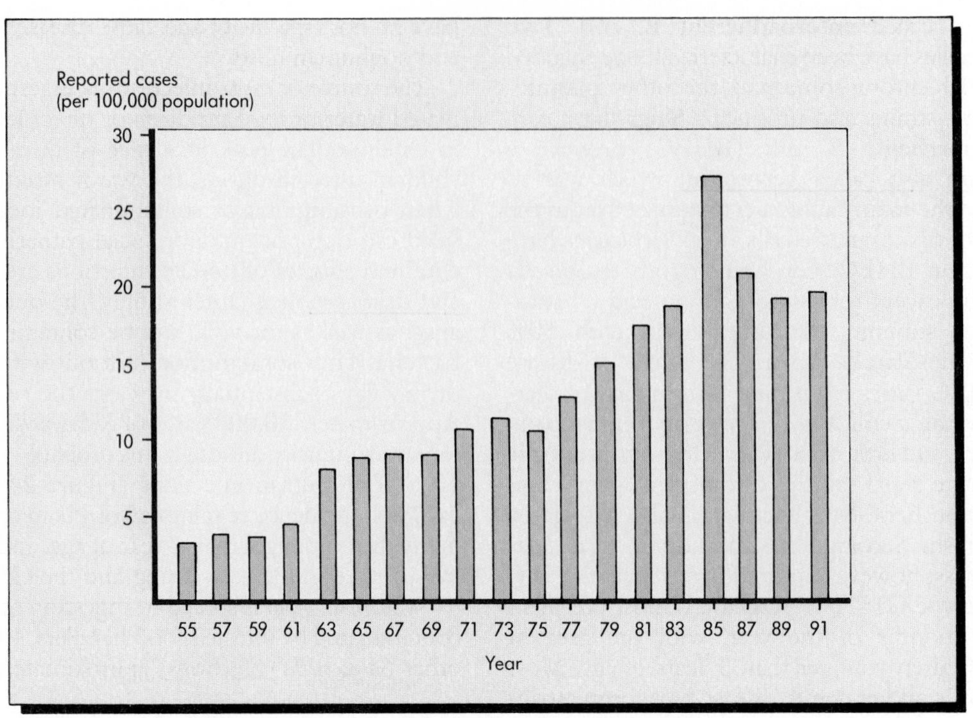

FIGURE 24-5 Annual reported incidence of *Salmonella* infection (excluding typhoid fever) in the United States from 1955 to 1990. (Redrawn from *MMWR*, 39:38, 1991.)

infections occur annually in the United States, with the majority associated with foreign travel.

Although exposure to *Salmonella* is frequent, a large inoculum (10^{6-8} bacteria) is required for the development of symptomatic disease. Disease occurs when the organism has an opportunity to multiply to a high density, such as in improperly refrigerated contaminated food products. The infectious dose is reduced for individuals at increased risk for disease because of age, immunosuppression or underlying disease (leukemia, lymphoma, sickle cell disease), or reduced gastric acidity.

Clinical Syndromes

Salmonella infections occur in one of four forms: enteritis, bacteremia, enteric fever, and asymptomatic colonization.

Enteritis

This is the most common form of salmonellosis (Figure 24-6). Symptoms generally appear 6 to 48 hours after consumption of the contaminated food or water, with the initial presentation of nausea, vomiting, and nonbloody diarrhea. Elevated temperature, abdominal cramps, myalgias, and headache are also common. Colonic involvement can be demonstrated in the acute form of disease. Symptoms can persist from 2 days to 1 week before spontaneous resolution.

Septicemia

All *Salmonella* can cause bacteremia, although infections with *S. choleraesuis, S. paratyphi, S. typhi,* and *S. dublin* more frequently lead to a bacteremic phase. Pediatric and geriatric patients, as well as AIDS patients, are at increased risk of developing *Salmonella* bacteremia. The clinical presentation of *Salmonella* bacteremia is like other gram-negative bacteremias. However, localized suppurative infections such as osteomyelitis, endocarditis, or arthritis can occur in as many as 10% of the patients.

Enteric Fever

S. typhi produces a febrile illness referred to as **typhoid fever**. A mild form of this disease, referred to as **paratyphoid fever**, is produced by *S. paratyphi A, S. schottmuelleri* (formerly *S. paratyphi B*), and *S. hirschfeldii* (formerly *S. paratyphi C*). After a 10- to 14-day incubation period following ingestion of the bacilli, the patient has a gradually increasing remittent fever with nonspecific complaints of headache, myalgias, malaise, and anorexia. These symptoms persist for a week or more and are followed by gastrointestinal symptoms. This cycle corresponds to an initial bacteremic phase followed by reinfection of the intestines (Figure 24-7).

Asymptomatic Carriage

The salmonella responsible for typhoid and paratyphoid fevers are maintained by human carriage. Chronic carriage for more than 1 year after symptomatic disease will develop in 1% to 5% of patients, with the gall bladder the reservoir in most patients. Chronic carriage with other *Salmonella* occurs in less than 1% of patients and does not represent a significant source of human infection.

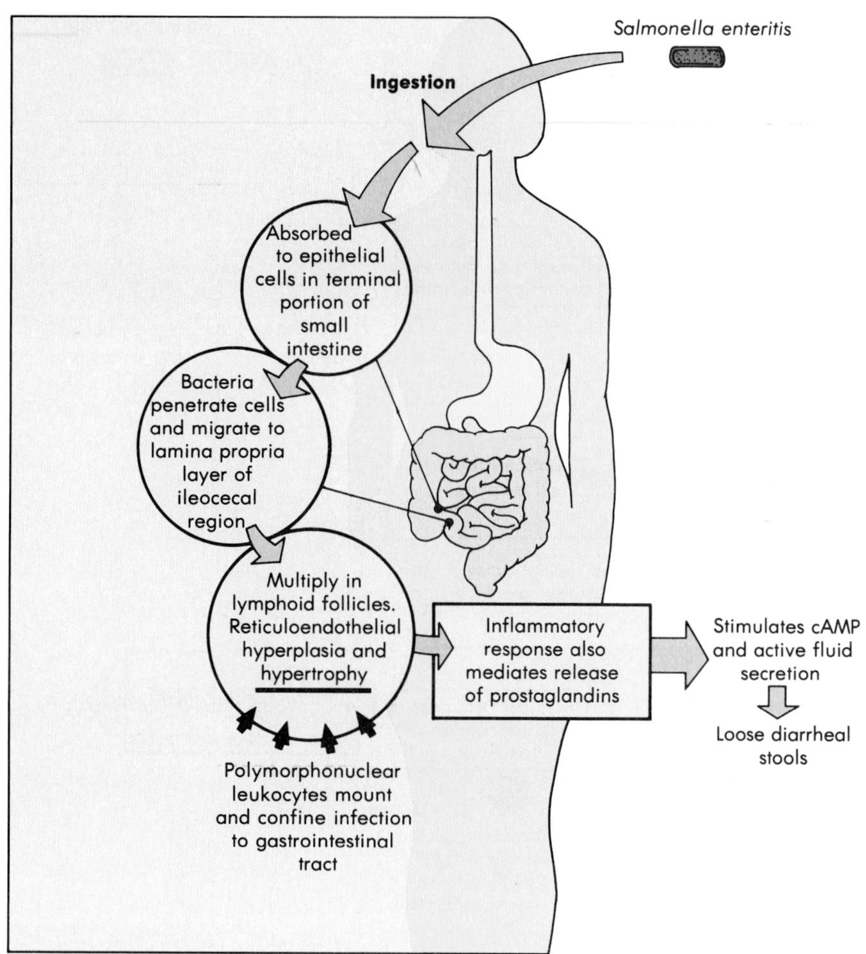

FIGURE 24-6 Gastroenteritis is the most common manifestation of *Salmonella* infection. After passage through the stomach, the bacteria absorb to the brush border of the epithelial cells lining the terminal small intestine and the colon. The bacteria migrate to the lamina propria layer, where they multiply in the lymphoid follicles, stimulating a leukocytic response. Stimulation of prostaglandin-mediated production of cyclic AMP and active fluid secretion also occurs.

SHIGELLA

Epidemiology

Unlike the genus *Salmonella*, the taxonomic classification of *Shigella* is quite simple (Box 24-5). Four species, consisting of approximately 38 O-antigen–based serotypes, have been described: *Shigella dysenteriae*, *Shigella flexneri*, *Shigella boydii*, and *Shigella sonnei*. *Shigella sonnei* is the most common cause of shigellosis in the industrial world, and *Shigella flexneri* is the most common in underdeveloped countries. More than 27,000 cases of *Shigella* were reported in the United States in 1990; however, this number greatly underestimates the true incidence of infection. Shigellosis is primarily a pediatric disease, with most infections in children from 6 months to 10 years of age. Endemic disease in adults is frequently due to contact with infected children. Infections in male homosexuals are also observed. Epidemic outbreaks of disease are associated with day-care centers, nurseries, and custodial institutions. Shigellosis is transmitted by the fecal-oral route, primarily by contaminated hands and less commonly in water or food. Bacilli can remain viable in contaminated water for as long as 6 months. In contrast to *Salmonella* infections, food-borne disease is uncommon. Because as few as 200 bacilli can establish disease, shigellosis spreads rapidly in communities where sanitary standards and the level of personal hygiene are low.

Clinical Syndrome

Shigellosis is characterized by abdominal cramps, diarrhea, fever, and bloody stools. Clinical signs and symptoms of shigellosis appear 1 to 3 days after the bacilli are ingested. The bacilli colonize the small intestine and begin to multiply within the first 12 hours. The initial sign of infection, profuse watery diarrhea without histologic evidence of mucosal invasion, is mediated by an enterotoxin. However, the cardinal feature of shigellosis is lower abdominal cramps and tenesmus, with abundant pus and

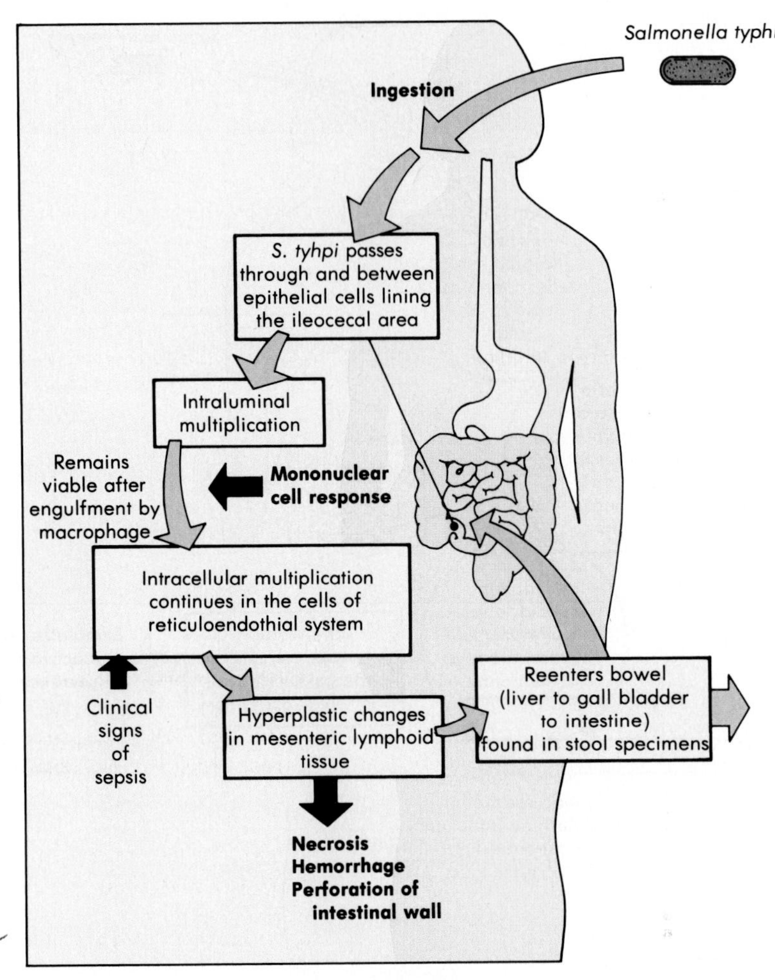

FIGURE 24-7 Pathogenesis of enteric fever. After ingestion of bacilli, *S. typhi* passes through the epithelial cells lining the terminal portion of the small intestine and the colon. The bacilli are engulfed by macrophages and then are carried to the cells of the reticuloendothelial system, where multiplication continues in the liver, spleen, and bone marrow. Signs of sepsis are seen after a 10- to 14-day incubation period. The bacilli will spread from the liver through the gall bladder and into the intestines. This stimulates gastrointestinal symptoms.

blood in the stool. This results from invasion of the colonic mucosa by the bacilli, destruction of the superficial mucosal layer, and production of mucosal ulcerations. Abundant neutrophils, erythrocytes, and mucus are found in the stool. The bacilli rarely penetrate beyond the mucosal layer, and bacteremia is uncommon. Infection is generally self-limited, although antibiotic treatment is recommended to reduce the risk of secondary spread to family members and other contacts. Asymptomatic carriage of the organism in the colon develops in a small number of patients and can represent a persistent reservoir for infection in a community.

YERSINIA

The genus *Yersinia* consists of seven species, of which *Yersinia pestis*, *Yersinia pseudotuberculosis*, and *Yersinia enterocolitica* are the best-known human pathogens. The other species can occasionally cause opportunistic human disease. Because the clinical presentation of *Y. pestis* is distinct, it will be considered separately.

Yersinia pestis

In contrast with other *Yersinia* species, growth of *Y. pestis* requires the presence of amino acids (e.g., L-methionine, L-phenylalanine, L-isoleucine, L-valine, and L-threonine), which limits the organism's ability to survive independently in nature. Virulence of *Y. pestis* is multifactorial and includes adaptation to intracellular survival, presence of a protein-polysaccharide capsule that is antiphagocytic (called fraction 1 antigen), production of an exotoxin (adrenergic antagonist) and endotoxin (as with other gram-negative bacteria), ability to absorb organic iron (by a siderophore-independent mechanism), and the presence of coagulase and fibrinolysin. The ability of the bacteria to cause disseminated infections is encoded on a 10-kd

BOX 24-5 Epidemiology of *Shigella* Infection

DISEASE/BACTERIAL FACTORS

Shigellosis
Numerous virulence factors (see Box 24-1)

TRANSMISSION

Person to person; primarily fecal-oral by contaminated hands
Consumption of contaminated food or water less important

WHO IS AT RISK?

Anyone exposed to carrier, particularly young children or those in day-care centers, nurseries, custodial institutions
Male homosexuals
Communities with poor sanitation and hygiene

GEOGRAPHY/SEASON

Worldwide
No seasonal incidence

MODES OF CONTROL

Antibiotic therapy used to decrease number of organisms and duration of carriage in symptomatic patients (thus reducing person-to-person spread)
Infection control procedures: hand washing, disposal of soiled linens

BOX 24-6 Epidemiology of *Yersinia* Infection

DISEASE/BACTERIAL FACTORS

Y. pestis: plague
Y. enterocolitica: enterocolitis, transfusion-related septicemia
Y. pseudotuberculosis: enterocolitis
Y. pestis: present in animal reservoir, fleas
Other *Yersinia:* present in domestic animals (GI tract) and contaminated food products
Numerous virulence factors (see Box 24-1)

TRANSMISSION

Y. pestis: spread from mammalian reservoir (rats, prairie dogs, dogs, mice, rabbits) via fleas or contact with contaminated animal tissues
Other *Yersinia:* ingestion of contaminated food products, infusion of contaminated blood products

WHO IS AT RISK?

Y. pestis: communities with endemic plague and exposure to infected animals
Y. enterocolitica: individuals eating contaminated food, recipients of contaminated blood products

GEOGRAPHY/SEASON

Y. pestis: primarily Asia and Africa
Y. pestis disease is cyclical, as reservoir population increases/decreases
Other *Yersinia:* infections worldwide but primarily in cold climates

MODES OF CONTROL

Y. pestis: control of rodent vector and improved hygiene vaccination, chemoprophylaxis
Y. enterocolitica: proper food preparation

plasmid (Pst plasmid); a 70-kd plasmid (Lcr or low calcium response plasmid) mediates the organism's requirement for calcium, which is believed to be important for the organism's intracellular survival; a 100-kd plasmid encodes for the fraction 1 antigen and exotoxin.

Epidemiology

One of the most devastating diseases in history was caused by *Yersinia pestis* (Box 24-6). During a 5-year period in the middle of the fourteenth century, epidemic plague (the "Black Death") claimed 25 million people—almost one fourth of the European population. Epidemics continued through the beginning of the twentieth century, and sporadic infections are still reported primarily from Asia and Africa. From 1950 through 1991, 336 cases of plague were reported in the United States (Figure 24-8); 13 states in the western United States reported disease, with 90% of the infections in New Mexico (56%), Arizona (14%), California (10%), and Colorado (10%).

Y. pestis infections are maintained in two epidemiologic forms: **urban plague,** the disease that was so devastating in the Middle Ages, and **sylvatic plague,** the disease that persists today in many countries, including the United States. Urban plague is maintained in rat populations and spread between rats or from rats to humans by infected fleas. Fleas become infected during a blood meal from a bacteremic rat. Following replication of the bacteria in the flea gut, the organisms can be transferred to another rodent or accidentally to humans. With effective control of rats and better hygiene, urban plague has been eliminated from most communities. In contrast, sylvatic plague will be difficult or impossible to eliminate because the mammalian reservoirs (prairie dogs, mice, rabbits, rats) and flea vectors are widespread. *Y. pestis* produces a fatal infection in the animal reservoir. Thus cyclic patterns of human disease are observed as the opportunity for contact with the reservoir population increases or decreases. Infections can also be acquired by ingestion of contaminated animals (by rodents, domestic cats or dogs, etc.) or handling contaminated animal tissues. Although the organism is highly infectious,

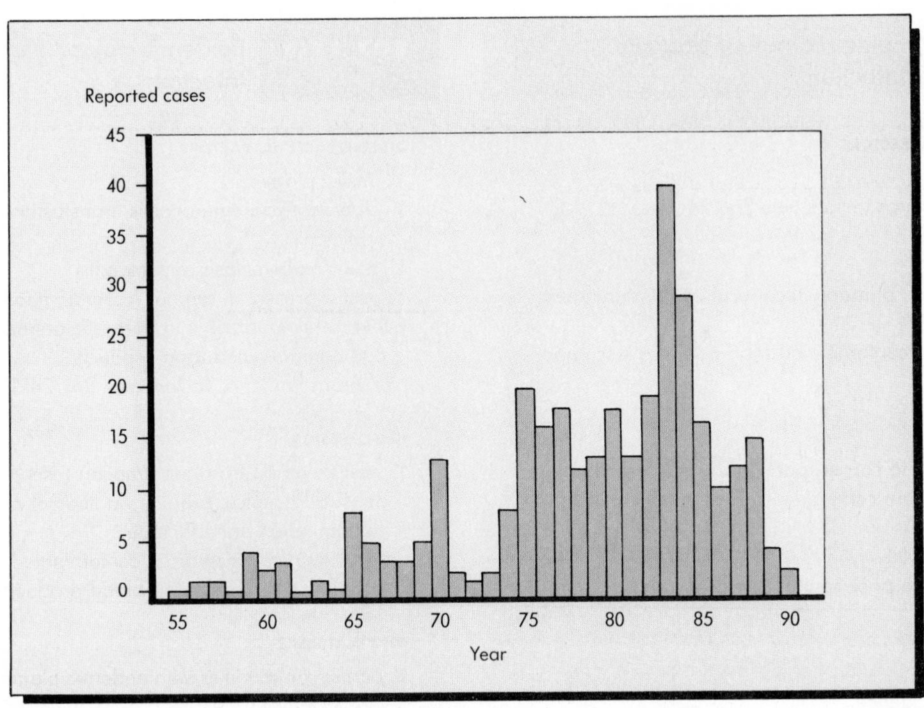

FIGURE 24-8 Annual incidence of *Yersinia pestis* infections (plague) in the United States from 1955 to 1990. (Redrawn from *MMWR* 39:35, 1991.)

human-to-human spread is uncommon unless the patient has pulmonary involvement.

Clinical Syndromes

Two forms of *Y. pestis* infections have been observed: bubonic plague and pneumonic plague. **Bubonic plague** is characterized by an incubation period of 7 days or less after a bite from an infected flea. Patients will have a high fever and a painful bubo (inflammatory swelling of lymph node) in the groin or axilla. In the absence of treatment patients will rapidly progress to bacteremia and as many as 75% will die. This was the form of plague that was so common during the pandemic of the Middle Ages. Patients with the second form of *Y. pestis* infection, **pneumonic plague,** experience a shorter incubation period (2 to 3 days), initially have fever and malaise, and then develop pulmonary signs within 1 day. The fatality rate with pneumonic plague is greater than 90% in untreated patients.

Yersinia enterocolitica

Epidemiology

Yersinia enterocolitica is a common cause of enterocolitis in Scandinavian and other European countries, as well as in the colder areas of North America (Box 24-6). Although most studies indicate that infections are more common during the cold months of the year, not all investigators have documented this observation. The speculation that *Y. enterocolitica* is clinically more active in cold climates is attractive because this parallels the increased metabolic activity of the organisms at 22° C to 25° C. Virulence with these organisms has also been associated with specific serotypes: O3 and O9 in Europe, Africa, Japan, and Canada, and O8 in the United States. *Y. enterocolitica* has been isolated in a variety of sources, including water, milk, and wild and domestic animals. Although an animal reservoir is generally considered to be important, the source of sporadic infections is rarely identified. Epidemic outbreaks have been associated with contaminated meat or milk.

Clinical Syndromes

Approximately two thirds of all *Y. enterocolitica* infections are enterocolitis, as the name would imply. The gastroenteritis is characterized by diarrhea, fever, and abdominal pain lasting for as long as 1 to 2 weeks, although a chronic form of the disease can develop and persist for months to more than 1 year. Disease involves the terminal ileum and, with enlargement of the mesenteric lymph nodes, can mimic acute appendicitis. *Yersinia* infections are most common in children, with pseudoappendicitis particularly troublesome in this age-group. *Y. pseudotuberculosis* can also produce a disease with this presentation. Other manifestations reported in adults include septicemia, arthritis, intraabdominal abscess, hepatitis, and osteomyelitis.

In 1987 *Y. enterocolitica* was first reported to cause blood-transfusion–related bacteremia and endotoxic shock. This problem has been observed in other medical centers and illustrates the problem with an organism that can survive and grow in nutritionally rich blood products that may be refrigerated for 3 weeks or more. At this time, there is no reliable method available for detecting contaminated blood products. Although use of products with a shorter storage period would probably eliminate the problem (organisms would not have the opportunity to grow to toxic levels), this is not practical with the current shortage of blood products. Fortunately this is a relatively uncommon problem (fewer than 15 cases to date).

OTHER ENTEROBACTERIACEAE

Klebsiella

Members of this genus have a prominent capsule that is responsible for the mucoid appearance of isolated colonies and enhanced virulence of the organisms in vivo. The most commonly isolated member of this genus is *Klebsiella pneumoniae,* which is associated with community-acquired primary lobar pneumonia. Alcoholics and individuals with compromised pulmonary function are at increased risk for pneumonia, particularly with *Klebsiella,* because of their inability to clear aspirated oral secretions from the lower respiratory tract. Pneumonia caused by *Klebsiella* is frequently associated with necrotic destruction of alveolar spaces, cavity formation, and the production of blood-tinged sputum. *Klebsiella* also cause wound, soft tissue, and urinary tract infections.

Proteus

Infection of the urinary tract by *Proteus mirabilis* is the most common disease produced by this genus. *Proteus* strains produce large quantities of urease, which splits urea into CO_2 and NH_3. This raises the urine pH and facilitates the formation of renal stones. The increased alkalinity of the urine is also toxic for the uroepithelium. Despite the serologic diversity of these organisms, infection has not been associated with any specific serotype. Furthermore, in contrast with *E. coli,* the presence of pili may actually decrease virulence of *Proteus* by enhancing phagocytosis of the bacilli.

Enterobacter, Citrobacter, Serratia, Providencia

Primary infections in immunocompetent patients are rarely caused by *Enterobacter, Citrobacter, Serratia,* or *Providencia* organisms. They are more commonly associated with hospital-acquired infections in patients with a compromised immune system. Antibiotic therapy can be complicated because resistance to multiple antibiotics is frequently seen. This is a particularly serious problem with *Enterobacter* isolates.

LABORATORY DIAGNOSIS

Culture

Members of the family Enterobacteriaceae grow readily when cultured in vitro. Specimens collected from normally sterile sources such as spinal fluid or tissue collected at surgery can be inoculated onto nonselective blood agar media. Selective media (e.g., MacConkey agar, Eosin Methylene Blue [EMB] agar) are used for specimens normally contaminated with other organisms (e.g., sputum, feces). The use of these selective differential agars has the advantage of separating lactose-fermenting Enterobacteriaceae from nonfermentative strains, information that can be used to guide empiric antimicrobial therapy. Highly selective or organism-specific media are useful for the recovery of organisms such as *Salmonella* in stool specimens, where large numbers of normal flora can obscure the presence of significant pathogens.

The recovery of *Yersinia enterocolitica* is complicated because this organism grows slowly at traditional incubation temperatures and prefers cooler temperatures where it is metabolically more active. This property has been exploited, however, in the clinical laboratory by mixing the fecal specimen with saline and then storing the specimen at 4° C for 2 weeks or more before it is subcultured to agar media. This **cold enrichment** permits the growth of *Yersinia* while inhibiting or killing other organisms present in the specimen. Although use of cold enrichment does not aid in the initial management of a patient with *Yersinia* gastroenteritis, it has helped elucidate the role of this organism in both acute and chronic intestinal disease.

Biochemical Identification

A large number of diverse species are present in the family Enterobacteriaceae. The references (particularly the *Manual of Clinical Microbiology*) listed at the end of this chapter provide additional information about biochemical identification. With increasing sophistication of biochemical test systems, virtually all members of the family can be accurately identified in 4 to 24 hours with one of a number of commercially available identification systems.

Serologic Classification

Serology is very useful for determining the clinical significance of an isolate (e.g., serotyping specific pathogenic strains such as *E. coli* Kl, *E. coli* O157:H7, *Y. enterocolitica* O:8) or for classifying isolates for epidemiological purposes (e.g., characterizing isolates in a suspected outbreak of salmonellosis). However, the usefulness of this procedure is limited by cross-reactions with antigenically related Enterobacteriaceae and other organisms.

TREATMENT, PREVENTION, AND CONTROL

Antibiotic therapy for infections with Enterobacteriaceae must be guided by in vitro susceptibility test results and clinical experience. Whereas some organisms such as *Escherichia coli* and *Proteus mirabilis* are susceptible to many antibiotics, others can be highly resistant. Furthermore, susceptible organisms can rapidly develop resistance when exposed to subtherapeutic concentrations of antibiotics in a hospital setting. In general, antibiotic resistance is more common in infections acquired in the hospital compared with community-acquired infections. Antibiotic therapy is not recommended for some infections. For example, symptomatic relief but not antibiotic treatment is usually recommended for *Salmonella* gastroenteritis because antibiotics can prolong fecal carriage of this organism.

Prevention of infections is difficult because the Enterobacteriaceae are a major part of the endogenous microbial population. However, some risk factors for infections should be avoided, including the unrestricted use of antibiotics that can select for resistant bacteria, performance of procedures that traumatize mucosal barriers without prophylactic antibiotic coverage, and use of urinary catheters. Unfortunately, many of these factors are present in patients at greatest risk for infection (e.g., immunocompromised individuals confined to the hospital for extensive periods).

Exogenous infection with Enterobacteriaceae is theoretically easier to control. The source of infections with organisms like *Salmonella* is well defined. However, these bacteria are ubiquitous in poultry and eggs. Unless care is used for the preparation and refrigeration of foods, little can be done to control *Salmonella* infections. Transmission of *Shigella* is predominantly in young children, and interruption of fecal-hand-mouth transmission in this population is difficult. Control can be effective only with education and introduction of appropriate infection control procedures (e.g., hand washing, proper disposal of soiled linens) in a setting with an identified outbreak.

Vaccination with formalin-killed *Yersinia pestis* has proved effective for those at high risk. Chemoprophylaxis with tetracycline has also proved useful for individuals in close contact with a patient with pneumonic plague. Live, attenuated *Salmonella typhi* vaccines have reduced typhoid fever by 50% in populations with a high endemic rate of disease. However, the duration of this protection is short lived. Inactivated whole-cell vaccines, as well as vaccination with purified Vi antigen, the polysaccharide capsular antigen of *Salmonella typhi* associated with virulence, are also protective.

CASE STUDY AND QUESTIONS

A 25-year-old, previously healthy woman entered the emergency room for evaluation of bloody diarrhea and diffuse abdominal pain of 24 hours' duration. She complained of nausea and had vomited twice. She denied a history of inflammatory bowel disease, previous diarrhea, or contact with other individuals with diarrhea. Onset of symptoms began 24 hours after eating an undercooked hamburger at a local fast food restaurant. Rectal examination revealed watery stool with gross blood present. Sigmoidoscopy showed diffuse mucosal erythema and petechiae with modest exudation but no ulceration or pseudomembranes. Cultures for *Salmonella*, *Shigella*, *Yersinia*, and *Campylobacter* were negative as was the examination for enteric parasites.

1. What is the most likely organism responsible for episodes of hemorrhagic colitis? Which other Enterobacteriaceae can present as colitis?
2. What are the five groups of *Escherichia* associated with gastroenteritis? What is the disease associated with these organisms, and what is the mechanism of pathogenesis?
3. What are the four forms of *Salmonella* infection?
4. Differentiate between disease caused by *Salmonella typhi* and *Shigella sonnei*.
5. Describe the epidemiology of *Yersinia pestis* infections.

Bibliography

Brubaker RR: Factors promoting acute and chronic diseases caused by Yersiniae, *Clin Microbiol Rev* 4:309-324, 1991.

Cantey JR: Infectious diarrhea: pathogenesis and risk factors, *Am J Med* 78(suppl 6B):65-75, 1985.

Cornelis G, Laroche Y, Balligand G et al: *Yersinia enterocolitica*, a primary model for bacterial invasiveness, *Rev Infect Dis* 9:64-87, 1987.

Cover TL and Aber RC: *Yersinia enterocolitica*, *N Engl J Med* 321:16-24, 1989.

Ewing WH: *Edwards and Ewing's identification of Enterobacteriaceae*, ed 4, New York, 1986, Elsevier Science.

Farmer JJ and Kelly MT: Enterobacteriaceae. In Balows A, Hausler WJ, Herrmann KL, Isenberg HD, and Shadomy HJ, editors: *Manual of clinical microbiology*, ed 6, Washington, DC, 1991, American Society for Microbiology.

Johnson JR: Virulence factors in *Escherichia coli* urinary tract infection, *Clin Microbiol Rev* 4:80-128, 1991.

Levine MM: *Escherichia coli* that cause diarrhea: enterotoxigenic, enteropathogenic, enteroinvasive, enterohemorrhagic and enteroadherent, *J Infect Dis* 155:377-389, 1987.

Moulder JW: Comparative biology of intracellular parasitism, *Microbiol Rev* 49:298-337, 1985.

Pajic JK and Davey RB, editors: The genus Yersinia: epidemiology, molecular biology, and pathogenesis. In *Contributions to microbiology and immunology*, vol 9, New York, 1987, Karger.

CHAPTER 25

Vibrionaceae

MEMBERS of the family Vibrionaceae are curved or straight bacilli, capable of aerobic or anaerobic growth, oxidase positive, and non–spore-formers. They are primarily found in water and are well known for their ability to produce gastrointestinal disease. The family includes three genera associated with human disease: *Vibrio*, *Aeromonas*, and *Plesiomonas*.

VIBRIO

The genus *Vibrio* is composed of gram-negative, curved bacilli that differ from Enterobacteriaceae by their positive oxidase reaction, polar flagella, and growth on alkaline media but not acidic media. Species pathogenic for humans are summarized in Table 25-1.

TABLE 25-1 *Vibrio* Species Associated With Human Disease

Vibrio species	Source of infection	Clinical disease
V. cholerae	Water or food	Gastroenteritis
V. parahaemolyticus	Shellfish	Gastroenteritis
V. vulnificus	Shellfish; seawater	Bacteremia; wound infection; cellulitis
V. alginolyticus	Fish; seawater	Soft tissue, wound, or external otitis infections; bacteremia
*V. hollisae**	Shellfish	Gastroenteritis
*V. damsela**	Seawater	Soft tissue infection
*V. mimicus**	Shellfish; seawater	Gastroenteritis; external otitis
*V. fluvialis**	Seafood	Gastroenteritis
*V. furnissii**	Seafood	Gastroenteritis
*V. metschnikovii**	—	Bacteremia
*V. cincinnatiensis**	—	Meningitis

*Isolates rarely associated with human infections.

Physiology and Structure

Vibrio species can grow aerobically or anaerobically on a variety of simple media, with a broad temperature range (from 18° C to 37° C) for optimal growth. *Vibrio cholerae*, the best-known member of the genus, can be serologically subdivided into six groups based on somatic O antigens. Most pathogens belong to the O1 group. Toxigenic *V. cholerae* non-O1 isolates can also cause human disease, although they are not associated with epidemics. *V. cholerae* O1 can be subdivided into two biotypes (el tor and cholerae), as well as two serologic subgroups (ogawa, inaba). Strains with both the ogawa and inaba antigens have been termed hikajima. These groups are important for the epidemiologic classification of isolates. *V. parahaemolyticus* can also be subdivided by differences in the somatic O antigens.

Pathogenesis

The mechanism by which *V. cholerae* causes cholera is well established. The **cholera enterotoxin** produced by the organism is a complex molecule (A-B toxin). The enterotoxin can bind to specific receptors in the small intestine, enter into the mucosal cells, and effect a series of reactions that result in the rapid secretion of sodium, potassium, and bicarbonate into the intestinal lumen (Figure 25-1). Severely infected patients can lose as much as 1 liter of fluid per hour during the height of disease. The tremendous loss of fluid would normally flush the organism out of the gastrointestinal tract; however, *V. cholerae* is able to penetrate through the mucus covering the surface of the intestine and adhere to the mucosal cell layer. Nonadherent strains are unable to establish infection. Similarly, toxin-negative strains of *V. cholerae* O1 are avirulent.

The means by which other *Vibrio* species cause disease is less clearly understood, although a variety of potential virulence factors have been identified (Table 25-2). Most virulent strains of *V. parahaemolyticus* produce a heat-stable hemolysin (**Kanagawa-positive** strains) that is cytotoxic and cardiotoxic in experimental animals. Virulent strains are also able to adhere to and invade the intestinal tissue (in contrast with *V. cholerae*, which is considered an adherent but noninvasive pathogen). The role of toxin production and tissue invasion in the

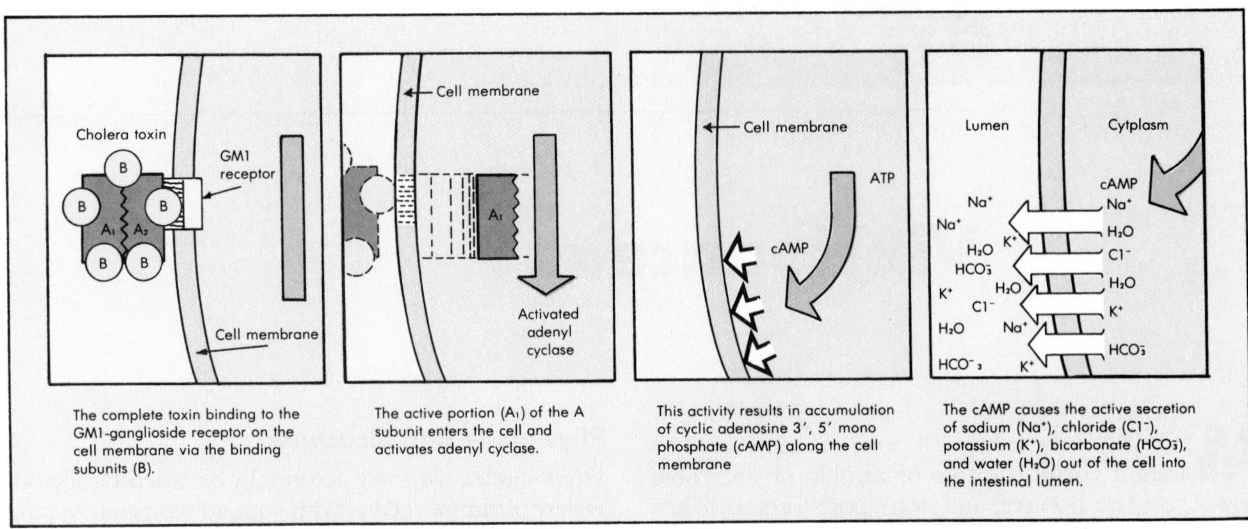

Cholera toxin
GM1 receptor
Cell membrane
Cell membrane
Activated adenyl cyclase
Cell membrane
ATP
cAMP
Lumen
Cytplasm
cAMP
The complete toxin binding to the GM1-ganglioside receptor on the cell membrane via the binding subunits (B).
The active portion (A₁) of the A subunit enters the cell and activates adenyl cyclase.
This activity results in accumulation of cyclic adenosine 3', 5' mono phosphate (cAMP) along the cell membrane
The cAMP causes the active secretion of sodium (Na⁺), chloride (Cl⁻), potassium (K⁺), bicarbonate (HCO₃⁻), and water (H₂O) out of the cell into the intestinal lumen.

FIGURE 25-1 Mechanism of cholera toxin action. The toxin molecule is composed of the A subunit, which determines biologic activity, and the B subunit, which binds the toxin to the GM1 ganglioside receptor on the membrane of intestinal cells. The A subunit consists of two peptides: A_1, with toxin activity, and A_2, which is a linking molecule to the B subunit. The B subunit consists of five identical peptides. After the toxin molecule binds to the cell receptor, the A subunit is transferred into the cell and the A_1 peptide is activated. Through a series of steps, adenyl cyclase activity is increased, with a corresponding increase in cyclic adenosine 3',5'-monophosphate (cAMP). The increased cAMP concentration mediates the active secretion of electrolytes and water into the lumen of the intestine.

TABLE 25-2 Virulence Factors Associated With *Vibrio* Species

Organism	Virulence factors
V. cholerae	Cholera enterotoxin, heat-stable and heat-labile enterotoxin, cytotoxin, flagellum, adhesions, mucinase
V. parahaemolyticus	Cytotoxin, hemolysin, adhesions, mucinase
V. vulnificus	Serum resistance, antiphagocytic polysaccharides, cytolysins, collagenase, protease, siderophore
V. alginolyticus	Collagenase
V. hollisae	Heat-stable and heat-labile enterotoxin, hemolysin
V. damsela	Cytolysin
V. mimicus	Enterotoxin, heat-stable and heat-labile enterotoxin, mucinase

development of gastroenteritis has not been delineated for *V. parahaemolyticus*.

Epidemiology

V. cholerae is found in freshwater ponds and estuaries in Asia, the Middle East, Africa, parts of Europe, and along the coastal areas of South, Central, and North America (Box 25-1). Although the major reservoir is believed to be human carriage, some evidence indicates that infected crustaceans may also be a significant source of infection. Disease is spread by contaminated water and food, most commonly during the warm months. Person-to-person spread is unusual because a high inoculum (e.g., 10^8 to 10^{10} organisms) is required to establish infection in an individual with normal gastric acidity. Achlorhydria or hypochlorhydria can reduce the infectious dose to 10^3 to 10^5 organisms. Cholera is usually seen in communities with poor sanitation. Once the reservoir for this organism is established, elimination is particularly difficult. For that reason sporadic disease has occurred for centuries, and seven major pandemics have been observed since 1817. The current pandemic began in Asia in 1961 with *V. cholerae* O1 (biotype el tor, serotype inaba) and spread to Africa, Europe, and Oceania in the 1970s and 1980s. Endemic disease with an unrelated strain of *V. cholerae* O1 has been reported sporadically in the Gulf of Mexico since 1973. In 1991 the pandemic strain spread to Peru and subsequently has involved most countries in South and Central America, as well as the United States and Canada (Figure 25-2). By the end of 1992 more than 600,000 cases had been reported in the Americas. Although cases are reported throughout the year, they are most prevalent during the warm months.

In contrast with *V. cholerae, V. parahaemolyticus, V. vulnificus*, and *V. alginolyticus* are halophilic marine vibrios that require salt for growth. These species are free-living vibrios that inhabit estuaries and coastal waters world-

BOX 25-1 Epidemiology of Cholera

DISEASE/BACTERIAL FACTORS

Enterotoxin causes rapid fluid loss (as much as 1 L/hr)
Adheres to mucosal cell layer; thus is not flushed from system
Two biotypes: *V. cholerae* O1 biotype cholerae causes more severe disease than *V. cholerae* O1 biotype el tor

TRANSMISSION

Major reservoir is humans
Ingestion of contaminated water and food
Very large inoculum of organisms is required for disease, except for patients with reduced gastric acidity

WHO IS AT RISK?

Individuals in communities with poor sanitation

GEOGRAPHY/SEASON

Freshwater ponds and estuaries in Asia, Middle East, Africa, parts of Europe, and coastal areas of South, Central, and North America
Disease more prevalent in warm months

MODES OF CONTROL

Fluid and electrolyte replacement is crucial
Antibiotic therapy of secondary value: tetracycline (drug of choice), erythromycin, chloramphenicol, trimethoprim-sulfamethoxazole, or fluoroquinolones
Improved hygiene
Killed cholera vaccine of limited value

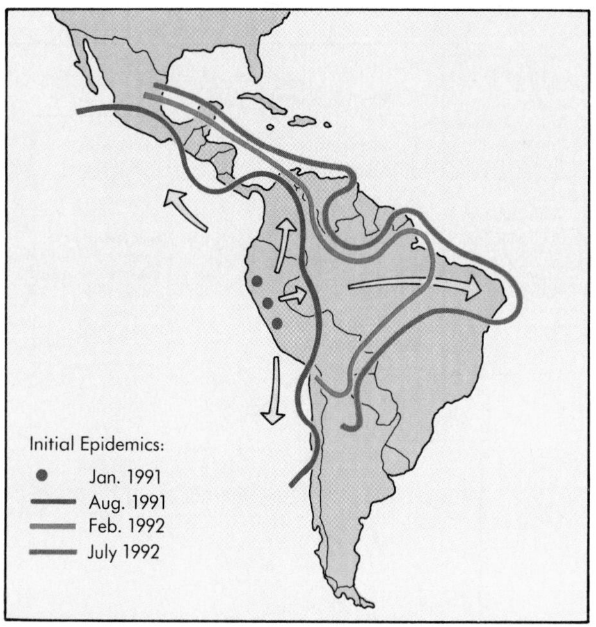

FIGURE 25-2 Spread of epidemic cholera in Latin America from January 1991 through July 1992. (Redrawn from *MMWR* 41:667, 1992.)

wide (Figure 25-3). Because they are also rapidly killed by gastric acids, the infectious dose of all vibrios is generally high. Gastroenteritis with *V. parahaemolyticus* and septicemia caused by *V. vulnificus* commonly follow ingestion of raw or improperly handled seafood such as oysters. *V. parahaemolyticus* is the major cause of diarrheal disease in Japan, where consumption of raw fish is common. Wound infections caused by *Vibrio* species are usually associated with exposure to seawater or laceration with a seashell.

Clinical Syndromes

Vibrio cholerae

Infection with *V. cholerae* can range from asymptomatic colonization or mild diarrheal disease to severe, potentially life-threatening diarrhea and vomiting (2% to 5% of all infections). Severe cholera will initially occur an average of 2 to 3 days after ingestion of the bacilli, with the abrupt onset of vomiting and severe watery diarrhea. The stool specimens are colorless and odorless, free of protein, and speckled with mucus flecks (rice-water stools). The severe fluid and electrolyte loss can lead to dehydration, metabolic acidosis and vomiting (bicarbonate loss), and hypokalemia and hypovolemic shock (potassium loss) with cardiac arrhythmia and renal failure. The mortality is 60% in untreated patients but less than 1% in patients promptly treated to replace lost fluids and electrolytes. Cholera will spontaneously resolve after a few days of symptoms. Disease caused by *V. cholerae* biotype cholerae is more severe than with biotype el tor. *V. cholerae* non-O1 causes a gastrointestinal disease similar to *V. cholerae* O1, although it is generally less severe and has not been associated with epidemic disease.

Vibrio parahaemolyticus

Gastroenteritis caused by *V. parahaemolyticus* can range from self-limiting diarrhea to a cholera-like illness. In general, the disease will present after a 5-hour to 92-hour incubation period (mean 24 hours) with an explosive, watery diarrhea. No gross blood or mucus is found in stool specimens except in very severe cases. Headache, abdominal cramps, nausea, vomiting, and low-grade fever may persist for 72 hours or more. Recovery is usually uneventful.

Vibrio vulnificus

V. vulnificus is a particularly virulent *Vibrio* species responsible for rapidly progressive wound infections after exposure to contaminated seawater and septicemia after consumption of raw oysters. The wound infections are characterized by initial swelling, erythema, and pain, followed by the development of vesicles or bullae and eventual tissue necrosis. Systemic signs of fever and chills are usually seen. Mortality caused by *V. vulnificus* septicemia can be as high as 50% unless antimicrobial

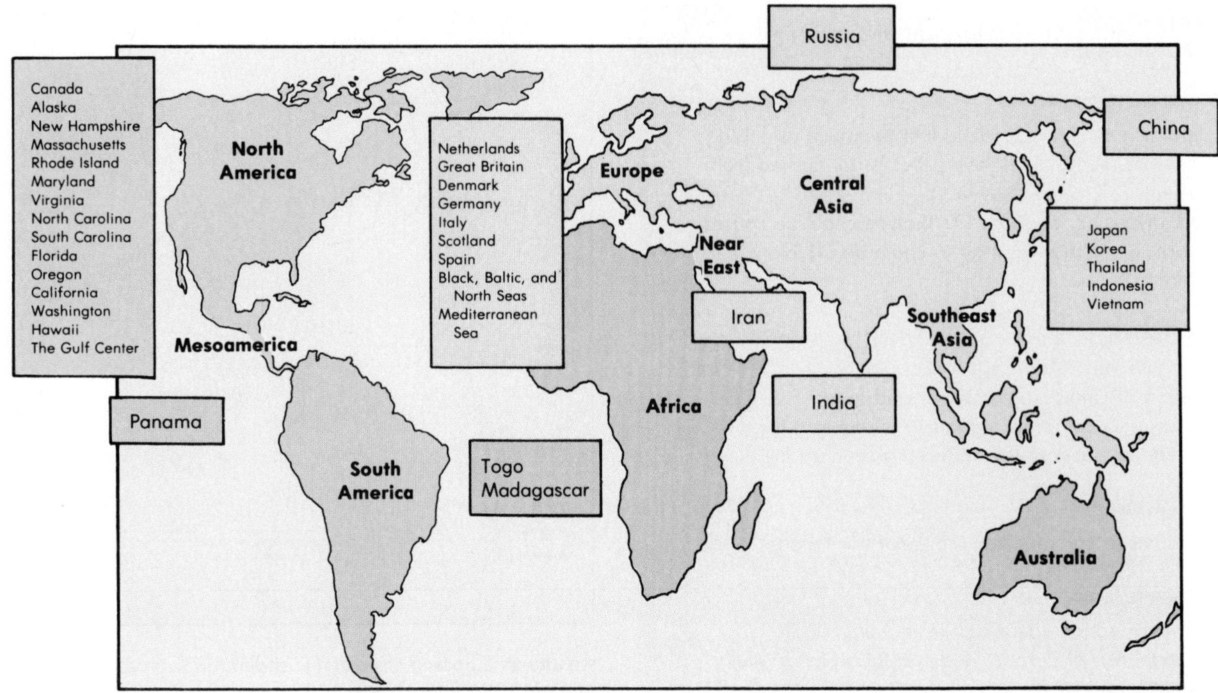

FIGURE 25-3 Worldwide distribution of *Vibrio parahaemolyticus.*

therapy is initiated rapidly. Infections are most severe for patients with hepatic disease, hematopoietic disease, chronic renal failure, or those receiving immunosuppressive drugs.

Other *Vibrio* Species

V. alginolyticus can cause infection in superficial wounds contaminated with seawater. Infections of the ear, eye, and gastrointestinal tract have also been rarely reported. *V. hollisae*, *V. fluvialis, V. furnissii*, and *V. mimicus* can cause a self-limited gastroenteritis, and *V. damsela* is responsible for soft-tissue wound infections. Single human infections have been reported with *V. metschnikovii* (bacteremia) and *V. cincinnatiensis* (meningitis).

Laboratory Diagnosis

Microscopy

Vibrio species are small (0.5 × 1.5 to 3 μm), curved, gram-negative bacilli. The organisms are rarely observed in Gram-stained stool or wound specimens; however, the detection of characteristic motile bacilli by an experienced observer using darkfield microscopy may be useful.

Culture

Vibrio survive poorly in an acidic or dry environment. Specimens must be collected early in the course of disease and cultured promptly onto appropriate media. If culturing is delayed, the specimen should be mixed in Cary-Blair transport medium and refrigerated. Vibrios survive poorly in buffered glycerol-saline, the transport medium used for most enteric pathogens.

Vibrios grow on most media used in clinical laboratories for stool cultures, including blood agar, MacConkey agar, and xylose-lysine-deoxycholate (XLD) agar. Special selective agar for vibrios (e.g., TCBS, or thiosulfate-citrate-bile-sucrose agar) can also be used (Table 25-3), as well as an enrichment broth (e.g., alkaline peptone broth, pH 8.6). Isolates are identified with selected biochemical tests and use of polyvalent antisera. Tests with halophilic vibrios will require supplementation of the media with 1% sodium chloride.

Treatment, Prevention, and Control

Cholera must be promptly treated with fluid and electrolyte replacement before massive fluid loss results in hypovolemic shock. Antibiotic therapy, although of secondary value, can reduce exotoxin production and more rapidly eliminate the organism. Tetracycline is the drug of choice, but vibrios are also usually susceptible to erythromycin, chloramphenicol, trimethoprim-sulfamethoxazole, and the fluoroquinolones. *V. parahaemolyticus* gastroenteritis is usually a self-limited disease, although antibiotic therapy can be used to supplement fluid and electrolyte therapy in severe infections. *V. vulnificus* wound infections and septicemia must be promptly treated with antibiotic therapy. Tetracycline is the most effective drug in vivo, although some success has been reported with aminoglycosides.

Because vibrios are free-living in freshwater and marine reservoirs and human carriage of *V. cholerae* can range from 1% to 20% in previously infected patients, it is unlikely that the reservoir for this organism will be

TABLE 25-3 Isolation of *Vibrio* Species on TCBS Agar

Vibrio Species	Sucrose Fermentation	Colony
V. cholerae O1	Positive	Yellow
V. cholerae non-01	Positive	Yellow
V. alginolyticus	Positive	Yellow
V. parahaemolyticus	Negative	Dark blue-green
V. vulnificus	Negative	Dark blue-green

eradicated. Disease can be controlled effectively only by improved hygiene. This involves adequate sewage management and water purification systems to eliminate contamination of the water supply and appropriate steps to prevent contamination of food.

Although a killed cholera vaccine is available, the protection is short-lived and useful only for individuals who will be in an endemic area for less than 6 months. Currently the vaccine is not recommended for individuals traveling to areas with endemic disease. Tetracycline prophylaxis has also been used to reduce the risk of infection in endemic areas but has not prevented spread of cholera. Because the infectious dose of *V. cholerae* is high, antibiotic prophylaxis is generally unnecessary if appropriate hygiene is used.

AEROMONAS

Aeromonas is a gram-negative aerobic and facultative anaerobic bacillus that morphologically resembles members of the Enterobacteriaceae. However, *Aeromonas* can be readily differentiated by positive oxidase reactivity and the presence of polar flagellum. As the name implies, the most commonly isolated species, *Aeromonas hydrophila*, is found in fresh and brackish water. Human infections caused by *A. hydrophila*, *A. sobria*, and possibly *A. caviae* follow exposure to untreated water, but disease has not been associated with consumption of shellfish or freshwater fish. Asymptomatic gastrointestinal carriage of this organism is less than 3%, with a peak in both carriage and disease during the warm months.

Although numerous potential virulence factors have been identified (e.g., endotoxin, hemolysins, enterotoxin, proteases, siderophores, adherence factors), the absence of an animal model of aeromonas infection has inhibited defining the role of these factors.

Aeromonas species cause opportunistic systemic disease in immunocompromised patients (particularly those with hepatobiliary disease or an underlying malignancy), diarrheal disease in otherwise healthy individuals (Table 25-4), and wound infections. Gastrointestinal disease in children is usually an acute, severe illness, whereas adults tend to have chronic diarrhea.

TABLE 25-4 Characteristics of *Aeromonas* and *Plesiomonas* Gastroenteritis

Epidemiological and clinical features	*Aeromonas*	*Plesiomonas*
Natural habitat	Fresh or brackish water	Fresh or brackish water
Source of infection	Contaminated water	Uncooked shellfish
Clinical presentation		
Diarrhea	Present	Present
Vomiting	Present	Present
Abdominal cramps	Present	Present
Fever	Absent	Absent
Blood and PMNs in stool	Absent	Present
Pathogenesis	Enterotoxin (?)	Invasive

Aeromonas wound infections have recently been recognized with the use of medicinal leeches. The leeches, which are colonized with *Aeromonas*, maintain vascular supply following microvascular or plastic surgery by their enzymatic digestion of clots. As the use of these leeches has increased, aeromonas infections have become more common. Acute diarrheal disease is self-limited and only supportive care is indicated. Chronic diarrheal disease or systemic infection requires antimicrobial therapy. *Aeromonas* is resistant to penicillins, cephalosporins, and erythromycin, with only gentamicin, tetracycline, trimethoprim-sulfamethoxazole, and chloramphenicol consistently active.

PLESIOMONAS

Plesiomonas is a facultative anaerobic gram-negative bacillus that is oxidase-positive, has multiple polar flagella, and is differentiated from *Aeromonas* by selected biochemical reactions. *Plesiomonas shigelloides*, the species responsible for human disease, is serologically related to *Shigella sonnei*. The organism is found in brackish water and is acquired by consumption of uncooked shellfish, particularly oysters and shrimp. Disease has also been associated with foreign travel, usually to Mexico, the Caribbean, or Southeast Asia.

As with *Aeromonas* the absence of an animal model has inhibited our ability to define the pathogenic mechanisms of *Plesiomonas* disease. The primary disease caused by *P. shigelloides* is self-limiting gastroenteritis (e.g., secretory form, colitis form, or chronic form), with the onset of disease 48 hours after exposure to the organism. Other diseases include perinatal bacteremia with or without meningitis, cholecystitis, pseudoappendicitis, arthritis, cellulitis, and osteomyelitis.

When antibiotic therapy is indicated, the organism has been found to be susceptible to chloramphenicol, cephalothin, imipenem, aztreonam, trimethoprim-sulfamethoxazole, and fluoroquinolones, but not ampicillin, carbenicillin, erythromycin, and many aminoglycosides.

CASE STUDY AND QUESTIONS

A 57-year-old man was hospitalized in New York City with a 2-day history of severe, watery diarrhea. The illness began 1 day after returning from Ecuador. The patient was dehydrated with electrolyte imbalance (acidosis, hypokalemia). After fluid and electrolyte replacement to compensate for the watery diarrhea, the patient made an uneventful recovery. Stool cultures were positive for *Vibrio cholerae*.

1. What clinical signs are characteristic of cholera? What virulence factors mediate this disease? What is the mode of their action?
2. How did this patient acquire this infection? How does this differ from infections caused by *Vibrio parahaemolyticus* or *V. vulnificus*?
3. How can cholera be controlled in areas where infection is endemic?

Bibliography

Blake PA: Diseases of humans (other than cholera) caused by vibrios, *Ann Rev Microbiol* 34:341, 1980.

Craig JP, Hardegree MC, Pierce NF, and Richardson SH: The structure and functions of enterotoxins. A workshop held at the National Institutes of Health, *J Infect Dis* 133(suppl):5-156, 1976.

Holmberg SD and Farmer JJ III: *Aeromonas hydrophila* and *Plesiomonas shigelloides* as causes of intestinal infections, *Rev Infect Dis* 6:633, 1984.

Holmberg SD, Schell WL, Fanning GR et al: *Aeromonas* intestinal infections in the United States, *Ann Intern Med* 105:683, 1986.

Holmberg SD, Wachsmuth IK, Hickman-Brenner FW et al: *Plesiomonas* enteric infections in the United States, *Ann Intern Med* 105:690, 1986.

Janda JM: Recent advances in the study of the taxonomy, pathogenicity, and infectious syndromes associated with the genus *Aeromonas*, *Clin Microbiol Rev* 4:397-410, 1991.

Janda JM, Powers C, Bryant RG, and Abbott SL: Current perspectives on the epidemiology and pathogenesis of clinically significant *Vibrio* spp., *Clin Microbiol Rev* 1:245-267, 1988.

Joseph SW, Colwell RR, and Kaper JB: *Vibrio parahaemolyticus* and related halophilic vibrios, *CRC Crit Rev Microbiol* 10:77, 1982.

Morris JG and Black RE: Cholera and other vibrios in the United States, *N Engl J Med* 312:343, 1983.

Scully RE, Mark EJ, McNeely WF, and McNeely BU. Weekly clinicopathological exercises, *N Engl J Med* 321:1029-1038, 1989.

Swerdlow DL and Ries AA: Cholera in the Americas: guidelines for the clinician, *JAMA* 267:1495-1499, 1992.

Tison DL and Kelly MT: *Vibrio* species of medical importance, *Diagn Microbiol Infect Dis* 2:263, 1984.

CHAPTER 26

Campylobacter and *Helicobacter*

THE classification of bacteria in these genera has undergone a number of changes since they were first isolated at the beginning of this century. The organisms that are now recognized as campylobacters were originally classified as *Vibrio* species based on their curved shape. More recently discovered species (e.g., *Campylobacter curvus*, *C. rectus*) were originally classified as *Wolinella* species, and the helicobacters were first placed in the *Campylobacter* genus. Through the use of 16S rRNA sequencing, the classification scheme for these bacteria has been resolved (Box 26-1). The *Campylobacter* and *Helicobacter* species most commonly involved with human infections are discussed in this chapter. See the Bibliography at the end of this chapter for additional information about the other related bacteria.

BOX 26-1 Taxonomic Classification of *Campylobacter, Helicobacter,* and Related Genera

Campylobacter species
- *C. jejuni* ssp. *jejuni*
- *C. jejuni* ssp. *doylei*
- *C. coli*
- *C. fetus* ssp. *fetus*
- *C. fetus* ssp. *venerealis*
- *C. hyointestinalis*
- *C. sputorum* (3 biovars)
- *C. lari*
- *C. concisus*
- *C. mucosalis*
- *C. curvus*
- *C. rectus*
- *C. upsaliensis*

Arcobacter nitrofigilis
Arcobacter cryaerophilus
Wolinella succinogenes
Helicobacter species (previously *Campylobacter*)
- *H. pylori*
- *H. cinaedi*
- *H. fennelliae*
- *H. mustelae*

CAMPYLOBACTER

The genus *Campylobacter*, from the Greek word *campylo* for curved, consists of comma-shaped, gram-negative bacilli that are oxidase-positive and catalase-positive, motile by means of a polar flagella, and require a microaerophilic atmosphere for growth. Eleven species and seven subspecies or biovars are now recognized (Box 26-1).

Campylobacter jejuni is the most common cause of bacterial gastroenteritis in the United States. *Campylobacter coli* is responsible for 2% to 5% of campylobacter gastroenteritis, although it is reported to be more common in underdeveloped countries. *C. lari* and *C. upsaliensis* have also been associated with diarrheal disease in humans. These species are primarily restricted to the gastrointestinal tract, with bacteremia observed in fewer than 1% of the infections. In contrast with other species, *Campylobacter fetus* ssp. *fetus* is most commonly responsible for systemic infections such as bacteremia, septic thrombophlebitis, arthritis, septic abortion, and meningitis.

Physiology and Structure

Campylobacter has a typical gram-negative cell wall structure. The major antigen of the genus is the lipopolysaccharide of the outer membrane. Serologic heterogeneity of *C. jejuni* isolates is common, with more than 90 different somatic O polysaccharide antigens recognized and 50 capsular and flagellar antigens.

Recognition of the role of campylobacters in gastrointestinal disease was delayed because the organisms grow best in an atmosphere of reduced oxygen (5% to 7%) and increased carbon dioxide (5% to 10%). In addition, *C. jejuni* grows better at 42° C vs. 37° C. These growth properties have now been exploited in the selective isolation of pathogenic campylobacters in stool specimens. The small size of the organisms (0.3 to 0.6 μm in diameter) has also been used to recover the bacteria by filtering stool specimens (campylobacters pass through 0.45 μm filters, whereas other bacteria are retained).

Pathogenesis and Immunity

The major factors associated with the development of disease are the infectious dose of organisms and the level of specific immunity. Patients exposed to a large number of organisms, or who lack gastric acids, are more likely to develop disease. Individuals in a population of high endemic disease develop measurable levels of specific serum and secretory antibodies and have less severe disease. Patients with hypogammaglobulinemia have prolonged, severe disease with *C. jejuni*.

The pathogenesis of *C. jejuni* gastrointestinal disease is not completely understood. Disease is characterized by destruction of the mucosal surfaces of the jejunum (as implied by the name), ileum, and colon. On gross examination, the mucosal surface appears edematous and bloody. Histologic examination reveals ulceration of the mucosal surface, crypt abscesses in the epithelial glands, and infiltration into the lamina propria, with neutrophils, mononuclear cells, and eosinophils. This inflammatory process is consistent with invasion of the organisms into the intestinal tissue. Enterotoxins, cytopathic toxins, and endotoxic activity have been detected in *C. jejuni* isolates. However, the precise roles of these factors in disease have not been defined. For example, strains lacking enterotoxin activity are still fully virulent.

Campylobacter fetus has a propensity to spread from the gastrointestinal tract to the bloodstream and distal foci. This is particularly common in debilitated and immunocompromised patients such as those with liver disease, diabetes mellitus, chronic alcoholism, or a malignancy. In vitro studies have demonstrated that *C. fetus* is resistant to complement-mediated and antibody-mediated serum killing, whereas *C. jejuni* is rapidly killed. *C. fetus* is covered with a protein (**S protein**) that prevents complement-mediated killing in serum (inhibits C3b binding to the bacteria).

Epidemiology

Campylobacters are commensals of cattle, sheep, dogs, cats, rodents, and fowl (Box 26-2). Lifelong asymptomatic carriage in animals, following an initial symptomatic phase, represents an important reservoir for human disease. Human infections result from consumption of contaminated food, milk, or water. Contaminated poultry is responsible for more than half of the campylobacter infections in developed countries. Food products that neutralize gastric acids (e.g., milk) effectively reduce the infectious dose. Fecal-oral transmission from person to person may also occur, but transmission from food handlers is uncommon.

The actual incidence of campylobacter infections is unknown because disease is not systematically reported to public health officials. However, it has been estimated that more than 2 million *C. jejuni* infections occur annually and such infections are more common than *Salmonella* and *Shigella* infections combined (Figure 26-1). Disease is most common in the warm months but does occur throughout the year. The peak incidence of disease is in young adults. In underdeveloped countries, symptomatic disease occurs in young children, and persistent carriage is observed in adults.

C. fetus infections are relatively uncommon, with fewer than 250 cases reported. In contrast with *C. jejuni*, *C. fetus* infects immunocompromised, elderly individuals.

BOX 26-2 Epidemiology of *Campylobacter jejuni* Infection

DISEASE/BACTERIAL FACTORS

C. jejuni is most common cause of bacterial gastroenteritis in the United States

C. jejuni destroys mucosal surfaces of jejunum

TRANSMISSION

Ingestion of contaminated food (especially poultry), milk, or water

Asymptomatic carriage in animals is important reservoir for humans

Fecal-oral transmission, person to person also possible

WHO IS AT RISK?

Patients exposed to large numbers of *C. jejuni* (e.g., via undercooked poultry) or who lack gastric acids at increased risk

Patients with hypogammaglobulinemia have more severe disease

GEOGRAPHY/SEASON

Worldwide

Disease more common in warm months

MODES OF CONTROL

Erythromycin (drug of choice), tetracyclines, aminoglycosides, chloramphenicol, and clindamycin

Control by proper preparation of food, consumption of pasteurized milk, and prevention of contamination of water supplies

Clinical Syndromes

C. jejuni infections are seen most commonly as acute enteritis with diarrhea, malaise, fever, and abdominal pain. Ten or more bowel movements per day can occur during the peak of disease, and grossly bloody stools may be present. The disease is generally self-limiting, although symptoms may last for 1 week or longer. The range of clinical manifestations can include colitis, acute abdominal pain, and bacteremia. *C. fetus* infection is most commonly seen as septicemia with dissemination to

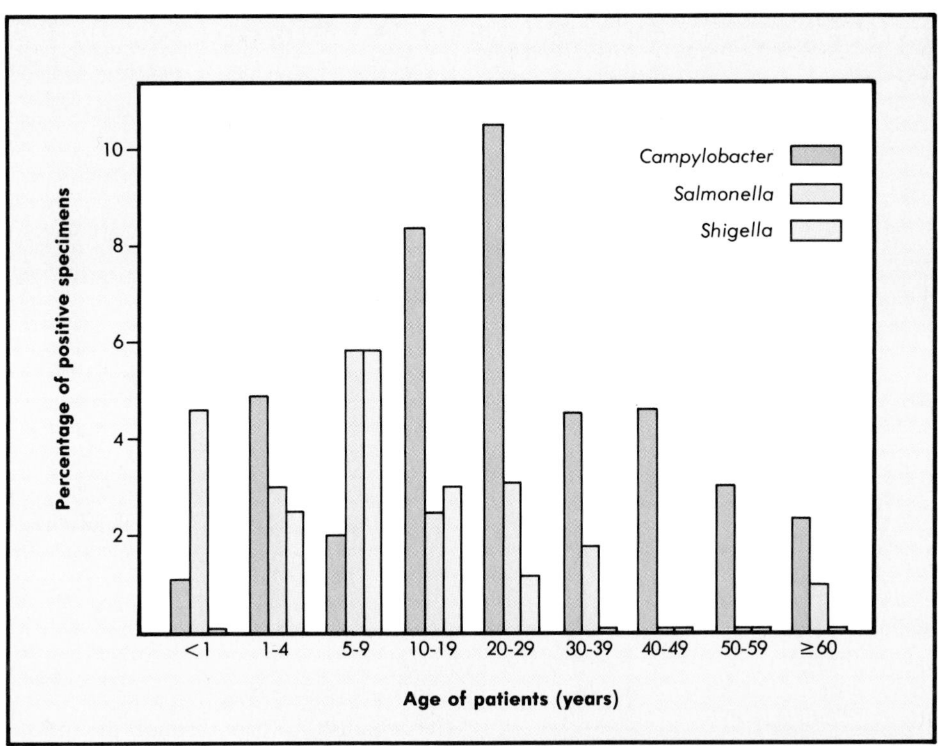

FIGURE 26-1 Age distribution for diarrheal disease caused by *Campylobacter*, *Salmonella*, and *Shigella* organisms.

multiple organs, although the initial presentation may be referable to the gastrointestinal tract or abdomen. Endovascular localization is reported.

Laboratory Diagnosis

Microscopy

C. jejuni is thin (0.3 mm) and cannot be easily seen in Gram-stained specimens. When observed, the organisms appear as small, curved bacilli. Pairs of bacteria resemble the wings of a seagull. The organism, with its characteristic darting motility, can be detected in freshly collected stool specimens when examined by darkfield or phase-contrast microscopy.

Culture

C. jejuni was unrecognized for many years because isolation requires growth in a microaerophilic atmosphere (e.g., 5% to 7% oxygen, 5% to 7% carbon dioxide, and the balance nitrogen), elevated incubation temperature (e.g., 42° C), and selective media. The selective media contain blood or charcoal to remove toxic oxygen radicals and antibiotics to inhibit the growth of contaminating organisms. Campylobacters are slow-growing organisms, usually requiring incubation for 48 to 72 hours or longer. *C. fetus* is not thermophilic and cannot grow at 42° C. However, a microaerophilic atmosphere is still required for isolation.

Identification

Preliminary identification of isolates is based on growth under selective conditions, typical microscopic morphology, and detection of oxidase and catalase activity. Definitive identification of all isolates is guided by the reactions summarized in Table 26-1.

Treatment, Prevention, and Control

Campylobacters are susceptible to a wide variety of antibiotics, including erythromycin, tetracyclines, aminoglycosides, chloramphenicol, and clindamycin. Most isolates are resistant to penicillins, cephalosporins, and sulfonamide antibiotics. Erythromycin is the antibiotic of choice and is used to treat enteritis when indicated; an aminoglycoside is generally used for systemic infections.

Campylobacter gastroenteritis is prevented by the proper preparation of food, particularly poultry, consumption of pasteurized milk, and safeguards to prevent contamination of water supplies. Elimination of campylobacter carriage in animal reservoirs is unlikely.

HELICOBACTER

In 1982 spiral-shaped bacilli, resembling campylobacters, were observed associated with type B gastritis. The organisms were originally classified as *Campylobacter* but were subsequently reclassified as a new genus, *Helicobacter*. *Helicobacter pylori* is the species associated with

TABLE 26-1 Identification Test for *Campylobacter* and *Helicobacter*

Test reactions	*C. jejuni*	*C. coli*	*C. fetus* ssp. *fetus*	*H. pylori**	*H. cinaedi*†	*H. fennelliae*‡
Growth at:						
25°C	−	−	+	−	−	−
37°C	+	+	+	+	+	+
42°C	+	+	±	−	−	−
Oxidase	+	+	+	+	+	+
Catalase	+	+	+	+	+	+
Urease	−	−	−	+	−	−
Nitrate reduction	+	+	+	−	+	−
Hippurate hydrolysis	+	−	−	−	−	−
Susceptibility to:						
Nalidixic acid	S	S	R	R	S	S
Cephalothin	R	R	S	S	S	S

Modified from Balows A et al: *Manual of clinical microbiology,* 1990.
*Previously *Campylobacter pylori.*
†Previously *Campylobacter cinaedi.*
‡Previously *Campylobacter fennelliae.*

BOX 26-3 *Helicobacter pylori* Virulence Factors

- Urease
- Motility
- Adherence factors
- Heat-labile cytotoxin
- Gastric mucin protease
- Hemolysin
- Lipopolysaccharide

gastritis, and more recently it has been implicated in gastric and duodenal ulcers, as well as gastric cancer. Other bacteria that have now been classified in the genus *Helicobacter* include *H. cinaedi* and *H. fennelliae* (isolated from homosexual men with proctitis, proctocolitis, or enteritis) and *H. mustelae* (isolated from ferrets).

Physiology and Structure

Members of the genus *Helicobacter* are characterized by sequence analysis of 16S rRNA, their cellular fatty acids, presence of one or more polar, sheathed flagella, and selected biochemical tests (e.g., positive oxidase and catalase reactions, negative hippurate hydrolysis). *H. pylori* is highly motile (corkscrew motility) and produces an abundance of urease.

Pathogenesis and Immunity

A number of factors have been identified as potential virulence factors in *H. pylori* disease (Box 26-3). The most important factors are believed to be urease production (produces a cloud of ammonia that protects the organism from gastric acids), motility and mucinase activity (allows the organism to pass through the mucous layer rapidly), and adherence factors (anchors the bacteria at the intracellular junction of enteric cells). The gastric tissue associated with *H. pylori* infection is invariably inflamed with infiltration of mononuclear cells into the lamina propria. A hypothetical model of *H. pylori* infection is illustrated in Figure 26-2. Antibody response to *H. pylori* infection is common; however, the organism is able to evade elimination in its protected location in the gastric mucosa.

Epidemiology

Serologic studies in the United States have documented that the incidence of *H. pylori* infection in healthy individuals is relatively low during childhood but increases to approximately 50% in older adults (Box 26-4). Infection appears earlier in individuals in a low socioeconomic class and in developing nations. *H. pylori* is identified in 70% to 100% of patients with gastritis, gastric ulcers, and duodenal ulcers but is infrequently isolated from patients without histologic evidence of gastritis. No animal reservoir has been identified and infection via food or water has not been demonstrated. Although the mechanism of transmission is not known, family clustering has been recognized. Humans are most likely the main reservoir for infection, which is probably spread person to person.

Clinical Syndromes

The clinical evidence is now overwhelming that *H. pylori* is the etiologic agent for virtually all cases of type B gastritis. Evidence includes virtually 100% association between gastritis and infection with the bacterium,

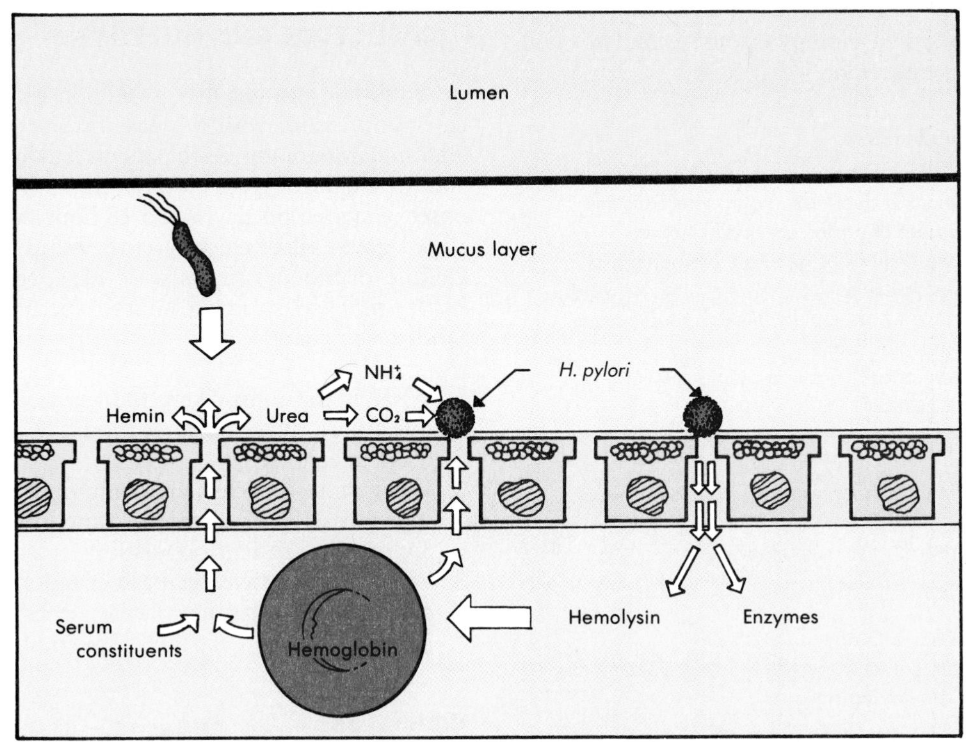

FIGURE 26-2 Diagrammatic representation of *H. pylori* colonization of gastric mucosa. The motile organism moves rapidly through the viscous mucus toward chemotactic growth factors, urea and hemin, present in the gastric pits. The stomach acidity is neutralized by the urease activity, and hemin stimulates growth of *H. pylori*. Infiltration of inflammatory cells and release of hydrolytic enzymes in response to the proliferating organism leads to gastritis. (Redrawn from Hazell SL et al: *J Infect Dis* 153:658, 1986.)

experimental infection in both animals and humans, and histological resolution of pathology when specific therapy is used to eradicate the organism. Strong evidence also implicates *H. pylori* in gastric and duodenal ulcers, where elimination of the organism leads to healing of the ulcers and significantly reduced recurrences. Since gastritis precedes the development of gastric adenocarcinomas, extensive epidemiological and experimental studies are underway to determine the role of *H. pylori* in the pathogenesis of this malignancy.

Laboratory Diagnosis

Histopathology

H. pylori is detected by histological examination of gastric biopsies. Although the organism can be seen in specimens with hematoxylin and eosin stain or Gram stain, the Warthin-Starry silver stain is the most sensitive.

Urease Test

The urease test is the most rapid method for detecting *H. pylori*. This can be measured either directly in the clinical specimen or after an organism has been isolated. The abundance of urease produced by the organism permits detection of the alkaline by-product within 1 to 2 hours.

Culture

Growth of the organism requires supplementation of enriched medium with blood, hemin, or charcoal. Such supplementation protects the bacteria from oxygen free radicals, hydrogen peroxide, and fatty acids present in the media (as with *Campylobacter*). Culture has not proven to be sensitive unless multiple biopsy specimens collected from the gastric mucosa are processed. This is due to the heterogeneous distribution of organisms, as well as the inhibitory effects of antibiotics, antiseptics, or other bacteriostatic agents used during endoscopy.

Identification

Preliminary identification of isolates is based on growth under selective conditions, typical microscopic morphology, and rapid detection of oxidase, catalase, and urease activity. Definitive identification of *H. pylori* and related bacteria is guided by the reactions summarized in Table 26-1.

Serology

As indicated above, infection with *H. pylori* stimulates a humoral immune reaction that will persist (presumably caused by continuous exposure to the bacteria). Although

BOX 26-4 Epidemiology of *Helicobacter* Infection

DISEASE/BACTERIAL FACTORS

H. pylori responsible for type B gastritis; strongly implicated in gastric and duodenal ulcers; infections precede development of gastric adenocarcinomas

Urease-producing organisms generate ammonia that neutralizes gastric acids

Motile organism can pass rapidly through mucus layer, thus avoiding elimination

Adherence factors anchor bacteria at intracellular junction of enteric cells

TRANSMISSION

Not clearly defined, although person-to-person spread most likely

Humans are probably the main reservoir

WHO IS AT RISK?

Incidence increases with age

Infection appears earlier in people in low socioeconomic class and in developing nations

GEOGRAPHY/SEASON

Ubiquitous and worldwide

No seasonal incidence

MODES OF CONTROL

Preliminary studies indicate elimination of organisms with antibiotics combined with bismuth

tests are currently available for detecting these specific antibodies, they are not clinically useful. Because the antibody titers persist for many years, the test cannot be used to discriminate between past and current infection. Furthermore, the titer of antibodies does not correlate with severity of disease or response to therapy.

Treatment, Prevention, and Control

Antibiotics alone are generally ineffective in eradicating *H. pylori*. However, when antibiotics are combined with bismuth, successful elimination of the organism has been reported in preliminary studies. Clinical trials are underway to determine the most efficacious approach to the management of *H. pylori* disease. Current therapy includes the use of bismuth salt with nitroimidazole and either amoxicillin or tetracycline. If the organism is found to be resistant to nitroimidazole, then therapy is usually unsuccessful. Prevention and control of *H. pylori* disease are difficult because the organism is ubiquitous.

CASE STUDY AND QUESTIONS

A mother and her 4-year-old son came to the local emergency room with a 1-day history of diarrhea and abdominal cramping. Both patients had low-grade fevers, and the child had gross blood in the stool specimen. The onset of symptoms developed 18 hours after a dinner of mixed green salad, chicken, corn, bread, and apple pie. Culture of blood samples were negative, but *Campylobacter jejuni* was isolated from stool specimens of both the mother and child.

1. What is the most likely food responsible for these infections? What measures should be used to prevent these infections?
2. What campylobacters are commonly found in blood specimens? What disease is caused by this organism and in what patient populations?
3. What diseases have been associated with *Helicobacter pylori*? What virulence factors does this organism possess, and what are their biological effects?

Bibliography

Blaser MJ: *Helicobacter pylori*: its role in disease, *Clin Infect Dis* 15:386-393, 1992.

Blaser MJ and Reller LB: *Campylobacter* enteritis, *N Engl J Med* 305:1444-1452, 1981.

Blaser MJ, Wells JG, Feldman RA et al: *Campylobacter* enteritis in the United States: a multicenter study, *Ann Intern Med* 98:360-365, 1983.

Buck GE: *Campylobacter pylori* and gastroduodenal disease, *Clin Microbiol Rev* 3:1-12, 1990.

Cover TL and Blaser MJ: *Helicobacter pylori* and gastroduodenal disease, *Ann Rev Med* 43:135-45, 1992.

Dick JD: *Helicobacter (Campylobacter) pylori*: a new twist to an old disease, *Ann Rev Microbiol* 44:249-269, 1990.

Guerrant RL, Lahita RG, Winn WC Jr, and Roberts RB: Campylobacteriosis in man: pathogenic mechanisms and review of 91 bloodstream infections, *Am J Med* 65:584-595, 1978.

Morgan DR: Symposium on *Helicobacter pylori*: a cause of gastroduodenal disease, *Rev Infect Dis* 8(suppl 13): 655-722,1991.

Penner JL: The genus *Campylobacter*: a decade of progress, *Clin Microbiol Rev* 1:157-172, 1988.

Peterson WL: *Helicobacter pylori* and peptic ulcer disease, *N Engl J Med* 324:1043-1047, 1991.

Totten PA, Fennell CL, Tenover FC et al: *Campylobacter cinaedi* and *Campylobacter fennelliae:* two new *Campylobacter* species associated with enteric disease in homosexual men, *J Infect Dis* 151:131-138, 1985.

Vandamme P and De Ley J: Proposal for a new family, Campylobacteraceae, *Int J System Bacteriol* 41:451-455, 1991.

Vandamme P, Falsen E, Rossau R et al: Revision of *Campylobacter*, *Helicobacter*, and *Wolinella* taxonomy: emendation of generic descriptions and proposal of *Arcobacter* gen. nov. *Int J System Bacteriol* 41:88-103, 1991.

CHAPTER 27

Pseudomonas and Related Nonfermenters

CLINICALLY important aerobic gram-negative bacilli can be artificially classified into four general groups: (1) facultatively anaerobic fermenters (e.g., Enterobacteriaceae), (2) obligately aerobic nonfermenters (e.g., Pseudomonadaceae), (3) *Haemophilus* and related genera, and (4) unusual bacilli. Of the bacilli isolated in clinical specimens, 68% to 78% are members of the first group, 12% to 16% are in the second group, 8% to 15% are haemophilic bacilli, and fewer than 1% are classified in the unusual bacilli group. The focus of this chapter is *Pseudomonas* and related nonfermentative gram-negative bacilli, whereas *Haemophilus* and the unusual bacilli are discussed in Chapters 28 to 30.

Pseudomonas and related bacilli are a complex mixture of opportunistic pathogens of plants, animals, and humans. A partial listing of clinically significant nonfermentative organisms is summarized in Box 27-1. Despite the large number of genera, relatively few are isolated with any frequency. *Pseudomonas aeruginosa*, *Xanthomonas maltophilia*, *Acinetobacter baumannii*, and *Moraxella catarrhalis* represent more than 75% of all isolates.

PSEUDOMONAS

Pseudomonads are ubiquitous organisms found in soil, decaying organic matter, vegetation, and water. They are also, unfortunately, found throughout the hospital environment in moist reservoirs such as food, cut flowers, sinks, toilets, floor mops, respiratory therapy equipment, and even disinfectant solutions. Persistent carriage as part of the normal microbial flora in humans is uncommon (less than 6% carriage rate in healthy individuals), unless the individual is hospitalized (38% carriage rate) or is an ambulatory, immunocompromised host (78% carriage rate). The broad environmental distribution of *Pseudomonas* is afforded by their simple growth requirements. More than 30 organic compounds can be used as a source of carbon and nitrogen, and some strains can even grow in distilled water by using trace nutrients. *Pseudomonas* also possess a number of structural factors and toxins that enhance the virulence potential of the organism, as well as render them resistant to most commonly used antibiotics. Indeed, it is surprising that these organisms are not more common pathogens, with their ubiquitous presence, ability to grow in virtually any environment, virulence properties, and broad-based antimicrobial resistance. Instead, *Pseudomonas* infections are primarily opportunistic (i.e., restricted to patients with compromised host defenses).

BOX 27-1 Clinically Significant Nonfermentative Gram-Negative Bacilli

Achromobacter	*Flavobacterium*
Acinetobacter	*Moraxella*
Agrobacterium	*Oligella*
Alcaligenes	*Pseudomonas*
Chryseomonas	*Skewanella*
Comamonas	*Weeksella*
Eikenella	*Xanthomonas*
Flavimonas	

Physiology and Structure

Pseudomonads are straight or slightly curved gram-negative bacilli (0.5-1.0 × 1.5-5.0 μm) and motile by means of polar flagella. The organisms are nonfermentative and use relatively few carbohydrates (e.g., glucose, ribose, gluconate) by oxidative metabolism. Oxygen is the terminal electron acceptor, and the presence of cytochrome oxidase in *Pseudomonas* is used to differentiate this group from the Enterobacteriaceae. Although these organisms are defined as obligate aerobes, anaerobic growth can occur with nitrate used as an alternate electron acceptor. Some strains appear mucoid because of the abundance of a polysaccharide capsule; these strains are particularly common in cystic fibrosis patients. Some pseudomonads produce diffusible pigments (e.g., pyocyanin [blue], fluorescein [yellow], or pyorubin [red-brown]). The genus consists of a number of different species subdivided by biochemical and genetic differences. The species of *Pseudomonas* and closely related

TABLE 27-1 Clinically Important Pseudomonas Species and Other Nonfermenters

rRNA homology group	Group	Genus and species
RNA group I	*P. fluorescens* group	*P. aeruginosa* *P. fluorescens* *P. putida*
	P. stutzeri group	*P. stutzeri* *P. medocina* CDC Group Vb-3
	P. alcaligenes group	*P. alcaligenes* *P. pseudoalcaligenes*
RNA group II	*P. solanacearum* group	*P. pseudomallei* *P. mallei* *P. cepacia* *P. gladioli* *P. pickettii*
RNA group III	*Comamonas acidovorans* group	*C. acidovorans* *C. testosteroni* *C. terrigena*
	P. facilis-delafieldii group	*P. delafieldii*
RNA group IV	*P. diminuta* group	*P. diminuta* *P. vesicularis*
RNA group V	*Xanthomonas* group	*X. maltophilia*
Uncertain affiliation		*P. paucimobilis* *P. pertucinogena* *Pseudomonas*-like group 2 CDC group 1 *Chryseomonas luteola* *Flavimonas oryzihabitans* *Shewanella putrefaciens*

From Gilardi GL: *Pseudomonas* and related genera. In Balows A, Hausler W, Herrmann K, et al., editors: *Manual of clinical microbiology*, Washington, DC, 1991, American Society of Microbiology.

genera that have been associated with human infections are summarized in Table 27-1. *Pseudomonas aeruginosa* is the most common clinically significant pseudomonad and the best-characterized member of the genus.

Pathogenesis

Pseudomonads have a number of virulence factors, including structural components, toxins, and enzymes (Table 27-2). Defining the role each factor plays in disease caused by these organisms is difficult, and most experts in this field believe *Pseudomonas* virulence is multifactorial.

TABLE 27-2 Virulence Factors Associated With *Pseudomonas*

Virulence factors	Biological effects
Pili	Adherence to respiratory epithelium
Polysaccharide capsule	Adherence to tracheal epithelium; antiphagocytic
Endotoxin	Sepsis syndrome: fever, shock, oliguria, leukopenia or leukocytosis, disseminated intravascular coagulation, metabolic abnormalities
Exotoxin A	Inhibition of protein synthesis
Exoenzyme S	Inhibition of protein synthesis
Elastase	Vascular tissue damage; inhibition of neutrophil function
Alkaline protease	Tissue damage; anticomplementary; inactivation of IgG; inhibition of neutrophil function
Phospholipase C	Tissue damage
Leukocidin	Inhibition of neutrophil and lymphocyte function

Pili or Fimbriae

These hairlike structures mediate adherence of the bacterium to the respiratory epithelium.

Polysaccharide Capsule

The surface of *P. aeruginosa* is covered with a polysaccharide layer that protects the organism from phagocytosis. This layer can also anchor the bacteria to cell surfaces, particularly in patients with cystic fibrosis or other chronic respiratory diseases who are predisposed to colonization with mucoid strains of *P. aeruginosa.*

Endotoxin

As is true with other gram-negative bacilli, pseudomonads possess a lipopolysaccharide endotoxin as a major cell wall antigen. The lipid A component of endotoxin mediates the various biological effects of the sepsis syndrome.

Exotoxin A

One of the most important virulence factors produced by pathogenic strains of *P. aeruginosa* is exotoxin A (Figure 27-1). This toxin blocks eukaryotic cell protein synthesis in a manner similar to that described for diphtheria toxin (Chapter 22). However, these toxins are structurally and immunologically different, and exotoxin A is less potent than diphtheria toxin.

Exoenzyme S

This extracellular toxin is produced by one third of the clinical isolates of *P. aeruginosa* and can inhibit protein

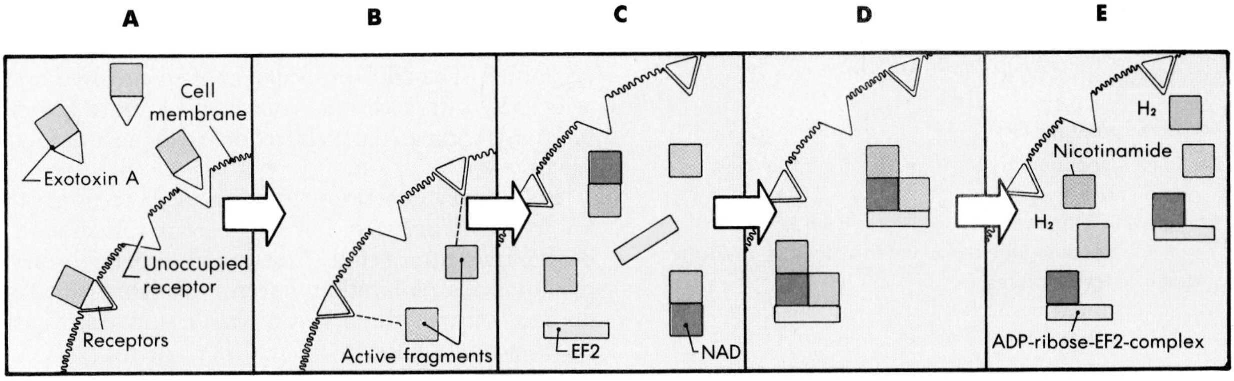

FIGURE 27-1 Mode of action of exotoxin A. **A,** Exotoxin A, composed of fragments A and B, inhibits eukaryotic cell protein synthesis by binding to specific receptors in the cell membrane. **B,** After fragment B binds to a cell receptor, fragment A enters the cell. **C,** Fragment A catalyzes the binding of nicotinamide adenine dinucleotide (NAD) to Elongation Factor 2 (EF2), which is required for translocation of nascent polypeptide chains on eukaryotic ribosomes. **D** and **E,** The reaction terminates in the irreversible formation of an adenosine diphosphate ribose. EF2 diphosphate—EF2 complex with the release of nicotinamide and hydrogen.

synthesis. Both exotoxin A and exoenzyme S are ADP-ribosyltransferases, but they are distinguished by the heat stability of exoenzyme S.

Elastase

This enzyme can catalyze the destruction of the elastic fiber in blood vessel walls, resulting in hemorrhagic lesions **(ecthyma gangrenosum)** associated with disseminated *P. aeruginosa* infections.

Other Proteases

Other proteases have been described in pseudomonads that mediate tissue destruction, inactivation of antibodies, and inhibition of neutrophils.

Phospholipase C

Phospholipase C breaks down lipids and lecithin, facilitating tissue destruction. The exact role of this enzyme in infections of the respiratory and urinary tracts is unclear, although a significant association exists between hemolysin production and disease at these sites.

Epidemiology

Pseudomonads are opportunistic pathogens present in a variety of environmental habitats (Box 27-2). The ability to isolate these organisms from moist surfaces may be limited only by one's interest in searching for the organism. Pseudomonads have minimal nutritional requirements, can tolerate a wide range of temperatures (4° C to 42° C), and are resistant to many antibiotics and disinfectants. Indeed, the simple recovery of *Pseudomonas* from an environmental source (e.g., hospital sink or floor) means very little without epidemiological evidence that the contaminated site is a reservoir for infection. Furthermore, isolation of *Pseudomonas* from a hospitalized patient is worrisome but does not normally justify therapeutic intervention without evidence of disease. It is important to note that recovery of *Pseudomonas,* particularly species other than *P. aeruginosa,* from a clinical specimen may represent contamination of the specimen during collection or laboratory processing. Because these organisms are opportunistic pathogens, the significance of an isolate must be measured by assessing the clinical presentation of the patient.

Similar to other *Pseudomonas* species, *P. pseudomallei* is an environmental organism that causes opportunistic infections. However, these infections (**melioidosis**) can occur in previously healthy individuals as either an acute suppurative infection or as a chronic pulmonary infection. Particularly important is that disease can occur from a few days to many years after exposure. For these reasons it is important to know *P. pseudomallei* is a saprophyte found in soil, water, and vegetation, with worldwide distribution but particularly in Southeast Asia, India, Africa, and Australia (Figure 27-2). Although the organism is rarely isolated in the Western hemisphere, latent disease occurs in persons who have been in endemic areas.

Clinical Syndromes

Pseudomonas aeruginosa

Many of the serious infections caused by *P. aeruginosa* are listed in Box 27-3.

Bacteremia and endocarditis. Bacteremia caused by *P. aeruginosa* is clinically indistinguishable from other gram-negative infections, although the mortality rate is higher. This is due in part to the predilection of this organism for immunocompromised patients and in part to the inherent virulence of *Pseudomonas. P. aeruginosa* bacteremia is particularly common in patients with neutropenia, diabetes mellitus, extensive burns, and hematological malignancies. Most *Pseudomonas* bacteremias originate from infections of the lower respiratory tract,

BOX 27-2 Epidemiology of *Pseudomonas aeruginosa* Infection

DISEASE/BACTERIAL FACTORS

Ubiquitous opportunistic pathogen of plants, animals, and humans
Can grow in virtually any environment because of minimal nutritional requirements and tolerance of a wide range of temperatures
Found throughout hospitals in moist reservoirs (respiratory therapy equipment, sinks, cut flowers, etc.)
Organisms have broad range of antimicrobial resistance
Numerous virulence factors (see Table 27-2)

TRANSMISSION

Endogenous spread from colonized body site to normally sterile areas of the body
Patient-to-patient spread related to antibiotic overuse
Persistent carriage uncommon in healthy humans, but more common in hospitalized patients and ambulatory immunocompromised patients

WHO IS AT RISK?

Immuncompromised patients
Burn patients
IV drug users (contaminated paraphernalia)
Note: Because organism is so widespread, recovery of *Pseudomonas* from patient does not justify therapy without clinical evidence of disease

GEOGRAPHY/SEASON

Worldwide
No seasonal incidence

MODES OF CONTROL

Combined use of aminoglycoside and β-lactam antibiotic with proven effectiveness against isolate
In immunocompromised patients, hyperimmune globulin and granulocyte transfusions may have benefits in selected cases
In hospitals, infection control efforts should concentrate on preventing contamination of sterile medical equipment and cross-contamination of patients by medical personnel
Avoid unnecessary use of broad-spectrum antibiotics

urinary tract, and skin and soft tissue (particularly burn wound infections). Although seen in a minority of patients, characteristic skin lesions (**ecthyma gangrenosum**) may develop. The lesions are seen initially as erythematous vesicles that progress to hemorrhage, necrosis, and ulceration. Microscopic examination of the lesion shows abundant organisms with vascular destruction (which explains the hemorrhagic nature of the lesions) and the absence of neutrophils as would be expected in neutropenic patients.

Pseudomonas endocarditis is most commonly observed in intravenous drug abusers; the source of infection is drug paraphernalia contaminated with the water-borne organisms. The tricuspid valve is often involved and is associated with a chronic course and a more favorable prognosis compared with infections of the aortic or mitral valves.

Pulmonary infections. *P. aeruginosa* infections of the lower respiratory tract can range from colonization or benign tracheobronchitis to severe necrotizing bronchopneumonia. Colonization is seen in patients with cystic fibrosis, other chronic lung diseases, and neutropenia. *Pseudomonas* pulmonary infection in patients with cystic fibrosis has been associated with exacerbation of the underlying disease, as well as invasive disease in pulmonary parenchyma. Neutropenic and other immunocompromised patients are frequently exposed to *Pseudomonas* following use of contaminated respiratory therapy equipment. Invasive disease in this population is characterized by a diffuse, typically bilateral bronchopneumonia with microabscess formation and tissue necrosis. Bacteremia, with an associated high mortality rate, can be observed in severe infections.

Ear infections. External otitis is most frequently due to *P. aeruginosa,* with swimming **(swimmer's ear)** a significant risk factor. Although this localized infection can be managed with topical antibiotics and drying agents, a more virulent form of disease **(malignant external otitis)** can invade the underlying tissues and be life threatening. Aggressive antimicrobial and surgical intervention is required for this latter disease. *P. aeruginosa* is also associated with chronic otitis media.

Burn infections. *P. aeruginosa* colonization of a burn wound, followed by localized vascular damage and tissue necrosis, and ultimately bacteremia, is not uncommon in patients who have sustained severe burns. The moist surface of the burn and absence of neutrophilic response to tissue invasion predispose patients to *Pseudomonas* infections. Use of topical creams and wound management has controlled *Pseudomonas* colonization with only limited success.

Other infections. *P. aeruginosa* is associated with a variety of other infections, including those localized in the gastrointestinal and urinary tracts, eye, central nervous system, and musculoskeletal system. The underlying conditions required for most *Pseudomonas* infections are the presence of the organism in a moist reservoir and the circumvention or absence of host defenses (e.g., cutaneous trauma, elimination of normal microbial flora by injudicious use of antibiotics, neutropenia). *Pseudomonas* urinary tract infections are observed in patients with indwelling urinary catheters.

Pseudomonas pseudomallei

Melioidosis has protean manifestations. Most individuals exposed to *P. pseudomallei* remain asymptomatic. Some with cutaneous exposure develop a localized suppurative infection with regional lymphadenitis, fever, and malaise. This form of disease can resolve without incidence or

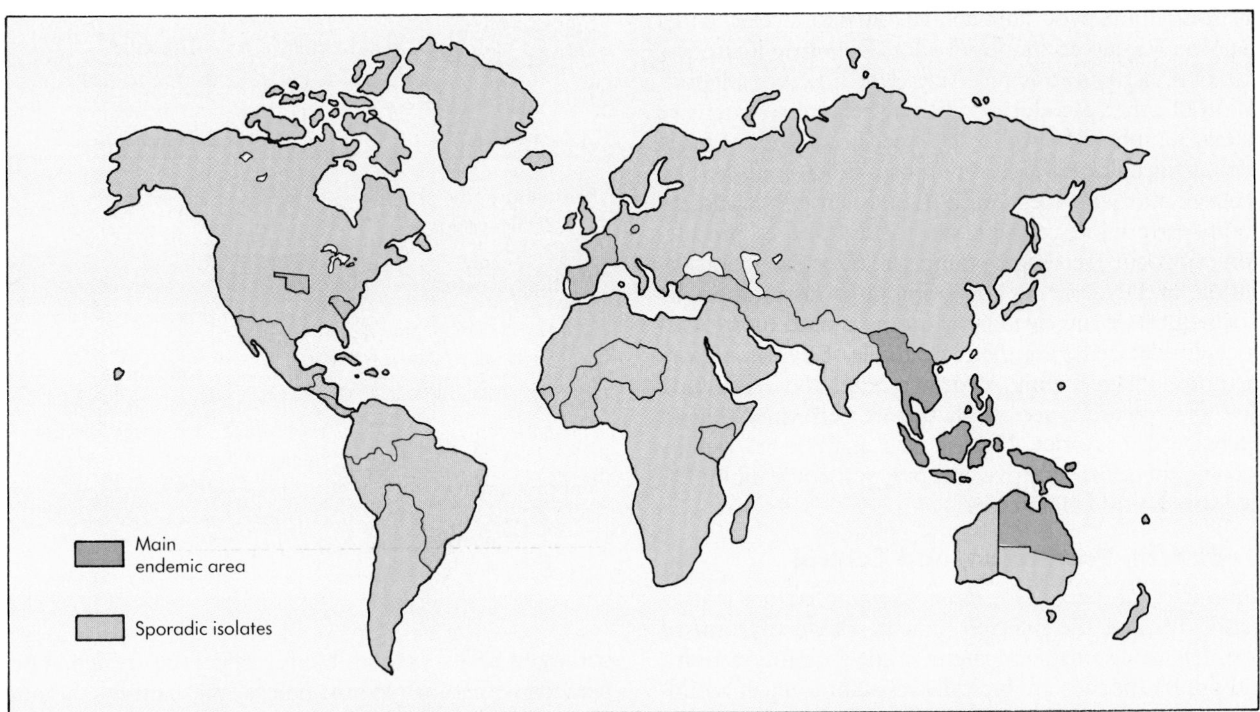

FIGURE 27-2 Geographical distribution of *Pseudomonas pseudomallei.* Shaded area, main endemic area; hatched areas, sporadic isolates. (Modified from Dance D., *Clin Microbiol Rev* 4:52-60, 1991.)

rapidly progress to overwhelming sepsis. The third form of infection is pulmonary disease, which may range from mild bronchitis to necrotizing pneumonia. Cavitation can develop in the absence of appropriate antimicrobial therapy. Isolation of *P. pseudomallei* for diagnostic purposes should be approached carefully because the organism is considered highly infectious.

Other Pseudomonads

The *Pseudomonas* species and related organisms listed in Table 27-1 are all capable of opportunistic infections in immunocompromised patients. The majority of true infections with these organisms have been localized to the respiratory tract in patients with underlying pulmonary disease or to the urinary tract following instrumentation or catheterization. *P. cepacia* is a particularly common respiratory pathogen in cystic fibrosis patients.

The clinical significance of an isolate is often difficult to assess because specific signs and symptoms of disease may be absent in patients and the organism may be an insignificant water-borne contaminant.

BOX 27-3 *Pseudomonas aeruginosa* Infections

- Bacteremia
- Endocarditis
- Pulmonary infections
  - Tracheobronchitis
  - Necrotizing bronchopneumonia
- Ear infections
  - Chronic external otitis
  - Malignant external otitis
  - Chronic otitis media
- Burn wound infections
- Urinary tract infections
- Gastroenteritis
- Eye infections
- Musculoskeletal infections

Laboratory Diagnosis

Culture

Because pseudomonads have simple nutritional requirements, they grow easily on common isolation media such as blood agar or MacConkey agar. Aerobic incubation is required (unless nitrate is available), so growth in broth is generally confined to the broth-air interface.

Identification

The colonial morphology (colony size, hemolytic activity, pigmentation, odor) combined with selected rapid biochemical tests (e.g., positive oxidase reaction) are used for the preliminary identification of isolates. For example, *P. aeruginosa* grows rapidly and has flat colonies with a spreading border, green pigmentation (caused by production of blue pyocyanin and yellow fluorescein), and a characteristic sweet, grapelike odor. Definitive identification of *P. aeruginosa* is relatively easy; however, identification of other pseudomonads may require an extensive battery of physiological tests. Specific classification of isolates for epidemiological purposes is accomplished by determination of biochemical profiles, antibiotic susceptibility patterns, susceptibility to bacteriophages, production of pyocins, serologic typing, or molecular characterization of DNA or rRNA. Although classification by biochemical or susceptibility patterns is used most often in clinical laboratories, these are the least discriminatory methods. Phage typing, pyocin typing, and serotyping have all been used successfully but are performed only in reference laboratories. Nucleic acid analysis has rapidly become the most sensitive and practical epidemiological tool for clinical laboratories.

Treatment, Prevention, and Control

Antimicrobial therapy for *Pseudomonas* infections is frustrating because the infected patient with compromised host defenses is unable to augment the antibiotic activity, and pseudomonads are typically resistant to most antibiotics (Table 27-3). Even in susceptible organisms resistance can develop during therapy by the induction of antibiotic inactivating enzymes (e.g., β-lactamases) or the transfer of plasmid-mediated resistance from a resistant organism to a susceptible one. Furthermore, some groups of antibiotics such as the aminoglycosides are ineffective at the site of infection (poor activity in the acidic environment of an abscess). Successful therapy for serious infections generally requires the combined use of aminoglycoside and β-lactam antibiotics, which have documented activity against the isolate. *P. cepacia* differs from *P. aeruginosa* and most other *Pseudomonas* species in that the isolates are generally susceptible to sulfonamide antibiotics. Augmentation of compromised immune function with hyperimmune globulin and granulocyte transfusions may have beneficial effects with selected patients who have *Pseudomonas* infections.

Attempts to eliminate *Pseudomonas* from the hospital environment are practically useless given the ubiquitous presence of the organism in water supplies. Effective infection-control practices should concentrate on prevention of contamination of sterile equipment such as respiratory therapy machines, and cross-contamination of patients by medical personnel. The inappropriate use of broad-spectrum antibiotics should be avoided, because this practice can suppress the normal microbial flora and permit the overgrowth of resistant pseudomonads.

TABLE 27-3 Mechanisms of Antibiotic Resistance in *Pseudomonas*

Antibiotic	Resistance mechanisms
Penicillins and cephalosporins	β-lactamase hydrolysis, altered binding proteins, decreased permeability
Aminoglycosides	Enzymatic hydrolysis by acetylation, adenylation, or phosphorylation; decreased permeability; altered ribosomal target
Chloramphenicol	Enzymatic hydrolysis by acetyltransferase; decreased permeability
Fluoroquinolones	Altered target (DNA gyrase); decreased permeability

XANTHOMONAS MALTOPHILIA

X. maltophilia is recognized as the second most commonly isolated, nonfermentative, gram-negative bacilli. This organism was originally classified as *Pseudomonas maltophilia*. It is an important opportunistic nosocomial pathogen and is responsible for infections in debilitated patients with impaired host-defense mechanisms. Because *X. maltophilia* is resistant to most commonly used β-lactam and aminoglycoside antibiotics, patients receiving long-term antibiotic therapy are particularly at risk for developing infections with this organism.

The spectrum of nosocomial infections with *X. maltophilia* is broad, including bacteremia, pneumonia, meningitis, wound infections, and urinary tract infections. Hospital epidemics with this organism have been traced to contaminated disinfectant solutions, respiratory therapy or monitoring equipment, and contaminated ice machines.

Antimicrobial therapy is complicated because the organism is resistant to aminoglycosides, penicillins, imipenem, and fluoroquinolones. Trimethoprim-sulfamethaxazole is the most active antibiotic, with good activity also seen with chloramphenicol and ceftazidime.

ACINETOBACTER

The genus *Acinetobacter* is currently undergoing taxonomic reorganization. Whereas one species, *A. calcoaceticus*, with two subspecies (var. *anitratus* and var. *lwoffi*) were previously recognized, additional species have been defined by DNA homology analysis. However, phenotypic separation of the species is problematic, and it has been proposed that the human pathogens should be called either *A. baumannii* or *A. calcoaceticus-A. baumannii* complex.

Acinetobacters are nonfermentative, opportunistic pathogens, most commonly responsible for nosocomial respiratory infections. Like the pseudomonads, these organisms thrive in moist environments and have been found as common contaminants of respiratory therapy equipment and monitoring devices. The organism is also part of the normal oropharyngeal flora of a small

BOX 27-4 *Moraxella* species

M. bovis	*M. lacunata*
M. catarrhalis	*M. nonliquefaciens*
M. caviae	*M. ovis*
M. cuniculi	

proportion of healthy individuals and can proliferate to large numbers during hospitalization.

Acinetobacters are resistant to many antibiotics, although infections can be successfully treated with selected aminoglycosides, broad spectrum cephalosporins, or imipenem.

MORAXELLA

The genus *Moraxella* has also been reorganized based upon DNA-rRNA hybridization analysis. Currently, seven species are included in this genus (Box 27-4), with *M. catarrhalis* the most important species. During the past 20 years, *M. catarrhalis* has been classified as *Neisseria catarrhalis* and *Branhamella catarrhalis*, nomenclature that is still commonly found in the literature.

M. catarrhalis is part of the normal oropharyngeal population and is a common cause of bronchitis and bronchopneumonia (in patients with chronic pulmonary disease), sinusitis, and otitis. Infections are most frequently observed in previously healthy individuals but are also seen in hospitalized patients. Most isolates produce β-lactamases and are penicillin resistant. These isolates are uniformly susceptible to erythromycin, tetracycline, trimethoprim-sulfamethoxazole, and the combination of ampicillin with a β-lactamase inhibitor (e.g., clavulanic acid).

CASE STUDY AND QUESTIONS

A 63-year-old man had been hospitalized for the previous 21 days for management of newly diagnosed leukemia. During the period of hospitalization the patient had developed a urinary tract infection with *E. coli* and was treated for 14 days with broad spectrum antibiotics. On hospital day 21 the patient developed fever and shaking chills. Within 24 hours the patient became hypotensive, and ecthymic skin lesions appeared. Despite aggressive therapy with antibiotics, the patient expired. Multiple blood cultures were positive for *Pseudomonas aeruginosa*.

1. What factors made this man at increased risk for infection with *P. aeruginosa*? What are the epidemiological characteristics of this organism?
2. What virulence factors possessed by the organism make it a particularly serious pathogen? What is the biological effect of these factors?
3. What measures could be used to manage this infection in this patient? What control measures should be used to prevent additional infections in other patients in the hospital unit?
4. What diseases are caused by *Xanthomonas maltophilia*? *Acinetobacter baumannii*? *Moraxella catarrhalis*? What antibiotics can be used to treat these infections? What antibiotics can be used to treat *P. aeruginosa* infections?

Bibliography

Bisbe J, Gatell JM, Puig J et al.: *Pseudomonas aeruginosa* bacteremia: univariate and multivariate analyses of factors influencing the prognosis in 133 episodes, *Rev Infect Dis* 10:629-635, 1988.

Bodey GP, Jadeja L, and Elting L: *Pseudomonas* bacteremia: retrospective analysis of 410 episodes, *Arch Intern Med* 145:1621-1629, 1985.

Bouvet PJM and Grimont PAD: Taxonomy of the genus *Acinetobacter* with the recognition of *Acinetobacter baumannii* sp. nov., *Acinetobacter haemolyticus* sp. nov., *Acinetobacter johnsonii* sp. nov., and *Acinetobacter junii* sp. nov., and emended descriptions of *Acinetobacter calcoaceticus* and *Acinetobacter lwoffi*, *Int J Syst Bacteriol* 36:228-240, 1986.

Catlin BW: *Branhamella catarrhalis*: an organism gaining respect as a pathogen, *Clin Microbiol Rev* 3:293-320, 1990.

Dance DAB: Melioidosis: the tip of the iceberg, *Clin Microbiol Rev* 4:52-60, 1991.

Gustafson TL, Band JD, Hutcheson RH Jr, and Schaffner W: *Pseudomonas* folliculitis: an outbreak and review, *Rev Infect Dis* 5:1-8, 1983.

Marshall WF, Keating MR, Anhalt JP, and Steckelberg JM: *Xanthomonas maltophilia*: an emerging nosocomial pathogen, *Mayo Clin Rev* 64:1097-1104, 1989.

Pruitt BA Jr and McManus AT: Opportunistic infections in severely burned patients, *Am J Med* 76(suppl):146-154, 1984.

Rossau R, Van Landschoot A, Gillis M, and De Ley J: Taxonomy of *Moraxellaceae* fam. nov., a new bacterial family to accommodate the genera *Moraxella*, *Acinetobacter*, and *Psychrobacter* and related organisms, *Int J Syst Bacteriol* 41:310-319, 1991.

Sadoff JC and Sanford JP: Symposium on *Pseudomonas aeruginosa* infections, *Rev Infect Dis* 5(suppl):833-1004, 1983.

Vandenbroucke-Grauls C, Kerver A, Rommes JH et al.: Endemic *Acinetobacter anitratus* in a surgical intensive care unit: mechanical ventilators as reservoir, *Eur J Clin Microbiol Infect Dis* 7:485-489, 1988.

Vauterin L, Swings J, Kersters K et al.: Towards an improved taxonomy of *Xanthomonas*, *Int J Syst Bacter* 40:312-316, 1990.

Wick MJ, Frank DW, Storey DG, and Iglewski BH: Structure, function, and regulation of *Pseudomonas aeruginosa* exotoxin A, *Annu Rev Microbiol* 44:335-363, 1990.

Young LS: The role of exotoxins in the pathogenesis of *Pseudomonas aeruginosa* infections, *J Infect Dis* 142:626-630, 1980.

CHAPTER 28

Haemophilus, Actinobacillus, and Pasteurella

THE family Pasteurellaceae consists of three genera: *Haemophilus, Actinobacillus,* and *Pasteurella,* with *Haemophilus* the most common human pathogen (Table 28-1). Members of the family are small (0.2 × 0.3 to 2.0 μm), gram-negative bacilli, non–spore-forming, nonmotile, and aerobic or facultative anaerobic. Most have fastidious growth habits, requiring enriched media for isolation.

HAEMOPHILUS

Haemophilus are small, sometimes pleomorphic, gram-negative bacilli that are obligate parasites present on the mucous membranes of humans and animal species. *Haemophilus influenzae* is the species most commonly associated with disease. Although less frequently isolated *H. ducreyi* is well-recognized as the etiological agent of the sexually transmitted disease, **soft chancre** or **chancroid**. DNA homology studies indicate *H. ducreyi* has been misclassified as a *Haemophilus* species, but reclassification into a new genus has not occurred at this time.

TABLE 28-1 Most Common Pasteurellaceae Associated With Human Disease

Organism	Primary diseases
Haemophilus influenzae	Meningitis, epiglottitis, cellulitis, otitis, sinusitis, pneumonia, conjunctivitis, bacteremia
H. parainfluenzae	Bacteremia, endocarditis, opportunistic infections
H. ducreyi	Chancroid
H. haemolyticus	Opportunistic infections
H. parahaemolyticus	Opportunistic infections
H. segnis	Opportunistic infections
H. aphrophilus	Endocarditis, opportunistic infections
H. paraphrophilus	Opportunistic infections
Actinobacillus actinomycetemcomitans	Juvenile periodontitis, endocarditis
Pasteurella multocida	Soft tissue infections, respiratory infections, bacteremia

Physiology and Structure

Most species of *Haemophilus* (from the Greek words for blood loving) require supplementation of media with growth-stimulating factors, specifically **X factor** (hematin) and/or **V factor** (nicotinamide adenine dinucleotide [NAD]). Although both factors are present in blood-enriched media, the blood must be gently heated to release the factors and destroy inhibitors of V factor. For this reason heated blood agar (i.e., chocolate agar) is used for the in vitro isolation of *Haemophilus*. In contrast with other *Haemophilus* species, *H. ducreyi* is very difficult to grow in vitro.

The cell wall structure of *Haemophilus* is typical of other gram-negative bacilli. Lipopolysaccharide endotoxin activity is present in the cell wall, and strain-specific and species-specific proteins are found in the outer membrane (Figure 28-1). The surface of many but not all strains of *H. influenzae* is covered with a polysaccharide capsule, with six antigenic serotypes (a through f) recognized. Before the introduction of vaccines directed against *H. influenzae* type b antigen, this serotype was responsible for more than 95% of all invasive *Haemophilus* infections. Other species of *Haemophilus* do not have capsules. In addition to the serologic differentiation of *H. influenzae*, the species is subdivided into nine biotypes (biotypes I to VIII and *H. aegyptius*) by three biochemical reactions: indole production, urease activity, and ornithine decarboxylase activity. *H. aegyptius* and *H. influenzae* biotype III have identical biochemical profiles; however, they can be distinguished by clinical disease, in vitro growth properties, and outer membrane protein profiles.

Pathogenesis and Immunity

Haemophilus species, particularly *H. parainfluenzae* and nonencapsulated *H. influenzae,* colonize the upper respiratory tract in virtually all individuals within the first few

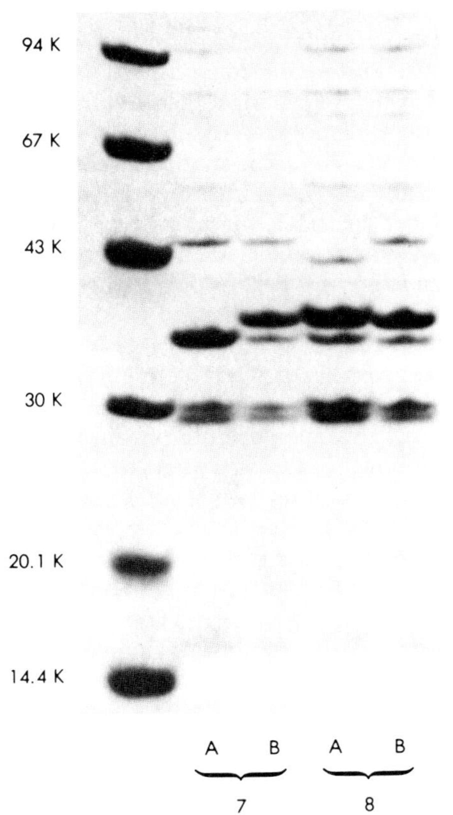

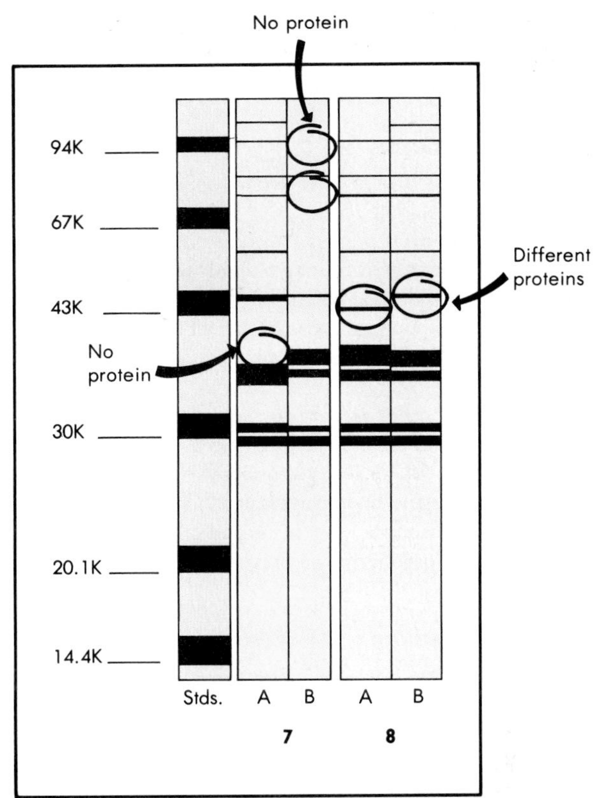

FIGURE 28-1 Migration patterns of *H. influenzae* type b outer membrane protein preparations on sodium dodecyl sulfate-polyacrylamide gels can be used to classify isolates for epidemiological investigations. The outer membrane protein profiles of four isolates from two day care centers (*7* and *8*) are demonstrated here. The isolates from each center have distinct profiles and therefore are not epidemiologically related. The first lane has six molecular weight standards. (From Barenkamp SJ et al: *J Infect Dis* 144:210, 1981.)

months of life. These organisms can spread locally and cause disease in the ears (otitis media), sinuses (sinusitis), and lower respiratory tract (bronchitis, pneumonia). Disseminated disease, however, is relatively uncommon. In contrast, encapsulated *H. influenzae* (particularly serogroup b) is infrequently present in the upper respiratory tract but has been a common cause of epiglottitis and pediatric meningitis. The organism is able to penetrate the nasopharyngeal submucosa and enter the bloodstream. In the absence of specific opsonic antibodies directed against the polysaccharide capsule, high-grade bacteremia can develop, with dissemination to the meninges or other distal foci.

The major virulence factor in *H. influenzae* type b is the antiphagocytic polysaccharide capsule, which contains ribose, ribitol, and phosphate (commonly referred to as **PRP** or **polyribitol phosphate**). Bacterial phagocytosis and complement-mediated bactericidal activity are greatly stimulated by antibodies directed against the capsule. These antibodies develop as the result of natural infection, passive transfer of maternal antibodies, or following vaccination with the purified PRP. Systemic disease is inversely related to the rate of clearance of bacteria from the bloodstream. The risk of meningitis and epiglottitis is significantly greater in patients with no anti-PRP antibodies, with depletion of complement, or after splenectomy. The lipopolysaccharide lipid A component induces meningeal inflammation in an animal model and may be responsible for initiating this response in human disease. The roles of other membrane antigens and pili are poorly defined but are not believed to be significant virulence factors. IgA1-specific proteases are produced by *H. influenzae* (both encapsulated and nonencapsulated strains) and may facilitate colonization of mucosal surfaces.

Epidemiology

The human species of *Haemophilus* comprise more than 10% of the bacteria in the oral cavity of healthy individuals (Box 28-1). The most common species are *H. parainfluenzae* and nonencapsulated strains of *H. influenzae*. Although *H. influenzae* type b is the most common species responsible for systemic disease, it is rarely isolated in healthy children (a fact that emphasizes the virulence of this bacterium).

The epidemiology of *Haemophilus* disease is in dramatic transition. The incidence of invasive *Haemophilus* disease had increased gradually during the last 50 years,

BOX 28-1 Epidemiology of *Haemophilus* Infection

DISEASE/BACTERIAL FACTORS

H. influenzae type b causes meningitis, epiglottitis, cellulitis, arthritis, conjunctivitis

H. influenzae type b is primarily a pediatric pathogen (children younger than 5 years old), although the incidence is rapidly decreasing with immunization

H. ducreyi is an important cause of genital ulcers

Nonencapsulated *H. influenzae* type b causes otitis media, sinusitis, bronchitis

The type b polysaccharide capsule is antiphagocytic

Increased exposure to *H. influenzae* type b is associated with increased risk for invasive disease

Increased exposure to nonencapsulated *Haemophilus* strains is *not* associated with increased infections because these organisms are ubiquitous and have a low virulence

TRANSMISSION

Endogenous spread from upper respiratory tract through the blood to meninges, epiglottis, skin, joints; or direct extension to eye, inner ear, sinuses, or lower respiratory tract

H. ducreyi: sexually transmitted

WHO IS AT RISK?

Children younger than 5 years old without protective antibodies against type B capsular polysaccharide

Patients with depleted complement or after splenectomy

Elderly at greatest risk for pulmonary disease, particularly those with obstructive pulmonary disease or conditions predisposing to aspiration

GEOGRAPHY/SEASON

H. influenzae infections occur worldwide

H. ducreyi causes genital ulcers in Africa and Asia, less commonly in Europe and North America

No seasonal incidence

MODES OF CONTROL

Severe infection: treat with β-lactamase–resistant cephalosporin with good CSF penetration (e.g., ceftriaxone) or chloramphenicol

Mild infection: ampicillin (if susceptible), trimethoprim-sulfamethoxazole, or cefaclor

Systemic spread of *H. influenzae* type b: drugs that penetrate to CNS

Active immunization with purified capsular PRP conjugated to protein carrier is best prevention against *H. influenzae* type b, especially in infants 2 months old or older

Passive immunization with hyperimmune globulins active against *H. influenzae* type b has some use in protecting high-risk children after exposure to organism

Rifampin prophylaxis useful to eliminate carriage of *H. influenzae* type b in children at high risk for disease

with an estimated 15,000 cases reported annually. Two thirds of the infections were meningitis, and the majority were observed in children younger than 1 year of age. As noted previously, the primary risk factor for invasive *Haemophilus* disease is the absence of protective antibodies directed against the polysaccharide capsule. The first vaccines developed against *H. influenzae* type b were not protective for children younger than 18 months of age (the population at greatest risk for disease) because there is a natural delay in the maturation of the immune response to polysaccharide antigens. However, use of purified PRP antigens conjugated to protein carriers can elicit a protective antibody response in infants 2 months of age and older. Thus with the use of this conjugated vaccine, we are now witnessing a dramatic decrease in both disease and colonization with *H. influenzae* type b in immunized populations. It can be anticipated that systemic *Haemophilus* disease as recognized in the past will be restricted to pediatric populations with limited access to health care or when genetic defects interfere with production of protective levels of immunoglobulins.

The epidemiology of disease caused by nonencapsulated *H. influenzae* and other *Haemophilus* species is distinct. Increased exposure to *H. influenzae* type b is associated with increased risk for invasive disease. In contrast, disease caused by nonencapsulated *Haemophilus* strains is not increased in crowded communities because of the ubiquitous presence of the organisms and their decreased virulence. Invasive disease is less common, and infections are not restricted to young children. Ear and sinus infections caused by these organisms are primarily pediatric diseases but can be observed in adults. Pulmonary disease is most commonly observed in the elderly, particularly those with a history of underlying obstructive pulmonary disease or conditions predisposing to aspiration (e.g., alcoholism, altered mental state).

H. ducreyi is an important cause of genital ulcers in Africa and Asia but is less commonly implicated in Europe and North America. Between 4000 and 5000 cases are reported in the United States each year (Figure 28-2), with clusters of disease in California, Texas, New York, Florida, and Georgia. The Centers for Disease Control have documented that chancroid is significantly underreported, so the true incidence of this disease is unknown.

Clinical Syndromes

The clinical syndromes that accompany infections of *H. influenzae* are illustrated in Figure 28-3. A discussion of disease caused by all *Haemophilus* species follows.

Meningitis

H. influenzae type b was the most common cause of pediatric meningitis, although this has changed rapidly with the widespread use of effective conjugated vaccines. Disease in nonimmune patients follows bacteremic spread from the nasopharynx and cannot be differentiated clinically from other causes of bacterial meningitis. The

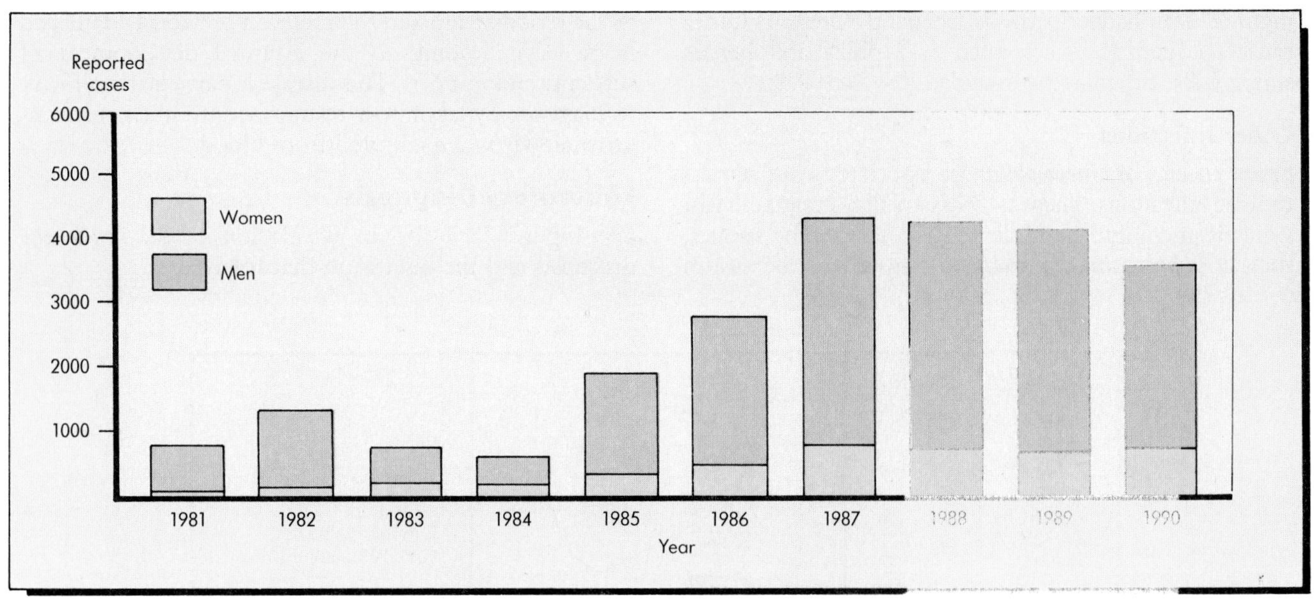

FIGURE 28-2 *Haemophilus ducreyi* disease in the United States from 1981 [illegible] from *MMWR* 41:61, 1992.)

initial presentation is generally preceded by a 1- to 3-day history of mild upper respiratory disease. With prompt therapeutic intervention, mortality is less than 10%, and carefully designed studies have documented a low incidence of serious neurological sequelae (in contrast with initial studies that reported as many as 50% of the children with severe residual damage).

Epiglottitis

This disease, characterized by cellulitis and swelling of the supraglottic tissues, represents a life-threatening emergency. Although epiglottitis is a pediatric disease, the peak incidence of disease in the prevaccine era was primarily in children from 2 to 4 years of age; this is in contrast with meningitis, which peaked in children from 3 to 18 months of age. Children with epiglottitis have pharyngitis, fever, and breathing difficulties, which can rapidly progress to complete obstruction of the airway and death.

Cellulitis

This disease is seen in very young children. Patients have fever and cellulitis characterized by a reddish-blue color on the cheek or periorbital area. The etiological diagnosis is strongly suggested by the typical clinical presentation, proximity to the oral mucosa, and age of the child.

Arthritis

Infection of single large joints, secondary to bacteremic spread of *H. influenzae* type b, was the most common form of arthritis seen in children younger than 2 years of age before the use of conjugated vaccines. Disease in older children and adults is reported, but it is very uncommon and generally occurs in joints with preexisting damage or in immunocompromised patients.

Conjunctivitis and [illegible] ver

Epidemic, as well as [illegible] an be caused by *H. influenzae,* [illegible] nerly called *Haemophilus aegyptius* [illegible] is organism has also been associa[illegible] puric fever. This fulminant pedia[illegible] erized by an initial conjunctivitis, f[illegible] r by an acute onset of fever, vomiti[illegible] in, and then the rapid development [illegible] a, shock, and death. The pathogenes[illegible] ric fever and the specific virulence [illegible] he etiological agent are poorly unders[illegible]

Otitis, Sinusitis, and [illegible] Tract Disease

Nonencapsulated strai[illegible] e opportunistic pathogens that can [illegible] he upper and lower airways. Most st[illegible] *H. influenzae* and *Streptococcus pneum*[illegible] ost common causes of both acute [illegible] and sinusitis. Primary pneumonia is [illegible] n in children and adults who have no[illegible] nction. However, these organisms c[illegible] patients who have chronic pulmon[illegible] frequently are associated with exacerba[illegible] s well as frank pneumonia.

Chancroid

Chancroid is a sexually [illegible] e and is most commonly diagnosed [illegible] ably because asymptomatic or inappa[illegible] ur in women. Approximately 5 to 7 da[illegible] tender papule with an erythematous [illegible] e genitalia or perianal area. The lesion [illegible] nful ulcer, and inguinal lymphadenopathy is frequently present. Other causes of genital ulcers, such as syphilis and herpes simplex disease, must be excluded.

Other Infections

Other species of *Haemophilus* are associated with opportunistic infections, such as otitis media, conjunctivitis, sinusitis, meningitis, and dental abscesses. Some species, such as *H. aphrophilus*, are able to spread from the mouth to the bloodstream and then infect a previously damaged heart valve, leading to the eventual development of subacute endocarditis. This disease is particularly difficult to diagnose by laboratory testing because the organisms grow slowly when cultured from blood.

Laboratory Diagnosis

See Figure 28-3 for an illustration of *H. influenzae* diagnosis and the discussion that follows.

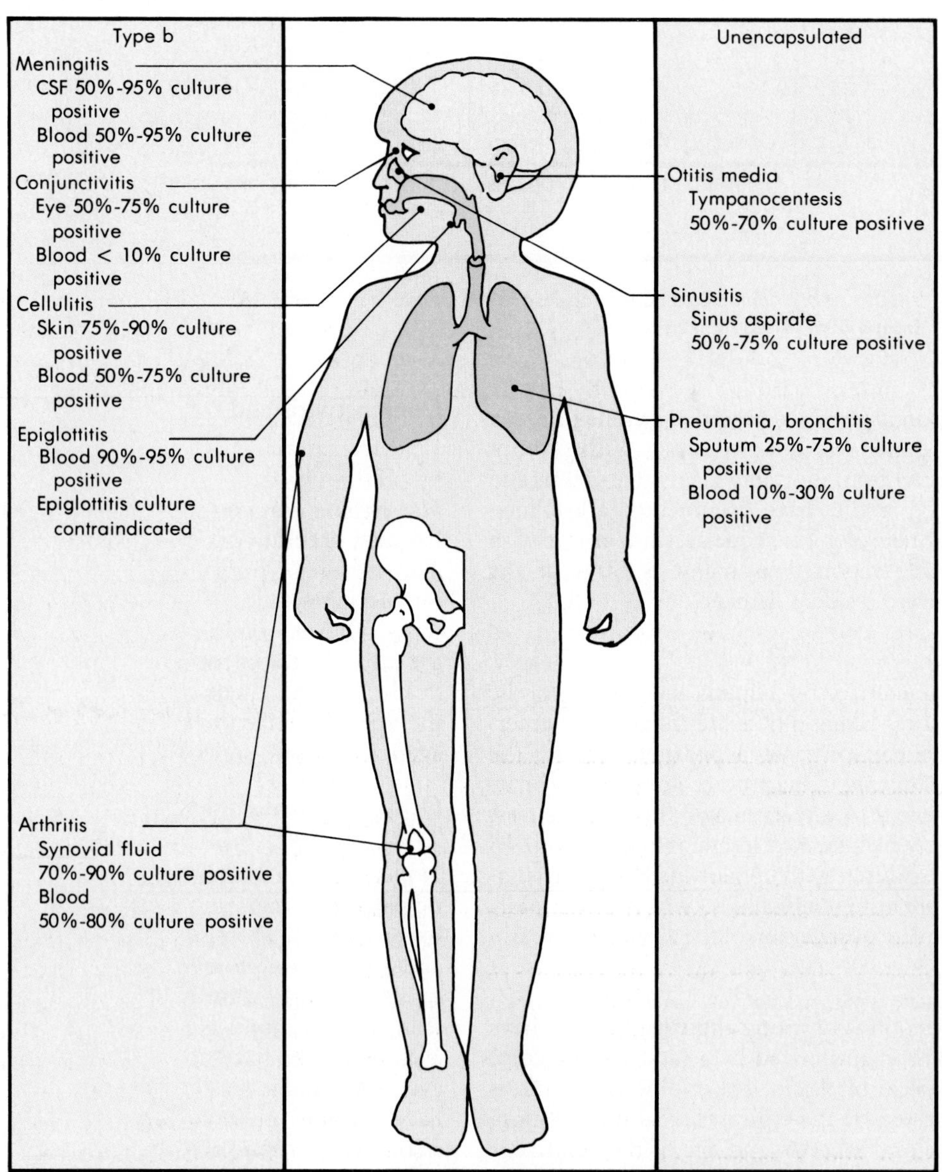

FIGURE 28-3 Infections caused by *H. influenzae* type b are usually invasive, and meningitis, epiglottitis, cellulitis, arthritis, and conjunctivitis are reported most commonly. Cultures of cerebrospinal fluid and blood in patients with meningitis are almost always positive unless the patient has been pretreated with antibiotics. Blood cultures are also usually positive for patients with epiglottitis, arthritis, and cellulitis. In contrast, unencapsulated strains of *H. influenzae* usually cause localized diseases that are diagnostic problems, because blood cultures are usually negative and appropriate respiratory specimens or aspirates from the middle ear or sinuses are difficult to collect.

Specimen Collection and Transport

The specific diagnosis of *Haemophilus* meningitis requires collection of cerebrospinal fluid and blood. In untreated meningitis, the concentration of organisms is approximately 10^7 bacteria/ml CSF; therefore 1 to 2 ml of fluid is generally adequate for microscopy, culture, and antigen detection tests. Blood should also be cultured for the diagnosis of epiglottitis, cellulitis, arthritis, and pneumonia. These cultures are less useful for patients with localized upper respiratory diseases (e.g., sinusitis, otitis), for whom direct needle aspiration is required for definitive microbiological confirmation. Specimens should not be collected from the posterior pharynx for the specific diagnosis of epiglottitis because the procedure may stimulate coughing and complete obstruction of the airway. Specimens for *H. ducreyi* should be collected with a moistened swab from the base or margin of the ulcer.

Microscopy

The direct microscopic detection of *Haemophilus* in clinical specimens is a sensitive and specific test when performed carefully. Small gram-negative coccobacilli can be detected in greater than 80% of cerebrospinal fluid specimens from patients with untreated *Haemophilus* meningitis. Gram-stained specimens are also useful for the rapid diagnosis of arthritis and lower respiratory disease.

Culture

Isolation of *H. influenzae* from clinical specimens is relatively easy if media supplemented with growth factors are inoculated. Chocolate agar or Levinthal agar is used in most laboratories. If chocolate agar is overheated during preparation, V factor is destroyed and *Haemophilus* species requiring this growth factor will not grow; thus each preparation of medium must be quality controlled. The bacteria appear as 1- to 2-mm smooth opaque colonies after 24 hours of incubation. Growth on unheated blood agar plates can also be detected surrounding colonies of *Staphylococcus aureus* **(satellite phenomenon).** The staphylococci provide required growth factors by lysing the erythrocytes in the medium and releasing intracellular V factor. The size of the colonies of *H. influenzae* is much smaller than on chocolate agar because the V factor inhibitors are not inactivated.

Growth of *Haemophilus* in blood cultures is generally delayed because most commercially prepared blood culture broths are not supplemented with optimum concentrations of X and V factors. Furthermore, the growth factors are released when the blood cells lyse, but inhibitors of V factor present in the medium can delay recovery of the bacteria. Isolates of *H. influenzae* frequently grow better in anaerobically incubated blood cultures, because under these conditions the organisms do not require X factor for growth.

Both *H. aegyptius* and *H. ducreyi* are fastidious and require specialized growth conditions. *H. aegyptius* grows best on chocolate agar supplemented with 1% IsoVitaleX, with growth detected after incubation in a CO_2 atmosphere for 2 to 4 days. Recovery of *H. ducreyi* in culture is relatively insensitive (less than 85% positive cultures under optimal conditions) but reportedly best on GC agar supplemented with 1% to 2% hemoglobin, 5% fetal bovine serum, 10% CVA enrichment, and vancomycin (3 μg/ml). Cultures should be incubated for 7 days or more at 33° C in 5% to 10% CO_2.

Antigen Detection

The immunological detection of *H. influenzae* antigen, specifically the PRP capsule, is a rapid and sensitive method for diagnosing *Haemophilus* disease. PRP can be detected by counterimmunoelectrophoresis or particle agglutination, with the latter procedure 5 to 10 times more sensitive (able to detect less than 1 ng/ml PRP compared with 5 to 10 ng/ml by CIE). Antibody-coated latex particles are mixed with the clinical specimen, and—in the presence of PRP—agglutination occurs. Antigen can be detected in both cerebrospinal fluid and urine (where the antigen is eliminated in intact form). This test has a sensitivity comparable to the Gram stain and is useful for diagnosis of disease in patients pretreated with antibiotics.

Identification

H. influenzae is readily identified by demonstrating a requirement for both X and V factors and the specific biochemical properties summarized in Table 28-2. Further subgrouping of *H. influenzae* can be made by electrophoretic characterization of membrane protein antigens (see Figure 28-1).

Treatment, Prevention, and Control

Unless prompt antimicrobial therapy is initiated, mortality with *H. influenzae* meningitis and epiglottitis approaches 100%. Historically, all isolates were susceptible to either ampicillin or chloramphenicol; however, resistance to these antibiotics is now widely recognized. In 1974 the first strains resistant to ampicillin were reported. This resistance was mediated by a TEM-1 **β-lactamase,** which is present on a transmissible plasmid and commonly found in other gram-negative bacilli such as *Escherichia coli*. Unfortunately, this β-lactamase is now ubiquitous (found in more than 30% of type b strains and 20% of nonencapsulated strains of *H. influenzae*). A second β-lactamase (designated ROB-1) has also been found in rare strains of *H. influenzae*. Finally, less than 1% of strains are resistant to beta-lactam antibiotics by alterations of the penicillin-binding proteins (the target of antibiotic activity). As a result of these changes, ampicillin cannot be reliably used as empirical therapy for severe *H. influenzae* infections. Chloramphenicol resistance, mediated by strains producing **chloramphenicol acetyltransferase,** has also been recognized but is relatively uncommon (less than 1% of all *H.*

TABLE 28-2 Differential Characteristics of Common Members of the Family Pasteurellaceae

Organism	Growth factor requirement: X	Growth factor requirement: V	Hemolysis	Enhanced growth with CO_2	Catalase	Fermentation of: Glucose	Fermentation of: Sucrose	Fermentation of: Lactose	Fermentation of: Mannose
Haemophilus									
H. influenzae	+	+	−	−	+	+	−	−	−
H. haemolyticus	+	+	+	−	+	+	−	−	−
H. parainfluenzae	−	+	−	−	±	+	+	−	+
H. parahaemolyticus	−	+	+	+	+	+	+	−	+
H. aphrophilus	−	−	−	+	−	+	+	+	+
H. paraphrophilus	−	+	−	+	+	+	+	+	+
H. ducreyi	+	−	−	−	−	−	−	−	−
Actinobacillus actinomycetemcomitans	−	−	−	+	+	+	−	−	+
Pasteurella multocida	−	−	−	−	+	+	+	−	+

influenzae). Thus infections can be treated either with this antibiotic or a β-lactamase–resistant cephalosporin with good penetration into the cerebrospinal fluid (e.g., ceftriaxone). Less severe infections such as sinusitis or otitis can be treated with ampicillin (if susceptible), trimethoprim-sulfamethoxazole, or cefaclor. Because localized infections with *H. influenzae* type b (e.g., cellulitis) can spread via the bloodstream into the central nervous system, all of these infections should be treated with active antibiotics that penetrate into these sites.

The major approach to prevention of *Haemophilus* disease is active immunization with purified capsular PRP. As discussed previously, the use of conjugated vaccines (combination of *H. influenzae* type b PRP with diphtheria toxoid or *N. meningitidis* outer membrane protein) has been remarkably successful in reducing both *H. influenzae* type b disease and colonization.

Limited use of passive immunization with hyperimmune globulins active against *H. influenzae* type b has been successful in protecting high-risk children after exposure to the organism. Further trials are necessary to define when this should be administered.

Antibiotic chemoprophylaxis is used to eliminate carriage of *H. influenzae* type b in children at high risk for disease (e.g., children younger than 2 years of age in a family or day care center where systemic disease is documented). Rifampin prophylaxis has been used in these settings.

ACTINOBACILLUS

Actinobacillus species are small, facultative anaerobic, gram-negative bacilli that grow slowly (generally requiring 2 to 3 days of incubation) and need carbon dioxide for growth in vitro on chocolate agar or blood agar media. Five species of *Actinobacillus* have been described, with *A. actinomycetemcomitans* the only significant human pathogen. The cumbersome name is derived from the fact this organism is frequently associated with (comitans is Latin for "accompanying") *Actinomyces*. *Actinobacillus* is part of the normal oropharyngeal population, detectable in approximately 20% of healthy individuals. *A. actinomycetemcomitans* is associated with juvenile and adult periodontitis and subacute endocarditis. Underlying cardiac disease and spread of the organism from the oral cavity following dental procedures or in patients with periodontitis are reported for virtually all patients with *Actinobacillus* endocarditis. Most serious infections are treated with ampicillin alone or in combination with an aminoglycoside.

PASTEURELLA

Six species of *Pasteurella* are currently recognized; *Pasteurella multocida* is the most common human pathogen. The natural reservoir of *P. multocida* is the upper respiratory tract of such domestic animals as dogs and cats, with human infection related to animal exposure (e.g., animal bite, cat scratch). Three general forms of disease are reported: (1) localized cellulitis and lymphadenitis following an animal bite or scratch; (2) exacerbation of chronic respiratory disease in patients with underlying pulmonary dysfunction (presumably related to colonization of the patients' oropharynx followed by aspiration of oral secretions); and (3) systemic infection in immunocompromised patients, particularly those with underlying hepatic disease.

P. multocida can be readily isolated on either blood agar or chocolate agar but not MacConkey agar. Large buttery colonies will grow after overnight incubation and have a characteristic musty odor caused by indole production. Identification can be readily accomplished, as indicated in Table 28-2. The organism is susceptible to a variety of antibiotics; penicillin is the antibiotic of choice, and tetracycline or a cephalosporin are acceptable alternatives.

CASE STUDY AND QUESTIONS

A previously healthy 18-month-old boy woke from his sleep with a severe headache and stiff neck. Because the child had a fever of 39.4° C and appeared quite ill, the mother took him to a local emergency room. At the time cerebrospinal fluid was collected, it appeared cloudy with 400 WBCs/mm^3 (95% polymorphonuclear neutrophils) present, protein of 75 mg/dl, and glucose of 20 mg/dl. Small gram-negative bacilli were observed on Gram stain of the CSF, and culture of CSF and blood was positive for *Haemophilus influenzae*.

1. Discuss the epidemiology of *Haemophilus influenzae* meningitis, and compare this with meningitis caused by *Streptococcus pneumoniae* (Chapter 20) and *Neisseria meningitidis* (Chapter 23).
2. Why is it now unusual to find *H. influenzae* infections in young children? What other diseases are caused by this organism?
3. Why is chocolate agar needed for the isolation of *Haemophilus*? What other techniques can be used to isolate this organism in culture?
4. What diseases are caused by *Actinobacillus*? What is the source of this organism?
5. What diseases are caused by *Pasteurella multocida*? What is the source of this organism?

Bibliography

Albritton WL: Infections due to *Haemophilus* species other than *H. influenzae, Ann Rev Microbiol* 36:199-216, 1982.

Brenner DJ, Mayer LW, Carlone GM et al.: Biochemical, genetic, and epidemiologic characterization of *Haemophilus influenzae* biogroup *aegyptius* (Haemophilus aegyptius) strains associated with Brazilian purpuric fever, *J Clin Microbiol* 26:1524-1534, 1988.

Campos J, Garcia-Tornel S, Roca J, and Iriondo M: Rifampin for eradicating carriage of multiply resistant *Haemophilus influenzae* b, *Pediatr Infect Dis J* 6:719-721, 1987.

Daum RS, Granoff DM, Makela PH et al.: Epidemiology, pathogenesis, and prevention of *Haemophilus influenzae* disease, *J Infect Dis* 165(suppl):1-206, 1992.

Farley MM, Stephens DS, Brachman PS et al.: Invasive *Haemophilus influenzae* disease in adults: a prospective, population-based surveillance, *Ann Intern Med* 116:806-812, 1992.

Hansen EJ, McCracken GH, and Syrogiannopoulos G: *Haemophilus influenzae* type b lipooligosaccharide induces meningeal inflammation, *Pediatr Infect Dis J 6:1150, 1987.*

Kaplan AH, Weber DJ, Oddone EZ, and Perfect JR: Infection due to *Actinobacillus actinomycetemcomitans*: 15 cases and review, *Rev Infect Dis* 11:46-63, 1989.

Morse SA: Chancroid and *Haemophilus ducreyi*, *Clin Microbiol Rev* 2:137-157, 1989.

Murphy TF and Apicella MA: Nontypable *Haemophilus influenzae:* a review of clinical aspects, surface antigens, and the human immune response to infection, *Rev Infect Dis* 9:1-15, 1987.

Taylor HG, Mills EL, Ciampi A et al.: The sequelae of *Haemophilus influenzae* meningitis in school age children, *N Engl J Med* 323:1657-1663, 1990.

Wallace RJ, Musher DM, Septimus EJ et al: *Haemophilus influenzae* infections in adults: characterization of strains by serotypes, biotypes, and β-lactamase production, *J Infect Dis* 144:101-106, 1981.

CHAPTER 29

Bordetella, Francisella, and Brucella

A number of gram-negative bacilli are classified together as genera of uncertain affiliation. Three clinically significant members are *Bordetella, Francisella,* and *Brucella* (Table 29-1).

BORDETELLA

Bordetella are extremely small (0.2 to 0.5 × 1 μm), strictly aerobic, gram-negative coccobacilli. Three species have been associated with human disease: *B. pertussis* (Latin for "severe cough"; the agent responsible for **pertussis,** or **whooping cough**), *B. parapertussis* (Latin for "like pertussis"; responsible for a milder form of pertussis), and *B. bronchiseptica* (responsible for respiratory disease in dogs, swine, laboratory animals, and occasionally humans).

Physiology and Structure

Differentiation of the species is based on growth characteristics, biochemical reactivity, and antigenic properties (Table 29-2). Despite these phenotypic differences, genetic studies indicate that these are closely related or identical species, differing only in the expression of virulence genes. However, at this time the species have not been reclassified and will be considered as distinct.

B. pertussis does not grow on common laboratory media, requiring supplementation with charcoal, starch, blood, or albumin to absorb toxic substances present in agar. Nicotinamide is also required for growth. The organism is nonmotile and oxidizes amino acids but does not ferment carbohydrates. The other *Bordetella* are less fastidious and can grow on blood and MacConkey agars. *Bordetella* species possess a genus-specific O antigen and strain-specific, heat-labile K antigens.

Pathogenesis

Infection with *B. pertussis* and the development of whooping cough require exposure to the organism, bacterial attachment to the ciliated epithelial cells of the bronchial tree, proliferation of the bacteria, and the production of localized tissue damage, and systemic toxicity. Unlike with other bacteria, fimbriae present on the bacterial surface are not primarily involved in attachment to ciliated epithelial cells. Instead, this is mediated by two bacterial virulence factors: filamentous

TABLE 29-1 Human Pathogens

Genus	Species	Disease
Bordetella	*pertussis*	Pertussis
	parapertussis	Pertussis
	bronchiseptica	Bronchopulmonary disease
Francisella	*tularensis*	Tularemia
Brucella	*melitensis*	Brucellosis
	abortus	Brucellosis
	suis	Brucellosis
	canis	Brucellosis

TABLE 29-2 Differential Characteristics of *Bordatella* Species

	Bordatella species		
Characteristics	*B. pertussis*	*B. parapertussis*	*B. bronchiseptica*
Oxidase	+	−	+
Urease	−	+	+
Motility	−	−	+
Browning on Mueller-Hinton agar	−	+	−
Growth on:			
Sheep blood agar	−	+	+
MacConkey agar	−	+	+

Modified from Lennette EH, Balows A, Hausler WJ Jr: *Manual of clinical microbiology,* ed 5, Washington, D.C., 1991, American Society for Microbiology.

hemagglutinin and pertussis toxin. Other toxins, such as those listed in Table 29-3 and discussed here, are responsible for the clinical manifestations of whooping cough. The clinical signs and symptoms of pertussis result from the coordinated expression of multiple toxins.

Pertussis Toxin

Consistent with the multiple biological properties associated with this toxin, pertussis toxin has also been called histamine sensitizing factor, lymphocytosis promoting factor, islet cell activating protein, and pertussigen. The heat-labile pertussis toxin is an A-B toxin, consisting of six protein subunits (five of which are unique). Subunit 1 is the A (active) portion of the toxin molecule, whereas pentameric subunits 2 through 5 (two molecules of subunit 4 are present) are the B or binding portion of the molecule. The B portion binds to specific cell receptors, permitting transfer of the A portion to the internal cellular target. The A portion has ADP-ribosylating activity for membrane surface proteins and is responsible for interference with the transfer of signals from cell-surface receptors (guanine nucleotide–binding proteins) to intracellular mediator systems (homeostatic inhibitory regulation of adenylate cyclase activity). Pertussis toxin can also block immune effector cells, including neutrophils, monocytes, macrophages, and natural killer cells. Finally, the toxin is believed to be important for bacterial binding to ciliated epithelial cells, because bacterial attachment is reduced when the toxin is not produced. Antibodies to pertussis toxin confer immunity.

Adenylate Cyclase Toxin

This toxin, released during exponential cell growth, is activated by intracellular calmodulin and catalyzes the conversion of endogenous ATP to cAMP in eukaryotic cells. Adenylate cyclase toxin interferes with immune effector cell function at the site of bacterial activity with inhibition of leukocyte chemotaxis, phagocytosis, and killing; oxidative activity of alveolar macrophages; and cell lysis by natural killer cells. This toxin may be important for the initial protection of the bacteria during the early stages of disease.

Tracheal Cytotoxin

The tracheal cytotoxin is a low molecular weight cell wall peptidoglycan monomer. It has a specific affinity for ciliated epithelial cells, which at low concentrations cause ciliostasis (inhibition of cilia movement) and at the higher concentrations produced later in the infection are responsible for extrusion of the ciliated cells. Tracheal cytotoxin specifically interferes with DNA synthesis, leading to impaired regeneration of damaged cells. This process disrupts the normal clearance mechanisms in the respiratory tree and leads to the characteristic cough associated with pertussis. Nonciliated cells are spared in infections with *B. pertussis.*

TABLE 29-3 Virulence Factors Associated With *Bordatella pertussis*

Virulence factors	Biological effects
Pertussis toxin	ADP-ribosylation of guanine nucleotide-binding proteins, lymphocytosis, hypoglycemia, mediates attachment to respiratory epithelium
Adenylate cyclase toxin	Impairment of leukocyte chemotaxis and killing, local edema
Tracheal cytotoxin	Ciliastasis and then extrusion of ciliated epithelial cells
Dermonecrotic toxin	Vascular smooth muscle contraction and ischemic necrosis
Filamentous hemagglutinin	Mediates attachment to ciliated epithelial cells, agglutinates erythrocytes
Lipopolysaccharide	Exotoxin activity

Dermonecrotic Toxin

This heat-labile toxin can cause vasoconstriction of peripheral blood vessels in an animal model, with localized ischemia, movement of leukocytes to extravascular spaces, and hemorrhage. The toxin probably is responsible for localized tissue destruction in pertussis, although further work is required to confirm this.

Filamentous Hemagglutinin

The hemagglutinin can agglutinate a variety of animal erythrocytes and is believed to be important in attachment of *B. pertussis* to ciliated cells. Antibodies directed against the filamentous hemagglutinin interfere with bacterial attachment and are protective.

Lipopolysaccharide

The lipopolysaccharide consists of two lipids (lipid A and lipid X) and two distinct polysaccharides. Endotoxin activity is associated with lipid X, whereas lipid A has reduced pyrogenicity and toxicity.

Epidemiology

Pertussis, a disease with worldwide endemicity, has been recognized for centuries (Box 29-1). The incidence of disease, with its associated morbidity and mortality, has been reduced in recent years with the widespread availability of effective vaccines. Most infections now are associated with inadequately immunized children (Figure 29-1). *B. pertussis* has no animal or environmental reservoir, so it must be spread from patients with clinically apparent pertussis or with subclinical infections. In theory, use of the vaccine could eliminate *B. pertussis* in the same manner smallpox virus was eradicated. Unfortunately, widespread acceptance of the vaccine has not been

BOX 29-1 Epidemiology of Pertussis

DISEASE/BACTERIAL FACTORS

Whooping cough

Filamentous hemagglutinin and pertussis toxin are responsible for bacterial attachment to ciliated epithelial cells

Multiple toxins (see Table 29-3): pertussis toxin, adenylate cyclase toxin, tracheal cytotoxin, dermonecrotic toxin, filamentous hemagglutinin, lipopolysaccharide

TRANSMISSION

Person-to-person spread via inhalation of infectious aerosols

WHO IS AT RISK?

Inadequately immunized children

GEOGRAPHY/SEASON

Worldwide; in the United States, most infections occur in California, Massachusetts, New York, and Illinois

No seasonal incidence

MODES OF CONTROL

Treatment is primarily supportive

Erythromycin of limited value because illness is usually unrecognized when drug would be most effective

Vaccines have reduced incidence of disease

Currently whole-cell inactivated vaccine is administered with vaccines for diphtheria and tetanus (DPT)

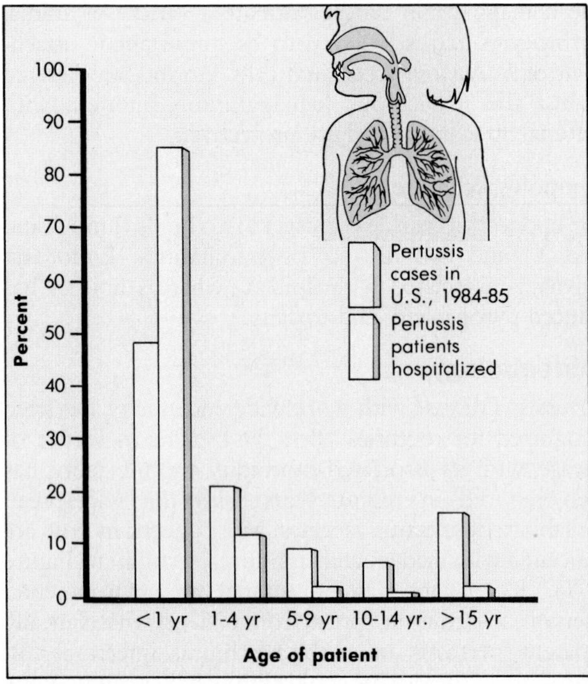

FIGURE 29-1 Age distribution and severity of illness reported for pertussis infection during 1984 and 1985.

achieved because of fears of vaccine-related toxicity and reports of decreased efficacy. Unfortunately, the limited use of the vaccine in Sweden, Japan, and areas in the United States has caused an increase of the incidence of pertussis and its complications. Although pertussis had steadily decreased in the United States from 1960 through 1980, the incidence of disease has increased during the last decade (Figure 29-2), with 4570 cases reported in 1990. The highest number of cases was reported in California, Massachusetts, New York, and Illinois.

Clinical Syndromes

Infection is initiated by inhalation of infectious aerosol droplets and attachment and proliferation of the bacteria on ciliated epithelial cells. After a 7- to 10-day incubation the patient will experience the first of three stages (Figure 29-3). The **catarrhal stage** resembles a common cold, with serous rhinorrhea, sneezing, malaise, anorexia, and a low-grade fever. Because the peak production of bacteria is during this stage and the cause of the disease is unrecognized, patients in the catarrhal stage pose the highest risk to their contacts. After 1 to 2 weeks the **paroxysmal stage** begins, corresponding to the extrusion of ciliated epithelial cells from the respiratory tract and impaired clearance of mucus. This stage is characterized by the classic whooping cough paroxysms (i.e., a series of repetitive coughs followed by an inspiratory whoop). Mucus production in the respiratory tract is common and is partially responsible for the restricted airway. The paroxysms are frequently terminated with vomiting and exhaustion. A marked lymphocytosis is also prominent during this stage. As many as 40 to 50 daily paroxysms may occur during the height of the illness. After 2 to 4 weeks the disease enters the **convalescent stage** when the paroxysms diminish in number and severity, but secondary complications can occur.

Laboratory Diagnosis

Specimen Collection and Transport

B. pertussis is extremely sensitive to drying and does not survive unless care is used for collection and transport to the laboratory. The optimal diagnostic specimen is a nasopharyngeal aspirate. Pernasal or oropharyngeal swabs have a lower yield and require use of synthetic fiber swabs (e.g., calcium alginate or Dacron). Fatty acids present in cotton swabs are toxic to *B. pertussis*, and these swabs must be avoided.

The most important factor affecting recovery of *Bordetella* is the speed with which the specimen is cultured. The specimen must be either directly inoculated at the patient's bedside onto freshly prepared isolation media (e.g., Regan-Lowe medium, Bordet-Gengou medium) or placed in a suitable transport medium (e.g., Regan-Lowe transport medium). Specimens cannot be transported to the laboratory before processing because the organism does not survive in traditional transport media. Inoculated culture media must be kept moist, or

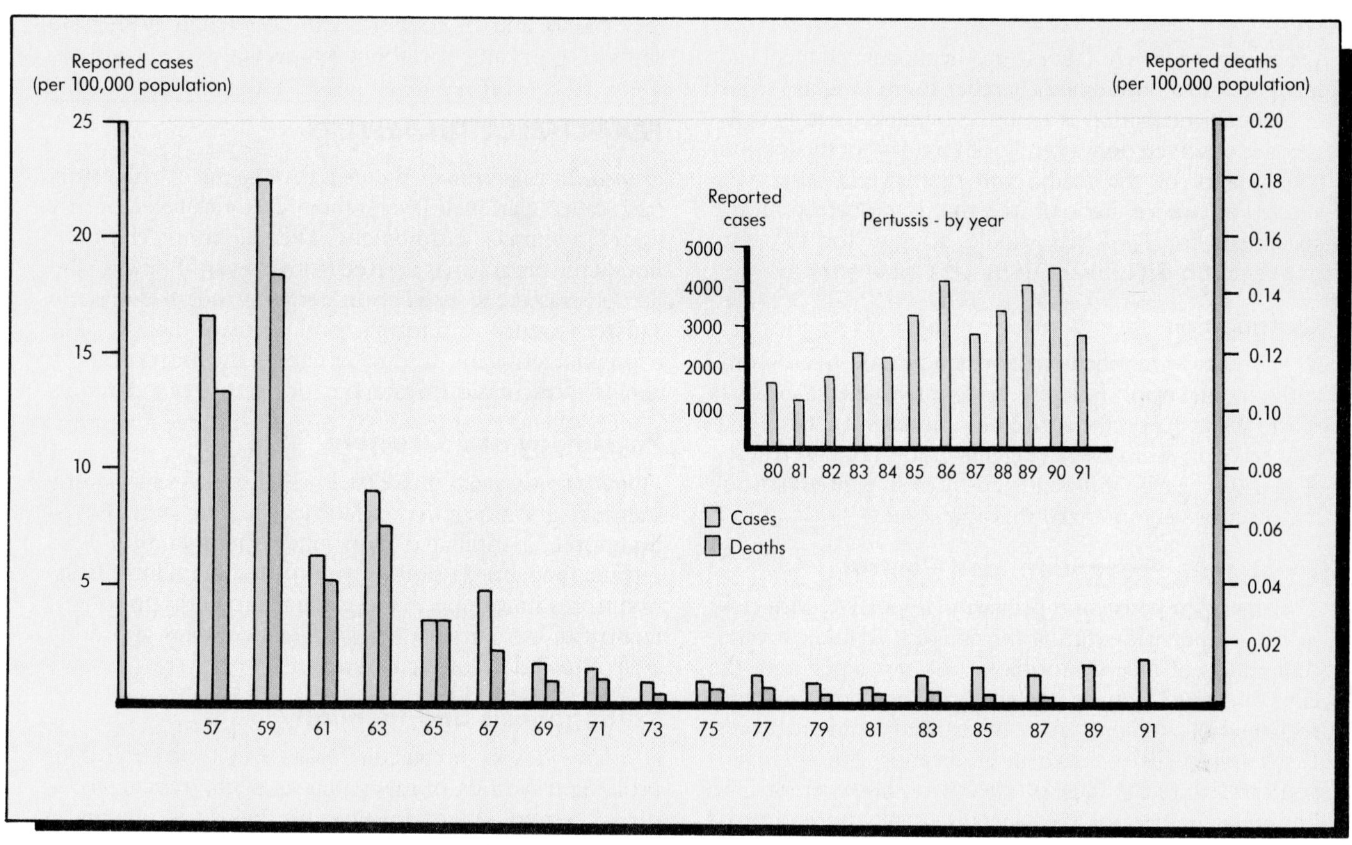

FIGURE 29-2 Incidence of pertussis in the United States from 1957 to 1990. Data not available for 1989-1990. (Redrawn from *MMWR* 39:33, 1991).

	Incubation	Catarrhal	Paroxysmal	Convalescent
Duration	7-10 days	1-2 weeks	2-4 weeks	3-4 weeks (or longer)
Symptoms	None	Rhinorrhea, malaise, fever sneezing, anorexia	Repetitive cough with whoops, vomiting, leukocytosis	Diminished paroxysmal cough, development of secondary complications (pneumonia, seizures, encephalopathy)
Bacterial culture				

FIGURE 29-3. Clinical presentation of *Bordetella pertussis* disease.

drying will kill the organisms. A portion of the specimen can also be used for microscopic examination.

Microscopy

Specimens can be examined by a direct fluorescent antibody (DFA) procedure, in which the aspirated specimen is smeared onto a microscopic slide, air-dried and heat-fixed, and then stained with fluorescein-labeled antibodies directed against *B. pertussis.* Antibodies against *B. parapertussis* should also be used to detect mild forms of pertussis caused by this organism. DFA will be positive in slightly more than half of the patients with pertussis.

Culture

When received in the laboratory, the inoculated media are incubated in a humidified chamber for as long as 7 days. Prolonged incubation is required because the tiny colonies are observed only after 3 or more days of incubation. The quality of the media will dramatically affect the success of culture. Laboratories that infrequently culture specimens for *Bordetella* should arrange for the state public health department to process these tests.

Identification

B. pertussis is identified by its characteristic microscopic and colonial morphology on selective media and its reactivity with specific antiserum (either in an agglutination reaction or with the reagents used in the DFA test). *B. pertussis* can be differentiated from *B. parapertussis* by the reactions summarized in Table 29-2.

Treatment, Prevention, and Control

Treatment for pertussis is primarily supportive, with close nursing supervision during the paroxysmal and convalescent stages of illness. Antibiotics do not ameliorate the clinical course because convalescence is correlated with regeneration of the layer of ciliated epithelial cells. Erythromycin is effective in eradicating the organisms and can reduce the stage of infectivity; however, this has limited value because the illness is usually unrecognized during the height of contagiousness.

The currently available whole-cell, inactivated vaccine is administered in conjunction with vaccines for diphtheria and tetanus (DPT vaccine) and is effective in eliminating symptomatic pertussis. However, concern about the associated complications has limited the acceptance of the current vaccine in some countries. Acellular pertussis vaccines have been developed, using components believed to evoke protective immunity, such as filamentous hemagglutinin, pertussis toxin, fimbriae agglutinins, and a recently identified 69-kd outer membrane protein. Clinical trials performed in Japan have demonstrated protective immunity and a lower incidence of side effects with acellular vaccines when administered to children older than 2 years of age. However, insufficient data exist for younger children who are at greatest risk for serious disease, and clinical trials have not compared the acellular vaccines with whole-cell vaccines.

Because pertussis is highly contagious in a susceptible population and unrecognized infections in family members of a symptomatic patient can maintain disease in a community, erythromycin has been used for prophylaxis in select instances.

Other *Bordetella*

B. parapertussis is responsible for 10% to 20% of the cases of pertussis seen annually in the United States. *B. bronchiseptica* causes respiratory disease primarily in animals but has been associated with human respiratory colonization and bronchopulmonary disease. Both organisms can be readily isolated on conventional laboratory media and in contrast with *B. pertussis* both have easily recognizable metabolic properties.

FRANCISELLA TULARENSIS

Francisella tularensis is the causative agent of **tularemia** (also called glandular fever, rabbit fever, tick fever, deerfly fever) in animals and humans. The taxonomic classification of the organism is derived from Edward Francis, who demonstrated the association between rodent disease in Tulare County, California, and human disease. The colloquial terms for the disease refer to the most common clinical presentation, reservoir, or vectors of tularemia.

Physiology and Structure

F. tularensis is a very small (0.2 × 0.2 to 0.7 μm), faintly staining, gram-negative coccobacillus. The organism is nonmotile, nonpiliated, surrounded with a thin lipid capsule, and has fastidious growth requirements. Isolation from clinical specimens generally requires prolonged incubation on enriched media, with colonies appearing after 2 to 3 days of incubation.

Pathogenesis and Immunity

F. tularensis is an intracellular parasite that can survive for prolonged periods in macrophages of the reticuloendothelial system. An antiphagocytic capsule is present in pathogenic strains, and loss of the capsule is associated with decreased virulence. Like all gram-negative bacilli, this organism has endotoxin activity.

Epidemiology

F. tularensis has worldwide distribution, although the prevalence of the two biochemical varieties (biovars tularensis and palaearctica) is somewhat restricted (Box 29-2 and Table 29-4). The organism is found in a large number of wild mammals, domestic animals, birds, fish, and blood-sucking arthropods, as well as in contaminated water. The most common reservoirs of *F. tularensis* in the United States are rabbits and ticks, as well as muskrats. Human tularemia is acquired most often after the bite of an infected arthropod or contact with an infected animal or domestic pet that has caught an infected animal (e.g., rabbit). However, disease can also be acquired after consumption of contaminated meat or water, or inhalation of an infectious aerosol (most commonly in a laboratory or during dressing an infected animal). Infection with *F. tularensis* requires as few as 10 organisms when exposure is by an arthropod bite or contamination of unbroken skin, 50 organisms when inhaled, and 10^8 organisms when ingested.

The reported incidence of disease is low (Figure 29-4), with fewer than 200 cases each year in the United States. Disease is reported most commonly in Arkansas, Missouri, and Oklahoma. The largest number of infections occur during the summer (when exposure to infected ticks is highest) and the winter (when hunters are exposed to infected rabbits). However, the actual number of

BOX 29-2 Epidemiology of Tularemia

DISEASE/BACTERIAL FACTORS

Ulceroglandular, glandular, typhoidal, oculoglandular, and oropharyngeal tularemia
F. tularensis is a facultative intracellular pathogen and can survive for prolonged periods in macrophages of the reticuloendothelial system
Antiphagocytic capsule is present in pathogenic strains
Most common reservoirs in the United States are rabbits, ticks, and muskrats

TRANSMISSION

Bite from infected tick or contact with infected animals
Infection also acquired after ingestion of contaminated meat or water, or inhalation of an infectious aerosol

WHO IS AT RISK?

Hunters
Persons exposed to ticks
Laboratory personnel

GEOGRAPHY/SEASON

Worldwide; in the United States most infections are in Arkansas, Missouri, and Oklahoma
Disease most frequent during summer and winter

MODES OF CONTROL

Streptomycin (drug of choice), gentamicin
Avoid reservoirs and vectors of infection (e.g., rabbits, ticks)
Live, attenuated vaccines reduce severity of disease
Lab personnel: use of gloves and biohazard hood when handling specimens

TABLE 29-4 Differentiation Between *Francisella tularensis*, Biovar Tularensis, and Biovar Palaearctica

Characteristic	Biovar tularensis	Biovar palaearctica
Name	Jellison A; nearctica	Jellison B
Geographic distribution	North America	Europe, Asia, the Americas
Biochemical properties		
Glycerol fermentation	Positive	Negative
Citrulline-ureidase	Positive	Negative
Source of infection	Ticks, rabbits	Contaminated water or rodents
Human disease	Severe	Mild

infections is likely to be much higher because tularemia is frequently unsuspected or difficult to confirm by laboratory tests. Persons at greatest risk for infection include hunters, those exposed to ticks, and laboratory personnel. In endemic areas it is said that if a rabbit is moving so slowly that it can be shot by a hunter or caught by a pet, then the rabbit could be infected.

Clinical Syndromes

After a 3- to 5-day incubation period, tularemia symptoms include an abrupt onset of fever, chills, malaise, and fatigue. The clinical classification of *F. tularensis* disease is based on the site of infection and the presence of skin ulcers and lymphadenopathy; thus tularemia can be subdivided into several manifestations (Table 29-5). In the ulceroglandular type of tularemia, axillary adenopathy is generally present after exposure to infected rabbits (presumably resulting from infection of the hands), and inguinal adenopathy is common with tick-borne disease (related to tick bites on the lower extremities). *F. tularensis* pneumonia is present in the majority of patients with typhoidal disease. Focal necrosis in the liver and spleen can also be found.

Laboratory Diagnosis

Specimen Collection

Collection and processing of specimens for the isolation of *F. tularensis* is extremely hazardous for both the physician and laboratory worker. The organism, by virtue of its small size, can penetrate through the skin and mucous membranes during collection of the sample or be inhaled if aerosols are produced. Tularemia is the third most commonly reported laboratory-acquired bacterial infection. Gloves should be worn during collection of the specimen (e.g., aspiration of an ulcer or lymph node), and all processing should be performed in a biohazard hood.

Microscopy

The detection of *F. tularensis* in Gram-stained aspirates from infected nodes or ulcers is almost always unsuccessful because the organism is extremely small and stains faintly. A more sensitive and specific approach is direct staining of the clinical specimen with fluorescein-labeled antibodies directed against the organism.

Culture

It is stated that *F. tularensis* cannot be isolated on common laboratory media because the organism requires sulfhydryl-containing substances (e.g., cysteine) for growth. However, chocolate blood agar plates that are used in most laboratories are supplemented with cysteine, and *F. tularensis* will grow on this medium. Specialized media such as cysteine blood agar or glucose cysteine agar are usually not required for most isolates. If infection with *F. tularensis* is suspected, the laboratory should be notified. *F. tularensis* grows slowly and will be overlooked unless the cultures are incubated for a prolonged period. Blood cultures are generally negative, whereas cultures of

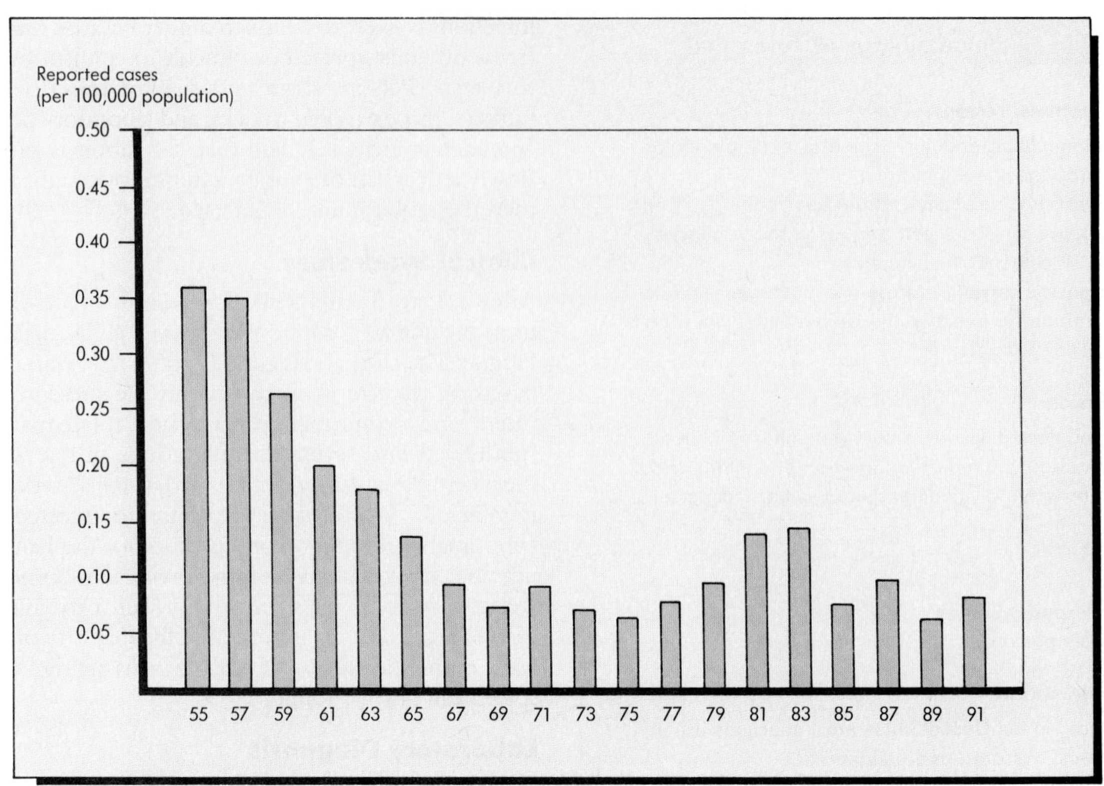

FIGURE 29-4. Incidence of tularemia in the United States from 1955 to 1990. (Redrawn from *MMWR* 39:48, 1991).

TABLE 29-5 Manifestations of Tularemia

Type of disease	Infections (%)	Characteristics
Ulceroglandular	75-85	Ulcers at the site of exposure and adenopathy of the draining lymph nodes
Glandular	5-10	Adenopathy but no ulcers
Typhoidal	5-15	Systemic signs but no adenopathy or ulcers
Oculoglandular	1-2	Eye involvement
Oropharyngeal	<1	Oropharyngeal involvement

sputum and aspirates of lymph nodes or draining sinuses are usually positive.

Identification

F. tularensis is strictly aerobic, weakly catalase positive, and oxidase negative. Biochemical characterization of the organism has little value. Identification is confirmed given evidence of reactivity with specific antisera in fluorescent antibody or agglutination tests. Only one serotype of *F. tularensis* has been identified.

Serology

Most cases of tularemia are diagnosed by a fourfold or greater increase in antibodies during the course of the illness (Figure 29-5). A fourfold increase in titer or a single titer of 160 or greater is considered diagnostic. However, antibodies (including IgG, IgM, and IgA) can persist for many years, preventing differentiation between past and current disease. Antibodies directed against *Brucella* can also cross-react with *Francisella*.

Treatment, Prevention, and Control

Streptomycin is the antibiotic of choice for all forms of tularemia. Gentamicin is an acceptable alternative, although less clinical experience exists with this drug. Tetracycline and chloramphenicol have been used to treat infections; however, these are associated with an unacceptably high rate of relapse. *F. tularensis* strains produce β-lactamase, rendering penicillins and cephalosporins ineffective. The mortality rate is less than 1% when appropriate antibiotic therapy is initiated promptly.

Prevention is accomplished by avoiding the reservoirs and vectors of infection (e.g., rabbits, ticks), although this is frequently difficult. At a minimum, ill-appearing rabbits should not be handled, and gloves should be worn when animals are skinned and eviscerated. Ticks should be promptly removed. Because the organism is present in the arthropod's feces and not saliva, the tick

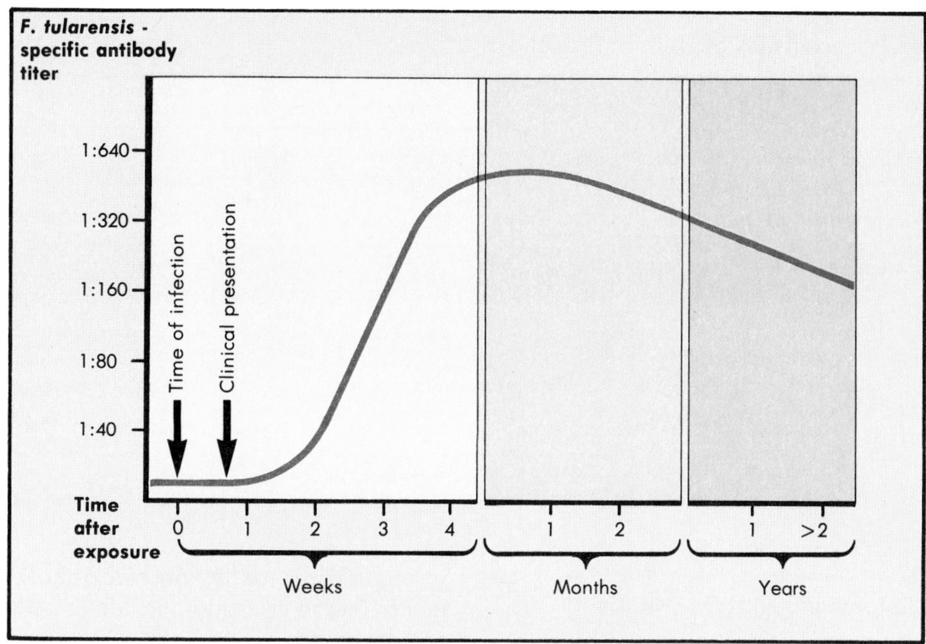

FIGURE 29-5. Antibody response to *Francisella tularensis* infections.

must feed for a prolonged time before the infection is transmitted.

Use of live, attenuated vaccines is not completely effective but does reduce the severity of disease. Inactivated vaccines are not protective.

BRUCELLA

The genus *Brucella* consists of six species, four of which are associated with human **brucellosis:** *B. abortus, B. melitensis, B. suis,* and *B. canis.* However, nucleic acid hybridization studies indicate that only one species of *Brucella* exists, with the current species biovars of *B. melitensis*. Until the nomenclature for this genus is changed, the species designation for the individual groups will be retained.

Brucellosis has a number of names based on the original microbiologists who isolated and described the organisms (Sir David Bruce and Bernhard Bang; Bang's disease), the clinical presentation (undulant fever), or the site of recognized outbreaks (Malta fever, Mediterranean remittent fever, rock fever of Gibraltar, county fever of Constantinople, fever of Crete).

Physiology and Structure

The individual species are distinguished by their reservoir host, growth properties, biochemical reactivities, and cell wall fatty acid composition. *Brucella* are small (0.5 × 0.6 to 1.5 μm), nonmotile, nonencapsulated gram-negative coccobacilli. The organism grows slowly on culture, is aerobic with some strains requiring supplemental carbon dioxide for growth, and does not ferment carbohydrates. Human isolates are catalase and oxidase positive, reduce nitrate, and have variable urease activity. *B. abortus, B. melitensis,* and *B. suis* share two surface antigens; the highest concentration of A antigen is found in *B. abortus*, and the M antigen is in *B. melitensis. B. canis* is antigenically distinct. Some characteristics of the four species that cause human disease are summarized in Table 29-6.

Pathogenesis and Immunity

Like *Francisella*, *Brucella* is an intracellular parasite of the reticuloendothelial system that is able to evade the patient's humoral immune response to infection. Intracellular survival can be prolonged unless specific cellular immunity develops. Survival is mediated by inhibition of polymorphonuclear leukocyte degranulation. *B. melitensis* is the species most able to resist the bactericidal effect of serum and phagocytic killing, consistent with the increased virulence of this species.

Epidemiology

Brucella infections have a worldwide distribution; more than 500,000 documented cases are reported annually (Box 29-3). However, the incidence of disease in the United States is much lower (85 reported infections in 1990), with approximately one reported case per 1 million individuals (Figure 29-6). The reason for the paucity of cases in the United States is related to control of disease in the animal reservoir.

Brucella causes mild or asymptomatic disease in the natural host: *B abortus* in cattle, *B. melitensis* in goats and sheep, *B. suis* in swine, and *B. canis* in dogs, foxes, and coyotes. The organism has a predilection for organs rich in erythritol, which is metabolized by many *Brucella*

TABLE 29-6 Characteristics of Human Brucellosis

Species	Animal reservoir	CO_2 required	Growth on dyes: Basic fuchsin	Growth on dyes: Thionin	Clinical disease
B. melitensis	Goats, sheep	−	+	+	Severe, acute disease with complications common
B. abortus	Cattle	+	+	−	Mild disease with suppurative complications uncommon
B. suis	Swine	−	±	+	Suppurative, destructive disease with chronic manifestations
B. canis	Dogs	−	−	+	Mild disease with suppurative complications uncommon

BOX 29-3 Epidemiology of Brucellosis

DISEASE/BACTERIAL FACTORS

Brucella is a facultative intracellular pathogen and can survive for prolonged periods in macrophages of reticuloendothelial system

Reservoirs are animals: cattle, goats, sheep, swine, dogs, foxes, and coyotes

TRANSMISSION

Ingestion of contaminated milk or cheese

Contact with infected animals

WHO IS AT RISK?

Persons in direct contact with infected animals: veterinarians, meat handlers, farmers

Persons eating unpasteurized milk or cheese

Laboratory personnel

GEOGRAPHY/SEASON

Worldwide; in the United States, most common in California and Texas; less disease in the United States attributable to control of disease in animals

No seasonal incidence

MODES OF CONTROL

Tetracycline combined with streptomycin or with gentamicin

Long-term therapy with high doses of trimethoprim-sulfamethoxazole

Control of disease in animal reservoir

Avoidance of unpasteurized dairy products

Protective clothing when working with animals or specimens

strains in preference to glucose. Animal (but not human) tissues rich in erythritol include breast, uterus, placenta, and epididymis. Thus *Brucella* localizes in these tissues in the nonhuman reservoirs and can cause sterility, abortions, or asymptomatic carriage. Human disease occurs in persons in direct contact with infected animals (veterinarians, slaughterhouse workers, farmers) or their products (consumption of unpasteurized milk or cheese). Laboratory personnel are also at significant risk for infection through direct contact or inhalation of the organism. The areas in the United States with the highest number of reported cases are California and Texas.

Clinical Syndromes

The disease spectrum of brucellosis is influenced by the infecting organism. *B. abortus* and *B. canis* tend to produce mild disease with rare suppurative complications. In contrast, *B. suis* is associated with destructive lesions and a prolonged course. *B. melitensis,* the most common cause of brucellosis, also causes severe disease with a high incidence of serious complications because it is able to survive in phagocytic cells and multiply to high concentrations.

After exposure to the organism, one can develop a localized abscess at the site of inoculation, which is followed by bacteremia. Organisms are phagocytized by macrophages and monocytes and then localized in tissues of the reticuloendothelial system (e.g., spleen, liver, bone marrow, lymph nodes, and kidneys). Infection may remain subclinical, with an increase in *Brucella*-specific antibodies the only evidence of disease, or may be seen clinically in a subacute or acute form. Severe toxic disease is particularly common with *B. melitensis*, again consistent with this species' increased virulence. The subacute and chronic manifestations of brucellosis can initially include malaise, chills, sweats, fatigue, weakness, myalgias, weight loss, arthralgias, and nonproductive cough. Fever is found in almost all patients and can be intermittent (hence the name undulant fever).

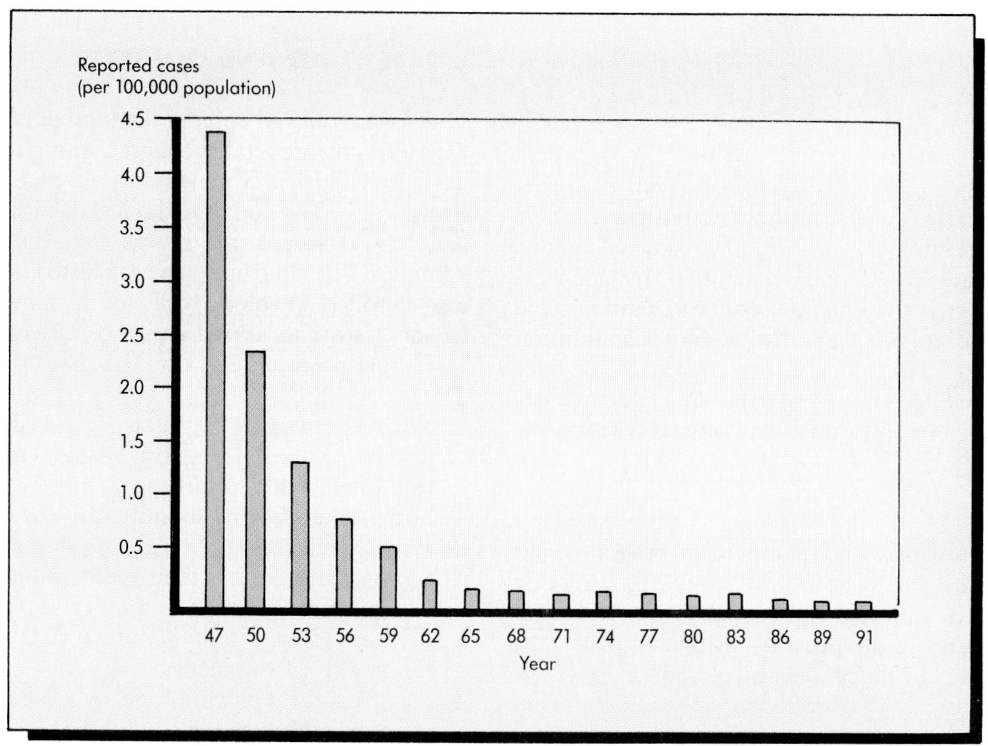

FIGURE 29-6. Incidence of brucellosis in the United States from 1945 to 1990. (Redrawn from *MMWR* 39:21, 1991).

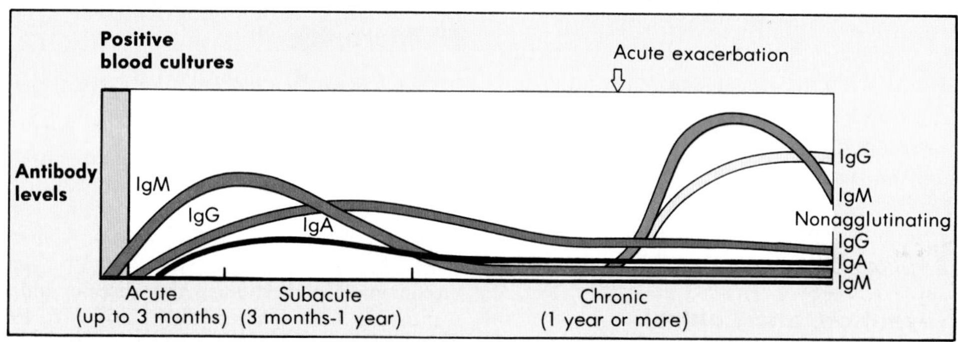

FIGURE 29-7. Antibody responses in untreated brucellosis. (From Mandell GL, Douglas RG Jr, Bennett JE: Principles and practice of infectious diseases, ed 2, New York, 1985, Churchill Livingstone.)

The subacute and chronic forms of brucellosis make diagnosis difficult because specific localizing signs are frequently absent. Granuloma formation in the liver, spleen, and bone marrow, as well as destructive changes in many other organs, have been observed.

Laboratory Diagnosis

Specimen Collection

Multiple blood samples should be collected for both culture and serologic testing. Bone marrow cultures may also be useful, as well as cultures of infected tissues. Care should be exercised in the handling of specimens. The laboratory should be notified if brucellosis is suspected because specialized growth conditions are required for the isolation of the pathogen.

Microscopy

Although *Brucella* organisms stain readily by conventional techniques, their small size makes them difficult to detect in clinical specimens. The direct fluorescent antibody technique has proved useful, but the test reagents are not readily available.

Culture

Brucella are slow-growing, fastidious organisms on primary isolation. Isolates will grow on most enriched blood agar and occasionally on MacConkey agar; however, incubation for 3 or more days may be required. The isolation from blood cultures can take as long as 4 to 6 weeks, although growth is faster when the blood culture is transferred to agar media (e.g., in biphasic cultures).

Incubation in a le enriched atmosphere is required for *B. a*

Identification

An isolate can be p y identified as *Brucella* by its microscopic and orphology, positive oxidase reaction, and react h antibodies directed against *Brucella*. Species ide ion is determined by biochemical reactivity, growt the presence of the dyes basic fuchsin and thionin, an agglutination in specific antisera. However, most laboratories in the United States refer isolates to reference centers because they infrequently isolate these bacteria and are unable to identify the specific species.

Serology

Subclinical brucellosis and many cases of acute and chronic diseases are identified by a specific antibody response in the infected individual. Antibodies are detected in virtually all patients, with an initial IgM response followed by the production of both IgG and IgA antibodies (Figure 29-7). Antibodies can persist for many months or years, so a significant increase in antibody titer is required for definitive serologic evidence of current disease. A presumptive diagnosis can be made with a fourfold increase in titer or a single titer greater than or equal to 160. The antigen used in the *Brucella* agglutination test is from *B. abortus*. Antibodies directed against *B. melitensis* or *B. suis* will cross-react with this antigen; however, there is no cross-reactivity with *B. canis*. The specific use of *B. canis* antigen is required for the diagnosis of this infection. Cross-reactivity with *B. abortus* antigen is also reported with *Yersinia enterocolitica, Francisella tularensis,* and specific serotypes of *Salmonella, Vibrio cholerae,* and *Escherichia coli.*

Treatment, Prevention, and Control

Tetracycline is generally active against most strains of *Brucella;* however, this is a bacteriostatic drug, and relapse is common after an initial successful response. The combination of tetracycline with either streptomycin or gentamicin has proved effective, with a low incidence of relapse. Long-term therapy with high doses of trimethoprim-sulfamethoxazole is an acceptable alternative regimen, and the addition of rifampin is useful for central nervous system disease.

Control of human brucellosis is accomplished by controlling disease in livestock, which has been demonstrated in the United States. This requires the systematic identification and elimination of infected herds and animal vaccination. Further efforts to prevent brucellosis include protective clothing for abattoir workers and the avoidance of unpasteurized dairy products. Vaccination of high-risk individuals has limited usefulness.

CASE STUDY AND QUESTIONS

A 5-year-old girl entered the local public health clinic with a severe, intractable cough. During the previous 10 days the child had a persistent cold that grew progressively worse. The cough had developed the previous day and was so severe that it was frequently followed by vomiting. The child appeared exhausted from the coughing episodes. A blood cell count showed a marked leukocytosis with a predominance of lymphocytes. The examining physician suspects the child has pertussis.

1. What laboratory tests can be performed to confirm the physician's clinical diagnosis? What is the sensitivity of the tests? What specimens should be collected, and how should they be submitted to the laboratory?
2. What virulence factors are produced by *Bordetella pertussis*, and what is their biological effect(s)?
3. What is the natural progression and prognosis of this disease? How can it be prevented? What are the limitations of vaccination?
4. Describe the epidemiology of *Francisella tularensis* infections. How is the clinical diagnosis confirmed in the laboratory?
5. Describe the epidemiology of the brucellosis.

Bibliography

Ariza J, Pellicer T, Pallares R et al.: Specific antibody profile in human brucellosis, *Clin Infect Dis* 14:131-140, 1992.

Biellik RJ, Patriarca RA, Mullen JR et al.: Risk factors for community and household acquired pertussis during a large scale outbreak in central Wisconsin, *J Infect Dis* 157: 1134-1141, 1988.

Goodnow RA: Biology of *Bordetella bronchiseptica, Microbiol Rev* 44:722-738, 1980.

Friedman RL: Pertussis: the disease and new diagnostic methods, *Clin Microbiol Rev* 1:365-376, 1988.

Pertussis surveillance—United States 1984 and 1985, *MMWR* 36:2013-2014, 1987.

Sutter RW and Cochi SL: Pertussis hospitalizations and mortality in the United States, 1985-1988: evaluation of the completeness of national reporting, *JAMA* 267:386-391, 1992.

Weiss AA and Hewlett EL: Virulence factors of *Bordetella pertussis*, *Ann Rev Microbiol* 40:661-686, 1986.

Woolfrey BF and Moody JA: Human infections associated with *Bordetella bronchiseptica*, *Clin Microbiol Rev* 4:243-255, 1991.

Young EJ: Human brucellosis, *Rev Infect Dis* 5:821-842, 1983.

Young EJ: Serologic diagnosis of human brucellosis: analysis of 214 cases by agglutination tests and review of the literature, *Rev Infect Dis* 13:359-372, 1991.

Young EJ and Corbel MJ: *Brucellosis: clinical and laboratory aspects*, Boca Raton, Fla., 1989, CRC Press.

CHAPTER 30

Legionella and Other Miscellaneous Gram-Negative Bacilli

GRAM-NEGATIVE bacilli are an extremely diverse group of organisms that may be only superficially related. In this chapter, miscellaneous groups of organisms responsible for human disease are discussed (Table 30-1).

LEGIONELLACEAE

In the summer of 1976 public attention focused on an outbreak of severe pneumonia that had a high mortality rate for members of the American Legion convention in Philadelphia. After months of intensive investigations the etiological agent, a previously unknown gram-negative bacillus, was isolated. In subsequent studies this organism, named *Legionella pneumophila*, has been associated with at least four epidemics before 1976 and multiple epidemic and sporadic infections after 1976. The existence of this organism was previously unappreciated because it stains poorly with conventional dyes and does not grow on common laboratory media. Despite the initial problems with the isolation of *Legionella,* it is now recognized to be a ubiquitous aquatic saprophyte and a common cause of human respiratory disease.

Taxonomic studies have demonstrated that the family Legionellaceae consists of three genera (*Legionella*, *Tatlockia*, and *Fluoribacter*), 34 species, 3 subspecies, and 21 serogroups. New members of this family continue to be added rapidly while older species are consolidated or renamed. Despite the taxonomic confusion observed with this family, the number of species responsible for human disease is limited to approximately 14, with the others found primarily in environmental sources. *Legionella pneumophila* is responsible for almost 85% of all infections, with serotype 1 isolated most commonly (Figure 30-1). Differentiation of the species is based on determination of DNA homology and analysis of branched cell wall fatty acids— procedures that are impractical for most clinical laboratories. Immunological serotyping further subdivides individual isolates.

TABLE 30-1 Miscellaneous Gram-Negative Bacilli and Their Diseases

Organism	Disease
Legionellaceae	Legionnaires' disease; Pontiac fever
Afipia felis	Cat scratch disease (?)
Bartonella bacilliformis	Oroya fever; verruga
Calymmatobacterium granulomatis	Granuloma inguinale
Cardiobacterium hominis	Endocarditis
Eikenella corrodens	Opportunistic infections
Flavobacterium species	Opportunistic infections
Streptobacillus moniliformis	Rat-bite fever
Spirillum minor	Rat-bite fever

Physiology and Structure

Members of the genus are slender, pleomorphic, gram-negative bacilli, 0.3 to 0.9 μm wide and 2 to 5 μm long. The organisms characteristically appear as short coccobacilli in tissue but are very pleomorphic when cultured on artificial media (Figure 30-2). *Legionella* in clinical specimens do not stain with common reagents but can be seen in tissues stained with the Dieterle silver stain. One species, *Legionella micdadei*, can also be stained with weak acid-fast stains, but this property is lost when the organism is isolated in culture and is not observed with other *Legionella* species. The cell wall of *Legionella* is typical of gram-negative bacilli, with a periplasmic space separating the inner and outer membranes. Although the peptidoglycan layer is difficult to visualize, the bacilli contain diaminopimelic acid and 2-keto-3-deoxyoctonate (components of peptidoglycan and lipopolysaccharide).

Legionellae are nutritionally fastidious, with growth enhanced with iron salts and dependent on supplementation of media with L-cysteine. The organisms are nonfermentative and derive energy from metabolism of amino acids. Most species are motile, catalase positive,

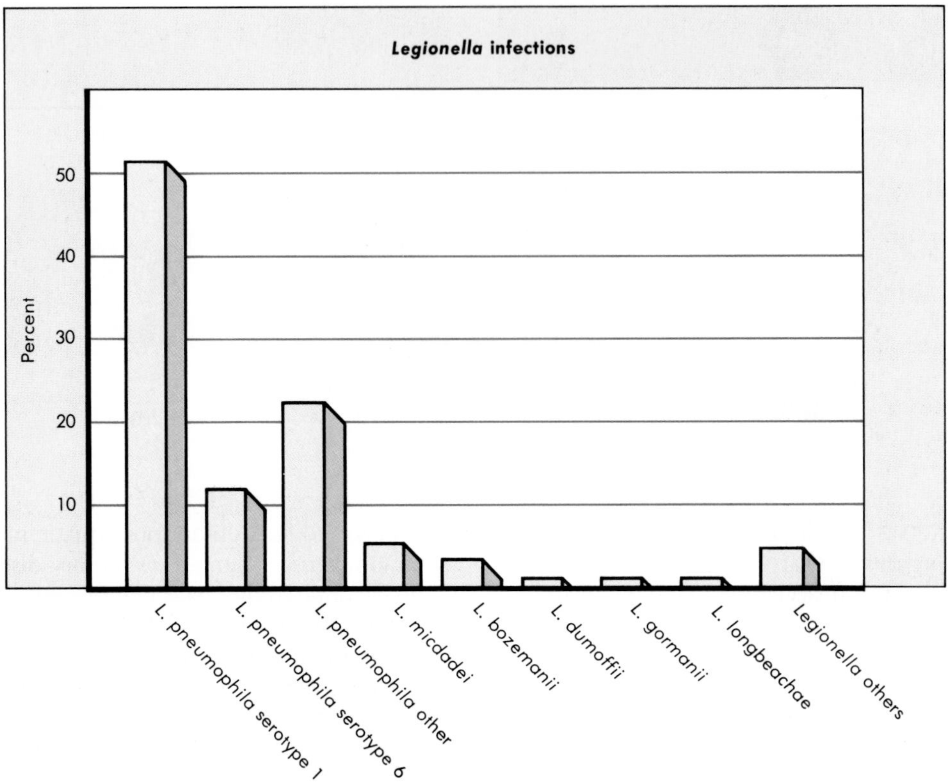

FIGURE 30-1 *Legionella* species associated with human disease.

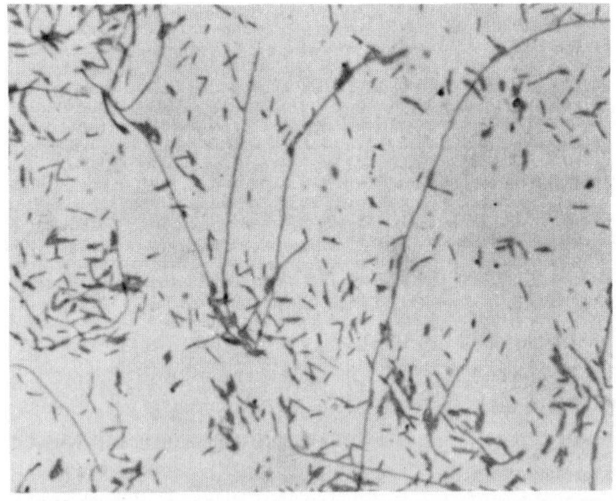

FIGURE 30-2 *Legionella pneumophila* grown on charcoal-yeast extract agar. Note the pleomorphic bacilli with short coccobacilli and very long filaments. (From Holt JG, editor: *Bergey's manual of systematic bacteriology*, vol 1, New York, 1984, Williams & Wilkins.)

liquify gelatin (except *L. micdadei* and *L. feeleii*), and do not reduce nitrate or hydrolyze urea. The selective growth properties of this family have been used for the preliminary identification of clinical isolates.

Pathogenesis and Immunity

Respiratory disease caused by *Legionella* follows inhalation of infectious aerosols by susceptible individuals. *Legionella* are facultative intracellular parasites, capable of multiplication in alveolar macrophages and monocytes. The replicative cycle is initiated by binding complement and depositing C3b on the bacterial surface. This permits the bacteria to bind to CR3 receptors on mononuclear phagocytes, followed by penetration into the cell by endocytosis. Intracellular killing by exposure to toxic superoxide, hydrogen peroxide, and hydroxyl radicals is avoided by inhibition of phagolysosome fusion. Proliferation of the bacilli ensues, with eventual killing of the host cell by the production of proteolytic enzymes, phosphatase, lipase, and nuclease. Immunity to disease is primarily cell mediated, with humoral immunity playing a minor role. Intracellular killing is effectively avoided until sensitized T-cells activate the parasitized macrophages.

Despite extensive examination of the relationship between *Legionella* and the infected host, why the majority of *Legionella* species are rarely responsible for human disease, whereas other species are more virulent, is unknown. Disease is particularly common in individuals with compromised cellular immunity (e.g., renal and cardiac transplant recipients) or pulmonary function (e.g., heavy smokers).

Epidemiology

Sporadic and epidemic legionellosis has a worldwide distribution (Box 30-1). The bacteria are commonly present in natural bodies of water such as lakes and streams, air conditioning cooling towers and condensers, and water systems (e.g., showers, vegetable misters in grocery stores). The organisms are capable of survival in moist environments for prolonged periods and at relatively high temperatures. Thus exposure to legionellae is a common event.

The incidence of infections caused by *Legionella* is unknown because documentation of disease is difficult. The number of cases has steadily increased during the last decade, with almost 1400 cases reported in 1990 (Figure 30-3). However, prospective studies have reported the proportion of pneumonias caused by *Legionella* ranges from less than 1% to greater than 30%, and it is estimated that between 25,000 and 50,000 cases of pulmonary legionellosis occur annually. In addition, serologic studies indicate a significant proportion of the population has developed immunity to this group of organisms. Based on these studies and the knowledge that *Legionella* are ubiquitous aquatic saprophytes, it is reasonable to conclude that contact with the organism and immunity following asymptomatic infection is common, and the incidence of true disease is certainly underestimated.

Although sporadic disease outbreaks are reported throughout the year, most epidemic infections occur in the late summer and fall, presumably because the organism proliferates in water reservoirs during the warm months. The elderly, with decreased cellular immunity and compromised pulmonary function, are at greatest risk for disease. Person-to-person spread has not been demonstrated, because disease is determined not by the opportunity of exposure but rather by the inoculum size, host immunity, and poorly defined virulence factors.

BOX 30-1 Epidemiology of Legionellosis

DISEASE/BACTERIAL FACTORS

Legionnaires' disease and Pontiac fever
Legionella is a facultative intracellular pathogen and can multiply in alveolar macrophages and monocytes
Intracellular killing avoided by inhibiting phagolysosome fusion
Organism can survive in moist environments and relatively high temperatures for prolonged periods

TRANSMISSION

Inhalation of aerosols

WHO IS AT RISK?

Elderly
Patients with compromised cellular immunity (e.g., renal and cardiac transplantation) or pulmonary function (e.g., smokers)

GEOGRAPHY/SEASON

Worldwide; common in lakes, streams, air conditioning cooling towers and condensers, and water systems
Most epidemics occur in late summer and fall

MODES OF CONTROL

Erythromycin (drug of choice), rifampin, and the fluoroquinolones
Hyperchlorination of water supply and higher water temperatures moderately successful in prevention

Clinical Syndromes

Asymptomatic *Legionella* infections are relatively common in many communities and can be detected by low levels of antibodies directed against the organism. Symptomatic infections primarily affect the lungs and are seen in one of two forms (Table 30-2): a flu-like illness (referred to as **Pontiac fever**) or a severe form of pneumonia (e.g., **Legionnaires' disease**).

Pontiac Fever

Legionella pneumophila was responsible for a self-limited, influenza-like, febrile illness in the Pontiac, Michigan Public Health Department in 1968. The disease was characterized by fever, chills, myalgia, malaise, and headache, but no clinical evidence of pneumonia. The symptoms developed over a 12-hour period, persisted for 2 to 5 days, and then resolved spontaneously, with minimal morbidity and no mortalities. Additional epidemics of Pontiac fever, with a high incidence of disease in exposed individuals, have been documented.

Legionnaires' Disease

Legionnaires' disease is characteristically more severe, with significant morbidity and mortality unless prompt therapy is initiated. After an incubation period of 2 to 10 days, patients experience an abrupt onset of fever, chills, dry nonproductive cough, headache, and systemic signs of an acute illness. Multiorgan disease with involvement of the gastrointestinal tract, central nervous system, and abnormality of liver and renal function is commonly observed. The primary manifestation of the disease is pneumonia with multilobe consolidation, and inflammation and microabscesses in lung tissue observed on histopathology. Untreated disease in susceptible patients is characterized by progressive deterioration of pulmonary function. The overall mortality is 15% to 20% but can be much higher in patients with severely depressed cell-mediated immunity (e.g., renal or cardiac transplant recipients).

Laboratory Diagnosis

The sensitivity and specificity of diagnostic tests for *Legionella pneumophila* is summarized in Table 30-3.

Microscopy

Legionellae in clinical specimens stain poorly with the Gram stain (Table 30-4). Nonspecific staining methods such as the Dieterle silver stain or Gimenez stain can be used to visualize the organisms but are of little value with specimens contaminated with normal oral bacteria. The most sensitive procedure for the microscopic detection of legionellae in clinical specimens is the direct fluorescent

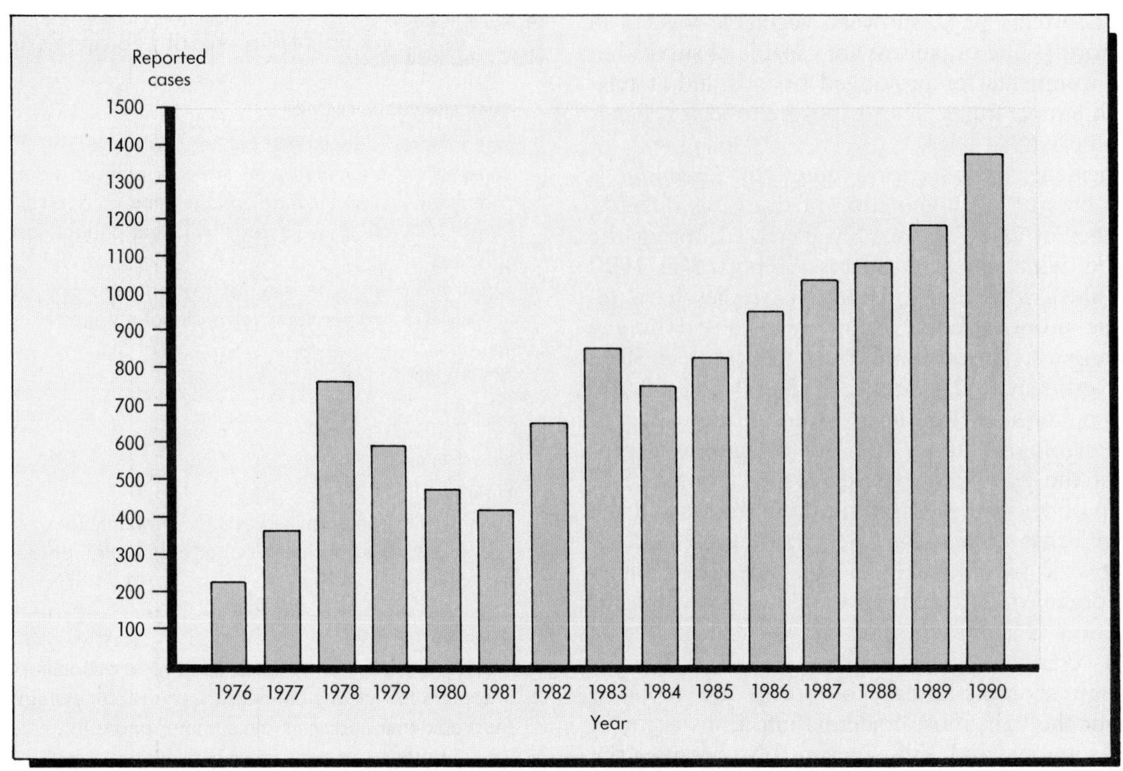

FIGURE 30-3 Number of reported cases of *Legionella* infections in the United States from 1976 to 1990. (Redrawn from *MMWR* 39:55-57, 1991.)

TABLE 30-2 Comparison of Diseases Caused by *Legionella*

	Legionnaires' disease	Pontiac fever
EPIDEMIOLOGY		
Presentation	Epidemic, sporadic	Epidemic
Attack rate	<5%	>90%
Person-to-person spread	No	No
Underlying pulmonary disease	Yes	No
Time of onset	Epidemic disease in late summer or fall; endemic disease throughout the year	Throughout year
CLINICAL MANIFESTATIONS		
Incubation period	2-10 days	1-2 days
Pneumonia	Yes	No
Course	Requires antibiotic therapy	Self-limited
Mortality	15% to 20%; higher if diagnosis is delayed	<1%

antibody (DFA) test, in which fluorescein-labeled monoclonal or polyclonal antibodies directed against *Legionella* species are used. The test is very specific; false-positive reactions are observed only rarely with *Pseudomonas, Bacteroides,* and other organisms. These cross-reactions appear to be limited to the polyclonal reagents. However, the sensitivity of the DFA test is low because the antibody preparations are serotype- or species-specific, and many organisms (e.g., 10^4 to 10^5 organisms per milliliter of specimen) must be present for detection. The latter problem is due to the relatively small size and predominantly intracellular location of the bacteria. Positive tests will revert to negative after about 4 days of treatment. The primary advantage of microscopy compared with other diagnostic tests is that a positive result can be obtained rapidly.

Culture

Although legionellae were initially difficult to grow in vitro, this can be readily accomplished now with commercially available media. Legionellae require L-cysteine, and growth is enhanced with iron (supplied in hemoglobin or ferric pyrophosphate). The medium must be carefully buffered at pH 6.9. The medium most commonly used for isolation of legionellae is buffered charcoal yeast extract (BCYE) agar, although other supplemented media have also been used. Antibiotics can be added to suppress rapidly growing contaminating bacteria. As an alternative, the specimen can be treated with potassium chloride–sodium chloride for the selective elimination of contaminating organisms. *Legionella* will grow in air or 3% to 5% carbon dioxide at 35° C after 3 to 5 days, appearing as small (1 to 3 mm) colonies with a ground-glass appearance.

Antigen Detection

Detection of *legionellae* in respiratory specimens or urine has been performed by enzyme-linked immunoassays, radioimmunoassays, agglutination of antibody-coated latex particles, and nucleic acid hybridization studies. Although the immunological assays are relatively sensitive, the serotype-specific reagents limit the clinical usefulness of the test. In addition, antigen excretion in urine may persist for as long as 1 year. Commercially prepared nucleic acid probe tests enjoyed some initial popularity. However, careful clinical evaluations of these products have demonstrated sensitivity problems. Additional developmental work will be required before these tests can be recommended.

TABLE 30-3 Summary of the Sensitivity and Specificity of Diagnostic Tests for *Legionella pneumophila**

Diagnostic tests	Sensitivity	Specificity
Microscopy		
Direct fluorescent antibody (DFA)	50%-75%	>95%
Antigen detection		
Respiratory specimens	80%	>99%
Urine specimens	70%	>99%
Culture	75%	100%
Serology		
Indirect fluorescent antibody (IFA)	75%	96%

**Legionella pneumophila* is responsible for approximately 85% of diseases caused by Legionella spp. With the exception of culture, the diagnostic tests listed here are specific for *L. pneumophila* or specific serotypes of this species. Thus the other diagnostic tests would not reliably detect the small proportion of legionelloses caused by other species. For optimal detection of *Legionella* infections, a combination of microscopy, culture, and serology should be used.

Serology

The diagnosis of legionellosis is commonly made by measuring a serologic response to infection with the indirect fluorescent antibody test. A fourfold or greater increase in antibody titer (to a level of 128 or greater) is considered to be diagnostic. However, the response may be delayed, with a significant serologic increase observed for only 20% to 40% of patients after 1 week of illness and 75% after 8 weeks. This limits the usefulness of the test for patient management. Antibody titers of 256 or higher are presumptive evidence of active infection, although high titers can occasionally persist for prolonged periods.

Identification

Identification of an isolate as *Legionella* can be easily accomplished by demonstrating typical morphology and specific growth requirements. Legionellae appear as weakly staining, pleomorphic, thin, gram-negative bacilli. Growth on BCYE, but not on BCYE without cysteine or on enriched blood agar media, is presumptive evidence the isolate is *Legionella*. Identification can be confirmed by specific staining with fluorescein-labeled antibodies. In contrast with the identification of the genus, species classification is problematic and generally relegated to reference laboratories. Although biochemical tests and the ability of bacilli to fluoresce under long-wave ultraviolet light are useful differential tests, definitive species classification is accomplished by analysis of the major branched-chain fatty acids in the cell wall and DNA homology.

Treatment, Prevention, and Control

In vitro susceptibility tests with legionellae are not routinely performed because growth is poor on media commonly used for these tests. However, the limited in vitro data and substantial clinical experience indicate erythromycin is the antibiotic of choice, with rifampin and the fluoroquinolones also active. β-lactam antibiotics are ineffective because most isolates produce β-lactamases. Erythromycin can substantially reduce the morbidity and

TABLE 30-4 Staining Reactions of Common *Legionella* Species in Smears and Tissue Sections

	Smears			Tissue sections		
Legionella	Gram	Gimenez	Modified acid-fast	Brown-Brenn	Kinyoun	Dieterle
L. pneumophilia	Negative	Positive	Negative	Negative	Negative	Positive
L. micdadei	Negative	Positive	Acid-fast*	Negative	Acid-fast*	Positive
L. bozemanii	Negative	Positive	Negative	Negative	Negative	Positive
L. dumoffii	Negative	Positive	Negative	Negative	Negative	Positive

*10% to 50% of bacilli will appear acid-fast.

mortality of Legionnaires' disease. Specific therapy for Pontiac fever is generally unnecessary because this is a self-limiting disease.

Prevention of legionellosis requires identification of the environmental source of the organism and reduction of the microbial burden. Hyperchlorination of the water supply and maintenance of elevated water temperatures have proved moderately successful. However, complete elimination of *Legionella* from a water supply is often difficult or impossible. Because the organism has a low potential for causing disease, reduction of the number of organisms in the water supply is frequently adequate for controlling infections.

AFIPIA

The newly formed genus, *Afipia* (from Air Force Institute of Pathology [AFIP]), consists of six species, with *Afipia felis* the type species. *A. felis* was originally isolated in clinical specimens from patients with **cat scratch disease**, a benign infection of children, characterized by chronic regional adenopathy of the lymph nodes draining the site of a cat scratch or bite. The diagnosis is suggested by a history of contact with a cat, clinical presentation, and the absence of common bacteria in cultures of aspirated lymph nodes. The diagnosis is confirmed by observation of the bacterium in histopathological specimens (using the Warthin-Starry silver stain) or in vitro isolation. Culture of the organism is difficult and has been accomplished in only a few laboratories. Unfortunately, the role of *A. felis* in cat scratch disease has been confounded by the fact that *Rochalimaea henselae*, a cause of septicemia, bacillary angiomatosis, and bacillary peliosis (see Chapter 38), has also been isolated in tissues from these patients. Most investigators now believe *A. felis* is an incidental finding. However, further studies must be performed to resolve the role of each organism in this disease.

BARTONELLA

Bartonella bacilliformis is a small (0.2 to 0.5 × 1 to 3 μm), poorly staining, gram-negative bacillus responsible for bartonellosis, an acute febrile illness characterized by severe anemia (**Oroya fever**) followed by a chronic cutaneous form (**verrugas**). Bartonellosis is restricted to Peru, Ecuador, and Colombia, the endemic regions of the sandfly vector, *Phlebotomus*. Following the bite of an infected sandfly, the bacteria enter the bloodstream, multiply, and penetrate into erythrocytes. This process increases the fragility of the infected cells and facilitates their clearance by the reticuloendothelial system, leading to acute anemia. Myalgias, arthralgias, and headaches are also commonly present. This stage of illness ends with the development of humoral immunity. The chronic stage of bartonellosis is characterized by the development of 1 to 2 cm cutaneous nodules, which appear over 1 to 2 months and may persist for months to years.

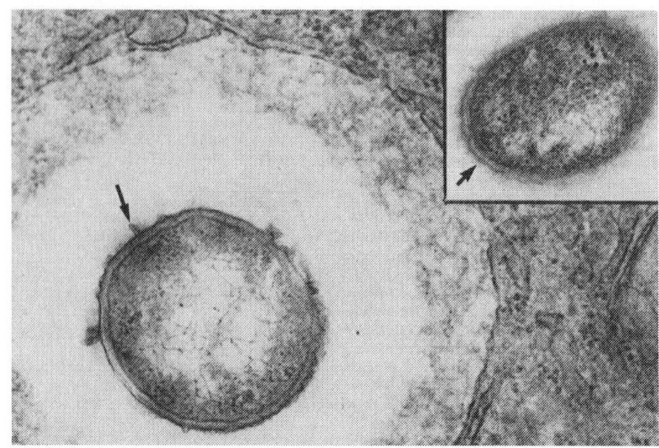

FIGURE 30-4 Electron micrograph of *Calymmatobacterium granulomatis* within a mononuclear cell phagosome. Note the prominent capsule surrounding the cell, surface projections (*arrow*), and typical gram-negative trilaminar membrane structure (*insert*). (From Kuberski T et al: *J Infect Dis* 142:744-749, 1980.)

The clinical diagnosis can be confirmed by observing infected erythrocytes in Giemsa-stained blood smears (primarily in the acute form of bartonellosis) or isolation of the bacteria from blood and from the cutaneous lesions. *B. bacilliformis* grows optimally at 30° C in nutrient agar supplemented with rabbit serum and rabbit hemoglobin.

Chloramphenicol or penicillin is used to treat bartonellosis, as well as blood transfusions when indicated for the anemia. Prevention and control of disease involves control of the sandfly vector.

CALYMMATOBACTERIUM

Calymmatobacterium (Donovania) *granulomatis* is the etiological agent of **granuloma inguinale,** a granulomatous disease of the genitalia and inguinal area. The organism was discovered by Donovan and subsequently renamed to reflect its appearance in tissues as encapsulated bacilli (*calymma* is Greek for sheathed; "sheathed bacterium"). *C. granulomatis* is not cultured in vitro, with the laboratory diagnosis made by staining infected tissues with a Wright or Giemsa stain. The organisms appear as small (0.5 to 1.0 × 1.5 μm) bacilli in the cytoplasm of histiocytes, polymorphonuclear leukocytes, and plasma cells. From 1 to 25 bacteria per phagocytic cell can be seen; a prominent capsule surrounds the organisms (Figure 30-4).

Granuloma inguinale is a rare disease in the United States but has been reported in tropical areas such as the Caribbean and New Guinea. Transmission after repeated exposure can occur by sexual intercourse or nonsexual trauma to the genitalia.

After a prolonged incubation of weeks to months subcutaneous nodules appear on the genitalia or in the inguinal area. The nodules subsequently break down, revealing one or more painless granulomatous lesions that can extend and coalesce.

Laboratory confirmation of granuloma inguinale is made by scraping the border of the lesion, spreading the collected tissue on a slide, and staining with Giemsa or Wright stain. Pathognomonic "Donovan bodies" are observed within mononuclear phagocytes.

Tetracycline, ampicillin, and trimethoprim-sulfamethoxazole has been used successfully for treatment. Antibiotic prophylaxis for prevention and control has not been proven effective.

CARDIOBACTERIUM

Cardiobacterium hominis, named for the predilection of this bacterium to cause endocarditis in humans, is the only member of the genus. *C. hominis* isolates are nonmotile, characteristically small (1 × 1 to 2 μm) but sometimes pleomorphic, gram-negative bacilli. The bacteria are fermentative, indole and oxidase positive, and catalase negative.

Endocarditis caused by *C. hominis* is uncommon, with less than 50 cases reported in the literature. However, many cases are unreported or undiagnosed because of the low virulence of this organism and its slow growth in vitro. *C. hominis* is present in the upper respiratory tract of almost 70% of healthy individuals.

Endocarditis is the only human disease caused by *C. hominis* (Box 30-2). Most patients with *C. hominis* endocarditis have a history of oral disease or dental procedures before clinical symptoms developed, as well as preexisting heart disease. The organism is able to enter the bloodstream from the oropharynx, adhere to the damaged heart tissue, and then slowly multiply. The course of disease is insidious and subacute, with a history of symptoms (fatigue, malaise, low-grade temperature) for months before the patient seeks medical care. Complications are rare, and complete recovery following appropriate antibiotic therapy is common.

Isolation of *C. hominis* from blood cultures confirms the diagnosis of endocarditis. The organism grows slowly in culture and requires 1 to 2 weeks before growth is detected, which is why infections with these organisms have not been confirmed in some patients. *C. hominis* appears in broth cultures as discrete clumps that can be easily overlooked when cultures are examined. The organism requires enhanced carbon dioxide and humidity for growth on agar media, with pinpoint (1 mm) colonies seen on blood or chocolate agar plates after 3 days of incubation. The organism does not grow on MacConkey agar or other selective media commonly used for gram-negative bacilli. *C. hominis* can be readily identified by its growth properties, microscopic morphology, and reactivity in biochemical tests.

C. hominis is susceptible to multiple antibiotics, and most infections are successfully treated with either penicillin or ampicillin for 2 to 6 weeks.

C. hominis endocarditis in individuals with preexisting heart disease is prevented by maintenance of good oral hygiene and use of antibiotic prophylaxis at the time of dental procedures. A long-acting penicillin is effective prophylaxis, but erythromycin should not be used because resistance is common.

BOX 30-2 Epidemiology of *Cardiobacterium* Infection

DISEASE/BACTERIAL FACTORS

Endocarditis
Present in upper respiratory tract of almost 70% of healthy people
Subacute course of disease

TRANSMISSION

Spread from oropharynx (caused by disease or dental procedure) into blood and to heart

WHO IS AT RISK?

Persons with oral disease or dental procedures
Persons with preexisting heart disease

GEOGRAPHY/SEASON

Worldwide
No seasonal incidence

MODES OF CONTROL

Penicillin or ampicillin for treatment
In patients with preexisting heart disease: good oral hygiene and antibiotic prophylaxis during dental manipulations
Long-acting penicillin for prophylaxis

EIKENELLA

Eikenella corrodens is a moderate-size (0.2 × 2 μm), nonmotile, non–spore-forming, faculatively anaerobic, gram-negative bacillus. The organism is named after Eiken, who characterized the bacterium and the ability of the organism to pit or "corrode" agar. *E. corrodens* is a normal inhabitant of the upper respiratory tract, although its fastidious growth characteristics make it difficult to detect without specific selective culture media. It is an opportunistic pathogen, causing infections in immunocompromised patients and in patients with diseases or trauma of the oral cavity (Box 30-3). *E. corrodens* has been associated with human bites or fistfight injuries (frequently complicated with septic arthritis or osteomyelitis if initially treated improperly), sinusitis, meningitis, brain abscesses, pneumonia, lung abscesses, and endocarditis. Because most infections originate from the oropharynx, polymicrobial mixtures of aerobic and anaerobic bacteria are frequently present. The etiological role of *Eikenella* in these infections is established by the failure to cure the infection unless specific therapy is administered.

BOX 30-3 Epidemiology of *Eikenella* Infection

DISEASE/BACTERIAL FACTORS

Human bite wound infection, sinusitis, meningitis, brain abscess, pneumonia, lung abscess, endocarditis
Normal inhabitant of upper respiratory tract

TRANSMISSION

Human bites
Spread of disease from oral cavity into blood to distant tissues

WHO IS AT RISK?

Persons with bite injuries
Persons with diseases or trauma of the oral cavity
Immunocompromised

GEOGRAPHY/SEASON

Worldwide
No seasonal incidence

MODES OF CONTROL

Penicillin or ampicillin

E. corrodens is a slow-growing, fastidious organism that requires 5% to 10% carbon dioxide for isolation. Small (0.5 to 1 mm) colonies are observed on common laboratory media after 48 hours of incubation. Pitting in agar is a useful differential characteristic but is seen in less than half of all isolates.

E. corrodens is susceptible to penicillin and ampicillin but resistant to oxacillin, first-generation cephalosporins, clindamycin, and the aminoglycosides. Unfortunately, this means *E. corrodens* is resistant to many antibiotics that are empirically selected to treat bite wound infections.

FLAVOBACTERIUM

The genus *Flavobacterium* consists of nine species that can cause opportunistic human diseases, of which *Flavobacterium* group IIb (also referred to as *F. indologenes*), *F. multivorum*, and *F. meningosepticum* are the best known. The organisms are small (0.5×1 to $2\ \mu m$), nonmotile, aerobic, gram-negative bacilli that grow on common laboratory media after 24 hours of incubation. Most strains are oxidase and catalase positive, acidify glucose, and fail to reduce nitrate or use citrate. The three indole-positive species (including *Flavobacterium* group IIb and *F. meningosepticum*) are strongly proteolytic, which may account for their increased virulence.

Flavobacteria are widely disseminated in nature, found in water, wet soil, and moist reservoirs in the hospital (e.g., sinks, faucets, humidifiers, respiratory therapy equipment). The organism is not part of the normal human microbial flora.

The flavobacteria are opportunistic pathogens in immunocompromised patients. As the name implies, *F. meningosepticum* has been associated with meningitis and septicemia, particularly in neonates. Other flavobacteria infections have developed following exposure to solutions contaminated with these organisms.

Flavobacterium species are resistant to many antibiotics, including aminoglycosides, penicillins, and cephalosporins. Effective therapy requires selection of specific agents that have proven in vitro activity against *Flavobacterium* and can reach therapeutic concentrations at the site of infection. Infection can be prevented through established infection control practices that reduce or eliminate exposure to contaminated water supplies and solutions.

STREPTOBACILLUS AND SPIRILLUM

Streptobacillus moniliforms and *Spirillum minor* are the etiological agents of two distinct diseases referred to collectively as **rat-bite fever** (Table 30-5). *S. moniliformis* is a long, thin (0.1 to 0.5×1 to $5\ \mu m$), gram-negative bacillus that tends to stain poorly and be more pleomorphic in older cultures. Granules and bulbous swellings, which resemble a string of beads, may be seen. *S. minor* is a spiral, gram-negative bacillus (0.2 to 0.5×3 to $5\ \mu m$) with a flagellum at each pole.

Both *Streptobacillus* and *Spirillum* are found in the nasopharynx of rats and other small rodents, as well as transiently in animals that feed on rodents (e.g., dogs, cats). Turkeys exposed to rats and mice, as well as contaminated water and milk, have also been implicated in *Streptobacillus* infections.

Although the epidemiology and clinical syndrome of recurrent fevers are similar for both *Streptobacillus* and *Spirillum* infections, distinct differences have been observed. *Streptobacillus* infections have a shorter incubation period and a clinical course that includes myalgias, arthralgias, and frank arthritis that is usually absent in *Spirillum* infections. One form of *S. moniliformis* infection, **Haverhill fever** or **erythema arthriticum epidemicum**, is characterized by fever, rash, arthralgia, chills, vomiting, and gastrointestinal and respiratory symptoms. Ulceration at the bite site with lymphadenopathy and lymphangitis is observed in *Spirillum* rat bite infections (also known as **Sodoku**). Recurrent febrile episodes are observed with both organisms in untreated disease.

S. moniliformis, but not *S. minor*, can be cultured in vitro. Blood and joint fluid should be collected, mixed with citrate to prevent clotting, and transported to the laboratory. Enriched media supplemented with 15% blood, 20% horse or calf serum, or 5% ascitic fluid will support growth of the organism. *S. moniliformis* is slow-growing, requiring 3 or more days for isolation. Growth in broth will appear as "puff balls"; small round colonies will appear on agar, as well as cell-wall defective forms with their typical fried-egg appearance. Identification is difficult because the organisms are relatively inactive, although acid is produced from glucose and other selected carbohydrates. Serologic tests for the detection of antibodies against *Streptobacillus* antigens are

TABLE 30-5 Comparison of *Streptobacillus* and *Spirillum*

	Streptobacillus moniliformis	***Spirillum minor***
Distribution	Worldwide	Worldwide, primarily Asia
Reservoir	Rats and other small rodents	Rats and other small rodents
Transmission	Bite of rat or other rodent; contact with animals that feed on rodents; consumption of water or other contaminated fluid or food	Bite of rat or other rodent; contact with animals that feed on rodents
Disease	Rat-bite fever (Haverhill fever)	Rat-bite fever (Sodoku)
Incubation period	Less than 10 days	2 weeks
Clinical presentation	Abrupt onset; high fever; chills, headache, myalgias, rash, arthritis/arthralgia; recurrent fevers if untreated	Abrupt onset; fever, chills, rash, lymphangitis, lymphadenopathy; recurrent fevers if untreated
Mortality	10% if untreated	6% if untreated
Treatment	Penicillin	Penicillin
Diagnosis	Culture; serology; false-positive syphilis serology	Darkfield; Wright or Giemsa stained blood smears; animal inoculation

available in reference laboratories. A titer greater than or equal to 80 or fourfold rise is considered diagnostic, although this test has not been standardized or extensively evaluated for cross-reactivity.

Spirillum minor, which is more common in countries outside the United States, has not been cultured in vitro. Detection of *S. minor* infections is by darkfield examination of blood, ulcer exudates, or lymph node aspirates. Blood smears can be stained with Giemsa or Wright stain. *S. minor* can also be detected in the blood of rodents 1 to 3 weeks after intraperitoneal inoculation with the clinical specimen.

Penicillin is the antibiotic of choice for treating rat-bite fever. Tetracycline can be used in penicillin-allergic patients.

CASE STUDY AND QUESTIONS

A 73-year-old man was admitted to the hospital with dyspnea, chest pain, chills, and fever of several days duration. He had been well until 1 week before admission when he noted the onset of a persistent headache and a productive cough. The patient had smoked 2 packs of cigarettes a day for more than 50 years, drank a six pack of beer daily, and had a history of bronchitis. Physical examination revealed an elderly man in severe respiratory distress with a temperature of 39.0° C, pulse, 120, respiratory rate, 36; and blood pressure, 145/95 mm Hg. Chest examination revealed an infiltrate in the middle and lower lobes of the right lung. The white blood cell count was 14,000 cells/mm^3 (80% PMNs). Gram stain of the sputum showed neutrophils but no bacteria, and routine bacterial cultures of sputum and blood were negative.

1. Infection with *Legionella pneumophila* is suspected. What laboratory tests can be used to confirm this? What are the limitations of these tests? Why was the routine culture and Gram stain negative for *Legionella*?
2. How is *Legionella* able to survive phagocytosis by the alveolar macrophages?
3. What environmental factors are implicated in spreading infections with *Legionella*? How can this risk be eliminated or minimized?
4. Compare Legionnaire's disease with Pontiac fever.
5. Describe the epidemiology of *Cardiobacterium* disease.

Bibliography

Brenner DJ, Hollis DG, Moss CW et al: Proposal of *Afipia* gen. nov., with *Afipia felis* sp. nov. (formerly the Cat Scratch Disease bacillus), *Afipia clevelandensis* sp. nov. (formerly the Cleveland Clinic Foundation strain), *Afipia broomeae* sp. nov., and three unnamed genospecies, *J Clin Microbiol* 29: 2450-2460, 1991.

Edelstein PH: Laboratory diagnosis of infections caused by Legionnellae, *Eur J Clin Microbiol* 6:4-10, 1987.

English CK, Wear DJ, Margileth AM et al: Cat-scratch disease: isolation and culture of the bacterial agent, *JAMA* 259:1347-1352, 1988.

Fallon RJ: The Legionellaceae, *Med Lab Sci* 43:64-71, 1986.

Fraser DW, Tsai TR, Orenstein W et al: Legionnaires' disease: description of an epidemic of pneumonia, *N Engl J Med* 297:1189-1197, 1977.

Kuberski T, Papadimitriou JM, and Phillips P: Ultrastructure of *Calymmatobacterium granulomatis* in lesions of granuloma inguinale, *J Infect Dis* 142:744-749, 1980.

McDade JE, Shepard CC, Fraser DW et al: Legionnaires' disease: isolation of a bacterium and demonstration of its role in other respiratory disease, *N Engl J Med* 297:1197-1203, 1977.

Reingold AL: Role of Legionnellae in acute infections of the lower respiratory tract, *Rev Infect Dis* 10:1018-1028, 1988.

Stoloff AL and Gillies ML: Infections with *Eikenella corrodens* in a general hospital: a report of 33 cases, *Rev Infect Dis* 8:50-53, 1986.

Wormser GP and Bottone EJ: *Cardiobacterium hominis:* review of microbiologic and clinical features, *Rev Infect Dis* 5:680-691, 1983.

CHAPTER 31

Anaerobic Gram-Positive Cocci and Non–Spore-Forming Bacilli

THE anaerobic gram-positive cocci and non–spore-forming bacilli are a heterogenous group of bacteria that characteristically colonize the skin and mucosal surfaces. These opportunistic pathogens are frequently recovered in mixed cultures and in the presence of a foreign body (e.g., catheter, prosthesis). They generally have fastidious nutritional requirements and grow slowly on laboratory media.

ANAEROBIC GRAM-POSITIVE COCCI

The taxonomic classification of anaerobic gram-positive cocci was extensively changed in 1983 (Box 31-1). *Peptococcus niger*, a species rarely isolated in clinical material, is currently the only member of the genus, with other peptococci transferred to the genus *Peptostreptococcus*. Organisms previously classified as *Gaffkya anaerobia* have also been reclassified as *Peptostreptococcus tetradius* (they are commonly arranged in tetrads). Unfortunately, reference to the older taxonomic nomenclature is still frequently found in the scientific literature. Three other genera of anaerobic gram-positive cocci are recognized (i.e., *Coprococcus*, *Ruminococcus*, and *Sarcina*). These organisms colonize the stomach and intestines of humans but are rarely isolated in clinical specimens and will not be discussed further.

More than 25% of the anaerobes isolated in clinical specimens are members of the genus *Peptostreptococcus*. These gram-positive cocci normally colonize the oral cavity, gastrointestinal tract, genitourinary tract, and skin, and cause infections by spread from these sites to adjacent sterile areas. Infections associated with the anaerobic gram-positive cocci include pleuropulmonary infections following aspiration of oral secretions, sinusitis and brain abscesses after spread of the organisms from the oropharynx or the lungs, intraabdominal sepsis with abscess formation after spread from the intestines, pelvic infections (endometritis, pelvic abscess, puerperal sepsis, salpingitis, bacterial vaginosis), soft tissue infections (e.g., Meleney's gangrene, synergistic necrotizing cellulitis), endocarditis, and osteomyelitis (Figure 31-1).

BOX 31-1 Anaerobic, Gram-Positive Cocci

Peptostreptococcus	*Coprococcus*
Peptococcus	*Ruminococcus*
Sarcinia	

Most infections are polymicrobial mixtures of aerobic and anaerobic bacteria. Only about 1% of all anaerobic bacteremias are caused by gram-positive cocci, with the majority of the bacteremias caused by peptostreptococci originating from the genital tract in women. This is because anaerobic gram-positive cocci are among the predominant organisms in the vagina, in contrast with other body sites colonized with anaerobes where gram-negative bacilli predominate. Bone and joint infections caused by anaerobes, particularly *Peptostreptococcus magnus,* are usually associated with surgical procedures (e.g., hip replacement), where bacteria residing on the skin contaminate prosthetic material and establish a chronic, indolent infection.

Laboratory confirmation of infections with *Peptostreptococcus* is complicated by three factors. First, care must be used to avoid contamination of the clinical specimen with peptostreptococci that normally colonize the mucosal surface. Second, transport of the collected specimen must be in an oxygen-free container to prevent loss of organisms. Finally, specimens should be cultured on nutritional enriched media for a prolonged period (i.e., 5 to 7 days).

Members of the genus *Peptostreptococcus* are usually susceptible to penicillin, the cephalosporins, imipenem, and chloramphenicol. They have intermediate susceptibility to clindamycin, erythromycin, the tetracyclines, and metronidazole, and are resistant to the aminoglycosides. Specific therapy is generally indicated in monomicrobic infections but may not be necessary in polymicrobic infections.

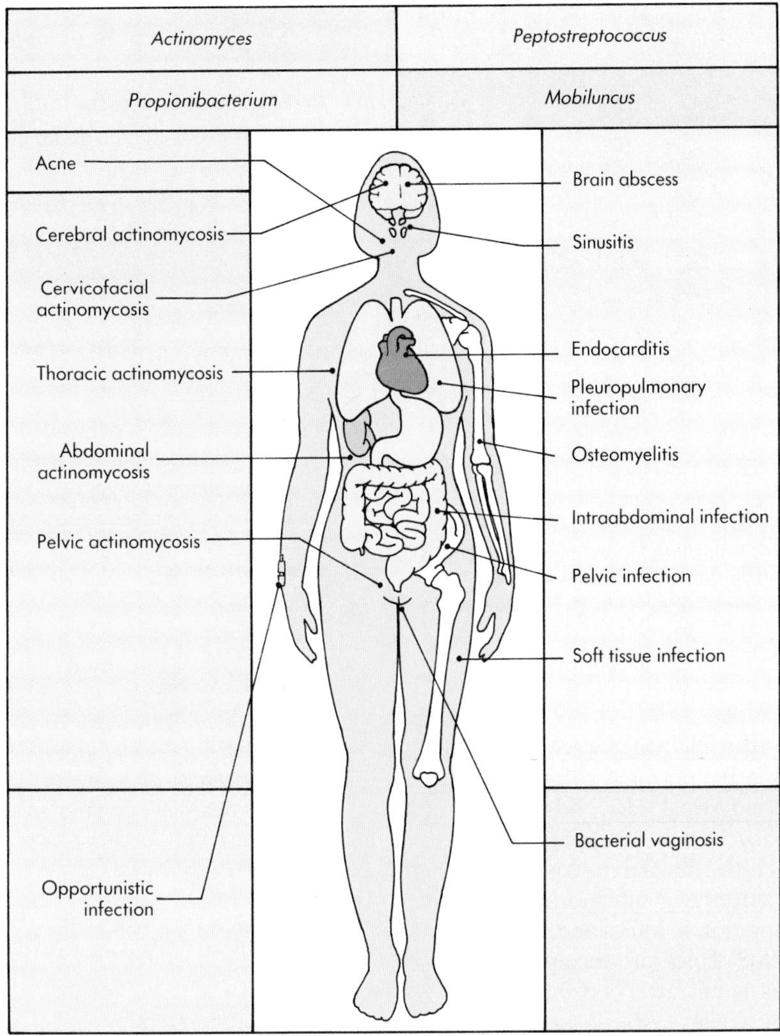

FIGURE 31-1 Diseases associated with *Peptostreptococcus, Actinomyces, Propionibacterium,* and *Mobiluncus.*

ANAEROBIC, NON–SPORE-FORMING, GRAM-POSITIVE BACILLI

The non–spore-forming, gram-positive bacilli are a diverse collection of facultative anaerobic or strict anaerobic bacteria that colonize the skin and mucosal surfaces (Box 31-2). *Actinomyces*, *Mobiluncus*, and *Propionibacterium* are well-recognized, opportunistic pathogens, whereas *Bifidobacterium*, *Eubacterium*, *Lactobacillus*, and *Rothia* are rarely responsible for human disease.

BOX 31-2 Anaerobic, Non–Spore-Forming, Gram-Positive Bacilli

Actinomyces
Propionibacterium
Mobulincus
Bifidobacterium
Eubacterium
Lactobacillus
Rothia

Actinomyces

Physiology and Structure

Actinomyces are facultative anaerobic or strict anaerobic, gram-positive bacilli. They are not acid-fast, grow slowly in culture, and tend to produce chronic, slowly developing infections. They typically form delicate filamentous forms or hyphae, similar to fungi when detected in clinical specimens or isolated in culture (Figure 31-2). In fact, the name *Actinomyces* is Greek for "ray fungus." However, these organisms are true bacteria: they lack mitochondria and a nuclear membrane, reproduce by fission, and are inhibited by penicillin but not antifungal antibiotics. Thirteen species are currently recognized, with *A. israelii, A. naeslundii, A. viscosus, A. odontolyticus, A. pyogenes*, and *A. meyeri* responsible for disease in humans.

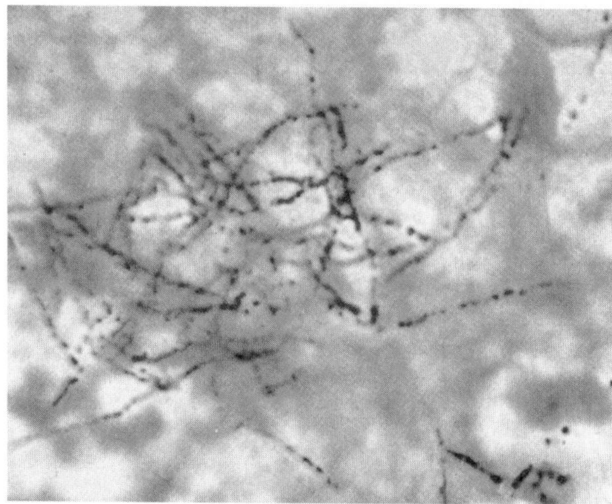

FIGURE 31-2 Gram stain of *Actinomyces* in pus, demonstrating irregularly stained, beaded, branching filaments. (From Smith EP. In HP Lambert and WE Farrar, editors: *Infectious diseases illustrated*, London, 1982, Gower Medical Publishing.)

Pathogenesis

Actinomycosis is a chronic infection produced by opportunistic organisms that normally colonize the upper respiratory tract, gastrointestinal tract, and female genital tract. The organisms have a low virulence potential and cause disease only when the normal mucosal barriers are disrupted by trauma, surgery, or infection. Actinomyces establish a chronic, suppurative infection that can spread unchecked through tissue planes, producing a multiorgan disease. Actinomycosis is characterized by multiple abscesses connected by sinus tracts. Macroscopic colonies of organisms can frequently be seen in the affected tissues and the sinus tracts. These colonies, called **sulfur granules** because they appear yellow or orange, are masses of filamentous organisms bound together by calcium phosphate. The areas of suppuration are commonly surrounded by fibrosing granulation tissue, which gives the surface overlying the involved tissues a hard or woody consistency.

BOX 31-3 Epidemiology of Actinomycosis

DISEASE/BACTERIAL FACTORS

Cervicofacial, thoracic, abdominal, pelvic, or CNS actinomycosis
Normally colonizes upper respiratory tract, GI tract, female genital tract
Infection occurs when mucosal barriers are disrupted

TRANSMISSION

Spread from endogenous site to normally sterile areas

WHO IS AT RISK?

Persons with poor oral hygiene
Persons undergoing oral therapy
Trauma patients
Women with intrauterine contraceptive devices (IUD)

GEOGRAPHY/SEASON

Worldwide
No seasonal incidence

MODES OF CONTROL

Surgical debridement combined with long-term antibiotics: penicillin (drug of choice), tetracycline, erythromycin, clindamycin
Good oral hygiene controls spread via oral mucosa
Antibiotic prophylaxis necessary when mouth or GI tract is penetrated

BOX 31-4 *Actinomyces* Infections

Cervicofacial actinomycosis
Thoracic actinomycosis
Abdominal actinomycosis
Pelvic actinomycosis
Central nervous system actinomycosis

Epidemiology

Actinomycosis is an endogenous infection (Box 31-3). There is no evidence of person-to-person spread or disease originating from an external source such as soil or water. All age-groups can be affected, and there is no seasonal or occupational predilection. Disease is classified by the organ systems involved (Box 31-4). *Cervicofacial* infections are seen in patients with poor oral hygiene or a history of an invasive dental procedure or oral trauma. Patients with *thoracic* infections generally have a history of aspiration, with establishment of disease in the lungs and then spread to adjoining tissues. *Abdominal* infections are most commonly preceded by surgery or trauma to the bowel. *Pelvic* infections can be a secondary manifestation of abdominal actinomycosis or may be a primary infection in women with intrauterine devices (Figure 31-3). *Central nervous system* infections usually represent secondary spread from another focus.

Clinical Syndromes

The majority of all cases of actinomycosis are cervicofacial. The disease may be seen either as an acute pyogenic infection or more commonly as a slowly evolving, relatively painless process. Tissue swelling with fibrosis and scarring, and open draining sinus tracts along the angle of the jaw and neck, should alert the physician to the possibility of actinomycosis. Symptoms of thoracic actinomycosis are nonspecific. Abscess formation in the lung tissue may be observed in early disease, with subsequent

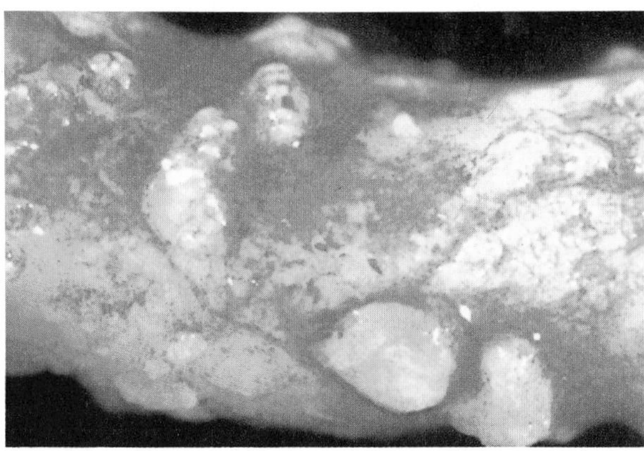

FIGURE 31-3 Pelvic actinomycosis. The female genital tract is normally colonized with *Actinomyces*. Although they rarely cause significant disease, the organisms can colonize the surface of an intrauterine device (IUD) and establish infection. Colonies of *Actinomyces israelii* cover the surface of this IUD. (From Smith EP. In Lambert HP and Farrar WE, editors: *Infectious diseases illustrated*, London, 1982, Gower Medical Publishing.)

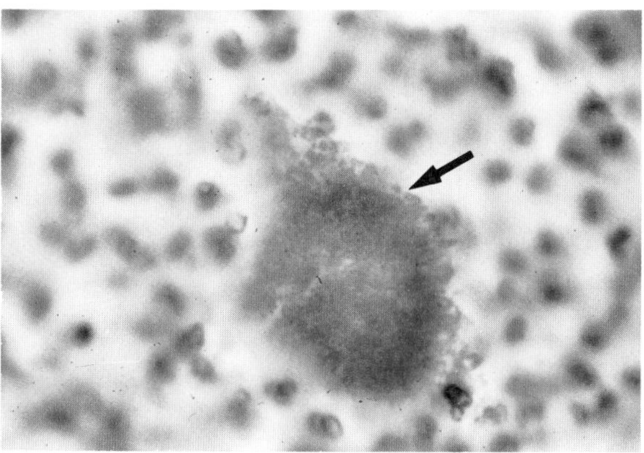

FIGURE 31-4 Sulfur granule collected from sinus tract in patient with actinomycosis. Note the delicate filamentous bacilli (arrow) at the periphery of the crushed granule.

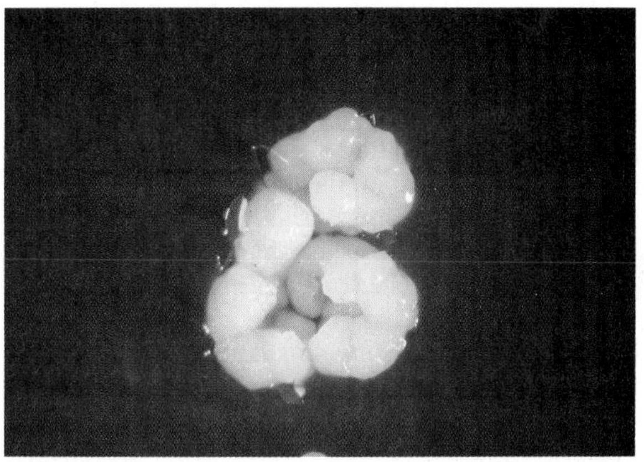

FIGURE 31-5. Molar tooth appearance of *Actinomyces israelii* after incubation for 1 week. This colonial morphology is consistent with the fact the bacteria are normally found in the mouth.

spread into adjoining tissues as the disease progresses. Abdominal actinomycosis can spread throughout the abdomen, involving virtually every organ system. Pelvic actinomycosis can occur as a relatively benign form of vaginitis or with more extensive tissue destruction, including tuboovarian abscess or ureteral obstruction. The most common manifestation of central nervous system actinomycosis is a solitary brain abscess, but meningitis, subdural empyema, or an epidural abscess can also be seen.

Laboratory Diagnosis

Laboratory confirmation of actinomycosis is frequently difficult. Care must be used when collecting clinical specimens to avoid contamination with actinomyces that are part of the normal bacterial population on mucosal surfaces, because the significance of isolating actinomyces from contaminated specimens cannot be determined. The most effective technique for specimen collection is to cleanse the surface of a sinus tract with povidone-iodine and then collect the specimen from deep in the sinus tract with a curette or syringe. Because the organisms are concentrated in sulfur granules and are sparsely distributed in the involved tissues, a large amount of tissue or pus should be collected. Swabs should not be used. If sulfur granules can be detected in a sinus tract or in tissue, then the granule should be crushed between two glass slides, stained, and examined microscopically. Thin, gram-positive branching bacilli along the periphery of the granules will be seen (Figure 31-4). Actinomyces are fastidious and grow slowly under anaerobic conditions; isolation requires incubation for 2 weeks or more. Colonies appear white, with a domed surface that can become irregular with incubation for a week or more, and resemble the top of a "molar" tooth (Figure 31-5).

Identification of actinomyces is accomplished by the selective use of differential biochemical tests. Although the organisms are biochemically active, their slow growth frequently delays definitive test results.

Treatment, Prevention, and Control

Treatment for actinomycosis involves the combination of surgical debridement of the involved tissues and prolonged administration of antibiotics. Actinomyces are uniformly susceptible to penicillin (considered the antibiotic of choice), as well as to tetracycline, erythromycin, and clindamycin. For infections that do not appear to respond to prolonged therapy (e.g., 4 to 12 months), an undrained focus should be suspected. Despite extensive tissue destruction by actinomyces, clinical response is generally good. Prevention of these endogenous infections is difficult. However, good oral hygiene should be maintained, and appropriate antibiotic prophylaxis should be used when the mouth or gastrointestinal tract is penetrated.

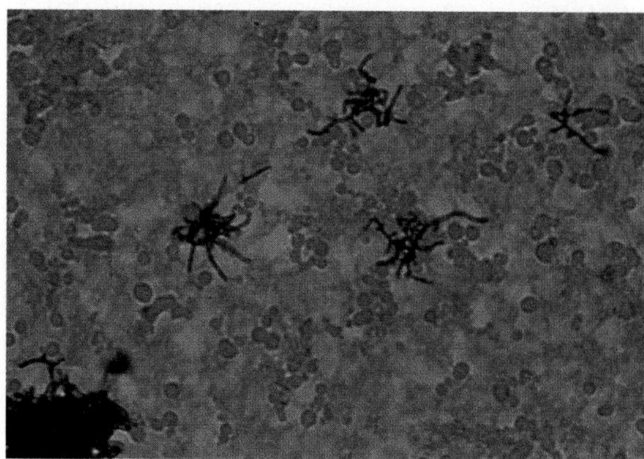

FIGURE 31-6 Gram stain of *Propionibacterium* recovered in a blood culture.

Propionibacterium

Propionibacteria are small gram-positive bacilli, frequently arranged in short chains or clumps (Figure 31-6). They are commonly found on the skin surface, conjunctiva, external ear, and in the oropharynx and female genital tract. The organisms are anaerobic or aerotolerant, nonmotile, catalase-positive, and ferment carbohydrates, producing propionic acid as their major by-product (hence the name). The two most commonly isolated species are *Propionibacterium acnes* and *Propionibacterium propionicus* (formerly *Arachnia propionica*).

Disease caused by *P. acnes* is observed in two populations: acne (as implied by the name) in teenagers and young adults and opportunistic infections in patients with prosthetic devices (e.g., artificial heart valves or joints) or intravascular lines (e.g., catheters, cerebrospinal shunts). Propionibacteria are also commonly isolated in blood cultures, but these usually represent contamination with bacteria on the skin of the phlebotomy site (Box 31-5).

The central role of *P. acnes* in acne is to stimulate an inflammatory response. Production of a low molecular weight peptide by the bacilli attracts leukocytes to the sebaceous follicles where they reside. Phagocytosis of the bacilli is followed by release of hydrolytic enzymes that, together with bacterial lipases, proteases, neuraminidase, and hyaluronidase, precipitates the inflammatory response leading to rupture of the follicle.

P. propionicus causes actinomycosis, lacrimal canaliculitis (inflammation of the tear duct), and abscesses when injected into experimental animals. Because of the role this organism plays in actinomycosis, some investigators have proposed that it belongs in the genus *Actinomyces*.

Propionibacteria will grow on most common media, although 2 to 5 days may be required before growth is observed. Care must be used to avoid contamination of the specimen with the organisms normally found on the skin surface. The significance of recovering an isolate must also be interpreted in light of the clinical presentation (e.g., a catheter or other foreign body can serve as a focus of infection for these opportunistic pathogens).

Acne is unrelated to the effectiveness of skin cleansing, because the lesion develops within the sebaceous follicles. For this reason, the primary management of acne is topical treatment with benzoyl peroxide and antibiotics. Antibiotics such as erythromycin and clindamycin have been used effectively. Oral antibiotic may be required for more persistent acne.

BOX 31-5 Epidemiology of *Propionibacterium* Infection

DISEASE/BACTERIAL FACTORS

Acne and opportunistic infections
P. acne stimulates an inflammatory response that results in rupture of sebaceous follicles
Release of hydrolytic enzymes (e.g., lipase, protease, neuraminidase, hyaluronidase)

TRANSMISSION

Spread from endogenous site to normally sterile areas

WHO IS AT RISK?

Teenagers and young adults (acne)
Patients with prosthetic devices or intravenous lines

GEOGRAPHY/SEASON

Worldwide
No seasonal incidence

MODES OF CONTROL

Acne: topical benzoyl peroxide and antibiotics (erythromycin, clindamycin)
Oral antibiotic used for persistent disease
Removal of contaminated prosthesis if possible

Mobiluncus

Members of the genus *Mobiluncus* are obligately anaerobic, gram-variable or gram-negative, curved, non–spore-forming bacilli with tapered ends. Despite their Gram-stain appearance, they are classified as gram-positive bacilli because they have a gram-positive cell wall, lack endotoxin, and are susceptible to vancomycin, clindamycin, erythromycin, and ampicillin but are resistant to colistin. The organisms are fastidious, growing slowly even on enriched media supplemented with rabbit or horse serum.

Two species, *Mobiluncus curtisii* and *Mobiluncus mulieris*, have been described in humans. The organisms colonize the genital tract in low numbers but are abundant in women with bacterial vaginosis (vaginitis). Their microscopic appearance is a useful marker for this disease. The precise role of these organisms in bacterial vaginosis is unclear.

Other Anaerobic Non–Spore-Forming, Gram-Positive Bacilli

Bifidobacterium and *Eubacterium* are commonly found in the large intestine, *Lactobacillus* in the urethra and female genital tract, and *Rothia* in the oropharynx. This group of bacteria can be isolated in clinical specimens but has a very low virulence potential and usually represents clinically insignificant contaminants. To demonstrate their etiological role in an infection, they should be isolated repeatedly in large numbers and in the absence of other pathogenic organisms. This is particularly true for lactobacilli, which are commonly isolated in large numbers in urine specimens contaminated with urethral bacteria.

CASE STUDY AND QUESTIONS

A 42-year-old man entered the University hospital for treatment of a chronically draining wound in the jaw. The patient had multiple tooth extractions 3 months before admission and had poor oral hygiene and fetid breath at the time of admission. Multiple pustular nodules were observed overlying the carious teeth and some nodules have ruptured. Drainage consisted of serosanguous fluid with small, hard granules present.

1. The diagnosis of actinomycosis is considered. How would you collect and transport specimens for confirmation of this diagnosis? What diagnosis tests can be performed?
2. Describe the epidemiology of actinomycosis. What is the risk factor for this patient?
3. What diseases are caused by *Propionibacterium*? What is the source of this organism?

Bibliography

Bourgault AM, Rosenblatt JE, and Fitzgerald RH: *Peptococcus magnus:* significant human pathogen, *Ann Intern Med* 93:244-248, 1980.

Brook I and Frazier EH: Infections caused by *Propionibacterium* species, *Rev Infect Dis* 13:819-822, 1991.

Ezaki T, Yamamoto N, Ninomiya K et al: Transfer of *Peptococcus indolicus, Peptococcus asaccharolyticus, Peptococcus prevotii,* and *Peptococcus magnus* to the genus *Peptostreptococcus* and proposal of *Peptostreptococcus tetradius* sp. nov., *Int J Syst Bacteriol* 33:683-698, 1983.

Finegold SM, Baron EJ, and Wexler HM: *A clinical guide to anaerobic infections*, Belmont, Calif., 1992, Star Publishing.

Hofstad T: Current taxonomy of medically important nonsporing anaerobes, *Rev Infect Dis* 12(suppl):122-126, 1990.

Pochi PE: The pathogenesis and treatment of acne, *Ann Rev Med* 41:187-198, 1990.

Smego RA: Actinomycosis of the central nervous system, *Rev Infect Dis*, 9:855-865, 1987.

Spiegel CA: Bacterial vaginosis, *Clin Microbiol Rev*, 4:485-502, 1991.

Topiel MS and Simon GL: *Peptococcaceae bacteremia*, *Diagn Microbiol Infect Dis* 4:109-119, 1986.

CHAPTER 32

Anaerobic Gram-Positive, Spore-Forming Bacilli

ALL medically important, anaerobic, gram-positive, spore-forming bacilli are classified in the genus *Clostridium* (Table 32-1). Unfortunately, the identification of many of these organisms poses a problem. The genus consists of more than 100 species that have diverse biochemical properties and limited genetic relatedness. Although most members of the genus are strict anaerobes, some are aerotolerant (e.g., *C. tertium, C. histolyticum*) and can grow on agar media exposed to air. Some clostridia can appear gram-negative (e.g., *C. ramosum, C. clostridiiforme*), and spores may not be observed in some species *(C. perfringens, C. ramosum)*. Thus classification of an isolate into the genus *Clostridium* must be accomplished by a combination of diagnostic tests, including demonstration of spores, optimal growth anaerobically, a complex pattern of biochemical reactivity, and analysis of metabolic by-products by gas chromatography. Fortunately, the majority of isolates fall within a limited number of species.

The organisms are ubiquitous, present in soil, water, sewage, and as part of the normal microbial flora in the gastrointestinal tract of animals and humans. Most clostridia are harmless saprophytes, although some are well-recognized human pathogens with a clearly documented history of causing diseases such as tetanus *(C. tetani)*, botulism *(C. botulinum)*, and gas gangrene (*C. perfringens, C. novyi, C. septicum,* and others). Despite the notoriety of these diseases, we now know that clostridia are more commonly associated with skin and soft tissue infections, food poisoning, and antibiotic-associated diarrhea and colitis. Their remarkable capacity for causing diseases is attributed to their ability to survive adverse environmental conditions by spore formation, rapid rate of growth in a nutritionally enriched, oxygen-deprived environment, and production of numerous histolytic toxins, enterotoxins, and neurotoxins. The most important human pathogens will be discussed in this chapter.

TABLE 32-1 Common *Clostridium* Species Associated With Human Disease

Organism	Disease
C. perfringens	Bacteremia; myonecrosis (gas gangrene); soft tissue infections (e.g., cellulitis, fasciitis); food poisoning; enteritis necroticans
C. tetani	Tetanus
C. botulinum	Food-borne botulism, infant botulism, wound botulism
C. difficile	Antibiotic-associated diarrhea, pseudomembranous colitis
Other *Clostridium* species (e.g., *C. septicum, C. ramosum, C. novyi, C. bifermentans*)	Bacteremia, myonecrosis, soft tissue infections

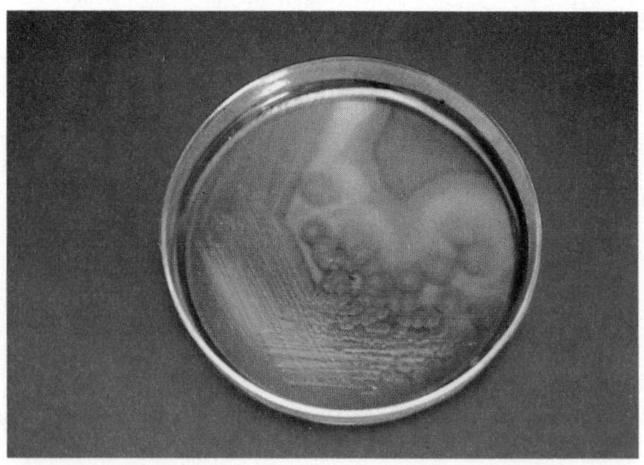

FIGURE 32-1 *C. perfringens* on sheep blood agar plates. Note the flat, rapidly spreading colonies and the hemolytic activity of the organisms. A preliminary identification of *C. perfringens* can be made by recognition of the zone of complete hemolysis (caused by the theta toxin) and a wider zone of partial hemolysis (caused by the alpha toxin), combined with their characteristic microscopic morphology (uniformly rectangular bacilli with no obvious spores).

CLOSTRIDIUM PERFRINGENS

Physiology and Structure

Clostridium perfringens, the clostridial species most frequently isolated in clinical specimens, either can be associated with simple colonization or can cause severe, life-threatening disease. *C. perfringens* is a large, rectangular, gram-positive bacillus, with spores rarely observed in vivo or following in vitro cultivation. The organism is one of the few nonmotile clostridia, but rapidly spreading growth on laboratory media (resembling growth of motile organisms) is characteristic (Figure 32-1). The organism grows rapidly both in tissues and in culture, is hemolytic, and is metabolically active, which facilitates the rapid identification of these organisms in the laboratory. Production of four major lethal toxins for *C. perfringens* (alpha, beta, epsilon, and iota toxins) is used to subdivide isolates into five types (A through E). Type A *C. perfringens*, the toxin type responsible for most human infections, is further subdivided into many epidemiological serotypes.

Pathogenesis

Clostridium perfringens can cause a spectrum of diseases, from self-limited gastroenteritis to overwhelming destruction of tissue (e.g., clostridial myonecrosis) with very high mortality despite early appropriate medical intervention. This pathogenic potential is attributed to the numerous toxins and enzymes produced by this organism (Table 32-2). **Alpha toxin,** the most important toxin that is produced by all *C. perfringens*, is a lecithinase (phospholipase C) that lyses erythrocytes, platelets, leukocytes, and endothelial cells (Figure 32-2). Increased vascular permeability with massive hemolysis and bleeding, tissue destruction (as found in myonecrosis), hepatic toxicity, and myocardial dysfunction (bradycardia, hypotension) are associated with this toxin. The largest quantities of alpha toxin are produced by *C. perfringens* type A. Beta toxin is responsible for the necrotic lesions in **necrotizing enterocolitis** (enteritis necroticans, pig-bel). Epsilon toxin is a prototoxin, activated by proteolytic enzymes, that increases vascular permeability of the gastrointestinal wall. Iota toxin, the fourth major lethal toxin of *C. perfringens*, has necrotic activity and increases vascular permeability.

Enterotoxin is a heat-labile protein produced in the colon and released during spore formation. Trypsin treatment enhances toxin activity threefold. The toxin is produced primarily by type A strains but also by a few type C and D strains. It disrupts ion transport in the ileum (primarily) and jejunum by inserting into the cell membrane and altering membrane permeability. A large number of vegetative cells must be ingested with the contaminated food to produce the enterotoxic effects. Antibodies to enterotoxin, indicating previous exposure, are commonly found in adults, although these are not protective.

The activities of the minor toxins of *C. perfringens* are summarized in Table 32-2.

TABLE 32-2 Virulence Factors Associated With *Clostridium perfringens*

Virulence factors	Biological activity
MAJOR TOXINS	
Alpha toxin	Phospholipase C; increase vascular permeability; hemolytic
Beta toxin	Necrotizing; induces hypertension by release of catecholamines
Epsilon toxin	Increases permeability of gastrointestinal wall
Iota toxin	Binary toxin responsible for necrotizing activity and increased vascular permeability
Enterotoxin	Alteration of membrane permeability (cytotoxic, enterotoxic)
MINOR TOXINS	
Delta toxin	Hemolytic
Theta toxin	Hemolytic cytolysin (also called perfringolysin O)
Kappa toxin	Collagenase, gelatinase
Lambda toxin	Protease
Mu	Hyaluronidase
Nu	DNase
Neuraminidase	Alters cell surface ganglioside receptors; promotes capillary thrombosis

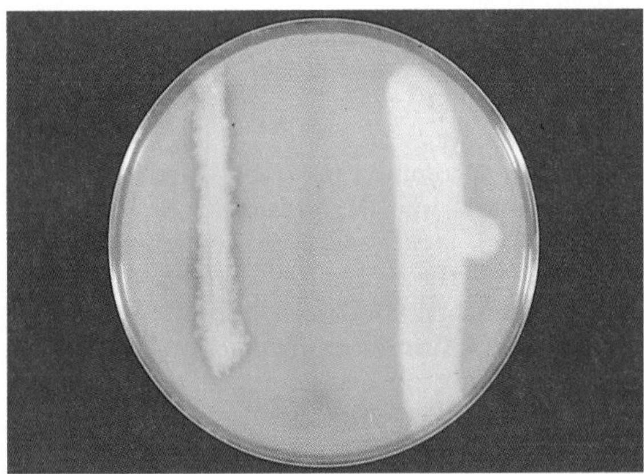

FIGURE 32-2 Growth of *C. perfringens* on egg yolk agar. The alpha toxin (lecithinase) produced by *C. perfringens* hydrolyzes phospholipids in serum and egg yolk, producing an increased turbidity (*right*). This precipitate is not observed when the organism is grown in the presence of antitoxin (*left*). This reaction (**Nagler reaction,** named after the microbiologist who first described it) can be used for the presumptive identification of *C. perfringens.* (From Howard BJ et al: *Clinical and pathogenic microbiology*, St. Louis, 1987, Mosby.)

BOX 32-1 Epidemiology of *Clostridium perfringens* Infection

DISEASE/BACTERIAL FACTORS

Bacteremia; myonecrosis; cellulitis, fasciitis, and other soft tissue infections; food poisoning; enteritis necroticans
Present in soil, water, sewage
Part of normal microbial flora of GI tract
Spore formation allows *C. perfringens* to survive harsh environment
Rapid growth in vivo
Production of numerous toxins including alpha, beta, epsilon, iota, and enterotoxin (see Table 32-2)

TRANSMISSION

Endogenous spread from GI tract into normally sterile areas
Inoculation through break in skin (trauma, surgery)
Ingestion of contaminated foods

WHO IS AT RISK?

Surgical/trauma patients
Persons ingesting contaminated meat products

GEOGRAPHY/SEASON

Ubiquitous and worldwide
No seasonal incidence

MODES OF CONTROL

Rapid treatment is essential
Systemic infection: surgical debridement and high-dose penicillin
Local infection: penicillin
Gastroenteritis: symptomatic treatment only
Proper wound care and prophylactic antibiotics

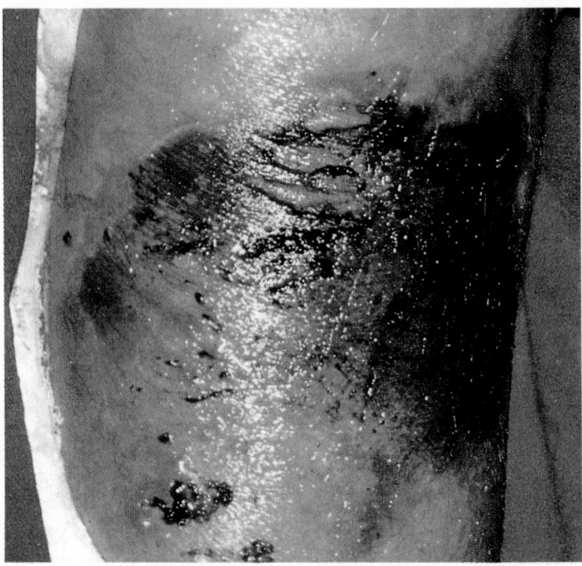

FIGURE 32-3 Clostridial cellulitis. Clostridia can be introduced into tissue following surgery or a traumatic injury. This patient suffered a compound fracture of the tibia. Five days after the injury, skin discoloration with bullae and necrosis and the presence of serosanguineous exudate revealed subcutaneous gas but no evidence of muscle necrosis. The patient made an uneventful recovery. (From Lambert HP and Farrar WE, editors: *Infectious diseases illustrated*, London, 1982, Gower Medical Publishing.)

Epidemiology

C. perfringens is a common inhabitant of the intestinal tract of humans and animals and is widely distributed in nature, particularly in soil and water contaminated with feces (Box 32-1). These organisms form spores under adverse environmental conditions and can survive for prolonged periods. Most environmental isolates are type A. Types B-E strains do not survive in soil but rather colonize the intestinal tract of animals and occasionally humans. Gas gangrene and food poisoning are primarily caused by *C. perfringens* type A, whereas enteritis necroticans is caused by type C.

Clinical Syndromes

Bacteremia

The isolation of *C. perfringens* or other clostridial species in blood cultures can be alarming. However, more than half of the isolates are clinically insignificant, representing transient bacteremia or, more likely, contamination of the culture with clostridia colonizing the skin surface. The significance of an isolate must be viewed in the light of other clinical findings.

Myonecrosis (Gas Gangrene)

This life-threatening disease illustrates the full virulence potential of histotoxic clostridia. The onset of disease, characterized by intense pain, generally begins within 1 week after clostridia are introduced into tissue by trauma or surgery. The progression from the time of onset through extensive muscle necrosis, shock, renal failure, and death is rapid, frequently occurring in less than 2 days. Macroscopic examination of muscle reveals devitalized necrotic tissue, with the presence of gas caused by the metabolic activity of the rapidly dividing bacteria (hence the name gas gangrene). Microscopically, abundant rectangular, gram-positive bacilli are seen in the absence of cellular material. Extensive hemolysis and bleeding caused by clostridial toxins are characteristic. Clostridial myonecrosis is most commonly caused by *C. perfringens,* although other species can also produce this disease (e.g., *C. septicum, C. histolyticum, C. bifermentans,* and *C. novyi*).

Cellulitis, Fasciitis, and Other Soft Tissue Infections

Clostridial species can colonize wounds and the skin surface with no clinical consequences. Indeed, most isolates of *C. perfringens* and other clostridial species from wound cultures are insignificant. However, these organisms can also initiate cellulitis (Figure 32-3) or a rapidly progressive, destructive process whereby the organisms spread through fascial planes (fasciitis), causing suppuration and gas formation. Fasciitis is distinguished from myonecrosis by the absence of muscle involvement, but it shares a dismal outcome. Surgical intervention is generally unsuccessful because of the rapidity with which the organisms spread. Most infections are caused by *C. perfringens, C. septicum,* or *C. ramosum.*

Food Poisoning

Clostridial food poisoning is characterized by a short incubation period (8 to 24 hours); clinical presentation of abdominal cramps and watery diarrhea in the absence of fever, nausea, or vomiting; and a clinical course of less than 24 hours. Disease is due to ingestion of meat products contaminated with large numbers (10^{8-9} organisms) of enterotoxin-producing type A *C. perfringens.* Clostridia are the third most common cause of food poisoning in the United States (behind *Salmonella* and *S. aureus*).

Enteritis Necroticans

This rare disease is an acute necrotizing process in the small intestine that is characterized by abdominal pain, bloody diarrhea, shock, and peritonitis. The incidence of death approaches 50%. Beta toxin–producing *C. perfringens* type C is responsible for this disease.

Laboratory Diagnosis

The laboratory performs a confirmatory role in the diagnosis of clostridial disease because therapy must be initiated immediately. The microscopic detection of gram-positive bacilli in clinical specimens, usually in the absence of leukocytes, can be very useful because these organisms have a characteristic morphology. Culture of the anaerobes is also relatively simple, with detection of *C. perfringens* accomplished on simple media after incubation for 1 day or less. Under appropriate conditions *C. perfringens* can divide every 8 minutes, so growth on agar media or in blood culture broths can be detected after incubation for only a few hours. The role of *C. perfringens* in food poisoning is documented by recovery of greater than 10^5 organisms per gram of food or 10^6 bacteria per gram of feces collected within 1 day of the onset of disease.

Treatment, Prevention, and Control

Treatment of systemic *C. perfringens* infections such as fasciitis and myonecrosis requires aggressive surgical debridement and high-dose penicillin therapy. The use of antiserum directed against alpha toxin (antitoxin) and treatment in a hyperbaric oxygen chamber (presumably to inhibit growth of the anaerobe) have poorly defined benefits. Despite all therapeutic efforts, the prognosis with these diseases is poor, with mortality reported from 40% to almost 100%. Less serious, localized clostridial diseases can be successfully treated with penicillin, with resistance only rarely reported for species other than *C. perfringens.* Antibiotic therapy for clostridial food poisoning is unnecessary.

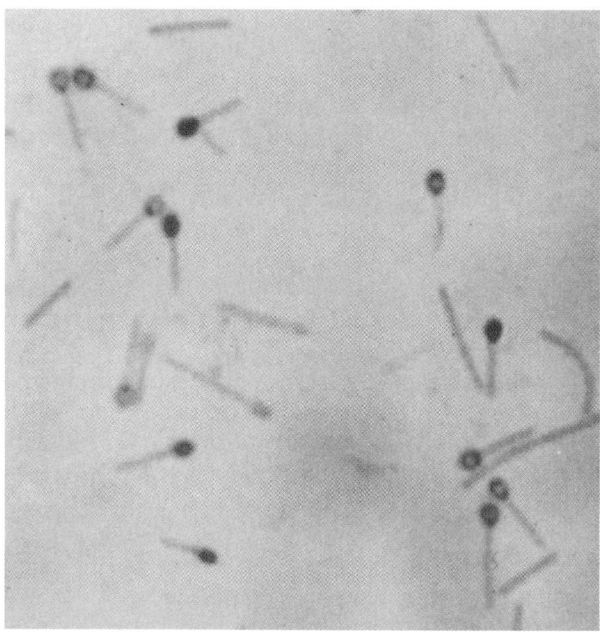

FIGURE 32-4 *Clostridium tetani.* Note the "drumstick" or "tennis racket" shape because of the terminal spore.

Prevention and control of *C. perfringens* infections is difficult because of the ubiquitous distribution of the organisms. Disease requires introduction of the organism into devitalized tissues and maintenance of an anaerobic environment favorable for bacterial growth. Thus most infections can be prevented by proper wound care and judicious use of prophylactic antibiotics.

CLOSTRIDIUM TETANI

Physiology and Structure

Clostridium tetani is a small, motile, spore-forming bacillus that frequently stains gram-negative. Round, terminal spores are produced that give the organisms a drumstick appearance (Figure 32-4). In contrast with *C. perfringens, C. tetani* is difficult to grow in vitro (because it is sensitive to oxygen toxicity) and is relatively inactive metabolically.

Pathogenesis

Tetanus is caused by a potent, heat-labile, neurotoxin (tetanospasmin) that is produced during the stationary phase of growth and released when cell lysis occurs (Table 32-3). Tetanospasmin (an A-B toxin) is synthesized as a single 150,000 d peptide that is cleaved into a light (A equivalent) and a heavy (B equivalent) chain by an endogenous protease when the neurotoxin is released from the cell. The two chains are held together by a disulfide bond and noncovalent forces. The carboxy-terminal portion of the heavy (100,000 d) chain binds to gangliosides (GT_1) on neuronal membranes. The light chain of the toxin is then internalized and moves from the peripheral nerve terminals to the central nervous system by retrograde axonal transport. It is released from the postsynaptic dendrites, crosses the synaptic cleft, and is localized within vesicles in the presynaptic nerve terminals (Figure 32-5). Tetanospasmin acts by blocking the release of neurotransmitters (e.g., gamma-aminobutyric acid [GABA], glycine) for inhibitory synapses, thus permitting unregulated excitatory synaptic activity (spastic paralysis).

C. tetani also produces an oxygen-labile hemolysin (**tetanolysin**) that is serologically related to some other clostridial hemolysins and streptolysin O. The clinical significance of this enzyme is unknown because it is inhibited by oxygen and serum cholesterol.

Epidemiology

Clostridium tetani is ubiquitous, found in fertile soil and colonizes the gastrointestinal tract of many animals, including humans (Box 32-2 and Figure 32-6). The vegetative forms of *C. tetani* are extremely susceptible to oxygen toxicity, but the organisms sporulate readily and can survive in nature for prolonged periods. Disease is relatively rare in the United States because of the high incidence of immunity following vaccination. However, tetanus is still responsible for significant mortality in underdeveloped areas where vaccination is unavailable or medical practices are lax. Tetanus in neonates and the unprotected elderly is associated with a high mortality rate. Fewer than 100 cases of tetanus are reported annually in the United States (Figure 32-7), with disease primarily restricted to the elderly (Figure 32-8). Virtually all patients with tetanus are inadequately immunized. Drug abusers who inject drugs subcutaneously ("skin poppers") are susceptible to tetanus.

TABLE 32-3 Virulence Factors Associated With *Clostridium tetani*

Virulence factors	Biological activity
Tetanospasmin	Neurotoxin blocks release of neurotransmitters for inhibitory synapses
Tetanolysin	Oxygen-labile hemolysin (unknown significance)
Spore formation	Able to persist in the environment for months to years

Clinical Syndromes

See Table 32-4 for a summary of clinical symptoms of tetanus. The incubation period for tetanus is variable, ranging from a few days to weeks. The length of the incubation period is directly related to the distance of the primary wound infection from the central nervous system.

Generalized tetanus is the most common form seen. Involvement of the masseter muscles (**trismus** or **lockjaw**) is the presenting sign in the majority of patients. The sardonic smile characteristic of sustained trismus is known as **"risus sardonicus"** (Figure 32-9). Other early signs include drooling, sweating, irritability, and persistent back spasms (**opisthotonos**; Figure 32-10). More severe disease is seen with involvement of the autonomic nervous system, with cardiac arrhythmias, fluctuations in blood pressure, profound sweating, and dehydration.

Another form of *C. tetani* disease is **localized tetanus** in which the disease remains confined to the musculature at the site of primary infection. A variant of localized tetanus is **cephalic tetanus** in which the primary site of infection is the head. In contrast with localized tetanus,

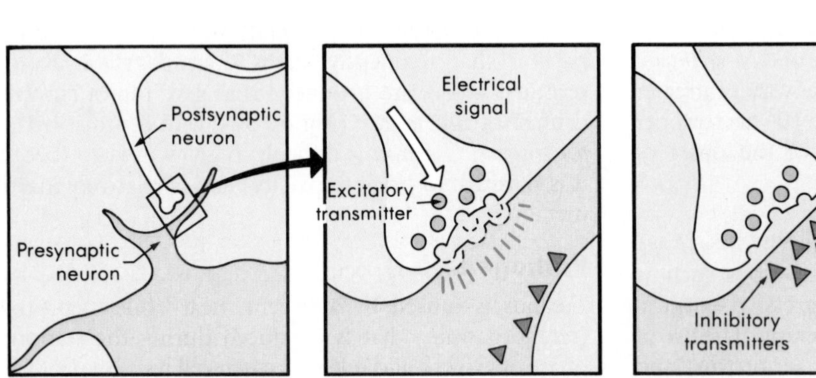

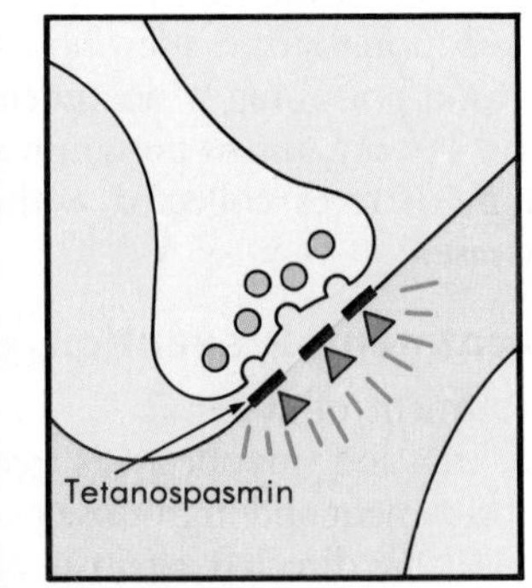

FIGURE 32-5 Mechanism of tetanospasmin activity. **A,** Neurotransmission is controlled by the balance between excitatory and inhibitory neurotransmitters. **B,** The inhibitory neurotransmitters (e.g., GABA, glycine) prevent depolarization of the postsynaptic membrane and conduction of the electrical signal. **C,** Tetanospasmin does not interfere with production or storage of GABA or glycine but rather their release (presynaptic activity). **D,** In the blockage of inhibitory neurotransmitters, excitation of the neuroaxon is unrestrained.

the prognosis for patients with cephalic tetanus is very poor.

Laboratory Diagnosis

The diagnosis of tetanus, like most other clostridial diseases, is made on the basis of clinical presentation. Microscopic detection or isolation of *C. tetani* is useful but frequently unsuccessful. Only about 30% of patients with tetanus have positive cultures because disease can be caused by relatively few organisms and the slow-growing bacteria are rapidly killed when exposed to air. Toxin production by an isolate is confirmed by tetanus antitoxin neutralization tests in mice (a procedure performed only in public health reference labs).

Treatment, Prevention, and Control

Mortality associated with tetanus has steadily decreased during the last century, caused in large part by the decreased incidence of tetanus in the United States. The highest incidence of mortality is in newborns and in patients who experience an incubation period of less than 1 week before the onset of disease.

Treatment of tetanus requires debridement of the primary wound (which may appear innocuous), administration of penicillin, passive immunization with human tetanus immunoglobulin, and vaccination with tetanus toxoid. Wound care and penicillin therapy eliminate vegetative bacteria that produce toxin, while the antitoxin antibodies bind free tetanospasmin molecules. The toxin bound to nerve endings is protected from antibodies. Thus the toxic effects must be controlled symptomatically until normal regulation of synaptic transmission is restored. Vaccination with a series of three doses of tetanus toxoid and booster doses every 10 years is highly effective in preventing tetanus.

BOX 32-2 Epidemiology of *Clostridium tetani* Infection

DISEASE/BACTERIAL FACTORS

Tetanus
Present in soil, water, sewage
Part of normal microbial flora of GI tract of many animals including humans (occasionally)
Spore formation allows *C. tetani* to exist in environment for prolonged periods
Neurotoxin (tetanospasmin) blocks release of neurotransmitters, permitting unregulated synaptic activity (spasm); binding to nerve endings protects it from antibodies

TRANSMISSION

Inoculation through break in skin

WHO IS AT RISK?

Persons with inadequate vaccine-induced immunity, particularly children and the elderly
Subcutaneous drug abusers

GEOGRAPHY/SEASON

Ubiquitous and worldwide; relatively rare in United States because of immunity after vaccination
Common in underdeveloped areas with poor vaccination compliance or where medical care is lax
No seasonal incidence

MODES OF CONTROL

Debridement of wound, penicillin, passive immunization with human tetanus immunoglobulin, and vaccination with tetanus toxoid
Vaccination with three doses of tetanus toxoid, with boosters every 10 years

CLOSTRIDIUM BOTULINUM

Microbial Physiology and Structure

Clostridium botulinum, the etiological agent of botulism, is a heterogeneous group of fastidious, spore-forming, anaerobic bacilli. The organisms are subdivided into four groups (I-IV) based on the type of toxin produced and their proteolytic activity. Most human disease is caused by types I and II strains. Seven antigenically distinct **botulinum toxins** (A, B, C alpha, D, E, F, and G) have been described, with human disease associated with types A, B, and E. Only one toxin is produced by most individual isolates. Like tetanus toxin, *Clostridium botulinum* toxin is a 150,000 d progenitor protein (A-B toxin) consisting of the neurotoxin subunit (light or A chain) and one or more nontoxic subunits (B or heavy chain). The nontoxic subunit(s) protects the neurotoxin from inactivation by stomach acids.

Pathogenesis

Botulinum is very specific for cholinergic nerves (Table 32-5). The toxin blocks neurotransmission at peripheral cholinergic synapses by preventing release of the neurotransmitter acetylcholine (Figure 32-11). Recovery of function requires regeneration of the nerve endings. *C. botulinum* also produces a binary toxin consisting of two components that combine to disrupt vascular permeability.

Epidemiology

Three forms of botulism have been identified: classical or food-borne, infant, and wound botulism (Box 32-3). Although *C. botulinum* is distributed worldwide, with spores commonly isolated in soil and water samples (Figure 32-12), disease is relatively uncommon in the United States (Figure 32-13). Fewer than 50 cases of food-borne botulism are seen annually, with most associated with home-canned foods and occasionally preserved fish (type E toxin). The food may or may not appear spoiled, but even a small taste can cause full-blown clinical disease. Botulism in infants is more common and

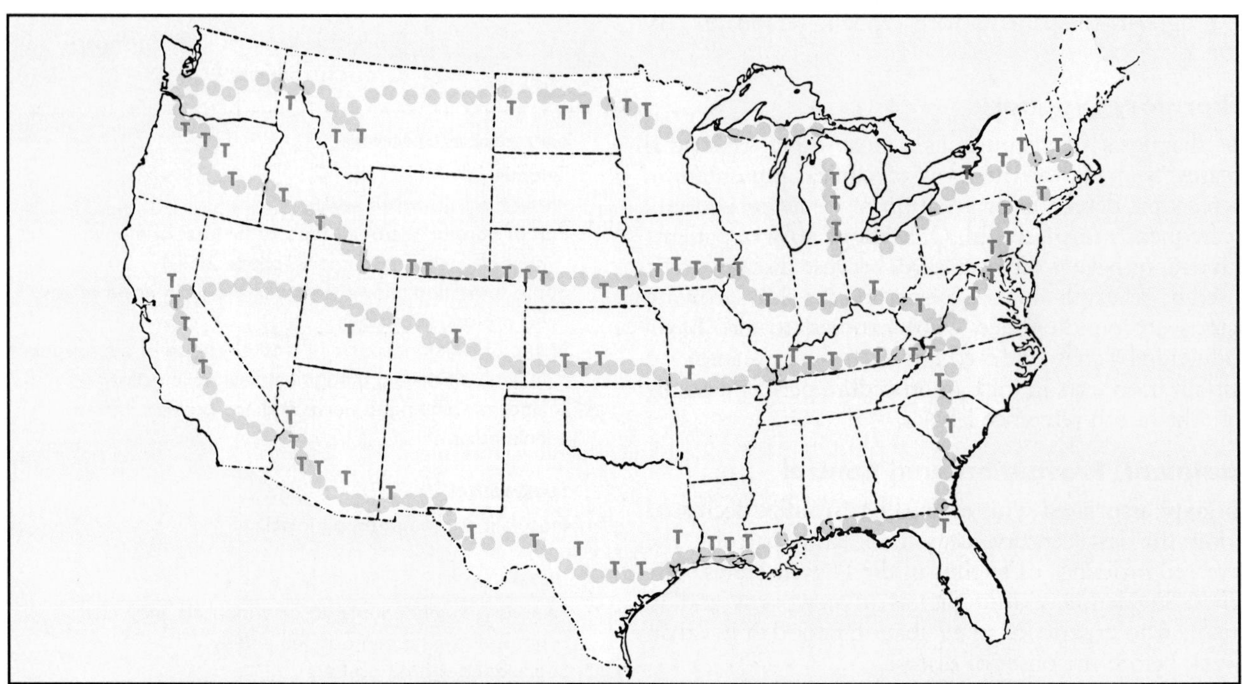

FIGURE 32-6 Distribution of *Clostridium tetani* in the soil of the United States. Soil samples were collected every 50 miles on four east-west transects across the United States. *C. tetani (T)* was present in 30% of the soil samples. (Modified from Smith LDS: *Health Lab Science* 15:74-80, 1978.)

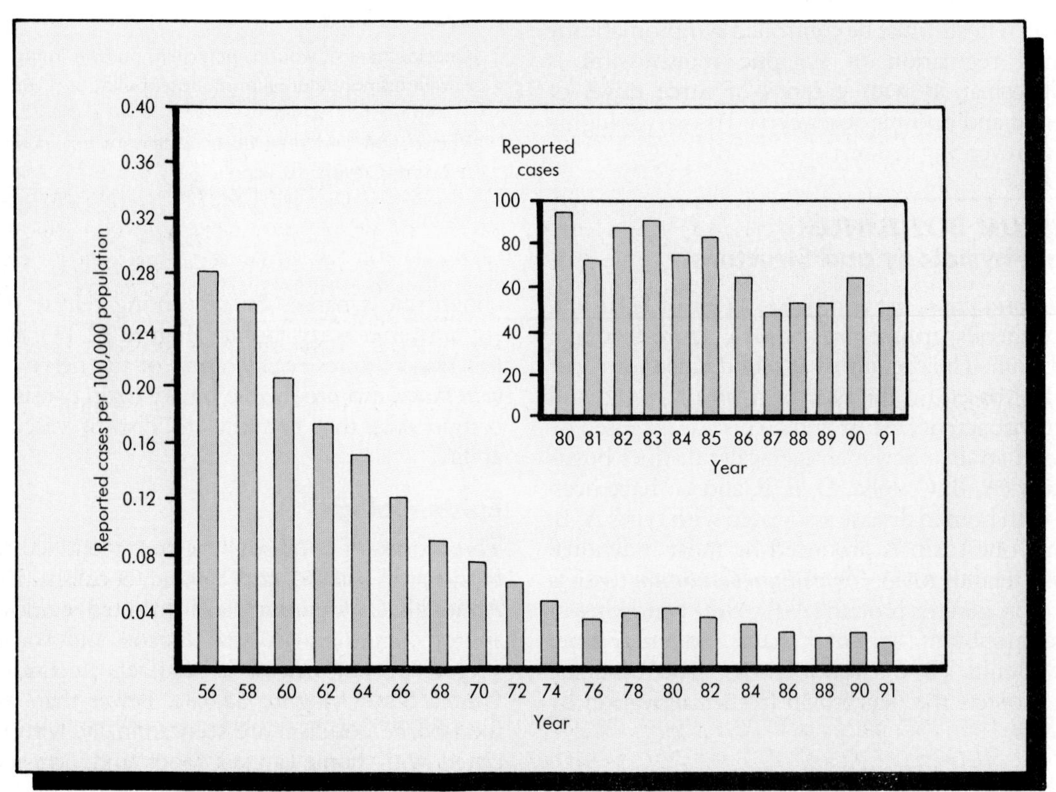

FIGURE 32-7 Incidence of tetanus in the United States from 1956 to 1991. (From *MMWR* 40:46, 1992.)

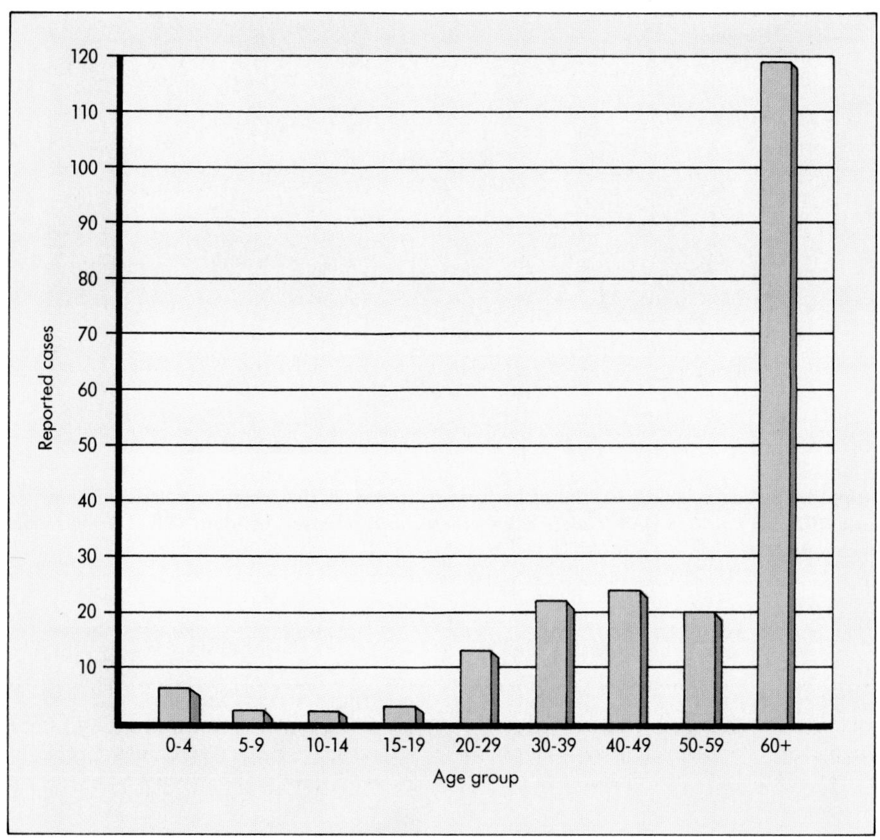

FIGURE 32-8 Age of patients with tetanus reported in the United States during a 4-year period from 1987 to 1990. (From *MMWR* 40:46, 1992.)

TABLE 32-4 Clinical Manifestations of Tetanus

Disease	Clinical manifestations
Generalized	Involvement of bulbar and paraspinal muscles (trismus or lockjaw, risus sardonicus, difficulty in swallowing, irritability, opisthotonos); involvement in the autonomic nervous system (sweating, hyperthermia, cardiac arrhythmias, fluctuations in blood pressure); disease in newborns called tetanus neonatorum; prognosis related to patient age, immune status, and site of primary infection
Cephalic	Primary infection in head, particularly ear; isolated or combined involvement of cranial nerves, particularly seventh cranial nerve; very poor prognosis
Localized	Involves muscles in area of primary injury; may precede generalized disease; favorable prognosis

has been associated with the consumption of honey contaminated with botulinal spores.

Clinical Syndromes

Food-Borne Botulism

After consumption of contaminated food and a 1- to 2-day incubation period, the patient develops weakness and dizziness. The initial signs of botulism include blurred vision with fixed dilated pupils, dry mouth (indicative of the anticholinergic effects of the toxin), constipation, and abdominal pain. Bilateral, descending weakness of the peripheral muscles develops in progressive disease **(flaccid paralysis),** with death most commonly attributed to respiratory paralysis. A clear sensorium is maintained throughout the course of disease. Despite aggressive management of the patient, the disease may continue to progress because of the neurotoxin's irreversible binding and long-term inhibitory activity on the release of excitatory neurotransmitters. Complete recovery in patients who survive this initial period frequently requires many months to years until the affected nerve endings regrow. Mortality, which once

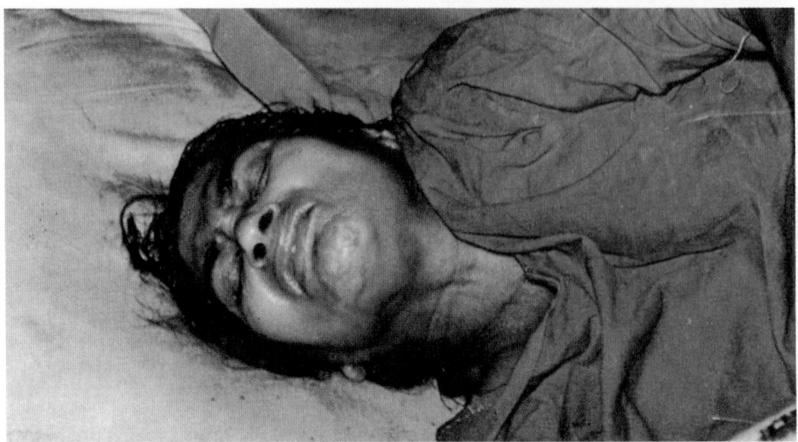

FIGURE 32-9 Risus sardonicus in tetanus because of spasms in the masseter muscles. (From Emond RTD and Rowland HAK: *Colour atlas of infectious diseases*, London, 1987, Wolfe Medical Publications).

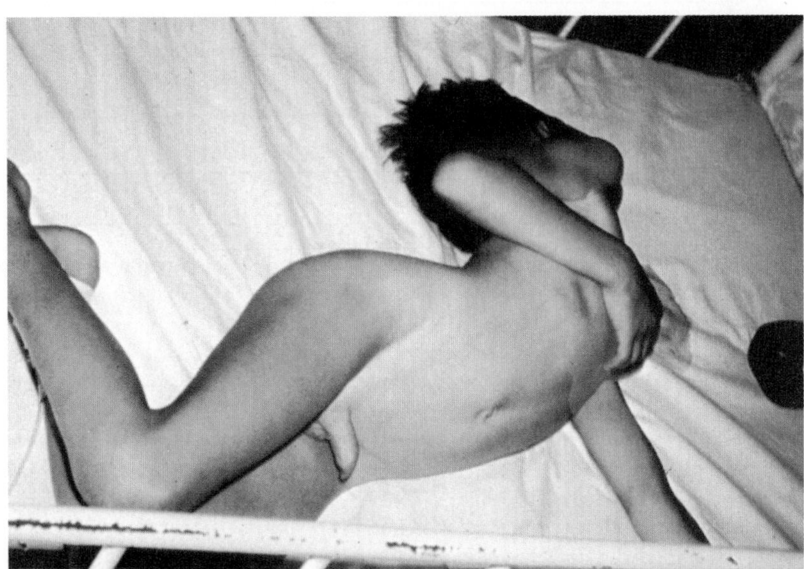

FIGURE 32-10 A child with tetanus and opisthotonus resulting from persistent spasms in the back muscles. (From Emond RTD and Rowland HAK: *Colour atlas of infectious diseases*, London, 1987, Wolfe Medical Publications.)

TABLE 32-5 Virulence Factors Associated With *Clostridium botulinum*

Virulence Factors	Biological activity
Neurotoxin (types A-G)	Blocks release of excitatory neurotransmitters for cholinergic nerves (acetylcholine)
Binary (C_2) toxin	Disrupts vascular permeability
Component I	ADP-ribosylating activity
Component II	Binds to cell surface
Spore formation	Able to persist in soil or vegetation for months to years and survive in contaminated food

approached 70%, has been reduced to 10% with the use of better supportive care, particularly in the management of respiratory complications.

Infant Botulism

Although this disease was first recognized in 1976, it is now the most common form of botulism seen in the United States (see Figure 32-13). In contrast with food-borne botulism, this disease is caused by the in vivo production of neurotoxin by *C. botulinum* colonizing the gastrointestinal tract of young infants. Disease is reported in infants younger than 1 year of age (most between 1 to 6 months) with the initial symptoms nonspecific (e.g., constipation or "failure to thrive"). Progressive disease with flaccid paralysis and respiratory arrest can develop, although the mortality rate in documented infant botu-

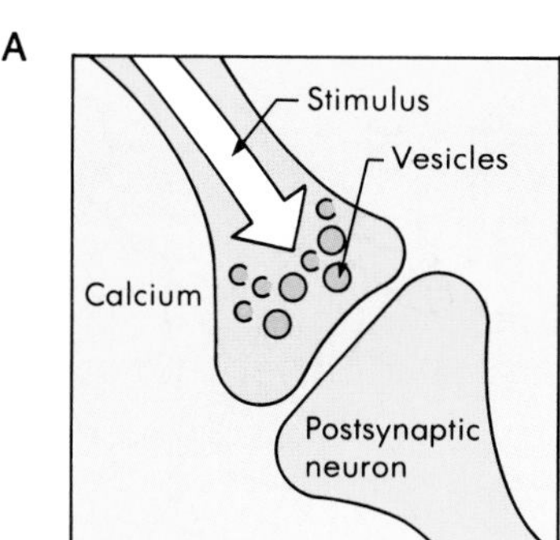

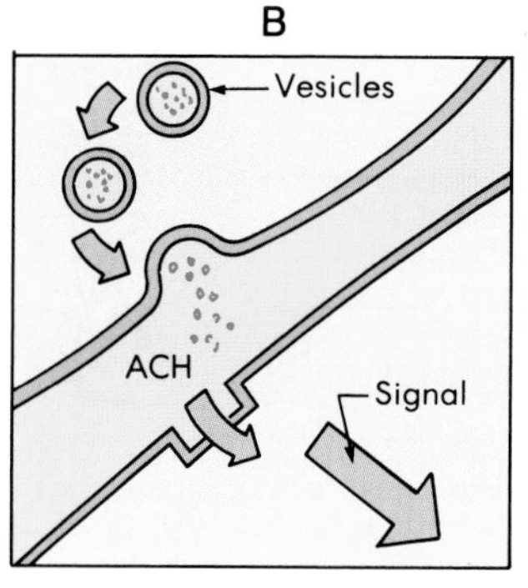

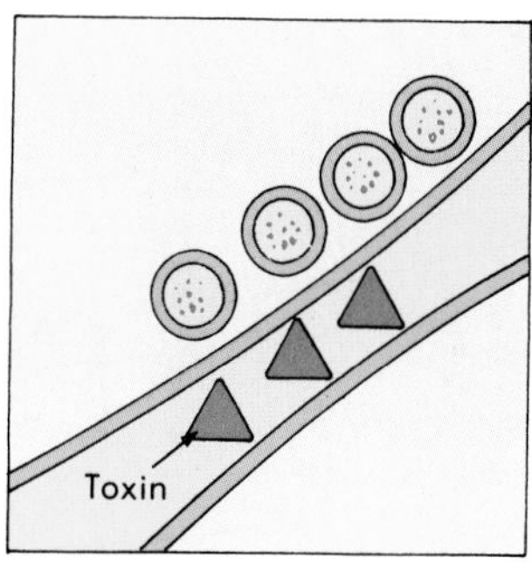

FIGURE 32-11 Mechanism of botulinum toxin activity. Synaptic activity at cholinergic synapses is mediated by the neurotransmitter acetylcholine (ACH). **A,** As a nerve stimulus enters the presynaptic nerve ending, an influx of calcium is stimulated. **B,** Calcium is required for the fusion of synaptic vesicles with the presynaptic membrane and release of ACH into the synaptic space. ACH crosses to the postsynaptic membrane and acts on specific receptors. ACH is rapidly hydrolzyed by acetylcholinesterase. The combined activity of many ACH-mediated stimuli produces an electrical potential change and transmission of the signal. **C,** Botulinum toxin interrupts this transmission by interfering with the release of ACH from the synaptic vesicles. The synthesis of ACH and its packaging in synaptic vesicles is not affected. The toxin binds to specific receptors (unique for each distinct neurotoxin type) on the nerve ending, and the active toxin (light or A chain) subunit is internalized where it interferes with ACH release.

BOX 32-3 Epidemiology of Botulism

DISEASE/BACTERIAL FACTORS

Botulism: food-borne, infant, wound
C. botulinum is present in soil, water, sewage
Spore formation allows *C. botulinum* to exist in environment for prolonged periods
Neurotoxin blocks peripheral cholinergic synapses by preventing release of acetylcholine
Nontoxic subunits protect neurotoxin from inactivation by stomach acids
Binary toxin disrupts vascular permeability

TRANSMISSION

Ingestion of toxin in contaminated food products (intoxication)
Inoculation of *C. botulinum* through skin with subsequent localized production of neurotoxin
In infants: ingestion of *C. botulinum* with subsequent production of neurotoxin in GI tract

WHO IS AT RISK?

Persons eating contaminated foods (particularly home-canned products)
Infants (particularly those eating honey)

GEOGRAPHY/SEASON

Ubiquitous and worldwide; disease in United States relatively rare
No seasonal incidence

MODES OF CONTROL

Treatment: penicillin, trivalent botulinum antitoxin, ventilatory support
Spore germination prevented by maintaining food in an acid pH or storing at 4° C or colder
Toxin destroyed by heating food for 20 minutes at 80° C
Infant botulism strongly associated with consumption of contaminated honey; thus honey should be avoided in infants younger than 1 year old

lism is very low (1% to 2%). Some infant deaths attributed to other conditions (e.g., sudden infant death syndrome) may be due to botulism.

Wound Botulism

This is the rarest form of botulism in the United States. As the name implies, wound botulism develops from in vivo toxin production by *C. botulinum* in contaminated wounds. The symptoms of disease are identical to those of food-borne disease; however, the incubation period is generally longer (4 days or more), and gastrointestinal symptoms are less prominent.

Laboratory Diagnosis

The clinical diagnosis of botulism is confirmed by isolating the organism or demonstrating toxin activity. In food-borne disease an attempt should be made to culture *C. botulinum* from the patient's feces and the implicated

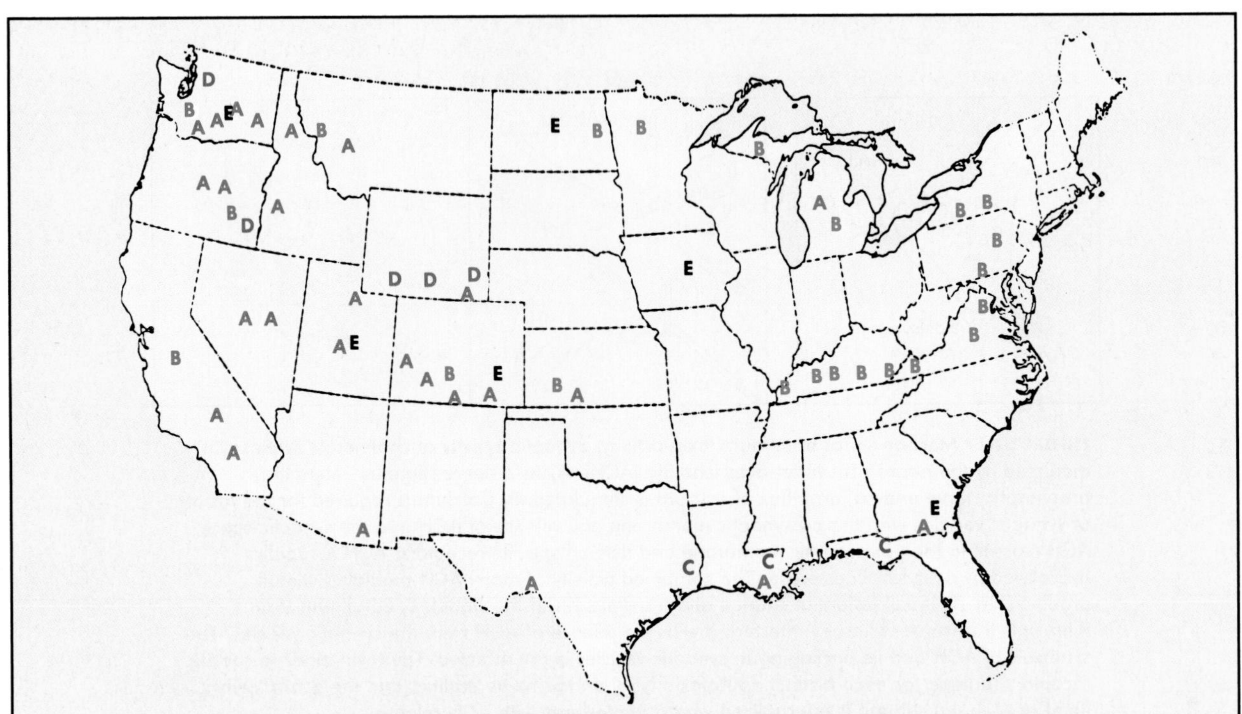

FIGURE 32-12 Distribution of *Clostridium botulinum* in soil samples collected in the United States. **A,** Type A strains were found mainly in neutral or alkaline soil in the western part of the United States. **B,** Type B strains were found primarily in the eastern part of the United States in rich, organic soil. **C,** Types C, D, and E were recovered less frequently, with type E mostly restricted to wet soil. (From Smith LDS: *Health Lab Sciences* 15:74-80, 1978.)

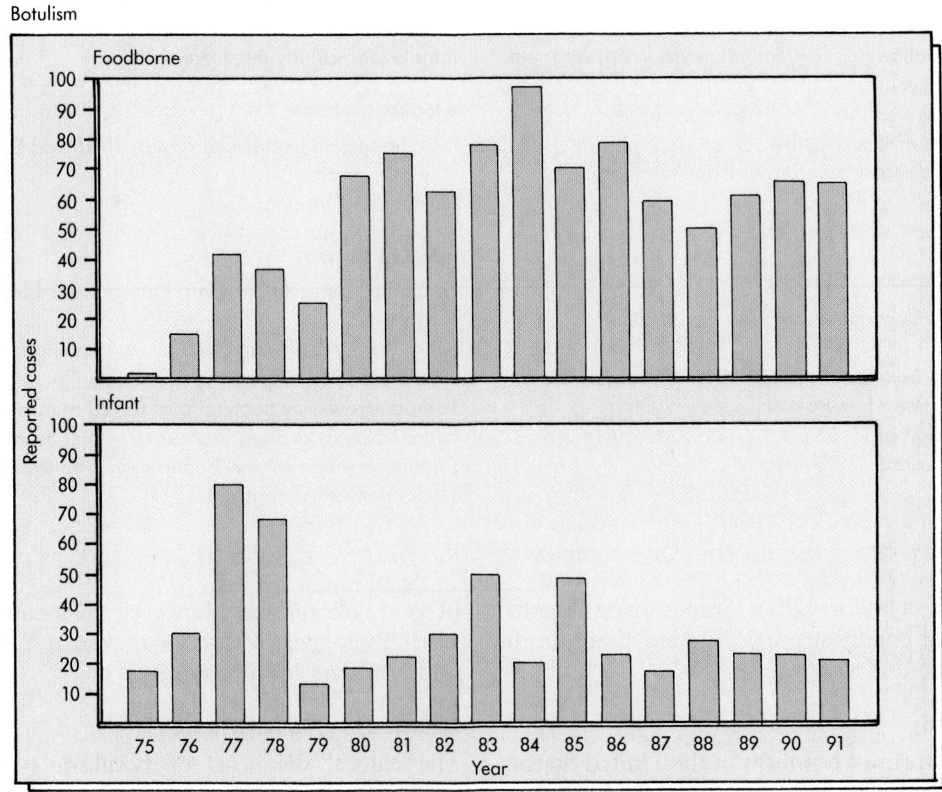

FIGURE 32-13 Incidence of food-borne and infant botulism in the United States from 1975 to 1991. Infant botulism was discovered in 1976. (From *MMWR* 40:21, 1992).

food if it is available (Figure 32-14). Isolation of *C. botulinum* from specimens contaminated with other organisms can be improved by heating the specimen for 10 minutes at 80° C to kill all vegetative cells. Culture of the heated specimen on nutritionally enriched anaerobic media permits the germination of the heat-resistant *C. botulinum* spores. *C. botulinum* produces lipase, which appears as an iridescent film on the colonies when grown on egg yolk agar.

The food, stool specimen, and patient's serum should also be tested for toxin activity by a mouse bioassay. The specimen is divided, and one portion is mixed with antitoxin. Both portions are then inoculated intraperitoneally into mice. If antitoxin treatment protects the mice, then toxin activity is confirmed.

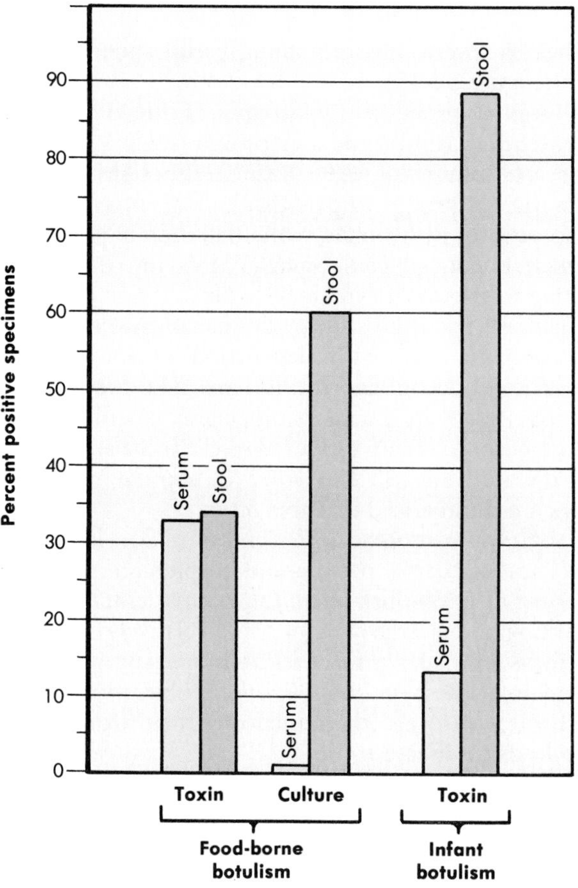

FIGURE 32-14 Detection of *Clostridium botulinum* and botulinal toxin in serum and stool specimens collected from patients with food-borne botulism and infants with botulism. Confirmation of food-borne disease requires testing the implicated food and the patient's serum and stool specimen for botulinal toxin activity, as well as culturing the food and stool specimen for the organism. No single test for food-borne botulism has a sensitivity greater than 60%. Serum and stool specimens from infants with botulism should be tested for toxin activity and the stool specimen cultured. (Data from Dowell VR et al: *JAMA* 238:1829, 1977, and Hatheway CL and McCroskey LM: *J Clin Microbiol* 25:2334, 1987.)

The diagnosis of infant botulism is supported by the isolation of *C. botulinum* from feces or detection of toxin activity in feces or serum. The organism can be isolated from stool cultures in virtually all patients, because carriage of the organism may persist for many months even after a baby has recovered. Wound botulism is confirmed by isolation of the organism in the wound or detection of toxin activity in wound exudate or serum.

Treatment, Prevention, and Control

Treatment of botulism requires adequate ventilatory support, elimination of the organism from the gastrointestinal tract by the judicious use of gastric lavage and penicillin therapy, and the use of trivalent botulinum antitoxin (vs. toxins A, B, and E) to bind toxin circulating in the bloodstream. Ventilatory support has had an unquestioned benefit in significantly reducing mortality.

Prevention of disease involves destruction of the spores in food products (virtually impossible for practical

BOX 32-4 Epidemiology of *Clostridium difficile* Infection

DISEASE/BACTERIAL FACTORS

Asymptomatic colonization, antibiotic-associated diarrhea, pseudomembranous colitis
Present in soil, water, sewage
Part of normal microbial flora of GI tract in some individuals
Enterotoxin induces hemorrhagic necrosis; hypersecretion of fluids
Cytotoxin destroys cellular cytoskeleton
Spore formation allows *C. difficile* to exist in environment for prolonged periods

TRANSMISSION

Endogenous because of overgrowth of normal enteric bacteria
Exogenous exposure via ingestion

WHO IS AT RISK?

Hospitalized patients receiving antibiotics, particularly the elderly
Exposure to antibiotics alters normal enteric flora, permitting overgrowth of *C. difficile*

GEOGRAPHY/SEASON

Ubiquitous and worldwide
No seasonal incidence

MODES OF CONTROL

Mild disease: discontinuation of antibiotic that is altering the GI flora
Serious disease: metronidazole or vancomycin
Relapse is common because of resistance of spores to antibiotics

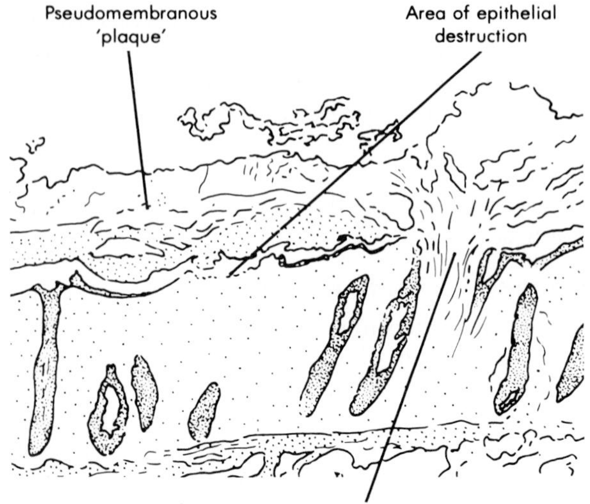

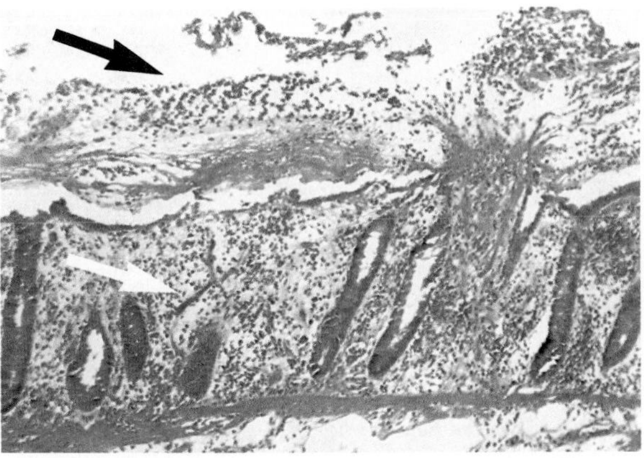

FIGURE 32-15 Antibiotic-associated colitis: histological section of colon showing intense inflammatory response with the characteristic "plaque" (*black arrow*) overlying the intact intestinal mucosa (*white arrow*). Hematoxylin and eosin stain. (Top from Lambert HP and Farrar WE, editors.: *Infectious diseases illustrated*, London, 1982, Gower Medical Publishing.)

reasons), prevention of spore germination (by maintaining the food in an acid pH or storage at 4° C or colder), or destruction of the preformed toxin (by heating the food for 20 minutes at 80° C). Infant botulism is strongly associated by consumption of honey contaminated with *C. botulinum* spores, so children younger than 1 year of age should not eat honey.

CLOSTRIDIUM DIFFICILE

Until the mid-1970s the clinical importance of *Clostridium difficile* was not appreciated. This organism was infrequently isolated in fecal cultures and rarely associated with human disease. However, systematic studies have now clearly demonstrated that toxin-producing *C. difficile* is responsible for antibiotic-associated gastrointestinal diseases ranging from relatively benign, self-limiting diarrhea to severe, life-threatening pseudomembranous colitis (Figure 32-15).

C. difficile produces two toxins (Table 32-6): an **enterotoxin** (toxin A) and a **cytotoxin** (toxin B). These toxins are immunologically distinct, although physical separation has proved to be difficult. The enterotoxin is chemotactic for neutrophils, with infiltration of polymorphonuclear neutrophil leukocytes (PMNs) into the ileum, resulting in release of cytokines, hypersecretion of fluid, and hemorrhagic necrosis. The cytotoxin causes depolymerization of actin with destruction of the cellular cytoskeleton both in vivo and in vitro. The precise role each toxin plays in disease pathogenesis is still unclear because both toxins are produced in clostridia associated with disease (Box 32-4). Other *C. difficile* virulence factors are summarized in Table 32-6.

TABLE 32-6 Virulence Factors Associated With *Clostridium difficile*

Virulence factors	Biological activity
Enterotoxin (toxin A)	Chemotaxis; induces cytokine production with hypersecretion of fluid; hemorrhagic necrosis
Cytotoxin (toxin B)	Induces depolymerization of actin with loss of cellular cytoskeleton
Adhesion factor	Binds specifically in vitro to human colonic cells
Hyaluronidase	Hydrolytic activity
Spore formation	Permits survival in hospital environment for months

C. difficile is part of the normal intestinal flora in a small proportion of healthy persons and hospitalized patients. Exposure to antibiotics alters the normal enteric flora, permitting the overgrowth of these relatively resistant organisms or making the patient more susceptible to exogenous acquisition of *C. difficile*. Proliferation of the organisms with localized production of their toxins in the colon leads to disease.

The specific diagnosis of *C. difficile* infection is accomplished by culture of feces on highly selective media, detection of the cytotoxin by an in vitro cytotoxicity assay with tissue culture cells, or detection of enterotoxin by immunoassays. The most specific test for *C. difficile* disease is the **cytotoxicity assay.** Maximal sensitivity for detecting colonization is accomplished by using a combination of diagnostic tests.

Discontinuation of the implicated antibiotic (e.g., ampicillin, clindamycin) is generally sufficient to alleviate mild disease. However, specific therapy with either metronidazole or vancomycin is required for serious disease. Relapses after completion of therapy may occur in as many as 20% to 30% of patients because spores of *C. difficile* are resistant to antibiotic treatment. Re-

TABLE 32-7 Virulence Factors Associated With Other Clostridial Species

Virulence factors	Biological activity
C. SEPTICUM	
Alpha toxin	Necrotizing, hemolytic
Beta toxin	Heat-stable DNase
Gamma toxin	Hyaluronidase
Delta toxin	Oxygen-labile hemolysin
Neuraminidase	Alters cell membrane glycoproteins
C. SORDELLII	
Lecithinase	Phospholipase C
Hemolysin	Oxygen-labile hemolytic activity
Fibrinolysin	Tissue destruction
Lethal (beta) toxin	Necrotic enterotoxin activity
Hemorrhagic (beta) toxin	Hemorrhagic cytotoxin activity
C. HISTOLYTICUM	
Alpha toxin	Necrotizing (not hemolytic)
Beta toxin	Collagenase
Gamma toxin	Protease
Delta toxin	Elastase
Epsilon toxin	Oxyge-labile hemolysin
C. NOVYI* AND *C. HAEMOLYTICUM	
Alpha toxin	Necrotizing
Beta toxin	Lecithinase; necrotizing; hemolytic
Gamma toxin	Lecithinase; necrotizing; hemolytic
Delta toxin	Oxgyen-labile hemolysin
Epsilon toxin	Lipase
Zeta toxin	Hemolysin
Eta toxin	Tropomyosinase
Theta toxin	Lecithinase

treatment with the same antibiotic is frequently successful. Prevention is difficult because the organism is commonly isolated in hospital environments, particularly in areas adjacent to infected patients. The spores of *C. difficile* are difficult to destroy; thus the organism can contaminate an environment for many months and be a major source of nosocomial hospital outbreaks of *C. difficile* disease.

OTHER CLOSTRIDIAL SPECIES

Many other clostridia have been associated with clinically significant disease. Their virulence is due to their ability to survive exposure to oxygen by formation of spores and production of many diverse toxins and enzymes. The virulence factors produced by some of the more important clostridia are summarized in Table 32-7. *C. septicum* is a particularly important pathogen because it is a cause of nontraumatic myonecrosis and frequently occurs in patients with occult colon cancer, acute leukemia, or diabetes. Compromised integrity of the bowel mucosa and the decreased ability of the patient to mount an effective response to the organism lead to spread of *C. septicum* into tissue and its rapid proliferation. Most patients have a fulminant course with death within 1 to 2 days after initial presentation.

CASE STUDY AND QUESTIONS

A 31-year-old woman with left-sided face pain visited the emergency department of a local hospital. She was unable to open her mouth because of facial muscle spasms and had been unable to eat for 4 days because of severe pain in her jaw. Her attending physician noted trismus and risus sardonicus. She reported that 1 week previously she had incurred a puncture wound to her toe while walking in her garden. The wound was cleaned and small pieces of wood removed, but she did not seek medical attention. Although she had received tetanus immunizations as a child, she had not received a booster vaccination since age 15. The presumptive diagnosis of tetanus was made.

1. How should this diagnosis be confirmed?
2. What is the recommended procedure for treating this patient? Should management wait until the laboratory results are available? What is the long-term prognosis for this patient?
3. Compare the mode of action of the toxins produced by *C. tetani* and *C. botulinum*.
4. What virulence factors are produced by *C. perfringens*? What diseases are caused by this organism?
5. What disease is produced by *C. difficile*? Why are infections caused by this organism difficult to manage (epidemiologically and for the individual patients)?

Bibliography

Allen SD and Baron EJ: Clostridium. In Balows A, Hausler W, Herrmann K, Isenberg H, and Shadomy HJ, editors: *Manual of clinical microbiology*, ed 5, Washington D.C., 1992, American Society for Microbiology.

Bizzini B: Tetanus toxin, *Microbiol Rev* 43:224-240, 1979.

Borriello SP, Davies HA, Kamiya S et al: Virulence factors of *Clostridium difficile*, *Rev Infect Dis* 12(suppl):185-191, 1990.

Dowell VR, McCroskey LM, Hatheway CL, et al: Coproexamination for botulinal toxin and *Clostridium botulinum*. A new procedure for laboratory diagnosis of botulism, *JAMA* 238:1829-1832, 1977.

Eidels L, Proia RL, and Hart DA: Membrane receptors for bacterial toxins, *Microbiol Rev* 47:596-620, 1983.

Hatheway CL: Toxigenic clostridia, *Clin Microbiol Rev* 3:66-98, 1990.

Hatheway CL and McCroskey LM: Examination of feces and serum for diagnosis of infant botulism in 336 patients, *J Clin Microbiol* 25:2334-2338, 1987.

Kornbluth AA, Danzid JB, and Bernstein LH: *Clostridium*

septicum infection and associated malignancy, *Medicine* 68:30-37, 1989.

Lyerly DM: Epidemiology of *Clostridium difficile* disease, *Clin Microbiol Newslett* 15:49-52, 1993.

Lyerly DM, Lockwood DE, Richardson SH, and Wilkins TD: Biological activities of toxins A and B of *Clostridium difficile*, *Infect Immun* 35:1147-1150, 1982.

Mellanby J and Green J: How does tetanus toxin act? *Neuroscience* 6:281-300, 1981.

Middlebrook JL and Dorland RB: Bacterial toxins: cellular mechanisms of action, *Microbiol Rev* 48:199-221, 1984.

Mills DC and Arnon SS: The large intestine as the site of *Clostridium botulinum* colonization in human infant botulism, *J Infect Dis* 156:997-998, 1987.

Smith LDS: The occurrence of *Clostridium botulinum* and *Clostridium tetani* in the soil of the United States, *Health Lab Sci* 15:74-80, 1978.

Stevens DL, Musher DM, Watson DA et al: Spontaneous, nontraumatic gangrene due to *Clostridium septicum*, *Rev Infect Dis* 12:286-296, 1990.

Sugiyama H: *Clostridium botulinum* neurotoxin, *Microbiol Rev* 44:419-447, 1980.

CHAPTER 33

Anaerobic Gram-Negative Bacteria

At least 28 species of anaerobic gram-negative bacilli and three genera of anaerobic gram-negative cocci colonize the human upper respiratory tract, gastrointestinal tract, or genitourinary tract. The taxonomic classification of these bacteria has been complicated recently, with many of the species previously placed within the genus *Bacteroides* now reclassified into other genera. Despite the abundance and diversity of these bacteria, the majority of infections are caused by relatively few genera (Table 33-1), which are the focus of this chapter.

BACTEROIDES

Physiology and Structure

At one time the genus *Bacteroides* consisted of almost 50 species but has now been restricted to anaerobes previously categorized in the *Bacteroides fragilis* group and some closely related species. The most common isolates are listed in Table 33-1. *B. fragilis*, the most important member of this genus, is pleomorphic in size and shape, resembling a mixed population of organisms in a casually examined Gram stain. Most members of the family stain weakly with the Gram reaction, so stained specimens must be carefully examined. Most current members of the genus grow rapidly in culture, in contrast with other anaerobic gram-negative bacilli. *Bacteroides* has a typical gram-negative cell wall structure (Figure 33-1), which can be surrounded by a polysaccharide capsule. A major component of the cell wall is a surface lipopolysaccharide (LPS). However, in contrast with LPS molecules in other gram-negative bacteria, the *Bacteroides* glycolipid has little or no endotoxin activity. This is because the lipid A component of LPS lacks phosphate groups on the glucosamine residues and the number of fatty acids linked to the amino sugars is reduced. Both factors are significantly correlated with loss of pyrogenic activity.

Pathogenesis and Immunity

Despite the variety of anaerobic species that colonize the human body, relatively few are responsible for disease. For example, *B. distasonis* and *B. thetaiotaomicron* are the predominant *Bacteroides* found in the gastrointestinal tract; however, more than 80% of intraabdominal infections are associated with *B. fragilis*, an organism that comprises less than 1% of the gastrointestinal flora. The enhanced virulence of this and other anaerobic bacteria has been carefully studied (Box 33-1).

Capsule

A polysaccharide capsule, detectable by staining and immunological techniques, is present in *B. fragilis* isolates but absent in most other *Bacteroides* species. The

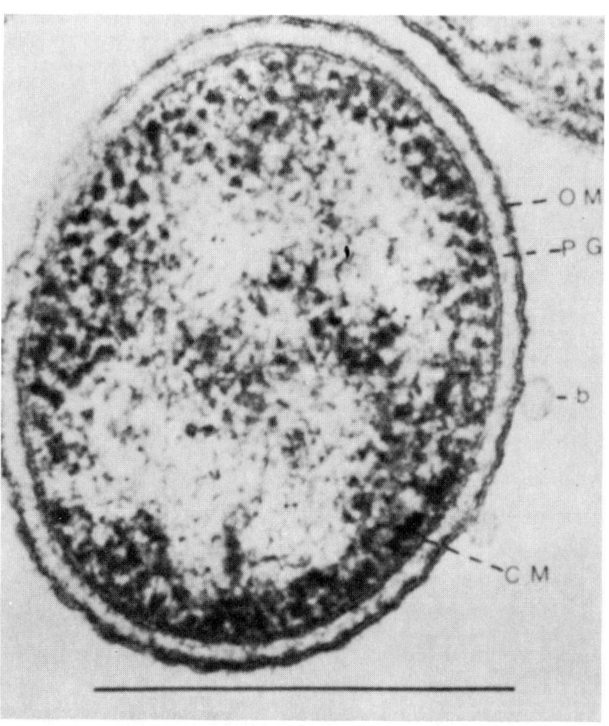

FIGURE 33-1 Electron micrograph of *Bacteroides fragilis*. Note the outer membrane *(OM)* and cytoplasmic membrane *(CM)* are separated by a periplasmic space and peptidoglycan layer *(PG)*. Blebs *(b)* of outer membrane are also seen. The bar is 1 μm. (From Kasper DL, et al: *Rev Infect Dis* 1:278, 1979.)

TABLE 33-1 Anaerobic Gram-Negative Bacteria of Clinical Interest

Anaerobes	Site(s) of colonization
GRAM-NEGATIVE BACILLI	
Bacteroides fragilis group	
B. caccae	Colon
B. distasonis	Colon
B. fragilis	Colon
B. ovatus	Colon
B. thetaiotaomicron	Colon
B. vulgatus	Colon
Other *Bacteroides* species	
B. eggerthii	Colon
B. ureolyticus	Oropharynx, intestines, urogenital tract
B. capillosus	Colon, oropharynx
PREVOTELLA	
P. bivia	Vagina
P. buccae	Oropharynx
P. buccalis	Oropharynx
P. denticola	Oropharynx
P. disiens	Vagina, oropharynx
P. intermedia	Oropharynx
P. loescheii	Oropharynx
P. melaninogenica	Oropharynx
P. oralis	Oropharynx
PORPHYROMONAS	
P. asaccharolytica	Oropharynx
P. endodontalis	Oropharynx
P. gingivalis	Oropharynx
FUSOBACTERIUM	
F. mortiferum	Colon
F. necrophorum	Oropharynx, colon
F. nucleatum	Oropharynx
F. varium	Colon
Bilophila wadsworthia	Colon
Leptotrichia buccalis	Oropharynx, vagina
Wolinella	Oropharynx
GRAM-NEGATIVE COCCI	
Acidaminococcus	Colon
Megasphaera	Colon
Veillonella	Oropharynx

capsule is antiphagocytic and promotes abscess formation (Figure 33-2).

Lipopolysaccharide

Although the *Bacteroides* LPS lacks classic endotoxin properties, it can stimulate leukocyte migration and chemotaxis. This is mediated by activation of the alternate complement pathway, with the subsequent cleavage of the complement component C5a, a strong inducer of leukocyte migration and chemotaxis.

BOX 33-1 Virulence Factors in *Bacteroides*

Polysaccharide capsule	Histolytic enzymes
Lipopolysaccharide	Oxygen tolerance
Agglutinins	β-lactamase

Agglutinins

Encapsulated *B. fragilis* strains can adhere to peritoneal surfaces more effectively than nonencapsulated strains. The role adherence plays in virulence is not known, although presumably this interferes with macrophage-mediated bacterial clearance.

Enzymes

A variety of enzymes have been associated with virulent *Bacteroides* species, including hyaluronidase, collagenase, chondroitin sulfatase, fibrinolysin, neuraminidase, heparinase, DNase, superoxide dismutase, and β-lactamase. Many of these enzymes are found in both virulent and avirulent isolates. Nonetheless, the ability to cause tissue destruction and inactivate immunoglobulins, as well as resist oxygen toxicity (superoxide dismutase) and hydrolyze antibiotics (β-lactamase), most likely plays an important role in anaerobic infections.

Oxygen Tolerance

Anaerobes capable of causing disease are generally able to tolerate exposure to oxygen. Catalase and superoxide dismutase, which inactivate hydrogen peroxide and the superoxide free radicals (O_2^-) respectively, are present in pathogenic strains of *Bacteroides*.

The ability of the patient to control bacterial proliferation and abscess formation is mediated by both humoral and cellular immune factors. Although *B. fragilis* is resistant to killing when exposed to serum, activation of the alternate complement pathway by LPS leads to C3 deposition on the bacterial surface. Exposure to naturally occurring IgM antibodies mediates phagocytosis and killing by neutrophils. In addition, a soluble immune T-cell factor regulates the cellular response to the *Bacteroides* capsular polysaccharide and thus abscess formation. In response to this immune reaction, the short-chain fatty acids produced during anaerobic metabolism inhibit phagocytosis and degranulation.

Epidemiology

The anaerobic gram-negative bacilli form a major component of the human microbial flora (Box 33-2). Anaerobes outnumber aerobic bacteria by roughly a factor of 10 in the oropharynx, 100 in the urogenital tract, and 1000 in the gastrointestinal tract. *B. fragilis* is

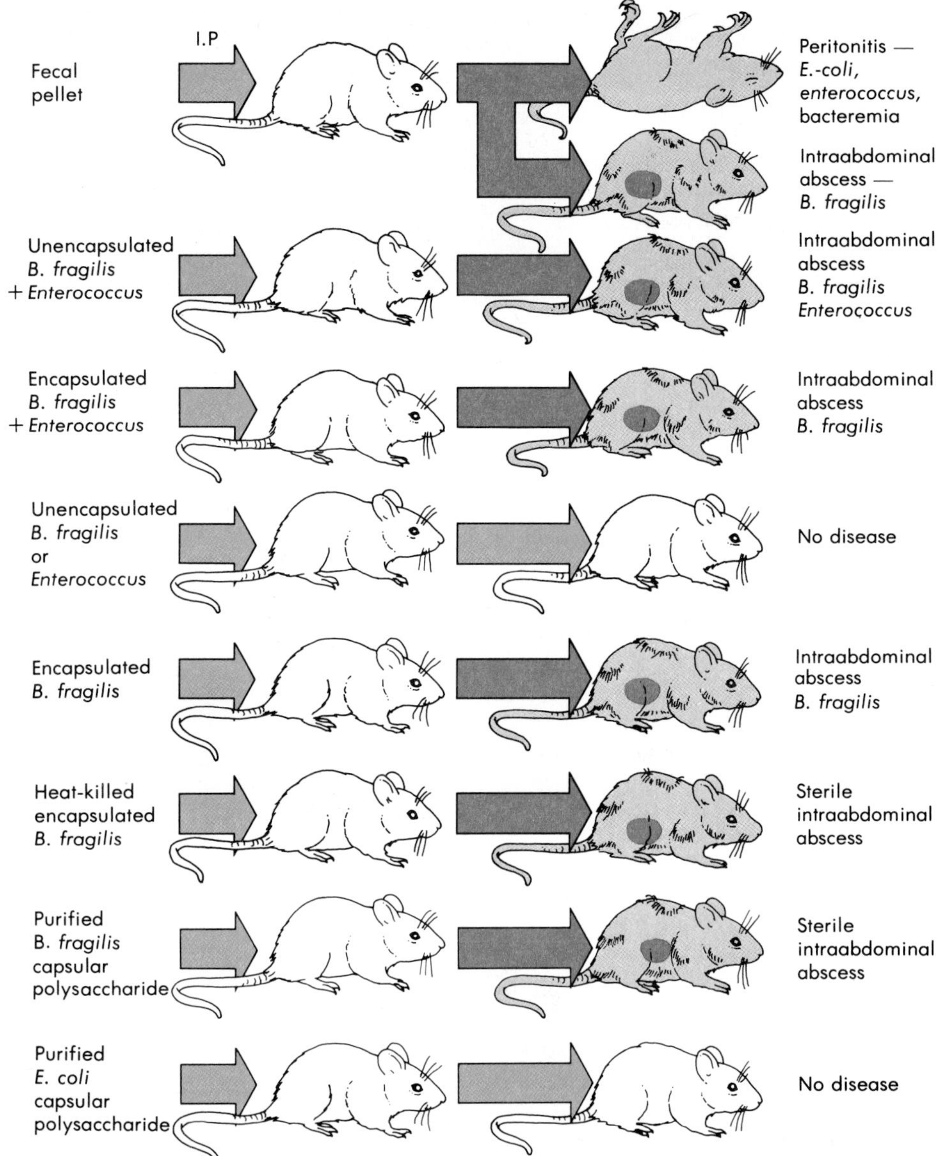

FIGURE 33-2 Demonstration of the role of encapsulation in *Bacteroides fragilis* virulence. In a series of experiments Kasper and associates were able to demonstrate that the capsule present in *Bacteroides fragilis* is responsible for abscess formation, which is characteristic of these infections. In the presence of multiple other bacterial species, abscess formation does not depend on encapsulated strains. However, in the absence of other bacteria (e.g., *Enterococcus* as depicted in this figure), abscess formation is rare, unless the *B. fragilis* strain possesses a capsule. Additional experiments demonstrated that sterile abscesses will develop if nonviable encapsulated *B. fragilis* strains or purified capsular material is injected intraperitoneally into mice or Wistar rats. This is not observed with rats inoculated with *Escherichia coli* capsular material or encapsulated *Streptococcus pneumoniae.*

commonly associated with pleuropulmonary, intraabdominal, and genital infections. However, the organism comprises less than 1% of the colonic flora and is rarely isolated from the oropharynx or genital tract of healthy persons unless highly selective techniques are used. The prominent role this organism plays in human disease is attributed to its enhanced virulence.

Clinical Syndromes

The cardinal features of infections with *Bacteroides* are (1) endogenous infections, (2) polymicrobic mixture of organisms, and (3) abscess formation. As the infection develops, the endogenous bacterial population is able to spread by trauma or disease from normally colonized mucosal surfaces to sterile tissues or fluids. Many organ-

BOX 33-2 Epidemiology of *Bacteroides fragilis* Group Infection

DISEASE/BACTERIAL FACTORS

Bacteremia; abscess formation in normally sterile sites
Capsule is antiphagocytic, promotes abscess formation
LPS stimulates leukocyte migration and chemotaxis
Agglutinins enhance adherence
Enzymes cause tissue destruction, inactivate immunoglobulins, and hydrolyze antibiotics
Bacteria tolerate oxygen exposure

TRANSMISSION

Endogenous spread to normally sterile tissues or fluids

WHO IS AT RISK?

Surgical /trauma patients
Patients with spontaneous peritonitis

GEOGRAPHY/SEASON

Ubiquitous and worldwide
No seasonal incidence

MODES OF CONTROL

Surgical intervention combined with antibiotics: carbenicillin, piperacillin, metronidazole, clindamycin, imipenem
Prophylactic antibiotics for planned procedures that disrupt mucosa

isms may be initially involved in the infection. However, the oxygen-susceptible and avirulent organisms are rapidly cleared by the host's defense mechanisms, with a resultant proliferation of virulent organisms and destruction of host tissue. Encapsulated bacteria such as *B. fragilis* are prominently featured in these infections and are typically associated with abscess formation. Thus infections are generally at body sites proximal to colonized mucosal surfaces. *B. fragilis* is isolated in 15% to 20% of anaerobic pleuropulmonary infections, two thirds or more of suppurative pelvic infections, and virtually all intraabdominal infections with abscess formation. More than 75% of all anaerobic gram-negative bacteremias are due to *B. fragilis*.

Laboratory Diagnosis

Microscopy

Microscopic examination of specimens from suspected anaerobic infections can be useful. Although the bacteria may stain faintly and irregularly (Figure 33-3) the presence of pleomorphic, gram-negative bacilli can be useful preliminary information.

Culture

Specimens should be collected and transported to the laboratory in an oxygen-free system, promptly inoculated onto specific media for the recovery of anaerobes, and incubated in an anaerobic environment. Because most anaerobe infections are endogenous, it is important to collect specimens in a manner that avoids contamination with the normal bacterial population on the adjacent mucosal surface. Specimens should also be maintained in a moist environment because significant bacterial loss is incurred with dried specimens. Most *Bacteroides* grow rapidly and should be detected within 2 days, although some strains may require prolonged incubation. In addition, the presence of different organisms in polymicrobic infections sometimes complicates the recovery of all clinically significant bacteria. The use of selective media has facilitated the recovery of most important anaerobes (Figure 33-4).

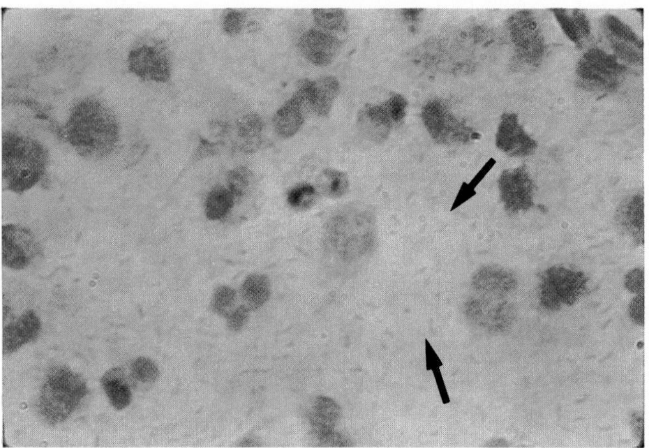

FIGURE 33-3 Bacteroides fragilis in an abscess. The organisms appear as faintly staining, pleomorphic gram-negative bacilli.

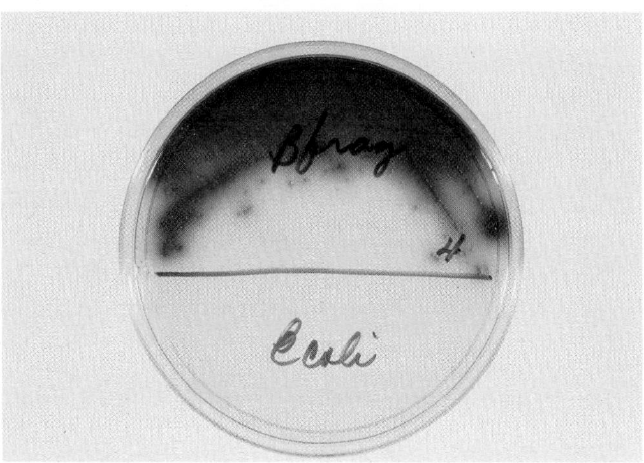

FIGURE 33-4 Growth of *Bacteroides fragilis* on *Bacteroides* bile esculin agar. Most aerobic and anaerobic bacteria are inhibited by bile and gentamicin in this medium, whereas the *B. fragilis* group of organisms is stimulated by bile, resistant to gentamicin, and able to hydrolyze esculin, producing a black precipitate.

Biochemical Identification

The *B. fragilis* group can be preliminarily identified by its Gram stain and colonial morphology, resistance to kanamycin, vancomycin, and colistin, and stimulated growth in 20% bile. Definitive identification of isolates can be accurately performed by use of commercially prepared biochemical systems that measure the activity of preformed enzymes. Occasionally the detection of metabolic by-products (short-chain fatty acids) by gas chromatography has proved to be a useful, simple technique to supplement biochemical testing.

Treatment, Prevention, and Control

Antibiotic therapy combined with surgical intervention is the main approach for managing serious anaerobic infections. B-lactamase is produced by virtually all members of the *B. fragilis* group, which render the bacteria resistant to penicillin and many cephalosporins. However, high concentrations of some penicillins (e.g., carbenicillin, piperacillin), use of β-lactamase inhibitors, and other selected β-lactam antibiotics (e.g., cefoxitin, imipenem) can be used to treat *Bacteroides* infections. Clindamycin resistance in *Bacteroides*, which is plasmid mediated, has increased in prevalence in recent years, with an average of 7% to 10% of the isolates in the United States resistant. Metronidazole is active against most *Bacteroides*.

Because *Bacteroides* form an important part of the normal microbial flora and infections are due to the endogenous spread of the organisms, disease is virtually impossible to control. However, it is important to recognize that diagnostic or surgical procedures that disrupt the natural barriers surrounding the mucosal surfaces can introduce these organisms into normally sterile sites. If these barriers are invaded, prophylactic treatment with antibiotics may be indicated.

OTHER ANAEROBIC, GRAM-NEGATIVE BACILLI

Three species of pigmented, asaccharolytic bacilli previously classified as *Bacteroides* now comprise the genus *Porphyromonas* (from the Greek adjective for purple). Sixteen additional species of pigmented or nonpigmented, saccharolytic, bile-sensitive bacilli were transferred from the genus *Bacteroides* to the new genus *Prevotella*. Other anaerobic gram-negative bacilli of medical interest include *Fusobacterium*, *Bilophila*, *Leptotrichia*, and *Wolinella* (Table 33-1). These bacteria are commonly found colonizing the oropharynx, gastrointestinal tract, and genitourinary tract. These anaerobes produce a variety of histolytic enzymes that are able to mediate tissue destruction, as well as β-lactamase, which can protect them from penicillin killing. In contrast with *B. fragilis* group, the lipopolysaccharide present in the cell wall of fusobacteria is biochemically and biologically similar to endotoxin present in aerobic gram-negative bacilli.

The spectrum of clinical diseases attributed to these anaerobes reflects their broad distribution in the human body. Organisms colonizing the oropharynx are associated with brain abscesses, oral infections, and pleuropulmonary infections; organisms in the gastrointestinal tract are associated with intraabdominal infections; and organisms colonizing the genitourinary tract (particularly *Prevotella bivia* and *P. disiens*) are involved with pelvic infections (e.g., abscesses, bacterial vaginosis). These infections, as is typical with most anaerobic infections, are usually polymicrobic mixtures of aerobic and anaerobic organisms.

Laboratory diagnosis relies upon microscopic examination of the clinical specimen and culture upon anaerobic media. Many of the non-*Bacteroides* gram-negative bacilli are oxygen sensitive and slow growing. Thus care must be used during transport of the specimens to the laboratory, and prolonged incubation is frequently required. Although these organisms historically were treated with penicillin, the widespread presence of β-lactamases in these species has limited the usefulness of this class of antibiotics. Penicillins combined with β-lactamase inhibitors or metronidazole still remain effective in most infections.

ANAEROBIC, GRAM-NEGATIVE COCCI

Three anaerobic cocci, *Acidaminococcus*, *Megasphaera*, and *Veillonella*, have been isolated from human infections. These bacteria are found in the oropharynx and colon, have a relatively low degree of virulence, and represent fewer than 1% of all anaerobes isolated in clinical specimens. Isolates are generally present in mixtures, and their clinical significance is difficult to assess. These cocci are usually susceptible to penicillin, cephalosporins, clindamycin, chloramphenicol, and metronidazole. However, specific therapy against them is often unnecessary.

CASE STUDY AND QUESTIONS

A 65-year-old man entered the emergency department of a local hospital appearing acutely ill with abdominal tenderness and a temperature of 40.0° C. Because appendicitis was suspected, the patient was taken to surgery. Laparotomy revealed a ruptured appendix surrounded by approximately 20 ml of gross, foul-smelling pus. The pus was drained and submitted for aerobic and anaerobic bacterial cultures, as well as Gram stain. Following surgery the patient was started on a course of antibiotic therapy. Gram stain revealed a polymicrobic mixture of organisms, and culture was positive for *Bacteroides fragilis, Escherichia coli*, and *Enterococcus faecalis*.

1. Which organism(s) is/are responsible for the abscess formation? What virulence factors are responsible for abscess formation?
2. *Bacteroides fragilis* causes infections at what other body sites?
3. What antibiotics should be selected to manage this polymicrobic infection?
4. What other anaerobic gram-negative bacilli can cause human disease?

Bibliography

Bjornson AB: Role of humoral factors in host resistance to the *Bacteroides fragilis* group, *Rev Infect Dis* 12: S161-168, 1990.

Cuchural GJ, Tally, FP, Jacobs NV et al: Susceptibility of the *Bacteroides fragilis* group in the United States: analysis by site of isolation, *Antimicrob Agents Chemother* 32:717-722, 1988.

Finegold SM: *Anaerobic bacteria in human disease*, New York, 1988, Academic Press.

Finegold SM, Baron EJ, and Wexler HM: *A clinical guide to anaerobic infections*, Belmont, Calif., 1992, Star Publishing.

Hofstad T: Pathogenicity of anaerobic gram-negative rods: possible mechanisms, *Rev Infect Dis* 6:189-199, 1984.

Hofstad T: Current taxonomy of medically important nonsporing anaerobes, *Rev Infect Dis* 12:S122-126.

Kasper DL, Hayes ME, Reinap BG et al: Isolation and identification of encapsulated strains of *Bacteroides fragilis*, *J Infect Dis* 136:75-81, 1977.

Kasper DL, Onderdonk AB, Pold BF, and Bartlett JG: Surface antigens as virulence factors in infection with *Bacteroides fragilis*, *Rev Infect Dis* 1:278-288, 1979.

Lindberg AA, Weintraub A, Zahringer U et al. Structure-activity relationships in lipopolysaccharides of *Bacteroides fragilis*, *Rev Infect Dis* 12:S133-140, 1990.

Styrt B and Gorbach SL: Recent developments in the understanding of the pathogenesis and treatment of anaerobic infection, *N Engl J Med* 321:240-246, 298-302, 1989.

CHAPTER 34

Nocardia and Related Actinomycetes

THE aerobic actinomycetes are gram-positive, catalase-positive bacilli found in soil, decaying vegetation, ventilation systems, and colonizing animals and humans. The most common members of this group, as well as their source and associated diseases, are listed in Table 34-1. Some actinomycetes (e.g., *Nocardia*) form delicate filamentous forms, or hyphae, similar to fungi when detected in clinical specimens or isolated in culture. However, the cell wall structure and antimicrobial susceptibility patterns are typical of bacteria. *Nocardia* and *Rhodococcus* characteristically stain irregularly in a beaded pattern when Gram stained and are partially acid-fast when decolorized with a weak acid solution. The spectrum of diseases associated with these organisms is extensive, including insignificant colonization (*Streptomyces* species), allergic pneumonitis (*Micropolysporas* and *Thermoactinomycetes*), mycetoma (*Actinomadura*, *Nocardiopsis*, *Streptomyces*, and *Nocardia*), pulmonary disease (*Nocardia*, *Rhodococcus*), and systemic infections (*Nocardia*, *Rhodococcus*). Of all these organisms, *Nocardia* is most commonly seen.

TABLE 34-1 Pathogenic Aerobic Actinomycetes

Organism	Source	Disease
Nocardia	Ubiquitous in soil, animals, and humans	Pulmonary, central nervous system, systemic, mycetoma
Rhodococcus	Ubiquitous in soil and plant material	Septicemia, generalized granulomatous, central nervous disease, pericarditis
Actinomadura	Ubiquitous in soil, plants, thorns, and decaying vegetation	Mycetoma
Nocardiopsis	Ubiquitous in soil	Mycetoma
Streptomyces	Ubiquitous in soil, thorns, plants, and decaying vegetation	Mycetoma; most nonpathogenic species
Micropolysporas	Ubiquitous in ventilation ducts, manure, and compost	Hypersensitivity pneumonitis ("farmer's lung")
Thermoactinomycetes	Ubiquitous in ventilation ducts, manure, compost, hay	Hypersensitivity pneumonitis ("farmer's lung")

NOCARDIA

Physiology and Structure

The genus *Nocardia* was named after Nocard, who first described bovine disease characterized by pyogenic pulmonary and cutaneous lesions. The genus consists of strict aerobic bacilli that form branched hyphae in both tissues and culture. The organisms are gram-positive, although many stain poorly and appear to be gram-negative with intracellular gram-positive beads (Figure 34-1). *Nocardia* organisms have a cell wall structure similar to mycobacteria with mycolic acids present, and, like the mycobacteria, are acid-fast (Figure 34-2). This acid-fastness is a helpful differential characteristic separating *Nocardia* from morphologically similar organisms such as *Actinomyces*. *Nocardia* species are catalase-positive, use carbohydrates oxidatively, and can grow on most nonselective

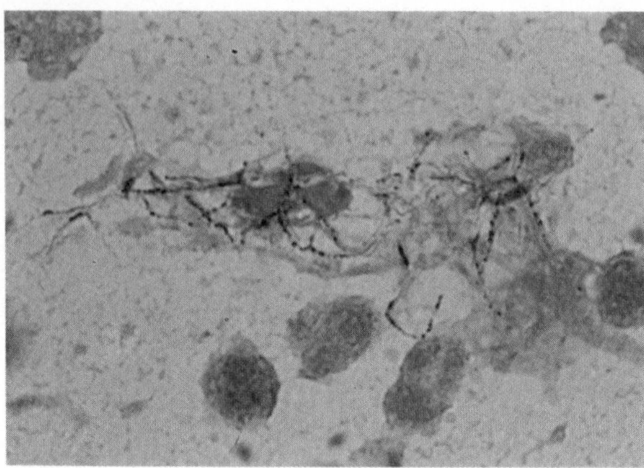

FIGURE 34-1 Gram stain of *N. asteroides* in expectorated sputum. Note that the delicate beaded filaments cannot be distinguished from *Actinomyces.*

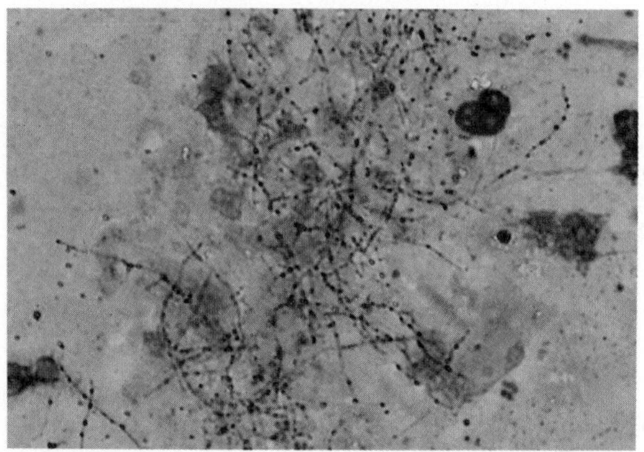

FIGURE 34-2 Acid-fast stain of *N. asteroides* in expectorated sputum.

laboratory media; however, isolation can require incubation for 1 week or more. Colonies vary in morphology from dry to waxy and from orange to white.

Pathogenesis

Nocardia asteroides, N. brasiliensis, and *N. otitidiscaviarum* (formerly *N. caviae*) are the most common human pathogens, capable of causing acute or chronic suppurative infections (Table 34-2). *N. asteroides* is the organism responsible for approximately 90% of human nocardial infections. It causes primarily bronchopulmonary disease, with a high predilection for hematogenous spread to the central nervous system or skin. *N. brasiliensis* and *N. otitidiscaviarum* are most commonly responsible for primary cutaneous infections with infrequent hematogenous dissemination. *Nocardia* are also a cause of actinomycotic **mycetoma** (a localized subcutaneous infection characterized by swelling, suppuration, formation of multiple sinus tracts, and occasionally the presence of granules in the draining purulent material).

Members of the genus *Nocardia* are found worldwide

TABLE 34-2 *Nocardia* Organisms Associated With Human Disease

Organism	Disease
N. asteroides	Bronchopulmonary disease with secondary dissemination to the central nervous system or skin
N. brasiliensis	Cutaneous disease with rare secondary dissemination
N. otitidiscaviarum	Same as *N. brasiliensis*

in soil rich with organic matter and only occasionally isolated as commensal organisms in humans. Localized infections, such as primary cutaneous nocardiosis and mycetoma, are observed in immunocompetent individuals. Pulmonary disease and disseminated infections are primarily restricted to patients with compromised immune function (particularly patients with T-cell deficiencies) produced by either disease (e.g., leukemia, AIDS) or immunosuppressive therapy (e.g., patients receiving corticosteroids). Renal and cardiac transplant recipients are particularly at risk for *Nocardia* infections. Patients infected with *N. brasiliensis* are usually immunocompetent.

Bronchopulmonary infections develop after the initial colonization of the oropharynx and then aspiration of oral secretions into the lower airways. Primary cutaneous nocardiosis develops after the traumatic introduction of organisms into subcutaneous tissues. Disease is characterized by necrosis and abscess formation, similar to that caused by other pyogenic bacteria. Chronic infections with sinus tract formation can be observed, particularly with some cutaneous infections. Although sulfur granules are observed with *Actinomyces*, these are uncommon with *Nocardia* and seen only with cutaneous involvement.

Epidemiology

Nocardia infections are exogenous (i.e., caused by organisms that are not part of the normal human flora [Box 34-1]). Despite the ubiquitous presence of the organism in nature and the abundance of immunocompromised patients in hospitals, nocardia infections are relatively uncommon. Estimates indicate that fewer than 1000 infections are seen annually in the United States.

Clinical Syndromes

Bronchopulmonary infections caused by *Nocardia* cannot be distinguished from infections caused by other pyogenic organisms. Signs such as cough, dyspnea, and fever are usually present but are not diagnostic. Cavitation and spread into the pleura are common. Although the clinical picture is not specific for *Nocardia*, these organisms should be considered when immunocompromised patients develop pneumonia with cavitation, particularly when evidence of dissemination to the central nervous

BOX 34-1 Epidemiology of *Nocardia* Infection

DISEASE/BACTERIAL FACTORS

Nocardiosis: bronchopulmonary; dissemination to skin or CNS; primary cutaneous; myetoma
Present in soil and vegetation

TRANSMISSION

Inhalation
Traumatic introduction into subcutaneous tissues

WHO IS AT RISK?

Immunocompromised patients, particularly renal and cardiac transplant recipients

GEOGRAPHY/SEASON

Ubiquitous and worldwide
No seasonal incidence

MODES OF CONTROL

Antibiotic therapy with sulfonamides
Proper wound care

system or skin exists. **Cutaneous infections** may be seen as cellulitis, pustules, pyoderma, subcutaneous abscesses, lymphocutaneous syndrome, or mycetoma. **Mycetoma** is a chronic, granulomatous disease most frequently present on the lower extremities where the etiological organism is traumatically introduced (Figure 34-3). The underlying connective tissues, muscle, and bone can be involved, and draining sinus tracts usually open on the skin surface. A variety of organisms can cause mycetoma, although *N. brasiliensis* is the most common cause in North, Central, and South America.

Central nervous system infections, most commonly single or multiple brain abscesses, can be observed in as many as one third of all patients with *N. asteroides* infections.

Laboratory Diagnosis

Collection of specimens for the isolation of *Nocardia* is dictated by the clinical presentation. Multiple early morning sputum specimens should be collected from patients with pulmonary disease because the slow growth of the organism makes recovery unreliable. Because *Nocardia* organisms are usually distributed throughout the tissue and abscess material, the microscopic detection and in vitro isolation of organisms in cutaneous or central nervous system disease is relatively easy. The delicate hyphae of *Nocardia* in tissues resemble *Actinomyces*; however, *Nocardia* Gram stain poorly, and most isolates are partially acid-fast (Figures 34-1 and 34-2). The organism grows on most laboratory media incubated in an atmosphere of 5% to 10% carbon dioxide, but the presence of this slow-growing organism may be obscured by more rapidly growing commensal bacteria. The organism occasionally survives the decontamination procedure used for the isolation of mycobacteria and will grow on mycobacterial media. However, this procedure is unreliable. If a specimen is received that is potentially contaminated with rapidly growing bacteria (e.g., sputum), then selective media should be inoculated. Success has been achieved with the medium used for the isolation of *Legionella* (BCYE agar), as well as some other media. It is important to notify the laboratory that nocardiosis is suspected, because most laboratories do not routinely incubate clinical specimens for more than 1 to 3 days. More time is required for the isolation of *Nocardia*, which should be incubated for as long as 1 week.

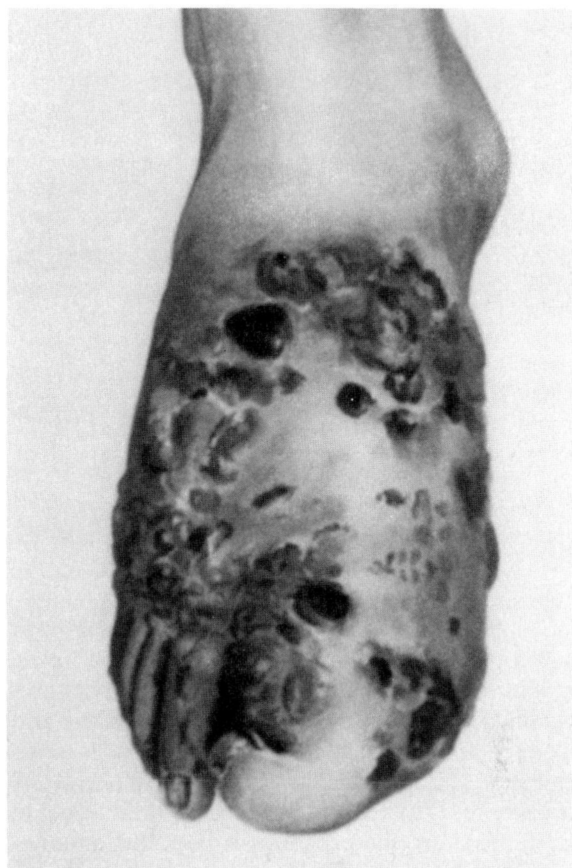

FIGURE 34-3 Mycetoma caused by *N. brasiliensis*. The foot is grossly enlarged and covered with multiple draining sinus tracts. (From Binford CH and Connor DH, editors: *Pathology of tropical and extraordinary diseases*, vol 2, Washington, DC, 1976, Armed Forces Institute of Pathology.)

Identification of *Nocardia* is uncomplicated. A preliminary classification can be made after demonstration of acid-fast hyphae. However, definitive identification is frequently delayed because *N. asteroides*, the species most commonly isolated, is nonreactive with most differential tests used for biochemical classification (Table 34-3).

TABLE 34-3 Identification of *Nocardia* Responsible for Human Diseases

	N. asteroides	*N. brasiliensis*	*N. otitidiscaviarum*
Decomposition of:			
Casein	−	+	−
Tyrosine	−	+	−
Xanthine	−	−	+
Urea	+	+	+
Gelatin	−	+	−
Acid from:			
Lactose	−	−	−
Xylose	−	−	−

Treatment, Prevention, and Control

Nocardia infections are treated with antibiotics combined with appropriate surgical intervention. Sulfonamides are the antibiotics of choice for treating nocardiosis. Tobramycin, amikacin, and some of the newer β-lactams also have good in vitro activity but unproven in vivo effectiveness. Antibiotic therapy should be extended for 6 weeks or more. Whereas clinical response is favorable in localized infections, the prognosis is poor for immunocompromised patients with disseminated disease.

Because nocardia are ubiquitous, exposure to the organisms cannot be avoided. However, bronchopulmonary disease is uncommon in immunocompetent persons, and primary cutaneous infections can be prevented by proper wound care. The complications associated with disseminated disease can be minimized by consideration of nocardiosis in the differential diagnosis for immunocompromised patients with cavitary pulmonary disease.

RHODOCOCCUS

The genus *Rhodococcus* ("red-pigmented coccus") consists of 12 species of gram-positive, obligate aerobic actinomycetes. The cell wall of these catalase-positive coccobacilli is similar to that of *Nocardia* and *Mycobacteria*—containing both mycolic acid and tuberculostearic acid, rendering the organisms acid-fast. *Rhodococcus* (formerly *Corynebacterium*) *equi* is a well-recognized veterinary pathogen, particularly in herbivores, and has been associated in recent years with disease in immunocompromised patients, including patients with AIDS and those receiving immunosuppressive drugs (Box 34-2). The recent increase in human infections is most likely related to the increase in patients with immunosuppressive diseases and enhanced awareness of the organism.

Rhodococcus is a soil organism commonly isolated in herbivore manure. Despite this association and the observation that this strict aerobic bacterium cannot survive in the anaerobic atmosphere of the human gut, most infected patients do not have a history of contact with grazing animals.

BOX 34-2 Epidemiology of *Rhodococcus* Infection

DISEASE/BACTERIAL FACTORS

Abscess formation in lungs, as well as lymph nodes, meninges, pericardium, skin
Present in soil and vegetation
Facultative intracellular pathogen in macrophages

TRANSMISSION

Inhalation

WHO IS AT RISK?

Immunocompromised patients, particularly AIDS patients

GEOGRAPHY/SEASON

Ubiquitous and worldwide
No seasonal incidence

MODES OF CONTROL

Prolonged therapy with rifampin and erythromycin

R. equi is a facultative intracellular organism that survives in macrophages and causes granulomatous inflammation, which leads to abscess formation. Although a number of putative virulence factors have been identified (Table 34-4), the precise pathophysiology of the infections is incompletely understood. Lesions are most commonly observed in the lungs, but lymph nodes, meninges, pericardium, and skin can also be involved in systemic disease.

Rhodococcus grows readily on aerobically incubated nonselective media, although the characteristic pigment may not be obvious for 4 days or more. The organism appears as pleomorphic coccobacilli that stain gram-positive, as well as acid-fast. The organism can be identified by biochemical tests although it is relatively inert.

Successful treatment of *Rhodococcus* infections requires use of multiple antibiotics with at least one lipophilic agent that can penetrate into the infected macrophages (e.g., prolonged therapy with rifampin and erythromycin).

ACTINOMADURA, NOCARDIOPSIS, AND *STREPTOMYCES*

Mycetoma can be caused by fungi, as well as by bacteria in the genera *Actinomadura*, *Nocardiopsis*, *Streptomyces*, and *Nocardia*. The precise etiology of this disease can be determined only by cultivation because many of these organisms resemble fungi when seen in tissue. Infection usually results from traumatic introduction of the bacteria or fungi into tissue, most commonly an extremity.

TABLE 34-4 Virulence Factors in *Rhodococcus equi*

Virulence factors	Biological activity
Capsular polysaccharide	Inhibits phagocytosis
"Equi factors" cholesterol oxidase Phospholipase C	May be responsible for eukaryotic cell membrane lysis
Mycolic acids	Stimulate granuloma formation
Unknown factors	Promote intracellular survival in macrophages by preventing phagolysome fusion; stimulate lysosomal degranulation with subsequent tissue destruction

Chronic cutaneous and subcutaneous infection, with abscess and sinus tract formation, will develop. These pathogens can be isolated on Sabouraud's dextrose agar (typically considered a fungal medium) or on nonselective bacterial media. Incubation for as long as 3 weeks may be required before growth of the organisms is apparent. Identification of the isolates is based upon morphological criteria and selected biochemical tests. Effective therapy includes both surgical debridement and appropriate antibiotics, such as trimethoprim-sulfamethoxazole, streptomycin, rifampin, diaminodiphenylsulfone (dapsone), or a combination of these agents. Because the clinical diagnosis is characteristic and the results of culture may be delayed for 3 weeks or more, empirical therapy must be initiated. Care should be used to select broad spectrum antibiotics that will be effective against both bacterial and fungal agents responsible for mycetoma.

MICROPOLYSPORAS AND *THERMOACTINOMYCETES*

Allergic pneumonitis ("farmer's lung") is a hypersensitivity reaction to repeated exposure to thermophilic actinomycetes commonly found in decaying vegetation. Disease is characterized by granulomatous changes in the lung with pulmonary edema, eosinophilia, and elevated IgE levels. Clinical diagnosis is confirmed by detecting specific precipitin antibodies in serum to these agents.

CASE STUDY AND QUESTIONS

A 47-year-old renal transplant recipient who had been receiving prednisone and azathioprine for 2 years was admitted to the University medical center. Two weeks previously the patient had developed a dry, persistent cough. Five days before admission the cough became productive, and pleuritic chest pain developed. One day before admission the patient was noted to be in mild respiratory arrest, and chest radiographs revealed a patchy right upper lobe infiltrate. Sputum specimens were initially sent for bacterial cultures, which after 2 days of incubation were reported as negative. Antibiotic therapy with cephalothin was ineffective, so additional cultures were collected for bacteria, mycobacteria, *Legionella*, and fungi. After 4 days of incubation, *Nocardia* was isolated on the media inoculated for mycobacteria, *Legionella*, and fungi.

1. Why did the organism fail to grow on media for bacteria? What can be done to correct this problem?
2. What is the most likely species of *Nocardia* involved with this infection? If this organism disseminates, what two target tissues are most likely to be involved?
3. What is the primary mode of acquisition of *Nocardia asteroides*? *N. brasiliensis*? *N. otitidiscaviarum*?
4. What disease is caused by *Rhodococcus* in immunocompromised patients? What diagnostic property does this organism share with *Nocardia*?
5. Which bacteria have been shown to cause mycetoma?

Bibliography

Arroyo JC, Nichols S, and Carroll GF: Disseminated *Nocardia caviae* infection, *Am J Med* 62:409-412, 1977.

Beaman BL, Burnside J, Edwards B, and Causey W: Nocardial infections in the United States, 1972-1974, *J Infect Dis* 134:286-289, 1976.

Frazier AR, Rosenow EC, and Roberts GD: Nocardiosis. A review of 25 cases occurring during 24 months, *Mayo Clin Proc* 50:657-663, 1975.

Harvey RL and Sunstrum JC: *Rhodococcus equi* infection in patients with and without human immunodeficiency virus infection, *Rev Infect Dis* 13:139-145, 1991.

Jones MR, Neale TJ, Say PJ, and Horne JG: *Rhodococcus equi*: an emerging opportunistic pathogen? *Aust N Z J Med* 19:103-107, 1989.

Land G, McGinnis M, Staneck J, and Gatson A: Aerobic pathogenic *Actinomycetales*. In Balows A, Hausler WJ, Herrmann KL, Isenberg HD, and Shadomy HJ: *Manual of clinical microbiology*, ed 5, Washington, DC, 1991, American Society for Microbiology.

Prescott JF: *Rhodococcus equi*: an animal and human pathogen, *Clin Microbiol Rev* 4:20-34, 1991.

Smego RA and Gallis HA: The clinical spectrum of *Nocardia brasiliensis* infection in the United States, *Rev Infect Dis* 6:164-180, 1984.

CHAPTER 35

Mycobacterium

THE genus *Mycobacterium* consists of nonmotile, non–spore-forming aerobic bacilli, 0.2 to 0.6 × 1 to 10 μm in size. The bacilli occasionally form branched filaments, but these can be readily disrupted. The cell wall is rich in lipids, making the surface hydrophobic and the mycobacteria resistant to many disinfectants, as well as to such common laboratory stains as the Gram and Giemsa. Once stained, the bacilli are also refractory to decolorization with acid solutions, hence the name **acid-fast bacilli.** Because the mycobacterial cell wall is complex and this group of organisms is fastidious, most mycobacteria grow slowly, dividing every 12 to 24 hours. Isolation of the "rapidly growing" mycobacteria requires incubation for 3 days or more; the slow-growing organisms (e.g., *Mycobacterium tuberculosis, M. avium-intracellulare*) can require 3 to 8 weeks of incubation. *M. leprae,* the etiological agent of leprosy, cannot be grown in cell-free cultures.

Mycobacteria are still a significant cause of morbidity and mortality, particularly in countries with limited medical resources. At least 41 species of mycobacteria have been described, with more than 27 species isolated in human clinical specimens (Table 35-1). Despite the abundance of mycobacterial species, more than 95% of all human infections are caused by six species or groups: *M. tuberculosis, M. avium-intracellulare complex, M. kansasii, M. fortuitum, M. chelonae,* and *M. leprae.*

PHYSIOLOGY AND STRUCTURE

Mycobacteria possess a complex cell wall. The structural foundation consists of the peptidoglycan skeleton with covalently linked arabinogalactan-mycolate molecules and is overlayed with free lipids and polypeptides (Figure 35-1).

The surface glycolipids, including species-specific mycosides (peptidoglycolipids, oligoliposaccharides) and phenolic glycolipids, are highly antigenic. They constitute 25% of the dry cell wall weight and contribute to the hydrophobic properties of mycobacteria. Another cell wall lipid, **cord factor** (6′6′-dimycolate of trehalose), is responsible for the parallel alignment of rows of bacilli ("cord" formation), a characteristic of virulent strains of *M. tuberculosis.*

The peptide chains in the outer layer comprise 15% of the cell wall weight and are biologically important

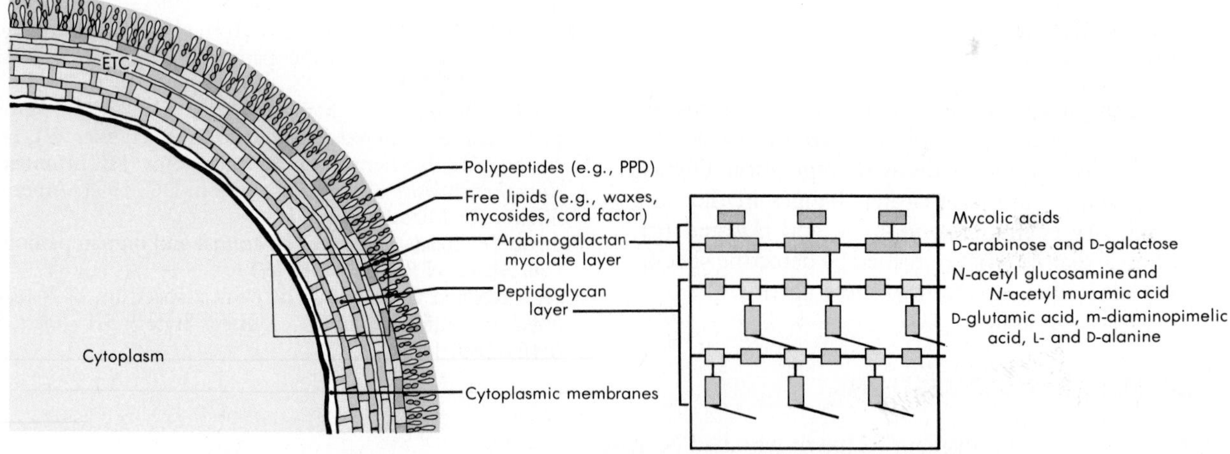

FIGURE 35-1 Structural arrangement of mycobacterial cell wall layers. Mycolic acid is attached to the arabinose-galactose layer at the arabinose side chain. Phosphodiester linkage binds the arabinogalactan layer to the underlying peptidoglycan layer at the muramic acid subunit. This linkage occurs at every tenth repeating arabinogalactan unit. (Redrawn from Kubica GP and Wayne LG, editors: *The mycobacteria: a sourcebook,* New York, 1984, Marcel Dekker.)

antigens, stimulating the patient's cellular immune response to infection. Extracted and partially purified preparations of these protein derivatives are used as a skin testing reagent to measure exposure to *M. tuberculosis.* Similar preparations from other mycobacteria have been used as species-specific skin testing reagents.

The peptidoglycan skeleton is relatively uniform in all mycobacterial species and forms the major component of the cell wall. As with other bacteria, intrapeptide bridges between the peptidoglycan chains bind the skeleton into a rigid structure. Attached to these chains by covalent bonds are mycolic acids linked to D-arabinose and D-galactose. The mycolic acids are the major lipids in the mycobacterial cell wall.

Growth properties and colonial morphology are used for the preliminary identification of mycobacteria. *M. tuberculosis* and closely related species are slow-growing bacteria, and the colonies are nonpigmented or buff-colored (Figure 35-2). Runyon classified the other mycobacteria into four groups based on their rate of growth and their ability to produce pigments in the presence or absence of light. The pigmented mycobacteria produce intense yellow pigmented carotenoids (Figure 35-3). **Photochromogens** (Runyon group I) are organisms that produce these pigments only after exposure to light, whereas the **scotochromogenic organisms** (Runyon group II) can produce the pigments in the dark as well as the light. The slow-growing, nonpigmented

TABLE 35-1 Classification of Mycobacteria Isolated in Humans

Organism	Pathogenicity	Frequency isolated in United States
MYCOBACTERIUM TUBERCULOSIS COMPLEX		
M. tuberculosis	Strictly pathogenic	Common
M. bovis	Strictly pathogenic	Uncommon
M. ulcerans	Strictly pathogenic	Uncommon
M. leprae	Strictly pathogenic	Uncommon
RUNYON GROUP I		
M. kansasii	Usually pathogenic	Common
M. marinum	Usually pathogenic	Uncommon
M. simiae	Usually pathogenic	Uncommon
M. asiaticum	Sometimes pathogenic	Uncommon
RUNYON GROUP II		
M. szulgae	Usually pathogenic	Uncommon
M. scrofulaceum	Sometimes pathogenic	Uncommon
M. xenopi	Sometimes pathogenic	Uncommon
M. gordonae	Nonpathogen	Common
M. flavescens	Nonpathogen	Uncommon
RUNYON GROUP III		
M. haemophilum	Strictly pathogenic	Uncommon
M. malmoense	Strictly pathogenic	Uncommon
M. shimoidei	Strictly pathogenic	Uncommon
M. avium	Usually pathogenic	Common
M. intracellulare	Usually pathogenic	Common
M. gastri	Nonpathogenic	Uncommon
M. nonchromogen	Nonpathogenic	Uncommon
M. terrae complex	Nonpathogenic	Uncommon
RUNYON GROUP IV		
M. abscessus	Sometimes pathogenic	Uncommon
M. fortuitum	Sometimes pathogenic	Common
M. chelonae	Sometimes pathogenic	Common
M. phlei	Nonpathogenic	Uncommon
M. smegmatis	Nonpathogenic	Uncommon
M. vaccae	Nonpathogenic	Uncommon

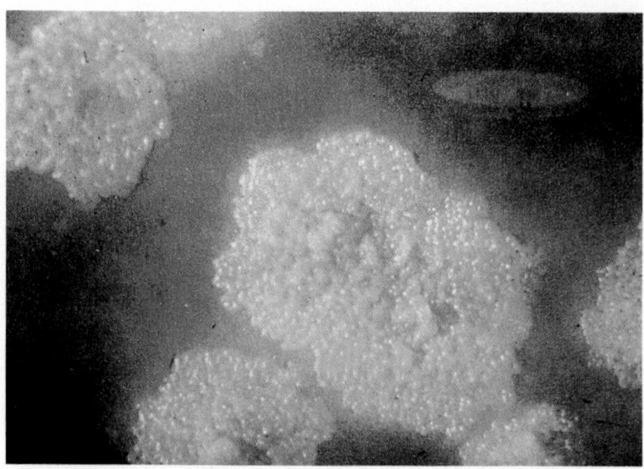

FIGURE 35-2 *M. tuberculosis* colonies on Lowenstein-Jensen agar after 8 weeks of incubation. (From Baron EJ and Finegold SM: *Bailey and Scott's diagnostic microbiology*, ed 7, St Louis, 1986, Mosby.)

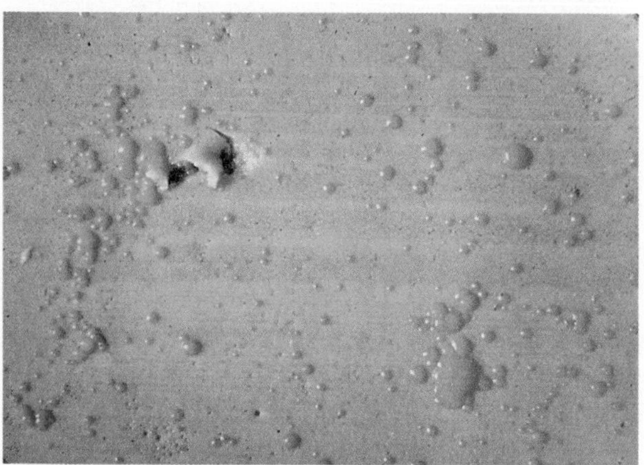

FIGURE 35-3 *M. kansasii* colonies on Middlebrook agar 1 day after exposure to light. (From Baron EJ and Finegold SM: *Bailey and Scott's diagnostic microbiology*, ed 7, St Louis, 1986, Mosby.)

mycobacteria are classified as Runyon group III, whereas the relatively rapidly growing, nonpigmented mycobacteria are classified as Runyon group IV. The **Runyon classification** can be used to differentiate the most common mycobacterial isolates (Table 35-1).

PATHOGENESIS AND IMMUNITY

Mycobacterium tuberculosis

Tissue destruction and fibrosis characteristically observed in mycobacterial disease is caused by the host response to infection; no known mycobacterial toxin or enzyme has been associated with tissue destruction. Because mycobacteria are intracellular pathogens, they are able to evade the natural immune response of the patient.

Tuberculosis is the classic human mycobacterial disease. The route of infection is inhalation of infectious aerosols, which are able to reach the terminal airways. Following engulfment by alveolar macrophages, these intracellular pathogens replicate freely in the cell because they evade phagocytic destruction by inhibiting phagolysosome fusion. The infected phagocytic cells are eventually destroyed. This process is followed by further cycles of phagocytosis by macrophages, mycobacterial replication, and cell lysis. Although phagocytosis is initiated by alveolar macrophages, circulating macrophages and lymphocytes are attracted to the infectious focus by the bacilli, cellular debris, and host chemotactic factors (e.g., complement component C5a). The histological characteristic of this focus is formation of multinucleated giant cells of fused macrophages, also called **"Langhans' cells."** Infected macrophages can also spread during the initial phase of disease to the local lymph nodes, as well as into the bloodstream and other tissues (e.g., bone marrow, spleen, kidneys, bone, central nervous system).

Two to four weeks after the process is initiated, CD4 T-cell derived cytokines activate the circulating macrophages, rendering them capable of bacterial killing. If a small antigenic burden is present at the time the macrophages are activated, then destruction of bacilli occurs with minimal tissue damage. However, if large numbers of bacilli are present, then the cellular immune response results in tissue necrosis. Multiple host factors are involved, including cytokine toxicity, local activation of the complement cascade, ischemia, and exposure to macrophage-derived hydrolytic enzymes and reactive oxygen intermediates. The effectiveness of bacillary elimination is in part related to the size of the focus of infection. Localized collections of activated macrophages (granulomas) prevent further spread of the bacilli. Macrophages can penetrate into small granulomas (less than 3 mm) and kill all bacilli. However, larger necrotic or caseous granulomas become encapsulated with fibrin, effectively protecting the bacilli from macrophage killing. The bacilli can remain dormant in this stage; however, quiescent bacilli can be reactivated years later when the patient's immunological responsiveness wanes, either because of old age or immunosuppressive disease or therapy.

Mycobacterium leprae

Leprosy or **Hansen's disease** is caused by *M. leprae*. The clinical presentation of leprosy is subdivided into tuberculoid leprosy and lepromatous leprosy, with intermediate forms also recognized. As observed with *M. tuberculosis*, the clinical manifestations of leprosy are due to the patient's immune reaction to the bacilli. Patients with **tuberculoid leprosy** have a strong delayed hypersensitivity reaction but a weak humoral antibody response. Infected foci are characterized by large numbers of lymphocytes and granulomas. Relatively few bacilli are seen in the tissues because production of cytokines (e.g., gamma interferon, interleukin-2) mediates macrophage activation, phagocytosis, and bacillary clearance. In contrast, patients with **lepromatous leprosy** have a strong antibody response but have a specific defect in their

BOX 35-1 Epidemiology of *Mycobacterium* Infection

DISEASE/BACTERIAL FACTORS

Localized pulmonary infections or dissemination to other body sites such as kidneys, meninges, skin, CNS; primary skin infections observed with some mycobacteria

Lipid-rich cell wall makes mycobacteria resistant to disinfectants

M. tuberculosis evades phagocytic destruction by inhibiting phagolysosome fusion

M. tuberculosis encapsulated with fibrin can remain dormant in tissue to be reactivated at a later time

Host's cellular immune response to the mycobacterium causes clinical disease

Humans are only natural reservoir for *M. tuberculosis*

TRANSMISSION

M. tuberculosis: person to person through inhalation of infectious aerosols

M. bovis: ingestion of contaminated milk

M. avium-intracellulare: inhalation or ingestion

M. leprae: person to person via inhalation or skin contact

M. fortuitum and *M. chelonae*: via trauma or IV catheters, contaminated wound dressings, contaminated prostheses

WHO IS AT RISK?

Anyone exposed to person with active tuberculosis, particularly immunocompromised patients (especially those with AIDS), the homeless, drug and alcohol abusers, and prisoners

M. avium-intracellulare infections in immunocompromised patients (e.g., AIDS) or persons with long-standing pulmonary disease

Persons exposed to *M. fortuitum* or *M. chelonae* through trauma

GEOGRAPHY/SEASON

Worldwide; frequency in the United States given in Table 35-1

No seasonal incidence

MODES OF CONTROL

Therapy for all infections must be prolonged (e.g., 6 months or longer)

Multiple antibiotics should be administered simultaneously to prevent development of resistance

M. tuberculosis: prophylaxis with isoniazid for 1 year in patients exposed to this species

M. leprae: dapsone, rifampin, and either clofazimine or ethionamide for a minimum of 2 years

M. fortuitum and *M. chelonae*: therapy with selected antibiotics and surgical intervention

Isolation and prophylactic antibiotics required only for close contacts of patients with *M. tuberculosis* complex infections

Vaccination with BCG used as immunoprophylaxis for human disease

For adequate control of tuberculosis, public health measures must be implemented to ensure patients receive a complete course of therapy

M. bovis: control of disease in herds reduces human exposure

cellular response to *M. leprae* antigens. Thus large numbers of bacilli are typically observed in dermal macrophages and Schwann cells of the peripheral nerves. This is the most infectious form of leprosy.

Other Mycobacteria

The histological hallmark of tuberculosis (granulomatous inflammation) is seen with other mycobacterial infections. Mycobacteria such as *M. kansasii* and *M. avium-intracellulare* can cause localized pulmonary infections clinically indistinguishable from *M. tuberculosis*, or disseminated infections with virtually every organ tissue infected. Overwhelming disseminated infections with *M. avium-intracellulare* is particularly common in AIDS patients in the terminal stages of their disease.

Infections with *M. marinum* and *M. ulcerans* are generally restricted to the skin surfaces because these organisms grow preferentially at cool temperatures. *M. haemophilum* also prefers growth in vitro at cooler temperatures and was initially associated with infections restricted to the skin surfaces. However, more recent evidence indicates that this organism can also cause disseminated infections. *M. fortuitum*, *M. chelonae*, and *M. abscessus* rarely cause disseminated infections because these mycobacteria are relatively avirulent.

EPIDEMIOLOGY

Mycobacterium tuberculosis

Tuberculosis can be established in primates and laboratory animals such as guinea pigs; however, humans are the only natural reservoir (Box 35-1). The disease is spread by close person-to-person contact through inhalation of infectious aerosols. Large particles are trapped on mucosal surfaces and removed by ciliary action of the respiratory tree. Small particles, however, containing 1 to 3 tubercle bacilli can reach the alveolar spaces. Although alveolar macrophages can engulf and destroy the bacilli, exposure to relatively few organisms (e.g., 5 to 200 organisms) can establish infection.

It is estimated that 1.7 billion people, including 10 million in the United States, are infected with *M. tuberculosis*. Eight million new cases of disease and 3 million deaths are reported worldwide. Since 1984 the downward trend of tuberculosis in the United States has reversed, with dramatic increases observed in recent years

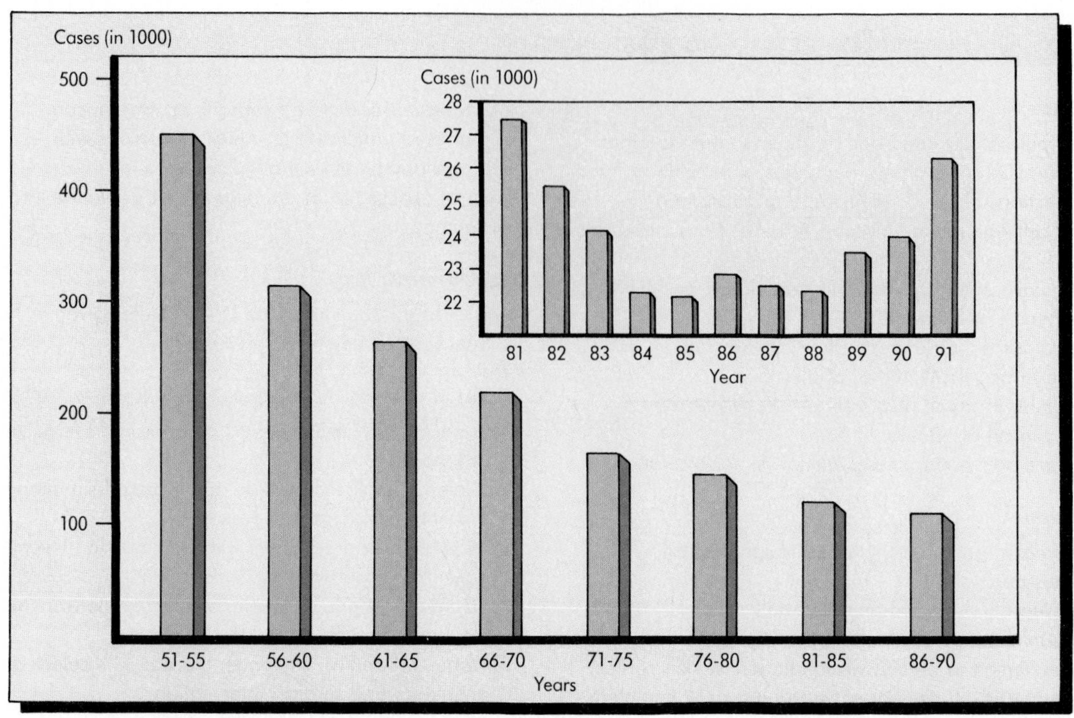

FIGURE 35-4 Incidence of new cases of *M. tuberculosis* in the United States since 1951; the annual incidence of disease since 1981 is summarized in the insert. (From *MMWR* 402:1992.)

(Figure 35-4). This problem is attributed to increased infections in the homeless, drug and alcohol abusers, prisoners, and AIDS patients. Because disease in these patients is difficult to eradicate, spread into other populations including health care workers poses a significant public health problem. This is particularly true with drug-resistant *M. tuberculosis,* in which inadequately treated patients may remain infectious for a prolonged period.

Mycobacterium bovis

M. bovis can infect a variety of animals, with cattle the most significant source of human exposure. Bovine tuberculosis is rarely seen in the United States because disease in animal herds is controlled by vaccination of healthy animals, quarantine and destruction of infected herds, and pasteurization of milk. In contrast with *M. tuberculosis,* most infections with *M. bovis* follow consumption of contaminated milk.

Mycobacterium avium-intracellulare Complex

These species are generally considered together because differentiation by physiological parameters is difficult and their diseases in humans are identical. The organisms are isolated in soil and water, as well as infected poultry, swine, and other animals. Although human exposure is common, significant human disease is rare, except in immunocompromised patients. Patients with AIDS are at particular risk for disseminated disease with these mycobacteria (Figure 35-5). Infection in patients with AIDS is believed to be primarily by ingestion of contaminated food or water. Disease initiated by inhalation of the organism is probably less common. Person-to-person spread does not occur.

Mycobacterium leprae

Leprosy is a relatively rare mycobacterial disease in the United States; approximately 250 cases are reported annually. More than 12 million cases worldwide are recognized, with 62% of these infections in Asia and 34% in Africa. Fewer than 10% of the infections in the United States are in native-born Americans, with most infections in immigrants from Mexico, Asia, the Pacific Islands, and Africa. The largest number of cases in the United States are reported in California, Hawaii, and Texas; leprosy is endemic in these states, as well as Louisiana. Endemic disease has also been demonstrated in armadillos.

Disease is spread by person-to-person contact. Although the most important route of infection is unknown, it is believed that *M. leprae* can be spread by either inhalation of infectious aerosols or skin contact with respiratory secretions, wound exudates, or arthropod vectors. Large numbers of *M. leprae* are observed in nasal secretions in patients with lepromatous leprosy.

Other Mycobacteria

Most other mycobacteria associated with human disease are isolated from environmental sources and acquired either by inhalation or trauma. Person-to-person spread is not observed.

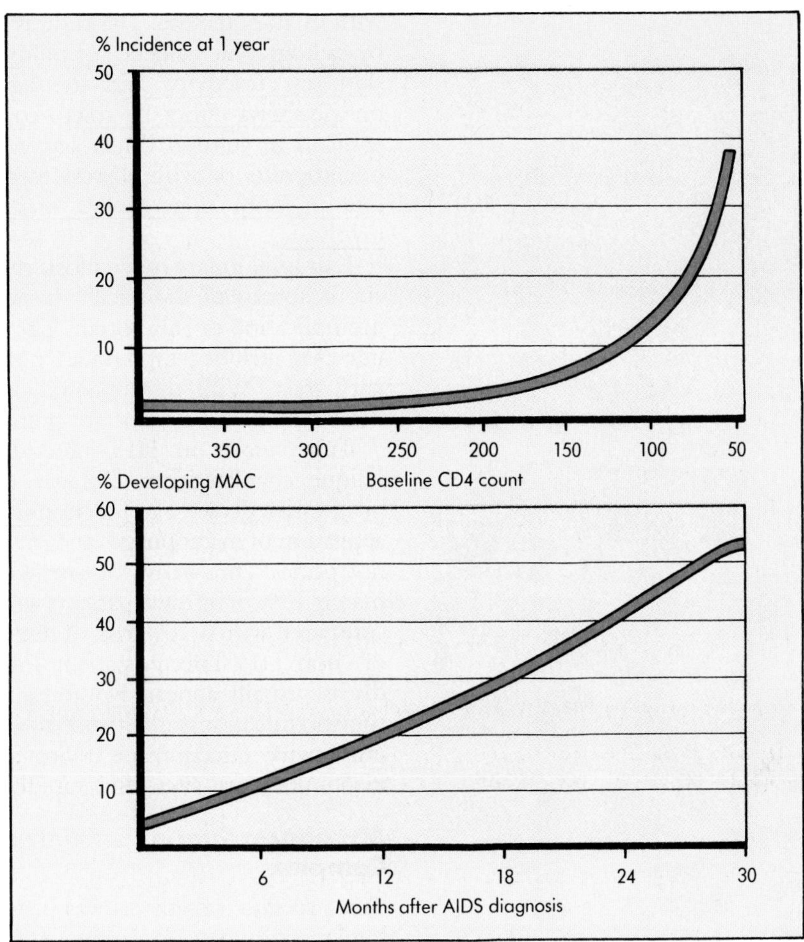

FIGURE 35-5 The incidence of *M. avium-intracellulare* infections in AIDS patients progressively increases as their CD4 lymphocyte counts decrease (*top*) and in the terminal stages of their illness (*bottom*). (Redrawn from Nightingale S. et al: *J Infect Dis* 165:1082, 1992).

CLINICAL SYNDROMES

Mycobacterium tuberculosis

Tuberculosis can involve any organ, although most infections are restricted to the lungs (Box 35-2). Infection is initiated after inhalation of contaminated aerosol droplets. The initial pulmonary focus is the middle or lower lung fields, where the tubercle bacilli can multiply freely. Within 3 to 6 weeks the patient's cellular immunity is activated and mycobacterial replication ceases in most patients. However, approximately 5% of patients exposed to *M. tuberculosis* will progress to active disease within 2 years, and another 5% to 10% will develop disease sometime later in life.

The clinical signs and symptoms of tuberculosis reflect the site of infection, with primary disease usually restricted to the lower respiratory tract. The onset is generally insidious, with nonspecific complaints of malaise, weight loss, cough, and night sweats. Sputum production may be scant or bloody and purulent. Sputum production and hemoptysis is usually associated

BOX 35-2 Clinical Syndromes

Mycobacterium tuberculosis
- Pulmonary tuberculosis
- Extrapulmonary tuberculosis
- Tuberculosis in HIV-infected patients

Mycobacterium avium-intracellulare complex
- Asymptomatic colonization
- Pulmonary disease
- Disseminated disease in HIV-infected patients

Mycobacterium leprae
- Tuberculoid leprosy
- Lepromatous leprosy

Other mycobacteria
- Pulmonary disease (e.g., *M. kansasii*)
- Cutaneous disease (e.g., *M. marinum, M. ulcerans, M. fortuitum-chelonae*)

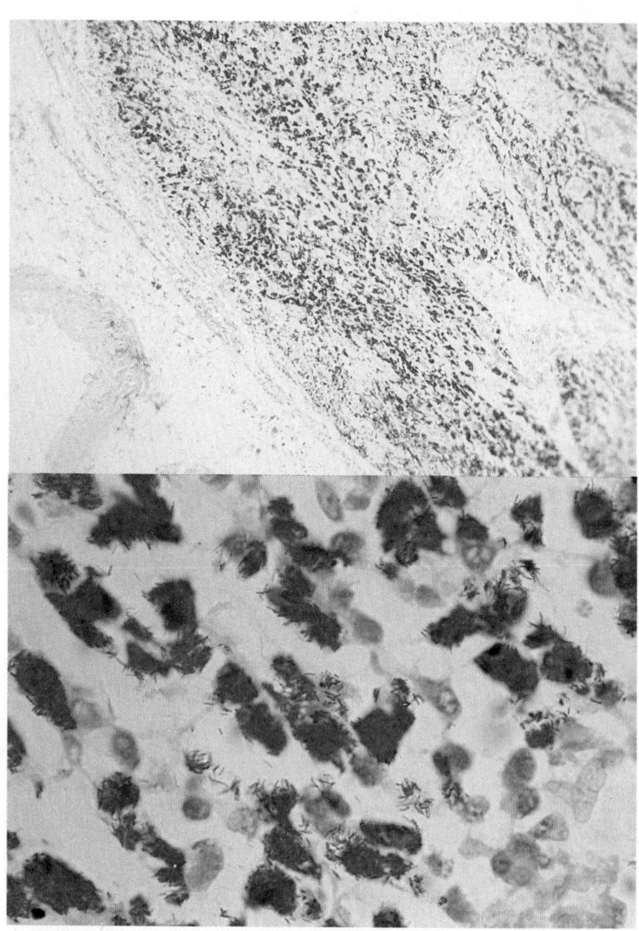

FIGURE 35-6 *M. avium-intracellulare*–infected tissue from an AIDS patient photographed under low (*top*) and high (*bottom*) magnification.

with cavitary disease. The clinical diagnosis is supported by radiographic evidence of pulmonary disease, positive skin test reactivity, and the laboratory detection of mycobacteria either by microscopy or isolation of organisms in culture. When active disease develops with pneumonitis or with abscess formation and cavitation, one or both upper lobes of the lungs are usually involved.

Extrapulmonary tuberculosis resulting from hematogenous spread of the bacilli during the initial phase of multiplication can also occur. The most common sites of infection include lymph nodes, pleura, and the genitourinary tract. With disseminated or miliary tuberculosis there may be no evidence of pulmonary disease.

Tuberculosis in HIV-infected patients has several unique characteristics. Because these patients have a progressive decrease in functioning CD4 T lymphocytes, activation of macrophages and mycobacterial killing does not occur. Thus active disease will develop in approximately 10% of infected patients within 1 year of exposure, compared with a 10% risk of disease during the lifetime of a non–HIV-infected patient. In HIV-infected patients, disease usually appears before the onset of other opportunistic infections, is difficult to distinguish from other pulmonary infections, is twice as likely to spread to extrapulmonary sites, and rapidly progresses to death.

Mycobacterium avium-intracellulare Complex

This group of organisms was historically an uncommon human pathogen. Isolation of *M. avium-intracellulare* frequently represented transient colonization in asymptomatic patients. When disease was observed, it was generally restricted to patients with compromised immune functions and was clinically identical to tuberculo-

TABLE 35-2 Clinical and Immunological Manifestations of Leprosy

	Tuberculoid	Lepromatous
Skin lesions	Few erythematous or hypopigmented plaques with flat centers and raised, demarcated borders; peripheral nerve damaged with complete sensory loss; nerves visibly enlarged	Many erythematous macules, papules, or nodules; extensive tissue destruction (e.g., nasal cartilage and bone, ears); diffuse nerve involvement with patchy sensory loss; nerves not enlarged
Histopathology	Infiltration of lymphocytes around center of epithelial cells; Langhans cells present; few or no acid-fast bacilli present	Predominantly "foamy" macrophages with few lymphocytes; Langhans cells absent; acid-fast bacilli abundant in skin lesions and internal organs
Infectivity	Low	High
Immune response		
Delayed hypersensitivity	Reactivity to lepromin	Nonreactive to lepromin
Immunoglobulin levels	Normal	Polyclonal hypergammaglobulinemia
Erythema nodosum leprosum	Absent	Usually present

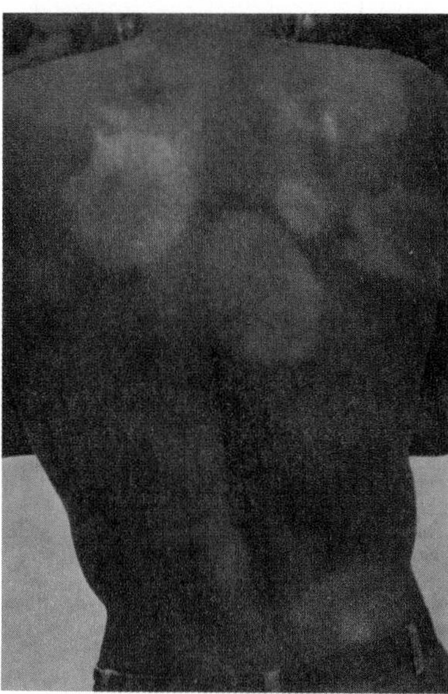

FIGURE 35-7 Tuberculoid leprosy. Early tuberculoid lesions are characterized by anesthetic macules with hypopigmentation. (From Peters W and Gilles HM: *A colour atlas of tropical medicine and parasitology,* ed 3, London, 1989, Wolfe Medical Publications.)

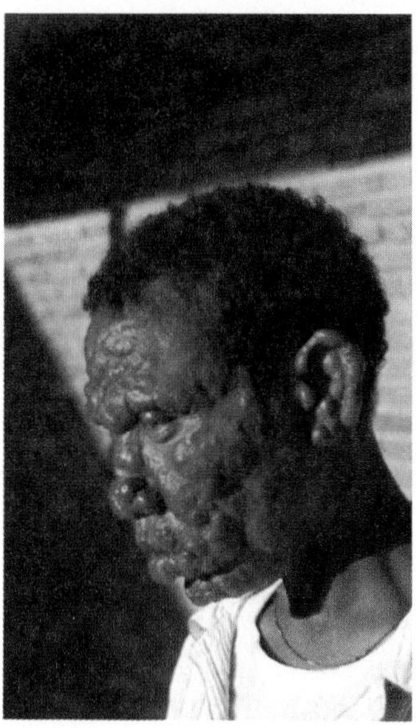

FIGURE 35-8 Lepromatous leprosy with extensive infiltration, edema, and corrugation of the face. Note the depilation of the eyebrows and face, and thickening of the ear. (From Peters W and Gilles HM: *A colour atlas of tropical medicine and parasitology,* ed 3, London, 1989, Wolfe Medical Publications.)

sis, with pulmonary disease seen most frequently. More recently these organisms have assumed increased importance. They are now the most common mycobacterial isolates in many clinical laboratories because they are the major mycobacterial pathogen in AIDS patients seen in the United States. In contrast with disease in other groups of patients, *M. avium-intracellulare* infection in AIDS patients is typically disseminated, with virtually no organ spared. The magnitude of these infections is remarkable, with the tissues of some patients literally filled with the mycobacteria (Figure 35-6) and hundreds to thousands of bacilli per milliliter of blood.

Mycobacterium leprae

The clinical presentation of leprosy ranges from the tuberculoid to the lepromatous forms, with characteristic clinical and immunological manifestations (Table 35-2; Figures 35-7 and 35-8). Lepromatous leprosy is the form characteristically associated with disfiguring skin lesions.

Other Mycobacteria

M. kansasii is the most common photochromogen responsible for human disease. Isolation from respiratory specimens can represent transient colonization or significant pulmonary disease. Chronic pulmonary disease is the most common presentation of *M. kansasii* infection, although disseminated disease in immunocompromised patients is also seen.

M. marinum and *M. ulcerans* grow preferentially at cooler temperatures; thus they usually cause disease restricted to the skin. *M. marinum* infections are acquired by contact with contaminated fresh water or salt water. For this reason these infections are termed **"swimming pool granulomas."** Cutaneous infection may be seen either as a nodular lesion that progresses to ulceration or as a series of nodular lesions along the lymphatics draining the area of primary ulceration. This latter appearance resembles cutaneous disease produced by the fungus *Sporothrix schenckii. M. ulcerans* infections are restricted primarily to Africa, Mexico, and Australia. The infection initially is seen as a subcutaneous nodule that ulcerates. The indolent infection can progress over a period of months, with involvement of the subcutaneous tissues and extensive ulceration.

The rapidly growing mycobacteria (e.g., *M. fortuitum* and *M. chelonae*) are most commonly associated with disease following the introduction of bacteria into the deep subcutaneous tissues by trauma or iatrogenically (e.g., infections introduced with a intravenous catheter, contaminated wound dressing, or prosthetic device such as a heart valve). Unfortunately, infections with these organisms are increasing as more invasive procedures are performed on hospitalized patients and advanced medical care is able to extend the survival of immunocompromised patients.

LABORATORY DIAGNOSIS

Skin Test

Reactivity to intradermal injection of mycobacterial antigens can differentiate between infected and noninfected individuals (Box 35-3). In most patients the only evidence of infection with mycobacteria is a lifelong

BOX 35-3 Laboratory Diagnosis

Skin test
Microscopy
- Carbol fuchsin stains
- Fluorochrome stains

Culture
- Agar and egg media
- Broth media

Nucleic acid probes
Preliminary identification using growth properties and morphology
Definitive identification
- Biochemical tests
- Chromatographic analysis of cell wall lipids

Serology

positive skin test and radiographic evidence of calcification of the initial active foci in the lungs or other organs. Tests with antigens extracted from *M. tuberculosis* have been used most commonly and are best standardized, although skin tests with species-specific antigens from other mycobacteria have also been developed.

The methods of antigen preparation and skin inoculation have undergone a number of changes since the tests were first developed. The currently recommended tuberculin antigen is the "purified protein derivative" **(PPD)** of the cell wall. Tuberculin can be inoculated into the intradermal layer of skin by either intradermal injection of a specific amount of antigen or by placing a drop of the antigen on the skin surface and then injecting the antigen via a multiprong inoculator **(tine test).** The latter test is not recommended because the amount of antigen injected into the intradermal layer cannot be accurately controlled.

Skin test reactivity is measured 48 hours after intradermal infection of 0.1 μg of PPD (5 tuberculin units). Although a reaction of 10 mm or more induration was previously considered positive for exposure to *M. tuberculosis*, the current definition of positive reactivity will vary in different populations (Table 35-3). A positive PPD reaction usually develops within 3 to 4 weeks after exposure. Exposure to other mycobacteria may lead to reactivity with tuberculin, but this is generally less than 10 mm induration. Patients infected with *M. tuberculosis* may not respond to tuberculin skin testing if they are anergic (particularly true in HIV-infected patients); thus control antigens should always be used with tuberculin tests.

TABLE 35-3 Criteria Defining Positive PPD Reactivity in Patients Exposed to *Mycobacterium tuberculosis*

Reactivity to PPD (mm of induration)	Populations
≥5 mm	Very high-risk persons including: HIV-infected patients* Persons with abnormal chest roentgenograms Recent contacts of patients with tuberculosis
≥10 mm	Other high-risk persons including: Foreign-born individuals HIV-negative intravenous drug users Medically underserved, low-income persons Residents of long-term care facilities Immunocompromised patients
≥15 mm	All other persons

*It has been proposed that ≥2 mm should be used for these patients.

Microscopy

The microscopic detection of acid-fast bacilli in clinical specimens is the most rapid method for confirming mycobacterial disease. The clinical specimen is stained with either carbol fuchsin (Ziehl-Neelsen and Kinyoun stains) or fluorochrome dyes (e.g., Truant auramine-rhodamine), decolorized with acid-alcohol solution, and then counterstained. The specimens are then examined with either a light microscope or, if fluorochrome dyes are used, a fluorescent microscope (Figures 35-9 and 35-10). The fluorochrome stain is more sensitive because the specimen can be rapidly scanned for fluorescence with low magnification and then confirmed using higher magnification.

Approximately one third to one half of all culture-positive specimens will have a positive acid-fast stain. The test sensitivity is improved with respiratory specimens (particularly from patients with radiographic evidence of cavitation) and specimens with large numbers of mycobacteria isolated in culture. The test specificity is greater than 95% when carefully performed.

Culture

Patients with pulmonary tuberculosis, particularly cavitary disease, can have large numbers of organisms in their respiratory secretions (e.g., 10^8 bacilli or more). A positive culture will be obtained in virtually all patients with active pulmonary disease if an early morning sputum is collected for 3 consecutive days. Recovery of *M. tuberculosis* from other sites in disseminated disease (e.g., genitourinary tract, cerebrospinal fluid) is more difficult and requires collection of additional cultures and processing a large volume of fluid.

Isolation of mycobacteria from clinical specimens is complicated by the fact that most isolates grow slowly and can be obscured by the rapidly growing bacteria normally present in clinical specimens. Thus specimens such as sputum are initially treated with a decontaminating

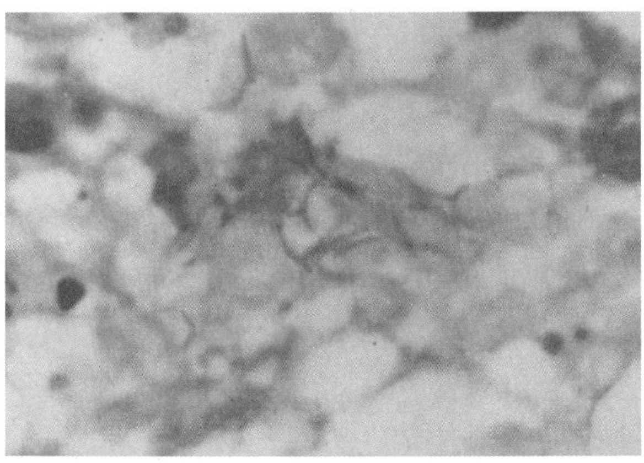

FIGURE 35-9 Acid-fast stain of *M. tuberculosis* stained by the Kinyoun method with carbolfuchsin.

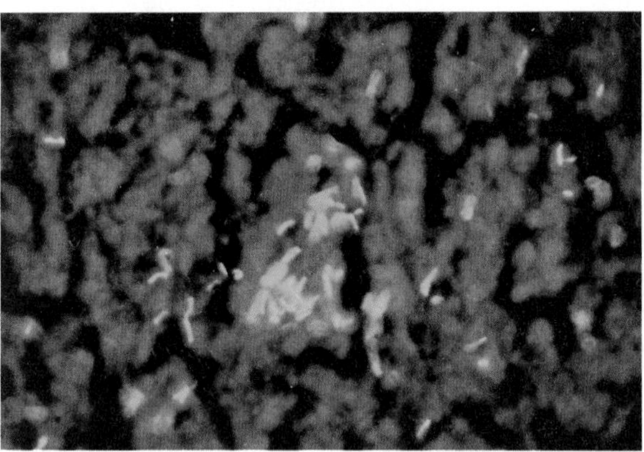

FIGURE 35-10 Acid-fast stain of *M. tuberculosis* stained by the Truant fluorochrome method with the fluorescent dyes auramine and rhodamine.

reagent (e.g., 2% sodium hydroxide). Because mycobacteria are tolerant to brief alkali treatment, this process kills the rapidly growing bacteria and permits the selective isolation of mycobacteria. Extended decontamination of the specimen will kill mycobacteria, so the procedure is not performed with normally sterile specimens or when small numbers of mycobacteria are expected.

Specimens traditionally are inoculated onto both egg-based (e.g., Lowenstein-Jensen) and agar-based (e.g., Middlebrook) media. Detection of *M. tuberculosis, M. avium-intracellulare,* and other important slow-growing mycobacteria on these solid media generally requires prolonged incubation. However, this detection time has recently been shortened by the use of specially formulated broth cultures in which the metabolism of palmitic acid and production of CO_2 can be detected (Figure 35-11).

Nucleic Acid Probes

Molecular probes have been developed to detect nucleic acid sequences specific for mycobacteria. This approach has been very successful for the identification of *M. tuberculosis* and *M. avium-intracellulare* isolated in culture. Through the use of gene amplification, it is anticipated that mycobacteria will soon be detected directly in clinical specimens.

Preliminary Identification

Growth properties and colonial morphology can be used for the preliminary identification of the most common species of mycobacteria. This is important because person-to-person transmission occurs only with mycobacteria in the *M. tuberculosis* complex. Thus isolation of patients and prophylactic antibiotics for close contacts are required only for infections with these organisms. The preliminary identification of an isolate can also be used to guide empirical antimicrobial therapy.

Definitive Identification

The definitive identification of many mycobacteria requires the use of selected biochemical tests (Table 35-4). Key tests for the identification of *M. tuberculosis* include production of niacin and nitrate reductase. Unfortunately, biochemical identification of mycobacteria requires 3 weeks or more before results are available. Mycobacterial species can also be identified by chromatographic analysis of their cell wall lipids. Characteristic lipids profiles have been determined for most species.

M. leprae cannot be grown in cell-free cultures. Thus laboratory confirmation of leprosy requires histopathology consistent with clinical disease and skin test reactivity to lepromin or the presence of acid-fast bacilli in the lesions.

Serology

A number of tests (e.g., RIA, ELISA, latex agglutination) have been developed for the serologic diagnosis of active mycobacterial disease. Unfortunately, tests for the detection of mycobacterial antigens or specific antibody are insensitive and nonspecific. Somewhat better success has been achieved with the use of highly purified antigens in the diagnosis of tuberculous meningitis. However, these tests are useful only in chronic, extensive disease. Further work is necessary before mycobacterial serology can be recommended as a diagnostic tool.

TREATMENT, PREVENTION, AND CONTROL

Treatment

Most mycobacteria are resistant to antibiotics used to treat other bacterial infections. Effective therapy for infection with *M. tuberculosis* requires use of multiple antimycobacterial agents to avoid the selection of resistant organisms during treatment. Because mycobacteria multiply slowly, treatment has traditionally been for 18 to 24 months, although recent studies indicate that therapy for 6 to 9 months is effective. The currently recommended treatment regimen is isoniazid (INH), rifampin, and pyrazinamide for 2 months followed by an additional 4 months of therapy with INH and rifampin alone. For

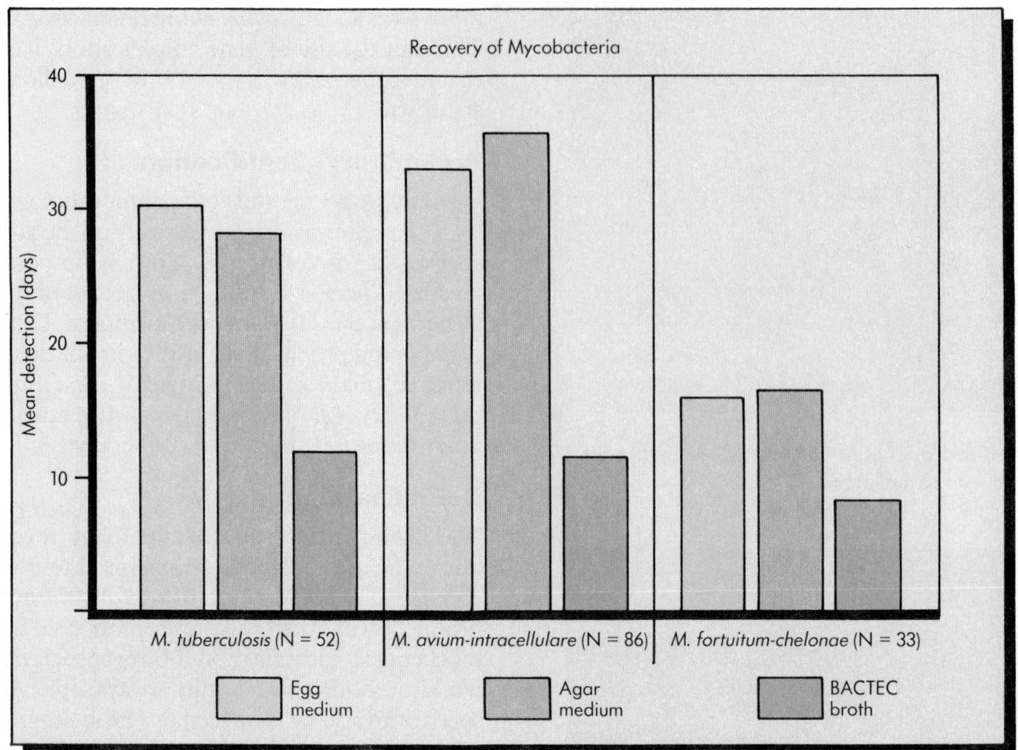

FIGURE 35-11 Detection of mycobacteria can occur 1 to 5 weeks faster in broth medium compared with solid-egg or agar media. This approach to culture became practical when methods were developed to inhibit the growth of contaminating organisms and detect the growth of mycobacteria. (*n*, number of isolates over a 9-month period at Barnes Hospital, St. Louis, Mo.)

TABLE 35-4 Selected Biochemical Reactions for Five Commonly Isolated Mycobacteria

Organism	Niacin	Nitrate reductase	Heat-stable catalase	Tween-80 hydrolysis	Iron uptake	Arylsulfatase	Urease
M. tuberculosis	+	+	−	−		−	+
M. kansasii	−	+	+	+		−	+
M. avium-intracellulare	−	−	±	−		−	−
M. fortuitum	−	+	+	V	+	+	+
M. chelonae	V*	−	V	V	−	+	+

Modified from Lennette EH, Balows A, Hausler WJ Jr, and Shadomy HJ, editors: *Manual of clinical microbiology*, ed 4, Washington DC, 1985, American Society for Microbiology.
**V*, variable.

treatment of HIV-infected patients, treatment with INH and rifampin should be extended for at least 3 more months. In 1990 the first outbreaks of multi–drug-resistant *M. tuberculosis* were reported in AIDS patients and the homeless in New York and Miami. Unless these strains can be eliminated, treatment of tuberculosis will become significantly more difficult.

M. avium-intracellulare is resistant to most common antimycobacterial agents. Effective therapy requires prolonged use of a combination of primary or secondary drugs demonstrated to be active in vitro. Unfortunately, the toxic effects of many of these therapeutic combinations are significant.

In contrast with related species, the rapidly growing mycobacteria associated with human disease (e.g., *M. fortuitum* and *M. chelonae*) are resistant to most commonly used antimycobacterial agents. However, they are susceptible to some aminoglycosides, cephalosporins, tetracyclines, and quinolones. The specific activity of these agents must be determined by in vitro tests. Because

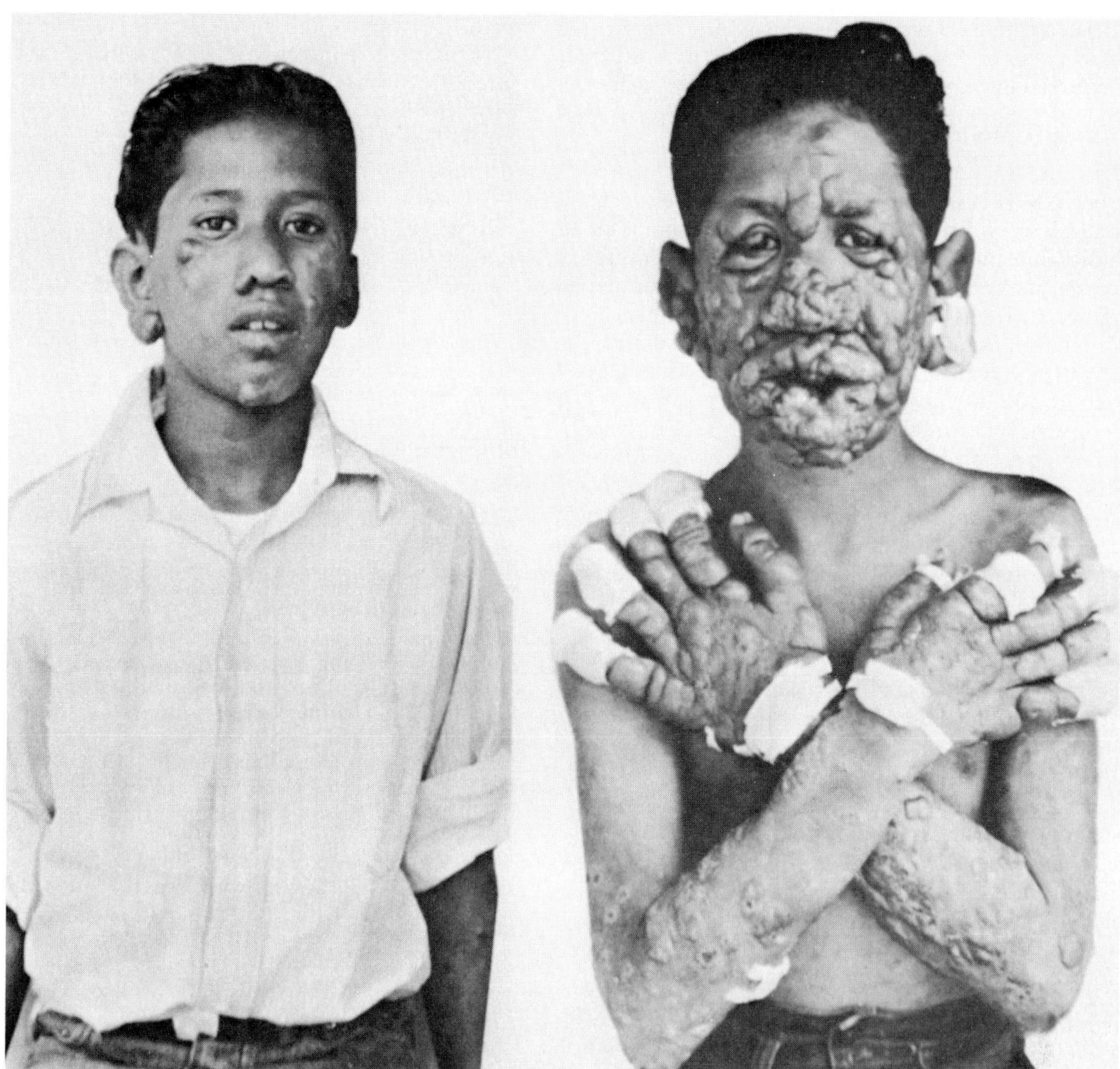

FIGURE 35-12 The photograph on the left shows the 13-year-old Hawaiian boy with leprosy in 1931. The photograph to the right was taken in 1933. If antibiotics had been available, the disease would not have progressed but would have regressed and probably become bacteriologically negative after several years of treatment. (From Binford CH and Connor DH: *Pathology of tropical and extraordinary diseases: an atlas*, Washington, DC, 1976, Armed Forces Institute of Pathology.)

infections with these mycobacteria are generally confined to the skin or associated with prosthetic devices, surgical intervention is also necessary.

Treatment of *M. leprae* infections is based on clinical experience because in vitro testing is not possible and in vivo testing with animal models (e.g., mouse foot pad inoculations) is not practical. Drug resistance develops rapidly if a single agent is used. Therefore it is recommended that primary therapy consist of dapsone, rifampin, and either clofazimine or ethionamide. If this disease is diagnosed early in its course and if treatment is initiated promptly, clinical response is satisfactory. However, delays in treatment can be devastating (Figure 35-12). Therapy is administered for a minimum of 2 years and can be lifelong in some patients.

Chemoprophylaxis

Prophylaxis with INH for 1 year is advocated for individuals with significant exposure to drug-susceptible *M. tuberculosis* or recent conversion of skin test reactivity. Prophylactic regimens for exposure to drug-resistant tuberculosis are being evaluated. In reality, this approach is aimed at treating subclinical infection rather than prophylaxis. Hepatotoxicity, particularly in older persons, is associated with INH prophylaxis. Chemoprophylaxis is unnecessary for persons exposed to patients with other mycobacterial infections.

Immunoprophylaxis

Vaccination with attenuated *M. bovis* (bacille Calmette-Guerin [**BCG**]) is commonly used in countries where tuberculosis is endemic and responsible for significant morbidity and mortality. This vaccination significantly reduces the incidence of tuberculosis if administered at a young age (it is less effective in adults). Unfortunately, BCG immunization cannot be used in immunocompromised patients (e.g., HIV-infected patients). Thus it is unlikely to be useful in controlling the spread of drug-resistant tuberculosis. An additional problem with BCG immunization is that all patients develop positive skin test reactivity; thus skin testing cannot be used to detect previous exposure to *M. tuberculosis.* For these reasons BCG is not in widespread use in the United States or in other countries where the incidence of tuberculosis is low.

Control

Public health projections estimated the elimination of tuberculosis in the United States by the end of the twentieth century. This seemed reasonable until the mid-1980s, when a dramatic change in the incidence of disease occurred (see Figure 35-4). With the prevalence of disease now increasing in immunocompromised patients, as well as in the homeless and abusers of drugs or alcohol, control of tuberculosis is both a medical and social problem. A high index of clinical suspicion combined with rapid diagnostic tests is required for the prompt initiation of appropriate therapy. Social changes will be required to ensure all patients are treated for a minimum of 6 to 9 months.

CASE STUDY AND QUESTIONS

A 35-year-old man with a history of intravenous drug use entered the local health clinic with complaints of a dry persistent cough, fever, malaise, and anorexia. Over the preceding 4 weeks the patient had lost 15 pounds and had experienced chills and sweats. The chest radiograph revealed patchy infiltrates throughout the lung fields. Because the patient had a nonproductive cough, sputum was induced and submitted for bacterial, fungal, and mycobacterial cultures, as well as examination for *Pneumocystis*. Blood cultures were performed, as well as serologic tests for HIV infection. The patient was HIV positive. *Pneumocystis* testing was negative, as were all cultures after 2 days of incubation; however, cultures were positive for *M. tuberculosis* after an additional 1 week of incubation.

1. How does the presentation of *M. tuberculosis* and *M. avium-intracellulare* infections differ in HIV-infected patients? Why is *M. tuberculosis* more virulent in HIV-infected patients compared with non–HIV-infected patients?
2. How does the composition of the mycobacterial cell wall affect the staining properties of this group of organisms?
3. What are the two clinical presentations of *M. leprae* infections? How do the diagnostic tests differ for these two presentations?
4. What is the definition of a positive skin test (PPD) for *M. tuberculosis*?
5. Why do mycobacterial infections have to be treated for 6 months or more?

Bibliography

Binford CH and Connor DH, editors: *Pathology of tropical and extraordinary diseases: an atlas,* Washington, DC, 1976, Armed Forces Institute of Pathology.

Brennan PJ: Structure of mycobacteria: recent developments in defining cell wall carbohydrates and proteins, *Rev Infect Dis* 11(suppl 2):420-430, 1989.

Brudney K and Dobkin J: Resurgent tuberculosis in New York City: human immunodeficiency virus, homeless, and the decline of tuberculosis control programs, *Am Rev Respir Dis* 144:745-749, 1991.

Chaisson RE and Slutkin G: Tuberculosis and human immunodeficiency virus infection, J Infect Dis 159:96-100.

Cohn ZA and Kaplan G: Hansen's disease, cell-mediated immunity, and recombinant lymphokines, *J Infect Dis* 163:1195-1200, 1991.

Collins FM: Mycobacterial disease, immunosuppressions, and acquired immunodeficiency syndrome, *Clin Microbiol Rev* 2:360-377, 1989.

Dannenberg AM: Immune mechanisms in the pathogenesis of pulmonary tuberculosis, *Rev Infect Dis* 11(suppl 2): 3369-3378, 1989.

Davidson PT: Tuberculosis: new views of an old disease, *N Engl J Med* 312:1514-1515, 1985.

Hastings RC, Gillis TP, Krahenbuhl JL, and Franzblau SG: Leprosy, *Clin Microbiol Rev* 1:330-348, 1988.

Havlik JA, Horsburgh CR, Metchock B, Williams PP, Fann SA, and Thompson SE: Disseminated *Mycobacterium avium* complex infection: clinical identification and epidemiologic trends, *J Infect Dis* 165:577-580, 1992.

Horsburgh CR: *Mycobacterium avium* complex infection in the acquired immunodeficiency syndrome, *N Engl J Med* 324:1332-1338.

Kim JH, Langston AA, and Gallis HA: Miliary tuberculosis: epidemiology, clinical manifestations, diagnosis, and outcome, *Rev Infect Dis* 12:583-590, 1990.

Kubica GP and Wayne LG: The mycobacteria: a sourcebook, New York, 1984, Marcel Dekker.

Lillo M, Orengo S, Cernoch P, and Harris RL: Pulmonary and disseminated infection due to *Mycobacterium kansasii*: a decade of experience, *Rev Infect Dis* 12:760-767, 1990.

Lipsky BA, Gates J, Tenover FC, and Plorde JJ: Factors affecting the clinical value of microscopy for acid-fast bacilli, *Rev Infect Dis* 6:214-222, 1984.

Neill MA, Hightower AW, and Broome CV: Leprosy in the United States, 1971-1981, *J Infect Dis* 152:1064-1069, 1985.

Onorato IM, McCray E, and the Field Services Branch: Prevalence of human immunodeficiency virus infection among patients attending tuberculosis clinics in the United States, *J Infect Dis* 165:87-92, 1992.

Styblo K: Overview and epidemiologic assessment of the current global tuberculosis situation with an emphasis on control in developing countries, *Rev Infect Dis* 11(suppl 2):339-346, 1989.

Van Scoy RE and Wilkowske CJ: Antituberculous agents, *Mayo Clin Proc* 67:179-187, 1992.

Wayne LG: The atypical mycobacteria: recognition and disease association, *CRC Crit Rev Microbiol* 12:185-222, 1986.

Wayne LG and Sramek HA: Agents of newly recognized or infrequently encountered mycobacterial diseases, *Clin Microbiol Rev* 5:1-25.

Wolinsky E: Nontuberculous mycobacteria and associated diseases, *Am Rev Resp Dis* 119:107-159, 1979.

Woods GL and Washington JA II: Mycobacteria other than *Mycobacterium tuberculosis:* review of microbiologic and clinical aspects, *Rev Infect Dis* 9:275-294, 1987.

CHAPTER 36

Treponema, Borrelia, and *Leptospira*

THE collection of bacteria in the order Spirochaetales has been grouped together based on their common morphological properties. These "spirochetes" are thin, helical (0.1 to 0.5 × 5 to 20 μm), gram-negative bacteria (Figures 36-1 and 36-2). The order Spirochaetales is subdivided into two families and seven genera, of which three *(Treponema, Borrelia,* and *Leptospira)* are responsible for human disease (Table 36-1).

TREPONEMA

The two treponemal species responsible for human disease are *T. pallidum* (with three subspecies) and *T. carateum*. All are morphologically identical, elicit the same serological response in humans (e.g., positive reactivity in the VDRL, FTA-ABS, MHA-TP tests), and are susceptible to penicillin. The organisms are distinguished by the epidemiology and clinical manifestations of their disease. *T. pallidum* subspecies *pallidum* (referred to as *T. pallidum* in this chapter) is the etiological agent of the venereal disease **syphilis**; *T. pallidum* ssp. *endemicum* is responsible for **bejel**; *T. pallidum* ssp. *pertenue* is responsible for **yaws**; and *T. carateum* is responsible for **pinta**. Bejel, yaws, and pinta are nonvenereal diseases. Syphilis will be discussed initially in this chapter, with the other treponemal diseases presented at the end of the section.

Physiology and Structure

Syphilis is a sexually transmitted disease that has plagued humans for centuries. The spirochete responsible for this disease is a strict human pathogen. Natural syphilis is not found in any other species, and experimental syphilis has been established only in rabbits. *T. pallidum* is a thin, coiled spirochete (0.1 × 5 to 15 μm) that cannot be grown in cell-free cultures. Limited growth has been achieved in cultured rabbit epithelial cells, but replication is slow (doubling time, 30 hours) and can be maintained only for a few generations. The spirochetes were once considered strict anaerobes; however, it is now known that they can utilize glucose oxidatively.

The spirochetes are too thin to be seen with light

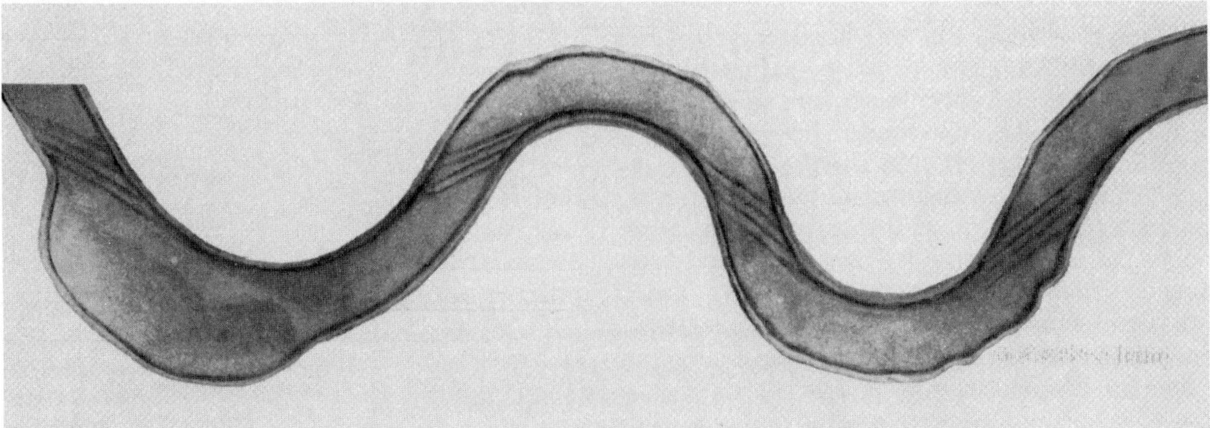

FIGURE 36-1 Helical arrangement of *Treponema pallidum*. The name "spirochete" is derived from the Greek words for "coiled hair." This is an appropriate term for bacteria longer than most others associated with human disease and that are frequently too thin to be seen by light microscopy. Note the periplasmic flagella that run along the length of the spirochete. (From Binford CH and Connor DH: *Pathology of tropical and extraordinary diseases,* vol 1, 1976, Washington, DC, 1976, Armed Forces Institute of Pathology.)

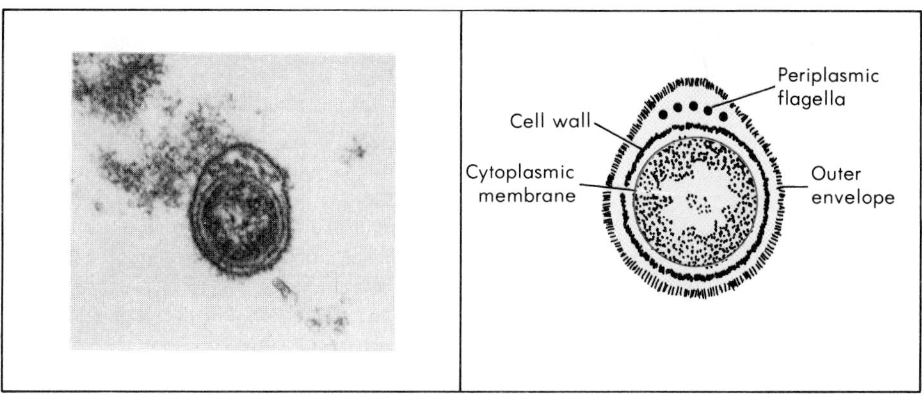

FIGURE 36-2 Electron micrograph of cross section through *Borrelia burgdorferi,* the agent responsible for Lyme borreliosis. The protoplasmic core of the bacterium is enclosed in a cytoplasmic membrane and conventional cell wall. This in turn is surrounded by an outer envelope, or sheath. Between the protoplasmic core and outer sheath are periplasmic flagella (also called axial fibrils), which are anchored at either end of the bacterium and wrap around the protoplasmic core. From two to more than 100 flagella are present, a number characteristic of individual species. These flagella are essential for motility. (From Steere AC et al: *N Engl J Med* 308:733-740, 1983.)

microscopy in specimens stained with Gram or Giemsa stains. Motile forms can be visualized by darkfield illumination or by staining with specific antitreponemal antibodies labeled with fluorescent dyes.

Pathogenesis and Immunity

The inability to grow *T. pallidum* to high concentrations in vitro has limited detection of specific virulence factors in this organism. However, several investigators have now successfully cloned *T. pallidum* genes in *E. coli* and isolated the protein products. Several gene products have been specifically associated with virulent strains, although their role in pathogenesis remains to be delineated. The outer membrane proteins are associated with adherence to the surface of host cells, and virulent spirochetes produce hyaluronidase, which may facilitate perivascular infiltration. Virulent spirochetes are also coated with host cell fibronectin, which can protect against phagocytosis.

Tissue destruction and lesions observed in syphilis are primarily the consequence of the patient's immune response to infection. The clinical course of syphilis evolves through three phases. The initial, or primary, phase is characterized by one or more skin lesions (chancres) at the site of spirochete penetration. Although dissemination of spirochetes in the bloodstream occurs soon after infection, the chancre represents the primary site of initial replication. Histological examination of the lesion reveals endarteritis and periarteritis (characteristic of syphilitic lesions at all stages) and infiltration of the ulcer with polymorphonuclear leukocytes and macrophages. Ingestion of spirochetes by the phagocytic cells is seen, but the organisms frequently survive. The secondary phase of syphilis heralds clinical signs of disseminated disease, with prominent skin lesions dispersed over the entire body surface (Figure 36-3). Spontaneous remission may occur after either the primary or secondary stages, or the patient may develop late manifestations of disease in which virtually all tissues may be involved. Each phase represents localized multiplication of the spirochete and tissue destruction. Although replication is slow, large

TABLE 36-1 Order Spirochaetales

Spirochaetales	Human diseases	Etiological agent
Genus *Cristispira*	None	
Genus *Leptonema*	None	
Genus *Serpula*	None	
Genus *Spirochaeta*	None	
Genus *Treponema*	Syphilis	*T. palladium,* ssp. *pallidum*
	Bejel	*T. pallidum,* ssp. *endemicum*
	Yaws	*T. pallidum,* ssp. *pertenue*
	Pinta	*T. carateum*
Genus *Borrelia*	Epidemic relapsing fever	*B. recurrentis*
	Endemic relapsing fever	Many *Borrelia* species
	Lyme borreliosis	*B. burgdorferi*
FAMILY LEPTOSPIRACEAE		
Genus *Leptospira*	Leptospirosis	*L. interrogans*

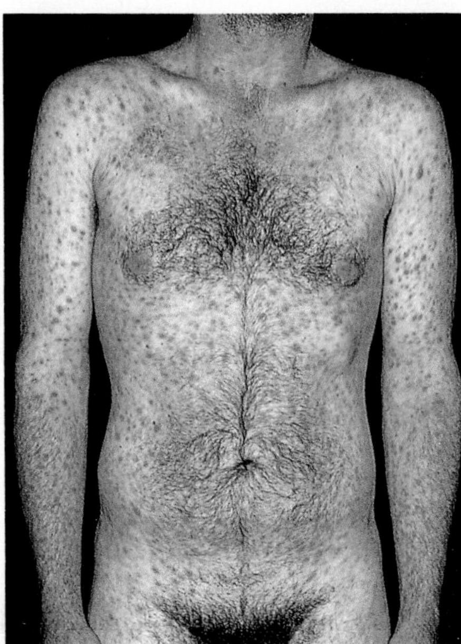

FIGURE 36-3 Disseminated rash in secondary syphilis. (From Habif TP, editor: *Clinical dermatology,* St Louis, 1985, Mosby.)

numbers of organisms are present in the initial chancre, as well as in the secondary lesions following dissemination of the spirochetes in the bloodstream.

Epidemiology

Syphilis is found worldwide and is the third most common sexually transmitted disease in the United States (after *Neisseria gonorrhoeae* and *Chlamydia* infections) (Box 36-1). Although the incidence of disease had steadily decreased since the early 1940s with the advent of penicillin therapy, this trend reversed in the mid-1980s (Figure 36-4). In 1990 more than 134,000 cases of syphilis, including 50,223 cases of primary and secondary disease, were reported in the United States. However, the large number of unreported infections contributes to a gross underestimation of the true incidence of this disease. The highest incidence of disease is reported in the southern and eastern states (Figure 36-5)and in the black and Hispanic populations.

Because natural syphilis is exclusive to humans and has no other known natural hosts, the most common method of spread is by direct sexual contact. *T. pallidum* is extremely labile, unable to survive exposure to drying or disinfectants. Thus inanimate objects such as toilet seats cannot contribute to the spread of syphilis. Direct person-to-person contact is required for transmission. This disease can also be acquired congenitally or by transfusion with contaminated blood. Syphilis is not highly contagious, with the risk of disease following a single sexual contact estimated to be 30%. However, contagiousness is influenced by the stage of disease in the infectious individual. As mentioned previously, the spirochetes are unable to survive on dry skin surfaces. Thus

BOX 36-1 Epidemiology of Syphilis

DISEASE/BACTERIAL FACTORS

Syphilis: primary, secondary, late, congenital
Outer membrane proteins promote adherence to host cells
Hyaluronidase may facilitate perivascular infiltration
Coating of fibronectin (from host cell) protects against phagocytosis
Tissue destruction primarily is due to host's immune response to infection

TRANSMISSION

Humans only natural host
Sexually transmitted through direct person-to-person contact
Congenitally acquired through infected birth canal
Transfusion with contaminated blood

WHO IS AT RISK?

People with multiple sexual partners
Newborns of infected mothers
Patients with AIDS at increased risk for neurosyphilis

GEOGRAPHY/SEASON

Worldwide; third most common STD in the United States
No seasonal incidence

MODES OF CONTROL

Penicillin (drug of choice); tetracycline, erythromycin, chloramphenicol if patient is allergic to penicillin
"Safe sex" techniques and treatment of sexual partners of infected patients

T. pallidum is transferred primarily during the early stages of disease when large numbers of organisms are present in moist cutaneous or mucosal lesions. Congenital transmission to the fetus can take place soon after the mother is infected because bacteremia characteristically occurs early during the course of the disease. A woman with untreated disease can have spontaneous bacteremia for as long as 8 years, transmitting the spirochetes to fetal tissues if she becomes pregnant during this period. After 8 years the disease can remain active, but bacteremia is not believed to occur.

With the advent of effective antimicrobial therapy, the incidence of late (tertiary) syphilis has markedly decreased. Although antibiotic therapy has decreased the length of infectivity in infected individuals, the incidence of primary and secondary syphilis has remained high because of sexual practices, particularly prostitution to support drug habits. The incidence of congenital syphilis corresponds to the pattern of syphilis in women of childbearing age (Figure 36-6).

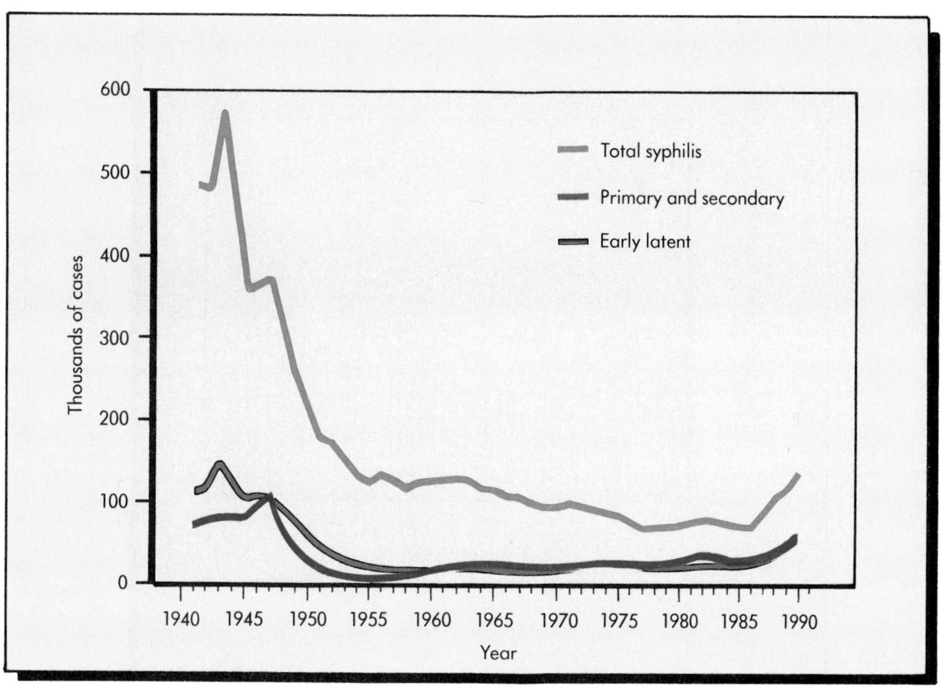

FIGURE 36-4 Incidence of syphilis in the United States from 1941 to 1990. (MMWR 40:42, 1992.)

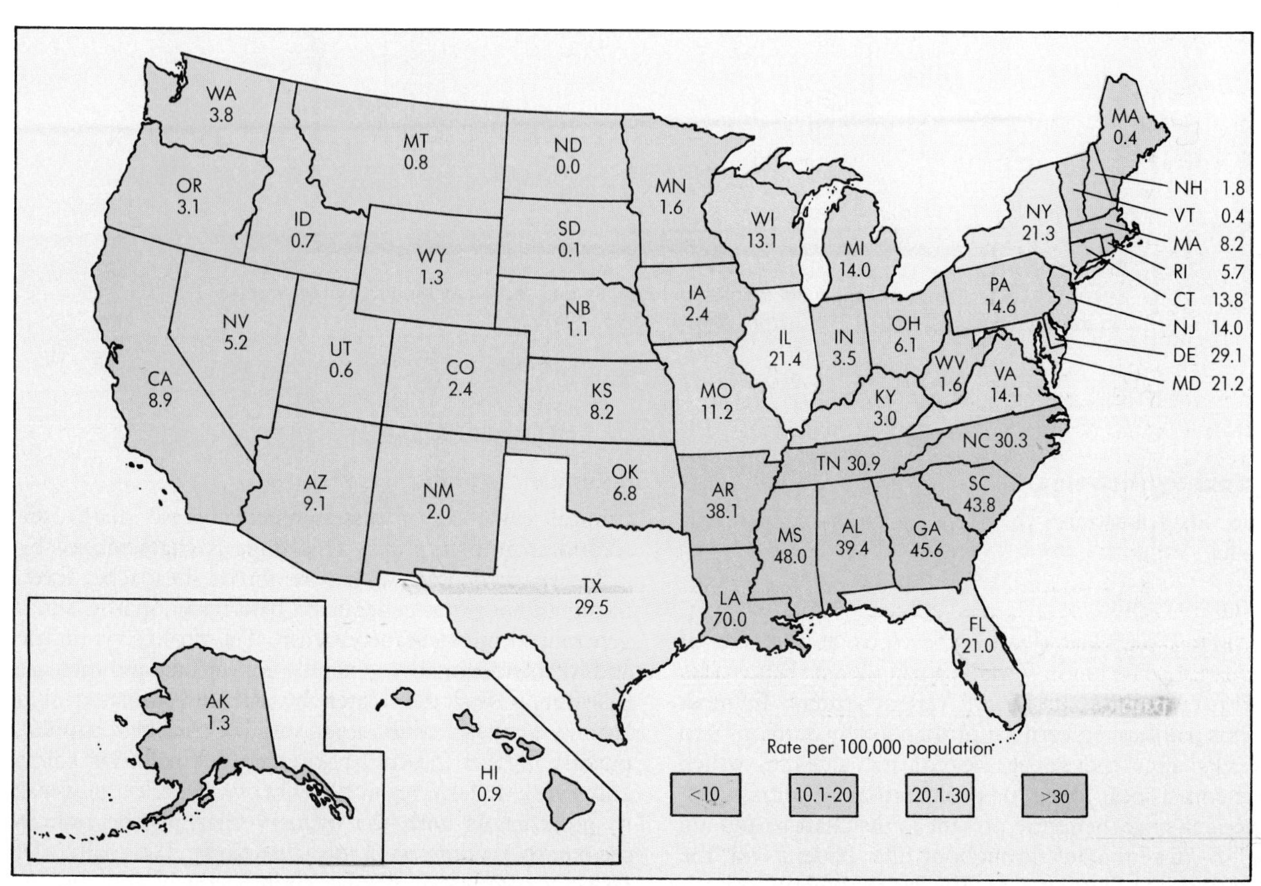

FIGURE 36-5 Total incidence of primary and secondary syphilis by state in the United States, 1990.

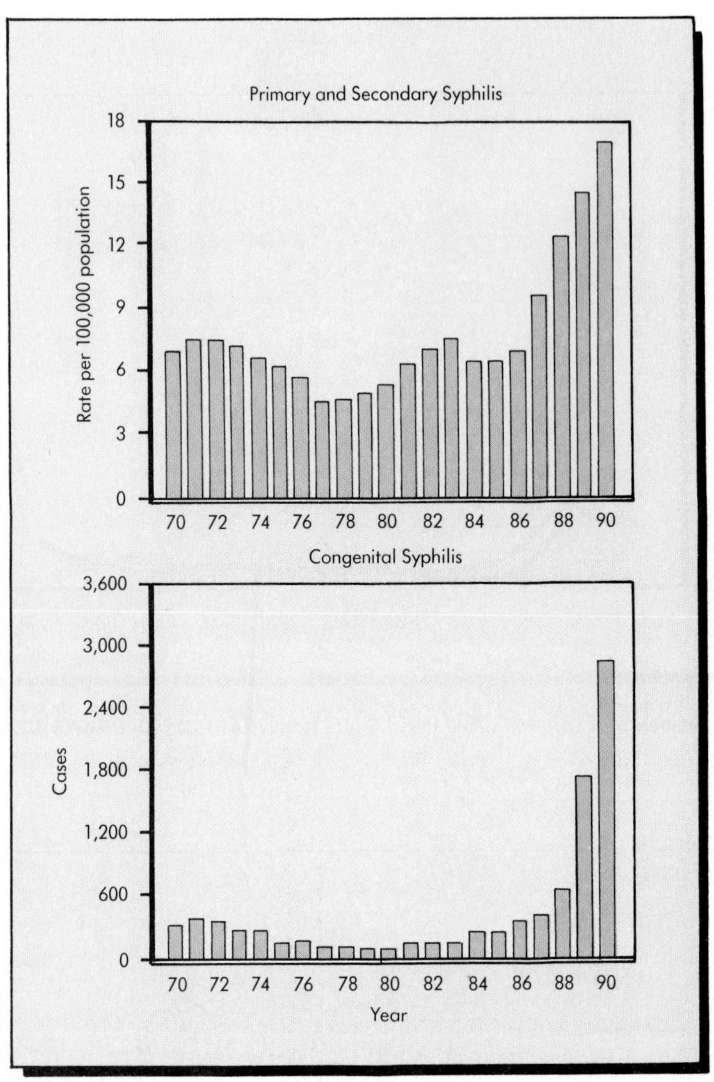

FIGURE 36-6 Incidence of congenital syphilis and primary and secondary syphilis among women in the United States, 1970-1991. (From *MMWR* 40:46, 1992).

Clinical Syndromes

Figure 36-7 illustrates the natural history of untreated syphilis.

Primary Syphilis

The initial syphilitic chancre develops at the site of inoculation. The lesion starts as a papule but then erodes to form a painless ulcer with raised borders. In most patients painless regional lymphadenopathy develops 1 to 2 weeks after the appearance of the chancre, which represents a local focus for proliferation of spirochetes. Abundant spirochetes are present in the chancre and are able to disseminate throughout the patient via the lymphatics and bloodstream. The fact that this ulcer heals spontaneously within 2 months gives the patient a false sense of relief.

Secondary Syphilis

Clinical evidence of disseminated disease marks the second stage of syphilis. This stage is characterized by a flu-like syndrome, with sore throat, headache, fever, myalgias, anorexia, generalized lymphadenopathy, and a generalized mucocutaneous rash. The flu-like syndrome and lymphadenopathy generally appear first and then are followed a few days later by the disseminated skin lesions. The rash can be quite variable (macular, papular, pustular), cover the entire skin surface (including palms and soles), and can resolve slowly over a period of weeks to months. As with the primary chancre, the rash in secondary syphilis is highly infectious. Gradually, the rash and symptoms resolve spontaneously and the patient enters the latent or clinically inactive stage of disease.

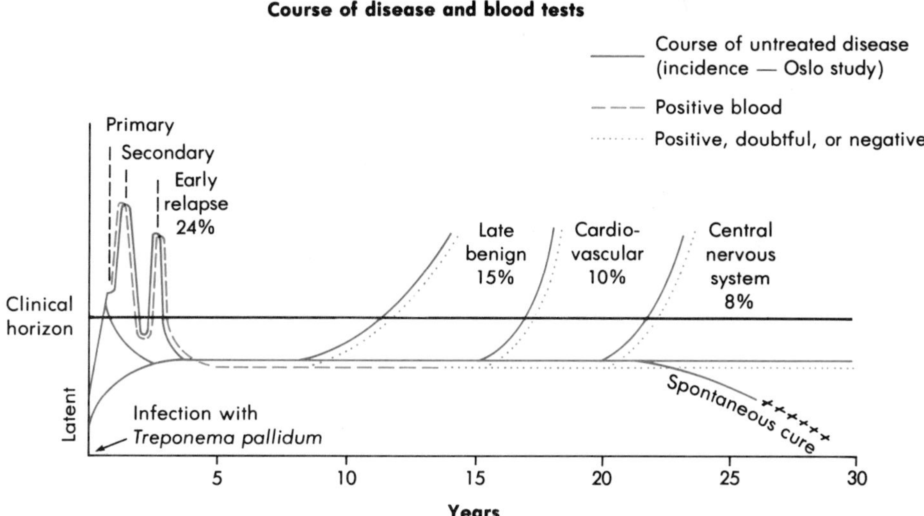

FIGURE 36-7 The natural history of untreated acquired syphilis was carefully chronicled at the University of Oslo, where almost 2200 untreated patients were studied. The incubation period from the time of infection to onset of primary disease varies from 10 to 90 days (average 21 days). Without treatment the chancre will heal in 3 to 6 weeks. Asymptomatic dissemination occurs during this period, and secondary lesions develop from 2 weeks to 6 months (average, 6 weeks) after the chancre initially appeared. These lesions will last 2 to 10 weeks. At the end of the secondary stage of syphilis, patients enter a latent phase from which they can undergo spontaneous cure or relapse into the secondary stage manifestations (observed in 24% of the patients). Tertiary syphilis can occur years later with the development of systemic granulomas (called gummas) in soft tissues (15% of the patients), cardiovascular disease (10%), or central nervous system lesions (8%). (Modified from *South Med J* 26:18, 1933; incidence data from Clark EG, Danbolt N: *J Chron Dis* 2:311, 1955.)

Late Syphilis

A small proportion of patients can progress to the tertiary stage of syphilis. The diffuse, chronic inflammation characteristic of late syphilis can cause devastating destruction of virtually any organ or tissue (e.g., arteritis, dementia, blindness). Granulomatous lesions **(gummas)** may be found in bone, skin, and other tissues. The nomenclature of late syphilis reflects the organs of primary involvement (e.g., neurosyphilis or cardiovascular syphilis). An increased incidence of neurosyphilis despite adequate therapy for early syphilis has been documented in patients with acquired immunodeficiency syndrome (AIDS).

Congenital Syphilis

In utero infections can lead to significant fetal disease, resulting in death, multiorgan malformations, or latent infections. Most infected infants are born without clinical evidence of disease but then develop rhinitis followed by a widespread desquamating maculopapular rash. Late bony destruction and cardiovascular syphilis are common in untreated infants who survive the initial course of disease.

Laboratory Diagnosis

Microscopy

The diagnosis of primary, secondary, or congenital syphilis can be made rapidly by darkfield examination of the exudate from skin lesions (Table 36-2 and Figure 36-8). However, the test is reliable only when clinical material with actively motile spirochetes is examined immediately by an experienced technologist. The spirochetes will not survive transport to the laboratory, and tissue debris can be mistaken for spirochetes. Material collected from oral lesions should not be examined because nonpathogenic, oral spirochetes can contaminate the specimen. Specific identification of *T. pallidum* can be made by use of fluorescein-labeled antitreponemal anti-

TABLE 36-2 Diagnostic Tests for Syphilis

Diagnostic test	Method or examination
Microscopy	Darkfield
	Direct fluorescent antibody staining
Culture	Not used
Serology	Nontreponemal tests
	VDRL ↳ detects IgA + IgG
	RPR
	Treponemal tests
	FTA-ABS
	MHA-TP

TABLE 36-3 Sensitivity of Serologic Tests in Untreated Syphilis

	Stage of disease			
	Primary	**Secondary**	**Latent**	**Late**
VDRL slide test	59-87	100	73-91	39-94
FTA-ABS test	86-100	99-100	96-99	96-100
MHA-TP	64-87	99-100	96-100	94-100

From Holmes KK, Mardh PA, Sparling PF, and Wiesner PJ: *Sexually transmitted diseases*, New York, 1984, McGraw-Hill.

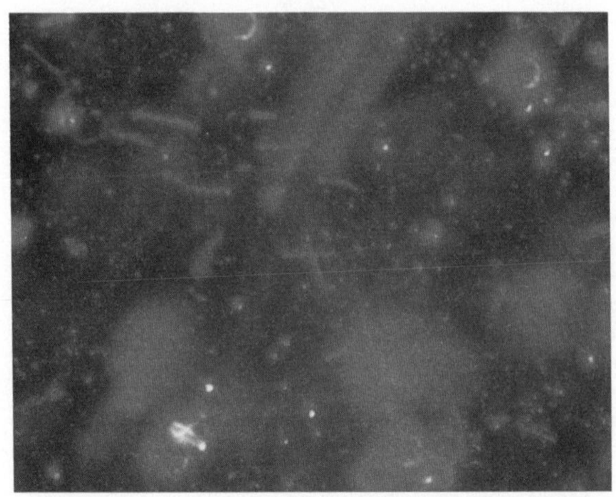

FIGURE 36-8 *Treponema pallidum* in darkfield microscopy. (From Peters W and Gilles HM: *A colour atlas of tropical medicine and parasitology*, ed 3, London, 1989, Wolfe Medical Publications.)

bodies. Histological staining of tissue lesions may be beneficial, with silver stains used most commonly.

Culture

Efforts to culture *T. pallidum* in vitro should not be attempted because the organism does not grow in artificial cultures.

Serology

The diagnosis of syphilis in most patients is made by serologic testing. The two general types of tests used are biologically nonspecific (nontreponemal) tests and the specific treponemal tests.

Nontreponemal tests measure IgG and IgM antibodies (also called **reagin** antibodies) developed against lipids released from damaged cells during the early stage of disease and also present on the cell surface of treponemes. The antigen used for the nontreponemal tests is cardiolipin, derived from beef heart. The two tests used most commonly are the Venereal Disease Research Laboratory **(VDRL)** test and the Rapid Plasma Reagin **(RPR)** test. Both tests measure flocculation of cardiolipin antigen by the patient's serum. Both tests are rapid, although complement in serum must be inactivated for 30 minutes before the VDRL test can be performed. Only the VDRL test should be used to test cerebrospinal fluid from patients with suspected neurosyphilis.

Treponemal tests are specific antibody tests used to confirm positive reactions with the VDRL or RPR tests. The treponemal tests can also be positive before the nontreponemal tests become positive in early syphilis, or remain positive when the nonspecific tests revert to negative in some patients who have late syphilis. The tests most commonly used are the Fluorescent Treponemal Antibody Absorption **(FTA-ABS)** test and the Microhemagglutination Test for *T. pallidum* **(MHA-TP).** The MHA-TP test is technically easier to perform and interpret than the FTA-ABS test. The Western Blot assay with whole cell *T. pallidum* as antigen recently has been used successfully as a confirmatory treponeme-specific test.

Because positive reactions with the nontreponemal tests develop late during the first phase of disease, many patients who initially have chancres will have negative serologic findings (Table 36-3). However, within 3 months all patients will develop positive serologic results that remain positive in untreated patients with secondary syphilis. The antibody titers in patients with untreated syphilis will slowly decrease, and approximately 25% of patients with late syphilis will have negative serology. Although treponemal tests generally remain positive for life, a negative test is unreliable for AIDS patients.

Successful treatment of primary or secondary syphilis, and to a lesser extent late syphilis, will lead to reduced titers with the VDRL and RPR tests (Figure 36-9). Thus these tests can be used to monitor therapy, although the rate of seroreversion is slowed by an advanced stage of disease, high initial titers, and a history of previous syphilis. The treponemal tests are influenced less by therapy, with seroconversion observed with fewer than 25% of the patients successfully treated during primary syphilis.

The specificity of the nontreponemal tests is 98% or greater. However, transient false-positive reactions are seen in patients with acute febrile diseases, following immunizations, and in pregnant women. Chronic false-positive reactions occur most often in patients with

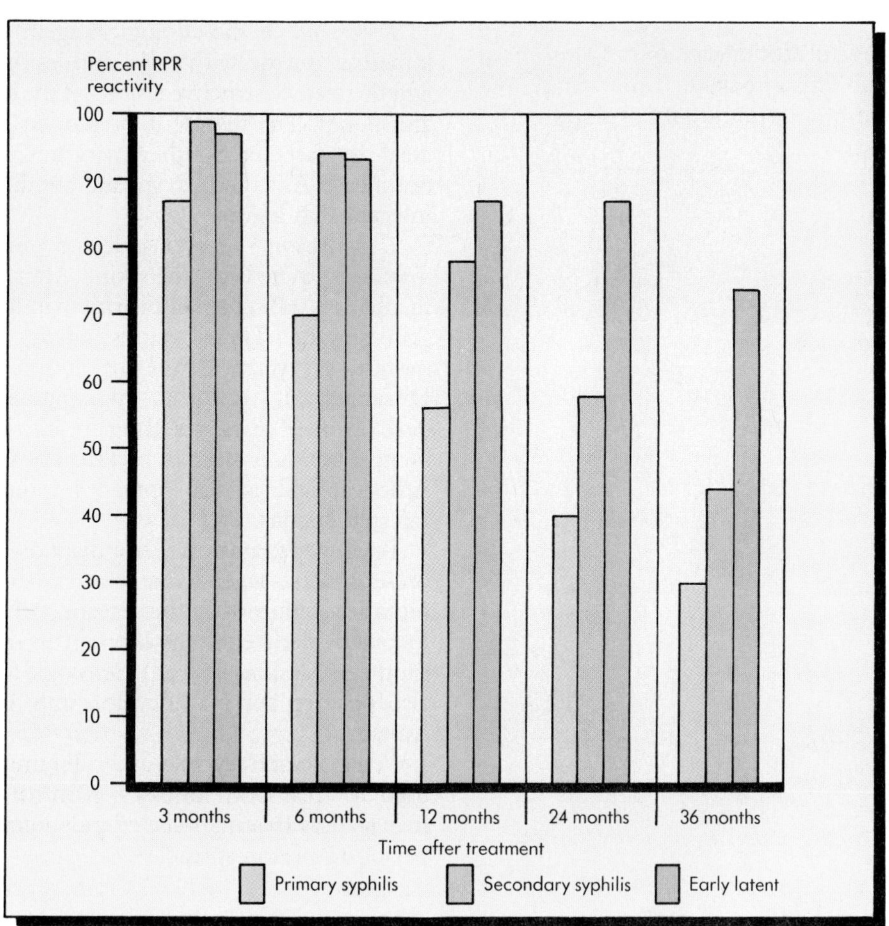

FIGURE 36-9 Effect of treatment for syphilis on Rapid Plasma Reagin (RPR) reactivity. (Data from Romanowski B et al: *Ann Intern Med* 114:1005-1009, 1991)

chronic autoimmune diseases or infections that involve the liver or cause extensive tissue destruction. The specificity of the treponemal tests is also 98% to 99%, with most false-positive reactions observed in patients with elevated gamma globulin levels and autoimmune diseases (Box 36-2). Many of the false-positive reactions can be resolved with the Western Blot assay, which may become the preferred confirmatory test.

Positive serologic tests in infants of infected mothers can represent passive transfer of antibodies or a specific immunological response to infection. These two possibilities are distinguished by collecting sera over a 6-month period. In noninfected infants the antibody titers will decrease to undetectable levels within 3 months of birth. The antibody titers will remain elevated in infants who have congenital syphilis.

Treatment, Prevention, and Control

Penicillin is the drug of choice for treating infections with *T. pallidum*. Long-acting benzathine penicillin is used for the early stages of syphilis, and penicillin G is recommended for congenital and late syphilis. Tetracycline, erythromycin, and chloramphenicol can be used as alternative antibiotics for patients allergic to penicillin. Only penicillin or chloramphenicol can be used for patients with neurosyphilis.

Because protective vaccines are not available, control of syphilis requires the practice of safe sex techniques and adequate contact and treatment of sex partners of patients who have documented infections. In recent years control of syphilis and other venereal diseases has been complicated by increases in prostitution in drug abusers.

OTHER TREPONEMES

Three other nonvenereal treponemal diseases are important: bejel, yaws, and pinta. The diseases are primarily observed in impoverished children.

T. pallidum ssp. *endemicum* is responsible for **bejel**, also called endemic syphilis. Disease is spread person-to-person by use of contaminated eating utensils. The initial oral lesions are rarely observed, but secondary lesions include oral papules and mucosal patches. Late manifestations consist of gummas of the skin, bones, and nasopharynx. The disease is present in Africa, Asia, and Australia (Figure 36-10).

BOX 36-2 Medical Conditions Associated With False-Positive Treponemal and Nontreponemal Serology Tests

NONTREPONEMAL TESTS

Viral infection
Collagen-vascular disease
Acute or chronic illness
Pregnancy
Recent immunization
Heroin addiction
Leprosy
Malaria

TREPONEMAL TESTS

Pyoderma
Skin neoplasm
Acne vulgaris
Mycoses
Crural ulceration
Rheumatoid arthritis
Psoriasis
Systemic lupus erythematosus
Pregnancy
Drug addiction
Herpes genitalis

T. pertenue is the etiological agent of **yaws**, a granulomatous disease with early skin lesions (Figure 36-11) and then late destructive lesions of the skin, lymph nodes, and bones. The disease is present in primitive, tropical areas in parts of South America, Central Africa, and Southeast Asia and is spread by direct contact with infected skin lesions.

T. carateum is responsible for **pinta**, a disease primarily restricted to the skin. After a 1- to 3-week incubation period small pruritic papules develop on the skin surface. These lesions enlarge and persist for months to years before resolution (Figure 36-12). Disseminated, recurrent, hypopigmented lesions can develop over years, resulting in scarring and disfigurement. Pinta is present in Mexico and Central and South America, and is also spread by direct contact with infected lesions.

Bejel, yaws, and pinta are diagnosed by their clinical presentation in an endemic area. The diagnoses of yaws or pinta are confirmed by the detection of spirochetes in skin lesions by darkfield microscopy (this test cannot be used for the oral lesions in bejel). Serologic tests for syphilis are also positive but may develop only late in the disease course.

Penicillin, tetracycline, and chloramphenicol have been used to treat both diseases. Control of the disease is managed by treating infected individuals and eliminating person-to-person spread.

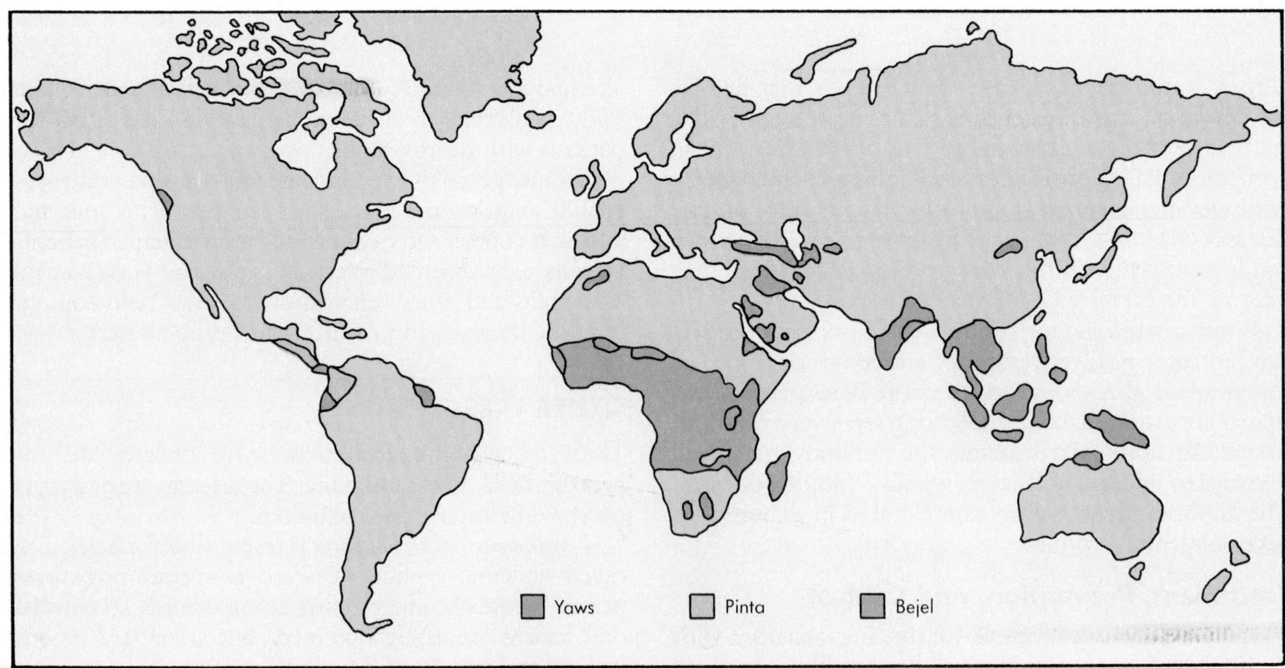

FIGURE 36-10 Geographic distribution of bejel, yaws, and pinta. (Redrawn from Mandell GL, Douglas RG Jr, and Bennett JE: *Principles and practices of infectious disease*, ed 3, New York, 1990, John Wiley & Sons.)

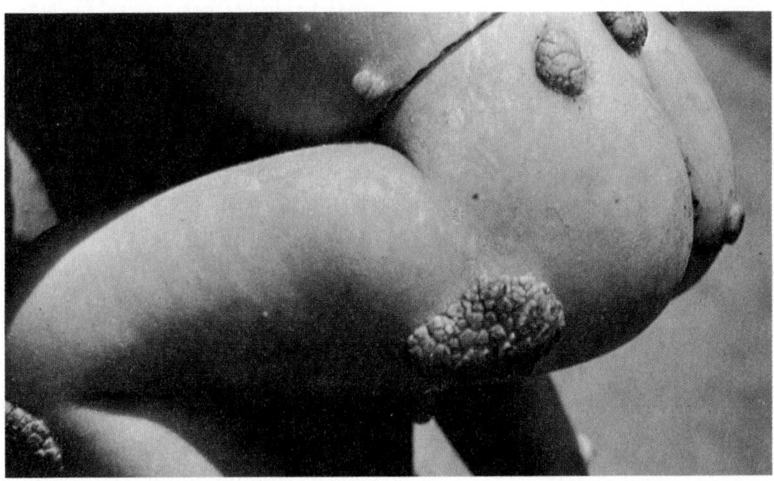

FIGURE 36-11 Yaws. The elevated papillomatous nodules characteristic of early yaws are widely distributed and painless. They contain numerous spirochetes easily demonstrable by darkfield examination. (From Peters W and Gilles HM: *A colour atlas of tropical medicine and parasitology,* ed 3, London, 1989, Wolfe Medical Publications.)

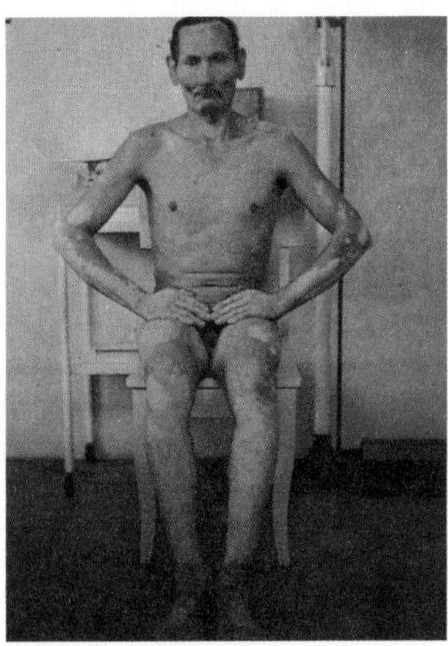

FIGURE 36-12 Depigmented lesions of pinta. Lesions start initially as papules, progress to plaques, and in the late stages become depigmented. Depigmentation is commonly seen as a late sequel of any of the treponemal diseases. (From Peters W and Gilles HM: *A colour atlas of tropical medicine and parasitology,* ed 3, London, 1989, Wolfe Medical Publications.)

BORRELIA

Members of the genus *Borrelia* are responsible for two important human diseases: relapsing fever and Lyme disease. **Relapsing fever** is a febrile illness characterized by recurrent episodes of fever and septicemia, separated by afebrile periods. Two forms of the disease are recognized. *Borrelia recurrentis* is the etiological agent of **epidemic** or **louse-borne relapsing fever** and is spread person-to-person by the human body louse *(Pediculus humanus)*. **Endemic relapsing fever** is caused by many species of borreliae and is spread by infected ticks.

In 1977 an unusual cluster of children with arthritis in Lyme, Connecticut was described. Five years later the spirochete responsible for this disease was discovered by Burgdorfer. **Lyme disease** is a tick-borne disease with protean manifestations, including dermatological, rheumatological, neurological, and cardiac abnormalities. The best clinical marker for the disease is the initial skin lesion, **erythema migrans**, that occurs in 60% to 70% of infected adults and less frequently in children. Until recently all cases of Lyme disease (or Lyme borreliosis) were believed to be caused by one organism, *B. burgdorferi*. More recent studies of DNA relatedness among isolates have identified at least three species: *B. burgdorferi* found in the United States and Europe, *B. garinii* found in Europe and Japan, and a third unnamed species also found in Europe and Japan. As additional isolates are characterized, it is likely that more species will be defined. For the purposes of this chapter, until the nomenclature is defined better, all strains will be referred to as *B. burgdorferi*.

Physiology and Structure

Members of the genus *Borrelia* are weakly staining, gram-negative bacilli that resemble other spirochetes. They tend to be larger (0.2 to 0.5 × 3 to 30 μm), stain well with aniline dyes (e.g., Giemsa, Wright), and can be easily seen in smears of peripheral blood collected from patients with relapsing fever (Figure 36-13). From 7 to 20 periplasmic flagella (depending on the individual species) are present between the periplasmic cylinder and the outer envelope and are responsible for the organism's twisting motility. Borreliae are microaerophilic and have complex nutritional requirements, making recovery in culture difficult. The species that have been successfully

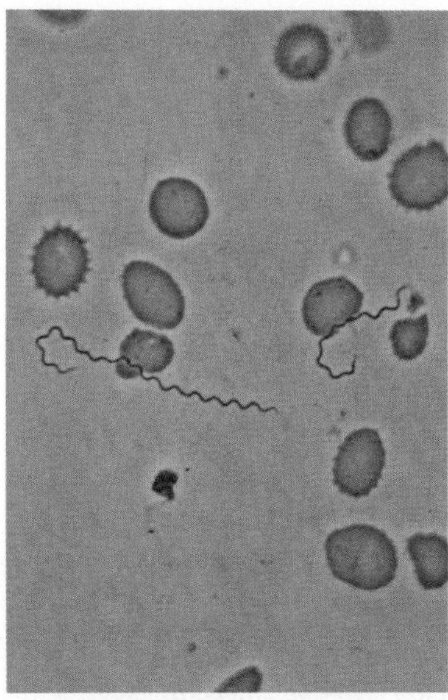

FIGURE 36-13 *Borrelia* present in the blood of a patient with endemic relapsing fever. Giemsa stain; phase contrast. (From Peters W and Gilles HM: *A colour atlas of tropical medicine and parasitology,* ed 3, London, 1989, Wolfe Medical Publications.)

cultured have generation times of 18 hours or longer. Because culture is generally unsuccessful, diagnosis of diseases caused by borreliae is by microscopy (relapsing fever) or serology (Lyme disease).

Pathogenesis and Immunity

After exposure to infected arthropods, borreliae are able to spread in the bloodstream to multiple organs. Members of the genus do not produce recognized toxins and are rapidly removed when a specific antibody response is mounted. The periodic febrile and afebrile cycles of relapsing fever are due to the ability of the borreliae to undergo antigenic variation. When specific IgM antibodies are formed, agglutination with complement-mediated lysis occurs and the borreliae are rapidly cleared from the bloodstream. However, organisms residing in internal tissues are able to alter their serotypespecific outer envelope proteins through gene rearrangement and emerge as antigenically novel organisms. Clinical manifestations of relapsing fever are in part a response to the release of endotoxin by the organism.

B. burgdorferi is present in low numbers in the skin tissues when erythema migrans develops. In the late manifestations of disease, spirochetes have also been isolated from clinical material. It is not known whether the viable organisms are responsible for these late manifestations of disease or if they represent immunological cross-reactivity to borrelia antigens. Although the initial immune response to the organism is depressed, antibodies develop over a period of months to years and are responsible for complement-mediated clearance of the borreliae.

Epidemiology

The vectors for relapsing fever are soft-shelled **ticks** (*Ornithodoros* species) and the human **body louse** (Box 36-3 and Figure 36-14). Humans are the only reservoir for *B. recurrentis*, the etiological agent of louse-borne epidemic relapsing fever. After lice are infected, the organisms pass through the wall of the gut and multiply in hemolymph. Infected lice do not survive for more than a few months, so maintenance of disease requires crowded, unsanitary conditions (wars, natural disasters) that permit frequent contact with infected lice. In contrast, tick-borne relapsing fever is a zoonotic disease, with rodents, small mammals, and ticks acting as the main reservoirs. Despite the fact the borreliae produce a disseminated infection in ticks, the arthropods are able to survive and maintain an endemic reservoir of infection by transovarian transmission. Furthermore, ticks can survive for months to years between feedings.

Louse-borne relapsing fever is endemic in both tropical and temperate regions of the world, particularly Central and Eastern Africa and South America. Tick-borne disease is widespread.

Despite the relatively recent recognition of Lyme disease in the United States, retrospective studies have demonstrated that the disease was present for many years in this and other countries. Lyme disease currently has been described on six continents, in at least 20 countries, and in 46 states of the United States. The incidence of disease has risen dramatically since 1982 when 497 cases were reported to 1990 with nearly 8000 cases reported. Lyme disease is the leading vector-borne disease in the United States. The three principal foci of infection in the United States are the Northeast (Massachusetts to Maryland), upper Midwest (Minnesota, Wisconsin, and Michigan), and Pacific West (California, Oregon, and Washington). Hard-shelled ticks are the major vectors of Lyme disease—*Ixodes dammini* in the Northeast and Midwest, and *I. pacificus* on the West Coast. *I. ricinus* is the major tick vector in Europe. The major reservoir hosts in the United States are the white-footed mouse and white-tail deer.

Only 30% of patients with Lyme disease recall a specific tick bite. The reason is that the nymph stages of the tick, as well as adult ticks, can transmit disease. The small nymph forms are responsible for the majority of infections. Most Lyme disease infections are reported from spring to fall, corresponding to activity of infected ticks. Person-to-person spread has not been reported.

Clinical Syndromes

Relapsing Fever

The clinical presentations of epidemic louse-borne and endemic tick-borne relapsing fever are essentially the same (Figure 36-15). After a 1-week incubation period, the abrupt onset of disease is heralded with shaking chills, fever, muscle aches, and headache. Splenomegaly and hepatomegaly are commonly present. The symptoms correspond to the bacteremic phase of the disease and are

BOX 36-3 Epidemiology of *Borrelia* Infection

DISEASE/BACTERIAL FACTORS

Borreliosis: relapsing fever, Lyme disease
Bacterium can undergo antigenic variation
Louse-borne relapsing fever requires crowded unsanitary conditions for maintenance of disease
Humans only reservoir for louse-borne epidemic relapsing fever
Rodents, small mammals, and ticks are reservoirs for tick-borne relapsing fever
Rodents, deer, domestic pets, and hard-shell ticks are reservoirs for Lyme disease

TRANSMISSION

Bite from infected arthropod (ticks, lice)

WHO IS AT RISK?

Relapsing fever: people in crowded, unsanitary environments (louse-borne disease) or people exposed to infected ticks (tick-borne disease)
Lyme disease: people exposed to infected ticks

GEOGRAPHY/SEASON

Relapsing fever: louse-borne disease: tropical and temperate regions (Central and Eastern Africa, South America); tick-borne disease: worldwide
Lyme disease: worldwide; leading vector-borne disease in United States; most common in United States in Northeast, upper Midwest, and Pacific West
Louse-borne relapsing fever occurs year-round; tick-borne disease occurs during period of greatest tick activity
Most Lyme disease infections reported from spring to fall

MODES OF CONTROL

Relapsing fever: tetracycline (drug of choice except for pregnant women and young children), chloramphenicol
Lyme disease: doxycycline, amoxicillin, erythromycin for early manifestations; ceftriaxone, penicillin, doxycycline, amoxicillin for late manifestations
Avoid ticks and their natural habitats, wear protective clothing, and use insect repellants
Control of rodents (epidemic relapsing fever)
Delousing sprays and improved hygiene important to control of epidemic louse-borne disease

Infection	Reservoir	Vector
Relapsing fever Epidemic (louse-borne)	Humans	Body louse 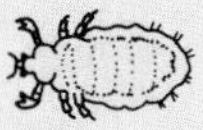
Replapsing fever Endemic (tick-borne)	Rodents, soft-shelled ticks	Soft-shelled tick 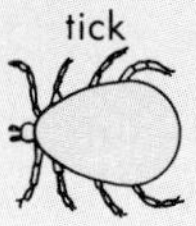
Lyme disease	Rodents, deer domestic pets, hard-shelled ticks	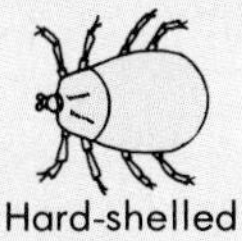 Hard-shelled tick

FIGURE 36-14 Epidemiology of *Borrelia* infections.

relieved after 3 to 7 days, when the borreliae are cleared from the blood. Bacteremia and fever return after a 1-week afebrile period. The clinical symptoms are generally milder and shorter during this and subsequent febrile episodes. Two or three relapses are common, although the number of relapses can be as many as 13. The clinical course and outcome of epidemic relapsing fever tend to be more severe than with endemic disease, but this may be related to the patient's underlying poor state of health. Mortality with endemic disease is less than 5% but can be from 4% to 40% in epidemic disease.

Lyme Disease

Clinical diagnosis of Lyme disease is complicated by the varied presentations of this disease and the lack of reliable diagnostic tests. The CDC clinical and laboratory definition of Lyme disease is summarized in Box 36-4.

After an incubation period of 3 to 30 days, one or more skin lesions develops at the site of the tick bite. The lesion (erythema migrans) begins as a small macule or papule and then enlarges over the next few weeks, covering an area ranging from 5 to more than 50 cm in diameter (Figure 36-16). As the lesion develops, it will typically appear with a red, flat border and central clearing; however, erythema, vesicle formation, and central necrosis can also be seen. Within weeks the lesion will fade and disappear, although new, transient lesions may subsequently appear. Other early signs and symptoms of Lyme disease include malaise, severe fatigue, headache, fever, chills, musculoskeletal pains, myalgias, and lymphadenopathy. These will last for an average of 4 weeks.

Late manifestations develop in almost 80% of untreated patients with Lyme disease; these occur within a week of the onset of disease to more than 2 years later. Two phases can be seen. The first involves neurological symptoms (meningitis, encephalitis, peripheral nerve neuropathy) and cardiac dysfunction (heart block, myopericarditis, congestive heart failure). These symptoms are seen in 10% to 15% of patients and can last for days to months. The second phase of late disease is characterized by arthralgias and arthritis. These complications can persist for months to years, during which spirochetes are only rarely visualized in the involved tissue or isolated in culture.

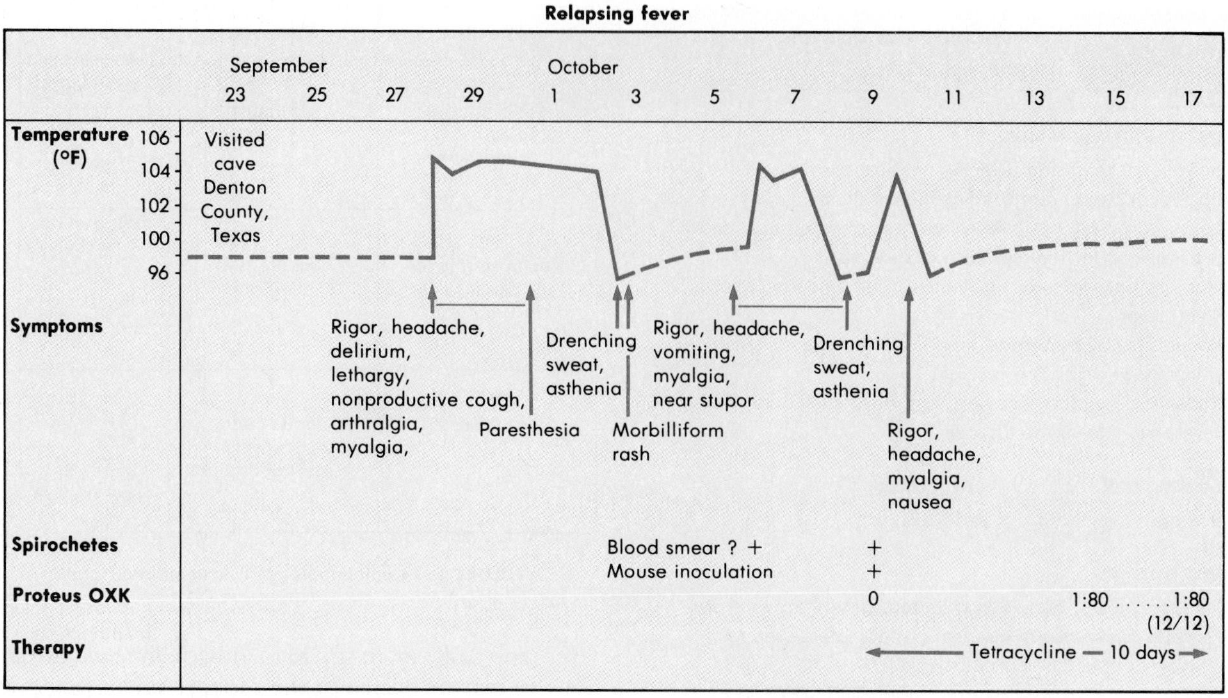

Relapsing fever

	September 23	25	27	29	October 1	3	5	7	9	11	13	15	17
Temperature (°F) 106, 104, 102, 100, 96	Visited cave Denton County, Texas												
Symptoms			Rigor, headache, delirium, lethargy, nonproductive cough, arthralgia, myalgia,	Paresthesia	Drenching sweat, asthenia	Morbilliform rash	Rigor, headache, vomiting, myalgia, near stupor		Drenching sweat, asthenia	Rigor, headache, myalgia, nausea			
Spirochetes						Blood smear ? + Mouse inoculation			+ +				
Proteus OXK									0			1:80 ...... 1:80 (12/12)	
Therapy									← Tetracycline — 10 days →				

FIGURE 36-15 The clinical evolution of tick-borne relapsing fever in a 14-year-old boy. The initial febrile episode is typically the most severe. Subsequent episodes tend to be shorter and less intense. Although nonspecific reactivity with Proteus OXK antigens are frequently observed, the specific diagnosis is made by observing borreliae in peripheral blood smears. These are positive only during the febrile periods. (Modified from Southern PM and Sanford JP: *Medicine* 48:129-149, 1969.)

BOX 36-4 Definition of Lyme Disease

CLINICAL CASE DEFINITION

Erythema migrans (≥5 cm in diameter), or
At least one late manifestation (i.e., musculoskeletal, nervous, or cardiovascular involvement) and laboratory confirmation of infection

LABORATORY CRITERIA FOR DIAGNOSIS

Isolation of *Borrelia burgdorferi*, or
Demonstration of diagnostic levels of IgM or IgG antibodies to the spirochetes, or
Significant increase in antibody titer between acute and convalescent serum samples

Laboratory Diagnosis

The sensitivity for the following diagnostic tests is summarized in Table 36-4.

Microscopy

Because of their relatively large size, the borreliae responsible for relapsing fever can be seen during the febrile period by preparing a Giemsa or Wright stain of the blood. Examination of Giemsa-stained blood smears is the most sensitive method for diagnosing relapsing fever; more than 70% of the patients may have positive smears. The test sensitivity can be improved by inoculating a mouse with blood from infected patients and then examining the mouse after 1 to 10 days for the presence of borreliae in the bloodstream.

In contrast, the microscopic examination of blood or tissues collected from patients with Lyme disease cannot be recommended because *B. burgdorferi* is rarely seen in clinical specimens.

Culture

Some borreliae including *B. recurrentis* and *B. hermsii* (a common cause of endemic relapsing fever in the United States) can be cultured in vitro on specialized media. However, the cultures are rarely performed in most clinical laboratories because the media are not readily available and the organisms grow slowly. Culture of *B. burgdorferi* has had limited success, although use of specialized media has improved the success of isolating the organism. However, the sensitivity of culture is low for all specimens except the initial skin lesion—where the lesion is pathognomonic and culture is rarely necessary.

Serology

Because the borreliae responsible for relapsing fever undergo antigenic phase variation, serologic tests are not

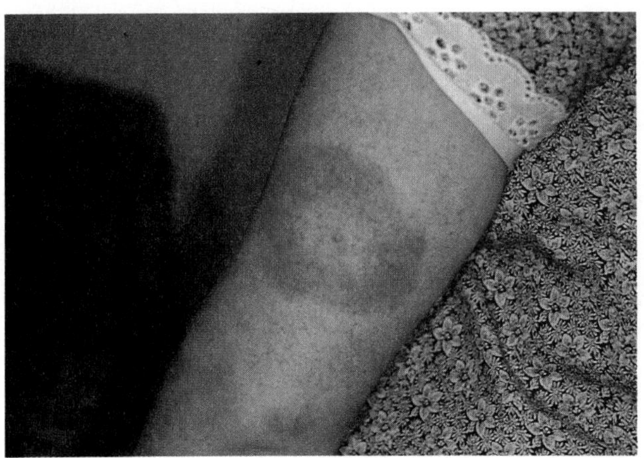

FIGURE 36-16 Erythema migrans rash on the arm of a patient with Lyme borreliosis.

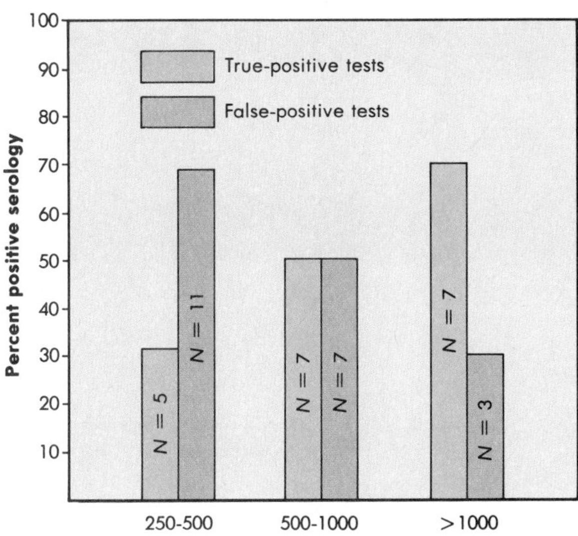

FIGURE 36-17 Predictive value of positive serologic tests for Lyme disease. A positive ELISA test unit of 250 is defined as positive for the test used in this study. Although false-positive tests are relatively uncommon, these can have a significant impact on the interpretation of a serologic test for a disease with a low prevalence. The majority of false-positive tests are from patients with other spirochetal infections, infectious mononucleosis, and autoimmune diseases. All positive ELISA tests should be confirmed with a second test, such as Western Blot. (Modified from *Mayo Clin Proc* 63:1116-1121, 1988.)

TABLE 36-4 Sensitivity of Diagnostic Tests for Borrelia Infections

	Test sensitivity	
Diagnostic test	**Relapsing fever**	**Lyme disease**
Microscopy	Good	Poor
Culture	Poor	Poor
Serology	Not available	Good

useful. In contrast, serologic testing is an important confirmatory test for patients suspected to have Lyme disease. The tests most commonly used are the immunofluorescence assay and the enzyme-linked immunosorbent assay (ELISA). ELISA is preferred because of its greater sensitivity and specificity for all stages of Lyme disease. Unfortunately, all serologic tests are relatively insensitive during the early acute stage of disease. In untreated patients IgM antibodies appear 2 to 4 weeks after the onset of erythema migrans, peak after 6 to 8 weeks of illness, and decline to a normal range after 4 to 6 months. In some patients with a persistent infection, the IgM level may remain elevated. The IgG antibodies appear later, peak after 4 to 6 months of illness, and persist during the late manifestations of the disease. Thus most patients who have late complications of Lyme disease have detectable antibodies to *B. burgdorferi,* although the antibody level may be ablated in patients treated with antibiotics. Detection of antibodies in CSF is strong evidence for neuroborreliosis.

Western blotting has been used to confirm the specificity of a positive ELISA reaction. The 41-kD flagellar antigen (common to many spirochetes) is the major target of IgM antibodies. IgG antibodies against other antigens (e.g., 31 kD Osp A [outer surface protein], 34 kD OspB, 60-kD common heat shock protein) develop late in disease. Specific reactions with antigens unique to *B. burgdorferi* need to be detected for this test to be considered useful. Preliminary studies have demonstrated that detection of borrelia-specific DNA amplified by the polymerase chain reaction may be an effective diagnostic test for Lyme disease.

Although cross-reactions are uncommon, positive serologic results must be interpreted carefully, particularly when the titers are low (Figure 36-17). Furthermore, if multiple borrelia species are found to be responsible for Lyme disease (as is likely to be the case), then interpretation of the ELISA and Western Blot tests needs to be carefully reassessed. At present, serologic tests should not be performed in the absence of an appropriate history and clinical symptoms of Lyme disease.

Treatment, Prevention, and Control

Relapsing fever has been treated most effectively with tetracycline or chloramphenicol. Tetracycline is the drug of choice except for pregnant women and young children, for whom the drug is contraindicated. A Jarisch-Herxheimer reaction (shock-like picture with an increase in temperature, decrease in blood pressure, rigors, and leukopenia) can occur within a few hours after therapy is started and must be carefully managed. This reaction corresponds to the rapid killing of borreliae and the possible release of toxic products such as endotoxin.

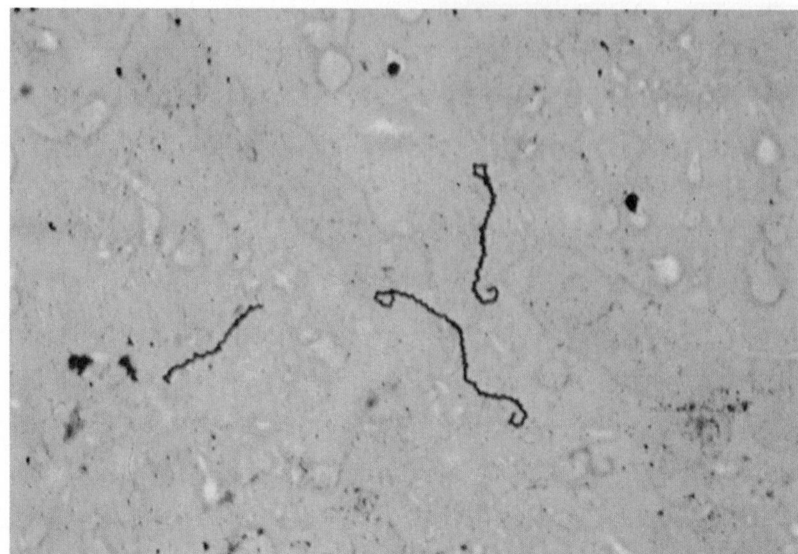

FIGURE 36-18 *Leptospira interrogans* serotype icterohaemorrhagiae. Silver stain of organisms grown in culture. Notice the tightly coiled body with hooked ends. (From Emond RTD and Rowland HAK: *A colour atlas of infectious diseases,* ed 2, London, 1987, Wolfe Medical Publications.)

The early manifestations of Lyme disease are effectively managed with doxycycline, amoxicillin or erythromycin. The incidence and severity of late complications are also ameliorated with therapy. Despite this intervention, Lyme arthritis and other complications can be seen in a small proportion of patients. For these manifestations, ceftriaxone, penicillin, doxycycline, or amoxicillin have been used.

Prevention of tick-borne borrelia diseases is attempted by avoiding ticks and their natural habitats, wearing protective clothing, and using insect repellants. Rodent control for endemic relapsing fever is also important. Epidemic louse-borne disease is controlled by the use of delousing sprays and improved hygienic conditions. Vaccines are currently not available for either relapsing fever or Lyme disease.

LEPTOSPIRA

Physiology and Structure

The genus *Leptospira* consists of two species: *Leptospira interrogans* (subdivided further into 19 serogroups and 172 serotypes) and *Leptospira biflexa* (38 serogroups and 65 serotypes). The species names are derived from the fact that *Leptospira* are thin, coiled bacilli (0.1 × 6 to 20 μm) with a hook at one or both ends ("interrogans" meaning shaped like a question mark; "biflexa" for twice bent; Figure 36-18). *L. interrogans* is pathogenic for many wild and domestic animals, as well as humans. *L. biflexa* is a free-living saprophyte found in moist environmental sites and is not associated with disease. About 22 serotypes of *L. interrogans* are responsible for human disease in the United States, with serotypes icterohaemorrhagiae, canicola, pomona, and autumnalis the most common. Some serotypes have been historically associated with specific clinical presentations (icterohaemorrhagiae, Weil's disease; pomona, Swineherd's disease; autumnalis, Fort Bragg fever or pretibial eruptions), but it is now recognized that the illnesses are not serotype-specific.

The pathogenic leptospires are obligatively aerobic and motile by means of two periplasmic flagella, each anchored at opposite ends of the bacterium. They utilize fatty acids or alcohols as sources of carbon and energy. The leptospires can be grown on specially formulated media enriched with rabbit serum or bovine serum albumin.

Pathogenesis and Immunity

L. interrogans can cause subclinical infection, a mild flu-like febrile illness, or severe systemic disease (Weil's disease), with renal and hepatic failure, extensive vasculitis, myocarditis, and death. The severity of disease is influenced by the number of infecting organisms, the host's immunological defenses, and the virulence of the infecting strain.

Because leptospires are thin and highly motile, they can penetrate intact mucous membranes or skin surfaces through small cuts or abrasions. They then are able to spread in the bloodstream into all tissues, including the central nervous system. Multiplication of *L. interrogans* proceeds rapidly and damages the endothelium of small blood vessels, which is responsible for the major clinical manifestations of disease (e.g., meningitis, hepatic and renal dysfunction, and hemorrhage). Organisms can be demonstrated in blood and cerebrospinal fluid early in the course of disease and in urine during the later stages.

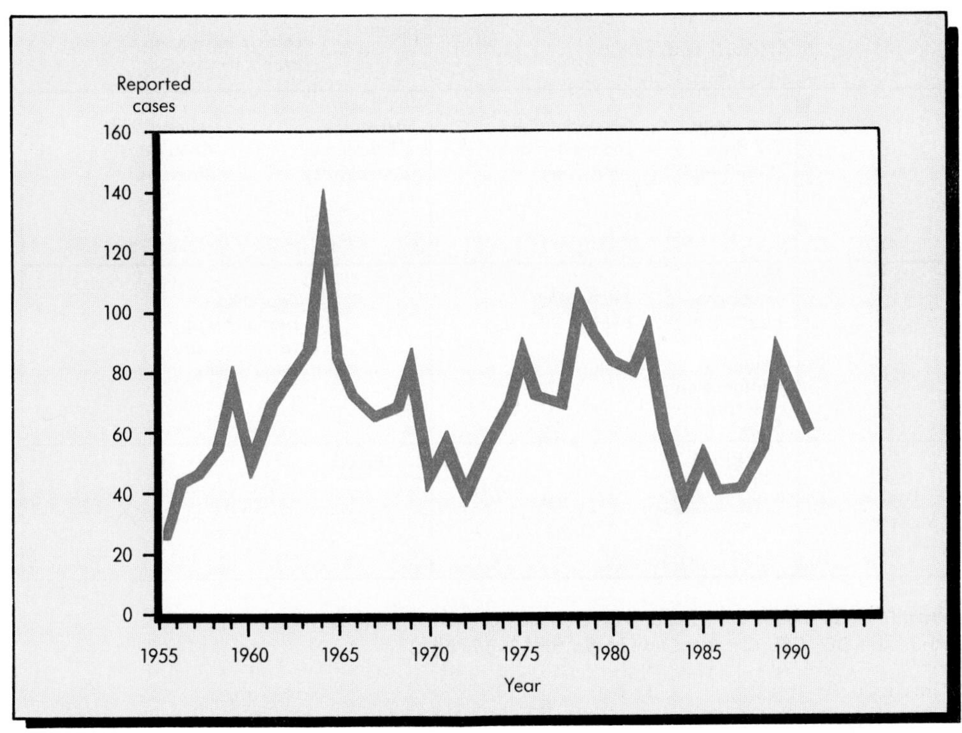

FIGURE 36-19 Leptospirosis in the United States from 1955 to 1991. (From *MMWR* 40:30, 1992.)

Clearance of leptospires occurs when humoral immunity develops. However, some clinical manifestations may be related to immunological reactions with the organisms. For example, meningitis develops after the organisms have been removed from the cerebrospinal fluid and immune complexes have been detected in renal lesions.

Epidemiology

Leptospirosis has worldwide distribution. Fewer than 100 human infections are normally documented in the United States each year (Figure 36-19), with 71% of the 224 cases observed between 1988-1990 reported from Hawaii (Box 36-5). However, the incidence of disease is significantly underestimated because most infections are mild and misdiagnosed as a "viral syndrome" or viral aseptic meningitis.

Many wild and domestic animals are colonized with leptospires, with as many as 10% to 50% of some species infected. Dogs, cattle, rodents, and wild animals are the most common sources for human disease in the United States. Chronic carriage in humans has not been demonstrated.

Leptospires usually cause asymptomatic infections in their reservoir host, where the spirochetes colonize the renal tubules and are shed in urine in large numbers. Streams, rivers, standing water, and moist soil can be contaminated with urine from infected animals and serve as a source for human infection, with organisms surviving for as long as 6 weeks. A moist, alkaline environment is

BOX 36-5 Epidemiology of Leptospirosis

DISEASE/BACTERIAL FACTORS

Leptospirosis, Weil's disease
Multiplication of *L. interrogans* causes clinical manifestations of disease
Dogs, cattle, rodents, and wild animals are reservoirs in United States

TRANSMISSION

Introduction of organism through break in skin after exposure to urine-contaminated water

WHO IS AT RISK?

People exposed to streams, rivers, and standing water contaminated with urine
Occupational exposure to infected animals: farmers, meat handlers, veterinarians

GEOGRAPHY/SEASON

Worldwide; rare in United States (see Figure 36-19)
Disease more common in warm months

MODES OF CONTROL

Treatment: penicillin, tetracycline, doxycycline
Prophylaxis: doxycycline
Vaccination of livestock and pets
Control of rodents

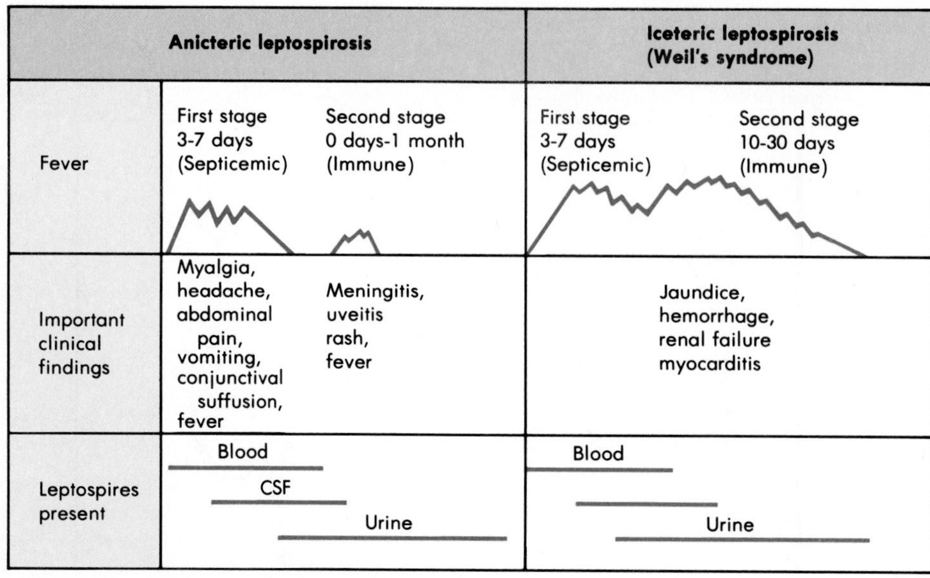

FIGURE 36-20 Stages of icteric and anicteric leptospirosis. (Redrawn from Feigin RD and Anderson DC: *CRC Crit Rev Clin Lab Sci* 5:413, 1975.)

required for survival of leptospires. Most human infections are due to either recreational exposure to contaminated water or occupational exposure to infected animals (farmers, slaughterhouse workers, veterinarians). Most human infections are reported during the warm months of the year when recreational exposure is greatest. Person-to-person spread has not been documented.

Clinical Syndromes

The majority of infections with *L. interrogans* are clinically inapparent and detected only by demonstration of specific antibodies. Symptomatic infections develop after a 1- to 2-week incubation period (Figure 36-20). The initial presentation is similar to a flu-like illness, with fever and myalgias. During this phase the patient is bacteremic with the leptospires, and the organisms can frequently be isolated in cerebrospinal fluid even though no meningeal symptoms are present. The fever and myalgias may remit after 1 week with no further difficulties, or the patient may progress to more advanced disease – including aseptic meningitis – or to a generalized illness, with headache, rash, vascular collapse, thrombocytopenia, hemorrhage, and hepatic and renal dysfunction **(Weil's disease)**.

Leptospirosis confined to the central nervous system can be mistaken for viral meningitis because the course of disease is generally uncomplicated with a very low mortality. Culture of the cerebrospinal fluid is usually negative at this stage. In contrast, the icteric form of generalized disease (approximately 10% of all symptomatic infections) is more severe and has a mortality approaching 10%. Although hepatic involvement with jaundice is striking in severe leptospirosis, hepatic necrosis is not seen and surviving patients do not suffer permanent hepatic damage. Similarly, most patients recover full renal function.

Congenital leptospirosis can also occur. The disease is characterized by a sudden onset with headache, fever, myalgias, and a diffuse rash.

Laboratory Diagnosis

The sensitivity for the diagnostic tests is summarized in Table 36-5.

Microscopy

Because leptospires are thin and at the limits of the resolving power of a light microscope, they cannot be seen easily by conventional light microscopy. Darkfield microscopy is also relatively insensitive and can be nonspecific. Although leptospires can be seen in blood specimens during the early course of disease, protein filaments from erythrocytes can be easily mistaken for organisms. Fluorescein-labeled antibody preparations have been used to stain leptospires but are not available in most clinical laboratories.

Culture

Leptospires can be readily cultured in vitro if specially formulated media (Fletcher's, EMJH, or Tween 80-albumin) are available; however, they grow slowly (generation time, 6 to 16 hours), requiring incubation at 28° C to 30° C for as long as 6 weeks. *L. interrogans* can be recovered in blood during the first week of infection and in urine thereafter for 3 months or more. The concentration of organisms in urine may be low, so multiple specimens should be collected if leptospirosis is considered. Organisms are also present in cerebrospinal

TABLE 36-5 Diagnostic Tests for Leptospirosis

Diagnostic test	Method	Sensitivity
Microscopy	Gram stain	Organisms cannot be seen
	Darkfield	Insensitive, nonspecific
	Direct fluorescent antibody	Insensitive, generally unavailable
Culture	Blood	Positive during first week
	CSF	Positive during first or second week
	Urine	Positive after first week
Serology	Microscopic agglutination	Sensitive, specific, positive after second week, peaks after 5 to 6 weeks, and may persist for months

fluid, but this is usually before the patient develops meningeal symptoms.

Serology

Because specialized media and prolonged incubation are needed, most laboratories do not attempt to culture leptospires and rely upon serologic techniques. The microscopic agglutination test (MAT) is used most often to detect specific antibodies directed against leptospires. Because the test is directed against specific serotypes, the use of pools of leptospiral antigens is necessary. If an infection is caused by a serotype of leptospire not contained in the antigen pool, then it would be undetected. Serial dilutions of the patient's serum are mixed with the test antigens and then examined microscopically for agglutination. Agglutinins appear in the blood of untreated patients during the second week of illness, although delayed response for as long as several months may occur. Infected patients have a titer of at least 1:100 and may be 1:25,000 or higher. Patients treated with antibiotics may have a diminished antibody response and nondiagnostic titers. The agglutinating antibodies are detectable in low titer for many years after the acute illness, so their presence in a treated patient may represent either a blunted antibody response in acute disease or residual antibodies from a distant, unrecognized infection with leptospires.

Treatment, Prevention, and Control

Leptospirosis is usually not fatal, particularly in the absence of icteric disease. Treatment with either penicillin or tetracycline can shorten the clinical symptoms and complications of leptospirosis. Doxycycline has also been used both to treat infections and to prevent disease in individuals exposed to infected animals or water contaminated with urine. The total eradication of leptospirosis is difficult because the disease is widespread in wild and domestic animals. However, vaccination of livestock and pets has proved successful in reducing disease in these populations and therefore subsequent human exposure. Rodent control is also effective in eliminating leptospirosis in communities.

CASE STUDY AND QUESTIONS

A 18-year-old woman spoke of knee pain that developed 2 weeks previously. Three months earlier, soon after vacationing in Connecticut, she noticed a circular area of redness, approximately 10 cm in diameter, on her lower leg. Over the next 2 weeks the area enlarged and the border became more clearly demarcated. However, the rash gradually disappeared. A few days later she experienced the onset of headaches, an inability to concentrate, and nausea. These symptoms also gradually decreased in intensity. Approximately 1 month later the pain in her knee developed for which she sought medical treatment. Upon examination of the knee, mild tenderness and pain was noted. A small amount of serous fluid was aspirated from the joint and found to have a WBC count of 45.0×10^7/ml. Antibodies to *Borrelia burgdorferi* were present in the patient's serum: titers of 32 and 1024 for IgM and IgG, respectively.

1. What are the initial and late manifestations of Lyme disease?
2. What are the limitations of the following diagnostic tests for Lyme disease: microscopy, culture, serology? How does this compare to diagnostic tests for other *Borrelia* infections?
3. Name examples of nontreponemal and treponemal syphilis tests. What reactions would you expect for those tests in primary, secondary, and late syphilis?
4. What are the reservoir and vectors for syphilis, epidemic and endemic relapsing fever, Lyme disease, and leptospirosis?
5. What diagnostic tests can be used for the diagnosis of leptospirosis?

Bibliography

Baranton G, Postic D, Girons IS et al: Delineation of *Borrelia burgdorferi* sensu stricto, *Borrelia garinii* sp. nov., and Group VS461 associated with Lyme borreliosis, *Int J Syst Bacteriol* 42:378-383, 1992.

Barbour AG: Laboratory aspects of Lyme borreliosis, *Clin Microbiol Rev* 1:399-414, 1988.

Barbour AG and Hayes SF: Biology of *Borrelia* species, *Microbiol Rev* 50:381-400, 1986.

Butler T, Hazen P, Wallace CK et al: Infection with *Borrelia recurrentis*: pathogenesis of fever and petechiae, *J Infect Dis* 140:665-672, 1979.

Canale-Parola E: Physiology and evolution of spirochetes, *Microbiol Rev* 41:181-204, 1977.

Coleman JL and Benach JL: Characterization of antigenic

determinants of *Borrelia burgdorferi* shared by other bacteria, *J Infect Dis* 165:658-666, 1992.

Feigen RD and Anderson DC: Human leptospirosis, *CRC Crit Rev Clin Lab Sci* 5:413-467, 1975.

Heath CW, Alexander AD, and Galton MM: Leptospirosis in the United States, analysis of 483 cases in man 1949-1961, *N Engl J Med* 273:857-864, 915-922, 1965.

Kaslow RA: Current perspective on Lyme borreliosis, *JAMA* 267:1381-1383, 1992.

Rahn DW and Malawista SE: Lyme disease: recommendations for diagnosis and treatment, *Ann Intern Med* 114:472-481, 1991.

Rolfs RT and Nakashima AK: Epidemiology of primary and secondary syphilis in the United States, 1981 through 1989, *JAMA* 264:1432-1437, 1990.

Romanowski B, Sutherland R, Fick GH et al: Serologic response to treatment of infectious syphilis, *Ann Intern Med* 114:1005-1009, 1991.

Southern PM and Sanford JP: Relapsing fever—a clinical and microbiological review, *Medicine* 48:129-149, 1969.

Welsh J, Pretzman C, Postic D et al: Genomic fingerprinting by arbitrarily primed polymerase chain reaction resolves *Borrelia burgdorferi* into three distinct phyletic groups, *Int J Syst Bacteriol* 42:370-377, 1992.

White DJ, Chang HG, Benach JL et al: The geographic spread and temporal increase of the Lyme disease epidemic, *JAMA* 266:1230-1236, 1991.

Zoller L, Burkard S, and Schafer H: Validity of Western immunoblot band patterns in the serodiagnosis of Lyme borreliosis, *J Clin Microbiol* 29:174-182, 1991.

CHAPTER 37

Mycoplasma and *Ureaplasma*

Two important members of the family Mycoplasmataceae are *Mycoplasma* with 69 recognized species and *Ureaplasma* with two species. Both genera will be referred to collectively as mycoplasmas in this text. Despite the ubiquity of the bacteria in plants and animals, only three species are definitively recognized as human pathogens (Table 37-1). *Mycoplasma pneumoniae* (also called **Eaton's agent** after the investigator who originally isolated it) is responsible for respiratory disease, and *M. hominis* and *Ureaplasma urealyticum* cause genitourinary tract diseases. These and other mycoplasmas that colonize humans have been associated with a variety of other maladies (e.g., infertility, spontaneous abortion, vaginitis, cervicitis, epididymitis, prostatitis). However, their etiological role in these diseases remains incompletely defined.

Physiology and Structure

Mycoplasma and *Ureaplasma* are the smallest free-living bacteria (Table 37-2). They form pleomorphic filaments with an average diameter of 0.2 to 0.8 μm. Many of these bacteria are able to pass through 0.45 μm filters that are used to remove bacteria. In addition, mycoplasmas do not have a cell wall or intracytoplasmic membrane; the cytoplasmic contents are enclosed only by a well-developed plasma membrane. The absence of the cell wall renders the organisms resistant to penicillins, cephalosporins, and other antibiotics that interfere with the integrity of the cell wall. For these reasons the mycoplasmas were thought originally to be viruses. However, the organisms divide by binary fission (typical of all bacteria) and are gram-negative. Most mycoplasmas are facultatively anaerobic (*M. pneumoniae* is a strict aerobe), grow on artificial cell-free media, and require exogenous sterols supplied by the addition of animal serum to the growth medium. The mycoplasmas grow slowly with a generation time of 1 to 6 hours and form small colonies that have a "fried egg" appearance (Figure 37-1). Colonies of *Ureaplasma* (also called **T-strains,** for tiny strains) are extremely small, 10 to 50 μm in diameter. The three human pathogens can be differentiated by their ability to metabolize glucose (*M. pneumoniae*), arginine (*M. hominis*), or urea (*U. urealyticum*).

Because these organisms do not have a cell wall, the major antigenic determinants are membrane glycolipids and proteins. Cross-reactivity of these antigens with human tissues and other bacteria is observed.

TABLE 37-1 Diseases Caused by *Mycoplasma* and *Ureaplasma*

Organism	Diseases
Mycoplasma pneumoniae	Pneumonia, tracheobronchitis, pharyngitis
Mycoplasma hominis	Pyelonephritis, pelvic inflammatory disease, postabortal fever, postpartum fever
Ureaplasma urealyticum	Nongonococcal urethritis

TABLE 37-2 Properties of *Mycoplasma* and *Ureaplasma*

Properties	Characteristics
Size	0.2 to 0.8 μm
Cell wall	Absent
Growth requirements	Sterols
Atmosphere requirements	Facultatively anaerobic*
Replication	Binary fission
Generation time	1 to 6 hours
Antibiotic susceptibility	
Penicillins	Resistant
Cephalosporins	Resistant
Tetracycline	Susceptible
Erythromycin	Susceptible†

**M. pneumoniae* is an obligate aerobe.
†*M. hominis* is resistant.

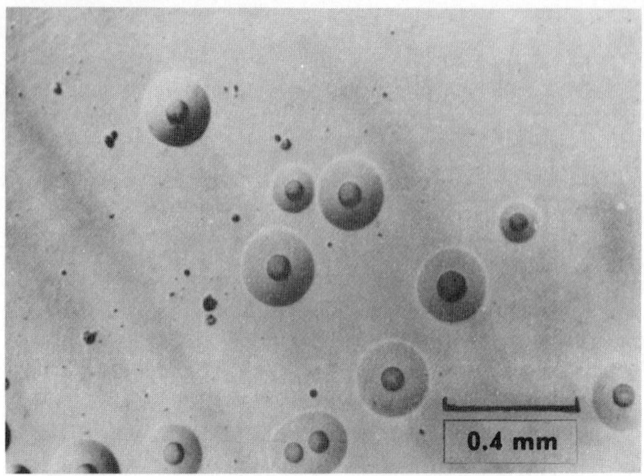

FIGURE 37-1 "Fried egg" colonies of mycoplasmas. This morphology is typically seen with all mycoplasmas except *M. pneumoniae. M. pneumoniae* has a strict aerobic atmosphere requirement, is one of the slowest growing mycoplasmas, and appears as homogeneous granular colonies after incubation for 1 week or more. The other mycoplasmas generally grow within 1 to 4 days. (From Razin S and Oliver O: *J Gen Microbiol* 24:225-237, 1961.)

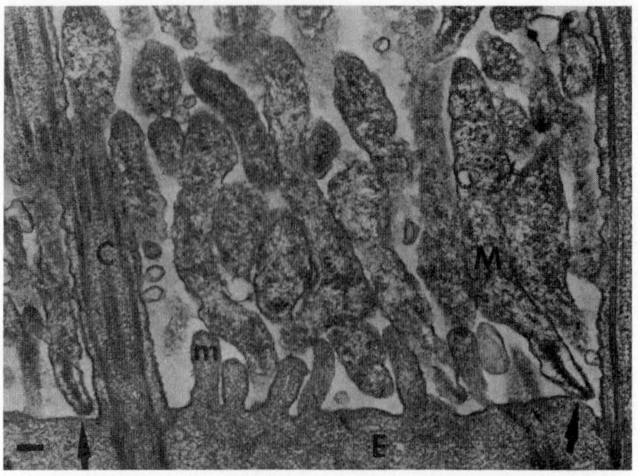

FIGURE 37-2 *M. pneumoniae* infection of a tracheal ring organ culture after 72 hours. Note the heavy parasitization of the mycoplasmas (*M*) with specialized tips (*arrows*) interacting with the epithelial cell (*E*) and in close apposition to the bases of the cilia (*C*) and microvilli (*m*). The bar marker represents 0.1 μm. (From Wilson MH and Collier AM: *J Bacteriol* 125:332-339, 1976.)

PATHOGENESIS AND IMMUNITY

M. pneumoniae is an extracellular pathogen that adheres to the respiratory epithelium by a specialized terminal protein attachment factor (Figure 37-2). This 168 kD adherence protein, called **P1,** interacts specifically with neuraminic acid residues on the epithelial cell surface. Ciliostasis occurs following attachment and then destruction of the superficial layer of epithelial cells. The mechanism of this cytopathic effect is unknown, but release of hydrogen peroxide and superoxide anion has been implicated. Because exposure to *M. pneumoniae* is common in childhood and disease is more severe in older individuals, the observed pathology may be due to the host's immune response. Dissemination to extrapulmonary sites is rare.

EPIDEMIOLOGY

Pneumonia caused by *M. pneumoniae* occurs worldwide throughout the year, with no consistent increased seasonal activity (Box 37-1 and Figure 37-3). However, because pneumonia caused by other infectious agents (e.g., *Streptococcus pneumoniae,* viruses) is frequently more common during the cold months of the year, *M. pneumoniae* disease is proportionally more common during the summer and fall. Epidemic disease is reported every 4 to 8 years. Disease is most common in school-age children and young adults (Figure 37-4), with disease uncommon in children younger than 5 years of age or adults older than 20 years of age. *M. pneumoniae* is the most common cause of pneumonia in children from 5 to 15 years of age.

In 1987 it was estimated that 11 to 15 million cases of *M. pneumoniae* infections occur annually. *M. pneumoniae* has been reported to cause an average of 15% to 20% of all community-acquired pneumonias. Infections in adults are more severe than in children; however, hospitalization is normally not required. Infection is spread by nasal secretions, requires close contact, and usually occurs among classmates or within a family. The attack rate is higher among children than adults (overall average approximately 60%). The incubation period and time of infectivity are prolonged. Thus disease can persist for months in a classroom or family.

Colonization of infants, particularly girls, with *M. hominis* and *Ureaplasma* occurs at birth, with *Ureaplasma* isolated more frequently. Carriage of these mycoplasmas usually does not persist, although a small proportion of prepubertal children will remain colonized. The incidence of genital mycoplasmas increases after puberty, corresponding to sexual activity. Approximately 15% of sexually active men and women are colonized with *M. hominis,* and 45% to 75% are colonized with *Ureaplasma*. The incidence of carriage in adults who are sexually inactive is no greater than in prepubertal children.

CLINICAL SYNDROMES

Three diseases associated with *M. pneumoniae* are pneumonia, tracheobronchitis, and pharyngitis. Pneumonia caused by this organism has been referred to as "primary atypical pneumonia" and "walking pneumonia" – indicative of the comparatively mild, although protracted, course of the disease (Figure 37-5). The onset of clinical pneumonia is insidious following a long incubation period. The initial symptoms include malaise, low-grade fever, and headache. These symptoms increase in severity, and after 2 to 4 days a nonproductive cough develops. Auscultation of the chest reveals rhonchi and rales, and patchy bronchopneumonia is seen on chest x-ray films. Myalgias are common, and a maculopapular rash may develop. Secondary complications can be seen that include otitis media, erythema multiforme, hemolytic anemia, myocarditis, pericarditis, and neurological abnormalities. Resolution of the disease is slow. Secondary infections can occur because immunity is incomplete.

Tracheobronchitis is a common form of mycoplasma disease, with an onset and symptoms similar to pneumonia. Disease primarily involves inflammation of the bronchials with peribronchial infiltration of lymphocytes and plasma cells. Pharyngitis either can be a complication of pneumonia or tracheobronchitis, or it can be the predominant manifestation. Fever, headache, sore throat, pharyngeal exudates, and cervical lymphadenopathy are common. *M. pneumoniae* pharyngitis is indistinguishable from pharyngitis caused by group A *Streptococcus,* Epstein-Barr virus, or other upper respiratory tract viruses.

M. hominis is associated with pyelonephritis, pelvic inflammatory disease, and postabortal and postpartum fevers. Although *M. hominis* commonly colonizes asymptomatic, sexually active individuals, the etiological role of this mycoplasma in disease is supported by isolation of the organism from the site of inflammation, as well as blood, and serologic response to infection. Similar evidence has supported the role of *Ureaplasma* in urethritis, in which

BOX 37-1 Epidemiology of *Mycoplasma pneumoniae*

DISEASE/BACTERIAL FACTORS

Pneumonia, tracheobronchitis, pharyngitis

Lack of cell wall renders organisms resistant to penicillins, cephalosporins, and other cell wall active antibiotics

Adherence protein (P1) for attachment to respiratory epithelium

TRANSMISSION

Inhalation of aerosolized droplets via close contact

WHO IS AT RISK?

School-age children and young adults

GEOGRAPHY/SEASON

Worldwide

No seasonal incidence; epidemics occur every 4 to 8 years

MODES OF CONTROL

Erythromycin and tetracycline equally effective (tetracycline used only in adults)

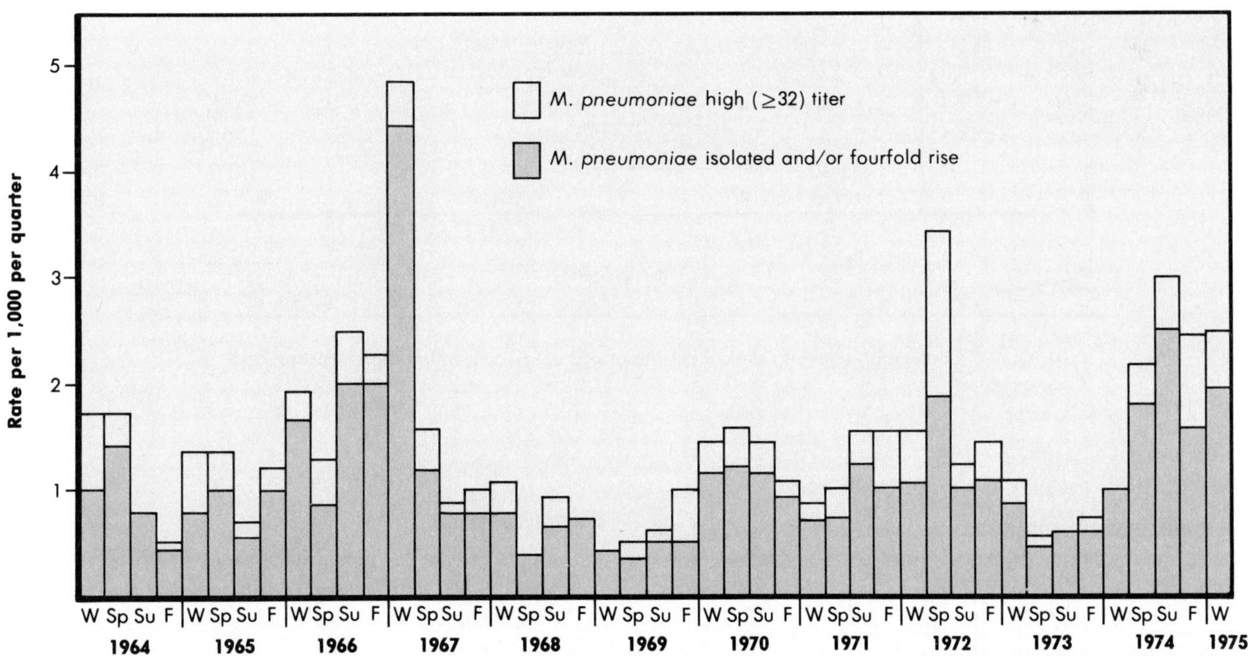

FIGURE 37-3 *Mycoplasma pneumoniae* infections in children younger than 15 years of age are seen throughout this 12-year study in Seattle. No seasonal increase is seen with endemic disease. (Redrawn from Foy HM et al: *J Infect Dis* 139:681-687, 1979.)

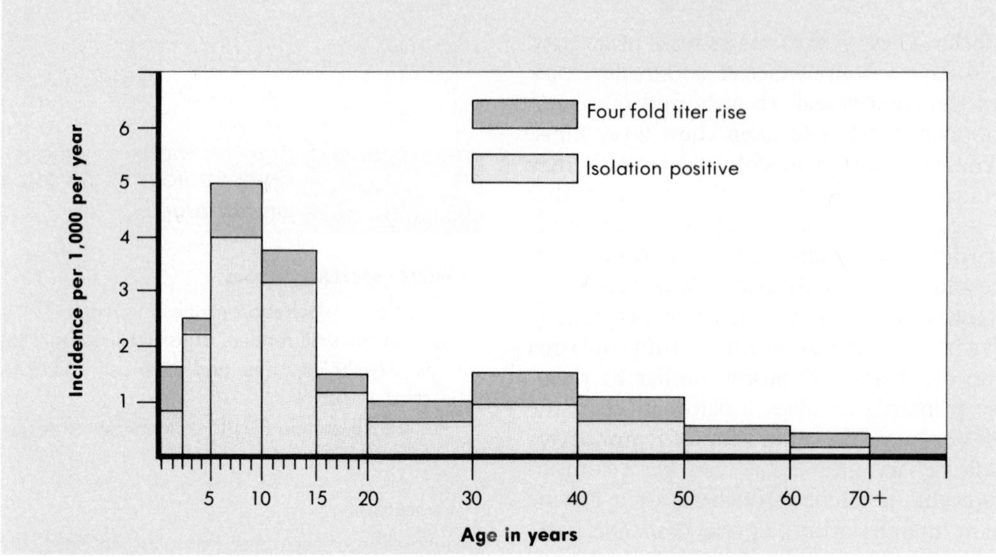

FIGURE 37-4 Incidence of pneumonia with *Mycoplasma pneumoniae* in different age-groups. The greatest proportion of infections is in patients from 5 to 15 years of age. (From Foy HM et al: *J Infect Dis* 139:681-687, 1979.)

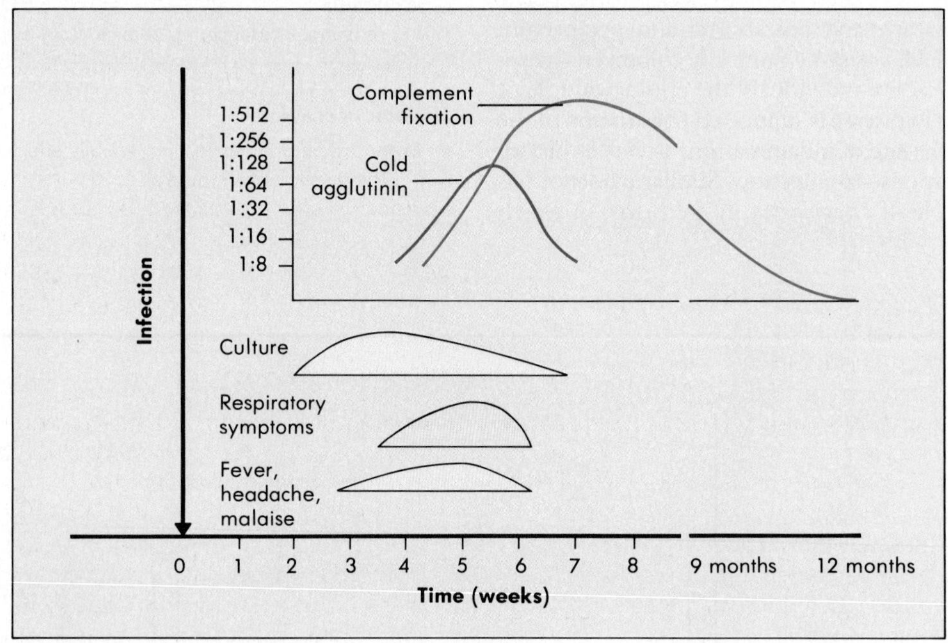

FIGURE 37-5 Correlation between clinical course of *Mycoplasma pneumoniae* infection and diagnostic tests.

this organism is implicated in as many as half of all urethral infections not caused by *Neisseria gonorrhoeae* or *Chlamydia*.

LABORATORY DIAGNOSIS

An assessment of the diagnostic tests for *M. pneumoniae* infections is summarized in Table 37-3.

Microscopy

Although mycoplasmas are taxonomically classified as gram-negative bacteria, they stain poorly because the cell wall is absent.

Culture

M. pneumoniae, unlike other mycoplasmas, is a strict aerobe. This mycoplasma can be isolated from throat washings or expectorated sputum, although most patients produce scant amounts of sputum. The specimen should be inoculated into special media supplemented with serum (provides cholesterol), yeast extract (for nucleic acid precursors), glucose, a pH indicator, and penicillin (to inhibit other bacteria). Growth in culture is slow, with a generation time of 6 hours, and relatively insensitive. In one well-designed study, 36% of the isolates were detected within 2 weeks, whereas the remaining isolates required incubation of cultures for as long as 6 weeks. In another study only 64% of the patients with serologic evidence of an acute mycoplasma infection had a positive culture.

Metabolism of glucose with a corresponding pH change indicates growth in culture. Colonies of *M. pneumoniae* are small and have a homogeneous granular appearance, unlike the "fried egg" morphology of other mycoplasmas. Identification of isolates can be confirmed by inhibition of growth with specific antisera.

M. hominis is a facultative anaerobe, grows within 1 to 4 days, and metabolizes arginine but not glucose. The colonies have a typical large fried-egg appearance (see Figure 37-1). Specific differentiation from other genital mycoplasmas is by inhibition of growth with specific antisera. *Ureaplasma* requires urea for growth but is inhibited by the increased alkalinity associated with metabolism of urea. Thus the growth medium must be both supplemented with urea and also highly buffered. Despite this, these mycoplasmas die rapidly after initial isolation.

Serology

Serologic tests are available only for *M. pneumoniae*. Detection of local production of IgA is generally not useful because the antibody rapidly disappears after onset of infection. Detection of IgG by complement fixation is more useful; the antibody is initially detected soon after onset of infection, peaks within 4 weeks, and persists for 6 to 12 months. This is the standard specific test for *M. pneumoniae* infections. One study reported that 90% of patients with a positive culture had a significant increase in antibody titers or initial titer of ≥32. Because the antibodies are directed against outer membrane glycolipids that are common to other organisms and tissues, false-positive reactions are reported with other mycoplasmas and some plant antigens, as well as in patients with bacterial meningitis, syphilis, and pancreatitis. Complement fixation tests are cumbersome, and tests such as ELISA or immunofluorescent assays are attractive. Preliminary work has demonstrated the ELISA IgM test is a sensitive and specific indicator of acute infection.

Nonspecific reactions to the outer membrane glycolipids can also be measured. The most useful is production of cold agglutinins (e.g., IgM antibodies that bind the I antigen on the surface of human erythrocytes at 4° C). A positive cold agglutinin assay is observed in approximately 65% of patients with *M. pneumoniae* infections, particularly in symptomatic patients. Because this test is not specific for *M. pneumoniae,* cross-reactions occur in respiratory diseases caused by other organisms (e.g., infectious mononucleosis, adenovirus). Strongly reactive cold agglutinin titers ≥128) or a significant increase in titer can provide presumptive evidence of mycoplasma disease.

TABLE 37-3 Diagnostic Tests for *Mycoplasma pneumoniae* Infections

Test	Assessment
Microscopic	Negative because of absence of cell wall
Culture	Slow (2 or more weeks for positive); not available in most labs
Serology	
Complement fixation	Titers peak within 4 weeks, persist for 6 to 12 months; diagnostic titer ≥32 or fourfold increase; good sensitivity and specificity
Cold agglutinins	Diagnostic titer ≥128 or fourfold increase; seroconversion in 34% to 68%; nonspecific
ELISA IgM	Sensitive and specific test for acute infection
Nucleic acid probes	Sensitive if sputum (77% to 82%) is used but not with throat swabs (30%); can be positive in asymptomatic carriers or patients on therapy

Nucleic Acid Probes

Genetic probes directed against *M. pneumoniae* have been commercially developed and appeared initially to be very promising for the rapid detection of *M. pneumoniae* in clinical specimens. The test sensitivity (77% to 82%) is reasonably good if expectorated sputum is used, but recent studies have documented that the probe test cannot be used with throat swabs (sensitivity, 30%) as originally recommended by the manufacturer. Furthermore, the test can detect asymptomatic carriers and patients receiving effective therapy, so a positive probe test must be carefully interpreted.

TREATMENT, PREVENTION, CONTROL

Both erythromycin and tetracycline are equally effective in treating *M. pneumoniae* infections, although tetracycline is reserved for treating adult infections. Tetracycline—which has the advantage of also being active against *Chlamydia,* a common cause of nongonococcal urethritis—is also active against *M. hominis* and *Ureaplasma.* For strains of *Ureaplasma* resistant to tetracycline, erythromycin or spectinomycin are active antibiotics. In contrast with the other mycoplasmas, *M. hominis* is resistant to erythromycin.

Prevention of mycoplasma disease is problematic. *M. pneumoniae* infections are spread by close contact; thus isolation of infected individuals could theoretically reduce the risk of infection. However, the prolonged infectivity of the patient, even while receiving appropriate antibiotics, makes this approach impractical. Inactivated vaccines, as well as attenuated live vaccines, have also been disappointing. Protective immunity has been low, and concern exists that disease in immunized persons may be more severe if the immune response participates in the pathogenesis of disease. Infections with *M. hominis* and *Ureaplasma* are transmitted by sexual contact. Thus the disease can be prevented by avoidance of sexual activity or use of proper barrier precautions.

CASE STUDY AND QUESTIONS

A 21-year-old student developed increasing lethargy, headache, cough, a low-grade fever, and chills and sweats at night. When she was seen at the student health center, she had a nonproductive cough and experienced dyspnea on exertion. Her pulse rate was 95 per minute, and respiratory rate was 28 per minute. Her pharynx was erythematous; scattered rhonchi and rales but no consolidation were noted by ascultation. A chest radiograph revealed patchy infiltrates. Gram stain of sputum revealed many WBCs but no organisms. Mycoplasma complement fixation titer upon admission was 8 and increased to 32 a week later. She was treated with erythromycin and responded slowly over the next 2 weeks.

1. Should cultures of induced sputum have been performed to confirm the serologic diagnosis? Why?
2. How does *Mycoplasma* differ from other bacteria?
3. Describe the epidemiology of *M. pneumoniae* infections. What is characteristic about this patient?
4. What other mycoplasmas cause human disease?

Bibliography

Barile MF, Razin S, Smith PF, and Tully JG: Current topics in mycoplasmology, *Rev Infect Dis* 4:1-277, 1982.

Cassell GH and Cole BC: *Mycoplasmas* as agents of human disease, *N Engl J Med* 304:80-89, 1981.

Foy HM, Kenny GE, Cooney MK, and Allen ID: Long-term epidemiology of infections with *Mycoplasma pneumoniae, J Infect Dis* 139:681-687, 1979.

Kenny GE, Kaiser GG, Cooney MK, and Foy HM: Diagnosis of *Mycoplasma pneumoniae* pneumonia: sensitivities and specificities of serology with lipid antigen and isolation of the organism on soy peptone medium for identification of infections, *J Clin Microbiol* 28:2087-2093, 1990.

Kleemola SRM, Karjalainen JE, and Raty RKH: Rapid diagnosis of *Mycoplasma pneumoniae* infection: clinical evaluation of a commercial probe test, *J Infect Dis* 162:70-75, 1990.

Luby JP: Pneumonia caused by *Mycoplasma pneumoniae* infection, *Clin Chest Med* 12:237-244, 1991.

McMahon DK, Dummer JS, and Pasculle AW: Extragenital *Mycoplasma hominis* infections in adults, *Amer J Med* 89:275-281, 1990.

Wilson HM and Collier AM: Ultrastructural study of *Mycoplasma pneumoniae* in organ culture, *J Bacteriol* 125:332-339, 1976.

CHAPTER 38

Rickettsiaceae

THE family Rickettsiaceae consists of aerobic, gram-negative bacilli that, with one exception *(Rochalimaea)*, are obligate intracellular parasites. Members of this family were originally thought to be viruses because they were small (0.3 × 1 to 2 μm), Gram stained poorly, and grew only in the cytoplasm of eukaryotic cells. However, they are now known to be structurally similar to gram-negative bacilli, to contain DNA and RNA, as well as enzymes for the Krebs cycle and ribosomes for protein synthesis, to multiply by binary fission, and to be inhibited by antibiotics (e.g., tetracycline, chloramphenicol).

Four genera *(Rickettsia, Coxiella, Rochalimaea,* and *Ehrlichia)* are associated with human disease. Originally *Rickettsia*, *Coxiella*, and *Rochalimaea* were classified in the tribe *Rickettsieae*, whereas *Ehrlichia* was classified in the tribe *Ehrlichieae*. However, analysis of 16S ribosomal RNA indicates that *Coxiella* is more closely related to *Legionella* than to either *Rickettsia* or *Rochalimaea*, and *Ehrlichia* is closely related to *Rickettsia prowazekii* but not to *Rochalimaea*. The precise taxonomic classification of these bacteria remains to be defined.

The pathogenic genera are maintained in animal and arthropod reservoirs and transmitted by arthropod vectors (e.g., ticks, mites, lice, fleas). Humans are accidental hosts. The pathogenic Rickettsiaceae can be subdivided into six groups: spotted fever, typhus, scrub typhus, Q (for "query") fever, trench fever, and ehrlichiosis, with each group associated with one or more diseases (Table 38-1).

PHYSIOLOGY AND STRUCTURE

The cell wall structure of Rickettsiaceae, with a peptidoglycan layer and lipopolysaccharide (LPS), is typical of

TABLE 38-1 Geographical Distribution of Rickettsiaceae Associated With Human Disease

Disease	Organism	Disease	Distribution
Spotted fever	*Rickettsia rickettsii*	Rocky Mountain spotted fever	Western hemisphere
	R. akari	Ricekttsialpox	United States, former USSR
	R. conorii	Boutonneuse fever	Mediteranean countries, Africa, India
	R. sibirica	Siberian tick typhus	Siberia, Mongolia
	R. australis	Australian tick typhus	Australia
Typhus	*R. prowazekii*	Epidemic typhus	South America, Africa, Asia
		Recrudescent typhus (Brill-Zinsser disease)	Worldwide
		Sporadic typhus	United States
	R. typhi	Murine typhus	Worldwide
Scrub typhus	*R. tsutsugamushi*	Scrub typhus	Asia, northern Australia, Pacific Islands
Q fever	*Coxiella burnetii*	Q fever	Worldwide
Trench fever	*Rochalimaea quintana*	Trench fever	Mexico, Europe, Middle East, North Africa (rare)
	R. henselae	Bacteremia, bacillary angiomatosis, parenchymal bacillary peliosis, cat scratch disease (?)	United States
Ehrlichiosis	*Ehrlichia sennetsu*	Sennetsu fever	Japan
	E. chaffeensis	Ehrlichiosis	United States

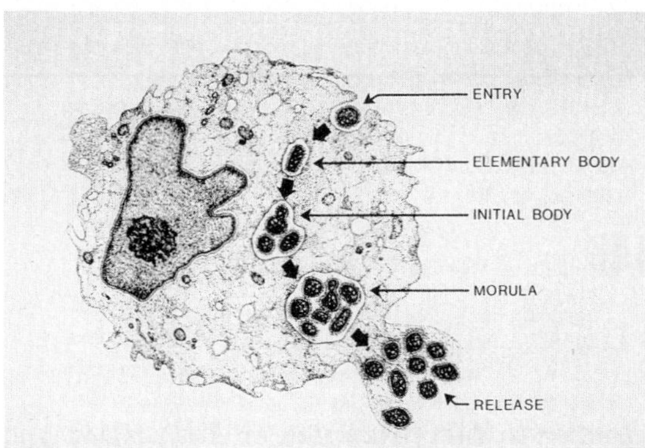

FIGURE 38-1 Schematic representation of the growth of *Ehrlichia* in an infected cell. (From McDade JE: *J Infect Dis* 161:610, 1990.)

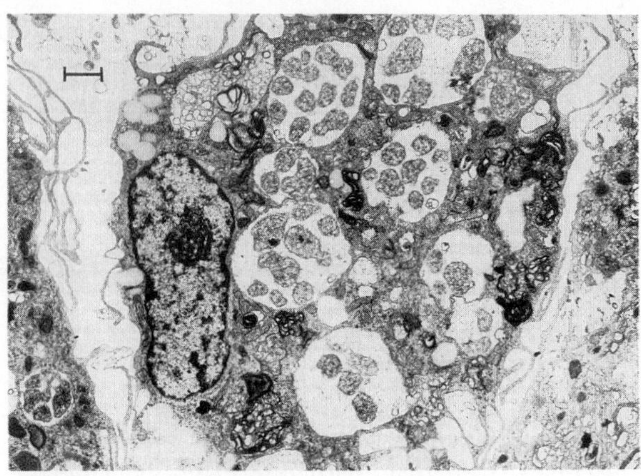

FIGURE 38-2 Electron micrograph of *Ehrlichia canis* in the cytoplasm of a canine monocyte (bar = 1 μm). (From McDade JE: *J Infect Dis* 161:610, 1990.)

gram-negative bacilli. However, the peptidoglycan layer is minimal in some bacteria, and the LPS has only weak endotoxin activity. The bacteria do not have flagella and are surrounded by a loosely adherent slime layer. All organisms are seen best with the Giemsa or Gimenez stains and react weakly with the Gram stain. With the exception of *Rochalimaea*, all bacteria are strict intracellular parasites. Their intracellular location varies: *Rickettsia* species are found free in the cytoplasm, whereas *Coxiella* and *Ehrlichia* multiply in cytoplasmic vacuoles. *Rochalimaea* multiplies readily on the surface of eukaryotic cells but rapidly dies following phagocytosis. The Rickettsiaceae can also grow to high concentrations in the yolk sac of embryonated eggs and in animal models.

The intracellular bacteria enter eukaryotic cells by "induced phagocytosis," or rickettsial-stimulated phagocytosis by nonprofessional phagocytes. After phagocytosis occurs, the *Rickettsia* species must degrade the phagosome membrane by production of phospholipase A and be released into the cytoplasm or the organisms will not survive. Multiplication by binary fission proceeds slowly (generation time, 9 to 12 hours). *R. prowazekii* will accumulate in the cell until it lyses; in contrast, *R. rickettsii* and *R. tsutsugamushi* will continually be released from cells through long cytoplasmic projections (filopodia).

After *Coxiella* enters the cell, it remains within the phagolysosome, where the organism has become adapted to growth in the acidic environment. In contrast, *Ehrlichia* species are killed if lysosomes fuse with their cytoplasmic vacuoles. Figure 38-1 illustrates the growth cycle of *Ehrlichia* with the progression through the three stages of growth: elementary body, initial body, and morula. Figure 38-2 is an electron micrograph of a canine monocyte infected with *E. canis*.

Why members of the Rickettsiaceae must grow inside eukaryotic cells is not completely understood. The bacteria are capable of protein synthesis and can produce ATP via the tricarboxylic acid cycle. It would appear that the bacteria are energy parasites that utilize the host cell ATP as long as it is available. They also use the host cell coenzyme A, nicotinamide adenine dinucleotide, and available amino acids.

Once released from the host cell, most of these bacteria are unstable and die quickly. The exception is *Coxiella*, which is highly resistant to desiccation and remains viable in the environment for months to years. This characteristic is extremely important in the epidemiology of *Coxiella* infections.

The following sections summarize the medically important Rickettsiaceae.

RICKETTSIA RICKETTSII

Pathogenesis

There is no evidence that *R. rickettsii* produces toxins or that the host's immune response is responsible for the pathology of **Rocky Mountain spotted fever**. The primary clinical manifestations appear to be due to the replication of the bacteria in the endothelial cells, with subsequent damage to the cells and leakage of the blood vessels. Hypovolemia and hypoproteinemia caused by the loss of plasma into the tissue can lead to reduced perfusion of various organs and organ failure.

Epidemiology

R. rickettsii is responsible for Rocky Mountain spotted fever, which is the most common rickettsial disease in the United States with 600 to 800 documented cases reported annually (Box 38-1, Figures 38-3 and 38-4). Although the disease was first described in Idaho and later in Montana, most cases are now reported in the Southeast Atlantic and South Central states (Figure 38-5). The reason for this shift is unknown, but it could result from either a reduction of the tick population or decrease in the

BOX 38-1 Epidemiology of *Rickettsia rickettsii*

DISEASE/BACTERIAL FACTORS

Rocky Mountain spotted fever

Strict intracellular parasite with multiplication in host-cell cytoplasm

TRANSMISSION

Ticks are primary reservoir and vector of human disease

WHO IS AT RISK?

Persons in contact with infected ticks; infection requires prolonged (24 to 48 hours) exposure to feeding tick

GEOGRAPHY/SEASON

Western hemisphere; most common in United States in Southeast Atlantic and South Central states (see Figure 38-5)

Disease most frequent April through September

MODES OF CONTROL

Prompt therapy with tetracyclines and chloramphenicol

Avoid tick-infested areas

Use protective clothing and insect repellant

Promptly remove attached ticks

proportion of infected ticks. The principle reservoir for *R. rickettsii* is infected ticks; wood ticks *(Dermacentor andersoni)* in Rocky Mountain states and the dog tick *(Dermacentor variabilis)* in Southeastern states and the West Coast. Other tick reservoirs are *Rhipicephalus sanguineus* in Mexico and *Amblyomma cajennense* in Central and South America. Whether the Lone Star tick *(Amblyomma americanum)* in the South Central states is a reservoir is unclear. The rickettsiae are maintained in the tick population by transovarian transmission. Mammals such as wild rodents can also serve as a reservoir, but this is considered an uncommon source for tick-to-human infections.

Rickettsial infections are spread to humans by the adult ticks when they feed. More than 90% of all infections occur from April through September, corresponding to the period of greatest tick activity. Effective transmission requires prolonged (e.g., 24 to 48 hours) exposure. The dormant avirulent rickettsii are activated by exposure to the warm blood meal and then must be released from the tick salivary glands and penetrate into the bloodstream of the human host. The incidence of Rocky Mountain spotted fever is highest in children and teenagers, but mortality is greatest in those older than 40 years of age.

Clinical Syndromes

Clinically symptomatic disease develops after an incubation period ranging from 2 to 14 days (average 7 days)

Disease	Organism	Vector	Reservoir
Rocky Mountain spotted fever	*R. rickettsii*	Tick-borne 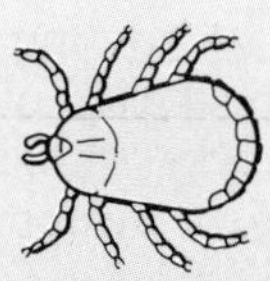	Ticks, wild rodents
Ehrlichiosis	*E. chaffeensis*		Ticks
Rickettsialpox	*R. akari*	Mite-borne 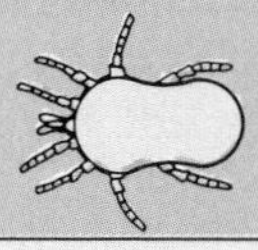	Mites, wild rodents
Scrub typhus	*R. tsutsugamushi*		Mites (chiggers), wild rodents
Epidemic typhus	*R. prowazekii*	Louse-borne 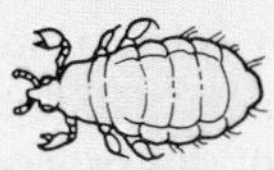	Humans, squirrel fleas, flying squirrels
Trench fever	*R. quintana*		Humans
Murine typhus	*R. typhi*	Flea-borne 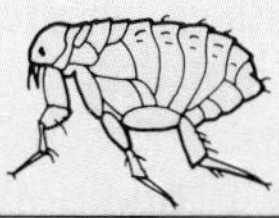	Wild rodents
Q fever	*C. burnetii*	None*	Cattle, sheep, goats, cats

*Tick vectors may be responsible for animal-to-animal transmission.

FIGURE 38-3 Epidemiology of common Rickettsiaceae infections.

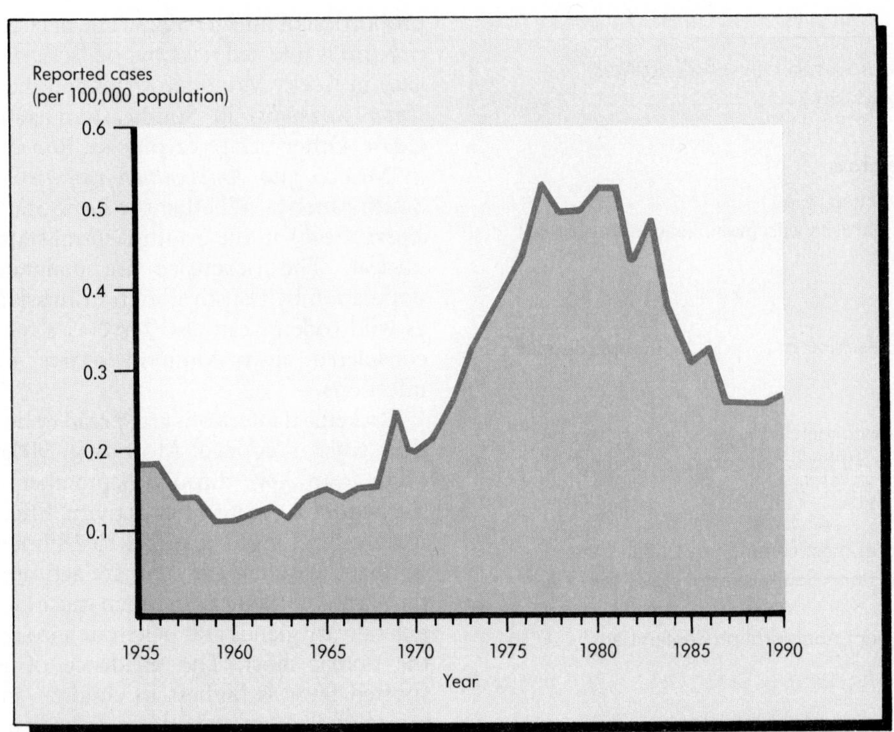

FIGURE 38-4 Annual incidence of Rocky Mountain spotted fever in the United States, 1955-1990. (Redrawn from *Morb Mort Ann Rep* 39:51, 1991.)

after the tick bite (Table 38-2). The patient may not recall the painless tick bite. The onset is heralded with fever, chills, headache, and myalgias. After 3 days or more a rash develops, which can evolve from macular to petechial (Figure 38-6). The rash can develop late during the disease process and is not observed in about 10% of the infected patients. Complications of Rocky Mountain spotted fever can include gastrointestinal symptoms, respiratory failure, encephalitis, and renal failure. Complications increase and the prognosis worsens when the characteristic rash fails to develop or develops late in the course of disease and the diagnosis is delayed.

Laboratory Diagnosis

Although the rickettsiae stain poorly with Gram stain, they can be stained with Giemsa or Gimenez stains. Specific fluorescein-labeled antibodies can be used to stain biopsied tissue; however, the sensitivity of this procedure is reduced if the patient has received effective antibiotics.

The rickettsiae can be isolated in tissue culture or embryonated eggs. However, bacterial isolation is primarily performed in reference laboratories because the bacteria grow slowly and their recovery is traditionally considered hazardous.

The primary diagnostic procedure for Rocky Mountain spotted fever is serology. Although the Weil-Felix test (differential agglutination of *Proteus* antigens) has been used historically for the diagnosis of rickettsial infections, this test is not currently recommended because it is both insensitive and nonspecific. Tests for detecting rickettsia-specific antibodies have been developed, including complement fixation (CF), indirect fluorescent antibody (IFA) test, and latex agglutination. The CF test is insensitive and develops slowly so it is rarely used. The IFA test is considered positive if a fourfold rise in antibodies is detected or an initial titer of ≥ 64. The initial antibody response is detected 2 to 3 weeks after onset, and antibodies will remain detectable for a prolonged time. The test is sensitive (94% to 100%) and specific (100%). The latex agglutination test is initially positive earlier than the IFA (e.g., 1 to 2 weeks after onset) but rapidly reverts to negative. The test may also be slightly less sensitive.

Treatment, Prevention, and Control

Rickettsia are susceptible to the tetracyclines and chloramphenicol. Prompt diagnosis and initiation of appropriate therapy usually result in a satisfactory prognosis. Unfortunately, key clinical signs (such as the rash) may develop late or not at all, and the serologic diagnosis frequently cannot be made until 2 to 4 weeks after onset of disease. Thus the mortality rate is high when the diagnosis or specific therapy is significantly delayed. No vaccine exists for Rocky Mountain spotted fever. Thus avoidance of tick-infested areas, use of protective clothing and insect repellants, and the prompt removal of attached ticks are the best preventive measures. Control is virtually impossible because the tick reservoir can survive for as long as 4 years without feeding.

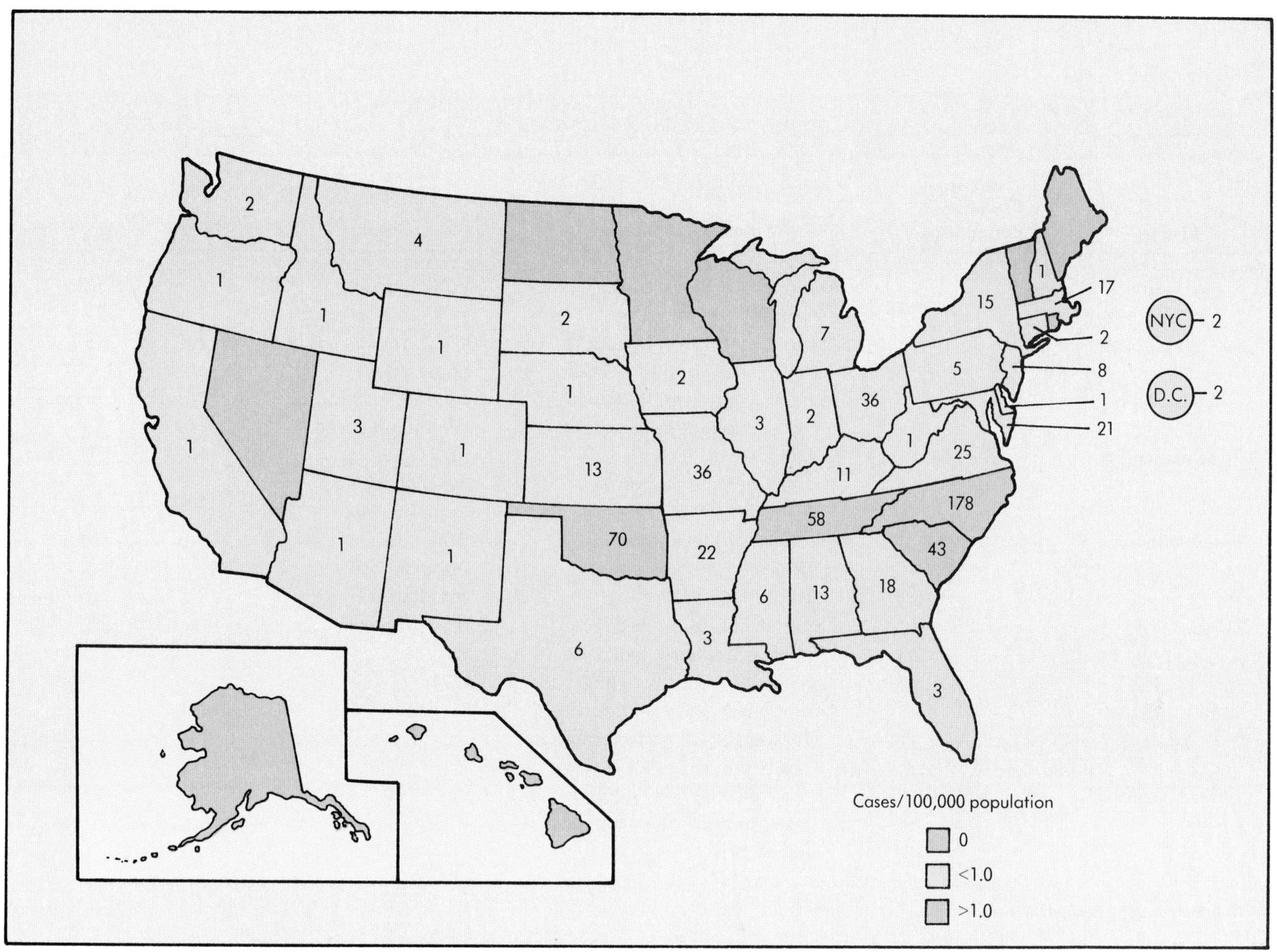

FIGURE 38-5 Distribution of Rocky Mountain spotted fever in the United States. 1990. (Redrawn from *MMWR* 27:452, 1991.)

OTHER SPOTTED FEVER RICKETTSIA

At least four other rickettsial species in the spotted fever group cause human disease (see Table 38-1) with *R. akari*, the agent responsible for **rickettsialpox**, occasionally isolated in the United States. Infections with *R. akari* are maintained in the rodent population by the bite of mouse ectoparasites (e.g., mites) and in mites by transovarian transmission. Humans are accidental hosts when bitten by infected mites.

Clinical infection with *R. akari* is biphasic. At first, as a result of localized multiplication of the rickettsiae, a papule develops at the site of contact with the infected mite. This occurs approximately 1 week after the bite and quickly progresses to ulceration and then eschar formation. During this period the rickettsiae spread systemically. After an incubation period of 7 to 24 days (average, 9 to 14 days), the second phase of disease develops abruptly with high fever, severe headache, chills, sweats, myalgias, and photophobia. Within 2 to 3 days a generalized papulovesicular rash forms. A "poxlike" progression of the rash is seen, with vesicle formation and then crusting. Despite the appearance of the disseminated rash, the course of rickettsialpox is usually mild and uncomplicated, with complete healing in untreated patients within 2 to 3 weeks. Specific therapy with tetracycline or chloramphenicol speeds this process.

RICKETTSIA PROWAZEKII
Epidemiology

R. prowazekii is the etiological agent of **epidemic typhus**, also called **louse-borne typhus**, and the principal vector is the human body louse, *Pediculus humanus* (Box 38-2). In contrast with most other rickettsial diseases, humans are the primary reservoir. Epidemic typhus is associated with crowded, unsanitary conditions that favor the spread of body lice, such as during wars, famines, and natural disasters. Lice die from their infection within 2 to 3 weeks, thus preventing transovarian transmission of *R. prowazekii*. The disease is currently reported in Central and South America, Africa, and less commonly in the

TABLE 38-2 Clinical Course of Common Rickettsial Diseases

Disease	Average incubation period (Days)	Clinical presentation	Rash	Eschar	Mortality
Rocky Mountain spotted fever	7	Abrupt onset; fever, chills, headache, myalgia	>90%, macular; centripetal spread	No	20%*
Rickettsialpox	9 to 14	Abrupt onset; fever, headache, chills, myalgia, photophobia	100%; papulovesicular; generalized	Yes	<1%
Epidemic typhus	8	Abrupt onset; fever, headache, chills, myalgia, arthralgia	40% to 80%; macular; centrifugal spread	No	Variable
Endemic typhus	7 to 14	Gradual onset; fever, headache, myalgia, cough	>55%; maculopapular rash on trunk	No	1 to 2%
Scrub typhus	10 to 12	Abrupt onset; fever, headache, myalgia	<50%; maculopapular rash; centrifugal	No	7%*
Ehrlichiosis	12	Abrupt onset; fever, headache, myalgia, malaise, leukopenic, thrombocytopenia	20%; nonspecific	No	5%
Q fever (acute)	20	Abrupt onset; fever, headache, chills, myalgia; granulomatous hepatitis	No	No	1%
Q fever (chronic)	Months to years	Chronic disease with subacute onset; endocarditis; hepatic dysfunction	No	No	High

*Mortality in untreated patients.

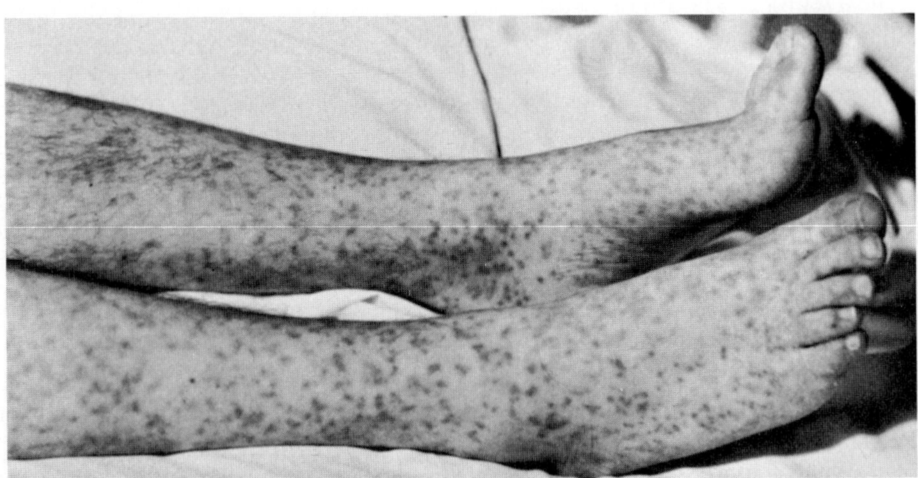

FIGURE 38-6 The rash of Rocky Mountain spotted fever consists of a generally distributed, sharply defined maculopapular rash that evolves to purpuric macules. Rash initially involves the extremities and then spreads to the trunk; palms and soles can be involved. (From Binford CH and Connor DH, editors: *Pathology of tropical and extraordinary diseases: an atlas,* vol 1, Washington, DC, 1976, Armed Forces Institute of Pathology.)

BOX 38-2 Epidemiology of *Rickettsia prowazekii*

DISEASE/BACTERIAL FACTORS

Louse-borne typhus, Brill-Zinsser disease (recrudescent typhus)
Principal vector is human body louse or (in sporadic disease in United States) squirrel fleas
Strict intracellular parasite with multiplication in host-cell cytoplasm
Recrudescent disease possible years after initial infection

TRANSMISSION

Humans are primary reservoir
Inoculation through break in skin via body louse

WHO IS AT RISK?

Persons in crowded, unsanitary conditions
Close contacts of infected persons

GEOGRAPHY/SEASON

Disease most common in Central and South America and Africa (see Figure 38-7)
No seasonal incidence

MODES OF CONTROL

Tetracyclines and chloramphenicol
Effective louse control measures

United States (Figure 38-7). For political and social reasons, the incidence of disease is significantly underreported. Sporadic disease in the United States is primarily restricted to rural areas of the Southeast. In this area flying squirrels, as well as squirrel fleas and lice, are infected with *R. prowazekii*. Squirrel lice do not feed on humans, but the fleas are less discriminating and may be responsible for transmission of the rickettsia from squirrels to humans (epidemiological and serologic evidence supports this hypothesis, but documented transmission has not been recorded).

Recrudescent disease with *R. prowazekii* **(Brill-Zinsser disease)** can occur years after the initial infection. Infected individuals in the United States are primarily Eastern European immigrants exposed to epidemic typhus during World War II.

Clinical Syndromes

In a recent study of epidemic typhus in Africa, clinical disease developed after a 2- to 30-day incubation (average, 8 days). The majority of patients presented initially with nonspecific symptoms and then within 1 to 3 days developed high fevers, severe headache, and other symptoms such as chills, myalgias, arthralgia, and anorexia. A petechial or macular rash was observed in fewer than 40% of the patients, although dark pigmented skin can obscure the rash. Complications of epidemic typhus can include myocarditis and central nervous system dysfunction; a mortality as high as 66% has been reported in some epidemics. The high mortality is undoubtedly due to the poor general health, nutrition, and hygiene of the population, and the lack of antibiotic therapy and proper supportive medical care. In uncomplicated disease the temperature returns to normal within 2 weeks, but complete convalescence may require 3 months or more.

Reactivation or recrudescent epidemic typhus (Brill-Zinsser disease) can occur years after the initial disease. The course is generally milder than with epidemic typhus, and convalescence is shorter.

Laboratory Diagnosis

CF testing with species-specific *R. prowazekii* antigens has been used but is insensitive. This test has been replaced now with IFA and agglutination tests.

Treatment, Prevention, and Control

The tetracyclines and chloramphenicol are highly effective in the treatment of epidemic typhus. However, antibiotic treatment must be combined with effective louse-control measures for the management of an epidemic. Live, attenuated vaccines have been effective, but the concern that the vaccine strain may revert to virulence has discouraged its use. Current vaccine efforts are now directed toward developing a subunit vaccine.

RICKETTSIA TYPHI

Epidemiology

Endemic or **murine typhus** is caused by *R. typhi*. Approximately 40 to 60 cases are reported annually in the United States (Figure 38-8) from the Southeast and Gulf states (especially Texas), and endemic disease continues to be reported in Africa, Asia, Australia, Europe, and South America (Box 38-3). Rodents are the primary reservoir worldwide, and the rat flea *(Xenopsylla cheopis)* is the principal vector. However, the cat flea (*Ctenocephalides felis*), which inhabits cats, opossums, raccoons, and skunks, is considered an important vector in disease seen in the United States. Most disease is reported during the warm months.

Clinical Syndromes

The incubation period for *R. typhi* disease is 7 to 14 days. The onset of symptoms is more gradual than that seen with epidemic typhus, but the symptoms include headache, myalgia, and fever. A nonproductive cough is also frequently seen. After 6 or more days a maculopapular rash develops in about half of the patients, primarily on the chest and abdomen. In a small proportion of patients the rash is more widespread. The course of disease is generally uncomplicated, lasting less than 3 weeks even in untreated patients.

Laboratory Diagnosis

A *R. typhi* specific IFA test is used to confirm the diagnosis of murine typhus. A fourfold increase in titer or a single

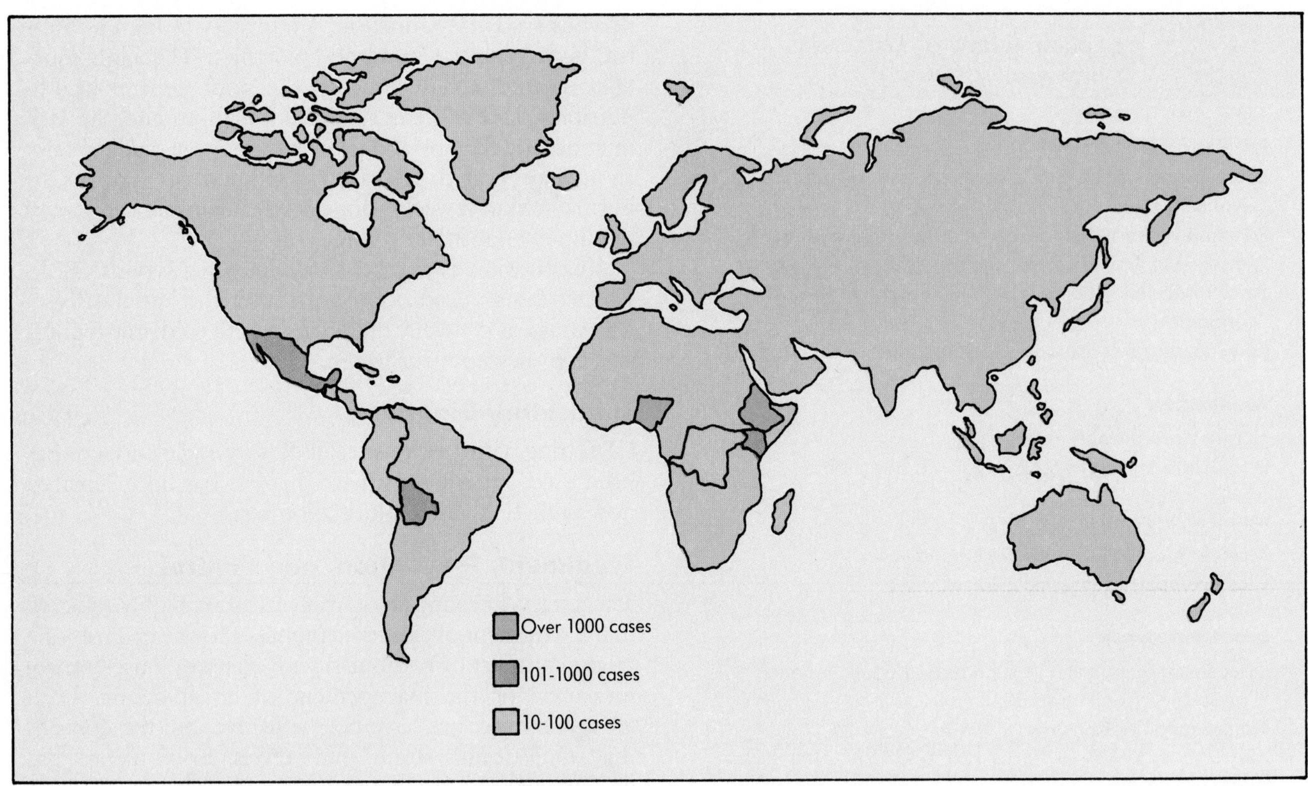

FIGURE 38-7 Geographic distribution of countries that reported 10 or more cases of epidemic typhus during the period 1981-1990. (Redrawn from Perine PL et al: *Clin Infect Dis* 14:1150, 1992.)

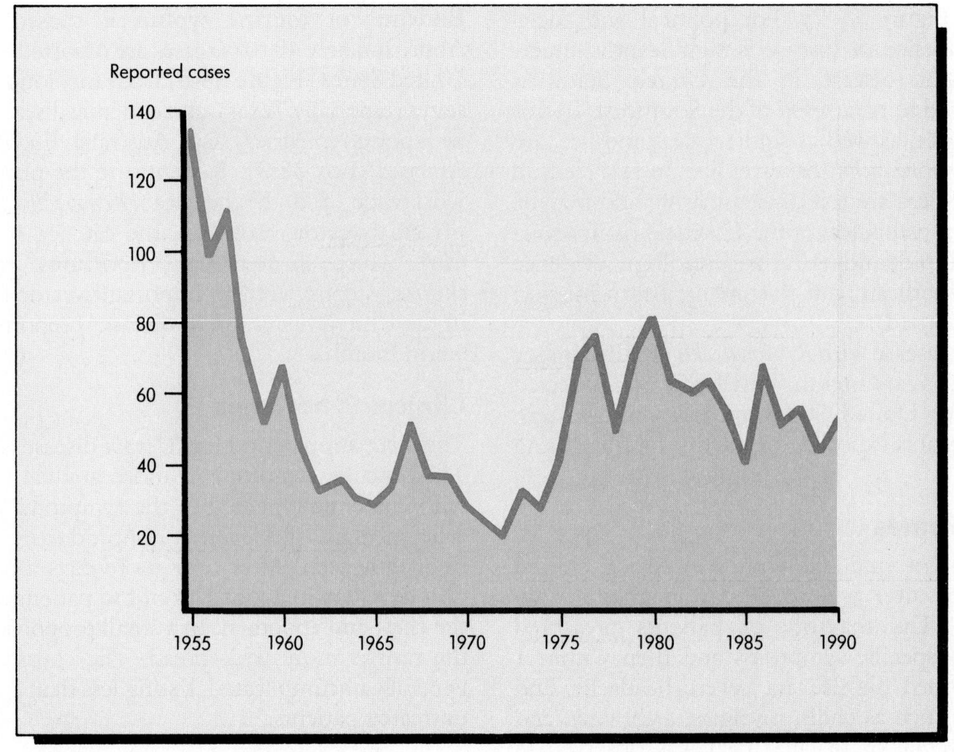

FIGURE 38-8 Annual incidence of endemic typhus in the United States, 1955-1990. (Redrawn from *Morb Mort Ann Rep,* 39:49, 1991.)

BOX 38-3 Epidemiology of *Rickettsia typhi*

DISEASE/BACTERIAL FACTORS

Endemic or murine typhus
R. typhi is a strict intracellular pathogen
Rodents cats, opossums, raccoons, and skunks are primary reservoir
Rat and cat fleas are principal vectors

TRANSMISSION

Inoculation through break in skin via infected flea

WHO IS AT RISK?

Persons in crowded areas infested with rodents

GEOGRAPHY/SEASON

Worldwide; most common in United States in Southeast and Gulf states
Disease more common in warm months

MODES OF CONTROL

Tetracycline, chloramphenicol
Control of rodent vector

titer ≥128 is diagnostic. Significant titers are usually detectable within 1 to 2 weeks of disease onset.

Treatment, Prevention, and Control

Response to either tetracycline or chloramphenicol is prompt and effective. Control and prevention of endemic typhus is difficult because of the widespread distribution of the reservoir and vector.

RICKETTSIA TSUTSUGAMUSHI

Epidemiology

R. tsutsugamushi is the etiological agent for **scrub typhus**, a disease transmitted to humans by mites (chiggers, red mites). The reservoir for this rickettsia is the mite population, where the rickettsiae are transmitted by transovarian means. Infection is also present in the rodent population, which can serve as a reservoir for mite infections. Disease is present in Eastern Asia, Australia, and Japan and other Western Pacific islands. Scrub typhus is also imported into the United States.

Clinical Syndromes

R. tsutsugamushi disease develops after a 6- to 18-day incubation (average, 10 to 12 days), appearing suddenly with severe headache, fever, and myalgias. A macular to papular rash develops on the trunk in fewer than half of the patients and spreads centrifugally to the extremities. Generalized lymphadenopathy, splenomegaly, central nervous system complications, and heart failure can occur. Fever in untreated patients will disappear after 2 to 3 weeks, whereas patients who receive appropriate treatment with tetracycline or chloramphenicol will respond promptly.

BOX 38-4 Epidemiology of *Coxiella burnetii*

DISEASE/BACTERIAL FACTORS

Q fever
Strict intracellular pathogen that multiplies in cytoplasmic vacuole
C. burnetii is extremely stable in harsh conditions
Many animals are reservoirs: wild mammals, birds, sheep, cattle, goats, ticks

TRANSMISSION

Inhalation of airborne particles from contaminated source
Ingestion of contaminated unpasteurized milk

WHO IS AT RISK?

Persons exposed to livestock: farmers, ranchers, veterinarians, meat handlers
Patients with prosthetic or damaged heart valve

GEOGRAPHY/SEASON

Worldwide; relatively rare in United States
No seasonal incidence

MODES OF CONTROL

Tetracyclines or chloramphenicol

COXIELLA BURNETII

Pathogenesis

Understanding of the pathogenesis of **Q fever** is limited because acute disease is rarely fatal. However, available studies indicate the pathogenesis of *C. burnetii* disease differs substantially from disease caused by other Rickettsiaceae. Human infection most commonly follows inhalation of airborne particles from a contaminated environmental source rather than from the bite of an arthropod vector. *Coxiella* then proliferate locally in the respiratory tract with subsequent dissemination to other organs. In severe, acute infections pneumonia develops, as well as granulomatous hepatitis.

Epidemiology

The epidemiology of Q fever is completely different from other rickettsial infections (Box 38-4). The etiological agent, *Coxiella burnetii,* is extremely stable in harsh environmental conditions and can survive in soil for months to years. A large number of wild mammals and birds are infected with these rickettsiae, as are sheep, cattle, and goats, the primary reservoirs associated with human disease. A number of different genera of ticks are also infected. Disease has also been associated with parturient cats in Canada and the northern United States.

The rickettsiae can reach high concentrations in the placenta of infected livestock. Dried placenta following parturition, feces, and urine, as well as tick feces, can contaminate soil, which in turn can serve as a focus for infection when airborne and then inhaled. *C. burnetii* is also excreted in urine, feces, and milk. Consumption of contaminated unpasteurized milk can cause human infection.

Q fever has a worldwide distribution. Although only 20 to 30 cases are reported annually in the United States, this is certainly an underestimation of the prevalence of this disease. Infection is common in the livestock in the United States, although actual disease is very rare. Human exposure, particularly for ranchers, veterinarians, and food handlers, is frequent, and experimental studies have demonstrated that the infectious dose of rickettsiae is small. Thus most human infections are mild or asymptomatic. In addition, *C. burnetii* is frequently not considered when patients have symptomatic disease.

Clinical Syndromes

Acute and chronic presentations of *C. burnetii* infections are recognized. Acute disease is characterized by a long incubation (average 20 days) followed by sudden onset with severe headache, high-grade fever, chills, and myalgias. Respiratory symptoms are generally mild but can be severe. Hepatosplenomegaly is present in approximately half of the patients. Histologically diffuse granulomas are seen in the liver of most patients who have acute Q fever. The most common presentation of chronic Q fever is chronic endocarditis, generally on a prosthetic or previously damaged heart valve. The incubation period for chronic Q fever can be months to years and the presentation insidious. Unfortunately, the progression of chronic disease is frequently unrelenting and the prognosis poor.

Laboratory Diagnosis

At present, the diagnosis can be made by culture (not commonly performed) or by specific serologic testing. *C. burnetii* differs from other rickettsiae by its ability to undergo phase variation, giving phase I and phase II antigens. The phase I antigens are only weakly antigenic. In acute Q fever, IgM and IgG antibodies develop primarily against phase II antigens. Diagnosis of acute Q fever disease is demonstrated by a fourfold increase in antibody titers, an IgM titer ≥ 64, or an IgG titer ≥ 256. The IgM complement fixation titer first appears positive after 2 weeks in untreated patients and reverts to negative after 12 weeks. The IgG titer is positive after 12 weeks and persists for more than 1 year in 90% of patients. Diagnosis of chronic Q fever disease is confirmed by demonstrating antibodies against both phase I and phase II antigens, with higher titers to the phase I antigen (ratio of phase I/phase II greater than 1). An indirect fluorescent antibody test for Q fever has recently become available and will likely replace CF testing in the future.

Treatment, Prevention, and Control

Acute Q fever infections can be managed with oral tetracyclines or chloramphenicol. Response to antibiotic therapy in chronic infections tends to be less satisfactory and the prognosis poor.

An inactivated vaccine for Q fever has been prepared but is not commercially available. Although it is protective for humans, the duration of immunity is unknown. The vaccine is poorly accepted for immunization of livestock herds, because infected animals are asymptomatic and it is unknown if animal immunizations will alter the incidence of human disease.

EHRLICHIA

Pathogenesis

Bacteria in the genus *Ehrlichia* (organisms named after Paul Ehrlich, one of the fathers of microbiology) are leukocytic rickettsiae that parasitize lymphocytes, neutrophils, and monocytes. Erythrocytes are spared.

Epidemiology

The genus *Ehrlichia* consists of five species including two known to cause human infections: *E. sennetsu* (primarily restricted to Japan; causes **Sennetsu fever**) and *E. chaffeensis* (isolated in army reservist at Fort Chaffee, Arkansas; agent of **human ehrlichiosis**) (Box 38-5). Tick-borne disease was first recognized in the United States in 1986. Disease was initially believed to be due to *E. canis*; however, it is now recognized that a new

BOX 38-5 Epidemiology of *Ehrlichia chaffeensis*

DISEASE/BACTERIAL FACTORS

Ehrlichiosis

Organism is a strict intracellular parasite (see Figure 38-1)

Reservoir may be Lone Star tick

TRANSMISSION

Inoculation through break in skin via infected tick

WHO IS AT RISK?

Persons exposed to infected ticks

GEOGRAPHY/SEASON

Common in Southeast, Mid-Atlantic and South Central areas of United States

Disease most common in May, June, July

MODES OF CONTROL

Tetracycline, chloramphenicol

Control of tick vector

serologically related species (*E. chaffeensis*) is the etiological agent. More than 260 infections have been reported from 1987 to 1991, predominantly in southeastern, mid-Atlantic, and south central areas of the United States (e.g., Oklahoma, Texas, Arkansas, Missouri, Georgia, South Carolina). This corresponds to the geographic distribution of the Lone Star tick (*Amblyomma americanum*), which may be the reservoir-vector responsible for transmission. The highest incidence of disease is between May and July, and most infections are in older males.

Clinical Syndromes

Sennetsu fever is characterized by an acute febrile illness with lethargy, cervical lymphadenopathy, and an increase in peripheral mononuclear cells and atypical lymphocytes.

Human ehrlichiosis in the United States is similar to Rocky Mountain spotted fever. Approximately 12 days after the tick bite (range, 1 to 3 weeks) the patient develops a high fever, headache, malaise, and myalgia. Leukopenia, caused by infection and destruction of leukocytes by the organisms, and thrombocytopenia are observed. In contrast with other Rickettsiaceae infections, a rash is observed only in 20% of the diseased patients. The absence of a rash has contributed to the difficulty in diagnosing this disease. However, the prognosis is generally good, with treatment and complete recovery normal.

Laboratory Diagnosis

An accurate estimate of the incidence of human ehrlichiosis was delayed by the inability to isolate the etiological agent; however, this has been recently rectified. Previous confirmation was obtained by measuring seroreactivity with *E. canis*, an organism that shares a 70 kD antigen with *E. chaffeensis*. Unfortunately it is now realized that not all patients with human ehrlichiosis reacted with the *E. canis* antigen preparation. Serologic testing with species-specific antigens should improve diagnosis, although two or more weeks after onset of disease may be required before positive serology (titer ≥ 64) is observed.

Treatment, Prevention, and Control

Response to tetracycline or chloramphenicol is generally prompt, with defervescence occurring within a few days and complete response within 1 week. Effective prevention and control must await additional epidemiological investigations. However, control of the tick vector, as in Rocky Mountain spotted fever, is critical.

ROCHALIMAEA

Two species of *Rochalimaea* have been associated with human disease: *R. quintana* (agent responsible for **trench fever**) and *R. henselae* (implicated in **septicemia, bacillary angiomatosis, parenchymal bacillary peliosis**, and possibly cat scratch disease).

R. quintana is the organism responsible for trench fever, a disease that was prevalent during World War I but is relatively uncommon now. The epidemiology of this disease is similar to that of epidemic typhus. Humans are the principal reservoir; the human body louse is the primary vector.

R. henselae is a recently described species that is responsible for the following diseases: bacillary (epithelioid) angiomatosis, a vascular proliferative disorder of the skin and visceral organs in HIV-infected or otherwise immunocompromised patients; bacillary peliosis hepatitis, a disease seen in immunocompromised patients and characterized by cystic, blood-filled spaces in the liver; and persistent bacteremia, observed in both immunocompetent and immunocompromised patients. Molecular analysis of 16S ribosomal RNA extracted from infected tissues demonstrates a close but distinct relationship with *R. quintana*. Subsequent experiments visualized the organism in tissue using the Warthin-Starry silver stain and isolated it in culture after prolonged incubation (5 to 15 days). Clearance of *R. henselae* from the bloodstream has been accomplished using prolonged therapy with erythromycin or chloramphenicol.

R. henselae has also been implicated as a cause of cat scratch disease. However, it is unrelated to *Afipia felis*, another gram-negative bacillus isolated from lymph nodes of patients with cat scratch disease. The role of *R. henselae* and *A. felis* in this disease remains to be defined.

CASE STUDY AND QUESTIONS

A 37-year-old man entered the local emergency room with fever, arthralgias, myalgias, and malaise. He was well until 4 days before admission when he developed a fever to 40° C, a diffuse headache, photophobia, nausea, and vomiting. His family doctor examined him and prescribed a cephalosporin antibiotic. The patient did not experience any relief in symptoms. Physical examination revealed a critically ill man with a temperature of 39.7° C, pulse 110/min, respiratory rate 28/min, and blood pressure 100/60mm Hg. A dermatological evaluation revealed no ulcerations, rashes, or petechiae. The patient recalled numerous tick bites 2 weeks before the onset of symptoms. Serologic tests for rickettsia were negative for all except *Ehrlichia*, which was positive with a titer of 64.

1. What Rickettsiaceae infections are observed in the United States? What are the responsible organisms, reservoirs, and vectors for each disease?
2. How are the following organisms able to survive phagocytosis: *Rickettsia, Coxiella, Ehrlichia*?
3. What are the major differences in clinical disease caused by *Rickettsia rickettsii* and *Ehrlichia chaffeensis*?
4. Describe the epidemiology of Q fever. How does the etiological agent differ from other Rickettsiaceae?
5. What diseases are caused by *Rochalimaea henselae*?

Bibliography

Anderson BE, Dawson JE, Jones DC, and Wilson KH: *Ehrlichia chaffeensis*, a new species associated with human ehrlichiosis, *J Clin Microbiol* 29:2838-2842, 1991.

Dumier JS, Taylor JP, and Walker DH: Clinical and laboratory features of murine typhus in South Texas, 1980 through 1987, *JAMA* 266:1365-1370, 1991.

Lucey D, Dolan MJ, Moss CW et al: Relapsing illness due to *Rochalimaea henselae* in immunocompetent hosts: implication for therapy and new epidemiological associations, *Clin Infect Dis* 14:683-688, 1992.

McDade JE: Ehrlichiosis—a disease of animals and humans, *J Infect Dis* 161:609-617, 1990.

Perine PL, Chandler BP, Krause DK et al: A clinico-epidemiological study of epidemic typhus in Africa, *Clin Infect Dis* 14:1149-1158, 1992.

Philip RN, Casper EA, MacCormack JN et al: A comparison of serologic methods for diagnosis of Rocky Mountain spotted fever, *Am J Epidemiol* 105:56-67, 1977.

Regnery RL, Anderson BE, Clarridge JE et al: Characterization of a novel *Rochalimaea* species, *R. henselae* sp. nov., isolated from blood of a febrile, human immunodeficiency virus-positive patient, *J Clin Microbiol* 30:265-274, 1992.

Rikihisa Y: The tribe *Ehrlichieae* and ehrlichial diseases, *Clin Microbiol Rev* 4:286-308, 1991.

Sawyer LA, Fishbein DB, and McDade JE: Q fever: current concepts, *Rev Infect Dis* 9:935-946, 1987.

Walker DH: *Biology of rickettsial diseases*, Boca Raton, Fla, 1988, CRC Press.

Walker DH: Rocky Mountain spotted fever: a disease in need of microbiological concern, *Clin Microbiol Rev* 2:227-240, 1989.

Weiss E: The biology of rickettsiae, *Ann Rev Microbiol* 36:345-370, 1982.

Welch DF, Pickett DA, Slater LN et al: *Rochalimaea henselae* sp. nov., a cause of septicemia, bacillary angiomatosis, and parenchymal bacillary peliosis, *J Clin Microbiol* 30:275-280, 1992.

Winkler HH: *Rickettsia* species, *Ann Rev Microbiol* 44:131-153, 1990.

CHAPTER 39

Chlamydiae

MEMBERS of the family Chlamydiaceae are obligate intracellular bacteria that were once regarded as viruses. Chlamydiae possess inner and outer membranes similar to those of gram-negative bacteria, contain both DNA and RNA, possess prokaryotic ribosomes, synthesize their own proteins, nucleic acids, and lipids, and are susceptible to numerous antibiotics. Unlike other gram-negative bacteria, however, chlamydiae lack a peptidoglycan layer between the inner and outer membranes and undergo a unique growth cycle. Chlamydiae are divided into three distinct species, *C. trachomatis, C. psittaci*, and *C. pneumoniae* (formerly TWAR strain). Properties that differentiate these species are summarized in Table 39-1.

PHYSIOLOGY AND STRUCTURE

Chlamydiae exist in two morphologically distinct forms: the small (300 to 400 nm) infectious **elementary body** (EB) and the larger (800 to 1000 nm) noninfectious **reticulate body** (RB) (Figure 39-1). The EB is rigid, resistant to disruption as a result of disulfide linkages among its outer membrane proteins, and never replicates. The RB is the metabolically active, replicating chlamydial form. RBs are osmotically fragile because of the paucity of cross-linked membrane proteins. Thus chlamydiae have compensated for the lack of structural rigidity provided by the peptidoglycan layer. The actively replicating, fragile RBs are protected in their intracellular location, and the rigidly stable EBs can survive extracellular cell to cell passage.

Other important structural components of chlamydiae include a heat-stable group-specific antigen that can be extracted from infected tissue with ether or detergents and has been used in the complement fixation test to diagnose chlamydial infections. Chlamydiae also possess a lipopolysaccharide (LPS) that contains a genus-specific determinant, as well as determinants that cross-react with LPS of gram-negative bacteria. Chlamydiae are nonmotile and nonpiliated. However, surface projections have been identified that presumably allow uptake of nutrients from the host cytoplasm.

Chlamydiae replicate via a unique growth cycle that

TABLE 39-1 Differentiation of *Chlamydia* Species

Property	*C. trachomatis*	*C. psittaci*	*C. pneumoniae*
Host range	Primarily human pathogen	Primarily animal pathogen; humans occasionally infected	Human pathogen
Human diseases	Lymphogranuloma venereum (LGV), trachoma, inclusion conjunctivitis, neonatal conjunctivitis, neonatal pneumonitis, urethritis, cervicitis, salpingitis, proctitis, epididymitis, asymptomatic infections	Psittacosis	Pharyngitis, bronchitis, pneumonia, sinusitis
Elementary body morphology	Round, narrow periplasmic space	Round, narrow periplasmic space	Pear-shaped, large periplasmic space
Inclusion body morphology	Round, vaculolar	Variable, dense	Round, dense
Glycogen in inclusions (positive iodine stain)	Yes	No	No
Susceptibility to sulfonamides	Yes	No	No
Plasmid DNA	Yes	Yes	No

occurs within susceptible host cells (Figure 39-2). The cycle is initiated by attachment of the infectious EB to microvilli of susceptible cells and active penetration into the host cell. After being internalized, the chlamydiae remain within cytoplasmic phagosomes where the replicative cycle proceeds. Fusion of cellular lysosomes with the EB-containing phagosome, which ordinarily would result in release of bactericidal substances into the phagosome, is specifically inhibited. If chlamydiae are inactivated with heat or coated with antibodies, they will be phagocytosed but rapidly eliminated following phagolysosomal fusion (an active humoral immune response in vivo regulates the efficacy of infection). In addition, if other bacteria are phagocytosed with the chlamydiae, they will be eliminated, so the protection is not a generalized phenomenon. Prevention of phagolysosomal fusion may be mediated by components of the chlamydial cell envelope.

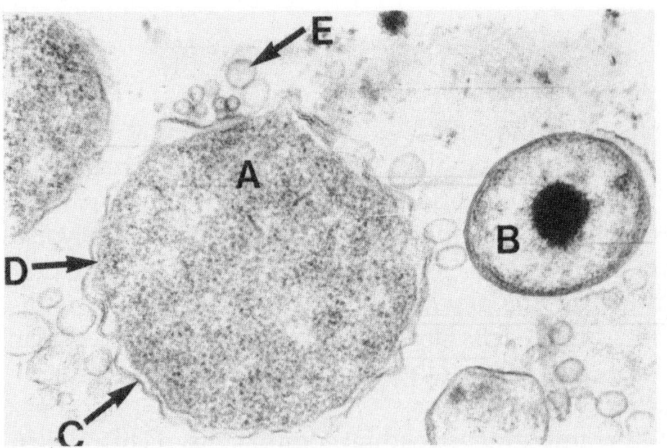

FIGURE 39-1 A transmission electron photomicrograph of *C. trachomatis*, showing a reticulate body *(A)* and a condensing form *(B)* that has nearly completed its transition to an elementary body. Note the electron-dense nucleic acid core in the condensing form. Separation between the outer membrane *(C)* and inner membrane *(D)* can be seen most clearly in the reticulate body. The smaller forms *(E)* are membrane blebs. (Courtesy Collett BA and Newhall WJ, Indiana University. From Batteiger BE and Jones RB: *Infect Dis Clin North Am* 1:55-81, 1987.)

Within 6 to 8 hours after entering the cell the EBs reorganize into the metabolically active RBs. RBs are able to synthesize their own DNA, RNA, and protein but lack the necessary metabolic pathways to produce their own high-energy phosphate compounds. They have been termed **"energy parasites"** because of this defect. The RBs repeatedly divide by binary fission. As replication proceeds, the phagosome is termed an **inclusion.** Approximately 18 to 24 hours after infection, the RBs reorganize into the smaller EBs. Between 48 to 72 hours the cell ruptures and infective EBs are released.

C. TRACHOMATIS

Chlamydia trachomatis has a very limited host range, with infections restricted to humans and one strain responsible for mouse pneumonitis. The species has been subdivided into 3 biovars: trachoma, LGV (lymphogranuloma venereum), and a third biovar that contains the mouse pneumonitis agent. The human biovars (Table 39-2) have been further divided into 15 serotypes (commonly

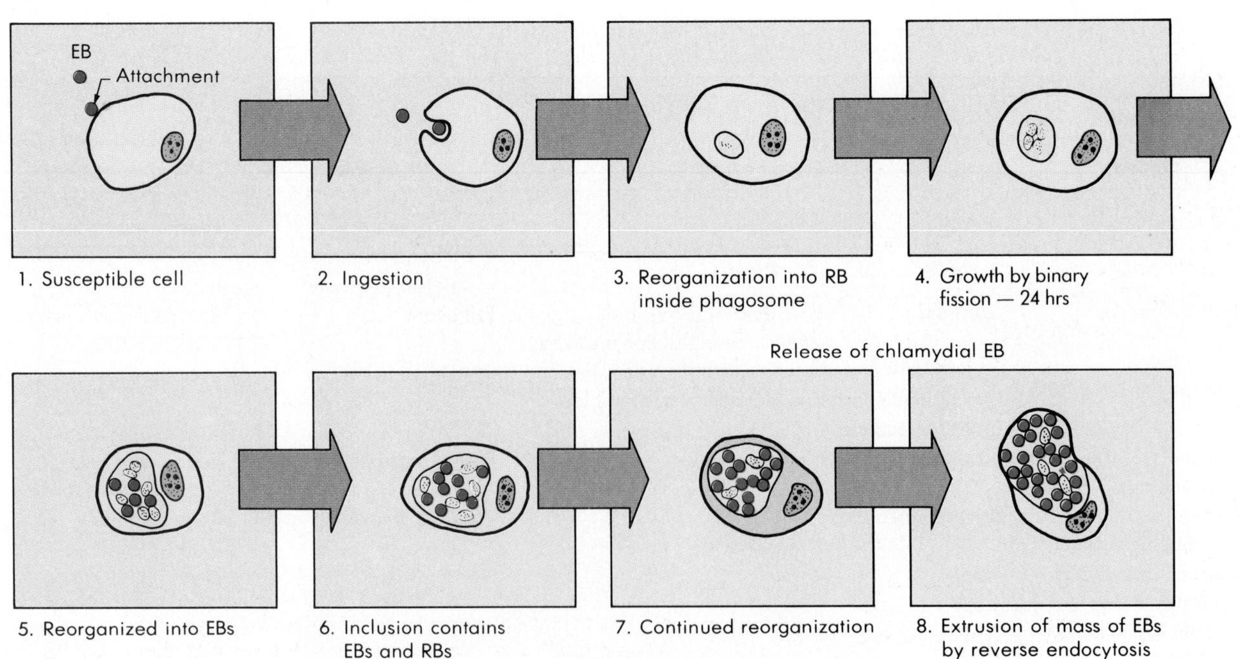

FIGURE 39-2 Schematic depiction of the growth cycle of *C. trachomatis.* (Redrawn from Batteiger BE and Jones RB: *Infect Dis Clin North Am* 1:55-81, 1987.)

TABLE 39-2 Clinical Spectrum of *Chlamydia trachomatis* Infections

Serovars	Host	Infection	Complication	Geographical distribution
A, B, Ba, C	Females, males, children	Trachoma	Blindness	Primarily endemic in Asia and Africa
B, D-K	Females	Cervicitis, urethritis, proctitis, conjunctivitis	Salpingitis, endometritis, perihepatitis, ectopic pregnancy, infertility, postpartum endometritis	Worldwide
B, D-K	Males	Urethritis, postgonococcal urethritis, proctitis, conjunctivitis	Epididymitis, Reiter's syndrome	Worldwide
B, D-K	Infants	Conjunctivitis, pneumonia, asymptomatic pharyngeal and gastrointestinal carriage; otitis media (?)		Worldwide
L_1, L_2, L_3	Females, males	Lymphogranuloma venereum	Rectal strictures, draining sinuses, lymphatic obstruction	Worldwide

Data from Bell TA, Grayston JT: Centers for Disease Control guidelines for prevention and control of *Chlamydia trachomatis* infections: summary and commentary, *Ann Intern Med* 104:524, 1986; Centers for Disease Control: *Chlamydia trachomatis* infections: policy guidelines for prevention and control, *MMWR* 34(suppl 3S):53S, 1985; Thompson SE, Washington AE: Epidemiology of sexually transmitted *Chlamydia trachomatis* infections, *Epidemiol Rev* 5:96, 1983; and Handsfield HH, editor: Sexually transmitted diseases, *Infect Dis Clin North Am* 1(1):62, 1987.
?, Relationship has not been conclusively established.

called serovars) based on antigenic differences among the strains. There are three serovars of the LGV biovar (L_1, L_2, L_3) and 12 serovars of the trachoma biovar: serotypes A, B, Ba, and C are associated with blinding trachoma; serotypes B and D through K are associated with oculogenital disease and pneumonias.

Pathogenesis and Immunity

C. trachomatis has a limited host range of cells that it is able to infect. Receptors for elementary bodies are primarily restricted to nonciliated columnar, cuboidal, or transitional epithelial cells, which are found on the mucous membranes of the urethra, endocervix, endometrium, fallopian tubes, anorectum, respiratory tract, and conjunctiva. Strains of LGV cause systemic infection by virtue of their ability to infect reticuloendothelial cells of the lymphatics. The clinical manifestations of these chlamydial infections are due to the direct destruction of cells during replication, as well as from the host inflammatory response.

Chlamydiae gain access through minute abrasions or lacerations. In LGV the lesions form in the lymph nodes, draining the site of primary infection (Figure 39-3). Abscesses are composed of aggregates of mononuclear cells surrounded by endothelial cells. The lesions may become necrotic, attract polymorphonuclear leukocytes, and cause spread of the inflammatory process to surrounding tissues. Subsequent rupture of the lymph node causes formation of abscesses, fissures, sinus tracts, or

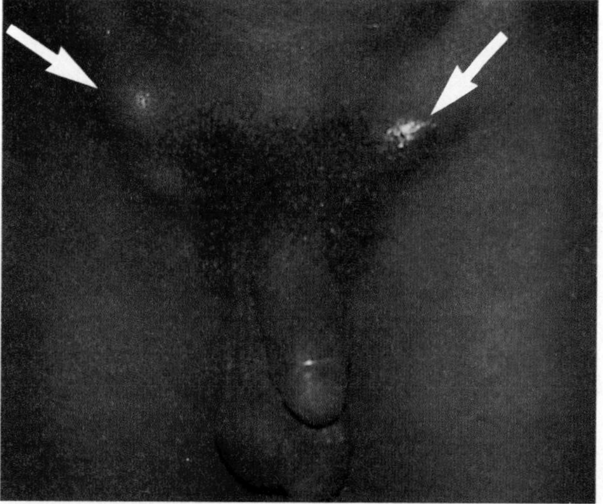

FIGURE 39-3 Lymphogranuloma venereum *(LGV)* showing bilateral inguinal buboes with adenopathy above and below the inguinal ligament on one side (the groove sign) and thinning of the skin over the adenopathy on the opposite side where the node is about to rupture. (From Holmes KK, Mardh PA, Sparling PF, Wiesner PJ: *Sexually transmitted diseases,* New York, 1984, McGraw-Hill.)

fistulas. Infection with non-LGV serotypes of *C. trachomatis* stimulates a severe inflammatory response consisting of neutrophils, lymphocytes, and plasma cells. True lymphoid follicles with germinal centers eventually are induced.

Clinical Syndromes

C. trachomatis is responsible for a wide range of clinical diseases (Box 39-1 and Table 39-2).

Trachoma

Trachoma is a chronic keratoconjunctivitis caused by serotypes A, B, Ba, and C. Trachoma is the leading cause of preventable blindness in developing countries, affecting an estimated 500 million individuals. This disease is seen initially as a follicular conjunctivitis with diffuse inflammation involving the entire conjunctiva. Progression of the disease leads to conjunctival scarring, producing inturned eyelids. The inturned eyelashes cause constant abrasion of the cornea, which eventually results in corneal ulceration, scarring, pannus formation (invasion of vessels into the cornea), and loss of vision.

Trachoma is endemic in the Middle East, North Africa, and India. Infections occur predominantly in children, who are the chief reservoir of *C. trachomatis* in endemic areas. The incidence of infection declines during late childhood and adolescence; however, the incidence of blindness continues to increase through adulthood as the disease progresses. Trachoma is transmitted eye-to-eye by droplet, hands, contaminated clothing, and by eye-seeking flies, which transmit ocular discharges to eyes of other children. Because a high percentage of children in endemic areas harbor *C. trachomatis* in the respiratory and gastrointestinal tracts, transmission may also occur by respiratory droplet or by fecal contamination. Communities in which trachoma is endemic generally are characterized by crowded living conditions, poor sanitation, and poor personal hygiene—risk factors that promote transmission of infections.

Trachoma recurrences are common after apparent healing. Inapparent or subclinical infection has been documented in children in endemic areas and in individuals who acquired trachoma in childhood and then emigrated to the United States.

Adult Inclusion Conjunctivitis

An acute follicular conjunctivitis caused by the *C. trachomatis* strains associated with genital infections has been documented in sexually active adults. The infection is characterized by mucopurulent discharge, keratitis, corneal infiltrates, and occasionally some corneal vascularization. In chronic cases corneal scarring has been reported. Most cases occur in individuals between the ages of 18 and 30, with genital infection probably occurring before eye involvement. Autoinoculation or oral-genital contact are believed to be the routes of transmission.

BOX 39-1 Epidemiology of *Chlamydia trachomatis* Infection

DISEASE/BACTERIAL FACTORS

Trachoma, adult inclusion conjunctivitis, neonatal conjunctivitis, infant pneumonia, urogenital infections, Reiter's syndrome, LGV
Infectious elementary body can survive extracellular cell-to-cell passage
Noninfectious reticular body is protected in the cell
Clinical signs relate to destruction of cells during replication and host's inflammatory response
Infectious patients can be asymptomatic
Male homosexuals major reservoir of LGV

TRANSMISSION

Sexually transmitted; most frequent STD in United States
Inoculation through break in skin or membranes
At birth via passage through infected birth canal
Trachoma: eye-to-eye by droplet, hands, contaminated clothes, flies

WHO IS AT RISK?

Persons with multiple sexual partners
Homosexuals more at risk for LGV
Newborn infants of infected mothers
Reiter's syndrome: young white males
Trachoma: children particularly those in crowded living conditions, poor sanitation, and poor hygiene

GEOGRAPHY/SEASON

Urogenital infections: Worldwide
LGV: highly prevalent in Africa, Asia, and South America
Trachoma: Endemic in Middle East, North Africa and India
No seasonal incidence

MODES OF CONTROL

Conjunctival disease: erythromycin in neonates and children, tetracycline in adults; surgical correction of lid deformities to minimize scarring
Urogenital disease: tetracycline, erythromycin; treatment of sexual partner; "safe sex" practices
LGV infection: drainage of fluctuant lymph nodes and antibiotic therapysurgical correction of complications "safe sex" practices
Improved personal hygiene

Neonatal Conjunctivitis

Inclusion conjunctivitis in the newborn is acquired by passage through an infected maternal birth canal. *C. trachomatis* conjunctivitis has been documented in 2% to 6% of neonates. It usually occurs 2 to 30 days after birth and is generally caused by the serotypes implicated in genital infections (serotypes D through K). After an incubation of 5 to 12 days, swelling of the lids, hyperemia, and copious purulent discharge appear. Untreated infections may run a course as long as 12 months, accompanied by conjunctival scarring and corneal vascularization. Without therapy or with topical therapy only, infants are at risk for development of *C. trachomatis* pneumonia.

Infant Pneumonia

Infants exposed to *C. trachomatis* at birth may develop a diffuse interstitial pneumonia. The incubation period is quite variable, but onset is generally 2 to 3 weeks after birth. Rhinitis is initially observed and is followed by the development of a distinctive staccato cough. The child remains afebrile throughout the clinical illness, which can last for several weeks. Radiographic signs of infection can persist for months.

Ocular Lymphogranuloma Venereum

The LGV serotypes of *C. trachomatis* have been implicated as a cause of Parinaud's oculoglandular conjunctivitis, which is a conjunctival inflammation associated with preauricular, submandibular, and cervical lymphadenopathy.

Urogenital Infections

C. trachomatis is the single most frequent cause of sexually transmitted disease in the United States, resulting in an estimated 3 to 4 million new cases per year (Table 39-3). The majority of genital tract infections are caused by serotypes D through K.

Most genital tract infections in women are asymptomatic but can nevertheless spread to cause symptomatic disease, including cervicitis, endometritis, urethritis, salpingitis, bartholinitis, and perihepatitis. Chlamydial infection may be overlooked in these asymptomatic patients. Women at high risk for chlamydial infection include female sex partners of men with **nongonococcal urethritis (NGU)** caused by chlamydia. Symptomatic infections produce mucopurulent discharge and hypertrophic ectopy and generally yield greater numbers of organisms on culture than do asymptomatic infections. Urethritis caused by *C. trachomatis* may occur with or without concurrent cervical infection.

The majority of genital infections in men caused by *C. trachomatis* are symptomatic; however, it has recently become apparent that as many as 25% of chlamydial infections in men may be asymptomatic (Figure 39-4). Approximately 35% to 50% of cases of nongonococcal urethritis are caused by *C. trachomatis*. Postgonococcal urethritis results from coinfection with both *Neisseria gonorrhoeae* and *C. trachomatis*, and symptomatic illness

TABLE 39-3 Clinical Urogenital Infections caused by *C. trachomatis*

Site of infection	Clinical syndrome
Men	
Urethra	Nongonococcal urethritis, postgonococcal urethritis
Epididymis	Epididymitis
Rectum	Proctitis
Conjunctiva	Conjunctivitis
Systemic	Reiter's syndrome
Women	
Urethra	Acute urethral syndrome
Bartholin's gland	Bartholinitis
Cervix	Cervicitis, cervical dysplasia (?)
Fallopian tube	Salpingitis
Conjunctiva	Conjunctivitis
Liver capsule	Perihepatitis
Systemic	Arthritis, dermatitis

From Holmes KK, Mardh PA, Sparling PF, and Wiesner PJ: *Sexually transmitted diseases*, New York, 1984, McGraw-Hill.

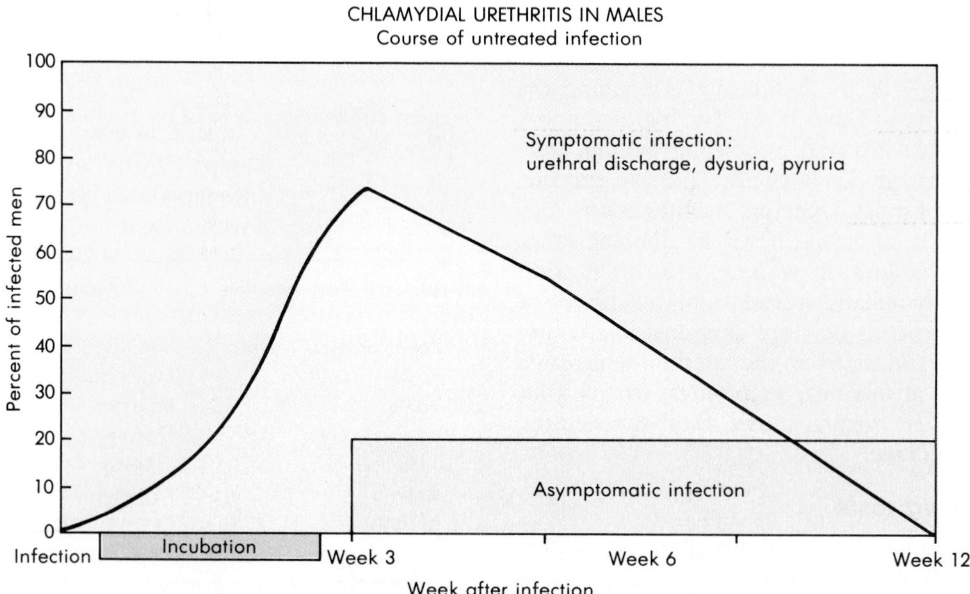

FIGURE 39-4 Time course of untreated chlamydial urethritis in men.

develops after successful treatment of the gonorrhea because of the longer incubation period of chlamydiae. Although chlamydial urethral infections are associated with less purulent exudate, infections in an individual patient cannot be differentiated from gonorrhea. *N. gonorrhoeae* and chlamydiae are the most common causes of epididymitis in sexually active males, whereas gram-negative bacilli (e.g., *E. coli*, *Pseudomonas*) are more common in males older than 35 years of age. As much as 15% of proctitis in homosexual men is caused by *C. trachomatis*.

Reiter's syndrome (urethritis, conjunctivitis, polyarthritis, and mucocutaneous lesions) is believed to be initiated by genital infection with *C. trachomatis*. Although chlamydiae have not been isolated from synovial fluid, elementary bodies have been observed in fluid or tissue from men with sexually acquired reactive arthritis. The disease usually occurs in young white males. Approximately 50% to 65% of patients with Reiter's syndrome have a chlamydial genital infection at the onset of arthritis, and serologic studies suggest that more than 80% of men with Reiter's syndrome have evidence of a preceding or concurrent infection with *C. trachomatis*.

Lymphogranuloma venereum (LGV) is a chronic sexually transmitted disease caused by *C. trachomatis* serotypes L_1, L_2, and L_3. LGV occurs sporadically in North America, Australia, and Europe, but it is highly prevalent in Africa, Asia, and South America. In the United States between 200 and 400 cases have been reported annually during the last decade, with male homosexuals the major reservoir of disease. Acute LGV is reported more frequently in men primarily because symptomatic infection is less common in women.

After an incubation of 1 to 4 weeks, a primary lesion appears at the site of infection (e.g., penis, urethra, glans, scrotum, vaginal wall, cervix, vulva). Small, painless, and inconspicuous, the lesion is often overlooked and heals rapidly. Fever, headache, and myalgia may accompany the lesion.

The second stage of infection is marked by inflammation and swelling of the lymph nodes draining the site of initial infection (Table 39-4). The inguinal nodes are most commonly involved, producing painful, fluctuant "buboes" that gradually enlarge and can rupture, forming draining fistulas. Systemic manifestations may include fever, chills, anorexia, headache, meningismus, myalgias, and arthralgias. In women, proctitis is common because of lymphatic spread from the cervix or vagina. In men, proctitis develops after anal intercourse or by lymphatic spread from the urethra. Untreated LGV may resolve at this stage or progress to a chronic ulcerative phase with genital ulcers, fistulas, strictures, or genital elephantiasis.

Laboratory Diagnosis

C. trachomatis can be diagnosed by cytology, culture, direct detection of antigen in clinical specimens, use of molecular probes, and serologic testing. The sensitivity of each method depends on the patient population examined, specimen site, and nature of disease. For example, symptomatic infections are generally easier to document than asymptomatic infections because higher numbers of chlamydiae are present in the specimen.

Cytology

Examination of Giemsa-stained cell scrapings for the presence of inclusions was the first method used for the diagnosis of *C. trachomatis*. However, this method is insensitive when compared with culture or direct immunofluorescence. Likewise, Papanicolaou staining of cervical material has been found to be insensitive and nonspecific.

Culture

Isolation of *C. trachomatis* in cell culture remains the most specific method of diagnosing *C. trachomatis* infections. The bacteria infect a restricted range of cell lines in vitro (e.g., HeLa-229, McCoy, BHK-21, Buffalo green monkey kidney cells), similar to their narrow range of infectivity in vivo. Modifications of the culture procedures have improved the test sensitivity. These changes include pretreatment with chemical inhibitors of host cell metabolism (e.g., cycloheximide), centrifugation of the specimen onto the cell monolayers (modifies the host cell), use of the shell vial technique (growth of the host cell monolayer on glass coverslips rather than in small microtiter wells), multiple passages or subcultures of infected cells, and detection of intracellular inclusions with iodine stains (Figure 39-5; stains glycogen containing *C. trachomatis* inclusions) or fluorescein-conjugated antibodies. Despite these improvements, the sensitivity of culture is compromised by collection of inadequate specimens and loss of chlamydial viability during transport. It has been estimated that a single endocervical specimen may have only a 70% to 80% sensitivity.

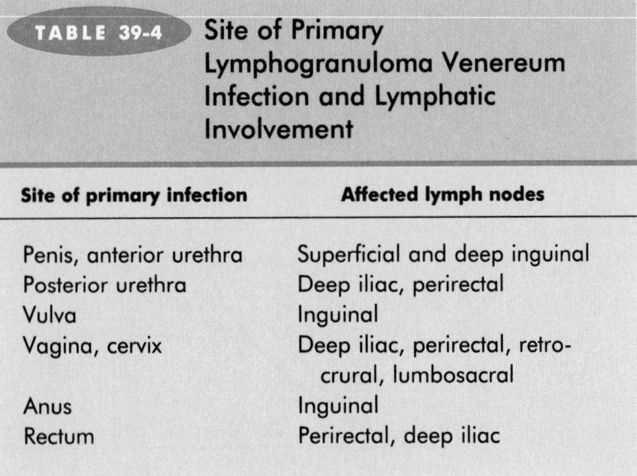

TABLE 39-4 Site of Primary Lymphogranuloma Venereum Infection and Lymphatic Involvement

Site of primary infection	Affected lymph nodes
Penis, anterior urethra	Superficial and deep inguinal
Posterior urethra	Deep iliac, perirectal
Vulva	Inguinal
Vagina, cervix	Deep iliac, perirectal, retrocrural, lumbosacral
Anus	Inguinal
Rectum	Perirectal, deep iliac

From Holmes KK, Mardh PA, Sparling PF, and Wiesner PJ: *Sexually transmitted diseases*, New York, 1984, McGraw-Hill.

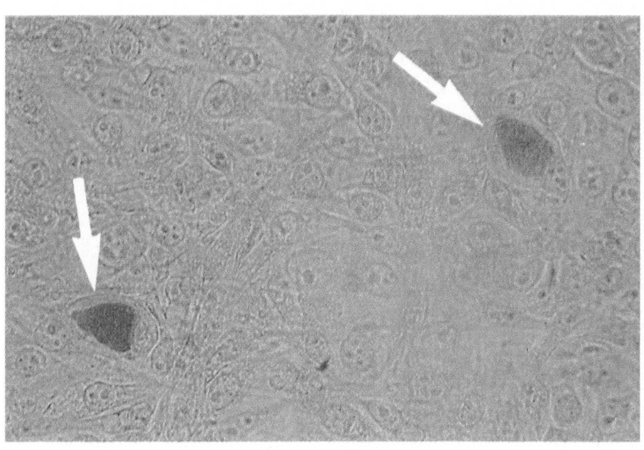

FIGURE 39-5 Iodine-stained *C. trachomatis* inclusion bodies *(arrows).*

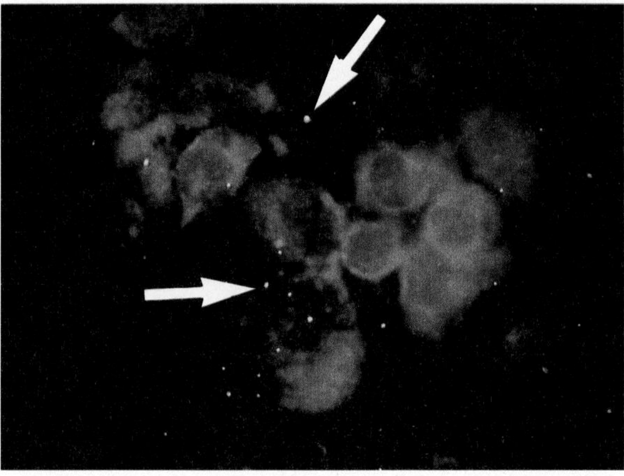

FIGURE 39-6 Fluorescent-stained elementary bodies *(arrows)* in a clinical sample.

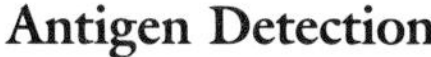

Antigen Detection

Two general approaches have been used to detect chlamydial antigens in clinical specimens: direct immunofluorescence (DFA) staining with fluorescein-conjugated monoclonal antibodies (Figure 39-6), and enzyme-linked immunoassays. In both assays, antibodies have been prepared against either the chlamydial major outer membrane protein (MOMP) or the cell wall lipopolysaccharide (LPS). Because antigenic determinants on LPS may be shared with other bacteria, particularly those in fecal specimens, antibody tests targeting the LPS antigen are considered less specific. The sensitivity of each assay method is difficult to evaluate, but neither is considered as sensitive as culture, particularly with male urethral specimens or specimens collected from asymptomatic patients in whom relatively few elementary bodies may be present.

Nucleic Acid Probes

Initial tests using molecular probes to detect chlamydial nucleic acids were insensitive. However, this problem has been rectified with the development of commercially prepared tests, particularly those using target amplification (e.g., PCR-based tests). It is likely that these tests will replace culture and antigen detection tests. The one reservation with this approach is that nonviable, as well as viable, chlamydia are detected, so nucleic acid probes may be unreliable for determining therapeutic response.

Serology

The skin test for LGV (**Frei test**) is of historical interest only because the test was found to be both insensitive and nonspecific. Diagnosis of LGV is currently based on the complement fixation (CF) test. The CF test measures complement-fixing antibodies directed against the LPS genus-specific antigen. Unfortunately, because this test will be positive in patients exposed to other strains of *C. trachomatis*, it is not specific for LGV. Serologic testing has limited value in the diagnosis of other chlamydial urogenital infections in adults because the test cannot differentiate between current and past infection. Most adults with infection have had a previous exposure to *C. trachomatis* and thus are seropositive. Although IgM may not always be produced, the presence of a high titer of IgM (e.g., ≥ 128) suggests a recent infection. A negative serologic test may exclude infection; however, antibodies are not detected early in the course of disease, and response may be diminished by antibiotic therapy. Detection of IgM to *C. trachomatis* is useful in the diagnosis of neonatal infection with *C. trachomatis*.

Treatment, Prevention, and Control

For neonatal conjunctivitis or disease in young children systemic erythromycin therapy is used. Systemic therapy with a tetracycline is recommended for treatment of ocular infections in older children and adults. However, in areas with endemic trachoma, antibiotic therapy without improved sanitation has limited value. Surgical correction of lid deformities reduces trachoma-induced blindness. Systemic therapy with tetracycline or erythromycin is recommended for treatment of urogenital infections. Treatment of the sexual partner is also recommended. LGV infections require aspiration of fluctuant lymph nodes in addition to antibiotic therapy. Complications of LGV, such as strictures, fistulas, and elephantiasis, require surgery.

Prevention of *C. trachomatis* infections is difficult because the population with endemic disease frequently has limited access to medical care. The blindness associated with advanced stages of this disease can be prevented only by prompt treatment of early disease and prevention of subsequent reexposure. Although treatment can be initiated, the eradication of disease within a population and prevention of reinfections are difficult.

Chlamydia conjunctivitis and genital infections are prevented by the use of safe sexual practices and the prompt treatment of both symptomatic patients and their contacts.

BOX 39-2 Epidemiology of Psittacosis

DISEASE/BACTERIAL FACTORS

Parrot fever
Infectious elementary body can survive extracellular cell to cell passage
Noninfectious reticular body is protected in the cell
Natural reservoir is birds

TRANSMISSION

Inhalation of dried bird excrement

WHO IS AT RISK?

Veterinarians
Zoo keepers
Pet shop workers
Poultry processing plant employees
Owners of infected pet birds

GEOGRAPHY/SEASON

Worldwide
No seasonal incidence

MODES OF CONTROL

Tetracycline, erythromycin
Control of infection in pet birds: treatment for 45 days with chlortetracycline HCl

C. PSITTACI

C. psittaci is the cause of psittacosis **(parrot fever),** which can be transmitted to humans. The disease was first described in parrots, thus the name psittacosis (Psittakos, Greek for parrot). The natural reservoir of *C. psittaci* is birds; virtually any species of birds, as well as reptiles and humans, can become infected. The organism is present in the blood, tissues, feces, and feathers of infected birds.

Epidemiology

Psittacosis is a notifiable disease in 42 states, and approximately 100 to 250 cases are reported annually, with most infections in adults (Box 39-2 and Figure 39-7). This number certainly is an underestimation of the prevalence of disease because human infections may be asymptomatic or mild, exposure to an infected bird may not be suspected, convalescent serum may not be collected to confirm the clinical diagnosis, and antibiotic therapy may blunt the antibody response.

Transmission to humans is usually by inhalation of dried bird excrement. The infected birds may be either ill appearing or asymptomatic. Person-to-person transmission is rare. Veterinarians, zoo keepers, pet shop workers, and poultry processing plant employees are at risk for this infection.

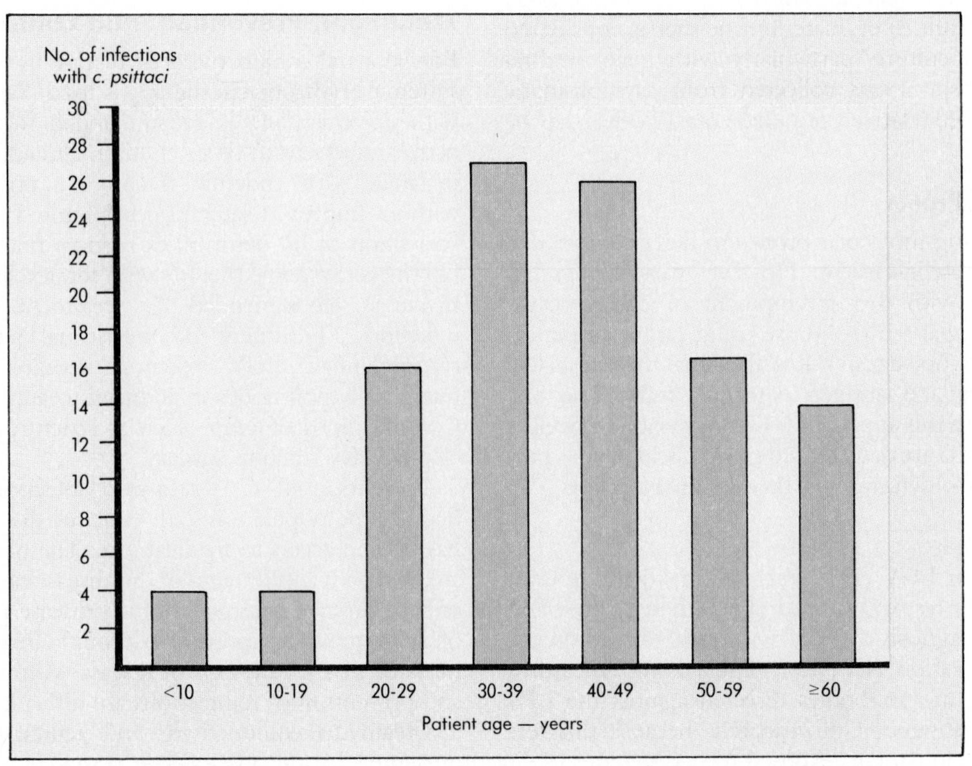

FIGURE 39-7 Age of patients with documented infections by *C. psittaci* in 1990. (Data from *MMWR* 39:1991.)

Pathogenesis and Immunity

Infection occurs via the respiratory tract, with subsequent spread to the reticuloendothelial cells of the liver and spleen. Multiplication of the organisms occurs in these sites, producing focal necrosis. The lung and other organs subsequently are seeded by hematogenous spread, causing a predominantly lymphocytic inflammatory response in both the alveolar and interstitial spaces. Edema, thickening of the alveolar wall, infiltration of macrophages, necrosis, and occasionally hemorrhage occur at these sites. Mucus plugs develop in the bronchioles, causing cyanosis and anoxia.

Clinical Syndromes

After an incubation of 7 to 15 days, onset of illness is usually manifested by headache, high fever, and chills (Figure 39-8). Other early manifestations include malaise, anorexia, myalgia, arthralgia, and occasionally a pale macular rash. Pulmonary signs include a nonproductive cough, rales, and consolidation. Central nervous system involvement is common, usually consisting of headache, but in severe cases encephalitis, convulsions, coma, and death may occur. Gastrointestinal symptoms such as nausea, vomiting, and diarrhea may be present. Other systemic symptoms include carditis, hepatomegaly, splenomegaly, and follicular keratoconjunctivitis.

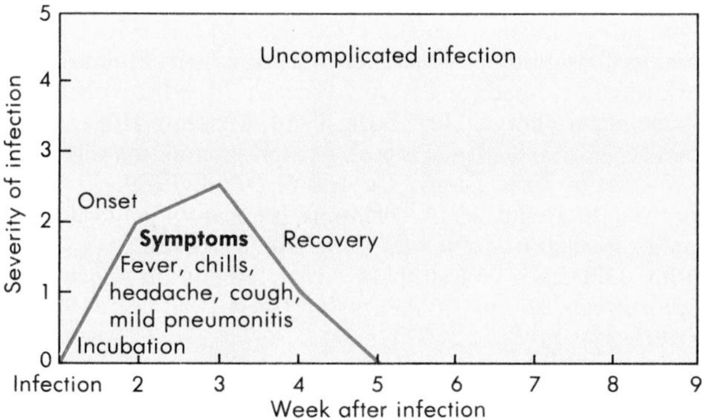

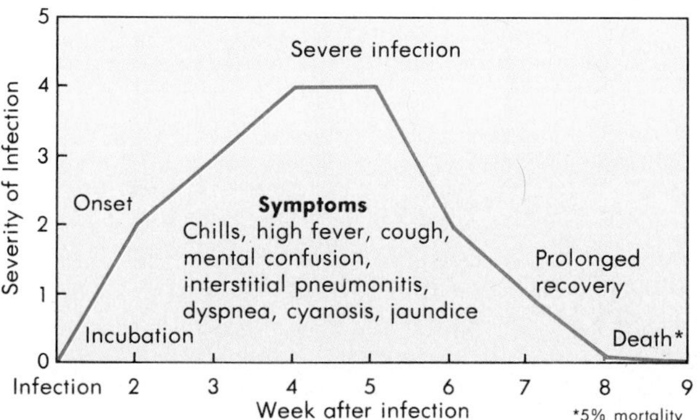

FIGURE 39-8 Time course of *Chlamydia psittaci* infection.

Laboratory Diagnosis

Psittacosis is usually diagnosed by serologic testing. A fourfold increase in titer by complement fixation (CF) testing of paired acute and convalescent phase sera is diagnostic. Titer increases are usually observed by the end of the second week of illness. A single CF titer of ≥ 32 is evidence of recent infection. *C. psittaci* can be isolated in cell culture (e.g., L cells) after 5 to 10 days of incubation, although this is rarely done in clinical labs. Genus-specific antigen tests and molecular probes can also be used to confirm the clinical diagnosis.

Treatment, Prevention, and Control

Infections can be treated successfully with tetracycline or erythromycin. Prevention of psittacosis requires control of infections in domestic and imported pet birds. This can be accomplished by treating birds for 45 days with chlortetracycline hydrochloride. No vaccine currently exists for this organism.

CHLAMYDIA PNEUMONIAE

Chlamydia pneumoniae was first isolated from the conjunctiva of a child in Taiwan. It was initially considered a psittacosis strain because of the morphology of the inclusions produced in cell culture. It was shown subsequently that the Taiwan isolate (TW-183) was serologically related to a pharyngeal isolate designated AR-39, and the strain was designated TWAR. DNA homology studies have demonstrated that the TWAR strain is a

BOX 39-3 Epidemiology of *Chlamydia pneumoniae* Infection

DISEASE/BACTERIAL FACTORS

Bronchitis, pneumonia, sinusitis
Infectious elementary body can survive extracellular cell to cell passage
Noninfectious reticular body is protected in the cell
No animal reservoir identified

TRANSMISSION

Person-to-person spread by inhalation of infectious aerosols

WHO IS AT RISK?

Disease most common in adults

GEOGRAPHY/SEASON

Worldwide
No seasonal incidence recognized

MODES OF CONTROL

Tetracycline or erythromycin for 10 to 14 days; treatment failures common species distinct from both *C. trachomatis* and *C. psittaci* and is now called *C. pneumoniae*. Only a single serotype has been identified. Infection appears to be transmitted by human contact; no animal reservoir has been identified.

C. pneumoniae is an important cause of bronchitis, pneumonia, sinusitis, and other respiratory infections (Box 39-3). Most *C. pneumoniae* infections are mild with a persistent cough and malaise and do not require hospitalization. Infection is believed to be common; an estimated 200,000 to 300,000 cases of *C. pneumoniae* pneumonia are reported annually, with disease most common in adults. As many as 50% of individuals have antibodies against the bacterium.

C. pneumoniae infections are diagnosed primarily by serology, although the bacterium can be cultured in selected cell lines (e.g., HL cells) and detected by antigen tests. Serologic diagnosis can be made by complement fixation or by microimmunofluorescence. The CF test uses a genus-specific antigen, and thus is not specific for *C. pneumoniae* infection; the microimmunofluorescence test uses *C. pneumoniae* elementary bodies as antigen. A fourfold titer increase in either IgM or IgG is diagnostic, whereas an IgM titer of ≥ 16 or an IgG titer of ≥ 512 are suggestive of recent infection. However, the microimmunofluorescence test is available only in a few specialized laboratories.

Tetracycline or erythromycin has been used to treat infections; however, treatment for 10 to 14 days is required, and failures are relatively common. Control of exposure to *C. pneumoniae* is likely to be difficult because the bacterium is ubiquitous.

CASE STUDY AND QUESTIONS

A 22-year-old man had a history of urethral pain and purulent discharge. This had developed after sexual contact with a prostitute. Gram stain of the discharge revealed abundant gram-negataive diplococci resembling *Neisseria*. The patient was treated with penicillin and sent home. Two days later the patient returned to the emergency room with a complaint of persistent watery urethral discharge. Abundant WBCs were observed on Gram stain but no organisms. Culture of the discharge was negative for *Neisseria gonorrhoeae* but positive for *Chlamydia trachomtis*.

1. Why was penicillin ineffective against Chlamydia? What antibiotic can be used to treat chlamydial infections in this patient?
2. Describe the growth cycle of chlamydia. What structural features make the elementary bodies and reticulate bodies well-suited for their environment?
3. Describe the differences among the three chlamydial species that cause human disease.
4. Describe the pathogenesis of trachoma? How does this differ from conjunctivitis seen in newborns and in adults?
5. Compare the epidemiology of psittacosis with respiratory infections caused by the other chlamydial species.

Bibliography

Barnes RC: Laboratory diagnosis of human chlamydial infections, *Clin Microbiol Rev* 2:119-136, 1989.

Batteiger BE, and Jones RB: Chlamydial infections, *Infect Dis Clin North Am* 1:55-81, 1987.

Grayston JT: *Chlamydia*, strain TWAR pneumonia, *Ann Rev Med* 43:317-323, 1992.

Kellogg JA: Clinical and laboratory considerations of culture vs. antigen assays for detection of *Chlamydia trachomatis* from genital specimens, *Arch Pathol Lab Med* 113:453-460, 1989.

Schacter J: Biology of *Chlamydia trachomatis*. In Holmes KK, Mardh PM, Sparling PF, and Wiesner PJ, editors: *Sexually transmitted diseases*, New York, 1984, McGraw-Hill.

Scieux C, Barnes R, Biachi A et al: Lymphogranuloma venereus: 27 cases in Paris, *J Infect Dis* 160:662-668, 1989.

Stamm WE: Diagnosis of *Chlamydia trachomatis* genitourinary infections, *Ann Intern Med* 108:710-717, 1988.

Thom DH and Grayston JT: Infections with *Chlamydia pneumoniae* strain TWAR, *Clin Chest Med* 12:245-256, 1991.

CHAPTER 40

Oral Microbiology

Most diseases of the oral cavity result directly from bacterial colonization and infections. However, other factors may also influence the course of oral diseases. The predominant etiological agents are colonized microorganisms and their products; this adherent mass on the teeth is collectively known as dental plaque.

The principal bacterial-associated diseases of the oral cavity are dental caries and periodontal diseases, both of which are considered among the most prevalent infections of humans.

Before delving into oral microbiology and related pathogenic factors in dental diseases, the potential niches of the oral cavity in which these bacteria reside will be reviewed. The oral cavity may be broadly subdivided into three major components: the teeth, the supporting structures of the teeth (periodontium), and other intraoral structures, including the lips, tongue, floor of the mouth, buccal mucosa, palate, temporomandibular joint, fauces, and the tonsils. This chapter focuses on the teeth and periodontium.

TEETH

Development

Humans experience two dentitions: deciduous and permanent (adult).

Deciduous Dentition

The deciduous dentition is composed of 20 teeth (Figure 40-1): 10 teeth for each dental arch (maxillary arch and mandibular arch). Eruption of the deciduous teeth usually begins between 6 and 7½ months of age with the lower central incisors. The second molars are the last deciduous teeth to erupt, occurring between 20 and 24 months of age. Along with eruption of the deciduous teeth is an ever-increasing complex of bacterial microflora.

Permanent Dentition

The permanent or adult dentition consists of 32 teeth (Figure 40-2). The integrity of the teeth in each dental

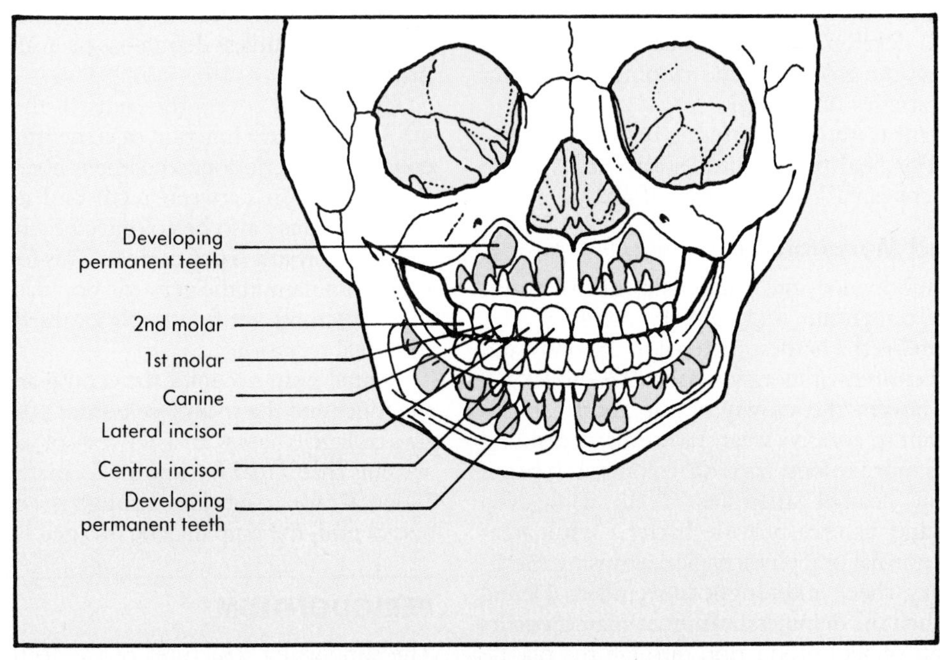

FIGURE 40-1 Dentition of 4-year-old child, anterior view.

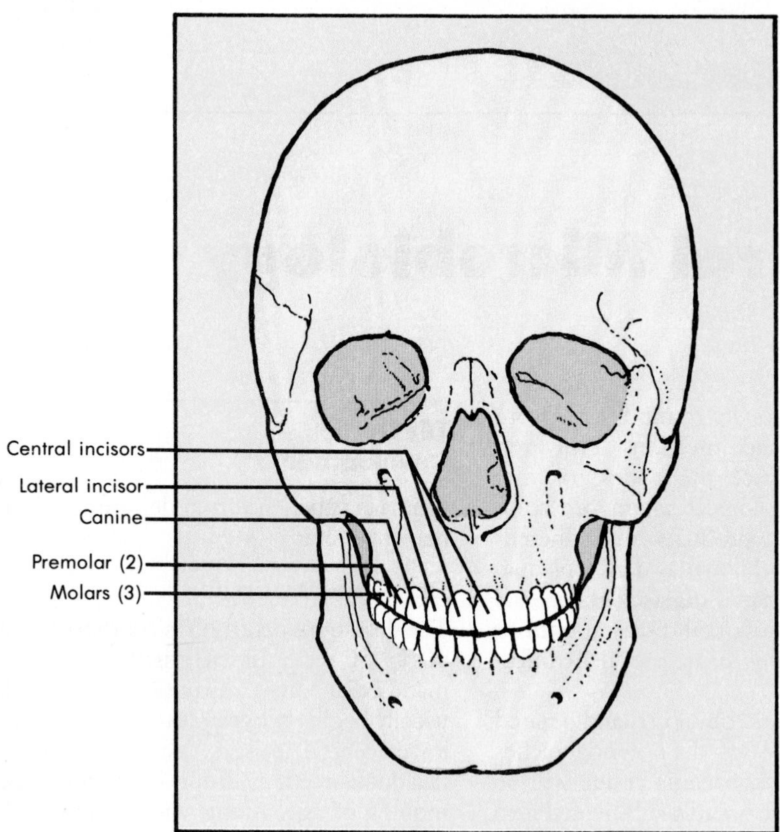

FIGURE 40-2 Dentition of adult, anterior view.

arch is contingent on the arrangement of the teeth, with each tooth in close contact with neighboring teeth. Malpositioning of the teeth permits greater bacterial colonization and growth because bacterial plaque-retentive areas develop. These plaque-retentive areas harbor and foster the growth and development of greater numbers and varieties of bacteria.

The permanent teeth begin erupting between 6 and 7 years of age. The final teeth, third molars or "wisdom teeth," erupt between 17 and 21 years of age.

Structure and Morphology

Teeth can be subdivided into four basic substructures: enamel, dentin, cementum, and pulp (Figure 40-3).

Dental **enamel** is the hardest material in the body and consists almost entirely of inorganic salts (97% to 98%). This material covers the crown of the tooth and is relatively resistant to abrasive wear. However, depending on the enamel's morphology, bacterial colonies can begin to act on basic enamel structures. Teeth with deep grooves, pits, and fissures provide bacteria with areas sheltered from normal oral physiological cleansing mechanisms, including cheek and tongue movements. Dental caries begins when the demineralization of enamel occurs as a direct result of acid production through the plaque constituents' metabolism of sugars (Figure 40-4).

Dentin (see Figure 40-3), which is approximately 65% to 70% inorganic salts, is the calcified tissue that forms the main structure of the tooth. Dentin is the second structure subjected to dental caries. Pain is generally not perceived by the patient unless dentin has been affected by the caries process.

Cementum covers the roots of the teeth (see Figure 40-3). A primary function of cementum is to incorporate collagenous periodontal ligament fibers and thus mediate the connection between teeth and alveolar bone. The cementum may also be colonized by bacteria, and dental caries may result (**root caries**). This form of dental caries is predominant in the geriatric population, among whom root structures are frequently exposed to the oral cavity (gingival recession).

Dental **pulp** occupies the central area of the crown of the tooth and the roots (see Figure 40-3). Pulp is primarily a collagen mass with a network of vascular and nervous systems that remains from the formative organ of dentin. If dental caries continues through the enamel, cementum, and dentin, the pulp may be invaded by microorganisms.

PERIODONTIUM

The supporting structures of the teeth include collagen fibers known as the **periodontal ligament**, as well as

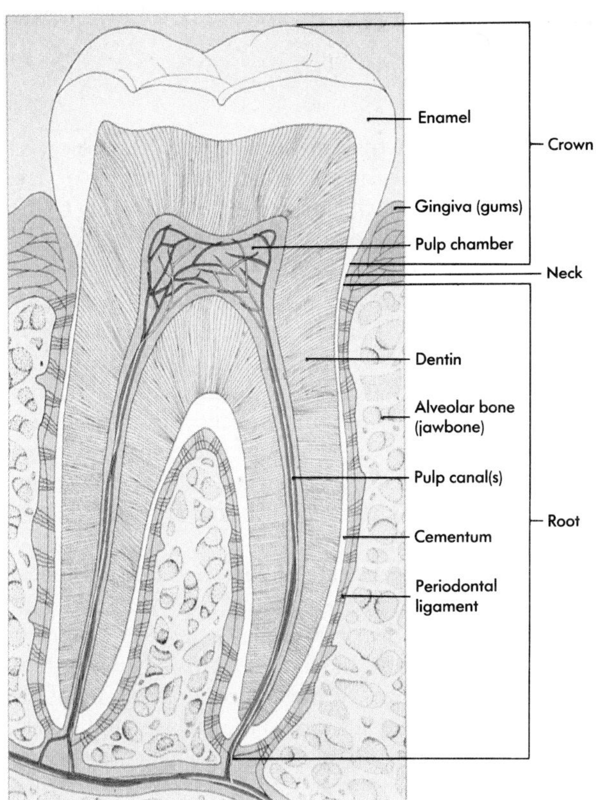

FIGURE 40-3 Cross-section of the tooth and its supporting structures.

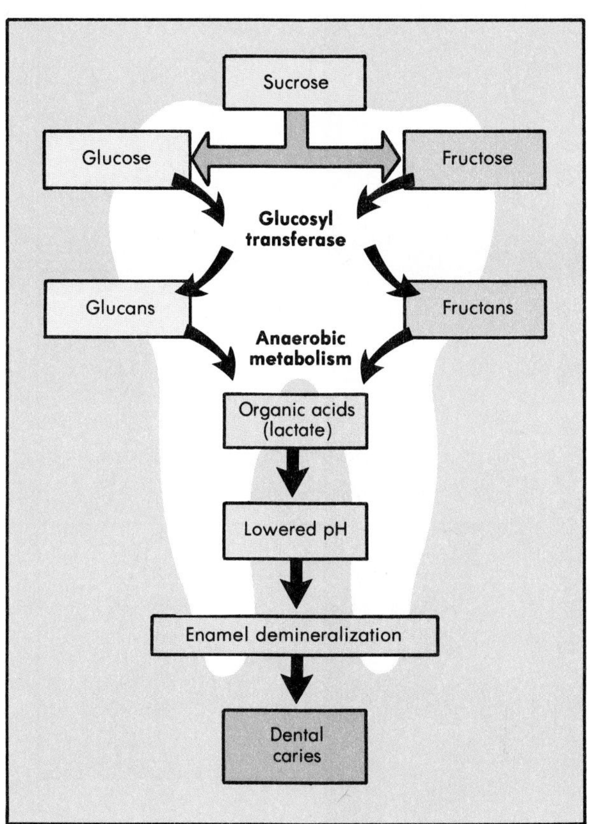

FIGURE 40-4 Dental plaque metabolism of sucrose.

cementum of the root and alveolar bone (Figure 40-5, *B*). These supporting structures are primarily responsible for maintaining the teeth in proper alignment for form and function within the maxilla and mandible, as well as adapting to occlusal (biting) forces. The specialized portion of the jaw bone surrounding the roots of the teeth is called the alveolar bone (Figure 40-5). Overlying the alveolar bone and periodontal ligament structures are the soft tissues known as the gingiva (Figure 40-5, *A*).

The **gingiva** (Figure 40-6) is attached to the tooth at the cementum of the roots and alveolar bone. It is usually pink and stippled (see Figure 40-5, *A*), with ethnic variations of melanin pigmentation possible. The gingiva is essential for the protection of the underlying structures: alveolar bone and periodontal ligament. An inadequate zone of gingiva may initiate or accelerate gingival recession.

The area of the gingiva between the teeth circumscribes a triangular space known as the **papilla** or interproximal zone (see Figure 40-6). This is a frequent site for the initiation of periodontal disease and may exhibit the earliest clinical signs of inflammation of the gingiva.

The nonkeratinized periodontal tissues adjacent to the gingiva are referred to as alveolar mucosa (see Figure 40-6). Alveolar mucosa has a thin layer of nonkeratinized epithelial cells and is transparent, covering the inside lining of the cheeks, vestibule areas of the dentition, and floor of the mouth. This mucosa is usually red and glistening, reflecting the absence of keratinized epithelial cells.

TOOTH-ASSOCIATED MATERIALS

The discussion of dental plaque should be put into proper perspective along with all tooth-associated materials. The tooth-associated materials collectively include food debris, acquired pellicle, materia alba, bacterial plaque, and calculus.

Food Debris

Food debris is retained in the mouth after mastication of food. The debris, unless wedged between the teeth or inside the periodontal-tooth interface, is usually removed by saliva or oral musculature action.

Pellicle

Acquired pellicle is a very thin (0.1 to 0.8 μm), primarily protein film that forms on surfaces of the teeth. The pellicle is derived from salivary components and is acquired very soon after the teeth are cleaned. It is basically acellular and bacteria free. The pellicle consists of high molecular-weight glycoproteins that are derived from the saliva and are selectively absorbed to the surfaces

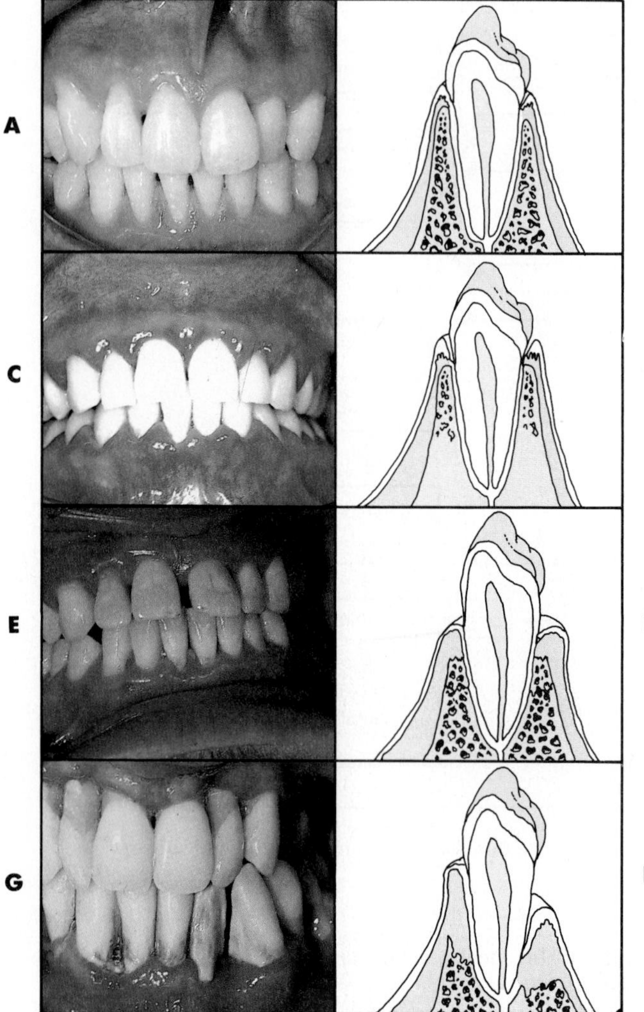

FIGURE 40-5 Progress of periodontal disease. **A** and **B**, Normal healthy gingiva. Healthy gingiva and bone anchor teeth firmly in place. **C** and **D**, Gingivitis. Plaque and its products irritate the gingiva, making it tender, inflamed, and likely to bleed. **E** and **F**, Early-moderate periodontitis. Unremoved, plaque hardens into calculus (tartar). As plaque and calculus continue to accumulate and pockets form between the teeth and gingiva, the gingiva may recede (pull away) from the teeth. **G** and **H**, Advanced periodontitis. More bone and the periodontal ligament are destroyed, and the gingiva recede farther. Teeth may become loose and require extraction.

of the teeth. The pellicle is re-formed within minutes of being removed from the surfaces of the teeth via brushing and flossing. It is not removed by even forceful rinsing. Acquired pellicle is considered the first stage in the formation of dental plaque because bacterial adherence and colonization quickly ensue.

Materia Alba

Materia alba, literally "white matter," is a mixture of salivary proteins, bacteria, desquamated epithelial cells, and dying leukocytes. Clinically, materia alba appears as a soft white structure that is loosely adherent to the surfaces of the teeth. Materia alba can usually be removed with rinsing or irrigation by fluids.

Bacterial Plaque

Bacterial plaque is a mat of densely packed, colonized microorganisms, growing and tenaciously attached to the teeth. It is embedded in a matrix of pellicle adhering to the surfaces of the teeth. Total bacterial counts are estimated to be approximately 10^8 to 10^{11} bacteria per gram of plaque. Bacterial plaque is not removed by rinsing or forceful spraying with fluids but is easily removed by mechanical means.

Subpopulations of the dental plaque develop further with varying compositions and metabolisms. An understanding of plaque development, and especially how bacteria inhabit the various niches of the teeth and periodontium, will enhance prevention of dental disease and improve treatment.

Factors enhancing the rate of bacterial colonization in the oral cavity include inadequate oral hygiene, a diet high in fermentable carbohydrates, malocclusion, malposed teeth, reduced oral immune factors, impaired saliva flow, and rough teeth surfaces. Without proper brushing of the teeth, colonies of bacteria form on the surfaces of the teeth within 1 to 3 days (Figure 40-7). The colonies are localized within the pits and fissures of the coronal (crown) portion of the tooth (see Figure 40-3) and are also found along the gingiva (see Figure 40-5, *D*, *F*, and *H*). Within a few days these bacterial colonies begin to coalesce and fuse to form a continuous "matlike" deposit.

Within approximately 7 to 10 days dental plaque increases in thickness on the surfaces of the teeth and in the region between the teeth and gingiva (sulcus). Streptococci and gram-positive bacilli form the predominant structures of early plaque development, which is located primarily supragingivally (at or above the gingiva). As dental plaque matures on the surfaces of the teeth, the bacterial mat becomes increasingly complex (see Figure 40-7, *D*).

Bacterial plaque, initially supragingival, continues to proliferate and extends underneath the gingiva (subgingival) (Figure 40-5, *F*). As bacteria continue to proliferate subgingivally, relatively low oxygen tension environments are created (Figure 40-5, *H*). In this niche below the gingiva, facultative and eventually strict anaerobic bacteria are favored for growth and development. Ultrastructurally, the subgingival plaque consists primarily of bacilli and filamentous bacteria (Figure 40-8).

The mixed, complex colonies contain more than 200 different species of bacteria. The types of bacteria found in dental plaque vary considerably among individuals with the age of the dental plaque mass itself and the area of the oral cavity from which it was collected.

Calculus

Dental calculus is a result of extremely mature plaque that has completed mineralization. It occurs as relatively hard, firmly adhering materials on the crowns and root surfaces

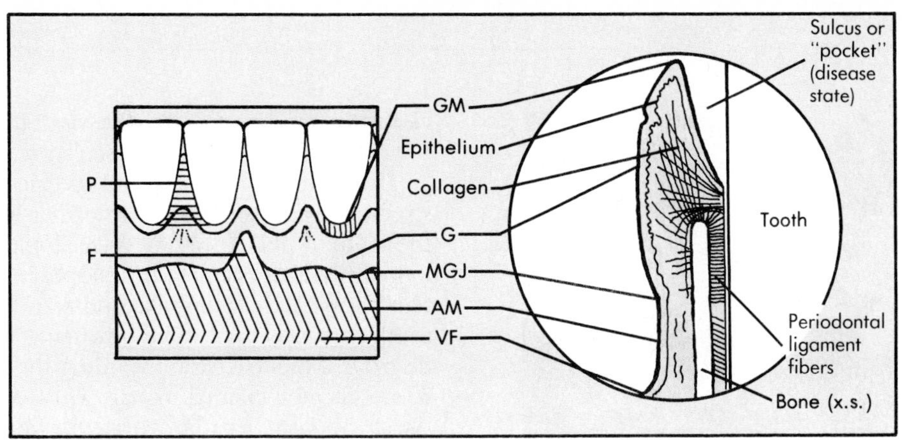

FIGURE 40-6 A diagram of surface characteristics of the clinically normal gingiva *P*, papilla; *F*, frenum; *GM*, gingival margin; *MGJ*, mucogingival junction; *AM*, alveolar mucosa; *VF*, vestibular fornix, *G*, gingiva.

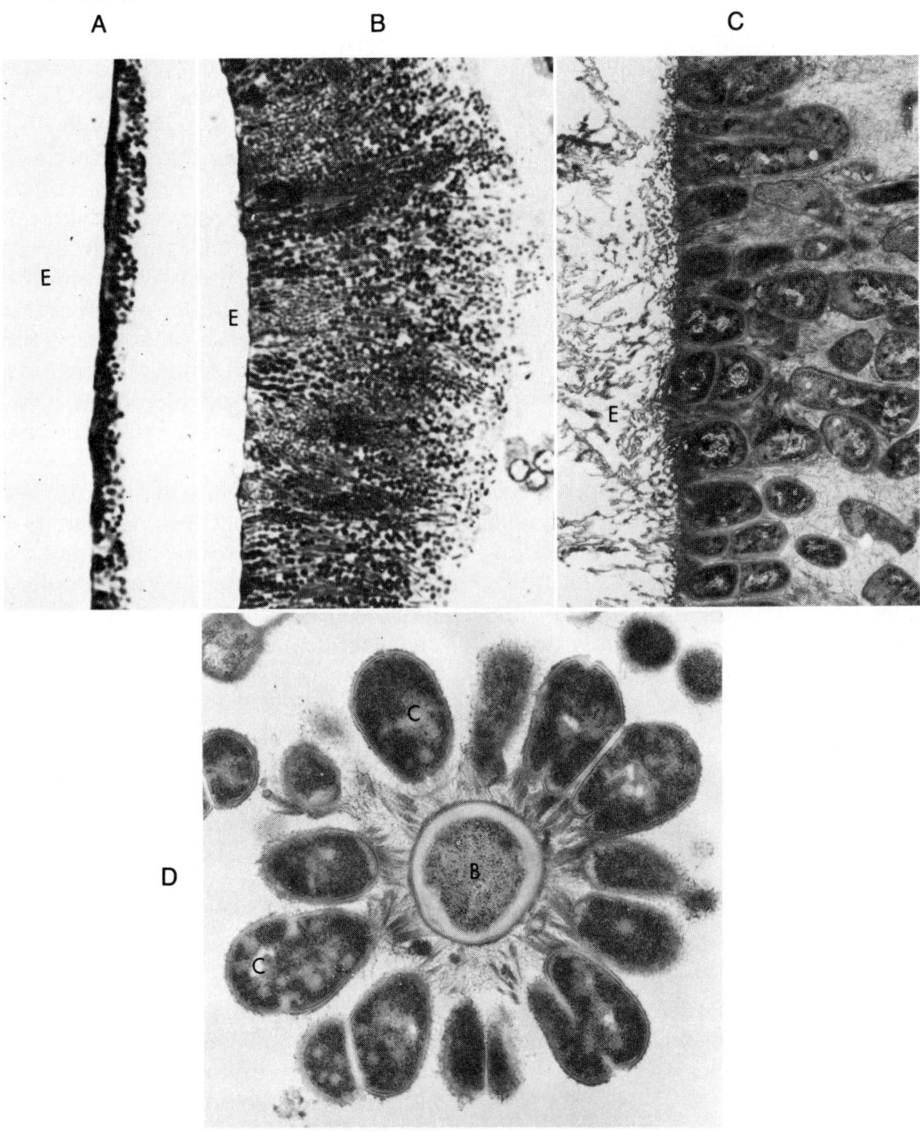

FIGURE 40-7 **A**, Initial colonization of cocci-shaped bacteria on a tooth surface immediately adjacent to healthy gingiva. *E*, enamel (×2000). **B,** Maturation of dental plaque colonies depicting thick layers of cocci-shaped bacteria on a tooth surface adjacent to healthy gingiva (×2000). **C**, Higher magnification using electron microscopy of **A**. Cocci-shaped bacteria are in contact with the pellicle (glycoprotein layer) of the enamel (×11,000). **D**, Formations of the cocci-shaped bacteria adherent to a central filament-shaped bacteria. These are often referred to as "corncob" structures (×23,000). (**A** and **C** from Grant DA, Stern IB, and Listgarten MA: *Periodontics*, St. Louis, 1988, Mosby; **B** from Listgarten MA: *J Periodontol* 47:1, 1976; **D** from Listgarten MA: *J Periodontol* 46:10, 1975.)

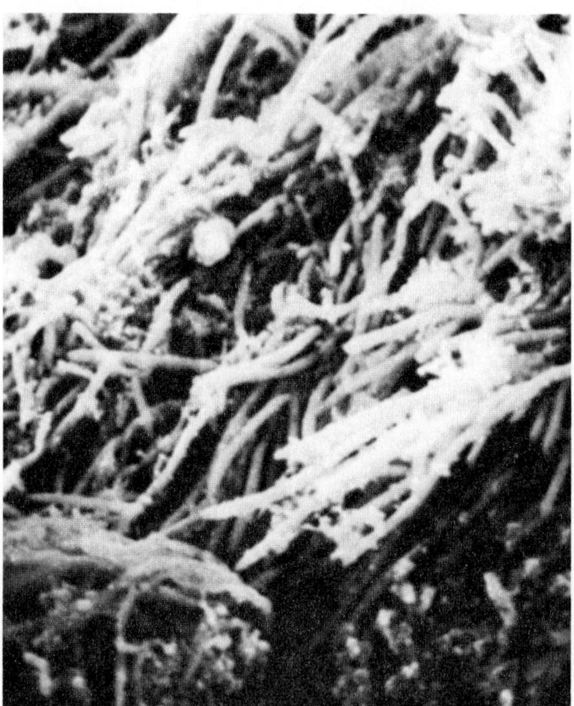

FIGURE 40-8 Maturation of plaque continuing for 4 days with scanning electron microscopy. Demonstrated are large colonies of filament-shaped bacteria at the tooth surface (×6000). (From Grant DA, Stern IB, and Listgarten MA: *Periodontics,* St. Louis, 1988, Mosby.)

of the teeth. Dental calculus is composed of permeable and toxic products from bacterial plaque associated with it, and these products are released into the local environment.

Calculus may also be classified by its location on the surfaces of the teeth. Supragingival calculus is usually quite abundant at the orifice of the major salivary glands and in particular on the lingual (tongue) surface of the lower anterior teeth. It may be enhanced by special intraoral situations such as malposed teeth, malocclusion, rough root surfaces, and improperly restored teeth.

Subgingival calculus is found underneath the gingival margin on the root surfaces of the teeth. The extent of subgingival plaque frequently correlates with the extent of the space created between the gingiva and tooth as a result of the disease process (periodontal "pocket"). The radius of infectivity of dental plaque and calculus is believed to be approximately 1 to 2 mm (i.e., the pathological processes in the periodontium are related to the location of the developing plaque and calculus).

PATHOGENESIS AND IMMUNITY

The pathogenesis of **dental caries** is initiated at selected sites in the dentition and usually includes the pits and fissures of the occlusal (biting) surfaces of the teeth, as well as the interproximal areas (between the teeth) of the dentition. These localized sites are protected from natural cleansing mechanisms of the oral cavity, such as the tongue, oral mucosa and musculature, and saliva.

The demineralization and decalcification of tooth structure by acids results in a "leather-like" consistency of the tooth. A pH of 4.6 or less (see Figure 40-4) can result in hydrolysis of enamel phosphoprotein by phosphoprotein phosphatase. Solubilization and demineralization of tooth enamel is accelerated by organic acids. As enamel is destroyed, oral bacteria, including the streptococci, penetrate into the enamel matrix. The acids formed during the metabolism of carbohydrates by oral bacteria in dental plaque are capable of dissolving the enamel structures of the teeth. The more frequently that acids form on the surfaces of the teeth and the longer acids remain there, the greater the likelihood of enamel demineralization.

Streptococci are present in the oral cavity in very large numbers and play a dominant role in the formation and pathogenesis of dental caries. The most frequently isolated bacterium associated with dental caries is *Streptococcus mutans.* Their numbers increase with initiation of dental caries and decrease when caries are treated, exhibiting a strong correlation with this disease process.

Dental caries extends through the enamel and into the dentin where the carious lesion must be restored (Figure 40-9, *A* to *C*). Without appropriate treatment at this time, the carious lesion may extend further through the dentin and into the dental pulp region (Figure 40-9, *D*). Sensitivity to heat and cold or sensitivity to percussion are possible symptoms related to extension of the caries to the pulp.

After bacterial involvement of the pulpal regions during caries pathogenesis, a periapical lesion (granuloma or abscess) may develop at the tip of the root (Fig. 40-9, *D*). Root canal therapy (endodontic therapy) is even more critical at this time and includes mechanical removal and debridement of the pulpal contents of the tooth. When this is performed, the periapical lesion frequently resolves without the use of antibiotic therapy.

Periodontitis is an inflammatory process that extends beyond the soft tissues and into the alveolar bone, periodontal ligament, and cementum (see Figure 40-5, *E* to *H*). Generally, during extension of bacterial plaque growth on the roots, the connective tissue fibers surrounding the teeth and connecting the teeth to alveolar bone are disrupted and in the process of dissolution.

The junctional epithelium, which connects the soft tissues to the root surfaces of the teeth, migrates downward, resulting in a relatively deep space (pocket) between the tooth and the gingiva. A pocket is the space around the teeth that is pathologically deepened by bacterial plaque colonization and maturation. This results directly from extension of the spread of inflammation caused by bacterial products (see Figure 40-5, *B, D, F, H*). Inflammatory cells may spread along the course of blood channels because of the loose connective tissue surrounding the neurovascular bundles. This area offers less resistance than the dense connective tissue fibers of the periodontal ligament and connective tissue. The

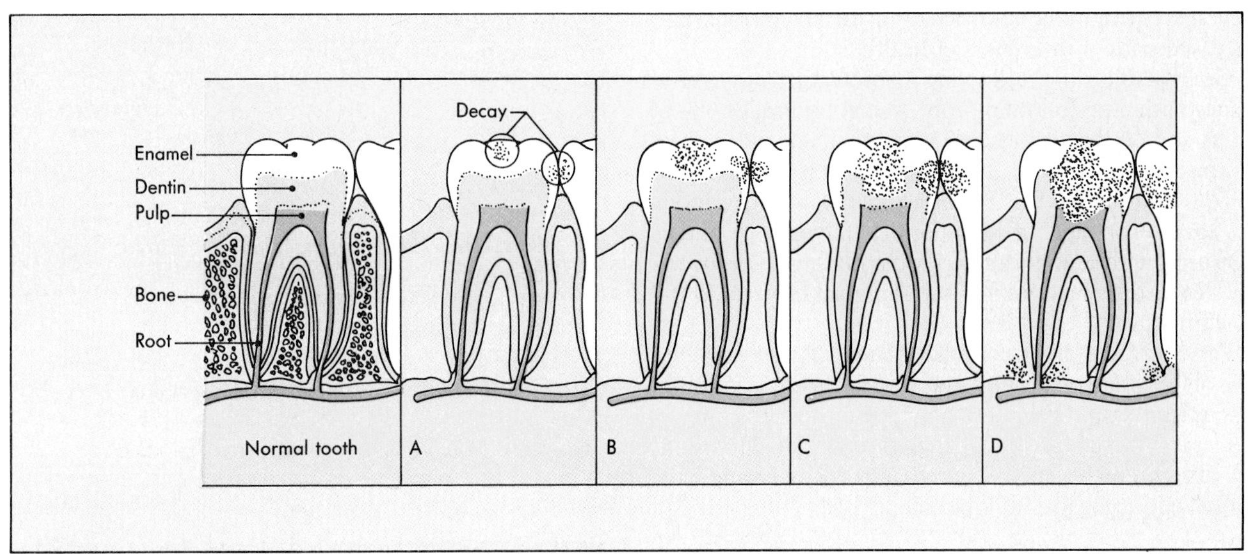

FIGURE 40-9 Dental caries. **A**, Decay often begins in hard-to- clean areas. **B**, Left untreated, an incipient carious lesion becomes larger. **C**, Decay spreads beneath the enamel to the dentin, destroying more tooth structure. **D**, Once decay enters the pulp, an abscess may occur. The tooth will need endodontic treatment or may need to be extracted.

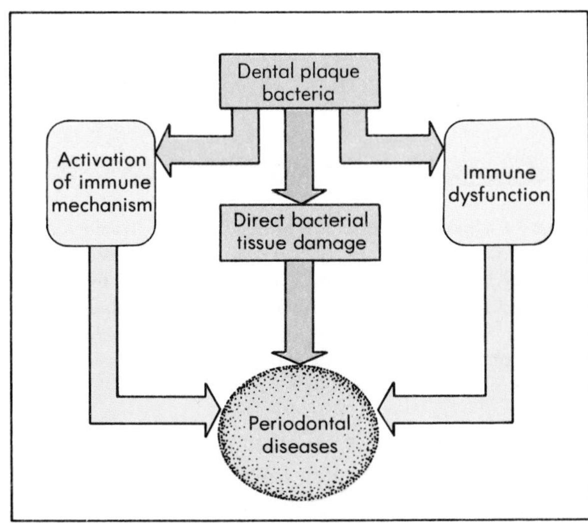

FIGURE 40-10 Pathogenic mechanisms of periodontal diseases.

location of the inflammation surrounding the alveolar bone depends on the course of inflammatory cells along the vascular channels. Frequently, the blood vessels extending on the alveolar crest between the teeth are the site of direct spread of inflammation into the periodontal ligament space. This inflammatory process is further driven by bacterial plaque as it develops in the pocket.

Selected bacteria within the periodontal pocket may penetrate or invade the contiguous epithelial and connective tissues. This pathogenic mechanism provides relative resistance to mechanical (by scaling) elimination of the bacteria. If the periodontal infection persists after treatment, these patients may have "refractory" periodontitis and suffer from recurrent disease.

The inflammatory process in the hard tissues around the teeth may result in marked osteoclastic activity, and the progressive extension results in alveolar bone destruction. Periodontitis is the loss of alveolar bone and clinical gingival attachment. This loss of bone can be observed radiographically (see Figures 40-13 and 40-14). The conversion clinically from gingivitis to periodontitis reflects the progression from the extension of inflammation from the soft tissues into the hard tissues. The reasons for this progression remain unclear but may represent colonization and infection by highly pathogenic plaque bacteria or reflect aberrations of host cell responsiveness to bacterial plaque, or both.

Three plausible hypotheses can be proposed for periodontal destruction (Figure 40-10): (1) direct destruction caused by bacterial plaque and metabolic products; (2) immune hyper-responsiveness precipitated by immune complexes, lymphocyte blastogenesis, or activation of complement pathways; or (3) immune deficiencies involving neutrophil function (chemotaxis, phagocytosis, superoxide radical formation), neutropenia, or the autologous mixed lymphocyte response (AMLR).

EPIDEMIOLOGY

Surveys completed by the Department of Health and Human Services in 1987 indicate a substantial reduction of dental caries (coronal) in adults compared with previous surveys. Factors responsible for this trend include fluoridation of drinking water, school-based preventive programs, knowledge of dietary factors, and increased patient awareness of health.

Gingival bleeding, following manipulation of gingival tissues with a periodontal probe, was found in 43.6% of adults and 46.9% of those 65 years of age or older. Loss of attachment (greater than 2 mm) was observed in 76.6% of adults and 95.1% of the older group. This index is a diagnostic sign of periodontitis (any form) and is measured with a periodontal probe. Gingivitis, a reversible dental disease, does not have gingival or periodontal attachment loss.

Periodontitis, an irreversible dental disease, involves loss of attachment around the teeth. Early periodontal destruction would have 2 to 4 mm of loss of attachment. Moderate periodontal destruction would have 4 to 6 mm loss of attachment, and advanced destruction would have 7 mm or greater loss of attachment.

TABLE 40-1 Classification of Gingivitis

Form	Primary etiology	Secondary etiology
1. Plaque-associated	Dental plaque	–
2. ANUG	Dental plaque	Stress, fatigue
3. Steroid hormone–influenced	Dental plaque	Steroids
4. Medication-influenced gingival overgrowth	Dental plaque	Medications (e.g., phenytoin, cyclosporins)
5. Miscellaneous	Dental plaque	Nutrition, other (?)

From Suzuki JB: *Dent Clin North Am* 32(2):195-216, 1988.

CLINICAL SYNDROMES

Dental Caries

Dental caries is a bacterial disease that can destroy the teeth. The normally hard tooth structure is converted to a soft, leather-like consistency. This is detected clinically with a sharp dental instrument (explorer) or with dental radiographs.

Periodontal Diseases

Periodontal infections cause the most common diseases of the periodontium and are among the most common of all diseases in humans. The periodontal diseases can be broadly subdivided into two main categories: gingivitis and periodontitis.

Gingivitis

Gingivitis is an inflammatory process precipitated by the accumulations of bacteria along the gingiva of the teeth. Gingivitis is primarily a reversible disease, and the removal of the bacteria from the teeth at the margin of the gingiva usually results in the resolution of inflammation. The inflammatory process in gingivitis is confined primarily to the gingiva (soft tissues) and is seen clinically as redness around the necks of the teeth. Bleeding of the gingiva (either spontaneous or induced) is a frequent accompanying sign.

The primary etiological agent of gingivitis is bacterial plaque. This forms the basis for a classification of gingivitis, with "plaque-associated" gingivitis being the most common form (Table 40-1). The primary bacteria involved in gingivitis are gram-positive cocci mixed with bacilli and filamentous forms.

Other modifying secondary etiological factors permit classification of other forms of gingivitis (Table 40-1). Acute necrotizing ulcerative gingival stomatitis (ANUG), commonly known as "**trench mouth**" or "Vincent's infection," has several secondary etiological factors and constitutes another form of gingivitis. Stress and anxiety are perhaps the most significant contributing factors. Other factors include fatigue, lowered resistance, nutritional impairment, smoking, mouth-breathing, calculus, and gross neglect of oral hygiene. However, the primary etiological agent for ANUG is bacterial plaque.

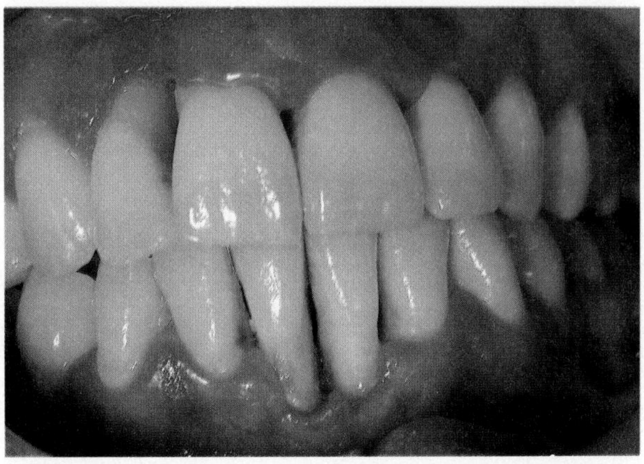

FIGURE 40-11 Clinical presentation of a systemically healthy 22-year-old female dental patient with acute necrotizing ulcerative gingivitis (ANUG) ("trench mouth"). The soft tissues of the gingiva around the teeth can be noted, with the diseased areas covered by a "pseudomembrane" of neutrophils, spirochetes and other motile bacteria, and sloughed epithelial cells.

The clinical features of ANUG are frequently seen by the practicing physician as periodontal tissues with gingival craters covered by a grayish-white pseudomembrane (Figure 40-11). In these areas of gingival necrosis, acute areas of inflammation contribute to the pain, bleeding, soreness, and sensitivity of these lesions. The extent of ANUG lesions may be isolated in the interproximal regions between the teeth, or they may be generalized throughout the entire dentition. This is one of the most painful and malodorous of the dental diseases. Boggy, edematous, keratinized gingiva is frequently present, with lymphadenopathy, malaise, and pyrexia as frequent accompanying signs. The primary bacteria involved in ANUG lesions are spirochetes, vibrios, and other filamentous forms.

A third form of gingivitis is **"steroid hormone–influenced gingivitis."** This disease results from the presence of steroid hormones that amplify the clinical inflammatory response of gingivitis. The increased levels of estrogens and progesterones associated with pregnancy, adolescence, or birth-control medication, enhance marginal gingival inflammation. The clinical signs and symptoms of this disease include acute gingival inflammation around one or more teeth, with spontaneous gingival bleeding or bleeding during gentle instrumentation by a dental clinician. Severe cases of steroid hormone–influenced gingivitis may progress to a pyrogenic granuloma, commonly known as a "pregnancy tumor," which is clinically apparent.

The fourth form of gingivitis is **"medication-influenced gingival overgrowth."** This form of gingivitis is complicated by phenytoin and cyclosporines, among other drugs, and frequently results in a hyperplastic type of tissue growth of the gingiva. The clinical signs and symptoms include gingival overgrowth in the form of a diffuse swelling of the interdental papilla or multiple tiny nodules on the gingiva of the anterior teeth (Figure 40-12). Other signs include moderate to acute inflammation, soreness, and tenderness of the gingiva.

"**Miscellaneous forms of gingivitis**" may be influenced by nutritional deprivation, mouth breathing, or HIV infections. The clinical signs and symptoms of nutritionally deficient patients are similar to the other forms of gingivitis.

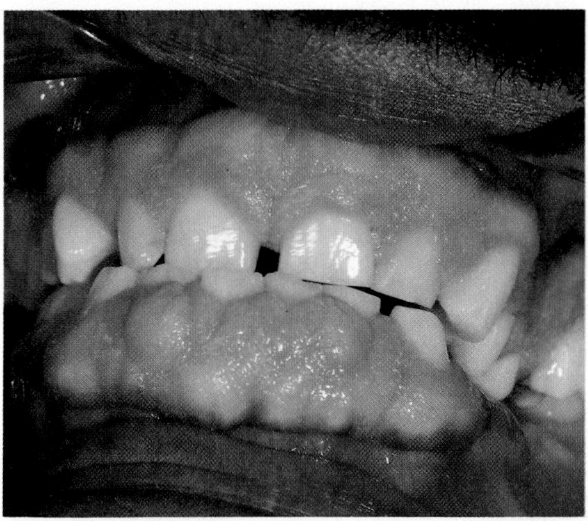

FIGURE 40-12 Clinical presentation of a dental patient with gingival overgrowth. This may result from a combination of dental plaque accumulation with systemic administration of medications such as phenytoin (Dilantin), cyclosporins, or nifedipine.

Periodontitis

Clinical observations, coupled with basic microbiology research, have permitted a descriptive classification of the various forms of periodontitis. These forms are generally associated with age of onset but also can be related to the types of bacteria present in the pockets surrounding the teeth (Table 40-2).

The most frequent cause of tooth loss in adults is due to adult periodontitis (Figure 40-13). Beyond 35 to 40 years of age the majority (70% to 90%) of the adult population of the United States exhibits some sign of periodontitis. The presence of bacterial plaque and calcified deposits (calculus or tartar) is usually related to the amount of destruction of gingiva and alveolar bone tissues.

The disease **adult periodontitis** progresses in a chronic fashion and generally takes years or perhaps decades to develop. Subgingival bacterial plaque formation and maturation cause the inflammatory process to extend to the hard tissues. Favorable environments for the development of subgingival anaerobic forms of bacteria are further established within the pockets surrounding the teeth.

The primary bacteria found in subgingival pockets in adult periodontitis patients are primarily gram-negative, motile, complex, and asaccharolytic forms. The associated microorganisms include *Bacteroides* species, *Eikenella corrodens*, *Fusobacterium nucleatum*, *Wolinella recta*, and *Eubacterium* species (Table 40-3).

The clinical dental characteristics associated with adult forms of periodontitis are bacterial and calcified deposits around the teeth commensurate with the disease.

Patients are generally older than 35 years. The destruction to the alveolar bone (seen radiographically in Figure 40-13) and gingiva in adult periodontitis patients (as well as all forms of periodontitis) is generally irreversible in nature.

TABLE 40-2 Classification and Clinical Features of Periodontitis

Form	Age	Clinical features
I. Adult	>35 years	Abundant plaque
II. Early onset		
Rapidly progressive	18-35 years	Variable plaque
Juvenile	12-26 years	Little plaque
Prepubertal	<12 years	Little plaque
III. Associated systemic disease	Any	Variable plaque
IV. Acute necrotizing periodontitis	<35 years	Abundant plaque
V. Refractory	Any	Variable plaque

Another form of periodontitis that occurs in younger adults between 18 and 35 years of age is referred to as **rapidly progressive periodontitis**. As the name states, a relatively rapid progression of disease occurs that may be related to abnormal host-defense mechanisms. The primary immune cells that may be incompetent include the neutrophils or lymphocytes.

It has been proposed that deficient host-defense mechanisms permit extremely pathogenic forms of bacteria and dental plaque to develop. These include *Porphyromonas* (previously *Bacteroides*) *gingivalis*, *Prevotella (previously Bacteroides) intermedia*, *Bacteroides forsythus*, *Actinobacillus actinomycetemcomitans*, *Eikenella corrodens*, and *Wolinella recta* (see Table 40-3). Frequently, gingival inflammation may be masked because of a deficient neutrophil chemotactic response. In addition, clinically evident deposits of plaque and calculus may not always be associated with rapidly progressive periodontitis. In this disease it is the *quality* of the bacterial plaque rather than the *quantity* of bacterial plaque that may be responsible for the rapid progression of disease in these younger individuals.

The third form of periodontitis is **juvenile periodontitis**, which affects persons between the ages of 12 and 26 years (Figure 40-14). Generally, only selected teeth are affected by this disease—specifically, the first molars and the incisor teeth. Ironically, usually no gross clinical dental deposits are observed with juvenile periodontitis. Genetic and host-defense mechanisms do, however, complicate the pathogenesis. The specific bacterium involved is *Actinobacillus actinomycetemcomitans*.

The most recently described form of periodontitis is **prepubertal periodontitis.** As the name implies, this form of periodontitis is confined to the mixed dentition or occurs during eruption of the primary teeth. Selected host-defense mechanisms (e.g., neutrophil adhesion) may be impaired in prepubertal periodontitis, permitting bacterial plaque to develop at a premature stage. The bacteria responsible for forms of prepubertal periodontitis include *Actinobacillus actinomycetemcomitans*, *Prevotella intermedia*, *Eikenella corrodens*, and *Capnocytophaga* species.

Collectively, rapidly progressive, juvenile, and prepubertal forms of periodontitis are currently referred to as "early onset periodontitis."

TABLE 40-3 Microbial Profile of Periodontitis

Form	Bacteria
Adult	*Bacteroides* species *Eikenella corrodens* *Fusobacterium nucleatum* *Wolinella recta* *Eubacterium* species
Rapidly progressive	*Porphyromonas (Bacteroides) gingivalis* *Prevotella (Bacteroides) intermedia* *Bacteroides forsythus* *Actinobacillus actinomycetemcomitans* *Eikenella corrodens* *Wolinella recta*
Juvenile	*Actinobacillus actinomycetemcomitans*
Prepubertal	*Actinobacillus actinomycetemcomitans* *Prevotella (Bacteroides) intermedia* *Eikenella corrodens* *Capnocytophaga* species

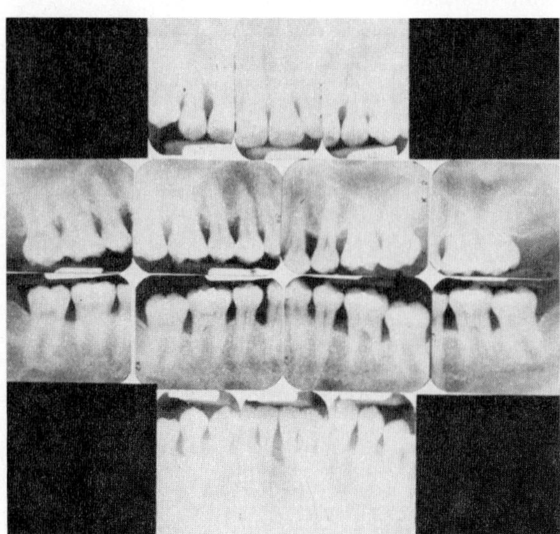

FIGURE 40-13 Adult periodontitis. Radiographs are from a male patient, age 52. (From Suzuki JB: *Dent Clin North Am* 32:195, 1988.)

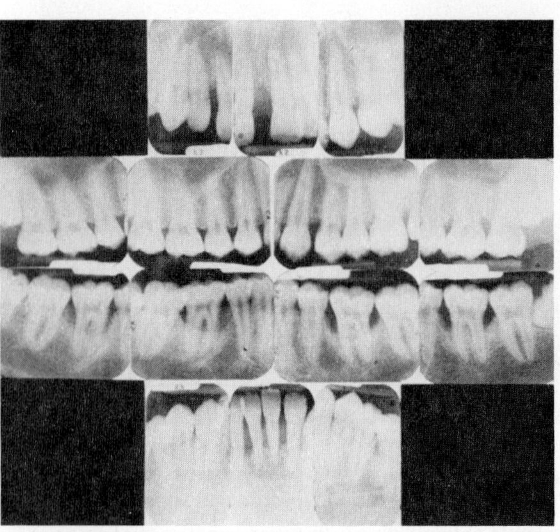

FIGURE 40-14 Juvenile periodontitis. Radiographs are from a female patient, age 13. (From Suzuki JB: *Dent Clin North Am* 32:195, 1988.)

Another type of periodontitis, which has been recently defined clinically but not as well documented microbially, is *periodontitis associated with systemic disease*. This type of periodontitis includes patients with systemic conditions that have periodontal manifestations (e.g., AIDS, diabetes mellitus, Down's syndrome). HIV-positive and AIDS patients generally display bright red inflamed gingiva coupled with rapid soft tissue necrosis and alveolar bone destruction. Other intraoral signs and symptoms of these patients include *Candida* infections, petechiae, lymphadenopathy (cervical, submandibular), herpes, Kaposi's sarcoma, and sialoadenitis.

Acute necrotizing periodontitis, related to ANUG, is a more extensive periodontal disease and affects the attachment apparatus (bone, periodontal ligament) of the teeth.

Refractory periodontitis, not fully characterized at this time, includes patients who do not respond to conventional periodontal treatment. Frequently, periodontal pockets continue to deepen and alveolar bone resorbs despite the clinician's best efforts of therapy.

LABORATORY DIAGNOSIS

Caries is detected by examination of the saliva for numbers of streptococci and lactobacilli; this ascertains which patients are "caries prone." However, these salivary tests have very limited application in clinical practice. Cultures of the caries lesion are not performed because the clinical diagnosis is fairly accurate.

The diagnosis of gingivitis is made primarily by clinical signs (specifically, gingival inflammation) and symptoms (bleeding or itching gums). Dental radiographs must be used to confirm no loss of alveolar bone structure around the teeth (which would indicate periodontitis). There are no laboratory diagnostic tests specifically for oral bacteria associated with gingivitis.

Clinical and radiographic observations remain the primary diagnostic criteria for periodontitis. Bone loss patterns and severity are related to the patient's age and systemic considerations. Recently, developments using anaerobic culture techniques, immunofluorescence, and DNA/RNA probes have permitted more accurate identification of the oral bacteria associated with periodontitis. Dental plaque samples are taken from the space (pocket) between the teeth and gingiva and submitted to a reference laboratory for analysis.

TREATMENT, PREVENTION, AND CONTROL

Dental Caries

Mechanical removal of the carious lesion is the treatment for most cases. This involves the use of a high-speed rotary instrument and hand instruments. The objective of the mechanical treatment is removal of the damaged enamel and dentin, as well as any bacteria contained within the lesion.

Extension of the carious lesion into the pulp of the tooth results in endodontic involvement (root canals). Mechanical removal and debridement of the pulpal contents is necessary.

Penicillin VK is frequently used as systemic antibiotic therapy for the management and control of periapical lesions resulting from pulpal involvement by caries. Erythromycin is used as an alternative to penicillin therapy. Warm compresses, both intraoral and extraoral, may improve the clinical problem created by an endodontically affected tooth.

Gingivitis

The treatment of the majority of forms of gingivitis involves improved oral hygiene, including brushing and flossing the teeth, scaling the calcified and soft tissue deposits around the teeth, and knowledge of possible secondary factors influencing the course of various gingivitis states.

Periodontitis

Treatment of adult periodontitis involves measures similar to those taken for the control of gingivitis. However, additional measures may be required to gain access to the deep pocket areas for removal of the deposits around the teeth, and surgical approaches may be necessary. Generally, systemic antibiotics are not required for management of adult periodontitis patients unless periodontal abscesses form. Systemic antibiotics such as penicillin, ampicillin, or the tetracyclines may be necessary in this situation.

Palliative therapy for ANUG ("trench mouth") and AIDS-associated periodontal patients includes gentle irrigation and intraoral rinsing with a mixture of warm water and hydrogen peroxide, diluted 50% each. This can be repeated four to eight times per day as needed. In addition, improved toothbrushing and interproximal cleaning such as flossing ameliorate the situation. Patients who have submandibular or cervical lymphadenopathy or who are febrile may require systemic antibiotics. The drug of choice is penicillin VK, with tetracycline as an alternative. Follow-up by a dental clinician is essential for scaling the teeth to remove the plaque and calcified deposits. In addition, soft tissue management (gingivoplasty or gingivectomy) may be necessary for more extensive regions of ANUG.

Treatment of rapidly progressive periodontitis is similar to treatment of the adult forms, with the addition of systemic antibiotics (usually tetracycline) during the initial stages of clinical management. Young adults who have rapidly progressive periodontitis may be more prone to acute periodontal abscesses and may require emergency dental care, which includes incision and drainage, scaling the affected teeth, irrigation of the pocket area, and a regimen of antibiotics (e.g., penicillin, metronidazole, augmentin, cephalosporins, ciprofloxacin, or a combination).

The treatment for juvenile periodontitis includes approaches similar to those for rapidly progressive periodontitis. In addition, innovative surgical techniques,

BOX 40-1 Conditions Affecting the Ability to Perform Effective Oral Hygiene

Mental impairment
Malposed teeth
Malocclusion
Extensive bridgework
Diet (high sucrose)
Lack of motivation
Orthodontic therapy
Orthognathic surgical therapy
Intermaxillary splinting (e.g., trauma)
Recurrent gingivitis
Periodontitis

including bone grafting (autografts, allografts, or synthetics) and other regenerative procedures may also be considered. Systemic antibiotics, including the tetracyclines, are becoming increasingly important for the management of juvenile periodontitis patients. Note that tetracyclines cause permanent staining of adult dentition if administered to patients younger than 8 years of age.

The treatment for prepubertal periodontitis includes improvement of oral hygiene measures, scaling and root planing of the teeth, curettage of the gingival lining of the pockets, and the use of systemic antibiotics such as amoxicillin.

Dental research is proceeding in the areas of antibiotic regimens and antiplaque agents because these seem to be the most useful in controlling dental diseases. These measures may be employed in debilitated dental patients, regardless of age, who are not able to perform normal oral hygiene procedures. Dental patients who may benefit from systemic antibiotics either have rapidly progressive, juvenile, or prepubertal forms of periodontitis, are myelosuppressed, or are experiencing exacerbations of the disease (e.g., abscesses, ANUG).

The antiplaque mouth rinses (e.g., 0.12% chlorhexidine) are among the newest applications of technology in the control of microflora associated with dental diseases. Dental patients who may benefit from antiplaque mouth rinses have conditions in the oral cavity favoring dental plaque development (Box 40-1).

Antiplaque mouth rinses should not be considered the primary recommendation for treatment and prevention of dental diseases caused by bacteria. They serve as adjunctive approaches to basic oral hygiene measures such as toothbrushing, flossing, and scaling of the teeth during routine dental appointments.

Dietary considerations aimed at reducing the production of acid from fermentable carbohydrates or reducing bacterial plaque growth may be a substantial means for prevention and control of oral diseases. The use of nonfermentable nutrition sweeteners (e.g., Aspartame) modifies bacterial metabolism relative to caries and periodontal disease.

CASE STUDY AND QUESTIONS

An 18-year-old white female college student was brought to the emergency room complaining of an extremely foul odor emanating from her mouth associated with a sour taste. She also complained that her neck and portions underneath her jaw bone were so tender that moving her neck was difficult.

The medical history was unremarkable. The social history indicated that she was in the middle of her first series of mid-term exams in college, coupled with preparations at her sorority house for multiple homecoming events. The patient was febrile (100° F) and had had malaise for the past 2 days. Submandibular lymphadenopathy was evident bilaterally, and the jaw was extremely sensitive to manipulation. Upon intraoral examination the foul odor was easily detected, and large amounts of dental plaque around the teeth were noted. In addition, the gingiva appeared quite inflamed, with selected (anterior) regions of tissue necrosis between the teeth. Serum chemistry tests and a complete blood count were within normal limits, except for an elevated WBC of 18,500 mm^3. The sedimentation rate (Westergren method) was also slightly elevated at 15 mm/hr.

1. What disease presentation is described in this patient?
2. Review the potential etiological agents for this form of dental disease.
3. A biopsy specimen taken of the areas affected by necrosis would show which types of microorganisms?
4. Describe preventive measures that would have promoted optimum oral health.

Bibliography

American Academy of Periodontology, World Workshop in Clinical Periodontitics, Chicago, 1989.

Department of Health and Human Services, United States Public Health Service, *Oral health of United States adults, national findings*, NIH publication No. 87-2868, Bethesda, Md, August 1987, National Institute of Dental Research.

Drake CW, Hunt RJ, Beck JD, and Zamdon JJ: The distribution and interrelationship of *Actinobacillus actinomycetemcomitans, Porphyromonas gingivalis, Prevotella interimedia,* and BANA scores among older adults, *J Periodontol* 64:89-94, 1993.

Genco RJ: Antibiotics in the treatment of periodontal diseases, *J Periodontol* 52:545, 1981.

Genco RJ, Goldman HM, and Cohen DW, editors: *Contemporary periodontics*, ed 6, St Louis, 1980, Mosby.

Gibbons RJ and Van Houte J: Bacterial adherence in oral microbial ecology, *Ann Rev Microbiol* 29:19, 1975.

Grant D, Stern I, and Listgarten M, editors: *Periodontics*, ed 3, St. Louis, 1988, Mosby.

Loesche WJ: Bacterial succession in dental plaque: role in dental disease. In Schlessinger D, editors: *Microbiology—1985*, Washington, DC, 1975, American Society of Microbiologists.

Moore WEC: Variation in periodontal floras, *Infect Immun* 46: 720, 1984.

Newbrun E: Dietary carbohydrates: their role in cariogenicity, *Med Clin North Am* 63:1069, 1979.

Newbrun E: Sugar and dental caries: a review of human studies, *Science* 217:418, 1982.

Newbrun E: *Cariology*, Baltimore, 1983, William & Wilkins.

Nolte W, editor: *Oral microbiology with basic microbiology and immunology*, St. Louis, 1982, Mosby.

Scheinin A and Odont D: Dietary carbohydrates and dental disorders, *Am J Clin Nutr* 40:19-65, 1982.

Suzuki JB: Diagnosis and classification of the periodontal diseases, *Dent Clin North Am* 32(2):195-216, 1988.

Suzuki JB et al.: Immunologic profile of localized and generalized juvenile periodontitis. II. Neutrophil chemotaxis, phagocytosis, and intracellular spore germination, *J Periodontol* 19:461, 1984.

Van Houte J: Bacterial specificity in the etiology of dental caries, *Int Dent J* 30:305, 1980.

CHAPTER 41

Role of Bacteria in Disease

THIS chapter summarizes the role of bacteria in human diseases. The preceding chapters (Chapters 19 through 40) have examined the biology of individual groups of bacteria. However, human diseases occur not as discrete groups of organisms but rather as pathogenic processes in one or more organ systems. Although an understanding of the mechanisms by which organisms precipitate an infectious process is vital, the clinical management of infections is predicated on the ability to develop a differential diagnosis. That is, knowledge of all organisms associated with a particular infectious process (e.g., bacteremia, pneumonia, gastroenteritis) is critical.

The development of an infection depends on the complex interactions of the host's susceptibility to infection, the organism's virulence potential, and the opportunity for interaction between host and organism. It is impossible to summarize in a single chapter these complex interactions leading to the development of

Text continued on p. 397

TABLE 41-1 Summary of Bacteria Associated With Human Disease

	Relative frequency of isolation	
Organ system affected	**Common pathogen**	**Uncommon pathogen**
Blood (bacteremia)	Coagulase-negative staphylococci, *Staphylococcus aureus, Streptococcus pneumoniae,* other *Streptococcus* species, *Enterococcus, Escherichia coli, Klebsiella pneumoniae, Enterobacter, Proteus mirabilis,* other Enterobacteriaceae, *Pseudomonas aeruginosa,* other *Pseudomonas* species, *Haemophilus influenzae, Bacteroides fragilis*	Many aerobic and anaerobic bacteria
Heart (endocarditis)		
Native valve	*Viridans* group streptococci, *Enterococcus, Staphylococcus aureus, Pseudomonas*	*Streptococcus pneumoniae,* HACEK group (*Haemophilus aphrophilus, Actinobacillus, Cardiobacterium, Eikenella, Kingella*), *Coxiella burnetii, Chlamydia psittaci*
Prosthetic valve	Coagulase-negative staphylococci, *Staphylococcus aureus, Enterococcus, Corynebacterium* species	*Streptococcus pneumoniae, Mycobacterium chelonae*
Central nervous system		
Acute meningitis	*Streptococcus pneumoniae, Neisseria meningitidis, Haemophilus influenzae,* group B *Streptococcus, Listeria monocytogenes, Escherichia coli*	*Leptospira, Staphylococcus aureus*
Chronic meningitis	*Mycobacterium tuberculosis, Nocardia, Treponema pallidum*	*Borrelia burgdorferi, Brucella,* other mycobacterial species
Brain abscess	*Viridans* group streptococci, mixed anaerobes (*Bacteroides, Fusobacterium, Porphyromonas, Prevotella, Peptostreptococcus*), *Staphylococcus aureus*	*Clostridium* species, *Haemophilus, Nocardia, Enterobacteriaceae*

TABLE 41-1 Summary of Bacteria Associated With Human Disease—cont'd

Organ system affected	Relative frequency of isolation: Common pathogen	Uncommon pathogen
Intraabdominal infection		
Spontaneous peritonitis	*Escherichia coli, Klebsiella pneumoniae, Streptococcus pneumoniae, Enterococcus*	*Staphylococcus aureus*, anaerobes, *Neisseria gonorrhoeae, Chlamydia trachomatis, Mycobacterium tuberculosis*
Secondary peritonitis	*Escherichia coli, Bacteroides fragilis*, other enteric anaerobes, *Enterococcus, Pseudomonas aeruginosa*	*Staphylococcus aureus, Neisseria gonorrhoeae, Mycobacterium tuberculosis*
Dialysis-associated peritonitis	Coagulase-negative *Staphylococcus, Staphylococcus aureus, Streptococcus* species, *Corynebacterium* species	*Escherichia coli, Klebsiella, Enterobacter, Proteus, Pseudomonas*
Intraabdominal abscess	*Bacteroides fragilis* group, *Escherichia coli, Enterococcus*	*Klebsiella, Enterobacter, Proteus, Pseudomonas, Staphylococcus aureus*
Upper respiratory tract		
Pharyngitis	Group A *Streptococcus*	Mixed anaerobes (Vincent's angina), *Neisseria gonorrhoeae, Corynebacterium diphtheriae, Corynebacterium ulcerans, Archanobacterium haemolyticum, Mycoplasma pneumoniae, Yersinia enterocolitica*
Tracheobronchitis		*M. pneumoniae*
Otitis externa	*Pseudomonas aeruginosa* (swimmer's ear)	*Staphylococcus aureus*, group A *Streptococcus*
Otitis media	*Streptococcus pneumoniae, Haemophilus influenzae, Moraxella catarrhalis*, anaerobes	*Staphylococcus aureus*, group A *Streptococcus*
Sinusitis	*Streptococcus pneumoniae, Haemophilus influenzae, Moraxella catarrhalis*, anaerobes	*Streptococcus aureus*, group A *Streptococcus*
Epiglottitis	*Haemophilus influenzae*	*Streptococcus pneumoniae, Staphylococcus aureus*, other *Haemophilus* species
Lower respiratory tract		
Bronchitis		*Mycoplasma pneumoniae, Bordetella pertussis, Chlamydia species*
Acute pneumonia	*Streptococcus pneumoniae, Staphylococcus aureus, Haemophilus influenzae, Klebsiella pneumoniae, Escherichia coli, Legionella, Pseudomonas aeruginosa*, mixed anaerobes, *Mycoplasma pneumoniae, Chlamydia*	*Acinetobacter, Moraxella catarrhalis, Neisseria meningitidis, Mycobacterium tuberculosis*, other *Mycobacterium* species, *Eikenella, Francisella, Nocardia, Pasteurella multocida, Pseudomonas pseudomallei, Yersinia pestis, Coxiella burnetii, Rickettsia, Bacillus anthracis*
Chronic pneumonia	Mixed anaerobes, *Mycobacterium tuberculosis, Nocardia*	*Actinomyces, Pseudomonas pseudomallei, Mycobacterium* species
Eye		
Conjunctivitis	*Streptococcus pneumoniae, Staphylococcus aureus*, coagulase-negative staphylococci, *Haemophilus influenzae (H. aegyptius), Neisseria gonorrhoeae, Chlamydia trachomatis*	
Keratitis	*Staphylococcus aureus, Streptococcus pneumoniae, Pseudomonas aeruginosa, Moraxella*	*Mycobacterium fortuitum-chelonae*
Endophthalmitis	*Staphylococcus aureus, Pseudomonas aeruginosa, Bacillus* species	

Continued on next page

TABLE 41-1 Summary of Bacteria Associated With Human Disease—cont'd

Organ system affected	Relative frequency of isolation: Common pathogen	Uncommon pathogen
Skin and soft tissue infections		
Impetigo	Group A *Streptococcus, Staphylococcus aureus*	
Furuncles and carbuncles	*Staphylococcus aureus*	
Paronychia	*Staphylococcus aureus*, group A *Streptococcus, Pseudomonas aeruginosa*	
Erysipelas	Group A *Streptococcus*	
Cellulitis	Group A *Streptococcus, Staphylococcus aureus, Haemophilus influenzae*	
Necrotizing cellulitis and fasciitis	Group A *Streptococcus, Clostridium perfringens*, other clostridial species, *Bacteroides fragilis*, other gram-negative anaerobes, *Peptostreptococcus*, Enterobacteriaceae, *Pseudomonas aeruginosa*	
Chancriform lesions	*Treponema pallidum, Haemophilus ducreyi*	*Bacillus anthracis, Francisella tularensis, Mycobacterium ulcerans, Mycobacterium marinum*
Wounds caused by trauma, burns, bites, etc.	Large variety of organisms including staphylococci, streptococci, Enterobacteriaceae, Pseudomondaceae, and other environmental bacteria	
Bone and joint		
Arthritis	*Staphlyococcus aureus, Neisseria gonorrhoeae, Streptococcus* species, *Haemophilus influenzae*	*Brucella, Nocardia, Mycobacterium* species
Osteomyelitis	*Staphylococcus aureus*, Enterobacteriaceae (*Salmonella, Escherichia, Klebsiella, Proteus*), *Pseudomonas*	*Mycobacterium tuberculosis*, other mycobacterial species, anaerobes
Prosthesis-associated infections	*Staphylcoccus aureus*, coagulase-negative staphylococci, *Streptococcus* species	*Peptostreptococcus*, miscellaneous aerobic gram-negative bacilli
Urinary tract		
Cystitis	*Escherichia coli, Proteus mirabilis, Klebsiella, Enterobacter, Pseudomonas, Enterococcus, Staphylococcus saprophyticus*	*Staphylococcus aureus, Corynebacterium ureolyticus, Clostridium* species, *Bacteroides fragilis, Ureaplasma urealyticum*
Pyelonephritis	*Escherichia coli, Proteus mirabilis, Klebsiella, Staphylococcus aureus*	*Enterococcus, Corynebacterium ureolyticus*
Prostatitis	*Escherichia coli, Klebsiella, Enterobacter, Proteus mirabilis, Enterococcus*	*Neisseria gonorrhoeae*
Genital		
Urethritis	*Neisseria gonorrhoeae, Chlamydia trachomatis*	*Ureaplasma urealyticum, Mycoplasma genitalum*
Bacterial vaginosis (vaginitis)	Synergistic infection with anaerobes (e.g., *Mobiluncus, Bacteroides* species, *Peptostreptococcus*) and possibly *Gardnerella vaginalis*	
Cervicitis	*Neisseria gonorrhoeae, Chlamydia trachomatis*	*Actinomyces, Mycobacterium tuberculosis*
Genital ulcers	*Treponema pallidum, Haemophilus ducreyi, Chlamydia trachomatis* (LGV)	

TABLE 41-1 Summary of Bacteria Associated With Human Disease—cont'd

Organ system affected	Relative frequency of isolation	
	Common pathogen	**Uncommon pathogen**
Gastrointestinal		
Intoxication (disease caused by toxin in food)	*Staphylococcus aureus, Bacillus cereus, Clostridium botulinum*	
Infection	*Campylobacter, Salmonella, Shigella, Clostridium difficile, Clostridium perfringens, Clostridium botulinum* (infant botulism), *Vibrio cholerae, Vibrio parahaemolyticus, Bacillus cereus*	*Escherichia coli* (enterotoxigenic, enteroinvasive, enteropathogenic, enterohemorrhagic), other toxin-producing Enterobacteriaceae), *Aeromonas, Plesiomonas, Yersinia enterocolitica*
Gastritis	*Helicobacter*	
Proctitis	*Neisseria gonorrhoeae, Chlamydia trachomatis, Treponema pallidum*	

disease in each organ system. That is the domain of texts in infectious disease. Rather, this chapter is intended to serve as a very broad overview of the bacteria most commonly associated with infections of specific body sites (Table 41-1). Because many factors will influence the relative frequency in which specific organisms cause disease (e.g., age, underlying disease, epidemiological factors, host immunity), no attempt is made to define all the factors associated with disease caused by specific organisms. Furthermore, the role of fungi, viruses, and parasites are not considered here but rather in their respective sections of this book. For additional information about organ-oriented infections, see the texts listed in the Bibliography.

Bibliography

Finegold SM, George WL: *Anaerobic infections in humans*, San Diego, 1989, Academic Press.

Kelley WN, DeVita VT, DuPont HL, et al: *Textbook of internal medicine*, Philadelphia, 1989, JB Lippincott.

Mandell GL, Douglas RG, Bennett JE: *Principles and practice of infectious diseases*, ed 3, New York, 1990, Churchill Livingstone.

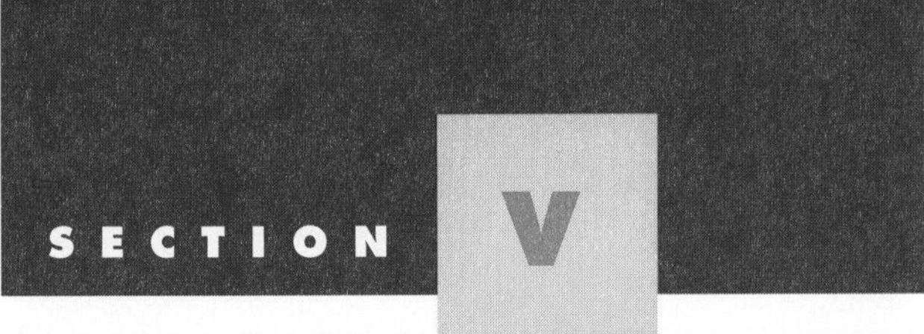

MYCOLOGY

CHAPTER 42

Clinical Syndromes and Laboratory Diagnosis of Fungal Diseases

CLINICAL SYNDROMES

Fungi are extremely common in nature where they exist as free-living saprobes. They frequently reside on body surfaces as transient environmental colonizers but obtain no obvious benefit from this relationship. Because they are so ubiquitous, they are occasionally cultured from clinical specimens. Determining what role they may be playing in an infection may be difficult. In addition, the effects of fungi on humans are numerous. From a medical viewpoint there are only three major categories of importance (Box 42-1).

Mycotoxicoses

Fungi are metabolically versatile organisms and sources of innumerable secondary metabolites such as alkaloids and other toxic compounds. The mycotoxicoses are most often the result of the accidental or recreational ingestion of fungi that produce these compounds. To determine what the source of the toxin might be, a good clinical history must be obtained from the patient. Unfortunately, in many cases the patient is comatose or delirious, and a history is not forthcoming. In the case of ingestion, emesis should be induced and supportive measures instituted consistent with the physiological signs exhibited by the patient. The clinical situation and laboratory diagnosis is much more complicated when material has been injected intravenously. Several examples will point out the positive and negative results on human health.

BOX 42-1 Medical Categories of Fungal Importance

Mycotoxicoses
Hypersensitivity diseases
Colonization of the host and resultant disease

Ergot Alkaloids

The pharmacological properties of ergot alkaloids, which are produced by *Claviceps purpurea* when it infects grain, have been known throughout history. During the Middle Ages epidemics of disease were associated with the consumption of bread and other bakery products made with contaminated rye and other grains. These epidemics were known as St. Anthony's fire. Symptoms consisted of inflammation of the infected tissues (cellular response to injury), followed by necrosis (cell death), and gangrene (death of large masses of tissue). Pharmacologically, we now know that the ergot alkaloids produce **alpha-adrenergic blockade,** which inhibits certain responses to epinephrine and 5-hydroxytryptamine. This creates marked peripheral vasoconstriction, which, if not corrected, restricts the flow of blood and results in necrosis and gangrene.

Another feature of the ergot alkaloids is their extensive activity in directly stimulating smooth muscle. Because of this, they have been used as oxytocic agents, promoting labor during childbirth by increasing the force and frequency of uterine contractions. The effects of ergot alkaloids on the central nervous system include stimulation of the hypothalamus and other sympathetic portions of the midbrain.

Psychotropic Agents

Toxic metabolites produced by fungi have also been used by primitive tribes for religious, magical, and social needs. In recent times problems involving toxins of fungi have been seen with the recreational use of psychotropic agents such as psilocybin and psilocin, as well as the semisynthetic derivative lysergic acid diethylamide (LSD).

Aflatoxins

Among the mycotoxicoses that have had a profound economic impact on society is contamination with *Aspergillus flavus.* This fungus produced the outbreak of "Turkey X" disease in the early 1960s in England and almost destroyed the turkey industry. Turkey poults consumed feed that was contaminated with *Aspergillus* and developed lethargy, anorexia, and muscle weakness followed by spasms and death. Postmortem studies on the birds revealed gross hemorrhage and necrosis of the liver. Further histopathological examination showed parenchymal cell degeneration and extensive proliferation of the bile duct epithelial cells. Biochemical and pharmacological studies showed that the etiological agents of the disease were toxins produced by *A. flavus* that belonged to a group of compounds called the **bisfuranocoumarin metabolites.** These compounds, the aflatoxins, have become known as potent carcinogens but have not been shown to play a specific role in human carcinogenesis.

Other Mycotoxicoses

Several other mycotoxicoses that have affected the well-being of humans have also been described. Among these are yellow rice toxicosis in Japan and alimentary toxic aleukia in the Soviet Union.

Hypersensitivity Diseases

One index used to measure the degree of air pollution is the "fungal spore count" because fungal spores are ubiquitous in nature, supply a good index of environmental contamination, and carry medical relevance. Humans are constantly bombarded by airborne spores and other fungal elements. These elements can be an antigenic stimulus and, depending on the immunological status of the individual, may induce a state of hypersensitivity resulting from the production of immunoglobulins or sensitized lymphocytes. In **hypersensitivity pneumonitis** the clinical manifestations of these reactions include rhinitis, bronchial asthma, alveolitis, and various forms of atopy. Growth of the fungus in tissues is not required, and the manifestations are seen only in sensitized patients when they are subsequently exposed to the fungus, its metabolites, or other cross-reactive materials. In patients who exhibit these symptoms, skin testing with various crude and purified fungal extracts **(allergens)** often identifies the basis of the hypersensitivity.

Colonization and Diseases

As stated previously, virtually all of the fungal organisms implicated in human disease processes are free living. In general, humans have a high level of innate immunity to fungi, and most of the infections they cause are mild and self-limiting. Intact skin serves as a primary barrier to any infection caused by fungi that primarily colonize the superficial, cutaneous, and subcutaneous layers of skin. The nature of mucosal surfaces discourages colonization by organisms that cause pulmonary infections. Fatty acid content, pH, epithelial turnover, and the normal bacterial flora of the skin appear to contribute to host resistance. Humoral factors such as transferrin have been shown to restrict the growth of several fungi by limiting the amount of available iron, but the role it plays in resistance has not been established.

A handful of fungi are capable of causing significant disease in otherwise healthy humans. Once established, these infections can be classified according to the tissue levels infected (Box 42-2).

In addition to these four categories of fungus infections, a fifth grouping has become increasingly important because of the acquired immunodeficiency syndrome (AIDS) epidemic and the increasing use of immunosuppressive therapy. These infectious problems include agents with low pathogenic potential, that produce disease only under unusual circumstances, mostly involving host debilitation. As a result of the many advances in medicine, these organisms, once thought to be innocuous saprobes, have gained prominence as etiological agents of disease. Among the unusual circumstances leading to infections by these fungi are changes in the normal microbial flora of the gut through the use of broad-spectrum antibacterial drugs, host debilitation produced by the use of therapeutic measures such as cytotoxins, x-irradiation, steroids, and other immunosuppressive drugs, and alteration of the host's immune system through underlying endocrine disorders (e.g., uncontrolled diabetes mellitus or suppression such as that caused by AIDS). The fungal infections that frequently accompany these situations are categorized as **opportunistic mycoses.** If they are not rapidly diagnosed, aggressively managed, and the underlying disorders brought under control, the infections become life threatening. Among the organisms causing these disorders are *Candida albicans,* a yeast that is found as part of the normal flora of the mouth, buccal mucosa, gastrointestinal tract, and vaginal vault; *Malassezia furfur,* a lipophilic yeast often isolated from areas rich in sebaceous glands; and other environmental fungi such as *Aspergillus* spp. and *Mucor* spp.

PATHOGENIC FUNGAL CHARACTERISTICS

In general, healthy, immunocompetent humans have a high innate resistance to fungi even though they are constantly exposed to infectious propagules produced by these organisms. Infection and disease occur when there

BOX 42-2 Classification of Fungal Disease According to Primary Sites of Infections

Superficial mycoses—infections limited to the outermost layers of the skin and hair
Cutaneous mycoses—infections that extend deeper into the epidermis, as well as invasive hair and nail diseases
Subcutaneous mycoses—infections involving the dermis, subcutaneous tissues, muscle, and fascia
Systemic mycoses—infections that originate primarily in the lung but may spread to many organ systems

are disruptions in the protective barriers of the skin and mucous membranes or when defects exist in the immune system that allow fungi to penetrate, colonize, and reproduce in the host. Although most of these encounters are accidental, many of the fungi that cause disease have developed mechanisms that make it easier for them to survive and reproduce within this hostile environment. Dermatophytes, for example, that colonize skin, hair, and nails, elaborate the enzyme keratinase, which hydrolyzes the structural protein keratin; yeasts belonging to the genus *Candida* become filamentous when they invade tissues; several of the agents causing the systemic mycoses are dimorphic in that they are molds in nature but adapt to a unicellular morphology when they parasitize tissues; and *Cryptococcus neoformans* elaborates an acidic mucopolysaccharide capsule, which is a virulence factor.

The fungal pathogens that colonize humans and cause disease possess features that allow categorization into groups according to primarily colonized tissues. The agents causing superficial infections (**superficial mycoses**), for example, tend to grow only on the outermost layers of the skin or cuticle of the hair shaft, rarely inducing an immune reaction. The **cutaneous mycoses** (**dermatophytes**) are also limited to keratinized tissues of the epidermis, hairs, and nails, but they do have greater invasive properties and, depending on the species involved, may evoke a highly inflammatory reaction from the host. The **subcutaneous mycoses** generally have a low degree of infectivity, and infections caused by these organisms are usually associated with some form of traumatic injury. The **systemic mycoses** all involve the respiratory tract, and they possess unique morphological features that contribute to the organism's ability to survive within the host.

DIAGNOSTIC PROCEDURES

The diagnosis of fungal infections caused by primary pathogens (e.g., *Histoplasma capsulatum, Blastomyces dermatitidis, Coccidioides immitis,* and others) can be made microscopically by visualizing the parasitic phase of the organism in clinical specimens or by growing the organism from tissues taken from the lesion. The situation is more complicated in the case of fungal infections caused by ubiquitous opportunistic agents such as *Aspergillus* spp., *Candida* spp., *Mucor,* and others, because these fungi are common in the environment and frequently found as contaminants in cultures. In this case it is of paramount importance that the same organism be isolated repeatedly from specimens taken from the lesion at different time intervals. Further support is given to the validity of these isolates if fungal elements are seen in material taken from the site of infection.

The methods used in collecting and handling clinical specimens are of considerable importance in the isolation and identification of fungi. Furthermore, the sampling procedures used will vary according to the area and type of tissue involved. Although selective media are available for the isolation and culture of most pathogenic fungi, it is important to use sterile techniques whenever possible. This is especially applicable to skin surfaces, nails, and hair that may be contaminated with saprobic fungi, bacteria, dirt and epithelial debris. The skin surface should be swabbed with 70% ethanol and allowed to air-dry before sampling, which involves simply scraping the surface to remove skin scales or hair that contain the fungus. A portion of this material should be examined microscopically to determine if hyphal elements are present. This is done by treating the specimen with 10% potassium hydroxide to destroy tissue elements. Because fungi contain chitin and various complex polysaccharides in their cell wall, they are refractory to the alkali treatment and can be easily visualized by light microscopy (Figure 42-1). In fact, several histological procedures that specifically stain fungi in tissue sections, such as Gomori's methenamine silver and the periodic acid Schiff's stains, are based on the presence of chitin and polysaccharides in their cell wall.

Whenever an infectious etiology is suspected, a portion of diseased tissue should be submitted to the pathologist for microscopic examination. Fungi can be stained preferentially because of the polysaccharide-rich properties of their cell walls. This procedure tells the clinician only that fungi are present in the tissue. For definitive identification of the organism, the fungus must be cultured on suitable medium and incubated at 25° C to 30° C. Specimens taken from blood, cerebrospinal fluid, and by surgical biopsy must be examined microscopically and cultured rapidly, because dessication, autolytic processes, and bacterial contamination can make the specimen unsuitable for diagnostic procedures.

A variety of media support the growth of fungi. Sabouraud's dextrose agar, which is composed of 4% dextrose, 1% peptone, and 2% agar adjusted to pH 5.5, is the most conventional medium used in diagnostic

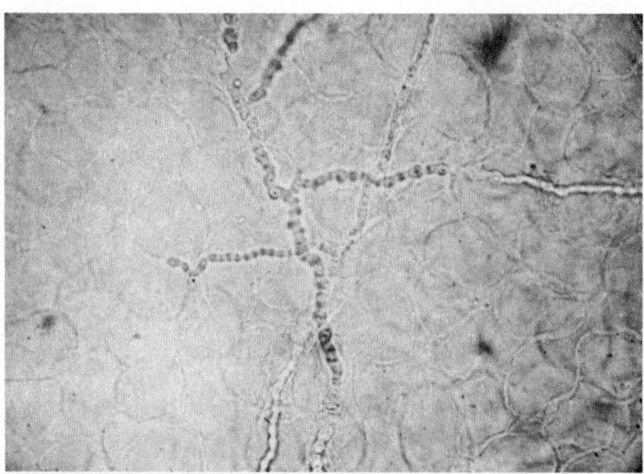

FIGURE 42-1 Skin scraping treated with 10% potassium hydroxide. Fungi are refractory to alkali treatment and appear as septate branching hyphal fragments.

laboratories for growth of fungi. It is selective for the growth of fungi because of its acidic pH and high sugar concentration. Unfortunately, saprobic fungi grow rapidly on this medium and often overgrow the surface, obscuring any pathogens that might be present. Therefore medium containing 2% glucose, 1% neopeptone, 2% agar supplemented with cycloheximide and chloramphenicol and adjusted to pH 7.0 is often used for primary isolation of dermatophytes and other pathogens. Chloramphenicol inhibits most bacteria and cycloheximide inhibits the growth of most saprobic fungi. It should be mentioned that some pathogens such as *C. neoformans* do not grow on this medium. Furthermore, all cultures should be incubated at 25° C to 30° C because the parasitic phase of some primary pathogens such as *H. capsulatum* do not grow at 37° C on this medium. Because opportunistic fungal infections caused by saprobic fungi have increased tremendously, clinical specimens taken from deep tissues should be cultured on media with and without antibiotics.

In general, the techniques used for the laboratory identification of yeast are similar to those used to identify bacteria. Although they are based on biochemical and physiological properties of the organism, the Gram stain plays no role in identifying the organisms because all fungi are Gram positive. Yeasts are unicellular, grow rapidly, and can be uniformly suspended in broth. On the other hand, molds are filamentous, produce specialized conidia, and grow slowly. They are identified microscopically according to the size and shape of the conidia and the way they develop. The morphological features of specialized structures such as chlamydospores and hyphae also aid in identification of molds. Identification of fungi requires a basic understanding and knowledge of different morphological features of fungi. See Chapters 43, 44, and 45, and the Bibliography for detailed description of their identifying features.

SUMMARY

The study of fungi is in the process of transition, and advances in medicine have placed a great deal of importance on the role these organisms play in infections of humans. Traditionally, medical mycology was almost entirely descriptive and taxonomically oriented, a result of its close and historical association with botany and dermatology. At present, medical mycology is enjoying a period of rapid growth and interest. Fungi are being employed as models for the elucidation of many molecular, genetic, and biological processes common to all living things. They are also being used as models to study cellular differentiation and adaptation, particularly concerning host-parasite interactions. The need for rapid identification of fungi in clinical material has been partially met with the development of specific molecular probes, and there is now an emphasis on discovering newer antifungals and novel therapeutic strategies to treat the increasing number of fungal infections that are occurring.

QUESTIONS

1. Fungi can be visualized in tissue sections by specific staining methods. What is the basis behind this technique?
2. Why are cultures for fungi held for at least 4 weeks before they are discarded as negative when bacterial cultures are usually discarded after 2 to 5 days?
3. The laboratory procedure employed in the identification of yeasts differs from that for molds. Why is this necessary?
4. In processing clinical material why are media with and without antibiotics used?
5. In contrast to bacteria, why is it unnecessary to use ×1000 magnification to visualize fungi in clinical material?
6. Why is a strong alkaline solution used to treat tissue specimens when fungi are suspected as being present?
7. In certain situations fungal cultures are incubated at both 25° C and 37° C. Why is this done?

Bibliography

Evans EGV and Gentles JC: *Essentials of medical mycology,* New York, 1985, Churchill Livingstone.

Howard DH, editor: *Fungi pathogenic for humans and animals.* Part A, Biology, New York, 1983, Marcel Dekker.

Kreger-van Rij NJW, editor: *The yeasts: a taxonomic study,* ed 3, Amsterdam, 1984, Elsevier Science Publishers.

Kwon-Chung KJ and Bennett JE: *Medical mycology,* Philadelphia, 1992, Lea & Febiger.

Lincoff G and Mitchel DH: *Toxic and hallucinogenic mushroom poisoning,* New York, 1977, Van Nostrand Reinhold.

Szaniszlo PJ, editor: *Fungal dimorphism: with emphasis on fungi pathogenic for humans,* New York, 1985, Plenum Press.

CHAPTER 43

Superficial, Cutaneous, and Subcutaneous Mycoses

As described previously, fungal infections can be classified according to the tissues that are initially colonized (see Box 42-2 in Chapter 42). Infections caused by (1) the **superficial mycoses** are limited to the outermost layers of the skin and hair; (2) the **cutaneous mycoses** include those that are deeper in the epidermis and its integuments, the hair and nails; and (3) the **subcutaneous mycoses** involve the dermis, subcutaneous tissues, muscle, and fascia.

In general, intact skin and mucosal surfaces serve as barriers to infection caused by the superficial, cutaneous, and subcutaneous mycotic agents. Fatty acid content, pH, epithelial turnover of the skin, and the normal bacterial flora contribute to host resistance. The mucosa and ciliary action of cells lining the respiratory tract help to eliminate organisms that are accidentally inhaled. Humoral factors such as transferrin have been shown to restrict the growth of several fungi in vitro by limiting the amount of available iron. Such factors may play a role in restricting the growth of dermatophytes to the outer layers of skin.

SUPERFICIAL MYCOSES

Superficial fungal infections are usually cosmetic problems that are easily diagnosed and treated. Four infections fall into this classification: two involve the skin (pityriasis versicolor and tinea nigra) and two the hair (black piedra and white piedra) (Figure 43-1). Infections of the skin are limited to the outermost layers of the stratum corneum. Those of hair involve only the cuticle. In general these

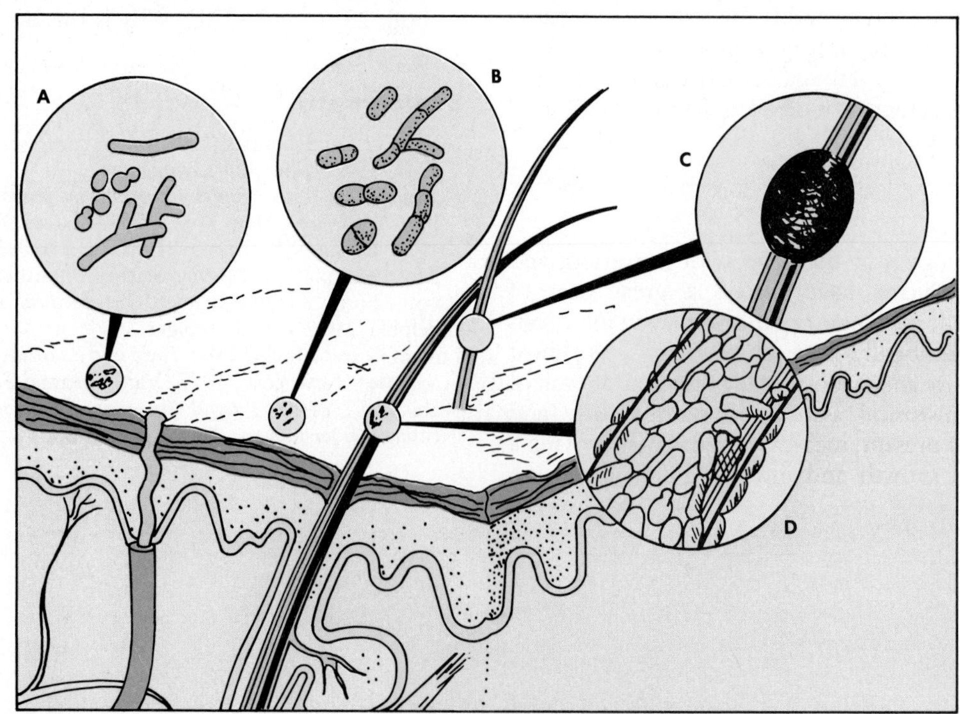

FIGURE 43-1 Schematic illustration of superficial fungal infection and tissue involvement. **A,** Pityriasis versicolor; **B,** tinea nigra; **C,** black piedra; **D,** white piedra.

superficial fungal organisms do not elicit a cellular response from the host because they colonize tissues that are not living. Furthermore, these infections cause no physical discomfort to the patient, and the condition is generally brought to the attention of the physician as an incidental finding or for cosmetic reasons. The diseases are easy to diagnose, and specific therapeutic measures usually result in good clinical responses (Table 43-1).

Etiology, Clinical Syndromes, and Diagnosis

Pityriasis Versicolor

This fungal infection (Figure 43-1, *A*) is caused by *Malassezia furfur (Pityrosporum orbiculare),* a lipophilic yeastlike organism. It is found in areas of the body rich in sebaceous glands and is part of the normal flora of the skin. This organism requires a medium supplemented with saturated or unsaturated fatty acids to support growth. The organism grows as budding yeasts, although hyphal forms are occasionally seen.

The lesions of pityriasis versicolor occur most commonly on the upper torso, arms, and abdomen as discrete hyper- or hypopigmented macular lesions (Figure 43-2). They scale very easily, giving the affected area a dry, chalky appearance. On rare occasions the lesions take on a papular (elevated) appearance, and in some cases where the hair follicle is involved the lesions can cause folliculitis. The clinical diagnosis of pityriasis versicolor is made microscopically by visualizing the characteristic "spaghetti and meatballs" appearance of the organism in potassium hydroxide–treated specimens (Figure 43-3).

Cultures are not routinely done to confirm the diagnosis, since the organism requires a special medium containing fatty acids.

Tinea Nigra

The etiological agent of tinea nigra (Figure 43-1, *B*), *Exophiala werneckii,* is a dimorphic fungus that produces melanin, imparting a brown to black color to the

TABLE 43-1 Important Features of the Organisms Causing the Superficial Mycoses

Organism	Disease	Tissue	Clinical features	Diagnostic procedures
Malassezia furfur	Pityriasis versicolor	Skin	Hyperpigmented or hypopigmented macular lesions that scale readily, giving it a chalky-branny apperance; occurs most frequently on the upper torso of the body	Direct microscopic examination of alkali-stain* treated skin scrapings reveals fungal elements having the classical "spaghetti and meatballs" appearance. Cultures not routinely done to confirm diagnosis. Organism requires fatty acid supplemented medium for growth.
Exophiala werneckii	Tinea nigra	Skin	Gray to black; well-demarcated macular lesions most frequently occurring on the palms of the hand	Direct microscopic examination of skin scrapings treated with alkali-stain.* Culture on Sabouraud's dextrose agar yields pigmented (brown to black) yeasts and hyphae (dimorphic).
Piedraia hortae	Black piedra	Hair	Hard, gritty, brown to black con- cretions that develop along the hair shaft; structures house the sexual phase (asci and ascospores) of the fungus	Direct microscopic examination of hairs. Culture yields asexual phase of the fungus.
Trichosporon beigelii	White piedra	Hair	Soft, white to creamy yellow granules that form a sleeve-like collarette along the hair shaft	Direct microscopic examination of hairs. Culture on Sabouraud's dextrose agar. Growth is dimorphic—hyphae, arthroconidia, and blastoconidia.

From Swartz JH and Lamkin B: *Arch Dermatol* 80:89.

*A useful alkaline dye containing clearing agent can be made from Parker Super Quick permanent blue-black ink by adding 10 g potassium hydroxide per 100 ml of ink. The solution is centrifuged to sediment the amorphous precipitate that forms. The clear blue supernatant should be decanted and stored in a plastic container to prevent insoluble carbonate precipitates from forming.

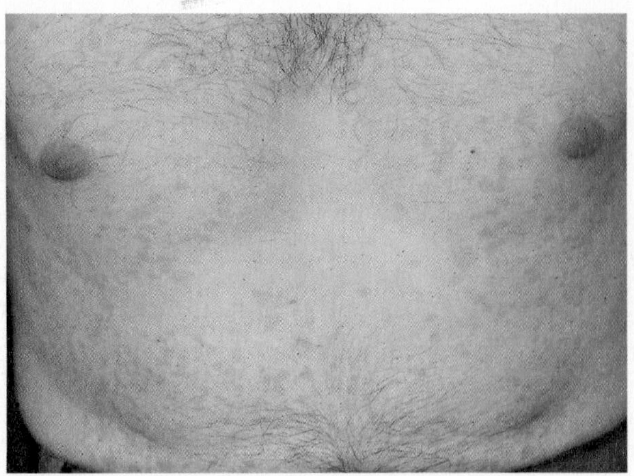

FIGURE 43-2 Clinical presentation of pityriasis versicolor.

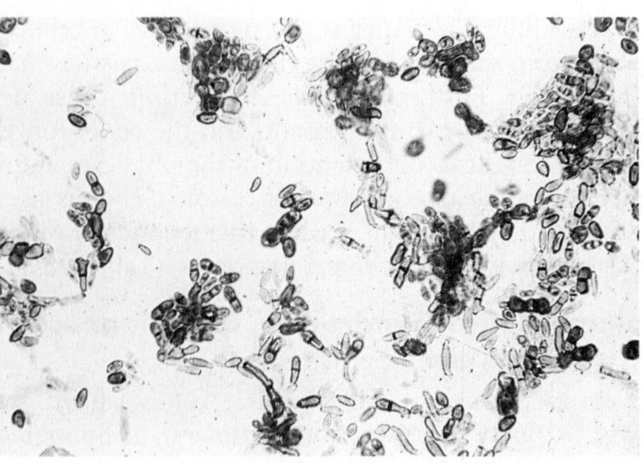

FIGURE 43-4 Yeastlike cells of *Exophiala werneckii,* the causative agent of tinea nigra.

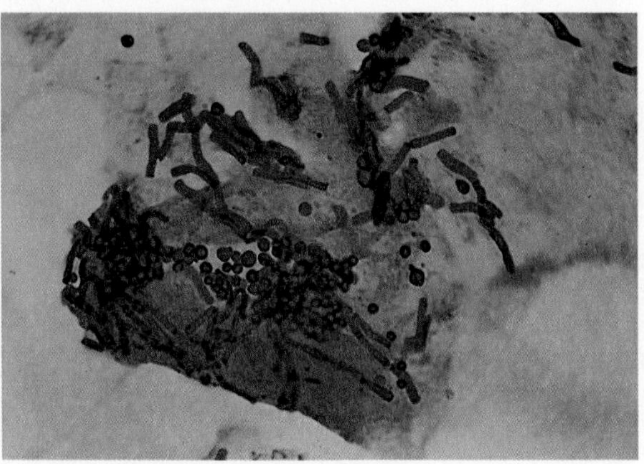

FIGURE 43-3 Skin scrapings stained with periodic-acid Schiff's stain showing typical yeastlike and hyphal fragments of *Malassezia furfur,* the etiological agent of pityriasis versicolor.

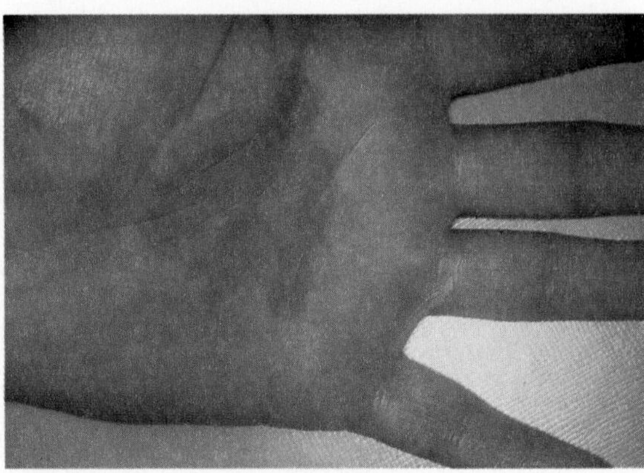

FIGURE 43-5 Clinical presentation of tinea nigra. Note dark pigmentation in the center of the palm.

organism. On primary isolation from clinical material it grows as yeasts with many cells in various stages of cell division, producing characteristic two-celled oval structures (Figure 43-4). As the colony ages, elongate hyphae develop, and in older cultures mycelia and conidia predominate.

The clinical manifestations of tinea nigra are usually asymptomatic and consist of well-demarcated macular lesions (discolored spots on the skin that are not raised above the surface) that enlarge by peripheral extension (Figure 43-5). The brown to black lesions are most often seen on the palms of the hands and soles of the feet but may occur on other areas of the body.

Diagnosis is made by visualizing the characteristic darkly pigmented yeastlike cells and hyphal fragments in microscopic examination of potassium hydroxide–treated scrapings taken from the affected areas; it is confirmed by culture.

Black Piedra

The cause of black piedra (Figure 43-1, *C*), a superficial hair infection, is *Piedraia hortae,* an organism that exists in the perfect (teleomorphic) state when it colonizes the hair shaft. Cultures taken from clinical material usually yield only the asexual (anamorphic) state of the fungus, which consists of slow-growing brown to reddish-black mycelia. The teleomorphic state is occasionally found in older cultures and consists of specialized structures within which asci containing spindle-shaped ascospores develop.

The major clinical feature of black piedra are the hard nodules, found along the infected hair shaft (Figure 43-6). The nodules have a hard carbonaceous consistency and house asci. The differential diagnosis includes ruling out nits of pediculosis and abnormal hair growth.

The infection is easily diagnosed by microscopic examination of affected hairs.

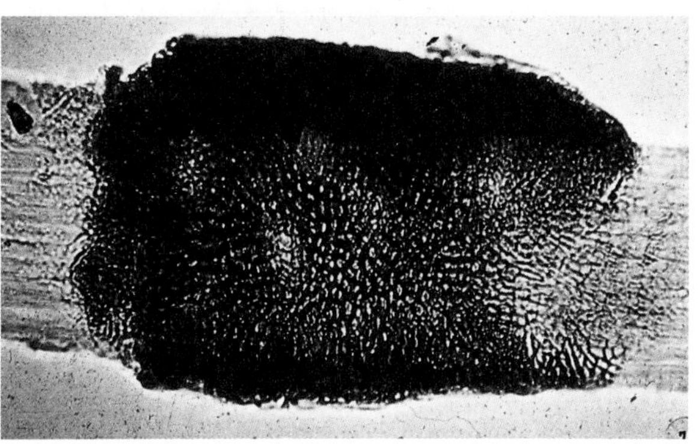

FIGURE 43-6 Hair infected with *Piedraia hortae.* The hard black nodule contains asci and ascospores, the sexual phase of the fungus.

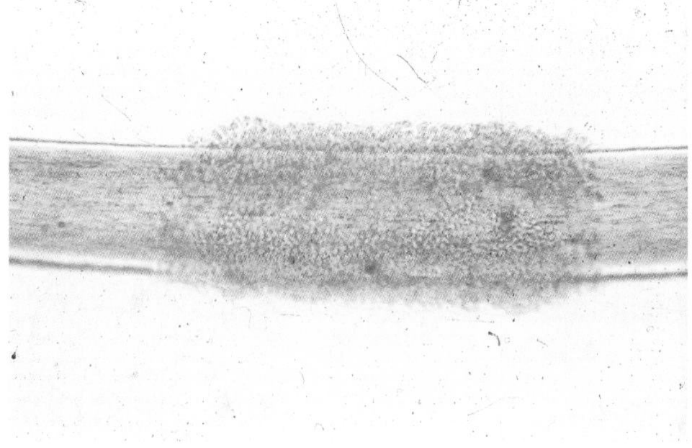

FIGURE 43-8 Clinical presentation of white piedra.

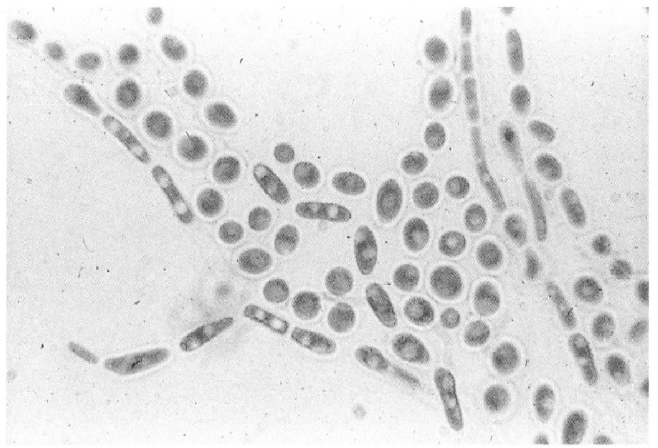

FIGURE 43-7 Hyphae, arthroconidia, and blastospores of *Trichosporon beigelii,* illustrating the dimorphic characteristics of the agent of white piedra.

White Piedra

This infection of the hair (Figure 43-1, *D*) is caused by the yeastlike organism *Trichosporon beigelii* (Figure 43-7). The organism grows well on all laboratory media except those containing cycloheximide, an antibiotic used in media for the selective isolation of most pathogenic fungi (e.g., Mycosel agar). Young cultures are white and have a pasty consistency. As the culture ages, colonies develop deep, radiating furrows and take on a yellowish coloration with a creamy texture. Microscopic examination reveals septate hyphae that fragment rapidly to form arthroconidia (see Figure 43-7). The arthroconidia rapidly round up, and many cells form blastoconidia.

White piedra affects hairs of the scalp, mustache, and beard. It is characterized by the development of cream-colored soft pasty growths along infected hair shafts (Figure 43-8). The growth occurs as a sleeve or collarette around the hair shaft and consists of mycelia that rapidly fragment into arthroconidia.

The organism is identified by various biochemical tests and its ability to assimilate certain carbohydrates. The differential diagnosis includes trichomycosis axillaris (caused by *Corynebacterium tenuis*) and the nits of pediculosis. The infection is diagnosed by microscopic examination of infected hairs and confirmed by culture.

Treatment

These infections in general are cosmetic and easily diagnosed. When proper therapy is instituted, the infections respond well, with no consequences. The general approach to treating pityriasis versicolor and tinea nigra is removal of the organism from the skin. This is accomplished by the topical use of keratolytic (chemicals that lyse keratin) agents. Preparations containing selenium disulfide, hyposulfite, thiosulfate, or salicylic acid accomplish this, but the disease may reoccur. Topical preparations containing miconazole nitrate, an antifungal that inhibits ergosterol synthesis (see Chapter 14), have been used effectively in eradicating the disease.

In hair infections caused by *P. hortae* and *T. beigelii,* effective therapy is achieved by shaving or cropping the infected hairs close to the scalp surface. These infections will not reoccur if proper personal hygiene is practiced.

CUTANEOUS MYCOSES

The cutaneous mycoses involve diseases of the skin, hair, and nails. They are generally restricted to the keratinized layers of the integument and its appendages (Figure 43-9). Unlike the superficial infections, various cellular immune responses may be evoked in cutaneous infections, causing pathological changes in the host that may be expressed in the deeper tissues of the skin. The severity of the response appears to be directly related to the immune status of the host and strain or species of fungus involved. The term **dermatophyte** has been used traditionally to describe these agents. However, the suffix "phyte" implies that these organisms are plants, which is

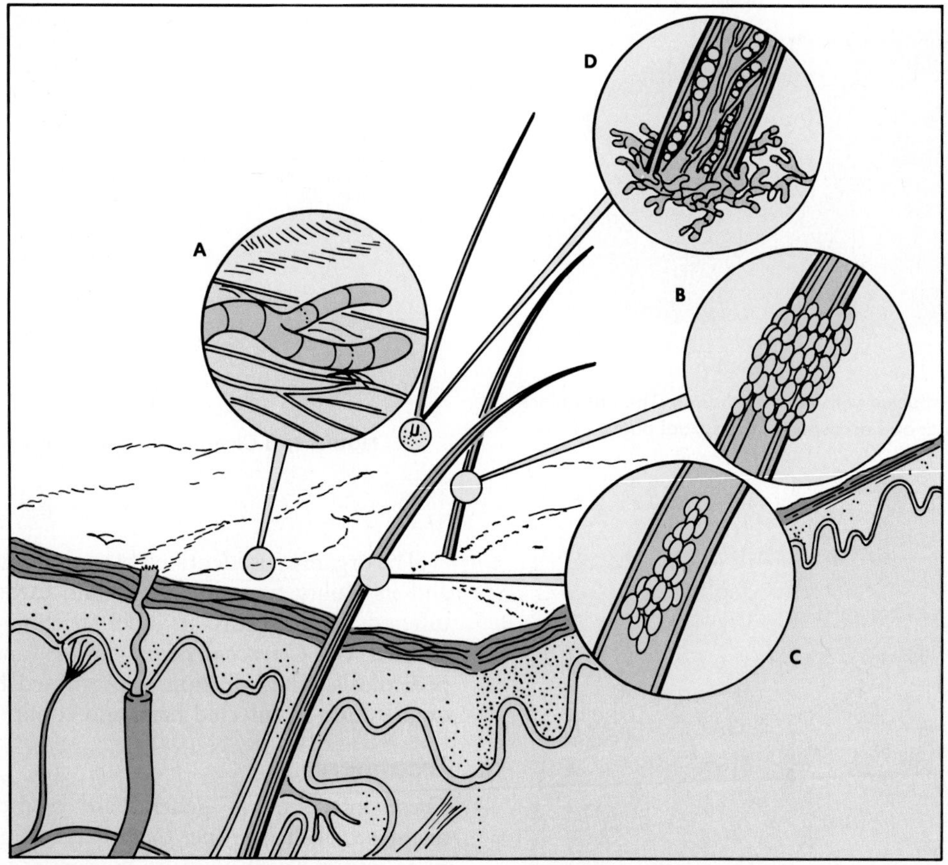

FIGURE 43-9 Schematic of tissues colonized by dermatophytes. **A,** Stratum corneum; **B,** ectothrix hair infection; **C,** endothrix hair infection; **D,** favic hair infection.

misleading because fungi are not phylogenetically related to plants. However, for historical reasons the term dermatophyte will be used in this section in reference to the organisms causing these diseases.

The clinical manifestations of these diseases are also referred to as **ringworm** or **tinea,** depending on the anatomical site involved (e.g., tinea pedis, feet; tinea capitis, scalp; tinea manus, hands; tinea unguium, nails; tinea corporis, body). In some cases they are given special names depending on what organism causes the disease (e.g., favus, *Trichophyton schoenleinii;* tokelau, *T. concentrichum*). The term *tinea* comes from Latin and means worm or moth. It is used descriptively because of the serpentine (snakelike) and annular (ringlike) lesions that occur on the skin, making it appear that a worm is burrowing at the margin (Figure 43-10).

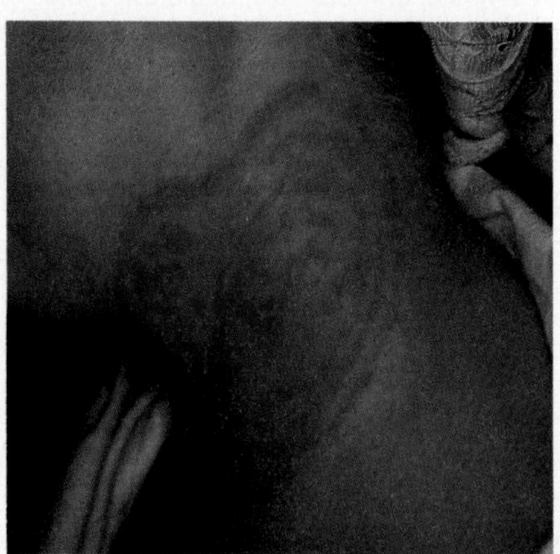

FIGURE 43-10 Clinical presentation of tinea corporis.

Etiology

The cutaneous mycoses are caused by a homogeneous group of closely related organisms known as the dermatophytes. Although more than 100 species have been described, only about 40 are considered valid and less than half of these are associated with human disease (Table 43-2). In the anamorphic state they are classified in three genera (i.e., *Microsporum, Trichophyton,* and *Epidermophyton*) on the basis of their sporulation patterns (Figure 43-11), certain morphological features of development, and nutritional requirements. The teleomorphic state of some of the organisms belonging to the genera *Microsporum* and *Trichophyton* are known. They are all Ascomycetes and have been reclassified in the genus *Arthroderma.* As yet, the sexual phase of *Epidermophyton* has not been observed.

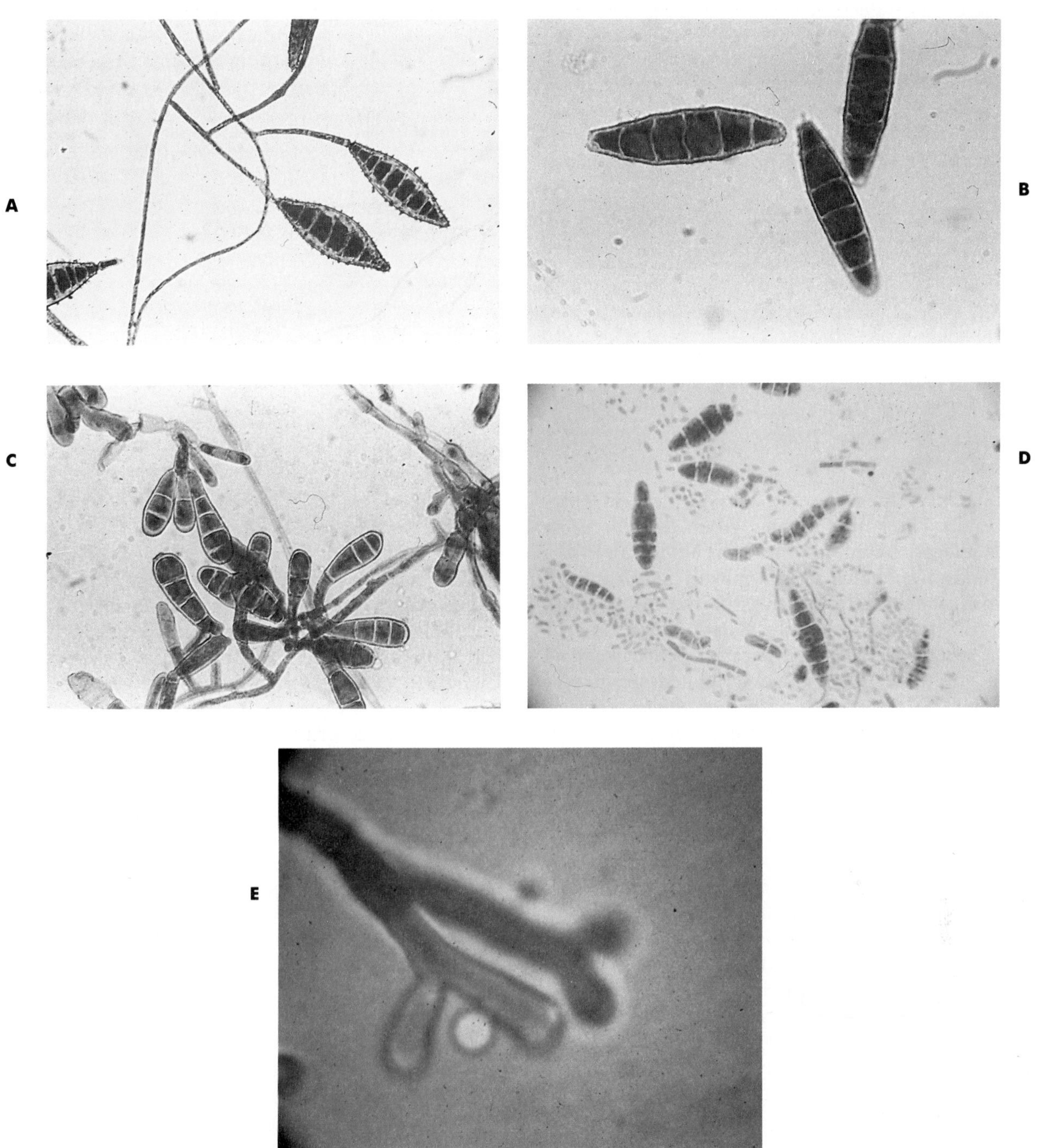

FIGURE 43-11 Sporulation pattern and identifying features of some dermatophytes. **A,** Macroconidia of *Microsporum canis;* **B,** macroconidia of *M. gypseum;* **C,** macroconidia of *Epidermophyton floccosum;* **D,** microconidia and macroconidia of *Trichophyton mentagrophytes;* **E,** favic chandelier of *Trichophyton schoenleinii.*

Ecology and Epidemiology

The isolation of different species of dermatophytes varies markedly from one ecological niche to another. Some species are frequently isolated from the soil and have been grouped as **geophilic dermatophytes.** Other species have been found most often in association with domestic and wild animals and birds. These are referred to as **zoophilic** dermatophytes. A third group, the **anthropophilic dermatophytes,** has been found almost exclusively in association with humans and their habitats. Table 43-3 summarizes the groupings of various species that are common throughout the world.

The clinical importance of identifying species of dermatophytes is to determine the possible source of

TABLE 43-2 Asexual (Anamorphic) State of Selected Dermatophytes*

Microsporum	*Trichophyton*	*Epidermophyton*
M. audouinii	*T. concentricum*	*E. floccosum*
M. canis	*T. equinum*	
M. cookei	*T. mentagrophytes* var. *interdigitale*	
M. equinum	*T. rubrum*	
M. fulvum	*T. tonsurans*	
M. gallinae	*T. verrucosum*	
M. gypseum	*T. violaceum*	
M. nanum		

*At present, 41 species of dermatophytes are recognized as etiological agents of disease.

TABLE 43-3 Classification of Dermatophytes According to Ecological Niche*

Anthropophilic dermatophytes	Zoophilic dermatophytes	Geophilic dermatophytes
M. audouinii	*M. canis*	*M. cookei*
T. mentagrophytes, var. *interdigitale*	*M. equinum*	*T. gypseum*
T. rubrum	*M. gallinae*	*M. fulvum*
T. tonsurans	*T. equinum*	*M. nanum*
T. violaceum	*T. mentagrophytes,* var. *mentagrophytes*	
E. floccosum		

*Includes only those species that are common throughout the world.

infection. There are also some considerations of prognostic value. The anthropophilic group tends to cause chronic infections and may be difficult to cure. The zoophilic and geophilic dermatophytes tend to cause inflammatory lesions, respond well to therapy, and may occasionally heal spontaneously.

Some species of dermatophytes are endemic in certain parts of the world and have a limited geographic distribution. At the present time, *T. yaoundei, T. gourvilli,* and *T. soudenense* are geographically restricted to Central and West Africa; in Japan and its surrounding areas *M. ferrugineum* predominates; and *T. concentricum* is confined to islands in the South Pacific and a small area of Central and South America. However, the increasing mobility of the world's population is disrupting several of these patterns. In recent times *T. tonsurans* has replaced *M. audouinii* as the principal agent of tinea capitis in the United States, a result of the mass migration of individuals from Mexico and other Latin American countries where *T. tonsurans* predominates. Less well understood are the epidemics of ringworm that occasionally occur.

The prevalence of dermatophytes and the incidence of disease are difficult to determine because they are not reportable. Fragmentary surveys from epidemiological studies and case reports indicate that the cutaneous mycoses are among the most common human diseases. Reports estimate that they are the third most common skin disorder in children younger than 12 years of age and the second most common in older populations. The occurrence of these diseases varies with age, sex, ethnic group, and cultural and social habits of the population.

The incidence of the cutaneous mycoses and clinical manifestations of the disease among various age-groups depend on the anatomical site of involvement and the species of dermatophyte involved. Tinea capitis is a problem of the pediatric population until puberty, when it spontaneously ceases to be a major infectious disorder. On the other hand, tinea pedis, which is rarely a disease in childhood, gradually becomes the predominant infection and remains so into adulthood.

The incidence of tinea capitis in black children in the United States is disproportionately high. In India tinea capitis occurs more often in the native children than in Europeans, whereas the Europeans have a higher incidence of tinea pedis than does the native population. Clinical surveys conducted during the war in Southeast Asia revealed that persons from the United States had a higher incidence of tinea pedis caused by *T. mentagrophytes* than did the native population. The indigenous population appeared to be highly susceptible to a distinctive strain of *T. rubrum.* Tinea capitis, tinea pedis, and tinea cruris are more common in men than women, whereas the reverse is true for tinea unguium (infections of the nail plate) of the hand. For nails of the feet it is seen more often in men.

The reasons for these observations are poorly understood. The incidence of cutaneous mycoses is related to customs associated with the type of clothing that is worn and how the feet are shod. Studies on institutionalized populations and family outbreaks of dermatophyte infections indicate that close and crowded living conditions are a factor in the spread of infections. There is evidence that natural resistance to these infections exists in certain individuals. Certain humoral factors are fungistatic, and cell-mediated immunity appears to be important in resistance to dermatophyte infections.

Pathogenesis

A delicate balance appears to operate between host and parasite in dermatophyte infections. Some of these fungi show an evolutionary development toward a parasitic existence. Those that have achieved a high level of coexistence with humans also exhibit a degree of specificity for the tissues that are colonized. These fungi are often referred to as **"keratinophilic fungi"** because they can use keratin as a substrate. Keratinases have been isolated from some of these fungi, but keratin is not an

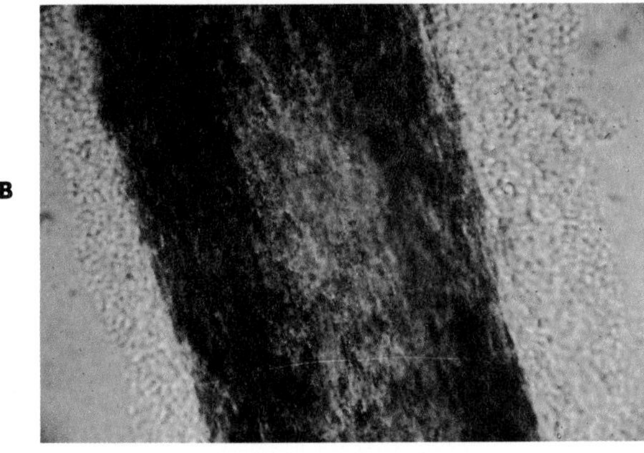

FIGURE 43-12 Fungal infections of the hair. **A,** Endothrix infection; **B,** ectothrix infection.

essential metabolite for them. The reason for the high degree of selectivity of tissues containing this protein for growth of the dermatophytes is unknown. As versatile as these fungi might appear, they seem unable to invade organs other than the keratinized layers of skin, hair, and nails.

Laboratory Diagnosis

The diagnosis of disease requires that fungal elements be seen in clinical specimens taken from the lesion and/or confirmed by culture. Skin and nail scrapings or hairs taken from areas suspected to be infected are examined microscopically. The procedure for processing these specimens is similar to the procedures described previously for examining clinical material from superficial fungal infections. The specimen is treated with an alkali solution to clear it of epithelial cells and other debris. Dermatophytes resist the caustic solution and will appear as branching septate hyphal elements in specimens taken from cutaneous lesions or nails. Fungus elements in infected hairs examined by this procedure will appear as spores inside (endothrix infection; Figure 43-12, *A*) or surrounding (ectothrix infection; Figure 43-12, *B*) the hair shaft.

An exception is the hair infection caused by *T. schoenleinii*. Disease caused by this organism is called

TABLE 43-4 General Characteristics of Macroconidia and Microconidia of Dermatophytes

Genus	Macroconidia	Microconidia
Microsporum	Numerous, thick-walled, rough*	Rare
Epidermophyton	Numerous, smooth-walled	Absent
Trichophyton	Rare, thin-walled, smooth	Abundant†

**M. audouinii* is an exception.
†*T. schoenleinii* is an exception.

favus, and the infected hair will have a waxy mass of hyphal elements (scutulum) surrounding the base of the hair follicle at the scalp line (Figure 43-9, *D*). Microscopic examination of the hair reveals degenerated hyphal elements coursing throughout the hair shaft (see Figure 43-9, *D*). Such hairs are called **favic** and are diagnostic of the infection.

Direct microscopic examination of clinical material will confirm only the diagnosis of a fungal infection. To identify the specific etiological agent, cultures must be taken.

The skin surface harbors many bacterial species and saprobic fungi as part of the normal flora or transient colonizers. Thus media such as Sabouraud's dextrose agar are not routinely used for primary culture because these organisms overgrow the culture and inhibit growth of the more slow-growing dermatophytes. For this reason selective media containing antibiotics are recommended when culturing specimens taken from the skin. A medium commonly used for the isolation of dermatophytes from clinical material is one that contains cycloheximide (to suppress saprobic fungal growth) and chloramphenicol (to inhibit growth of bacteria). Clinical material is seeded directly onto the medium and incubated at 25° C. Dermatophytes and most pathogenic fungi grow well on this medium when incubated at 25° C, whereas saprobic fungi and bacteria are inhibited.

Cultures are examined periodically, and all fungi that grow are identified microscopically and by physiological tests. In general, the mycelia of these fungi are undifferentiated, and species identification is based primarily on the conidia that are produced (Table 43-4). The conidia may be large (5 to 100 μm × 6 to 8 μm) and multicellular (macroconidia), or they may be small (3 μm × 10 μm) and unicellular (microconidia).

In addition to conidia, some dermatophytes produce spiral hyphae, chlamydospores, nodular bodies, racquet hyphae, and chandeliers. These structures are produced commonly by some species of dermatophytes and infrequently by others; however, they should not be considered distinguishing features of the species. Figure 43-11 illustrates the identifying features of some dermatophytes.

All cultures are routinely held for 4 weeks before being discarded as negative.

Treatment

The clinical nature of the dermatophyte infections frequently poses a challenge to the clinician. Skin infections generally are approached conservatively with topical treatment. The discovery of azole derivatives as effective antifungal agents has provided several new drugs that can be used topically, such as miconazole, clotrimazole, and econazole. All of the azole derivatives appear to work by interfering with the cytochrome P-450–dependent enzyme systems at the demethylation step from lanosterol to ergosterol.

For hair infections, griseofulvin, a secondary metabolite of the fungus *Penicillium griseofulvum,* is an effective and safe drug prescribed orally for the management of tinea capitis. This compound is fungistatic and appears to work by affecting the microtubular system of fungi. It interferes with the mitotic spindle and cytoplasmic microtubules. The molecular action of griseofulvin is different from that of other inhibitors, such as cholchicine and the vinca alkaloids, which bind to receptors on tubulin and inactivate the free subunits of microtubules.

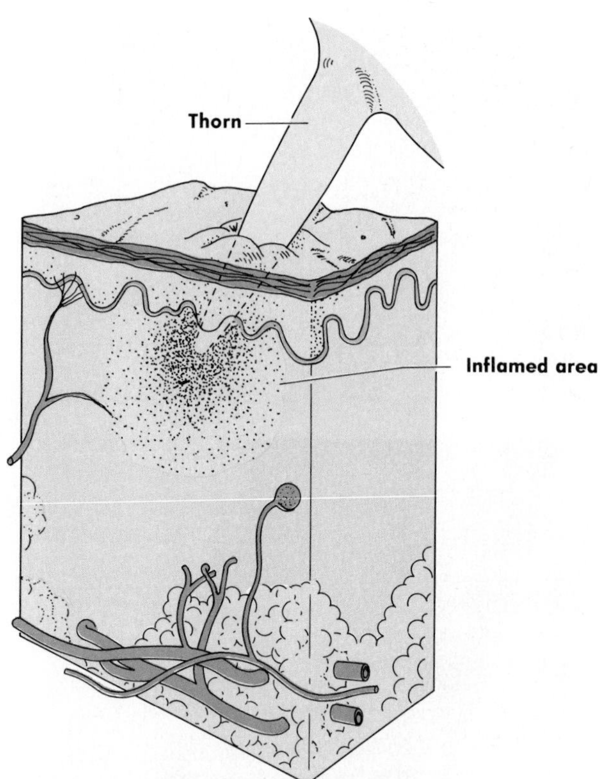

FIGURE 43-13 Schematic of tissue level colonized primarily by agents causing subcutaneous mycoses. The fungus gains access to the deeper layers of skin by traumatic implantation. The organisms implicated in these disease processes are usually common fungi found in the soil.

SUBCUTANEOUS MYCOSES

The subcutaneous mycoses include a wide spectrum of fungal infections characterized by the development of lesions, usually at sites of trauma where the organism is implanted in the tissue (Figure 43-13). The infections initially involve the deeper layers of the dermis, subcutaneous tissue, or bone. Most infections have a chronic and insidious growth pattern, eventually extending into the epidermis, and are expressed clinically as lesions on the skin surface. Several features are common about this group of infections. The patient can usually associate some form of trauma occurring at the sites of the infection before the lesions developed (e.g., a splinter, a thorn, the implantation of other foreign bodies, or a bite). The infections occur on parts of the body that are most prone to be traumatized (e.g., feet, legs, hands, arms, and buttocks). The etiological agents are usually organisms commonly found in the soil or on decaying vegetation. Several bacterial infections (e.g., actinomycotic mycetoma, botryomycosis, and atypical acid-fast disease) mimic the subcutaneous fungal infections. For this reason it is extremely important that the etiological agent be established, because most of the bacterial infections can be managed with antibiotics. Finally, with one or two exceptions, the subcutaneous mycoses are difficult to treat, and surgical intervention (i.e., excision or amputation) may be indicated.

Etiology and Clinical Syndromes

With the exception of lymphocutaneous sporotrichosis, most subcutaneous fungal infections are rare and considered exotic in the United States and other highly developed countries. The diseases that are less frequently or rarely seen are chromoblastomycosis, phaeohyphomycosis, chronic subcutaneous zygomycosis, and eumycotic mycetoma. Two diseases, lobomycosis and rhinosporidiosis, are considered possibly caused by fungi, but confirmation by culture is lacking.

The causative agents are a heterogeneous group of organisms with low pathogenic potential that are commonly isolated from soil or decaying vegetation. The clinical manifestations of these diseases appear to be an interplay between the etiological agent and host responses. In general, patients who develop disease have no underlying immunological defect.

Lymphocutaneous Sporotrichosis

This chronic infection is characterized by nodular and ulcerative lesions that develop along lymphatics that drain the primary site of inoculation (Figure 43-14). Other infrequently seen forms of sporotrichosis include fixed cutaneous lesions, primary and secondary pulmonary sporotrichosis, and disseminated disease. The causative agent is the dimorphic fungus *Sporothrix schenckii.*

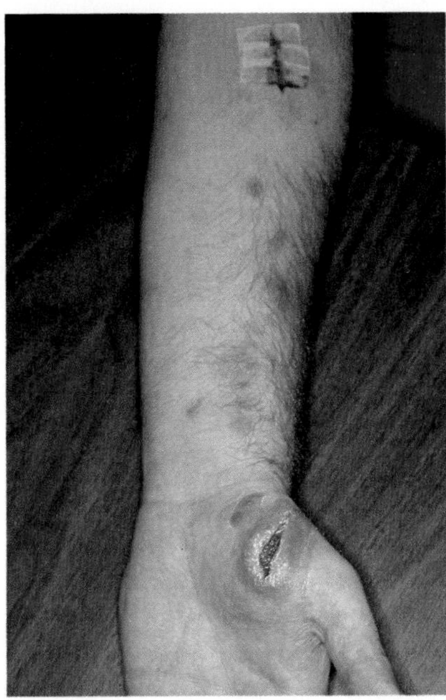

FIGURE 43-14 Clinical case of lymphocutaneous sporotrichosis, illustrating the characteristic pattern of lesions along the lymphatics that drain the site of the original lesion.

Chromoblastomycosis

This disease is characterized by the development of verrucous (warty) nodules that appear at sites of inoculation (Figure 43-15). As lesions progress they appear to vegetate and take on a "cauliflower-like" appearance. The organisms responsible for chromoblastomycosis are common soil inhabitants that are collectively called the **dematiaceous fungi.** The term "dematiaceous" is used to describe fungi that have brown to black melanin pigments in their cell wall (see also tinea nigra).

Phaeohyphomycosis

Another clinical disease caused by various dematiaceous fungi is phaeohyphomycosis, which is a heterogeneous group of cutaneous diseases caused by various dematiaceous fungi. The most common form described is phaeohyphomycotic cyst. The disease does not exhibit the intense hyperplasia seen in chromoblastomycosis, and when organisms are seen in histopathological examination of tissues they usually appear as pigmented septate hyphal fragments.

The taxonomy of the dematiaceous agents is currently undergoing careful scrutiny, and as yet complete agreement has not been reached. The dematiaceous fungi most often associated with chromoblastomycosis are *Fonsecaea pedrosoi, F. compacta, Cladosporium carrionii,* and *Phialophora verrucosa.* These organisms are identified according to the pattern and type of sporulation exhibited by the isolate. In many cases the isolate may exhibit more than one pattern of sporulation, and for this reason confusion and conflicts often arise concerning the correct taxonomic placement of the organism.

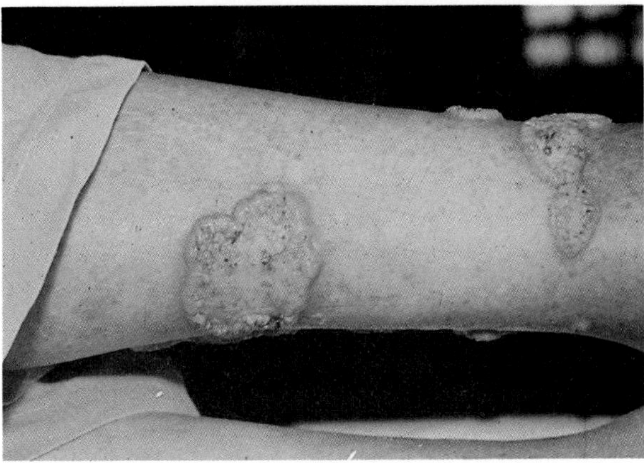

FIGURE 43-15 Clinical case of chromoblastomycosis, illustrating the characteristic verrucous vegetative lesions.

Similar taxonomic problems exist in the identification of agents implicated in phaeohyphomycosis, for which about 40 different organisms have been incriminated. Included in this large number of etiological agents are some fungi that are rare and no doubt reflect the exotic nature of some of these clinical entities.

Eumycotic Mycetoma

The term *mycetoma* is clinically descriptive and includes a wide spectrum of manifestations involving the skin and deeper tissues of the dermis and subcutaneous tissues. The disease is characterized by indolent, deforming, swollen lesions that contain numerous draining sinus tracts.

Other Subcutaneous Mycoses

Zygomycosis, lobomycosis, and rhinosporidiosis are rare clinical entities. A detailed description of these diseases is contained in references listed in the Bibliography at the end of the chapter.

Laboratory Diagnosis

Lymphocutaneous Sporotrichosis

In tissue and in cultures incubated at 37° C *Sporothrix schenckii* is a budding yeast cell. Cultures at 25° C develop as delicate radiating colonies that appear within 3 to 5 days on most media. The colonies are moist and white at first; with prolonged incubation they slowly develop a brown to black pigmentation. Microscopic examination reveals delicate branching hyphae, about 2 μm in diameter, with numerous conidia developing in a rosette pattern at the ends of conidiophores (Figure 43-16). Laboratory confirmation is established by converting the mycelial growth to the yeast morphology by subculture at 37° C.

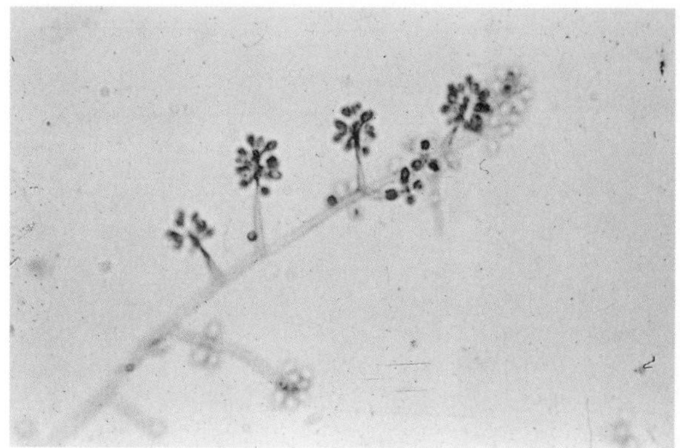

FIGURE 43-16 Microscopic examination illustrating "rosette pattern" of conidia in *Sporothrix schenckii.*

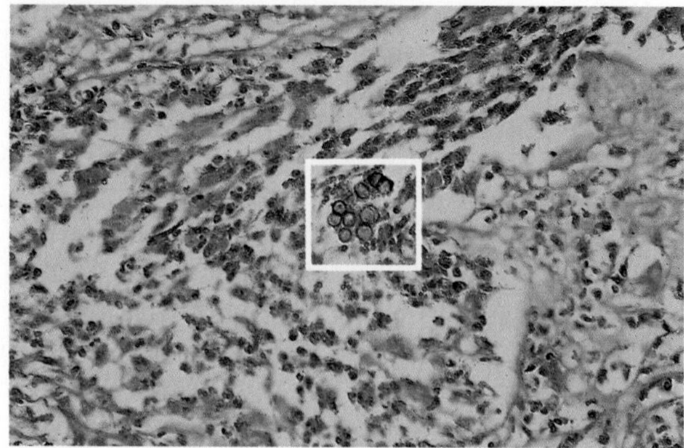

FIGURE 43-17 Tissue section taken from a case of chromoblastomycosis, illustrating the characteristic "sclerotic" cells.

Chromoblastomycosis

The diagnosis of chromoblastomycosis is usually made by histopathological examination of clinical material taken from the lesions. There is a characteristic tissue response termed *pseudoepitheliomatous hyperplasia,* which means that the tissue exhibits an epithelial overgrowth caused by an abnormal multiplication in the number of normal cells in normal arrangement in the tissue. In addition to the histopathology, copper-colored spherical cells in various stages of cell division are seen (Figure 43-17). These structures, called **sclerotic** or **Medlar bodies,** are the tissue forms of the fungus.

Eumycotic Mycetoma

Examination of the purulent fluid that exudes from the sinus tracts in eumycotic mycetoma often reveals small grains of fungal tissue. These elements may be white, brown, yellow, or black and can be well demonstrated on histopathological examination of tissue biopsies of the lesion (Figure 43-18). The etiological agents causing these diseases consist of various actinomycetes belonging to the genera *Actinomyces, Nocardia, Streptomyces,* and *Actinomadura,* as well as a whole host of fungi, including *Pseudallescheria boydii* and *Madurella grisea.* It is important to establish the cause of the disease by culturing specimens because the clinical management of the infection will vary depending on the causative organism.

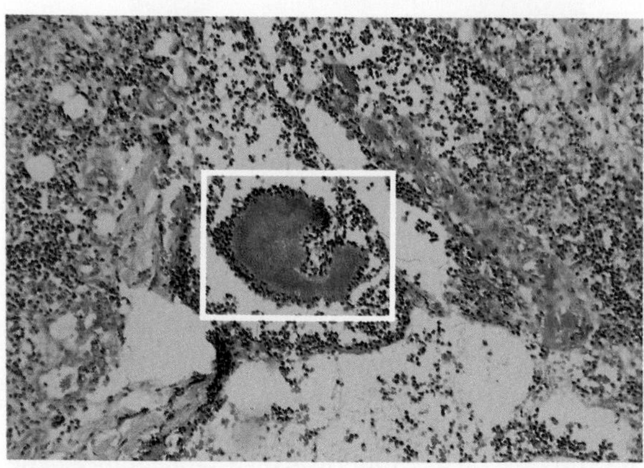

FIGURE 43-18 Histopathological section of tissue taken from mycetoma, illustrating a microcolony (often referred to as a granule).

Treatment

Subcutaneous lymphangitic sporotrichosis responds dramatically to a saturated solution of potassium iodide given orally. Adverse side effects include gastrointestinal upset and dermatological problems that are rapidly reversed by discontinuing therapy. Extracutaneous sporotrichosis invariably requires systemic therapy with amphotericin B.

Cautery and surgical removal of early lesions have been used in the treatment of chromoblastomycosis; however, most patients who seek help have advanced disease. The extensive tissue involvement is often not amenable to surgical intervention and requires chemotherapy. At present, the drug of choice for treating chromoblastomycosis is 5-fluorocytosine. This drug is given orally and acts by inhibiting RNA and DNA synthesis.

As stated previously, the clinical treatment of eumycotic mycetoma varies with the causative agent. In the case of actinomycotic mycetomas, several antibacterial antibiotics can be used. For example, infections caused by *Actinomyces israellii* respond to high doses of penicillin, and those caused by *Nocardia asteroides* respond to sulfa drugs in combination with streptomycin. However, if a fungal organism is the causative agent, the physician will frequently resort to total excision of the lesion or amputation of an affected limb if the disease is extensive because antifungal therapy in general is unsuccessful.

CASE STUDY AND QUESTIONS

The school nurse was informed that three first-grade boys had scaly patchy alopecia. She examined them for nits but did not find any, so she sent them home with instructions to be seen by their pediatrician. The pediatrician confirmed that nits were not the problem.

1. What should the pediatrician do to confirm the diagnosis of tinea capitis?
2. Should their siblings and the rest of the classroom be examined?
3. What are some interesting epidemiological and clinical features of the pathophysiology of tinea capitis, tinea pedis, and tineas caused by anthropophilic, zoophilic, and geophilic fungi?

Two healthy construction laborers were seen by a dermatologist after developing painless bilateral ulcerative lesions along the lymphatics of the forearms. On examination they were afebrile. There was regional lymphadenopathy, and the lesions extended up the lymphatics as tender erythematous subcutaneous nodules, some of which were fluctuant. Histories taken from the patients revealed that these lesions began to appear 2 to 3 weeks after they had demolished an attic as part of an urban renewal project. Both stated that they got splinters from carrying wood they had salvaged from the rafters. The only other comments elicited were that bats and pigeons had roosted in the attic and a lot of dust was raised during the salvage.

1. What is the most likely diagnosis, and how do you go about confirming your suspicions?
2. What generalizations can you make about subcutaneous mycotic infections?
3. What are the therapeutic strategies used in the various subcutaneous mycoses?

Bibliography

Kwon-Chung KJ and Bennett JE: *Medical mycology,* Philadelphia, 1992, Lea & Febiger.

Larone DH: *Medically important fungi: a guide to identification,* ed 2, New York, 1987, Elsevier Science Publishing.

McGinnis MR: *Laboratory handbook of medical mycology,* New York, 1980, Academic Press.

Rebell G and Taplin D: Dermatophytes: their recognition and identification, Coral Gables, Fla, 1979, University of Miami Press.

CHAPTER 44

Systemic Mycoses

THE organisms classified as systemic mycotic agents are inherently virulent and cause disease in healthy humans. Five fungi are included in this group (Box 44-1): *Histoplasma capsulatum, Blastomyces dermatitidis, Paracoccidioides brasiliensis, Coccidioides immitis,* and *Cryptococcus neoformans.* Each of these fungi exhibits biochemical and morphological features that enable it to evade host defenses.

Four of these pathogens (*H. capsulatum, B. dermatitidis, P. brasiliensis,* and *C. immitis*) are dimorphic. They grow as filamentous molds as saprobes and in culture at 25° C; however, when they infect humans or are cultured at 37° C, they transform to a unicellular morphology (Figure 44-1, *A* to *D*). Tissue infections caused by *H. capsulatum, B. dermatitidis,* and *P. brasiliensis* are characterized by the presence of budding yeast cells (Figure 44-1, *A* through *C*), whereas *C. immitis* infections are characterized by the presence of spherules (sporangium-like structures filled with endospores; Figure 44-1, *D*).

Unlike the dimorphic pathogens, *C. neoformans* is monomorphic. The organism grows as a yeast within infected tissue and in culture at 25° C or 37° C (Figure 44-1, *E*). A characteristic feature of *C. neoformans* is that it possesses an acidic mucopolysaccharide capsule.

The primary focus of infection for all five systemic fungi is the lung. In the vast majority of cases the respiratory infections are asymptomatic or of very short duration, resolve rapidly without therapy, and are accompanied in the host by a high degree of specific resistance to reinfection. In some cases a secondary spread occurs outside the lungs, with each organism exhibiting a characteristic pattern of secondary organ involvement. Frequently, it is the secondary spread of systemic disease that causes the patient to seek medical attention. The severity of infection depends on the organism and the host. If the host's immune status is compromised because of underlying disease or immunosuppressive therapy, the infection can be life threatening if therapy is not rapidly instituted and the underlying disorder corrected. In addition, immunosuppression may cause reactivation of latent infection.

Four of the systemic mycoses (i.e., **histoplasmosis, blastomycosis, paracoccidioidomycosis,** and **coccidioidomycosis**) tend to be restricted to particular geographical regions. However, ease of travel and increases in reactivation disease are starting to blur these distinctions.

BOX 44-1 Agents Causing the Systemic Mycoses

Histoplasma capsulatum
Blastomyces dermatitidis
Paracoccidioides brasiliensis
Coccidioides immitis
Cryptococcus neoformans

HISTOPLASMOSIS

Histoplasmosis results from the inhalation of conidia or hyphal fragments of *H. capsulatum* (Figure 44-2). It occurs worldwide and is particularly common in the Midwestern United States (Figure 44-3). In most cases it is asymptomatic, but in about 5% of the cases clinical symptoms of an acute pneumonia occur, followed less often by a progressive disseminated disease. It has also been known as **Darling's disease, reticuloendothelial cytomycosis, cave disease,** and **spelunker's disease** (Table 44-1).

Morphology

The mold phase of *H. capsulatum* is characterized by thin, branching, septate hyphae that produce microconidia and tuberculate macroconidia (Figure 44-4). The parasitic or tissue phase of *H. capsulatum* is a small budding yeast cell 2 to 5 μm in diameter and found almost exclusively within macrophages (Figure 44-5). The sexual state for *H. capsulatum* has been designated *Ajellomyces capsulatus* and is classified as an ascomycete.

Epidemiology

The etiological agent of histoplasmosis, *H. capsulatum* var. *capsulatum,* grows in soil with a high nitrogen content, especially in areas contaminated with the excreta of bats and birds (starlings and chickens in particular). Birds are not infected, whereas natural infection does occur in bats. The fungus has been isolated from soil samples taken from habitats associated with birds and bats

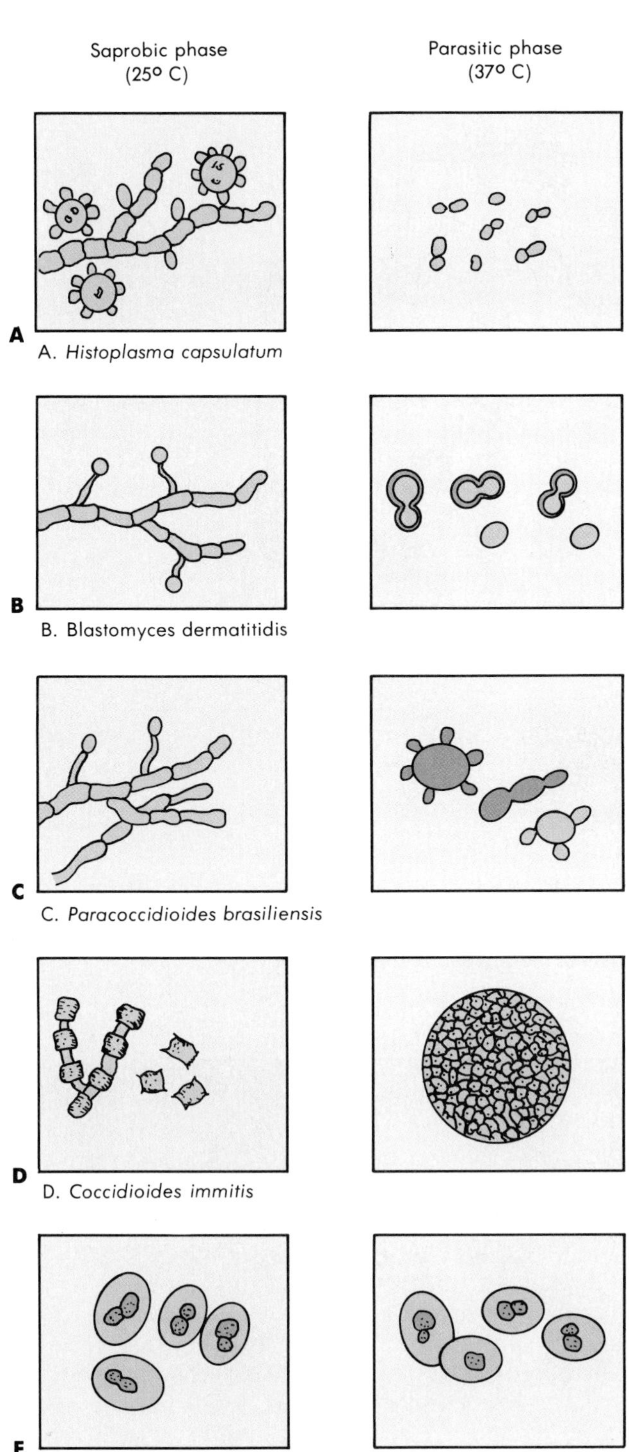

FIGURE 44-1 Schematic illustration of the saprobic and parasitic phases of systemic pathogenic fungi. **A,** *Histoplasma capsulatum,* **B,** *Blastomyces dermatitidis,* and **C,** *Paracoccidioides brasiliensis* exhibit mold-to-yeast transition when infecting susceptible species; **D,** *Coccidioides immitis* exhibits mold-to-spherule transition when it infects susceptible species; **E,** *Cryptococcus neoformans* is an encapsulated yeast at 25° C, 37° C, or in infected tissues.

(e.g., chicken coops, attics, barns, wood piles, caves, and roosting areas such as city parks and even schoolyards). Numerous well-documented epidemics of respiratory histoplasmosis have occurred when environments harboring the fungus have been disturbed by activities such as exploring caves (spelunking), demolishing old buildings during urban renewal, cleaning chicken coops, and setting up campsites. Researchers and epidemiologists have accidentally acquired the disease as a result of efforts to document the outbreaks when they explored suspected sites to take soil samples.

Histoplasmosis is widely distributed throughout the temperate, subtropical, and tropical zones of the world. Within these zones are areas of high endemicity, including the Ohio and Mississippi Valley regions of the United States, the southern fringes of the provinces of Ontario and Quebec in Canada, and scattered areas of Central and South America (see Figure 44-3). Surveys of skin test reactivity to histoplasmin indicate that 80% or more of the long-term residents in the Ohio and Mississippi River Valley have been infected with *H. capsulatum.* Serial studies of individuals living in an endemic area have shown that skin test reactivity can be lost and reacquired, suggesting that the high incidence of reactivity in these areas results from reinfection.

Cases of histoplasmosis have also been reported in Europe and Asia. A variant form of histoplasmosis occurs in Africa; the etiological agent of this disease has been designated *H. capsulatum* var. *duboisii.*

Clinical Syndromes

The lung is the usual portal of entry for infection. *H. capsulatum* conidia or hyphal fragments are inhaled, phagocytized by pulmonary macrophages, and then convert to yeasts, which are able to replicate in macrophages (see Figure 44-5). In the immunocompetent host, macrophages acquire fungicidal activity and contain the infection. Transient fungemia before the development of immunity accounts for the distribution of calcified granulomas in liver and spleen frequently seen at autopsy of patients from endemic areas. Viable organisms may persist in the host following resolution of uncomplicated histoplasmosis; they are the presumed source of disseminated disease in immunocompromised patients who do not have a history of recent exposure. The major clinical syndromes associated with *H. capsulatum* infection are summarized in Table 44-2.

An estimated 500,000 persons in the United States are exposed to *H. capsulatum* each year; however, most persons infected with *H. capsulatum* have a high degree of natural resistance to the organism. Few, if any, overt symptoms appear, and the disease resolves rapidly. Approximately 5% of infections result in symptomatic disease, usually an acute self-limited flu-like illness with varying degrees of pulmonary involvement. Symptoms usually resolve without specific antifungal therapy. Occasionally, an overly vigorous host immune response can result in complications such as mediastinal fibrosis

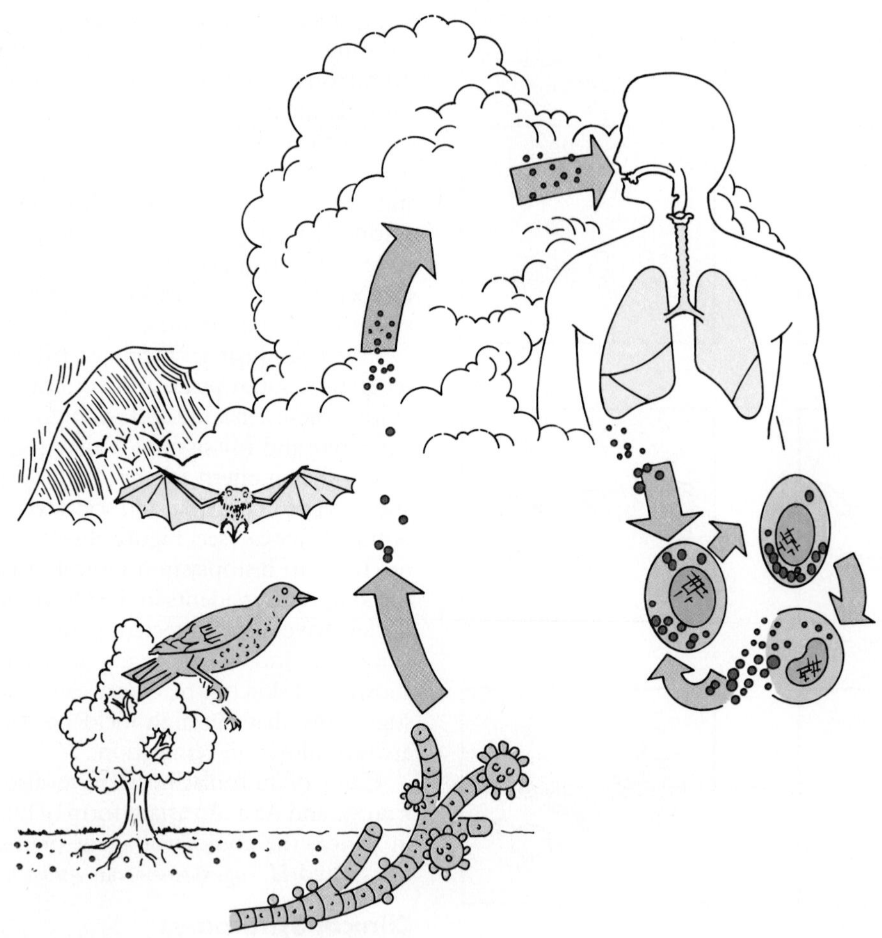

FIGURE 44-2 Schematic illustration of the natural history of the saprobic and parasitic cycles of *Histoplasma capsulatum.*

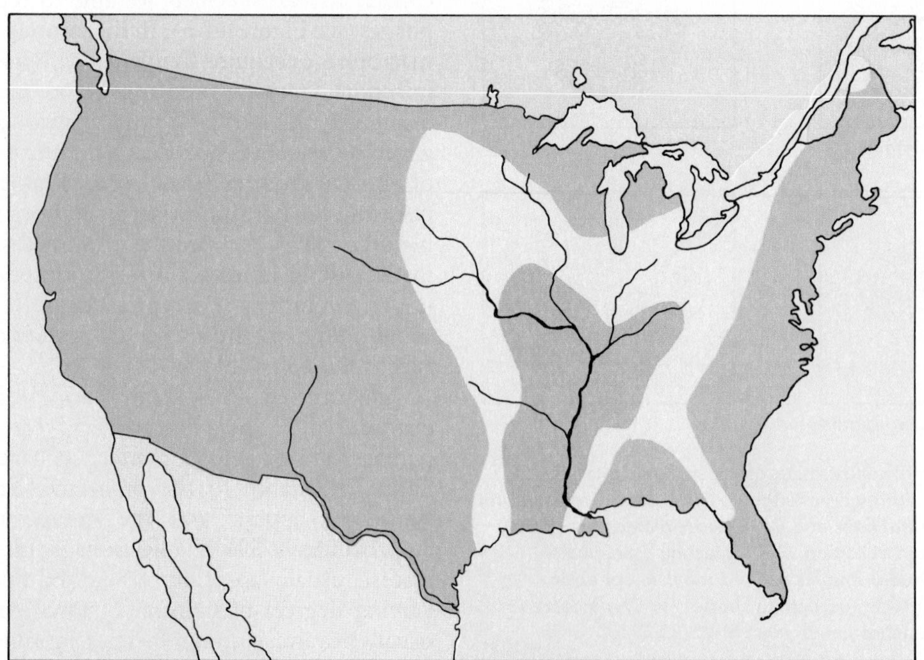

FIGURE 44-3 Endemic areas of histoplasmosis in North America (shaded).

TABLE 44-1 Summary of Histoplasmosis

Etiological agent	Mycology	Epidemiology and ecology	Clinical disease
Asexual phase: *Histoplasma capsulatum* Sexual phase: *Ajellomyces capsulatus*	Dimorphic; mycelia at 25° C; typical tuberculate macroconidia 8-14 μm in diameter; microconidia 2-4 μm in diameter. At 37° C and in tissue this organism is a budding yeast 2-3 × 3-4 μm in diameter. Found predominantly in histiocytes.	Occurs throughout temperate, subtropical, and tropical areas of the world. Endemic areas include the Ohio and Mississippi River Valleys and parts of Central and South America. The organism has been isolated from numerous soil samples, particularly those contaminated by bat, chicken, and starling droppings. Bats are naturally infected, but birds are not. A unique clinical form occurs in Africa caused by *H. capsulatum* var. *duboisii*.	The clinical symptoms vary depending on the degree of individual exposure and immunological state of the patient. About 95% of all primary cases are not referable to specific symptomology. Less than 1% of infections become progressive and require therapy. In this case there is usually an underlying condition of debilitation or immunosuppression that makes these individuals prone to life-threatening disease.

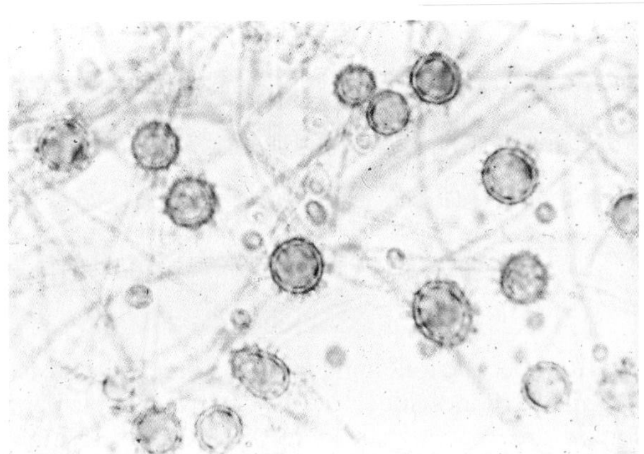

FIGURE 44-4 Tuberculate macroconidia and microconidia of *Histoplasma capsulatum.*

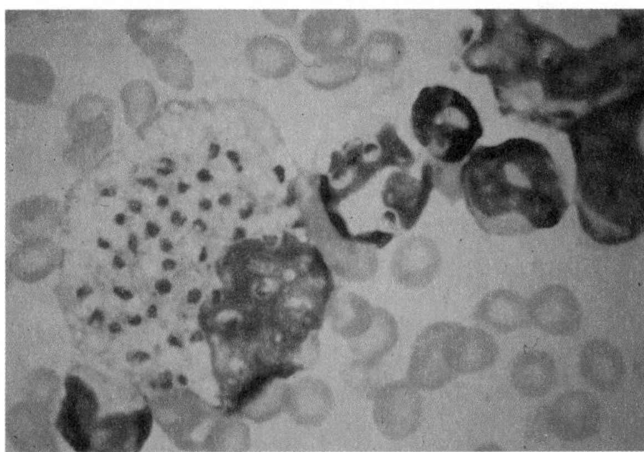

FIGURE 44-5 Yeast cells of *Histoplasma capsulatum* phagocytized by bone marrow mononuclear cells (Giemsa stained section).

(development of hard fibrous tissue in the upper mediastinum, causing compression, distortion, or obliteration of the superior vena cava and sometimes constriction of the bronchi and large pulmonary vessels).

H. capsulatum can also cause progressive and potentially fatal disease when host defenses are impaired. In a small number of cases the initial infection is not cleared and disease progresses to disseminated histoplasmosis. This condition is characterized by continued intracellular replication of *H. capsulatum* yeasts within macrophages, presumably caused by a defect in cell-mediated immunity. Clinically, infection ranges from acute, life-threatening, disseminated histoplasmosis to chronic, mild, disseminated histoplasmosis, depending on the extent of parasitization of the mononuclear phagocytic system. Patients frequently complain of fever, night sweats, and weight loss. Mucosal lesions are also common and may be the primary clinical finding in an otherwise healthy-appearing individual.

Severe progressive disseminated histoplasmosis is reported with increasing frequency in adults who have hematological malignancies, who are receiving immunosuppressive therapy (particularly chronic corticosteroid therapy), or who have acquired immunodeficiency syndrome (AIDS). In these settings disseminated histoplasmosis is best described as an opportunistic infection. Infection with the human immunodeficiency virus (HIV-1) may trigger reactivation of dormant *H. capsulatum.* Central nervous system involvement, an unusual complication of disseminated histoplasmosis, has also been reported in association with HIV infection.

TABLE 44-2 Classification of Histoplasmosis

Type of infection	Specific disorder	Comments
Histoplasmosis in normal hosts	Asymptomatic or mild flu-like illness	Occurs with normal exposure
	Acute pulmonary histoplasmosis	Occurs with heavy exposure
	Rare complications	Pericarditis, mediastinal fibrosis
Opportunistic infection	Disseminated histoplasmosis	Occurs in individuals who have an immune defect
	Chronic pulmonary histoplasmosis	Occurs in individuals who have a structural defect

Chronic pulmonary histoplasmosis is a disease most often seen in patients with underlying chronic obstructive pulmonary disease. As a result of structural defects in the lung, *H. capsulatum* can escape normal defense mechanisms and cause progressive, destructive lesions, similar to tuberculosis.

In Africa a distinct clinical form of histoplasmosis is seen that involves primarily the bone and subcutaneous tissues.

Laboratory Diagnosis

The diagnosis of histoplasmosis is based on serologic findings, direct histopathological examination of infected tissue, and culture. Diagnosis of disseminated histoplasmosis requires demonstration of the organism in extrapulmonary sites. This is best accomplished by a combination of culture and histopathological examination of tissue.

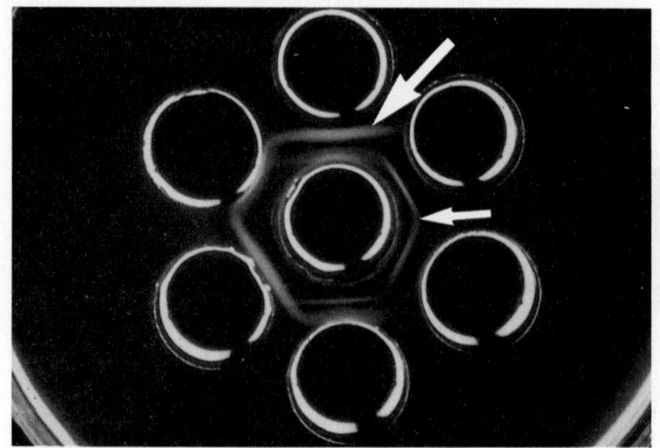

FIGURE 44-6 Immunodiffusion illustrating H *(short arrow)* and M *(long arrow)* precipitin bands that form when histoplasmin is tested against sera containing reactive antibodies.

The antigenic reagents used in the serologic tests for histoplasmosis are derived from two sources—the cell-free culture filtrate from the **mycelial phase** of growth *(histoplasmin)* and inactivated whole **yeast phase** cells. Both reagents are used because neither type of antigen detects antibodies in all cases.

In general, delayed skin test reactivity to histoplasmin develops within 2 weeks after exposure. This test is of little diagnostic or prognostic value and may be misleading, because in a significant percentage of the hypersensitive patients, serologic titers may become elevated as a result of skin testing with the reagent (anamnestic response). For this reason the skin test has no place in the diagnostic workup of a patient and should not be used.

Two serologic tests are frequently used to diagnose histoplasmosis. The complement fixation test is the standard test and is positive later in disease (6 weeks or longer after symptoms). Complement fixation tests, which measure antibodies directed against *H. capsulatum,* are performed using histoplasmin and intact formalin-treated yeast as the antigens. Serum complement fixation titers ≥ 16 or a fourfold rise in titer are suggestive of histoplasmosis; however, false-positive reactions can occur because of cross-reactive antibodies associated with other fungal infections and tuberculosis. Complement fixation titers decline following infection in normal hosts; fewer than 5% of individuals have a positive complement fixation in areas of high skin test positivity. A single serologic test does not allow a reliable diagnostic or prognostic interpretation and might cause a delay in instituting specific therapeutic measures. However, serologic tests on two or more serum specimens taken at suitable intervals during the acute and convalescent phases of infection yield information of great diagnostic and prognostic value.

The immunodiffusion test detects antibodies to **H** and **M antigens** of *H. capsulatum* (Figure 44-6) and is more specific but less sensitive than complement fixation. Serologic tests can aid in the diagnosis of histoplasmosis but do not distinguish disseminated disease from other forms of histoplasmosis. Furthermore, these tests can be negative in 25% or more of patients who have disseminated histoplasmosis.

In contrast to traditional serologic tests, direct detection of *H. capsulatum* antigens in blood or urine may prove valuable for the rapid diagnosis of disseminated disease. Intracellular yeast can often be seen by histopathologic examination of infected tissue, especially bone marrow, blood, and lung, using special stains, thus

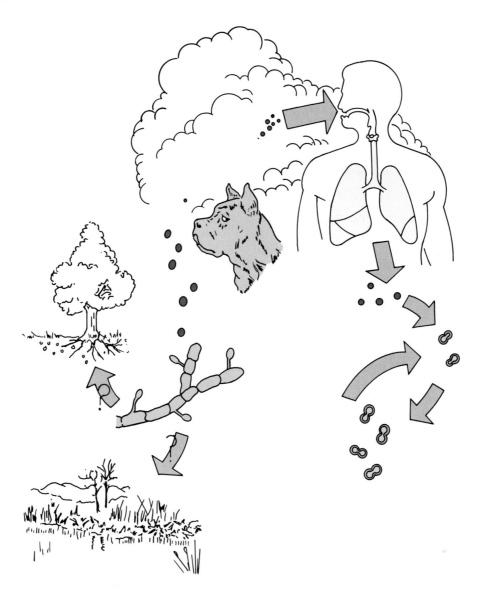

FIGURE 44-7 Schematic illustration of the natural history of the saprobic and parasitic cycle of *Blastomyces dermatitidis.*

permitting rapid diagnosis. *H. capsulatum* can be cultured from bone marrow or blood in more than 75% of cases of disseminated histoplasmosis. Sputum cultures are useful in the diagnosis of chronic pulmonary histoplasmosis but are usually negative in cases of acute self-limited disease. *H. capsulatum* usually takes 1 to 2 weeks to grow in culture. Preliminary identification of the isolate is based on morphological features, including delicate septate hyphae with tuberculate macroconidia (see Figure 44-4). In the past, confirmation was based on the ability to convert the culture from the mycelial to the yeast morphology, a process that can require weeks to months. Use of an **exoantigen test** now permits confirmation as soon as sufficient growth occurs. In the exoantigen test, antigens are extracted from the agar medium supporting growth of the fungus and reacted against antihistoplasma antibody in an immunodiffusion test. A positive identification is made when precipitin lines of identity form with control histoplasmin antigens.

Treatment

Amphotericin B remains the mainstay of treatment for disseminated histoplasmosis and other severe forms. However, in AIDS patients relapses following completion of therapy are a significant problem and lifelong suppressive therapy must be considered.

BLASTOMYCOSIS

Blastomycosis, also called **Chicago disease, Gilchrist's disease,** and **North American blastomycosis,** is caused by the inhalation of conidia of *B. dermatitidis* (Figure 44-7). Primary pulmonary infections are often inapparent and difficult to document even radiologically. The forms of disease most often seen clinically are ulcerative lesions of the skin and lytic bone lesions, both of which represent systemic or disseminated disease (Table 44-3).

Morphology

B. dermatitidis is closely related biochemically and serologically to *H. capsulatum.* The sexual phase of *B. dermatitidis* has been discovered, classified as an ascomycete, and designated *Ajellomyces dermatitidis,* the same genus as the sexual state of *H. capsulatum.*

Epidemiology

The geographical distribution of blastomycosis is limited to the North American continent and parts of Africa. Blastomycosis, like histoplasmosis, is endemic in the Ohio and Mississippi Valley region, and to a lesser extent in the Missouri and Arkansas River basins. Additional endemic sites have been found in Minnesota, Southern Manitoba, and Southwest Ontario, including the St. Lawrence River basin. Epidemics have occurred in Wisconsin, Minnesota, Illinois, and in the eastern states of Virginia and North Carolina. It has also been reported in a wide geographical area of Africa. In endemic areas natural disease exists among dogs and horses and is an important veterinary problem. The veterinary picture is similar to the clinical and pathological disease seen in human infections. Untreated, blastomycosis in animals may have a rapid and fatal course.

The natural reservoir for the agent of blastomycosis is not known. Unlike *H. capsulatum, B. dermatitidis* is rarely cultured from soil in endemic areas. It is believed that the organism is present in the soil but flourishes only in a narrow, as yet undefined, ecological niche.

Clinical Syndromes

The natural history of *B. dermatitidis* infections is less well documented than are infections caused by *H. capsulatum,* because of the lack of reliable serologic tests and characteristic radiographic findings. Symptomatic blastomycosis is an uncommon disease whose manifestations frequently indicate systemic spread. It is thought that large numbers of asymptomatic infections occur, analogous to histoplasmosis.

Inhalation of *B. dermatitidis* conidia produces a primary pulmonary infection in the host. As with *H. capsulatum, B. dermatitidis* conidia convert to yeast and are phagocytized by macrophages, which may carry them to other organs. The initial infection can be symptomatic or asymptomatic. Chest x-ray films may show nonspecific pulmonary infiltrates; however, unlike histoplasmosis, resolution of these lesions is not accompanied by calcifications. Primary pulmonary disease can have three outcomes: resolution without involvement of other organs, progressive pulmonary disease, or resolution of the pulmonary infection followed by systemic disease.

Laboratory Diagnosis

Serologic and immunological findings for blastomycosis are unclear. At present, two antigenic preparations are used in tests to detect the immune response to infection by *B. dermatitidis:* cell-free culture filtrate of the **mycelial phase (blastomycin)** and inactivated whole **yeast phase** cells. The data obtained from skin testing and serologic studies are difficult to interpret because of the poorly defined antigenic preparations that have been used. The reagents tend to have a high degree of cross-reactivity with other mycoses, particularly histoplasmosis and coccidioidomycosis.

An immunodiffusion test that appears to be specific for blastomycosis has been developed. It is based on the availability of a yeast phase culture filtrate, designated "A" antigen. Suitable control sera containing antibodies that react with "A" antigen must be included in immunodiffusion studies with patient sera.

TABLE 44-3 Summary of Blastomycosis

Etiological agent	Mycology	Epidemiology and ecology	Clinical disease
Asexual phase: *Blastomyces dermatitidis* Sexual phase: *Ajellomyces dermatitidis*	Dimorphic; mycelia at 25° C; typical pyriform microconidia 2-4 μm in diameter. At 37° C and in tissue this organism is a yeast 8-15 μm in diameter; buds produced singly are attached to parent cell by a broad base.	Geographically limited to North American continent and parts of Africa. The area of endemicity in the United States overlaps that for histoplasmosis. Blastomycosis is an important veterinary problem, and dogs develop a disease similar to that in humans. There are few reports of successful isolation of this organism from soil.	Primary infection in lung is often inapparent, although epidemics of respiratory blastomycosis have been documented. Chronic cutaneous and osseous diseases are the most common clinical presentation.

Diagnosis of blastomycosis requires identification of the organism in infected tissue or isolation in culture. Microscopic examination of potassium hydroxide–treated purulent fluid expressed from abscesses reveals characteristic broad-based budding yeast cells (Figure 44-8). Biopsies of stained skin lesions will reveal characteristic broad-based budding yeast. The organism grows readily in culture. Identification is based on conversion of the mycelial phase to the yeast phase or by the exoantigen test.

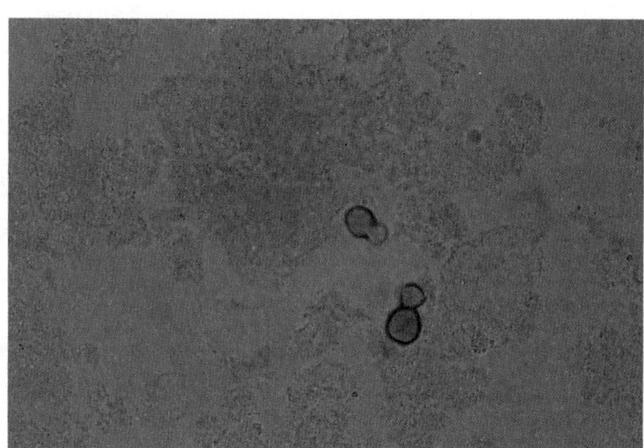

FIGURE 44-8 Broad-based budding yeast cells of *Blastomyces dermatitidis* seen in purulent material expressed from a microabcess.

Treatment

Amphotericin B remains the mainstay of therapy for patients with systemic disease or serious pulmonary disease, particularly in immunocompromised patients. Uncomplicated pulmonary disease may respond to ketoconazole.

PARACOCCIDIOIDOMYCOSIS

Paracoccidioidomycosis is a pulmonary disease resulting from the inhalation of infectious conidia of **P. brasiliensis** (Figure 44-9). Pulmonary infections are often asymptomatic; the form most often seen is ulcerative lesions of the oral and nasal cavity. The disease has been called **South American blastomycosis** and **Lutz-Splendore-Almeida's disease** (Table 44-4).

Morphology

P. brasiliensis is dimorphic, growing as a mold in the environment and as budding yeast in infected tissue. The yeast phase is characterized by multiple budding from a single cell (Figure 44-10). The transition from mold to yeast can be induced in vitro by raising the temperature from 25° C to 37° C. Recent studies have shown that as little as 10^{-10} M-17-beta-estradiol significantly inhibits

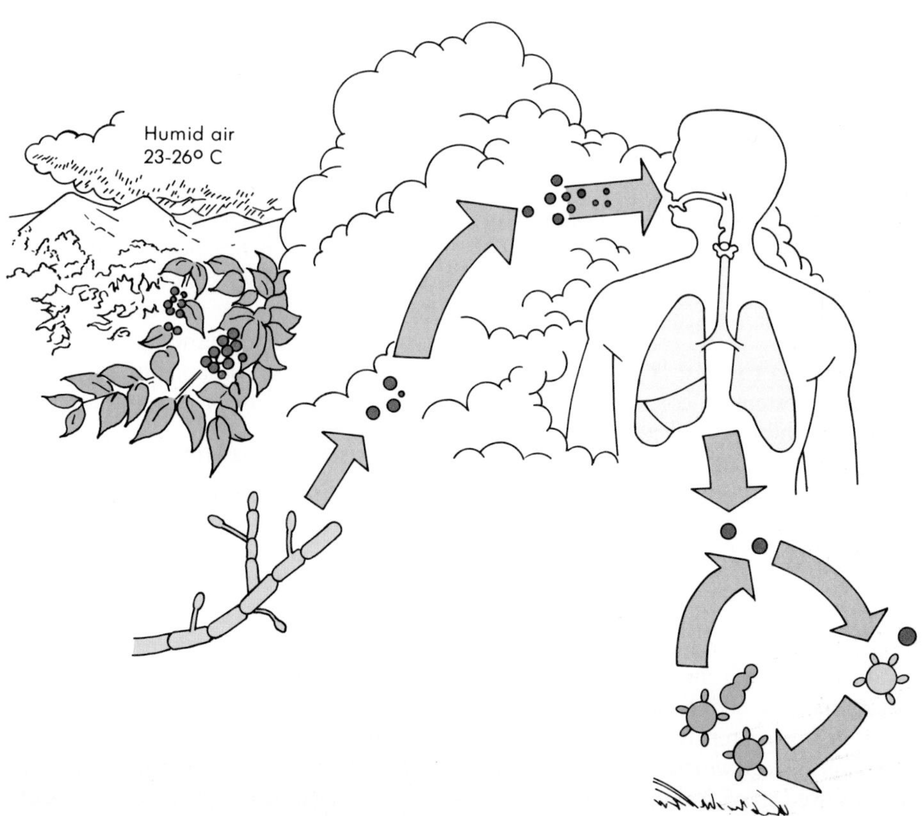

FIGURE 44-9 Schematic illustration of the natural history of the saprobic and parasitic cycle of *Paracoccidioides brasiliensis.*

TABLE 44-4 Summary of Paracoccidioidomycosis

Etiological agent	Mycology	Epidemiology and ecology	Clinical disease
Asexual phase: *Paracocciodes brasiliensis* Sexual phase: Not known	Dimorphic; mycelia at 25° C; no typical pattern of sporulation. At 37° C and in tissues the organism is a yeast with several budding cells attached to the parent cell, some in a "pilot's wheel" arrangement. Yeasts are 2-30 μm in diameter.	This disease is geographically limited to Central and South America. The major focus of the disease is Brazil. Females are as susceptible to infections as males, but the incidence of clinical disease is about 9 times higher in males. The organism has been isolated from the soil on rare occasions.	Primary pulmonary disease is often inapparent. Disseminated disease often causes ulcerative lesions of the buccal, nasal, and occasionally gastrointestinal mucosa.

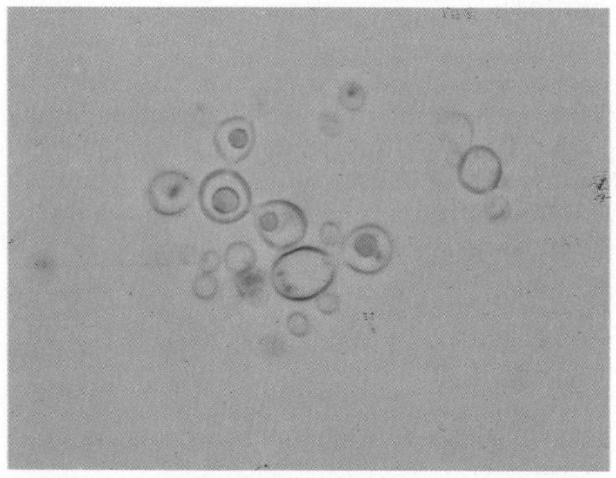

FIGURE 44-10 Multipolar budding characteristic of the yeast phase of *Paracoccidioides brasiliensis.*

the transformation of mycelia to yeast at the permissive temperature of 37° C. Testosterone, corticosterone, and 17-alpha-estradiol had no inhibitory effect on the mycelia to yeast transition at the elevated temperature. The findings may have clinical significance (see the following discussion on epidemiology). A sexual state for *P. brasiliensis* has not been described.

Epidemiology

This disease is geographically restricted to Central and South America and has a high incidence in Brazil, Venezuela, and Colombia. The endemic areas have been delineated by data taken from extensive skin test surveys and case reports. Like *B. dermatitidis, P. brasiliensis* cannot routinely be cultured from soil in endemic areas. Careful retrospective epidemiological studies and data taken from a report on the isolation of *P. brasiliensis* from soil samples suggest that the fungus resides in environments that have high humidity and average temperatures around 23° C.

Results of skin test surveys indicate an equal distribution of reactors among males and females. However, when data from clinically significant disease are analyzed, there is a disproportionate number of males affected (9:1 ratio). This difference has been attributed to factors that place males at higher risk, as well as underlying diseases, malnourishment, and hormonal differences. Inhibition of the mycelia to yeast transition by beta-estradiol may also account for the lower incidence of disseminated paracoccidioidomycosis in adult females.

Clinical Syndromes

Because of the prominence of oral and nasal lesions, infection was believed to result from local inoculation. However, it is now known that paracoccidioidomycosis resembles the other systemic mycoses in that the primary infection occurs in the lungs as a result of inhaling conidia. Primary pulmonary paracoccidioidomycosis is frequently asymptomatic but can develop into progressive pulmonary disease or disseminated disease.

Laboratory Diagnosis

As with histoplasmosis and coccidioidomycosis, diagnosis is based on detection of specific antibodies, visualization of the organism in histopathological material, and isolation of the organism in culture. Two antigenic preparations of *P. brasiliensis* are used for the serologic diagnosis: a cell-free culture filtrate of the **mycelial phase (paracoccidioidin)** and an inactivated whole **yeast phase** preparation. These serologic reagents are not routinely available in the United States. Specific antibodies are measured by complement fixation and immunodiffusion.

The organism can be seen in KOH preparations of infected material or in silver-stained histological sections. The presence of multiple small budding cells arranged around a large mature cell ("ship's wheel" pattern) is

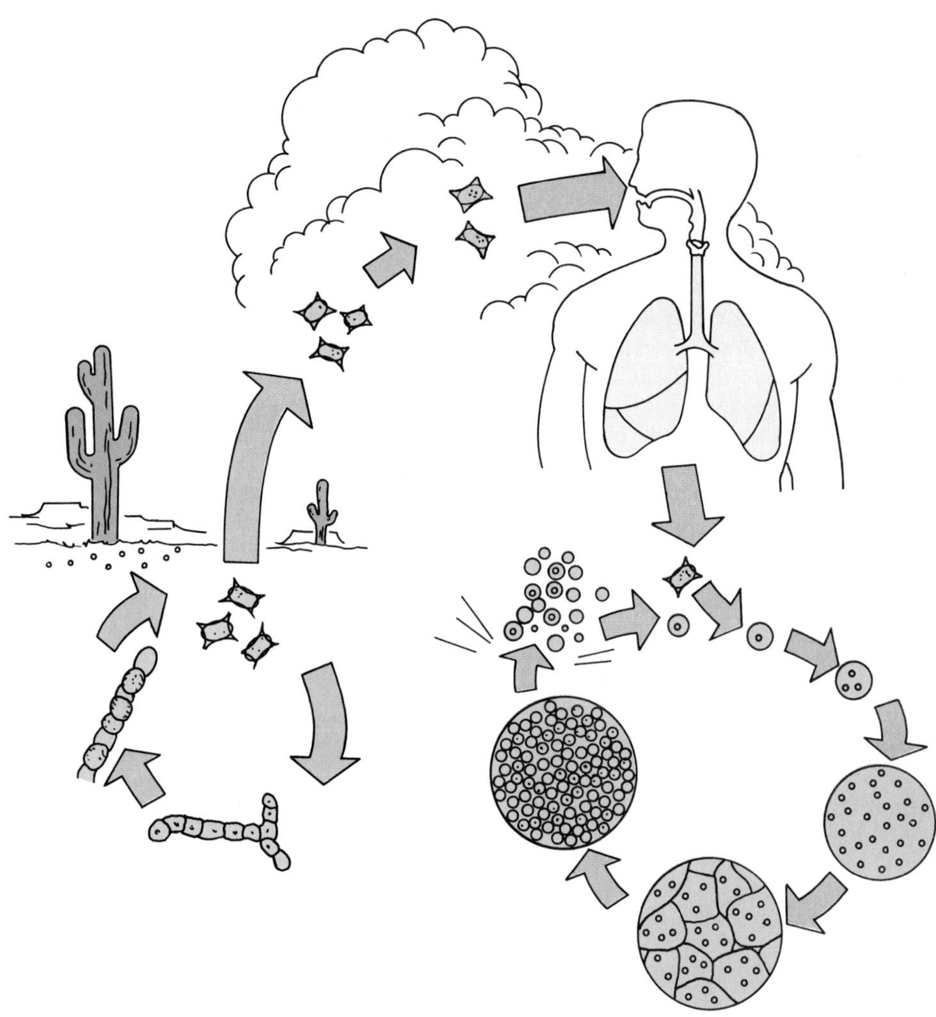

FIGURE 44-11 Schematic illustration of the natural history of the saprobic and parasitic cycle of *Coccidioides immitis.*

diagnostic of *P. brasiliensis* (see Figure 44-10); however, in the absence of buds the yeast of *P. brasiliensis* may be confused with immature spherules of *C. immitis* or the nonbudding yeast of *B. dermatitidis* or *H. capsulatum.* Clinical material cultured on medium and incubated at 25° C will yield a slow-growing white mold after 10 to 14 days of incubation. Microscopic examination of the growth is usually not diagnostic because *P. brasiliensis* does not sporulate readily. Transfer of the culture to incubation at 37° C will yield a yeastlike growth with characteristic multipolar budding cells.

Treatment

Successful treatment of paracoccidioidomycosis generally requires long-term therapy. Amphotericin B is effective against all forms of paracoccidioidomycosis, but because of toxicity and the difficulty of long-term administration it is usually reserved for severe cases. Sulfa drugs have been used for decades to treat disease; however, treatment failures can occur despite therapy that lasts years. Ketoconazole (and the newer azoles) are very active in vitro against *P. brasiliensis* and appear to be clinically effective.

COCCIDIOIDOMYCOSIS

Inhalation of arthroconidia of *C. immitis* causes an acute, self-limited, and usually benign respiratory infection. The condition may be asymptomatic or vary in severity from the level of a common cold to disseminated and life-threatening disease (Figure 44-11). Coccidioidomycosis has also been called **Posada's disease, San Joaquin Valley fever,** and **desert rheumatism** (Table 44-5).

Morphology

C. immitis is a dimorphic fungus that grows as a filamentous mold in the environment. The mycelia of *C. immitis* fragment to produce cylindrical arthroconidia (Figure 44-12). The tissue phase of *C. immitis* is the spherule (Figure 44-13), a multinucleated structure that undergoes internal cleavage to produce uninucleate

TABLE 44-5 Summary of Coccidioidomycosis

Etiological agent	Mycology	Epidemiology and ecology	Clinical disease
Asexual phase: *Coccidioides immitis* Sexual phase: Not known	Dimorphic; mycelia at 25° C; as the culture ages, the septate hyphae matures such that alternate cells develop into arthroconidia separated by vacuolized cells. The arthroconidia separate readily and have a "barrel-shaped" appearance. In tissue and at 37° C the organism develops into large spherical structures 10-60 μm in diaqmeter, called spherules (sporangia) that are filled with endospores, 2-5 μm in diameter.	This disease is geographically restricted to North, Central, and South America, where there are areas of high endemicity. In North America the disease is highly endemic in the San Joaquin Valley of California, the Southwestern part of the United States and the northern states of Mexico. Natural infection occurs in domestic and wild animals. The organism has been repeatedly isolated from soil samples taken from an endemic area.	Approximately 60% of these infections are asymptomatic. The most common symptoms of primary disease are cough, fever, and chest pain. Night sweats and joint pain are not unusual. An epidemiological history should be taken to find out if the patient has been in an endemic area.

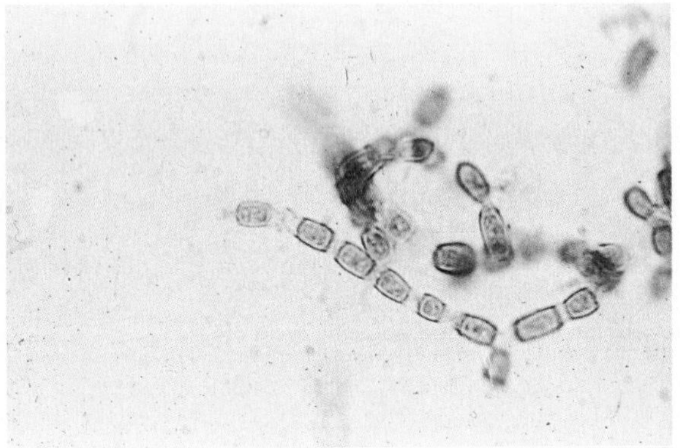

FIGURE 44-12 Hyphae and arthroconidia of *Coccidioides immitis.*

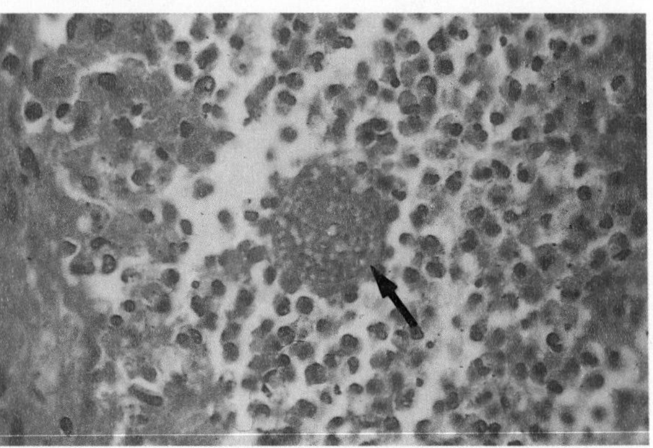

FIGURE 44-13 The spherule phase of *Coccidioides immitis* as seen in stained tissue section.

endospores that can then generate new spherules. A sexual state has not been observed for *C. immitis.*

Epidemiology

Coccidioidomycosis, which can be described as a disease of the "New World," is geographically limited to the North, Central, and South American continents (Figure 44-14). The areas of highest endemicity have a semiarid climate and include the central San Joaquin Valley in California, Maricopa and Pima Counties in Arizona, and several western and southwestern counties in Texas. The disease is also endemic in the northern states of Mexico and parts of Venezuela, Paraguay, and Argentina. Cases of coccidioidomycosis have also been reported in Central America. The organism can be routinely isolated from soil in areas of high endemicity. Although geographically restricted, the organism has on occasion spread extensively as a result of large dust storms.

Clinical Syndromes

The natural history of coccidioidomycosis has been well characterized because large groups of nonimmune individuals who have migrated to endemic areas could be studied (e.g., military personnel stationed in the San Joaquin Valley during World War II). In contrast to histoplasmosis, exposure to *C. immitis* causes a greater percentage of individuals to undergo a mild febrile to moderately severe respiratory disease. In general, however, a high degree of innate immunity exists in the adult population. Approximately 40% of individuals develop a symptomatic pulmonary infection following exposure to the organism. These primary infections are usually self-limited, but in a small proportion of patients *C. immitis* causes progressive pulmonary disease or disseminates to produce extrapulmonary disease, mainly involving the meninges and/or skin.

Laboratory Diagnosis

At present, two sources of antigen, both cell-free culture filtrates, are used in the preparation of serologic reagents: the **mycelial phase** of growth **(coccidioidin)** and the **spherule phase (spherulin).** Skin test reactivity to coccidioidin develops 2 to 4 weeks after symptoms. The tube precipitin and the complement fixation tests are the time-honored serologic procedures used to diagnose coccidioidomycosis. Precipitins appear early, between 2 to 4 weeks after symptoms, followed by the appearance of complement-fixing antibodies.

Other methods of detecting specific antibodies, such as latex particle agglutination and agar immunodiffusion, are now available. These tests have largely replaced the tube precipitin and complement fixation tests for routine screening because they are more sensitive in detecting infected individuals, are commercially available, and are easily performed. In the immunodiffusion test, two lines of precipitation appear to be significant. One line is associated with the antigen that detects precipitin and agglutinating antibodies, and another line is associated with the complement-fixing antibodies. Once the presence of an infection has been established, complement fixation titers can yield important prognostic information. High titers, or persistent or rising titers, indicate a high probability of disseminated disease. *C. immitis* spherules can be seen on infected tissue stained with hematoxylin and eosin. The organism can be cultured on conventional media; however, it must be handled with caution because *C. immitis* is a leading cause of laboratory-acquired infections. Although the mold phase of *C. immitis* is highly suggestive, arthroconidia are found in several saprobic fungi; therefore definitive identification is based on conversion to spherules or a specific exoantigen test.

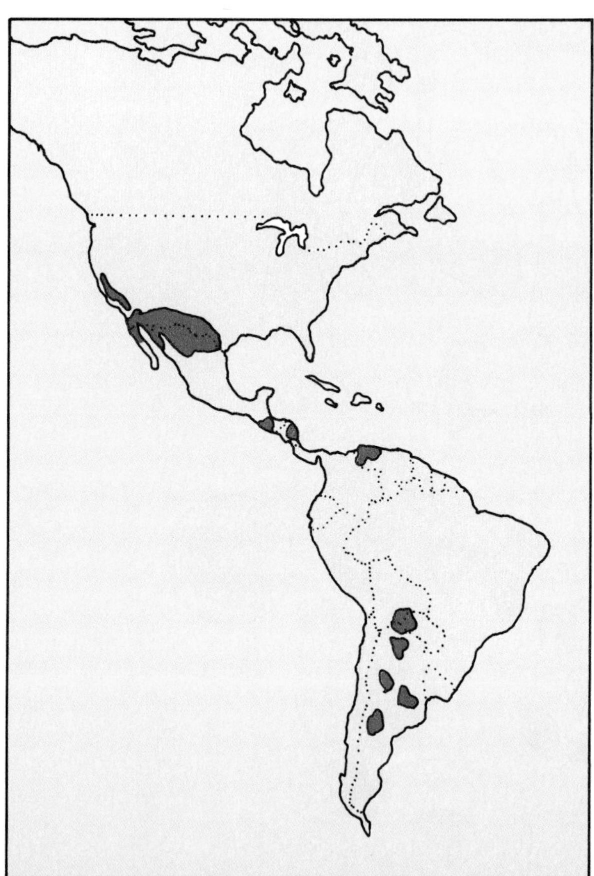

FIGURE 44-14 Geographical distribution of coccidioidomycosis in North, Central, and South America (shaded).

Treatment

Amphotericin B is the drug of choice for the treatment of serious coccidioidal infections. Meningeal infections are particularly difficult to treat, partly because of the poor penetration of amphotericin B into the cerebrospinal fluid. Ketoconazole is effective in suppressing infections, but relapses occur following cessation of therapy.

CRYPTOCOCCOSIS

Cryptococcosis, also called **Busse-Buschke's disease, torulosis,** or **European blastomycosis,** is a chronic-to-acute infection caused by *C. neoformans* (Table 44-6). There are two varieties of *C. neoformans: C. neoformans* var. *neoforman* (serotypes A and D) and *C. neoformans* var. *gatti* (serotypes B and C). In contrast to the other systemic mycotic agents dimorphism does not play a role in the pathogenesis of *C. neoformans* because it is an encapsulated yeast at 25° C, 37° C, and in tissues. In the case of *C. neoformans* several putative virulence factors have been identified. The capsular polysaccharide, for example, inhibits phagocytosis. Another virulence factor appears to be phenoloxidase, an enzyme that converts phenolic compounds to melanin. The lung is the primary site of infection; however, the organism has a high predilection for systemic spread to the brain and meninges (Figure 44-15). *C. neoformans* is the leading cause of fungal meningitis and is an important cause of morbidity and mortality in AIDS patients and transplant recipients. *C. neoformans* also produces systemic disease in patients who have no apparent underlying immunological disorder.

Morphology

Unlike the other systemic mycotic agents the asexual phase of *C. neoformans* is not dimorphic. It grows as a budding yeast in infected tissue and in culture at 25° C and 37° C. The most distinctive feature of *C. neoformans* is the presence of an acidic mucopolysaccharide capsule. This capsule is required for pathogenicity and is important diagnostically, both in terms of antigen detection and specific histolo-

TABLE 44-6 Summary of Cryptococcosis

Etiological agent	Mycology	Epidemiology and ecology	Clinical disease
Asexual phase: *Cryptococcus neoformans* Sexual phase: *Filobasidiella neoformans*	Monomorphic; this organism is a yeast at 25° C and 37° C. The unique feature of the yeast is the acidic mucopolysaccharide capsule.	This disease is worldwide in distribution. This yeast has been repeatedly isolated from sites inhabited by pigeons, particularly their roosts and droppings. Pigeons are not naturally infected.	Primary pulmonary cryptococcosis is usually inapparent but may be chronic, subacute, or acute. The clinical entity most often seen is cryptococcal meningitis. Osseous and cutaneous disease can be present without apparent neurological involvement.

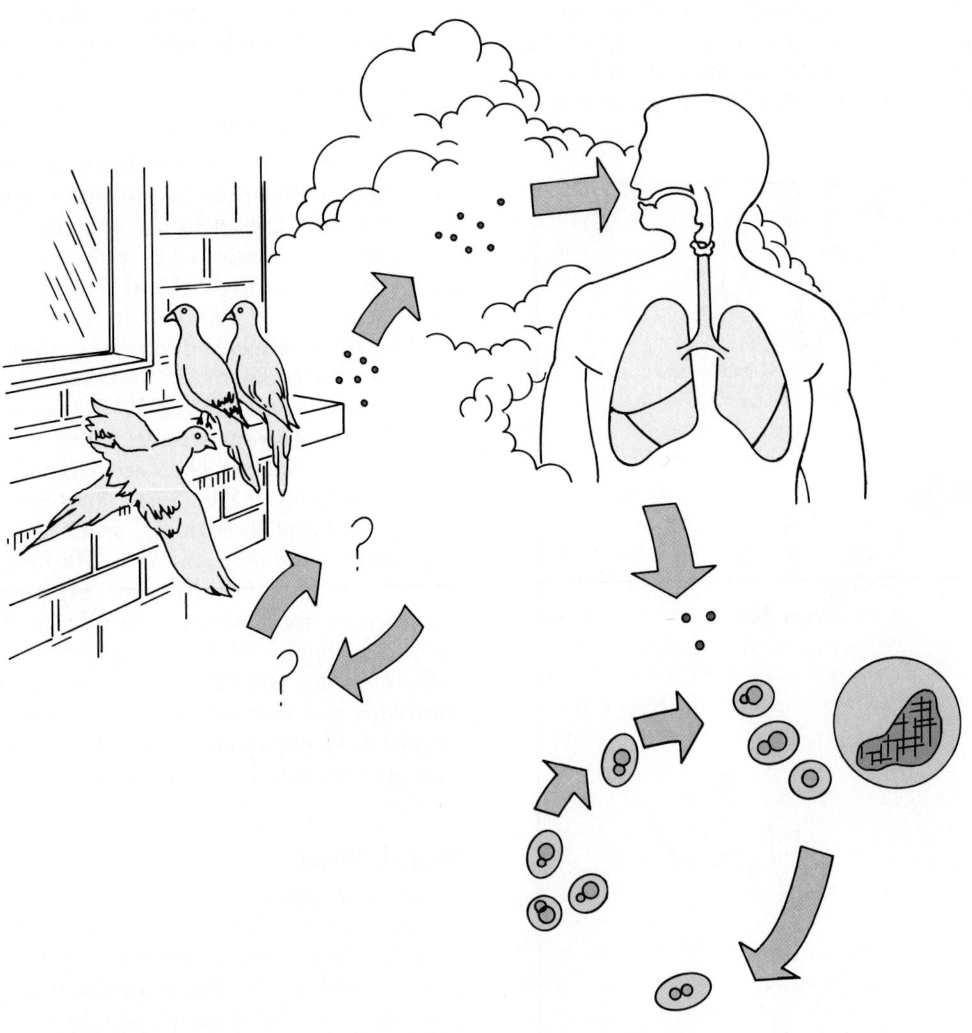

FIGURE 44-15 Schematic illustration of natural history of the saprobic and parasitic cycle of *Cryptococcus neoformans*.

gical staining. The sexual phase of *C. neoformans* has been discovered; it is named *Filobasidiella neoformans* and has been classified as a basidiomycete (see Chapter 5). There is speculation that the basidiospore may be the infectious propagule, but it has not been identified.

Epidemiology

C. neoformans serotypes A and D have been recovered in large numbers from the excreta and debris of pigeons. Thus it appears to survive well in a desiccated, alkaline, nitrogen-rich, and hypertonic environment. There is a close relationship to the habitats of pigeons, but the organism does not appear to naturally infect the bird. The natural reservoir of *C. neoformans* var. *gatti* (serotype B) was unknown until it was isolated recently from the tree sap of *Eucalyptus camaldulensis* (red gum). Cryptococcosis occurs throughout the world. The true prevalence of infection is unknown because of the lack of a reliable skin test or other serologic screening test, but subclinical infections are believed to be common. Symptomatic cryptococcal disease, mainly meningitis, is frequently seen in individuals who are debilitated, immunosuppressed, or otherwise compromised. However, a large number of patients who develop cryptococcal meningitis have no underlying immune or metabolic defects.

Clinical Syndromes

Primary pulmonary infections are frequently asymptomatic and may be detected as an incidental finding on a routine chest x-ray examination. The most common picture is that of a solitary pulmonary nodule that can mimic a carcinoma; the correct diagnosis is usually made when the mass is resected. *C. neoformans* can also produce a symptomatic pneumonia characterized by diffuse pulmonary infiltrates.

Cryptococcal meningitis, caused by hematogenous spread of yeast from the lungs to the meninges surrounding the brain, is the most frequently diagnosed form of cryptococcosis. Symptoms usually include combinations of headache, mental status changes, and fever lasting several weeks. Occasionally, cryptococcal disease of the central nervous system may take the form of an expanding intracerebral mass that causes focal neurological deficits. Other common manifestations of disseminated cryptococcosis include skin lesions and osteolytic bone lesions.

Laboratory Diagnosis

In contrast to the other systemic mycoses, the serologic procedures used in the diagnosis of cryptococcosis are based on the detection of antigen, not antibody. The latex agglutination test for detection of cryptococcal polysaccharide antigen in cerebrospinal fluid and serum is routinely used in clinical laboratories; it is sensitive, specific, and simple to perform. The test involves the use of latex particles that have been coated with rabbit anticryptococcal antibody. Capsular polysaccharide present in a clinical specimen binds to the antibodies and agglutinates the latex particles. Because the latex particles are coated with antibody, false positive reactions can be caused by rheumatoid factor (IgM antibodies that bind IgG). Therefore appropriate control tests must be performed in which the clinical specimen is mixed with latex particles coated with nonimmune rabbit antibodies. In addition, the patient's serum can be treated with a protease to destroy any proteins that might cause nonspecific agglutination of the latex particles. Rare cross-reactions occur with sera from patients with disseminated infections caused by *Trichosporon beigelii*. To evaluate the clinical progress of a patient during therapy, serial samples of cerebrospinal fluid are evaluated for the presence of cryptococcal antigen. A favorable prognosis is indicated by a decrease in the titer of antigen.

A rapid diagnosis of cryptococcal meningitis can often be made by examination of an India ink preparation of cerebrospinal fluid. *C. neoformans* appears as a single cell or budding yeast surrounded by a clear halo because of the exclusion of the ink particles by the polysaccharide capsule (Figure 44-16). Although diagnosis may be rapid, the India ink preparation is positive in only half of the cases of cryptococcal meningitis. Culture remains the definitive method for documenting infection. The organism grows well on standard nonselective mycological media but is inhibited by cycloheximide, which is an antibiotic used to suppress growth of saprobes. The identification of *C. neoformans* is based on the presence of a capsule, production of the enzyme urease, the assimilation pattern of carbon substrates, and other specific biochemical reactions.

Treatment

Whereas pulmonary cryptococcosis is frequently a self-limited infection or can be cured by surgical excision of a solitary nodule, disseminated cryptococcosis is almost always fatal if untreated. Cryptococcal meningitis remains the model for combination therapy with antifungal agents. Amphotericin B is active against *C. neoformans* but exhibits relatively poor penetration into cerebrospinal fluid. Although 5-fluorocytosine has good cerebrospinal

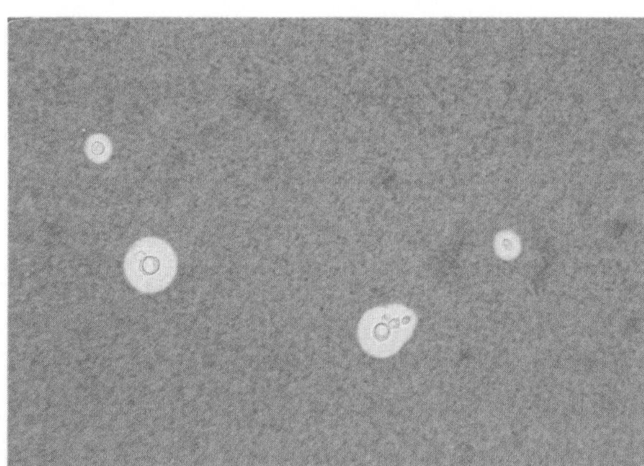

FIGURE 44-16 Encapsulated budding yeast cells of *Cryptococcus neoformans* highlighted with India ink.

fluid penetration, development of resistant cryptococci is a problem. Controlled clinical trials have shown that combination therapy with amphotericin B and 5-fluorocytosine for 6 weeks is as effective as amphotericin B alone for 10 weeks. Nonetheless, relapses following either treatment regimen remain a problem, particularly in AIDS patients.

CASE STUDY AND QUESTIONS

About 7 to 10 days after exploring a bat cave in Missouri, three of five members of a spelunkers' club who had gone on the expedition complained of flu-like symptoms and made appointments to see their internist. Patient #1 was febrile and had a nonproductive cough but was otherwise fine. Patient #2, who is HIV-positive, was febrile, complained of night sweats, chest pains, tender joints, and also had a very deep cough. Patient #3 could not get in to see his internist immediately and had to wait a week for his appointment. When patient #3 was seen, he was asymptomatic and said that after taking a couple of aspirins with a lot of water and getting 3 days of rest, he felt "fit as a fiddle." The remaining two spelunkers said that they felt fine and did not experience any of the described symptoms. During the course of examination, all of the spelunkers remarked that bats had roosted in the cave and a great deal of dust was raised during their exploration.

1. What is your diagnosis, and what should be done to confirm it?
2. What are the geographical distributions of and endemic areas for: (a) coccidioidomycosis; (b) histoplasmosis; (c) blastomycosis; (d) paracoccidioidomycosis; and (e) cryptococcosis?
3. What are the distinguishing morphological features of the etiological agents of the systemic mycoses: (a) in nature; and (b) in tissue?
4. What is interesting about the epidemiology of (a) paracoccidioidomycosis; (b) coccidioidomycosis; (c) histoplasmosis; (d) blastomycosis; and (e) cryptococcosis?
5. What concern should be shown for the patient who also has AIDS?

Bibliography

Drutz DJ, editor: Systemic fungal infections: diagnosis and treatment. I. *Med Clin North Am,* vol 3, 1988.

Drutz DJ, editor: Systemic fungal infections: diagnosis and treatment. II. *Med Clin North Am,* vol 4, 1989.

Kwon-Chung KJ and Bennett JE: *Medical mycology,* Philadelphia, 1992, Lea & Febiger.

Sarosi GA and Davies SF, editors: *Fungal diseases of the lung,* Orlando, Fla, 1986, Grune & Stratton.

Szaniszlo PJ, editor: *Fungal dimorphism: with emphasis on fungi pathogenic for humans,* New York, 1985, Plenum Press.

CHAPTER 45

Opportunistic Mycoses

As emphasized previously, humans are constantly exposed to viable fungal propagules. Most of us tolerate these exposures with no resulting sequela, except for some who develop an allergic hypersensitivity. There are at least two reasons for this. First, healthy immunologically competent humans have a high degree of innate resistance to fungal colonization, and second, the majority of fungi have a low inherent virulence. However, under conditions that lead to host debilitation, many individuals become susceptible to fungi. If the infection is not diagnosed rapidly, treated aggressively, and the underlying conditions causing host debilitation brought under control, the fungal infection may become life threatening. These infections, once considered to be rare and exotic, have become more common and of great medical significance. This has resulted because of the AIDS epidemic and increased use of radiation and cytotoxic drug therapy to treat patients who are recipients of organ transplants or those with malignancies. Because these fungi take advantage of the host's debilitated condition to become pathogens, they are commonly called **opportunistic fungi.**

A growing list of fungi have been implicated in opportunistic infections, but the vast majority are caused by various species of *Candida* (e.g., *C. albicans*), *Aspergillus fumigatus,* and *Rhizopus.* Although these organisms are called "opportunistic pathogens," the term is based on the clinical setting and has no taxonomic significance. Two of the most common ones, *C. albicans* and *A. fumigatus,* have very different biological properties and host interactions. In addition, pathogenicity is not an all-or-nothing phenomenon. Individual species within both *Candida* and *Aspergillus* exhibit a range of pathogenicity.

CANDIDIASIS

Several species of *Candida* have been implicated in candidiasis (Table 45-1). Candidiasis has been and continues to be a major disease problem of immunocompromised hosts. The clinical spectrum of manifestations ranges from superficial infections of the skin to systemic life-threatening infections. Under various conditions, *C. albicans, C. tropicalis, C. kefyr* (formerly *C. pseudotropicalis*), *C. glabrata* (formerly *Torulopsis glabrata*), and *C. parapsilosis* are found as part of the normal flora of humans. They can be isolated from healthy mucosal surfaces of the oral cavity, the vagina, the gastrointestinal tract, and the rectal area. As many as 80% of individuals may show colonization of these sites in the absence of disease. In contrast, the organism is rarely isolated from

TABLE 45-1 Species of *Candida*, Spectrum of Infections, and Conditions Leading to Increased Susceptibility in Candidiasis

Etiological agents	Clinical categories	Underlying conditions
C. albicans *C. stellatoidea* *C. tropicalis* *C. parapsilosis* *C. kefyr** *C. guilliermondii* *C. krusei* *C. glabrata*** *C. viswanathii* *C. lusitaniae*	Cutaneous: intertrigo, paronychia, onychomycosis Mucocutaneous: perleche, thrush, perianal Chronic: mucocutaneous candidiasis, granulomatous disease Systemic: fungemia, endocarditis, pulmonary infection, urinary tract, meningitis, endopthalmitis	Variable causes, mostly mechanical (e.g., trauma, occlusion); broad-spectrum antibacterial therapy; oral contraceptives AIDS; avitaminosis; pregnancy Defects in T-cell lymphocytes, macrophages Various conditions leading to immunosuppression (e.g., endocrinopathies, diabetes mellitus, burns), intravascular catheters, IV drug abuse

*Formerly called *Candida pseudotropicalis.*
**Formerly called *Torulopsis glabrata.*

the surface of normal human skin except sporadically from certain intertrigenous areas (skin surfaces that appose each other), as in the groin. Under certain circumstances these organisms gain hematogenous access from the oropharynx or gastrointestinal tract, when the mucosal barrier is breached (e.g., inflammation of mucous membranes secondary to chemotherapy) or through contaminated intravenous catheters and syringes. The organs most often involved include the lungs, spleen, kidney, liver, heart, and brain. *Candida* may produce an endophthalmitis (inflammation involving the eyes), which indicates there is hematogenous dissemination of *C. albicans* and possible involvement of multiple organs. Skin lesions may occur in 10% to 30% of patients who have disseminated infections. The early recognition of such lesions is important in diagnosis, because antemortem blood cultures are negative in a high percentage of patients with autopsy-proven systemic candidiasis.

Morphology

With one exception, a striking morphological feature of the yeasts in the genus *Candida* is that they multiply by forming blastospores, pseudohyphae and septate hyphae (see Chapter 5). *Candida glabrata,* a yeast implicated in urinary tract infections and systemic disease in debilitated individuals, is the exception, producing only yeast cells.

Clinical Syndromes

The spectrum of infections caused by organisms in the genus *Candida* includes the following: localized diseases of the skin and nails; diseases that affect the mucosal surfaces of the mouth, vagina, esophagus, and bronchial tree; and diseases that disseminate and involve multiple organ systems. The diseases involving skin and nails frequently mimic those seen with the dermatophytes. In all cases the diagnosis must be supported by microscopically observing fungi in specimens taken from the lesion and confirmed by culture. Factors leading to a predisposition to the various *Candida* infections are summarized in Table 45-1.

Chronic mucocutaneous candidiasis (CMC) is a heterogeneous group of clinical syndromes characterized by chronic, treatment-resistant superficial *Candida* infections of the skin, nails, and oropharynx (see discussion on immunity and host factors). Despite extensive cutaneous involvement there is virtually no propensity for disseminated visceral candidiasis to occur. In many cases there are narrow but specific abnormalities in T cell-mediated immunity. In others the defects are more general. Various underlying conditions such as hypoparathyroidism, hypoadrenalism, hypothyroidism, and the presence of circulating autoimmune antibodies have been associated with CMC. In adults CMC is often associated with a thymoma. When cutaneous candidiasis indicates the possibility of an immunological or endocrine disorder, efforts must be made to uncover and correct the underlying defect so that the fungal infection can be properly treated.

Disseminated candidiasis is usually spread through the bloodstream and therefore involves many organs. Severe neutropenia is considered to be the most significant predisposing factor for life-threatening infections. The incidence of this form of candidiasis is steadily rising as more patients with serious hematological malignancies are treated aggressively with potent immunosuppressive drugs and as more patients undergo bone marrow and organ transplants (Figure 45-1).

Whereas disseminated candidiasis continues to be a major problem in immunocompromised hosts, this is not the case in patients with AIDS. AIDS patients develop serious infections of the oropharynx and upper gastrointestinal tract but rarely experience systemic disease. The development of oral candidiasis in previously healthy adults not receiving corticosteroid therapy or broad-spectrum antibiotic therapy should strongly alert the physician to consider infection with the HIV (human immunodeficiency virus).

Immunity and Host Factors

Innate immunity to these organisms in the normal adult human appears to be very good. The immune mechanisms responsible for protection against *Candida* infections include both humoral and cell-mediated processes. Cell-mediated processes are considered to be more important in this regard, based on experiments with CMC, in which a defect in cell-mediated immunity leads to extensive superficial candidiasis despite normal, or even exaggerated, humoral defenses.

Production of serum antibody to the principal wall glycoprotein antigens of *Candida* occurs in low titers in normal individuals. The protective role of these antibodies, however, is controversial, and their presence may reflect only an immunological response to colonization of the gastrointestinal tract early in life. For this reason, the serodiagnosis of candidiasis is not routinely performed. In

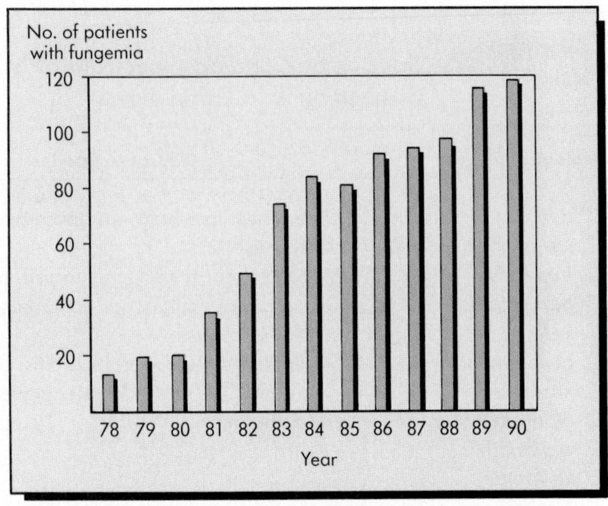

FIGURE 45-1 Incidence of culture proven *Candida* fungemia at Barnes Hospital (St. Louis, Mo.) for the period 1978 to 1990.

certain experimental studies, such as passive transfer of serum, a slight degree of protection may be provided. Yet, in the clinical setting, it is clear that patients with primarily B-cell deficiency states are not at high risk for infections by *Candida*. Evidence for the role of secretory IgA in limiting mucosal infections is confusing. It is probable that various innate, nonimmune host factors in conjunction with cell-mediated immunity and complement activation contribute more to host defense against *Candida* than does humoral immunity.

Laboratory Diagnosis

The species most often responsible for these infections include *C. albicans, C. tropicalis, C. kefyr, C. glabrata, C. krusei,* and *C. parapsilosis.* In histopathological sections and sputum, they may produce budding yeast cells, pseudohyphae, and septate hyphae (Figure 45-2). On solid media the organisms produce yeast and pseudohyphal cells, and the gross appearance of the colony is opaque and cream colored with a pasty consistency. All yeasts cultured from blood, cerebrospinal fluid, and surgical specimens should be identified as to species. Laboratory standards should be set for identification of yeasts from sputum, urine, and other nonsterile sources since yeasts may be part of the normal biota or transient colonizers. Several procedures are available for identification, most of which combine morphological, physiological, and biochemical tests. A rapid and reliable test to identify *C. albicans* is the germ tube test. Blastospores of *C. albicans* produce hyphal outgrowths (germ tubes) when they are suspended in serum and incubated at 37° C (Figure 45-3). For the test to be valid, the suspension must be examined within 2 to 3 hours after incubation because other species may form similar structures with longer incubation. A few isolates of *C. albicans* do not form germ tubes under these conditions. Therefore other tests are performed based on biochemical and physiological properties of the organisms, such as ability to assimilate various sugars or produce morphological structures (e.g., chlamydospores) (Figure 45-4) under certain growth conditions.

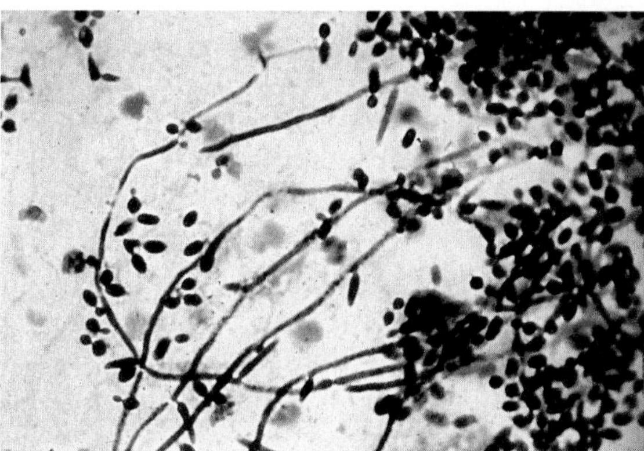

FIGURE 45-2 Sputum specimen illustrating budding yeast cells and pseudohyphae of *Candida.*

Treatment, Prevention, and Control (see also Chapter 14)

In the immunologically competent patient, topical treatment is usually preferred for cutaneous and mucocutaneous disease, and, except for disease of the nails, a good clinical response generally results when proper therapy is instituted. Therapy for systemic disease will vary depending on organ involvement and immune status. For systemic disease, amphotericin B alone or combined with 5-fluorocytosine may be indicated. Alternative therapy includes the use of the azole derivatives. Ketoconazole and fluconazole are preferred because they are active when given orally and less toxic than amphotericin B. However,

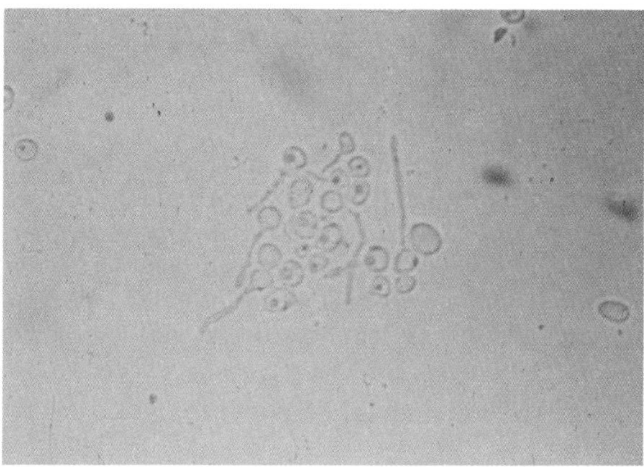

FIGURE 45-3 Development of germ tubes by *Candida albicans* yeast cells after incubation in serum for 2 hours at 37° C.

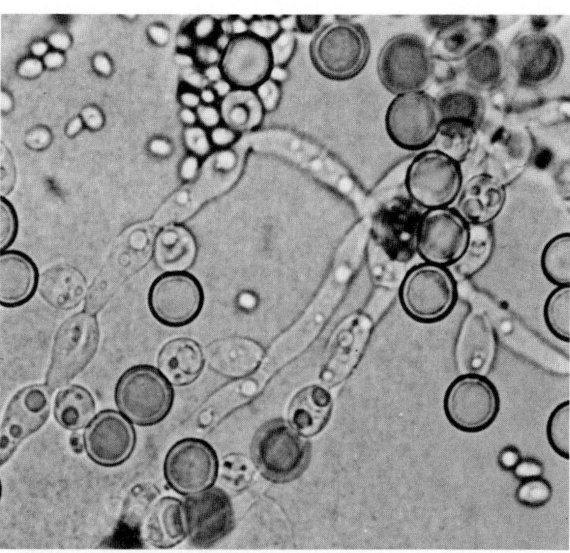

FIGURE 45-4 Formation of chlamydospores by *Candida albicans* when cultured on cornmeal agar at 25° C.

the azole derivatives are fungistatic, and in many cases the disease recurs once therapy is discontinued. Fungal infections in patients who are immunosuppressed pose a problem because the underlying conditions leading to immunosuppression must be corrected to obtain maximum response from the antifungal treatment. Patients who are intubated or are connected to various support catheters must be monitored closely; lines must be changed frequently so that they do not become contaminated and serve as foci for fungal colonization.

ASPERGILLOSIS

The spectrum of medical problems caused by various species of *Aspergillus* is broad (Table 45-2). Organisms belonging to this genus are extremely common in the environment. In contrast to most infections caused by *Candida,* aspergillosis is acquired from exogenous sources. As a result, assessing the significance of culture reports may be difficult unless the organism is seen in histopathological specimens.

Morphology

These organisms are identified in culture by their morphological features, the pattern of conidiophore development, and color of the formed conidia (Figure 45-5). Species of *Aspergillus* are extremely common in the environment, and several have been implicated as etiological agents. Of the approximately 900 described species, *A. fumigatus* and *A. flavus* have been most frequently associated with invasive disease.

Clinical Syndromes

The normal healthy individual is not susceptible to systemic aspergillosis. It is purely an opportunistic infection. As with candidiasis, the type of disease evoked depends on the local or general physiological and immunological state of the host. Factors that lead to host debilitation are also important in aspergillosis. In contrast to candidiasis, the etiological agents implicated in aspergillosis are ubiquitous in the environment and are not part of the normal flora of humans, although transient colonization may occur. These agents are involved in many animal diseases, such as mycotic abortion of sheep and cattle and pulmonary infections of birds, and their metabolites serve as carcinogenic agents in animals that have ingested contaminated feed. Because of their diverse involvement in both human and animal disease, they pose a great economic problem.

Allergic aspergillosis may initially occur as a benign process and then become severe as the patient grows older. With aging, respiratory distress increases, leading to bronchiectasis (chronic dilation of the air passages). Collapse of a segment of the lung eventually results in fibrosis (scarring).

In **secondary colonization,** a chronic clinical situation may exist with little distress except occasional bouts of hemoptysis (coughing up blood) and pathological changes in the lung that lead to the formation of a **"fungus ball"** (Figure 45-6). Histopathologically, the fungus ball is a spherical mass of intertwined septate-branching hyphal elements. These structures can also be

TABLE 45-2 Diseases That Are Associated With *Aspergillus*

Disease	Etiological factors
Mycotoxicoses	Ingestion of contaminated food products
Hypersensitivity pneumonitis	Allergic bronchopulmonary disease
Secondary colonization	Fungal colonization of preexisting cavity (e.g., pulmonary abscess) without invasion into contiguous tissues
Systemic disease	Invasive disease involving multiple organs

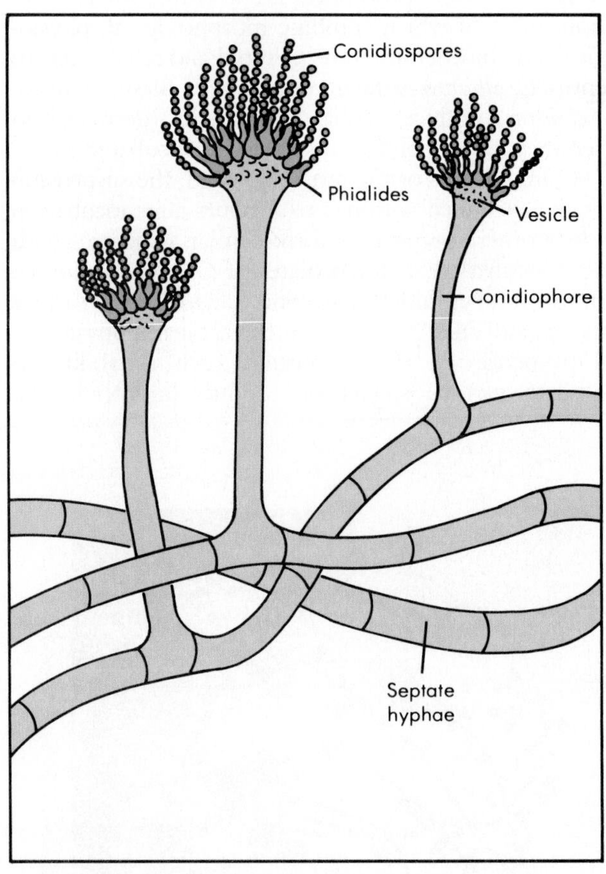

FIGURE 45-5 Asexual fruiting structure of *Aspergillus* species in culture, illustrating septate hyphae, conidiophore, vesicle, phialides, and conidiospores.

visualized radiologically as space-occupying spherical structures that move within the cavity as the patient's position is changed.

Systemic aspergillosis is an extremely serious disorder that is usually rapidly fatal unless diagnosed early and treated aggressively. In the immunosuppressed host the organism spreads from its primary site to contiguous tissues without regard to tissue planes, and lesions frequently contain hyphae within blood vessels, causing infarcts and hemorrhage. As in disseminated candidiasis, the physiological and immunological conditions that contribute to the host's increased susceptibility to the infection must be reversed for proper management.

Laboratory Diagnosis

The diagnosis of invasive aspergillosis is considered when septate hyphae that branch at regular intervals and tend to be oriented in the same direction are seen in clinical specimens (Figure 45-7). Confirmation of invasive aspergillosis is sometimes difficult, because cultures are not always performed or are often negative. Because these organisms exist everywhere in the environment, the clinical and histopathological diagnosis of invasive aspergillosis is strongly supported by repeated isolation of the organism in culture.

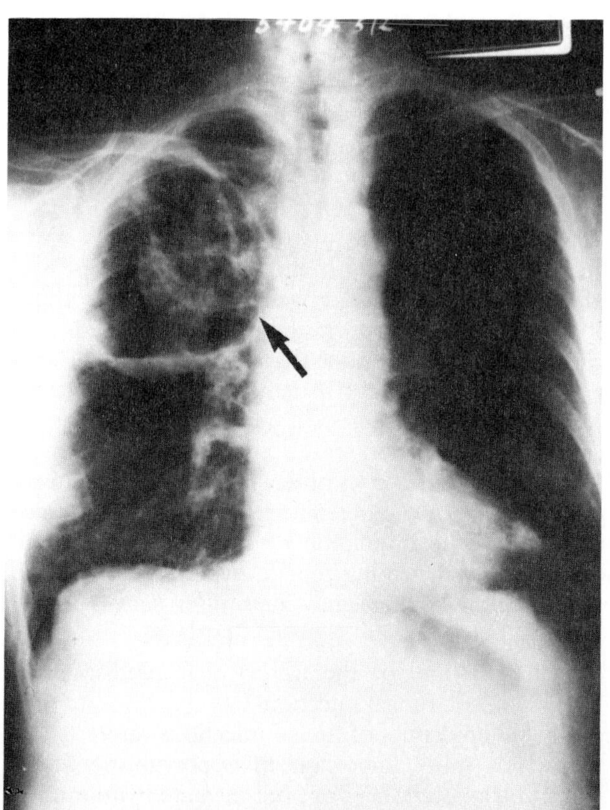

FIGURE 45-6 Chest film illustrating cavity in the upper right lobe *(arrow)* with an organizing fungus ball.

ZYGOMYCOSIS (MUCORMYCOSIS, PHYCOMYCOSIS)

Fungi belonging to the Zygomycetes are very common in the environment. The clinical entity zygomycosis, also termed mucormycosis or phycomycosis, encompasses a spectrum of infections similar to aspergillosis. Like candidiasis and aspergillosis, several underlying factors lead to increased susceptibility to fungi belonging to the class Zygomycetes. Most notable are metabolic acidosis, diabetes mellitus, leukopenia, and hyperglycemia.

Morphology

Fungi causing the zygomycoses grow rapidly on all laboratory media not containing cycloheximide. *Rhizopus, Absidia,* and *Mucor* have all been implicated in zygomycosis. They form coenocytic hyphae (i.e., not separated by cross walls) and reproduce asexually by producing sporangia within which develop sporangiospores (Figure 45-8). These organisms are ubiquitous in the environment and frequently encountered as contaminants. The relevance of the isolate may be difficult to establish if coenocytic hyphal elements are not seen in histopathological section. Repeated isolation of the organism from consecutive specimens provides strong evidence that the organism may be relevant, even though coenocytic hyphal elements are not seen in histopathological examination of tissue. A point to remember is that all fungi that have coenocytic hyphae are classified as zygomycetes, but not all zygomycetes are coenocytic.

Clinical Syndromes

Various diseases are caused by organisms belonging to the class zygomycetes order Mucorales. Rhinocerebral zygomycosis is the most common. This infection originates in the paranasal sinuses and can involve the ocular orbit and palate with extension into the brain. It usually occurs as a terminal event in acidotic patients who have metabolic disorders or uncontrolled diabetes mellitus.

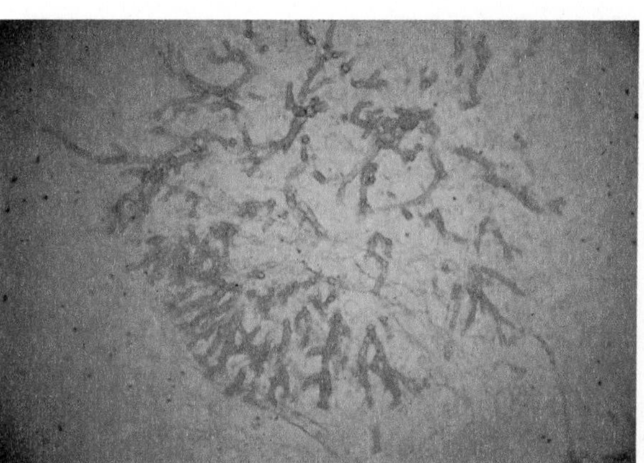

FIGURE 45-7 Dichotomous branching septate hyphae of *Aspergillus fumigatus* in tissue specimen.

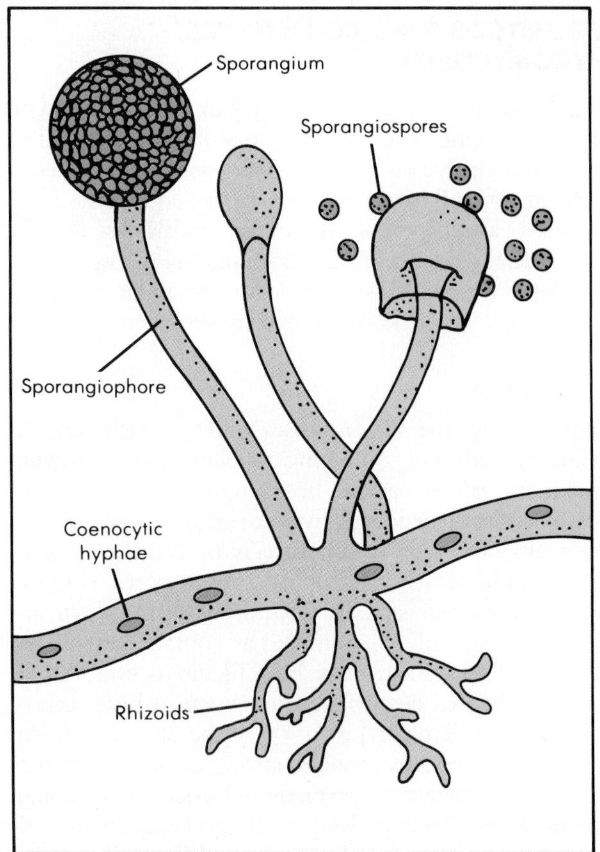

FIGURE 45-8 Asexual fruiting structure of *Rhizopus* species, illustrating sporangium, sporangiophore, sporagiospores, coenocytic hyphae, and rhizoids.

Other forms of zygomycosis seen in immunosuppressed or otherwise debilitated patients involve the lungs, the gastrointestinal tract, and subcutaneous tissues. In severely burned patients these organisms colonize the damaged tissues and tend to become invasive. In disseminated disease the organism shows a marked predilection for invading major blood vessels. The emboli (clots) that result cause ischemia (obstruction of blood vessels) and necrosis of adjacent tissues.

Laboratory Diagnosis

These organisms are filamentous, and their distinct morphology helps identify them in microscopic examination of pathological material. The hyphal filaments are coenocytic and have a ribbonlike appearance in tissue specimens (Figure 45-9). Cultures grown on medium not containing antibiotics are dense and have a "hairy" appearance. Microscopic examination of this growth confirms the coenocytic nature of the hyphae, and sporulating species produce characteristic sporangia (asexual fruiting bodies; Figure 45-8) that contain sporangiospores. The most frequently encountered agents of human disease are *R. arrhizus* and *A. corymbifera.* Assessing reports on the number and variety of species that may cause disease is often difficult because confirmation by culture is frequently lacking. Therefore the diagnosis is often based on histopathological examination of tissue.

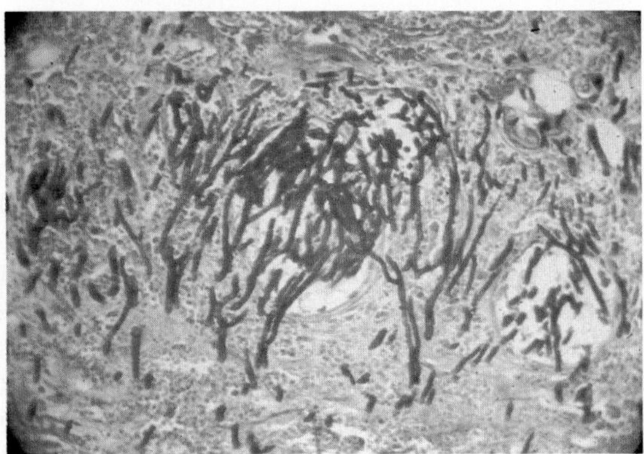

FIGURE 45-9 Histological section from a case of zygomycosis, illustrating coenocytic hyphae.

OTHER OPPORTUNISTIC FUNGAL INFECTIONS

Numerous fungi have been implicated as etiological agents of opportunistic infections of humans. A cursory examination of the literature supports the contention that the list of exotic and rare species of fungi causing infectious problems is large and continues to grow. For further details, see the Bibliography at the end of this chapter for specifics.

CASE STUDY AND QUESTIONS

A 42-year-old man with end-stage liver disease secondary to hepatitis B underwent orthoptic liver transplantation. Immunosuppression was maintained with cyclosporine and prednisone therapy. Four months after the surgical procedure the patient was readmitted to the hospital because of persistent fever and hypotension. Examination of the skin revealed echymotic lesions over the abdominal surface. Biopsies were taken for histological examination and culture. Microscopy revealed granulomatous inflammation of the deep dermis, and dichotomously branching septate hyphae were seen on special stains. Cultures grew *Aspergillus flavus.*

1. What are some of the factors that predispose to opportunistic fungal infections?
2. Why are epidemics of fungal infections rare?
3. Which is more important in opportunistic fungal infections: humoral- or cell-mediated immunity? Why?
4. Is contagion a problem (i.e., should the patient be placed on isolation)?

Bibliography

Drutz DJ, editor: Systemic fungal infections: diagnosis and treatment. I. *Med Clin North Am,* vol 3, 1988.

Drutz DJ, editor: Systemic fungal infections: diagnosis and treatment. II. *Med Clin North Am,* vol 4, 1989.

Gradon JD, Timpone JG, and Schnittman SM: Emergence of unusual opportunistic pathogens in AIDS: a review. *Clin Infect Dis* 15:134-157, 1992.

Kwon-Chung KJ and Bennett JE: *Medical mycology,* Philadelphia, 1992, Lea & Febiger.

Musial CE, Cockerill FR III, and Roberts GD: Fungal infections of the immunocompromised host: clinical and laboratory aspects, *Clin Microbiol Rev* 1:349-364, 1988.

Odds FC: *Candida and candidiasis,* London, 1988, Bailliere Tindall.

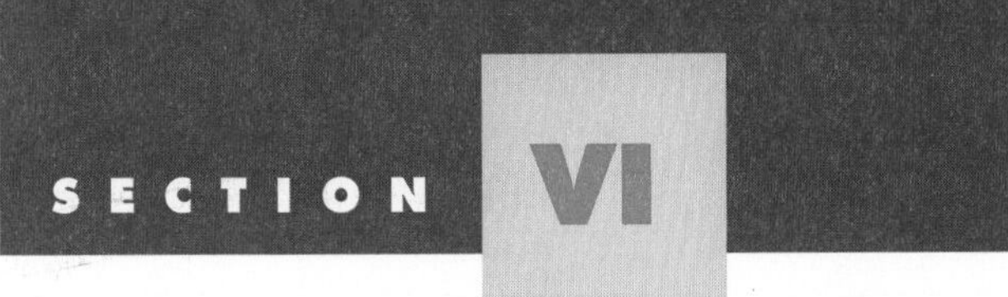

PARASITOLOGY

CHAPTER 46

Laboratory Diagnosis of Parasitic Diseases

THE diagnosis of parasitic infections may be quite difficult, particularly in the nonendemic setting. The clinical manifestations of parasitic diseases are seldom specific enough to raise the possibility of these processes in the mind of the clinician, and routine laboratory tests are seldom helpful. Although peripheral eosinophilia is widely recognized as a useful indicator of parasitic disease, this phenomenon is characteristic only of helminthic infection and even in these cases is frequently absent. Thus the physician must maintain a heightened index of suspicion and must rely on detailed travel, food intake, transfusion, and socioeconomic history to raise the possibility of parasitic disease. Proper diagnosis requires that (1) the physician consider the possibility of parasitic infection, (2) appropriate specimens be obtained and transported to the laboratory in a timely fashion, (3) the laboratory competently perform the appropriate procedures for recovery and identification of the etiological agent, (4) the laboratory results be effectively communicated to the physician, and (5) the results be correctly interpreted by the physician and applied to the care of the patient. In addition, for most parasitic diseases, appropriate test selection and interpretation is based on an understanding of the life cycle of the parasite, as well as the pathogenesis of the disease process in humans.

Numerous methods for diagnosis of parasitic diseases have been described (Box 46-1). Some are useful in detecting a wide variety of parasites, and others are particularly useful for one or a few parasites. Although the mainstay of diagnostic clinical microbiology is the isolation of the causative pathogen in culture, diagnosis of parasitic diseases is accomplished almost entirely by morphological (usually microscopic) demonstration of parasites in clinical material. Occasionally, demonstration of a specific antibody response (serodiagnosis) is helpful in establishing the diagnosis. Detection of parasite antigens in serum, urine, or stool may provide a rapid and sensitive means of diagnosing infection with certain organisms. Likewise, the recent development of nucleic acid probe–based assays may prove to be an excellent means of detecting and identifying a number of parasites in biological samples such as blood, stool, urine, sputum, or tissue biopsies obtained from infected patients. In general, it is better for the laboratory to offer a limited number of competently performed procedures than to offer a wide variety of infrequently and poorly performed tests.

This chapter provides a general description of the principles of specimen collection and processing necessary to diagnose most parasitic infections. Specific details of these and other procedures of general and limited usefulness may be found in several reference texts listed in the Bibliography.

THE PARASITE LIFE CYCLE AS AN AID IN DIAGNOSIS

Parasites may have complex life cycles involving single or multiple hosts. Understanding the life cycle of parasitic organisms is key to understanding important features of geographical distribution, transmission, and pathogenesis of many parasitic diseases. The life cycles of parasites often suggest useful clues for diagnosis as well. For example, in the life cycle of filariae that infect humans,

BOX 46-1 Laboratory Methods for the Diagnosis of Parasitic Diseases

- Macroscopic examination
- Microscopic examination
  - Wet mount
  - Permanent stains
  - Stool concentrates
- Serologic
  - Antibody response
  - Antigen detection
- Nucleic acid probes
  - Detection
  - Identification
- Culture
- Animal inoculation
- Xenodiagnosis

certain species such as *Wuchereria bancrofti* have a "nocturnal periodicity" in which greater numbers of microfilariae are found in the peripheral blood at night. Sampling the blood of such patients during daytime hours may fail to detect the microfilariae, whereas a blood specimen collected between 10 PM and 4 AM may demonstrate many microfilariae. Likewise, intestinal nematodes such as *Ascaris lumbricoides* and hookworm, which reside in the lumen of the intestine, produce large numbers of eggs that can be detected easily in the stool of an infected patient. In contrast, another intestinal nematode, *Strongyloides stercoralis*, lays its eggs in the bowel wall rather than in the intestinal lumen. As a result, eggs of *S. stercoralis* are rarely seen on stool examination, and to make the diagnosis the parasitologist must be alert for the presence of larvae. Finally, parasites may cause clinical symptoms at a time when diagnostic forms are not yet present in the usual site. For example, in certain intestinal nematode infections the migration of larvae through the tissues may cause intense symptomatology weeks before the characteristic eggs are present in the feces.

GENERAL DIAGNOSTIC CONSIDERATIONS

The importance of appropriate specimen collection, the number and timing of specimens, timely transport to the laboratory, and prompt examination by an experienced microscopist cannot be overemphasized. Because the vast majority of parasitological examinations and identifications are based entirely on recognizing the characteristic morphology of the organisms, any condition that may obscure or distort the morphological appearance of the parasite may result in an erroneous identification or missed diagnosis. As noted previously and in Box 46-1, there may be alternatives to microscopy for the detection and identification of certain parasites. These tests (antigen detection, nucleic acid probes), although presently uncommon, may become more widely applied in the future. They offer the promise of providing more rapid, sensitive, and specific diagnostic testing for parasitic diseases. These diagnostic test options would potentially expand the testing capabilities of many laboratories, allowing laboratories with limited proficiency in parasitology to offer diagnostic testing for certain parasitic diseases. A listing of common and uncommon diagnostic procedures and specimens to be collected for selected parasitic infections is provided in Table 46-1.

Intestinal and Urogenital Parasitic Infections

Protozoa and helminths may colonize or infect the intestinal and urogenital tract of humans. Most commonly these parasites are amebae, flagellates, or nematodes (Table 46-2). However, infection with trematodes, cestodes, ciliate, coccidian or microsporidian parasites may also be encountered.

In intestinal and urogenital infections, a simple wet mount or stained smear is often inadequate. Repeated specimens are often necessary to optimize the detection of organisms that are shed intermittently or in fluctuating numbers. Concentration of specimens by sedimentation or flotation techniques may be required to detect low numbers of ova (worms) and/or cysts (protozoa) present in fecal specimens. Occasionally, specimens other than stool or urine must be examined (see Table 46-1). Optimal detection of small bowel pathogens such as *Giardia lamblia* or *Strongyloides stercoralis* may require aspiration of duodenal contents or even small bowel biopsy. Likewise, the detection of colonic parasites such as *Entamoeba histolytica* and *Schistosoma mansoni* may necessitate proctoscopic or sigmoidoscopic examination with aspiration or biopsy of mucosal lesions. Sampling of the perianal skin is a useful means of recovering the eggs of *Enterobius vermicularis* (pinworm) or *Taenia* species (tapeworm).

Fecal Specimen Collection

Patients, clinicians, and laboratory personnel must be properly instructed on collection and handling of specimens. Fecal specimens should be collected in clean, widemouthed waterproof containers with a tight-fitting lid to ensure and maintain adequate moisture. Specimens must not be contaminated with water, soil, or urine because water and soil may contain free-living organisms that can be mistaken for human parasites and urine can destroy motile trophozoites and may cause helminth eggs to hatch. Stool specimens should not contain barium, bismuth, or medications containing mineral oil, antibiotics, antimalarials, or other chemical substances because they compromise the detection of intestinal parasites. Specimen collection should be delayed for 5 to 10 days to allow barium to clear and for at least 2 weeks to allow intestinal parasites to recover from the toxic (but not curative) effects of antibiotics such as tetracycline.

Purged specimens may be collected when organisms are not detected in normally passed fecal specimens; however, only certain purgatives (sodium sulfate and buffered phosphosoda) are satisfactory. One series of purged specimens may be examined in place of, or in addition to, a series of normally passed specimens.

Unpreserved formed fecal specimens should arrive in the laboratory within 2 hours after passage. If the stool is liquid, and thus more likely to contain trophozoites, it should reach the laboratory for examination within 30 minutes. Soft or loose stools should be examined within 1 hour of passage. All fresh fecal samples should be placed into preservatives such as 10% formalin, polyvinyl alcohol (PVA), merthiolate-iodine-formalin (MIF), or sodium acetate–formalin (SAF) if examination is not possible within the recommended time limits. Fecal specimens may be stored at 4° C but should not be incubated or frozen.

The number of specimens required to demonstrate intestinal parasites varies depending on the quality of the specimen submitted, the accuracy of the examination performed, the severity of the infection, and the purpose for which the examination is made. If the physician is

TABLE 46-1 Body Sites, Specimen Collection, and Diagnostic Procedures for Selected Parasitic Infections

Site of infection	Infecting organism	Specimen options	Collection methods	Diagnostic procedure
Blood	*Plasmodium* spp., *Babesia*, Filiaria,	Whole blood, anticoagulated	Venipuncture	Microscopic examination (Giemsa stain) Thin film Thick film Blood concentration (filaria) Serology Antibody Antigen
Bone marrow	*Leishmania* spp.	Aspirate, Serum	Sterile Venipuncture	Microscopic (Giemsa stain) Culture Serology (antibody)
Central nervous system	*Acanthamoeba*, *Naegleria*, Trypanosomes *Angiostrongylus cantonensis*	Spinal fluid, Serum	Sterile Venipuncture	Microscopic Wet mount Permanent stain Culture Serology (antibody)
Cutaneous ulcers	*Leishmania* spp.	Aspirate, Biopsy, Serum	Sterile plus smears Sterile; nonsterile to histology Venipuncture	Microscopic (Giemsa stain) Culture Serology (antibody)
Eye	*Acanthamoeba*	Corneal scrapings, Corneal biopsy	Sterile saline, air dried smear Sterile saline	Microscopic Wet mount Permanent stain Culture
Intestinal tract	*Entamoeba histolytica*	Fresh stool, Preserved stool, Sigmoidoscopy material, Serum	Waxed container Formalin, PVA Fresh, PVA, or Schaudinn's smears Venipuncture	Microscopic Wet mount Permanent stains Serology Antigen (stool) Antibody (serum) Culture
	Giardia	Fresh stool, Preserved stool, Duodenal contents	Waxed container Formalin, PVA Entero-Test or aspirate	Microscopic Wet mount Permanent stains Antigen IFA EIA Culture
	Cryptosporidium	Fresh stool, Preserved stool, Biopsy	Waxed container Formalin, PVA Saline	Microscopic (acid-fast) Antigen IFA EIA
	Microsporidia	Fresh stool, Perserved stool, Duodenal contents, Biopsy	Waxed container Formalin, PVA Aspirate Saline	Microscopic Giemsa stain Gram stain Chromotrope stain
	Pinworm	Anal impression smear	Cellophane tape	Macroscopic Microscopic (eggs)
	Helminths	Fresh stool, Preserved stool Serum	Waxed container Formalin, PVA Venipuncture	Macroscopic (adults) Microscopic (larvae and eggs) Serology (antibody) Culture (*Strongyloides*)

TABLE 46-1 Body Sites, Specimen Collection, and Diagnostic Procedures for Selected Parasitic Infections—cont'd

Site of infection	Infecting organism	Specimen options	Collection methods	Diagnostic procedure
Liver, spleen	*E. histolytica*, *Leishmania* spp.	Aspirates Biopsy Serum	Sterile, collected in four separate aliquots (liver) Sterile; nonsterile to histology Venipuncture	Microscopic Wet mount Permanent stains Serology Antigen Antibody Culture
Lung	*Pneumocystis carinii*, rarely amebae (*E. histolytica*), trematodes (*P. westermani*) larvae (*S. stercoralis*), or cestode hooklets	Sputum, Lavage Transbronchial aspirate, Brush biopsy Open lung biopsy	Induced, no preservative No preservative Air dried smears As above Fresh squash preparation, nonsterile to histology	Microscopic Giemsa stain Gram stain H&E Antigen IFA EIA Serum (antibody)
Muscle	*Trichinella spiralis* *Trypanosoma cruzi*	Biopsy Serum	Nonsterile to histology Venipuncture	Microscopic Permanent stains Serology Antibody Antigen
Skin	*Onchocerca volvulus*, *Leishmania* spp., migrans Cutaneous larval migrans	Scrapings, Skin snip, Biopsy, Serum	Aseptic, smear, or vial, No preservative, Nonsterile to histology Venipuncture	Microscopic Wet mount Permanent stains Serology (antibody) Culture (leishmania)
Urogenital system	*Trichomonas vaginalis*	Vaginal discharge Urethral discharge Prostatic secretions	Saline swab, culture medium As above	Microscopic Wet mount Permanent stains Antigen IFA Culture (*T. vaginalis*) Serology (antibody) Nucleic acid probes (*T. vaginalis*)
	Schistosoma haematobium	Urine Biopsy	Single unpreserved specimen Nonsterile to histology	Microscopic

interested only in determining the presence or absence of helminths, one or two examinations may suffice provided concentration methods are used. For a routine parasitic examination, a minimum of three fecal specimens is recommended. The examination of at least six specimens, using a combination of techniques, will ensure detection of approximately 90% of infections. For example, combining methods in the examination of six stool specimens for amebiasis increases the likelihood of detecting *E. histolytica*. With saline and iodine mounts only, 55% of the examples will reveal infection; when zinc sulfate concentrate is added to the mounts, the percentage of detection increases to approximately 75%; and the further addition of iron-hematoxylin stain will increase detection to more than 90%.

It is inappropriate for multiple specimens to be collected on the same patient on the same day. It is also not recommended for the three specimens to be submitted, one each day for 3 consecutive days. The series of three specimens should be collected within no more than 10 days and the series of six within no more than 14 days. Many parasites do not appear in fecal specimens in consistent numbers on a daily basis; therefore collection of specimens on alternate days tends to yield a higher percentage of positive findings.

In recent years it has become apparent that in the

TABLE 46-2 Most Commonly Identified Intestinal Parasites in State Public Health Departments—1987

Organism	Percentage of stool specimens with organism
Giardia lamblia	7.2
Blastocystis hominis	2.6
Hookworm	1.5
Trichuris trichiura	1.2
Entamoeba histolytica	0.9
Ascaris lumbricoides	0.8
Clonorchis/Opisthorchis	0.6
Dientamoeba fragilis	0.5
Strongyloides stercoralis	0.4
Enterobius vermicularis	0.4
Hymenolepsis nana	0.4
Cryptosporidium	0.2
Nonpathogenic protozoa	10.8

Modified from Kappus KK, Juranek DD, Roberts JM: *MMWR* 40:25-45, 1991.

United States submission of stool for parasitological examination from patients with hospital-acquired diarrhea (onset more than 3 days after admission) is usually inappropriate. This is because the frequency of acquisition of protozoan or helminthic parasites in a hospital is vanishingly rare. A request for stool examination for ova and parasites in a hospitalized patient should be accompanied by a clear statement of clinical indications and only after the more common causes of hospital-acquired diarrhea (e.g., antibiotic induced, etc.) have been ruled out.

Techniques of Stool Examination

Specimens should be examined systematically by a competent microscopist for both helminth eggs and larvae, as well as intestinal protozoa. For optimal detection of these various infectious agents a combination of several techniques of examination is required, including the following:

Macroscopic examination. The fecal specimen should be examined for consistency and for the presence of blood, mucus, worms, and proglottids.

Direct wet mount. Fresh stools should be examined under the microscope using the saline and iodine wet mount technique to detect any motile trophozoites or larvae (*Strongyloides*) that may be present. Both the saline and iodine wet mounts are also used to detect the presence of helminth eggs, protozoan cysts, and body cells such as leukocytes and red blood cells. This approach is also useful in examining material from sputum, urine, vaginal swabs, duodenal aspirates, sigmoidoscopy, abscesses, and tissue biopsies.

Concentration. All fecal specimens should be placed in 10% formalin to preserve parasite morphology and concentrated using a procedure such as formalin-ethyl acetate (or formalin-ether) sedimentation or zinc sulfate flotation. The purpose of these methods is to separate protozoan cysts and helminth eggs from the bulk of fecal material and thus enhance the ability to detect small numbers of organisms usually missed by using only a direct smear. After concentration the material is stained with iodine and examined microscopically.

Permanently stained slides. The detection and correct identification of intestinal protozoa often depend on the examination of the permanently stained smear. These slides serve to provide a permanent record of protozoan organisms identified. The cytological detail revealed by one of the permanent staining methods is essential for accurate identification, and most identification should be considered tentative until confirmed by the permanently stained slide. The common permanent stains used are the trichrome, the iron hematoxylin, and the phosphotungstic acid–hematoxylin. Slides are made either by preparing smears of fresh fecal material and placing them in Schaudinn's fixative solution or by fixing a small amount of fecal material in PVA fixative.

Collection and Examination of Specimens Other Than Stool

Frequently specimens other than fecal material must be collected and examined to diagnose infections caused by intestinal pathogens. These specimens include perianal samples, sigmoidoscopic material, aspirates of duodenal contents and liver abscesses, sputum, urine, and urogenital specimens.

Perianal specimens. The collection of perianal specimens is frequently necessary to diagnose pinworm (*Enterobius vermicularis*) and occasionally *Taenia* (tapeworm) infections. The methods include the preparation of a clear cellulose tape slide or an anal swab. The cellulose tape slide preparation is the method of choice for detection of pinworm eggs. Specimens collected by either method should be obtained in the morning before the patient bathes or goes to the bathroom. The tape method requires that the adhesive surface of the tape be pressed firmly against the right and left perianal folds and then spread onto the surface of a microscope slide. Likewise, the anal swab should be rubbed gently over the perianal area and transported to the laboratory for microscopic examination. With either collection method the slides or swabs should be kept at 4° C if transport to the laboratory is to be delayed.

Sigmoidoscopic material. Material from sigmoidoscopy can be helpful in the diagnosis of *Entamoeba histolytica* infection that has not been detected by routine fecal examinations. The specimens consist of scraped or aspirated material from the mucosal surface. At least six areas should be sampled. After collection, the material should be placed in a tube containing 0.85% saline and should be kept warm during transport to the laboratory. The specimens should be examined immediately for the presence of motile trophozoites.

Duodenal aspirates. Sampling and examination of duodenal contents is a means of recovering *Strongyloides* larvae, the eggs of *Clonorchis*, *Opisthorchis*, and *Fasciola*, and other small bowel parasites such as *Giardia*, *Isospora*, and *Cryptosporidium*. Specimens may be obtained by endoscopic intubation or by the use of the enteric capsule or string test (Entero-Test). Endoscopic biopsy of the small intestinal mucosa may reveal *Giardia*, *Cryptosporidium*, and microsporidia, as well as *Strongyloides* larvae. Specimens should be collected in saline and transported directly to the laboratory for microscopic examination.

Liver abscess aspirate. Suppurative lesions of the liver and subphrenic spaces may be caused by *Entamoeba histolytica* (extraintestinal amebiasis). Extraintestinal amebiasis may occur in the absence of any history of symptomatic intestinal infection. The specimen should be collected from the liver abscess margin instead of the necrotic center. The first portion removed is usually yellow-white in appearance and seldom contains amebae. Later portions, which are reddish in color, are more likely to contain organisms. A minimum of two separate portions of exudative material should be removed. Frequently following aspiration the collapse of the abscess and subsequent inflowing of blood release amebae from the tissue. Subsequent aspirations may have a greater chance of revealing organisms. The aspirated material should be transported immediately to the laboratory.

Sputum. Occasionally intestinal parasites may be detected in sputum. These organisms include the larvae of *Ascaris*, *Strongyloides*, and hookworm, cestode hooklets, and intestinal protozoa such as *E. histolytica* and *Cryptosporidium*. The specimen should be a deep sputum rather than a specimen composed primarily of saliva, and it should be delivered immediately to the laboratory. Microscopic examination should include both saline wet mount and permanent stain preparations.

Urine. Examination of urine specimens may be useful in diagnosing infections caused by *Schistosoma haematobium* (occasionally other species as well) and *Trichomonas vaginalis*. Detection of eggs in urine can be accomplished using direct detection or concentration using the sedimentation centrifugation technique. Eggs may be trapped in mucus or pus and are more frequently present in the last few drops of the specimen rather than the first portion. Production of *Schistosoma* eggs fluctuates; therefore daily exams should be performed for 3 consecutive days. *T. vaginalis* may be found in the urinary sediment of both males and females.

Urogenital specimens. Urogenital specimens are collected if infection with *Trichomonas vaginalis* is suspected. Identification is based on wet preparation examinations of vaginal and urethral discharges, prostatic secretions, or urine sediment. Specimens should be placed in a container with a small amount of 0.85% saline and sent immediately to the laboratory for examination. If no organisms are detected by direct wet mounts, culture may be used.

Blood and Tissue Parasitic Infections

Parasites localized within the blood and/or tissues of the host are more difficult to detect than intestinal and urogenital parasites. Microscopic examination of blood films is a direct and useful means of detecting malarial parasites, trypanosomes, and microfilariae. Unfortunately, the concentration of organisms often fluctuates and thus requires the collection of multiple specimens over several days. The preparation of both wet mounts (microfilariae and trypanosomes) and permanently stained thick and thin blood films are the mainstay of diagnosis. Examination of sputum may reveal helminth ova (lung flukes) or larvae (*Ascaris*, *Strongyloides*) following appropriate concentration techniques. Biopsy of skin (onchocerciasis) or muscle (trichinosis) may be required for the diagnosis of certain nematode infections (see Table 46-1).

Blood Films

The clinical diagnosis of parasitic diseases such as malaria, leishmaniasis, trypanosomiasis, and filariasis largely rests on the collection of appropriately timed blood samples and the expert microscopic examination of properly prepared and stained thick and thin blood films. The optimal time for obtaining blood for parasitological examination varies with the particular parasite expected. Because malaria is one of the few parasitic infections that can be life threatening, blood collection and examination of blood films should be performed immediately on suspicion of malaria. Laboratories offering this service should be prepared to do so on a 24-hour basis, 7 days a week. Because the levels of parasitemia may be low and/or fluctuating, it is recommended that repeat blood films be obtained and examined at 6, 12, and 24 hours after the initial sample. Detection of trypanosomes in blood is occasionally possible during the early acute phase of the disease. *T. cruzi* (Chagas' disease) may also be detected during subsequent febrile periods. After several months to a year the trypomastigotes of African trypanosomiasis (*T.b. rhodesiense* and *T.b. gambiense*) are better demonstrated in spinal fluid than blood. Blood films for the detection of nocturnal microfilariae (*Wuchereria bancrofti* and *Brugia malayi*) should be prepared between 10 PM and 4 AM, whereas for the diurnal *Loa loa*, films are prepared around noon.

Two types of blood films are prepared for diagnosis of blood parasite infections: thin films and thick films. Although wet preparations of blood films can be examined for the presence of motile parasites (microfilariae and trypanosomes), most laboratories proceed directly to the preparation of thick and thin films for staining. In the **thin film** the blood is spread over the slide in a thin (single cell) layer, and the red blood cells remain intact after staining. In the **thick film** the red cells are lysed before staining, and only the white blood cells, platelets, and parasites (if present) will be visible. Thick films allow a larger amount of blood to be examined, which increases the possibility of detecting light infections. Unfortunately, increased distortion of the parasites makes species identification using the thick film particularly difficult. Proper use of this technique usually requires a great deal of expertise and experience.

Occasionally, blood concentration procedures in addition to thick films may be useful in detecting light infections. Alternative concentration methods for detecting blood parasites include the use of microhematocrit centrifugation, examination of buffy coat preparations, a triple centrifugation technique for detection of low numbers of trypanosomes, and a membrane filtration technique for detection of microfilariae.

Once prepared, the blood films must be stained. The most dependable staining of blood parasites is obtained with Giemsa stain buffered to pH 7.0 to 7.2, although special stains may be used occasionally to identify species of microfilariae. Giemsa stain is particularly useful for staining of protozoa (malaria and trypanosomes); however, the sheath of microfilariae may not always stain with Giemsa. In this case hematoxylin-based stains such as hemalum may be used.

Specimens Other Than Blood

Examination of tissue and body fluids other than blood may be necessary based on clinical presentation and epidemiological considerations. Smears and concentrates of spinal fluid (CSF) are necessary to detect trophozoites of *Naegleria* and trypanosomes and larvae of *Angiostrongylus cantonensis* within the central nervous system. CSF must be examined promptly since the trophozoite forms of these parasites are very labile (trypanosomes) or tend to round up and become nonmotile (*Naegleria*). The examination of tissue impression smears of lymph nodes, liver biopsy material, spleen, or bone marrow stained with Giemsa stain is very useful in detecting intracellular parasites such as *Leishmania* or *Toxoplasma*. Likewise, biopsies of various tissues are an excellent means of detecting localized or disseminated infections caused by both protozoan and helminthic parasites. Saline mounts of superficial skin snips are very useful in detecting the microfilariae of *Onchocerca volvulus*. Examination of the sputum (induced) is indicated when there is a question of *Pneumocystis carinii* pneumonia, pulmonary paragonimiasis (lung fluke), or abscess formation with *E. histolytica*. *Strongyloides* larvae may be detected in sputum in hyperinfection syndrome.

Alternatives to Microscopy for the Diagnosis of Parasitic Infections

In the majority of cases the diagnosis of parasitic disease is made in the laboratory by microscopic detection and morphological identification of the parasite in clinical specimens. In some cases the parasite cannot be detected despite careful search because of low or absent levels of organisms in readily available clinical material. In such cases one may need to rely on alternative methods to search for a diagnosis based on detection of parasite-derived material (antigens or nucleic acids) or by the host response to parasitic invasion (antibodies). Additional approaches used in selected infections include culture, animal inoculation, and xenodiagnosis.

Immunodiagnostics

Immunodiagnostic methods have long been used as aids in the diagnosis of parasitic diseases. The majority of these serologic tests are based on the detection of specific antibody responses to the presence of the parasite. The analytical approaches include the use of classical agglutination, complement fixation, and gel diffusion methods, and more recently include immunofluorescence, enzyme immunoassay, and Western blot assays. Antibody detection is useful and indicated in the diagnosis of many protozoan (extraintestinal amebiasis, South American trypanosomiasis, leishmaniasis, transfusion-acquired malaria, and toxoplasmosis) and helminthic (clonorchiasis, cysticercosis, hydatidosis, lymphatic filariasis, schistosomiasis, trichinellosis, and toxocariasis) diseases. The problem with the detection of antibody as a means of diagnosis is the fact that because of the persistence of antibody for months to years after the acute infection, demonstration of antibody rarely can differentiate between acute and chronic infection.

In contrast to antibody detection, measurement of circulating parasite antigen in serum, urine, or feces may provide a more appropriate marker for the presence of active infection and may also indicate parasite load. Likewise, demonstrations of specific parasite antigen in lesion fluid such as material from an amebic abscess or fluid from a hydatid cyst may provide a definitive diagnosis of the infecting organism. Most common antigen detection assays employ an enzyme immunoassay (EIA) format; however, immunofluorescence, radioimmunoassay, and immunoblot methods have also proved useful. Several commercial assays for detection of parasite antigens are now available in kit form. These include EIA for detection of *Giardia* and *Cryptosporidium* in stool, EIA for detection of *Trichomonas vaginalis* in urogenital specimens, and immunofluorescent assays (IFA) for detection of *Pneumocystis carinii*, *Giardia*, *Cryptosporidium*, and *Trichomonas*. The reported sensitivity and specificity for most of these kits are quite good. The advantages to these approaches are labor savings and potential increase in the sensitivity of the parasite examination. The disadvantages are the loss of parasitological expertise and the fact that in each case the available assay tests for only a single organism, whereas conventional microscopic examination provides the opportunity to recognize many different parasites. Although antigen detection assays have been described for many other parasites, they are not widely available. The availability of a broader panel of antigen detection assays would make the use of an antigen screen a viable alternative to tedious microscopic examination.

Molecular Diagnostic Approaches

In addition to immunodiagnostic methods, the diagnosis of parasitic diseases has been enhanced considerably by the application of molecular diagnostic methods based on nucleic acid hybridization. This approach takes advantage of the fact that all organisms contain nucleic acid sequences, which may be used in a hybridization assay to distinguish among strains, species, and genera. Thus parasites may be simultaneously detected and identified in clinical material depending on the specificity of the nucleic acid probe employed. Another advantage of nucleic acid–based detection systems is that they are independent of the patients' immunological status or previous infection history, thereby identifying active infection. Finally, the development of target amplification techniques such as the polymerase chain reaction (PCR) provides exquisite sensitivity, allowing the detection of as little as one organism in a biological sample.

Nucleic acid probes can be used to detect parasites not only in clinical samples of blood, stool, or tissue from infected patients but also in their natural vector. The application of DNA fingerprinting allows precise identification of parasite or vector to the subspecies or strain level and has considerable value in epidemiological studies. Assay formats utilizing nucleic acid probes range from dot blot and Southern hybridization methods to in situ hybridization in tissue to PCR amplification coupled with solid or solution phase hybridization. The use of nonisotopic DNA labeling techniques greatly expands the potential applicability of these assays worldwide. Diagnostic kits based on these methods are not currently available; however, several are under development and may be available for clinical use in the near future.

Irrespective of the assay format, nucleic acid probes are now being used on a research basis for detection and identification of species and strains of *Plasmodium*, *Leishmania*, *Trypanosoma cruzi*, *Entamoeba histolytica*, *Schistosoma*, *Onchocerca*, *Brugia*, and *Taenia*. A simple nucleic acid–probe assay for *Trichomonas vaginalis* in urogenital specimens is currently in development and will be offered commercially in kit form for use in clinics and physicians' offices. It must be understood that the application of nucleic acid–probe methods to the diagnosis of parasitic diseases is still in its infancy. The widespread use of these techniques requires further development of simple procedures for sample handling and preparation and will require extensive clinical and field testing before they can be applied broadly to aid in clinical diagnosis.

Culture

Although culture is the standard for diagnosis of most infectious diseases, it is not commonly employed in the parasitology laboratory. Certain protozoan parasites such as *Trichomonas vaginalis*, *Entamoeba histolytica*, *Acanthamoeba* and *Naegleria*, *Leishmania* spp., *Trypanosoma cruzi*, and *Toxoplasma* can be cultured with relative ease. However, culture of most other parasites has not been successful or is too difficult or cumbersome to be of practical value in routine diagnostic efforts.

Animal Inoculation

Animal inoculation is a sensitive means of detecting infection caused by blood and tissue parasites such as *Trypanosoma brucei gambiense*, *T.b. rhodesiense*, *T. cruzi*, *Leishmania* spp., and *Toxoplasma gondii*. Although useful, this is not a practical approach for most diagnostic laboratories and is largely confined to research settings.

Xenodiagnosis

The technique of xenodiagnosis employs the use of laboratory raised arthropod vectors to detect low levels of parasites in infected individuals. Classically, this approach was used to diagnose Chagas' disease by allowing an uninfected reduviid bug to feed on an individual suspected of having the disease. Subsequently, the bug was dissected and examined microscopically for evidence of developmental stages of *T. cruzi*. Although this technique may be used in endemic areas, it is obviously not practical for most diagnostic laboratories.

QUESTIONS

1. Why is it important to understand the life cycle of parasites in approaching the diagnosis of parasitic diseases?
2. What factors may confound the use of microscopy in the diagnosis of parasitic disease?
3. Describe the important considerations in collecting and submitting a fecal specimen for parasitological examination.
4. Which parasites can be detected in blood?
5. What are the alternatives to microscopy for the diagnosis of parasitic infections?

Bibliography

Barker RH: DNA probe diagnosis of parasitic infections, *Exp Parasitol* 70:494-499, 1990.

Baron EJ and Finegold SM: *Bailey & Scott's diagnostic microbiology*, ed 8, St. Louis, 1990, Mosby.

Garcia LS, Bullock-Iacullo SL, Fritsche TR, Healy GR, Neimeister RP, Palmer J, Wolfe MS, and Wong J: *Slide preparation and staining of blood films for the laboratory diagnosis of parasitic diseases*, National Committee for Clinical Laboratory Standards document M15-T, 1992.

Hommel M: Impact of modern technologies on tropical medicine, *Trans Royal Soc Trop Med Hyg* 85:151-155, 1991.

Kappus KK, Juranek DD, Roberts JM: Results of testing for intestinal parasites by state diagnostic laboratories, United States, 1987, *MMWR* 40:25-45, 1991.

Maddison SE: Serodiagnosis of parasitic diseases, *Clin Microbiol Rev* 4:457-469, 1991.

Markell EK, Voge M, and John DT: *Medical parasitology*, ed 7, Philadelphia, 1992, WB Saunders.

Sawitz WG, Faust EC: The probability of detecting intestinal protozoa by successive stool examinations, *Am J Trop Med* 22:131-136, 1942.

Strickland GT: *Hunter's tropical medicine*, ed 7, Philadelphia, 1991, WB Saunders.

CHAPTER 47

Intestinal and Urogenital Protozoa

PROTOZOA may colonize and infect the oropharynx, duodenum and small bowel, colon, and urogenital tract of humans. The majority of these parasites belong to the amebae and flagellates; however, infection with ciliate, coccidian, or microsporidian parasites may also be encountered. These organisms are transmitted by the fecal-oral route. In the United States transmission of intestinal protozoa is particularly problematic in day-care centers, where several outbreaks of diarrhea caused by *Giardia* or *Cryptosporidium* have been well documented. In other parts of the world the spread of enteric protozoal infections may be controlled in part by improved sanitation and by chlorination and filtration of water supplies; however, this may be difficult or impossible in many developing countries.

AMEBAE

The amebae are primitive unicellular microorganisms. For most, their life cycle is relatively simple and divided into two stages: the actively motile feeding stage (**trophozoite**) and the quiescent, resistant, infective stage (**cyst**). Replication is accomplished by binary fission (splitting the trophozoite) or by the development of numerous trophozoites within the mature multinucleated cyst. Motility of amebae is accomplished by extension of a **pseudopod** ("false foot") with extrusion of the cellular ectoplasm, and then drawing up the rest of the cell in a snail-like movement to meet this pseudopod. The amebic trophozoites remain actively motile as long as the environment is favorable. The cyst form will develop when the environmental temperature or moisture level drops.

Most amebae found in humans are commensal organisms *(Entamoeba coli*, *Entamoeba hartmanni*, *Entamoeba gingivalis*, *Endolimax nana*, *Iodamoeba butschlii)*. However, *Entamoeba histolytica* is an important human pathogen. Other amebae, particularly *Entamoeba polecki,* can cause human disease but are rarely isolated. Some free-living amebae *(Naegleria fowleri*, *Acanthamoeba* species) are present in soil and in warm freshwater ponds or swimming pools and can be opportunistic human pathogens, causing meningoencephalitis or keratitis.

Entamoeba histolytica

Physiology and Structure

Cyst and trophozoite forms of *E. histolytica* are detected in fecal specimens from infected patients (Figure 47-1). Trophozoites can also be found in the crypts of the large intestine. In freshly passed stools actively motile trophozoites can be seen, whereas in formed stools the cysts are usually the only form recognized. To diagnose amebiasis, distinguishing between the *E. histolytica* trophozoites and cysts and those of commensal amebae is important.

Pathogenesis

Following ingestion the cysts pass through the stomach, where exposure to gastric acid stimulates release of the pathogenic trophozoite in the duodenum. The trophozoites divide and produce extensive local necrosis in the large intestine. The basis for this tissue destruction is incompletely understood, although it is attributed to production of a cytotoxin. Necrosis requires direct contact with the ameba, so lysosomal enzymes (e.g., phospholipase A_2) may be important. Recently the application of lectin binding, zymodeme analysis, and staining with specific monoclonal antibodies have been used as markers to identify invasive strains of *E. histolytica*. Flask-shaped ulcerations of the intestinal mucosa are present with inflammation, hemorrhage, and secondary bacterial infection. Invasion into the deeper mucosa with extension into the peritoneal cavity may occur. This can lead to secondary involvement of other organs, primarily the liver but also the lungs, brain, and heart. Extraintestinal amebiasis is associated with trophozoites. Amebae are found only in environments with a low Po_2 because the protozoa are killed by ambient oxygen concentrations.

Epidemiology

E. histolytica has a worldwide distribution. Although it is found in cold areas such as Alaska, Canada, and Eastern Europe, its incidence is highest in tropical and subtropical regions that have poor sanitation and contaminated water. The average prevalence of infection in these areas is 10% to 15%, with as many as 50% of the population infected in some areas. Many of the infected individuals are asymptomatic carriers, who represent a reservoir for

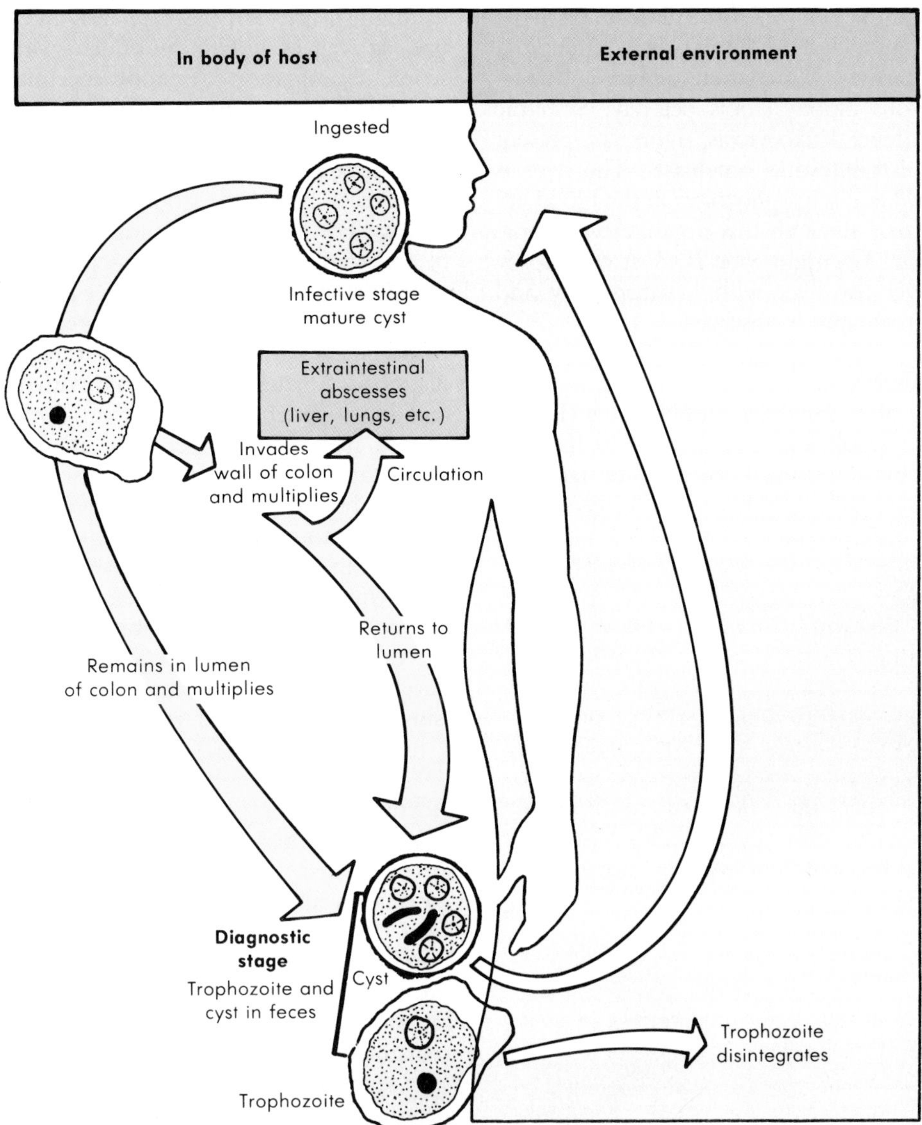

FIGURE 47-1 Life cycle of *Entamoeba histolytica.*

spread of *E. histolytica* to others. The prevalence of infection in the United States is 1% to 2%.

Patients infected with *E. histolytica* pass noninfectious trophozoites, as well as the infectious cysts, in their stools. The trophozoites cannot survive in the external environment or in transport through the stomach if ingested. Therefore the main source of water and food contamination is the asymptomatic carrier who passes cysts. This is a particular problem in hospitals for the mentally ill, military and refugee camps, prisons, and crowded day-care centers. Flies and cockroaches can also serve as vectors for the transmission of *E. histolytica* cysts. Sewage containing cysts can contaminate water systems, wells, springs, and agricultural areas where human waste is used as fertilizer. Finally, cysts can be transmitted by oral-anal sexual practices, with amebiasis prevalent in homosexual populations. Direct trophozoite transmission in sexual encounters can produce cutaneous amebiasis.

Clinical Syndromes

The outcome of infection may result in a carrier state, intestinal amebiasis, or extraintestinal amebiasis. If the strain of *E. histolytica* has a low virulence, if the inoculum is low, or if the patient's immune system is intact, the organisms may reproduce and cysts be passed in stool specimens with no clinical symptoms. Noninvasive strains of *E. histolytica* have been characterized by specific isoenzyme profiles (zymodemes), as well as their susceptibility to complement mediated lysis and failure to agglutinate in the presence of the lectin concanavalin A. Detection of carriers in areas with a low endemicity is important for epidemiological purposes.

Patients with intestinal amebiasis develop clinical

symptoms related to the localized tissue destruction in the large intestine. These include abdominal pain, cramping, and colitis with diarrhea. More severe disease is characterized by numerous bloody stools per day. Systemic signs of infection (fever, leukocytosis, rigors) are present in patients with extraintestinal amebiasis. The liver is primarily involved because trophozoites in the blood are removed as they pass through this organ. Abscess formation is common. The right lobe is most commonly involved. Pain over the liver with hepatomegaly and elevation of the diaphragm is observed.

Laboratory Diagnosis

The identification of *E. histolytica* trophozoites (Figure 47-2) and cysts in stools and trophozoites in tissue is diagnostic of amebic infection. Care must be taken to distinguish between these amebae and commensal amebae, as well as polymorphonuclear leukocytes. Microscopic examination of stool specimens is inherently insensitive because the protozoa are not usually distributed homogeneously in the specimen and the parasites are concentrated in the intestinal ulcers and at the margins of the abscess, not in the stool or the necrotic center of the abscess. For this reason multiple stool specimens should be collected. Extraintestinal amebiasis is sometimes diagnosed using scanning procedures for the liver and other organs. Specific serologic tests, together with microscopic examination of the abscess material, can confirm the diagnosis. Virtually all patients with hepatic amebiasis and most patients (greater than 80%) with intestinal disease have positive serology at the time of clinical presentation. This may be less useful in endemic areas where the prevalence of positive serologic results is higher. Examinations of stool specimens are frequently negative in extraintestinal disease. In addition to conventional microscopy and serology, several immunological tests for detection of fecal antigen and DNA-probe assays for detection of *E. histolytica* nucleic acids have been developed. These newer diagnostic approaches are promising but as yet are not widely available.

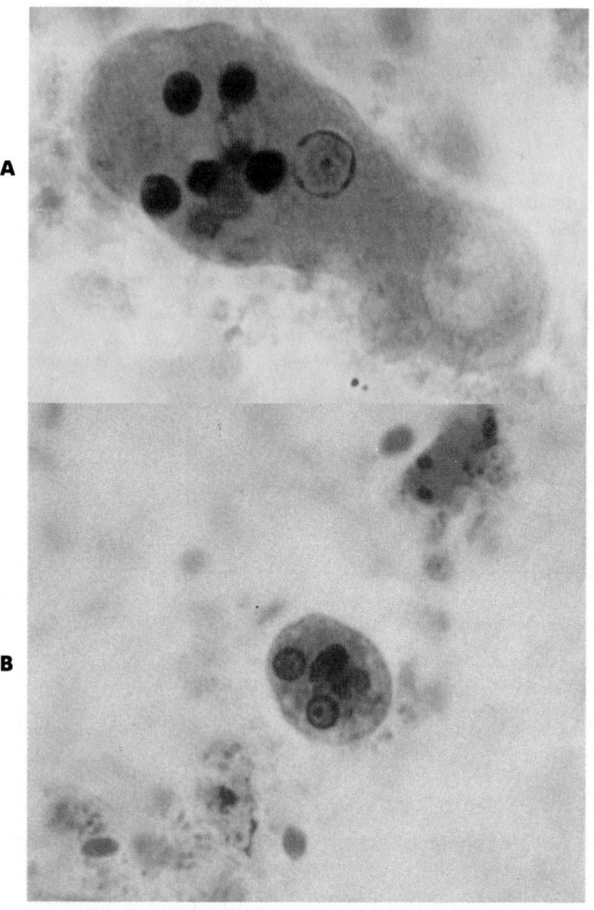

FIGURE 47-2 *Entamoeba histolytica* trophozoite **(A)** and cyst **(B)**. Trophozoites are motile and vary in size from 12 to 60 μm (average 15 to 30μm). The single nucleus in the cell is round with a central dot (karyosome) and an even distribution of chromatin granules around the nuclear membrane. Ingested erythrocytes may be in the cytoplasm. The cysts are smaller (11 to 20μm with an average size of 15 to 20μm) and contain one to four nuclei (usually four). Round chromatoidal bars may be in the cytoplasm. (From Lennette EH et al.: *Manual of clinical microbiology*, ed 5, Washington, DC, 1991, American Society for Microbiology.

Treatment, Prevention, and Control

Acute, fulminating amebiasis is treated with metronidazole followed by iodoquinol. Asymptomatic carriage can be eradicated with iodoquinol, diloxanide furoate, or paromomycin. Human infection results from ingestion of food or water contaminated with human feces, or as a result of specific sexual practices. The elimination of the cycle of infection requires introduction of adequate sanitation measures and education about the routes of transmission. Chlorination and filtration of water supplies may serve to limit the spread of these and other enteric protozoal infections but is not possible in many developing countries. Physicians should alert travelers to developing countries of the risks associated with consumption of water (including ice cubes), unpeeled fruits, and raw vegetables. Water should be boiled and fruits and vegetables thoroughly cleaned before consumption.

Other Intestinal Amebae

Other amebae that can parasitize the human gastrointestinal tract include *Entamoeba coli, Entamoeba hartmanni, Entamoeba polecki, Endolimax nana,* and *Iodamoeba butschlii.* Only *E. polecki,* which is primarily a parasite of pigs and monkeys, can cause human disease, a mild transient diarrhea. The diagnosis of *E. polecki* infection is confirmed by the microscopic detection of cysts in stool specimens. Treatment is the same as for *E. histolytica* infections.

The nonpathogenic intestinal amebae are important because they must be differentiated from *E. histolytica* and *E. polecki*. This is particularly true for *E. coli,* which is frequently detected in stool specimens collected from patients exposed to contaminated food or water. Accurate identification of intestinal amebae requires careful microscopic examination of the cyst and trophozoite forms present in stained and unstained stool specimens (Table 47-1).

Free-Living Amebae

Naegleria, *Acanthamoeba*, and other free-living amebae are found in soil and in contaminated lakes, streams, and other water environments. Most human infections with these amebae are acquired during the warm summer months by individuals exposed to the amebae while swimming in contaminated waters. Inhalation of cysts present in dust may account for some infections, whereas ocular infections with *Acanthamoeba* are associated with contamination of contact lenses with nonsterile cleaning solutions.

Clinical Syndromes

Naegleria are opportunistic pathogens. Although colonization of the nasal passages is usually asymptomatic, these amebae can invade the nasal mucosa and extend into the brain. Destruction of brain tissue is characterized by a fulminant, rapidly fatal **meningoencephalitis.** Symptoms include intense frontal headache, sore throat, fever, blocked nose with altered senses of taste and smell, stiff neck, and Kernig's sign. The cerebrospinal fluid is purulent and may contain many erythrocytes and motile amebae. Clinically, the course of the disease is rapid, with death usually occurring within 4 or 5 days. Postmortem findings show *Naegleria* trophozoites present in the brain but no evidence of cysts. Although all cases were fatal before 1970, survival has now been reported in a few cases in which the disease was rapidly diagnosed and treated.

In contrast to *Naegleria*, *Acanthamoeba* produces **granulomatous amebic encephalitis** primarily in immunocompromised individuals. The course of the disease is slower, with an incubation period of 10 days or more. The resulting disease is a chronic granulomatous encephalitis with edema of the brain tissue.

Eye and skin infection caused by *Acanthamoeba* may also occur. The **keratitis** is usually associated with trauma to the eye preceding contact with contaminated soil, dust, or water. The use of improperly cleaned contact lenses is also associated with this disease. Invasion of *Acanthamoeba* produces corneal ulceration and severe ocular pain. Cases of apparent disseminated cutaneous and subcutaneous infection with *Acanthamoeba* recently have been described in AIDS patients. These infections include multiple soft tissue nodules, which on biopsy contain *Acanthamoeba*. Central nervous system or deep tissue involvement may also be present with this form of infection.

Laboratory Diagnosis

For the diagnosis of *Naegleria* and *Acanthamoeba* infections, nasal discharge, cerebrospinal fluid, and, in the case of eye infections, corneal scrapings should be collected. The specimens should be examined by both a saline wet preparation and iodine-stained smears. *Naegleria* and *Acanthamoeba* are difficult to differentiate except by experienced microscopists. However, the observation of an ameba in a normally sterile tissue is diagnostic (Figure 47-3). The clinical specimens can be cultured on agar plates seeded with live gram-negative enteric bacilli. Amebae present in the specimens are able to use the bacteria as a nutritional source and can be detected within 1 or 2 days by the presence of trails on the agar surface formed as the amebae move.

Treatment, Prevention, and Control

The treatment of choice for *Naegleria* infections is amphotericin B combined with miconazole and rifampin. Experimental infections with *Acanthamoeba* appear to respond to sulfadiazine. Amebic keratitis and cutaneous

TABLE 47-1 Morphological Identification of *Entamoeba histolytica* and *Entamoeba coli*

	E. histolytica	*E. coli*
Size (μg diameter)		
Trophozoite	12-50	20-30
Cyst	10-20	10-30
Pattern of peripheral nuclear chromatin	Fine, dispersed ring	Coarse, clumped
Karyosome	Central, sharp	Eccentric, coarse
Ingested erythrocytes	+	0
Cyst structure		
Nuclei	1-4	1-8
Chromatid bars	Rounded ends	Splintered, frayed ends

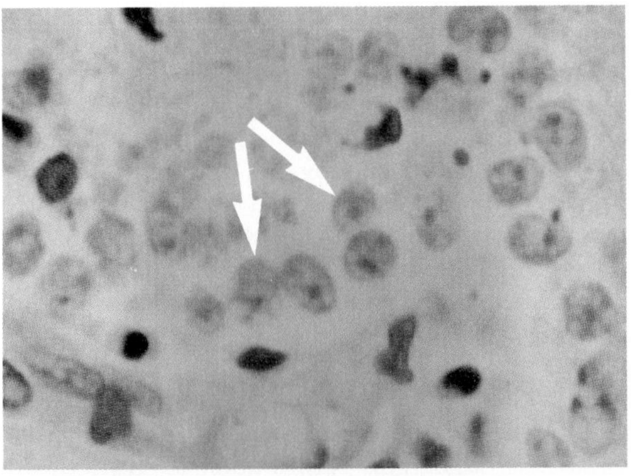

FIGURE 47-3 Numerous *Naegleria* trophozoites present in a section of spinal cord from a patient with amebic meningoencephalitis. (From Rothrock JF and Buchsbaum HW: *JAMA* 243:2329-2330.)

infections may respond to topical miconazole and propamidine isethionate. Treatment of amebic keratitis may require repeated corneal transplantation or, rarely, enucleation of the eye. The wide distribution of these organisms in fresh and brackish waters makes prevention and control of infection difficult. It has been suggested that known sources of infection be off-limits to bathing, diving, and water sports, although this is generally difficult to enforce. Swimming pools with cracks in the walls, allowing soil seepage, should be repaired to avoid creation of a source of infection.

FLAGELLATES

The flagellates of clinical significance include *Giardia lamblia, Dientamoeba fragilis,* and *Trichomonas vaginalis*. Nonpathogenic commensal flagellates such as *Chilomastix mesnili* (enteric) and *Trichomonas tenax* (oral) may also be observed. *Giardia,* like *E. histolytica,* has both cyst and trophozoite stages in its life cycle. In contrast, no cyst stage has been observed for either *Trichomonas* or *Dientamoeba*. Unlike the amebae, most flagellates move by the lashing of flagella that pull the organisms through fluid environments. Diseases produced by flagellates are primarily the result of mechanical irritation and inflammation. For example, *G. lamblia* attaches to the intestinal villi with an adhesive disk, resulting in localized tissue damage. The tissue invasion with extensive tissue destruction, as seen with the *E. histolytica,* is rare with flagellates.

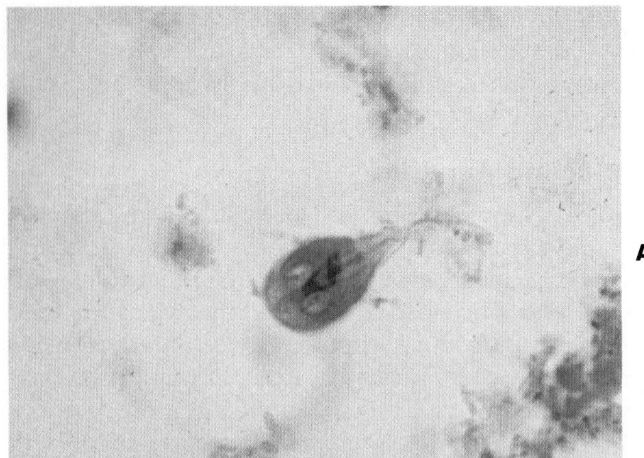

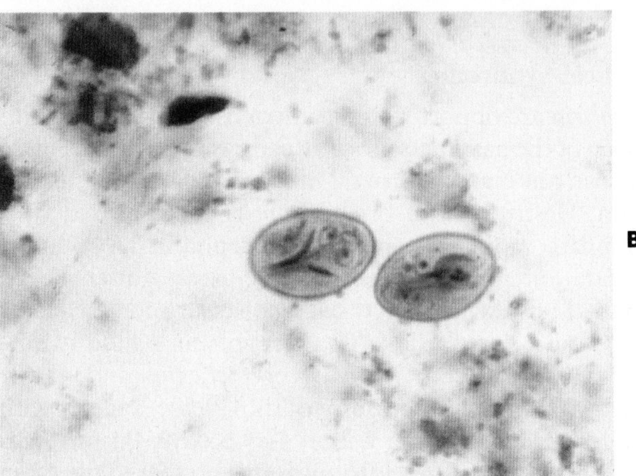

FIGURE 47-4 *Giardia lamblia* trophozoite **(A)** and cyst **(B)**. Trophozoites are 9 to 12 μm long and 5 to 15 μm wide. Flagella are present, as well as two nuclei with large central karyosomes, a large ventral sucking disk for attachment of the flagellate to the intestinal villi, and two oblong parabasal bodies below the nuclei. The morphology gives the appearance the trophozoites are looking back at the viewer. Cysts are smaller—8 to 12 μm long and 7 to 10 μm wide. Four nuclei and four parabasal bodies are present. (From Feingold SM and Baron EJ: *Bailey and Scott's diagnostic microbiology,* ed 7, St Louis, 1986, Mosby.)

Giardia lamblia

Physiology and Structure

Both cyst and trophozoite forms of *G. lamblia* are detected in fecal specimens from infected patients (Figure 47-4).

Pathogenesis

Infection with *G. lamblia* is initiated by ingestion of cysts (Figure 47-5). The minimum infective dose for humans is estimated to be 10 to 25 cysts. Gastric acid stimulates excystation with release of trophozoites in the duodenum and jejunum, where the organisms multiply by binary fission. The trophozoites can attach to the intestinal villi by a prominent ventral sucking disk. Although the tips of the villi may appear flattened and inflammation of the mucosa with hyperplasia of lymphoid follicles may be observed, frank tissue necrosis does not occur. In addition, metastatic spread of disease beyond the gastrointestinal tract is very rare.

Epidemiology

Giardia has worldwide distribution, and this flagellate has a sylvatic or "wilderness" distribution in many of our streams, lakes, and mountain resorts. This sylvatic distribution is maintained in reservoir animals such as beavers and muskrats. **Giardiasis** is acquired by drinking inadequately treated contaminated water, ingestion of contaminated uncooked vegetables or fruits, or person-to-person spread by the fecal-oral or oral-anal routes. The cyst stage is resistant to chlorine concentrations (1 to 2 parts per million) used in most water treatment facilities. Therefore adequate water treatment should include chemical treatment combined with filtration. Risk factors associated with *Giardia* infections include poor sanitary conditions, travel to known endemic areas, drinking inadequately treated water (e.g., from contaminated mountain streams), day-care centers, and oral-anal sexual practices. Infections may occur in outbreak and endemic forms within day-care centers and other institutional settings and among family members of infected children. Scrupulous attention to handwashing and treatment of all

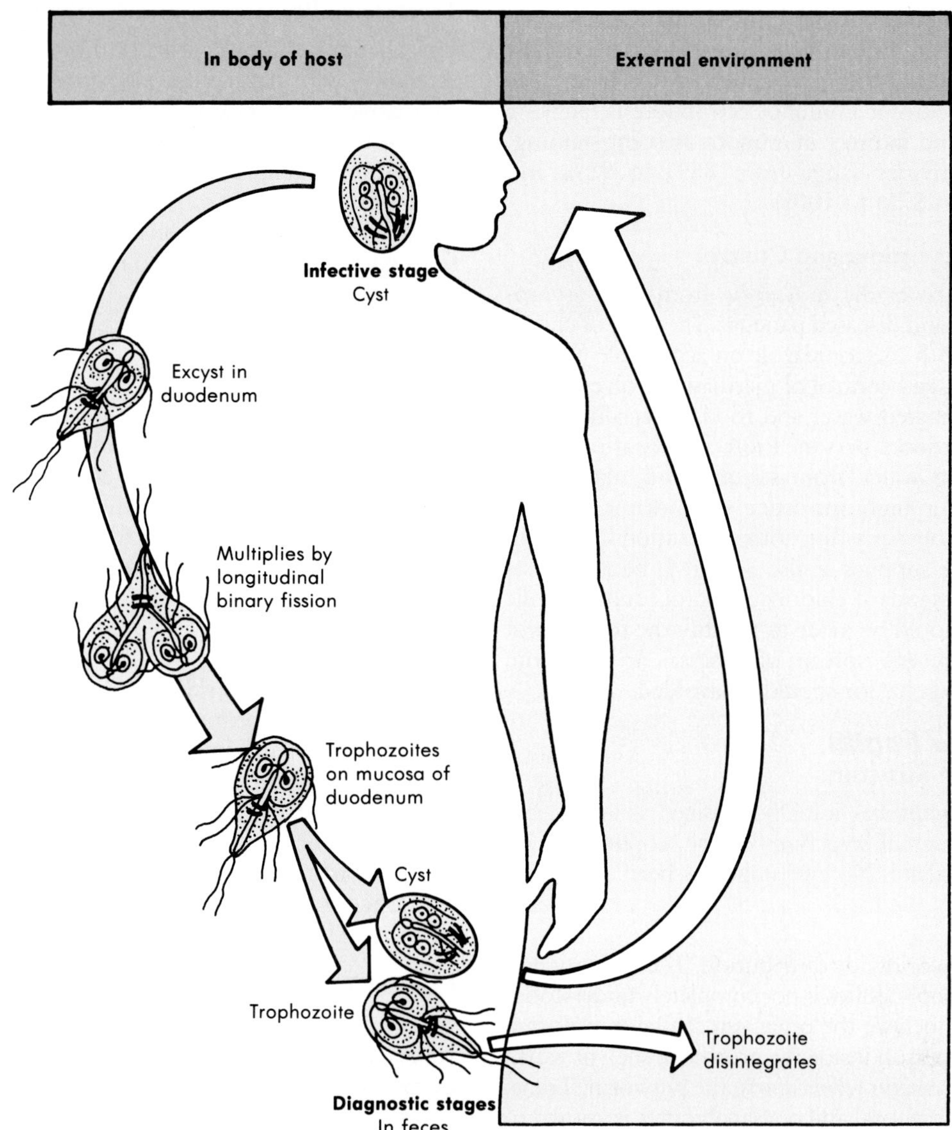

FIGURE 47-5 Life cycle of *Giardia lamblia.*

infected individuals are important in controlling the spread of infection in these settings.

Clinical Syndromes

Giardia infection can result in either asymptomatic carriage (observed in approximately 50% of infected individuals) or symptomatic disease, ranging from mild diarrhea to a severe **malabsorption syndrome.** The incubation period before symptomatic disease develops ranges from 1 to 4 weeks (average 10 days). The onset of disease is sudden, with foul-smelling, watery diarrhea, abdominal cramps, flatulence, and steatorrhea. Blood and pus are rarely present in stool specimens, consistent with the absence of tissue destruction. Spontaneous recovery generally occurs after 10 to 14 days, although a more chronic disease with multiple relapses may develop. This is particularly a problem for patients with IgA deficiency or intestinal diverticuli.

Laboratory Diagnosis

With the onset of diarrhea and abdominal discomfort, stool specimens should be examined for cysts and trophozoites (see Figure 47-4). *Giardia* may occur in "showers," with many organisms present in the stool on a given day and few or none detected on the next. For this reason, the physician should never accept a single negative stool specimen as conclusive that the patient is free of intestinal parasites. One stool specimen per day for 3 days should be examined. If stools remain persistently negative in a patient in whom giardiasis is highly suspected, additional specimens can be collected by duodenal aspiration, by the Entero-test or string test, or biopsy of the upper small intestine. In addition to conventional microscopy, several immunological tests for detection of fecal antigen are available commercially. These tests include countercurrent immunoelectrophoresis, enzyme immunoassay, and indirect immunofluorescent staining. Reported sensitivities range from 88% to 98% and specificities from 87% to 100%.

Treatment, Prevention, and Control

It is important to eradicate *Giardia* from both asymptomatic carriers and diseased patients. The drug of choice is quinacrine, with metronidazole an acceptable alternative. Prevention and control of giardiasis involves avoidance of contaminated water and food, especially by the traveler and outdoors person. Protection is afforded by boiling drinking water from streams and lakes or in countries with a high incidence of endemic disease. Maintenance of properly functioning filtration systems in municipal water supplies is also required, because cysts are resistant to standard chlorination procedures. Public health efforts should be made to identify the reservoir of infection to prevent spread of disease. In addition, high-risk sexual behavior should be avoided.

Dientamoeba fragilis

Physiology and Structure

Dientamoeba fragilis was initially classified as an ameba; however, the internal structures of the trophozoite are typical of a flagellate. No cyst stage has been described.

Epidemiology

D. fragilis has a worldwide distribution. The transmission of the delicate trophozoites is not completely understood. Some observers believe the organism can be transported from person to person inside the protective shell of worm eggs such as *Enterobius vermicularis,* the pinworm. Transmission by the fecal-oral and oral-anal routes is known to occur.

Clinical Syndromes

Most infections with *D. fragilis* are asymptomatic, with colonization of the cecum and upper colon. However, some patients may develop symptomatic disease, with abdominal discomfort, flatulence, intermittent diarrhea, anorexia, and weight loss. There is no evidence of tissue invasion with this flagellate, although irritation of the intestinal mucosa occurs.

Laboratory Diagnosis

Infection is confirmed by the microscopic examination of stool specimens in which typical trophozoites can be seen. The trophozoite is small (5 to 12 μm), with one or two nuclei. The central karyosome consists of four to six discrete granules. The excretion of the parasite may fluctuate markedly from day to day, and thus collection of several stool samples may be necessary. Examination of a purged stool sample may also be useful.

Treatment, Prevention, and Control

The therapy of choice for *D. fragilis* infection is iodoquinol, with tetracycline or paromomycin acceptable alternatives. The reservoir for this flagellate and the organism's life cycle are unknown. Thus specific recommendations for prevention and control are difficult. However, infections can be avoided by maintaining adequate sanitary conditions. The eradication of infections with *Enterobius* may also reduce the transmission of *Dientamoeba.*

Trichomonas vaginalis

Physiology and Structure

Trichomonas vaginalis is not an intestinal protozoan but rather the cause of urogenital infections. The flagellate possesses four flagella and a short undulating membrane that are responsible for motility. *T. vaginalis* exists only as a trophozoite and is found in the urethras and vaginas of women and the urethras and prostate glands of men.

Epidemiology

This parasite has worldwide distribution, with sexual intercourse as the primary mode of transmission (Figure 47-6). Occasionally, infections have been transmitted by fomites (toilet articles, clothing), although this transmission is limited by the lability of the trophozoite form. Infants may be infected by passage through the mother's infected birth canal. The prevalence of this flagellate in developed countries is reported to be from 5% to 20% in women and from 2% to 10% in men.

Clinical Syndromes

Most infected women are asymptomatic or have a scant, watery vaginal discharge. Vaginitis may occur with more extensive inflammation and erosion of the epithelial lining, associated with itching, burning, and painful urination. Men are primarily asymptomatic carriers who serve as a reservoir for infections in women. However, men occasionally experience urethritis, prostatitis, and other urinary tract problems.

Laboratory Diagnosis

The microscopic examination of vaginal or urethral discharge for characteristic trophozoites is the diagnostic method of choice (Figure 47-7). Stained (Giemsa, Papanicolaou) or unstained smears can be examined. The diagnostic yield may be improved by culturing the organism (93% sensitivity) or using monoclonal fluorescent antibody staining (86% sensitivity). A nucleic acid–probe assay is also under development. Serologic tests may be useful in epidemiological surveillance.

Treatment, Prevention, and Control

The drug of choice is metronidazole. Both male and female sex partners must be treated to avoid reinfection. Resistance to metronidazole has been reported and may require retreatment with higher doses. Personal hygiene,

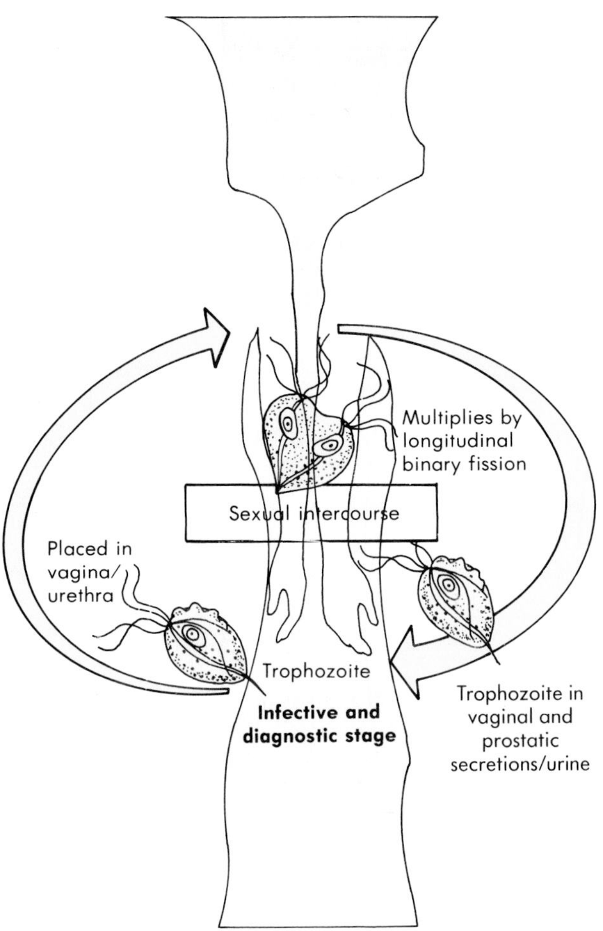

FIGURE 47-6 *Trichomonas vaginalis* life cycle.

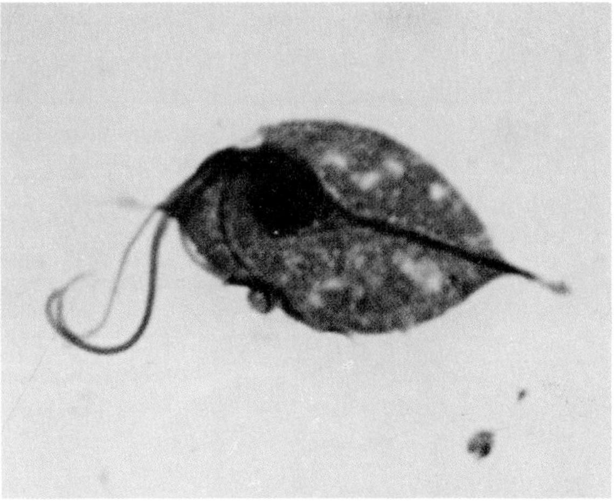

FIGURE 47-7 *Trichomonas vaginalis* trophozoite. The trophozoite is 7 to 23 μm long and 6 to 8 μm wide (average 13 by 7 μm; flagella and a short undulating membrane are present at one side, and an axostyle extends through the center of the parasite). (From Ash LR and Orihel TC: *Atlas of human parasitology*, ed 2, Chicago, 1984, American Society of Clinical Pathologists Press.)

avoidance of shared toilet articles and clothing, and safe sexual practices are important preventive actions. Elimination of carriage in men is critical for the eradication of disease.

CILIATES

The intestinal protozoan *Balantidium coli* is the only member of the ciliate group that is pathogenic for humans. Disease produced by *B. coli* is similar to amebiasis because the organisms elaborate proteolytic and cytotoxic substances that mediate tissue invasion and intestinal ulceration.

Balantidium coli

Physiology and Structure

The life cycle is simple, involving ingestion of infectious cysts, excystation, and invasion of trophozoites into the mucosal lining of the large intestine, cecum, and terminal ileum (Figure 47-8). The trophozoite is covered with rows of hairlike cilia that aid in motility. Morphologically more complex than amebae, *B. coli* has a funnel-like primitive mouth called a *cytostome*, a large and small nucleus involved in reproduction, food vacuoles, and two contractile vacuoles.

Epidemiology

B. coli is distributed worldwide. Swine and (less commonly) monkeys are the most important reservoirs. Infections are transmitted by the fecal-oral route; outbreaks are associated with contamination of water supplies with pig feces. Person-to-person spread, including food handlers, has been implicated in outbreaks. Risk factors associated with human disease include contact with swine and substandard hygienic conditions.

Clinical Syndromes

As with other protozoan parasites, asymptomatic carriage of *B. coli* can exist. Symptomatic disease is characterized by abdominal pain and tenderness, tenesmus, nausea, anorexia, and watery stools with blood and pus. Ulceration of the intestinal mucosa, as with amebiasis, can be seen, as well as secondary complication caused by bacterial invasion into the eroded intestinal mucosa. Extraintestinal invasion of other organs is extremely rare in balantidiasis.

Laboratory Diagnosis

Microscopic examination of feces for trophozoites and cysts is performed. The trophozoite is very large, varying in length from 50 to 200 μm and in width from 40 to 70 μm. The surface is covered with cilia, and the prominent internal structure is a macronucleus. A micronucleus is also present. Two pulsating contractile vacuoles are also seen in fresh preparation of the trophozoites. The cyst is smaller (40 to 60 μm in diameter), surrounded by a clear

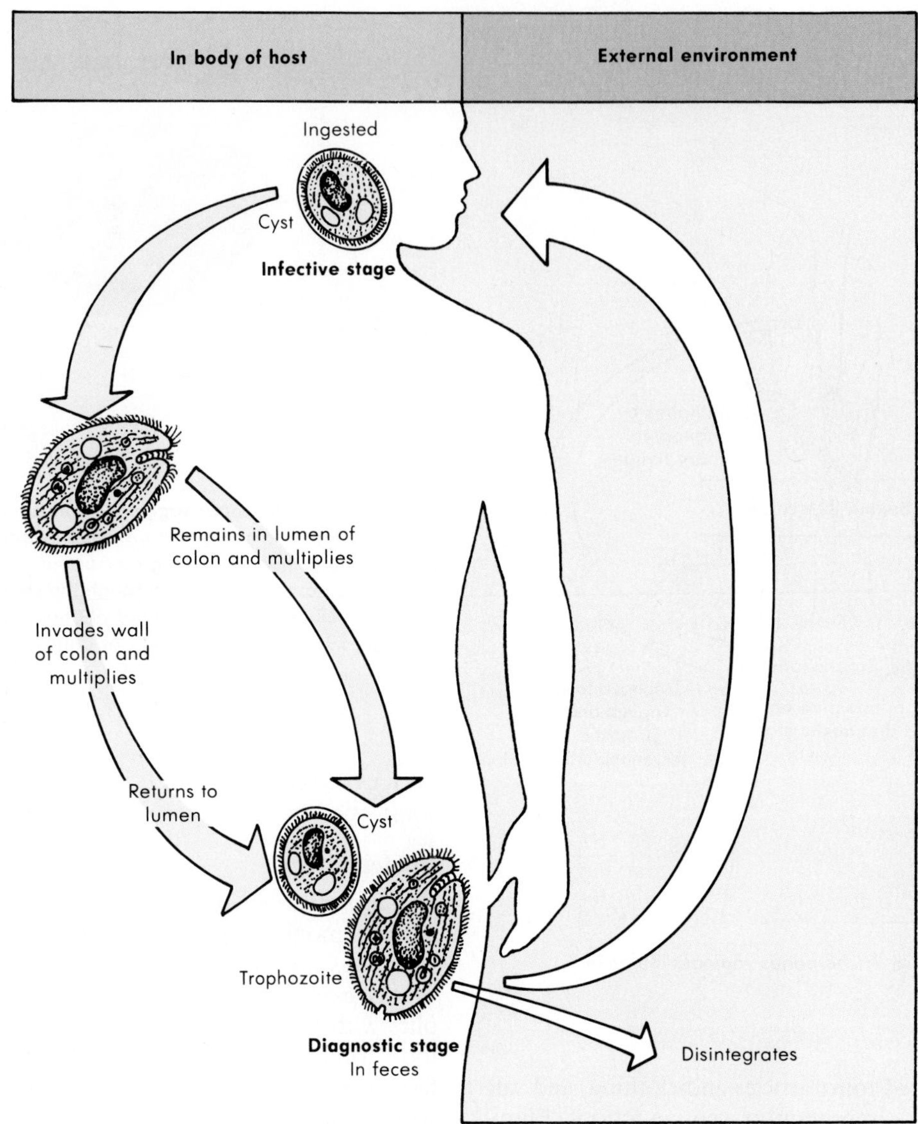

FIGURE 47-8 *Balantidium coli* life cycle.

refractile wall and has a single nucleus in the cytoplasm. *B. coli* is a large organism compared with other intestinal protozoa and is readily detected in fresh, wet microscopic preparations.

Treatment, Prevention, and Control

The drug of choice is tetracycline; iodoquinol or metronidazole are alternative antimicrobials. Prevention and control are similar to that used for amebiasis. Appropriate personal hygiene, maintenance of sanitary conditions, and the careful monitoring of pig feces are all important preventive measures.

COCCIDIA

Coccidia comprise a very large group called *Apicomplexa,* some members of which are discussed in this section with the intestinal parasites and others with the blood and tissue parasites. All coccidia demonstrate typical characteristics, especially the existence of both asexual (schizogony) and sexual (gametogony) reproduction. Most members of the group also share alternative hosts. A familiar example of this is with malaria, for which mosquitoes harbor the sexual cycle and humans the asexual cycle. The coccidia that are discussed in this chapter are *Isospora*, *Sarcocystis*, *Cryptosporidium,* and *Blastocystis.*

Isospora belli

Physiology and Structure

Isospora belli is a coccidian parasite of the intestinal epithelium. Both sexual and asexual reproduction in the intestinal epithelium can occur, resulting in tissue damage (Figure 47-9). The end product of gametogenesis is the

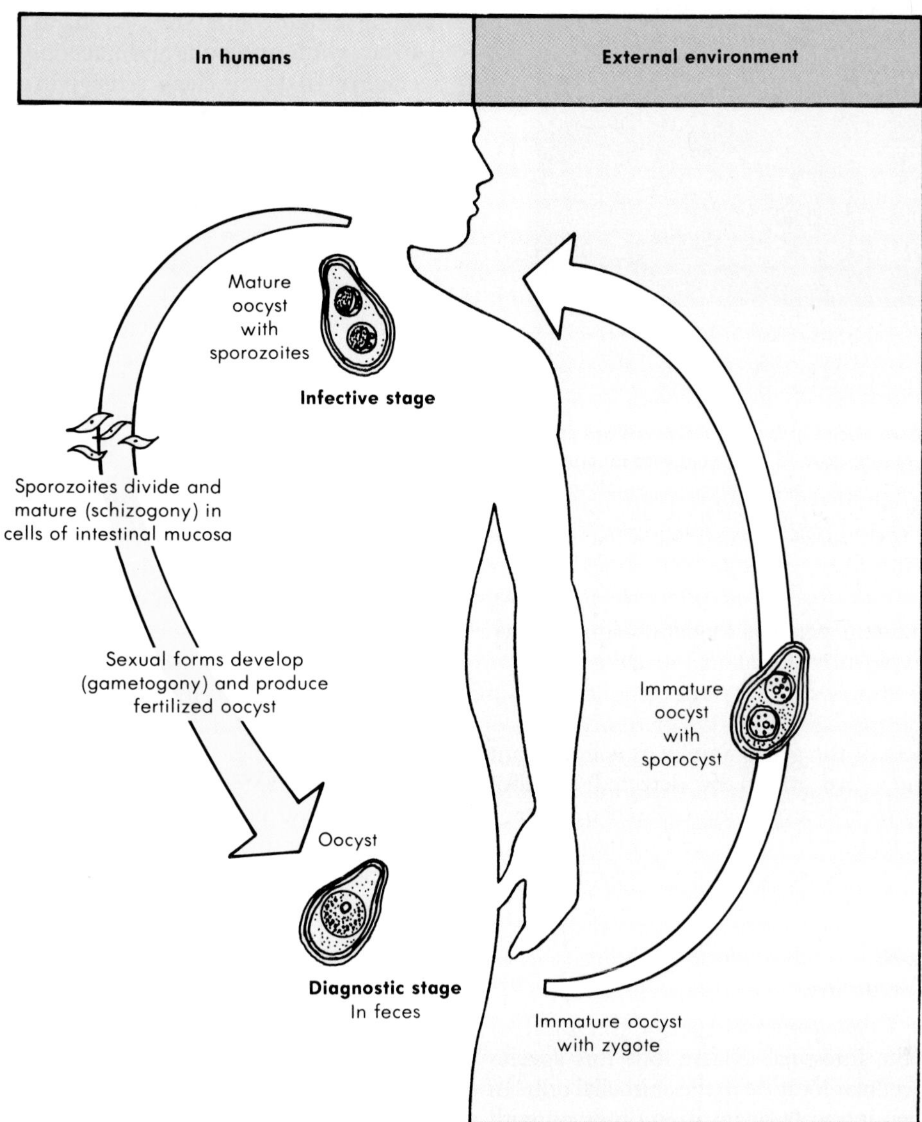

FIGURE 47-9 *Isospora* life cycle.

oocyst, which is the diagnostic stage present in fecal specimens.

Epidemiology

Isospora is distributed worldwide but has been infrequently detected in stool specimens. Recently, however, this parasite has been reported with increasing frequency in both normal and immunocompromised patients. This is likely due to the increased awareness of disease caused by *Isospora* in AIDS patients. Infection with this organism follows ingestion of contaminated food or water, or oral-anal sexual contact.

Clinical Syndromes

Infected individuals may be asymptomatic carriers or suffer gastrointestinal disease ranging from mild to severe. Disease most commonly mimics giardiasis, with a malabsorption syndrome characterized by loose, foul-smelling stools. Chronic diarrhea with weight loss, anorexia, malaise, and fatigue can be seen, although it is difficult to separate this presentation from the patient's underlying disease.

Laboratory Diagnosis

Careful examination of concentrated stool sediment and special staining with either iodine or a modified acid-fast procedure will reveal the parasite (Figure 47-10). Small bowel biopsy has been used to establish the diagnosis when stool specimens are negative.

Treatment, Prevention, and Control

The drug of choice is trimethoprim sulfamethoxazole, with the combination of pyrimethamine and sulfadiazine an acceptable alternative. Prevention and control is

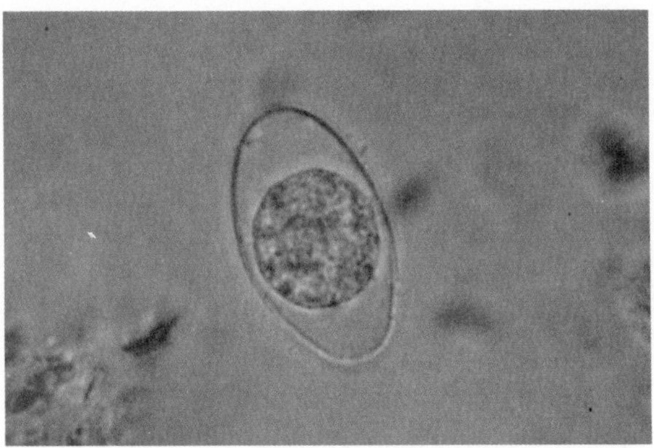

FIGURE 47-10 Immature oocyst of *Isospora.* Oocysts are ovoid (approximately 25 μm long and 15 μm wide) with tapering ends. A developing sporocyst is seen within the cytoplasm. (From Lennette EH et al: *Manual of clinical microbiology*, ed 4, Washington, DC, 1985, American Society for Microbiology.)

effected by maintaining personal hygiene, high sanitary conditions, and avoidance of oral-anal sexual contact.

Sarcocystis

Physician awareness of the genus *Sarcocystis* is important only in recognition that it can be detected in stool specimens. *Sarcocystis* species can be isolated from pigs and cattle and are identical in all aspects to *Isospora* with one exception: *Sarcocystis* oocysts rupture before passage in stool specimens, and only sporocysts will be present.

Cryptosporidium

Physiology and Structure

The life cycle of *Cryptosporidium* species is typical of coccidians, as is the intestinal disease, but this species differs in the intracellular location in the epithelial cells. In contrast to the deep intracellular invasion observed with *Isospora*, *Cryptosporidium* is found just within the brush border of the intestinal epithelium. The coccidia attach to the surface of the cells and replicate by a process that involves schizogony (Figure 47-11).

Epidemiology

Cryptosporidium species are distributed worldwide. Infection is reported in a wide variety of animals, including mammals, reptiles, and fish. Zoonotic spread from animal reservoirs to humans, as well as person-to-person spread by fecal-oral and oral-anal routes, are the most common means of infection. Veterinary personnel, animal handlers, and homosexuals are at particularly high risk for infection. Many outbreaks have now been described in day-care centers where fecal-oral transmission is common.

Clinical Syndromes

As with other protozoan infections, exposure to *Cryptosporidium* may result in asymptomatic carriage. Disease in previously healthy individuals is usually a mild self-limiting enterocolitis that is characterized by watery diarrhea without blood. Spontaneous remission after an average of 10 days is characteristic. In contrast, disease in immunocompromised patients (e.g., AIDS patients), characterized by 50 or more stools per day and tremendous fluid loss, can be severe and last for months to years. In some AIDS patients disseminated *Cryptosporidium* infections have been reported.

Laboratory Diagnosis

Cryptosporidium may be detected in large numbers in unconcentrated stool specimens obtained from immunocompromised individuals with diarrhea. Oocysts may be concentrated with the modified zinc sulfate centrifugal flotation technique or by Sheather's sugar flotation procedure. Specimens may be stained using the modified acid-fast method (Figure 47-12) or by an indirect immunofluorescence assay. An enzyme immunoassay for detecting fecal antigen is also available commercially. The number of oocysts shed in stool may fluctuate; therefore a minimum of three specimens should be examined. Serologic procedures for diagnosing and monitoring infections are under investigation but are not widely available at present.

Treatment, Prevention, and Control

Unfortunately, no broadly effective therapy has been developed for managing *Cryptosporidium* infections in immunocompromised patients. No controlled studies have been published, and all therapeutic information is based on isolated reports and anecdotal information. Spiramycin may help control the diarrhea in some patients with cryptosporidiosis in the early stages of AIDS but is ineffective in patients who have progressed to the later stages of AIDS. Spiramycin was no more effective than placebo in treating cryptosporidial diarrhea in infants. Reports concerning efficacy of oral paromomycin are promising, but these need confirmation. Therapy consists primarily of supportive measures to restore the tremendous fluid loss from the watery diarrhea.

Because of the widespread distribution of this organism in humans and other animals, preventing infection is difficult. The same methods of improved personal hygiene and sanitation used for other intestinal protozoa should be maintained for this disease. Contaminated water supplies should be treated with both chlorination and filtration. In addition, avoidance of high-risk sexual activities is critical.

Blastocystis hominis

Blastocystis hominis, previously regarded as a nonpathogenic yeast, is now the center of considerable controversy concerning its taxonomic position and its pathogenicity. The organism (Figure 47-13) is found in stool specimens from asymptomatic individuals, as well as from persons with persistent diarrhea. It has been suggested that the presence of large numbers of these parasites (five or more per oil immersion microscopic field) in the absence of

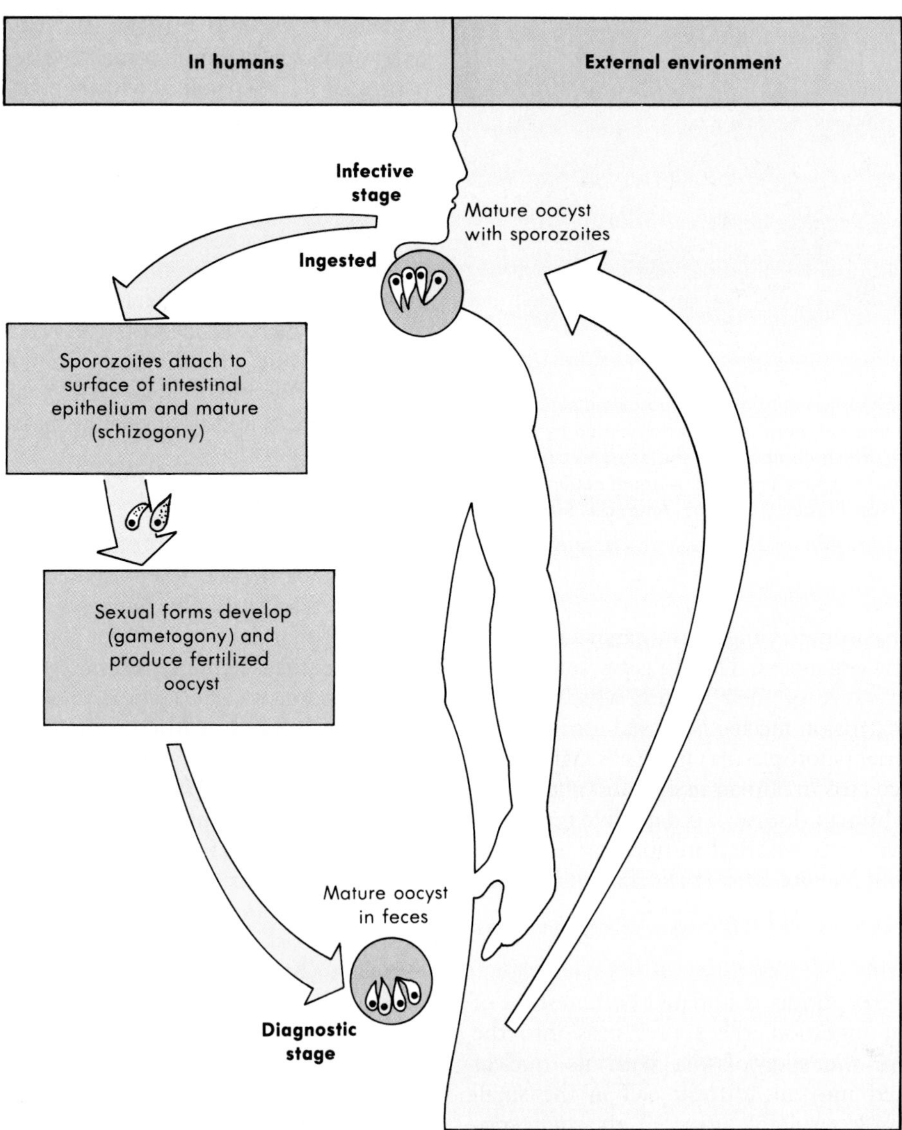

FIGURE 47-11 *Cryptosporidium* life cycle.

other intestinal pathogens is consistent with its role in disease. Other investigators have concluded that "symptomatic blastocystosis" is attributable to either an undetected pathogen or functional bowel problems. The organism may be detected in wet mounts or trichrome-stained smears of fecal specimens. Treatment with iodoquinol or metronidazole has been successful in eradicating the organisms from the intestine and alleviating symptoms. However, the definitive role of this organism in disease remains to be demonstrated.

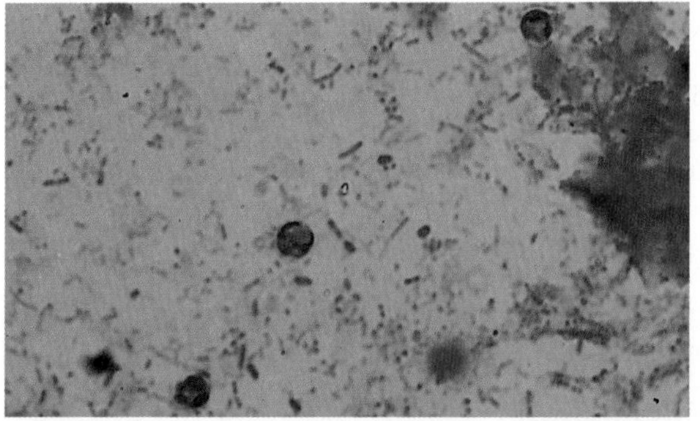

FIGURE 47-12 Acid-fast stained *Cryptosporidium* oocysts (approximately 5 to 7 μm in diameter).

MICROSPORIDIA

Physiology and Structure

Microsporidia are obligate intracellular pathogens belonging to the phylum Microspora. They are considered to be primitive eukaryotic organisms because they lack

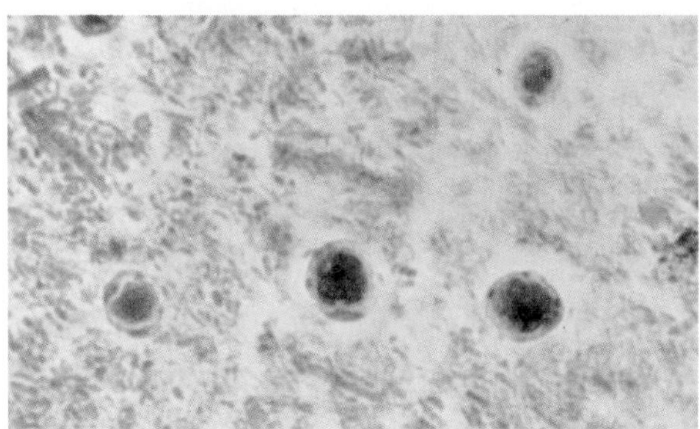

FIGURE 47-13 *Blastocystis hominis* oocysts. Approximately 8 to 10 μm in diameter; the internal morphology is dominated by the large central vacuole, which displaces the nucleus and cytoplasm to the periphery. (From Lennette EH et al.: *Manual of clinical microbiology*, ed 4, Washington, DC, 1985, American Society for Microbiology.)

mitochondria, peroxisomes, Golgi membranes, and other typically eukaryotic organelles. The parasites are characterized by the structure of their spores, which have a complex tubular extrusion mechanism used for injecting the infective material (sporoplasma) into cells. Microsporidia have been detected in human tissues and implicated as participants in human disease. To date, five genera of microsporidia have been reported in humans: *Encephalitozoon*, *Pleistophora*, *Nosema*, *Microsporidium*, and *Enterocytozoon*.

Pathogenesis

Infection with microsporidia is initiated by ingestion of spores. Following ingestion, the spores pass into the duodenum, where the sporoplasma with its nuclear material is injected into an adjacent cell in the small intestine. Once inside a suitable host cell, the microsporidia multiply extensively either within a parasitophorous vacuole or free within the cytoplasm. The intracellular multiplication includes a phase of repeated divisions by binary fission (merogony) and a phase culminating in spore formation (sporogony). The parasites spread from cell to cell, causing cell death and local inflammation. Although some species are highly selective in the cell type that they invade, collectively the Microspora are capable of infecting every organ of the body and disseminated infections have been described in severely immunocompromised individuals. Following sporogony the mature spores containing the infective sporoplasm may be excreted into the environment, thus continuing the cycle.

Epidemiology

Microsporidia are distributed worldwide and have a wide host range among invertebrate and vertebrate animals. Of the five genera, only *Enterocytozoon* is unique to humans. *Enterocytozoon bieneusi* has gained increasing attention as a cause of chronic diarrhea in patients with AIDS. *Encephalitozoon*-like organisms have been reported in the tissues of AIDS patients with hepatitis and peritonitis. *Pleistophora* was the cause of myositis in an individual with AIDS. *Nosema* has caused localized keratitis, as well as disseminated infection in a child with severe combined immunodeficiency. *Microsporidium* has caused infection of the human cornea.

Although the reservoir for human infection is unknown, transmission is likely accomplished by ingestion of spores that have been shed in the urine and feces of infected animals or individuals. As with cryptosporidial infection, individuals with AIDS and other cellular immune defects appear to be at increased risk for infection with microsporidia.

Clinical Syndromes

Clinical signs and symptoms of microsporidiosis are quite variable in the few human cases reported. Intestinal infection caused by *Enterocytozoon bieneusi* in AIDS patients is marked by persistent and debilitating diarrhea similar to that seen in patients with cryptosporidiosis and isosporiasis. The clinical presentation of infection with other species of Microspora depends on the organ system involved and ranges from localized ocular pain and loss of vision (*Microsporidium* and *Nosema* species) to neurological disturbances and hepatitis (*Encephalitozoon cuniculi*) to a more generalized picture of dissemination with fever, vomiting, diarrhea, and malabsorption (*Nosema*). In a report of disseminated infection with *Nosema connori*, the organism was observed involving the muscles of the stomach, bowel, arteries, diaphragm, and heart and the parenchymal cells of the liver, lungs, and adrenals.

Laboratory Diagnosis

Diagnosis of microsporidial infection may be made by detection of the organisms in biopsy material and by light microscopic examination of cerebrospinal fluid and urine. Spores measuring between 1.0 and 2.0 μm may be visualized by Gram (gram-positive), acid fast, periodic acid-Schiff, immunochemical, and Giemsa staining techniques (Figure 47-14). Recently a new chromotrope-based staining technique for light-microscopic detection of *E. bieneusi* spores in stool and duodenal aspirates was described (Figure 47-15). Electron microscopy is considered the gold standard for diagnostic confirmation of microsporidiosis; however, its sensitivity is unknown. Additional diagnostic techniques including culture and serologic testing are currently under investigation. These techniques are not considered reliable enough for routine diagnosis at the present time.

Treatment, Prevention, and Control

There is no known effective treatment for microsporidium infections. Treatment with metronidazole has resulted in temporary improvement in patients with intes-

CHAPTER 48

Blood and Tissue Protozoa

THE protozoa of blood and tissues are closely related to the intestinal protozoan parasites in practically all aspects except for their sites of infection (Box 48-1). The malaria parasites (*Plasmodium*) infect both blood and tissues and will be discussed first.

PLASMODIUM

Plasmodia are coccidian or sporozoan parasites of blood cells, and—as is seen with other coccidia—they require two hosts: the mosquito for the sexual reproductive stages, and humans and other animals for the asexual reproductive stages.

The four species of plasmodia that infect humans are *P. vivax*, *P. ovale*, *P. malariae*, and *P. falciparum* (Table 48-1). These species share a common life cycle, as illustrated in Figure 48-1. Human infection is initiated by the bite of an *Anopheles* mosquito, which introduces infectious plasmodia sporozoites via its saliva into the circulatory system. The sporozoites are carried to the parenchymal cells of the liver, where asexual reproduction (schizogony) occurs. This phase of growth is termed the *exoerythrocytic cycle* and will last for 8 to 25 days, depending on the plasmodial species. Some species (e.g., *P. vivax* and *P. ovale*) can establish a dormant hepatic phase in which the sporozoites (called **hypnozoites** or "sleeping forms") do not divide. The presence of these viable plasmodia can lead to relapse of infections months to years after the initial clinical disease (**relapsing malaria**). The hepatocytes eventually rupture, liberating the plasmodia (termed **merozoites** at this stage), which in turn attach to specific receptors on the surface of erythrocytes and enter the cells, thus initiating the erythrocytic cycle. Asexual replication progresses through a series of stages (ring, trophozoite, schizont) that culminates in the rupture of the erythrocyte, releasing up to 24 merozoites, which initiates another cycle of replication by infecting other erythrocytes. Some merozoites also develop within erythrocytes into male and female gametocytes. If a mosquito ingests mature male and female gametocytes during a blood meal, the sexual reproductive cycle of malaria can be initiated, with the eventual production of sporozoites infectious for humans. This sexual reproductive stage within the mosquito is necessary for maintenance of malaria within a population.

Most malaria seen in the United States is acquired by visitors or residents from countries with endemic disease (**imported malaria**). However, the appropriate vector *Anopheles* mosquito is found in several sections of the United States, and domestic transmission of disease has been observed (**introduced malaria**). In addition to transmission by mosquitos, malaria can also be acquired by blood transfusions from an infected donor (**transfusion malaria**). This type of transmission can also occur among narcotic addicts who share needles and syringes (**"mainline" malaria**). Congenital acquisition, although rare, is also a possible mode of transmission (**congenital malaria**).

Plasmodium vivax

Physiology and Structure

P. vivax (Figure 48-2) is selective in that it invades only young, immature erythrocytes. In infections caused by *P. vivax*, infected red blood cells are usually enlarged and contain numerous pink granules or Schüffner's dots, the trophozoite is ring shaped but ameboid in appearance,

BOX 48-1 Medically Important Blood and Tissue Protozoa

Plasmodium	*Pneumocystis*
Babesia	*Leishmania*
Toxoplasma	*Trypanosoma*
Sarcocystis	

TABLE 48-1 Human Malarial Parasites

Parasite	Disease
Plasmodium vivax	Benign tertian malaria
Plasmodium ovale	Benign tertian or ovale malaria
Plasmodium malariae	Quartan or malarial malaria
Plasmodium falciparum	Malignant tertian malaria

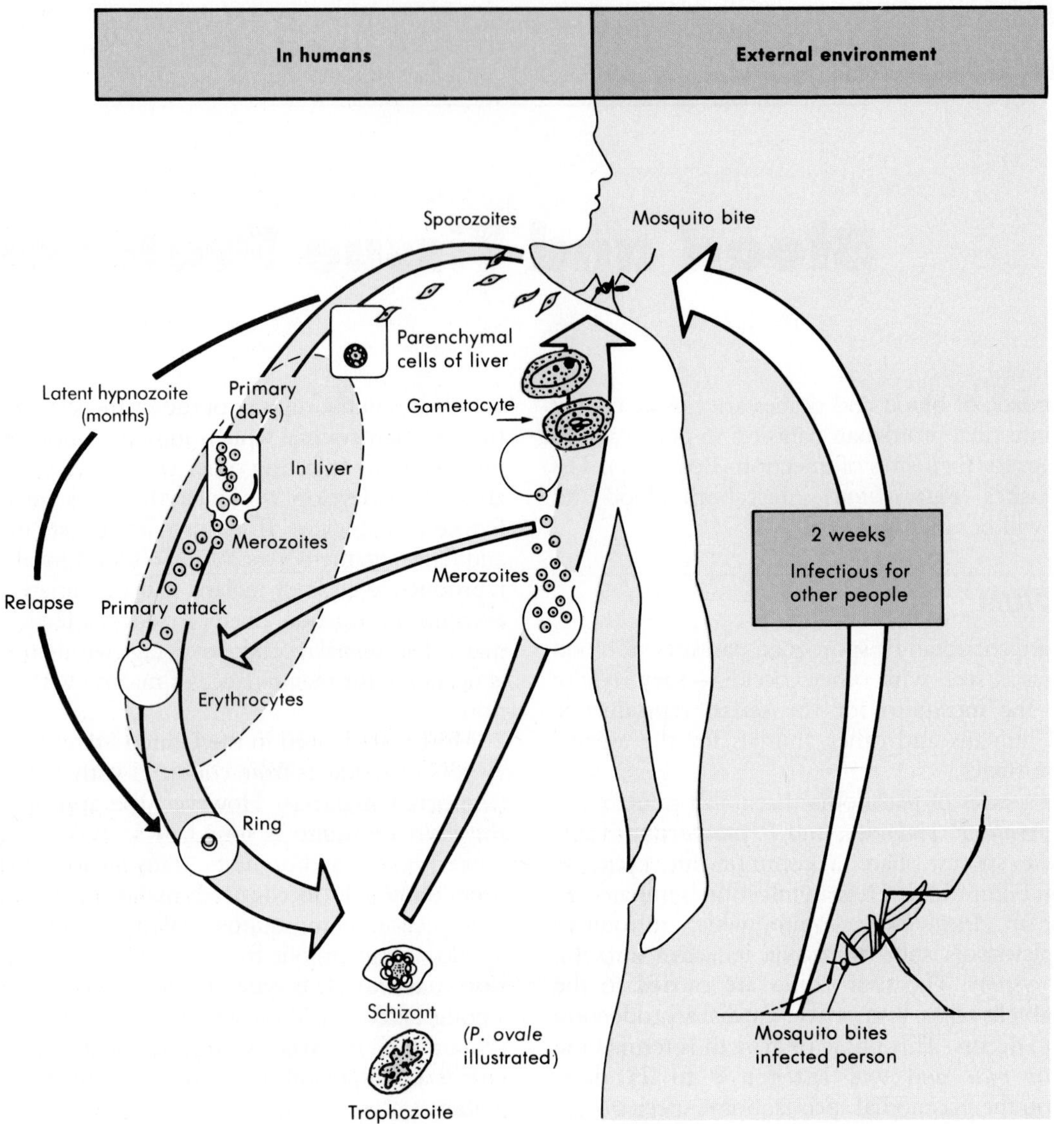

FIGURE 48-1 Life cycle of *Plasmodium* species.

more mature trophozoites and erythrocytic schizonts containing up to 24 merozoites are present, and the gametocytes are round. These characteristics are helpful in identification of the specific plasmodial species, which is important for the treatment of malaria.

Epidemiology

P. vivax is the most prevalent of the human plasmodia with the widest geographical distribution, including the tropics, subtropics, and temperate regions.

Clinical Syndromes

After an incubation period (usually 10 to 17 days) the patient experiences vague flu-like symptoms with headache, muscle pains, photophobia, anorexia, nausea, and vomiting.

As the infection progresses, increased numbers of rupturing erythrocytes liberate merozoites, as well as toxic cellular debris and hemoglobin, into the circulation. Together these produce the typical pattern of chills, fever, and malarial rigors. These paroxysms usually reappear periodically (generally every 48 hours) as the cycle of infection, replication, and cell lysis progresses. The paroxysms may remain relatively mild or progress to severe attacks, with hours of sweating, chills, shaking, persistently high temperatures (103° F to 106° F), and exhaustion.

P. vivax causes **"benign tertian malaria,"** which refers to the cycle of paroxysms every 48 hours (in untreated patients) and the fact that most patients tolerate the attacks and can survive for years without treatment. If left untreated, however, chronic *P. vivax* infections can lead to brain, kidney, and liver damage as a result of the malarial pigment, cellular debris, and

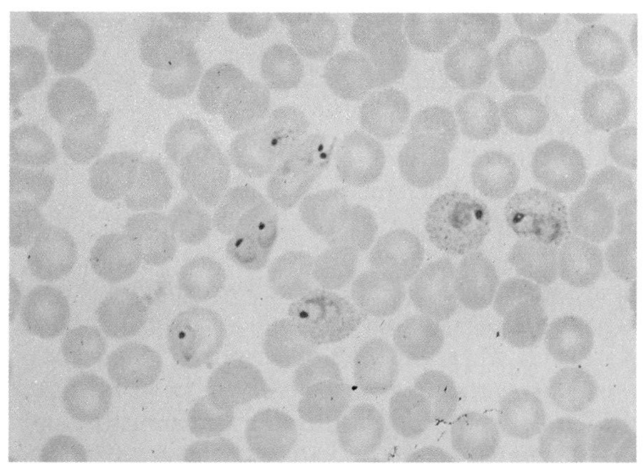

FIGURE 48-2 *Plasmodium vivax* ring forms and young trophozoites. Note the multiple stages of the parasite seen in the peripheral blood smear, enlarged parasitized erythrocytes, and presence of Schüffner's dots with the trophozoite form. These are characteristic of *P. vivax* infections.

capillary plugging of these organs by masses of adherent erythrocytes.

Laboratory Diagnosis

Microscopic examination of both thick and thin films of blood is the method of choice for confirming the clinical diagnosis of malaria and identifying the specific species responsible for disease. The thick film is a concentration method and may be used to detect the presence of organisms. With training, thick films may be used to diagnose the species as well. The thin film is most useful for establishing species identification. Blood films can be taken at any time over the course of the infection, but the best time is midway between paroxysms of chills and fever, when the greatest number of intracellular organisms will be present. It may be necessary to take repeated films at intervals of 4 to 6 hours.

Serologic procedures are available, but they are used primarily for epidemiological surveys or for screening blood donors. Serologic findings usually remain positive for approximately a year, even after complete treatment of the infection.

Treatment, Prevention and Control

The treatment of *P. vivax* infection involves a combination of supportive measures and chemotherapy. Bed rest, relief of fever and headache, regulation of fluid balance, and in some cases blood transfusion are supportive therapies.

The chemotherapeutic regimens are as follows:

Suppressive—a form of prophylaxis to avoid infection and clinical symptoms

Therapeutic—aimed at eradicating the erythrocytic cycle

Radical cure—aimed at eradicating the exoerythrocytic cycle in the liver

Gametocidal—aimed at destruction of erythrocytic gametocytes to prevent mosquito transmission

Chloroquine is the drug of choice for suppression and therapeutic treatment of *P. vivax,* followed by primaquine for radical cure and elimination of gametocytes. Recent reports suggest the emergence of chloroquine-resistant forms of *P. vivax* in Indonesia and New Guinea. Patients infected with chloroquine-resistant *P. vivax* may be treated with other agents including mefloquine, quinine, Fansidar (pyrimethamine-sulfadoxine) or doxycycline. Primaquine is especially effective in preventing relapse from latent forms of *P. vivax* in the liver. Because antimalarial drugs are potentially toxic, it is imperative that physicians carefully review the recommended therapeutic regimens.

Chemoprophylaxis and prompt eradication of infections are critical in breaking the mosquito-human transmission cycle. Control of mosquito breeding and protection of individuals by screening, netting, protective clothing, and insect repellents are also essential. Immigrants from and travelers to endemic areas must be carefully screened, using blood films or serologic tests to detect possible infection. The development of vaccines to protect persons living in or traveling to endemic areas is actively under investigation.

Plasmodium ovale

Physiology and Structure

P. ovale is similar to *P. vivax* in many respects, including its selectivity for young, pliable erythrocytes. As a consequence, the host cell becomes enlarged and distorted, usually in an oval form. Schüffner's dots appear as pale pink granules, and the cell border is frequently fimbriated or ragged. The schizont of *P. ovale*, when mature, contains about half the number of merozoites seen in *P. vivax.*

Epidemiology

P. ovale is distributed primarily in tropical Africa, where it is often more prevalent than *P. vivax.* It is also found in Asia and South America.

Clinical Syndromes

The clinical picture of tertian attacks for *P. ovale* (**benign tertian** or **ovale malaria**) infection is similar to that for *P. vivax.* Untreated infections last only about a year instead of the several years for *P. vivax.* Both relapse and recrudescence phases are similar to *P. vivax.*

Laboratory Diagnosis

As with *P. vivax,* both thick and thin blood films are examined for the typical oval-shaped host cell with Schüffner's dots and a ragged cell wall. Serologic tests reveal cross-reaction with *P. vivax* and other plasmodia.

Treatment, Prevention, and Control

The treatment regimen, including the use of primaquine to prevent relapse from latent liver forms, is similar to that used for *P. vivax* infections. Preventing *P. ovale* infection involves the same measures as for *P. vivax* and the other plasmodia.

Plasmodium malariae

Physiology and Structure

In contrast with *P. vivax* and *P. ovale*, *P. malariae* is able to infect only mature erythrocytes with relatively rigid cell membranes. As a result, the parasite's growth must conform to the size and shape of the red cell. This produces no red cell enlargement or distortion, as seen in *P. vivax* and *P. ovale,* but does result in distinctive shapes of the parasite seen in the host cell—"band and bar forms," as well as very compact, dark-staining forms. The schizont of *P. malariae* shows no red cell enlargement or distortion and is usually composed of eight merozoites appearing in a rosette formation. Occasionally, reddish granules called Ziemann's dots appear in the host cell.

Unlike *P. vivax* and *P. ovale*, hypnozoites for *P. malariae* are not found in the liver, and relapse does not occur. Recrudescence does occur, and attacks may develop after apparent abatement of symptoms.

Epidemiology

P. malariae infection occurs primarily in the same subtropical and temperate regions as the other plasmodia but is less prevalent.

Clinical Syndromes

The incubation period for *P. malariae* is the longest of the plasmodia, usually lasting 18 to 40 days, but possibly several months to years. The early symptoms are flu-like, with fever patterns of 72 hours (**quartan** or **malarial malaria**) in periodicity. Attacks are moderate to severe and last several hours. Untreated infections may last as long as 20 years.

Laboratory Diagnosis

Searching thick and thin films of blood for the characteristic bar and band forms, as well as the "rosette" schizont, will establish the diagnosis of *P. malariae* infection. As noted previously, serologic tests cross-react with other plasmodia.

Treatment, Prevention, and Control

Treatment is similar to that for *P. vivax* and *P. ovale* infections and must be undertaken to prevent recrudescent infections. However, treatment to prevent relapse caused by latent liver forms is not required, because these forms do not develop with *P. malariae*. Preventive and controlling mechanisms are as discussed for *P. vivax* and *P. ovale.*

Plasmodium falciparum

Physiology and Structure

P. falciparum demonstrates no selectivity in host erythrocytes and will invade any red blood cell at any stage in its existence. Also, multiple sporozoites can infect a single erythrocyte. Thus three or even four small rings may be seen in an infected cell. *P. falciparum* is often seen in the host cell at the very edge or periphery of the cell membrane, appearing almost as if it were stuck on the outside of the cell. This is called the appliqué or accolé position and is distinctive for this species.

Growing trophozoite stages and schizonts of *P. falciparum* are rarely seen in blood films because their forms are sequestered in the liver and spleen. Only in very heavy infections will they be found in the peripheral circulation. Thus examination of peripheral blood smears from patients with *P. falciparum* malaria characteristically contains only young ring forms and occasionally gametocytes. The typical crescentic gametocytes are diagnostic for the species. Infected red cells do not enlarge and become distorted, as for *P. vivax* and *P. ovale,* and only occasionally will reddish granules known for *P. falciparum* as Maurer's dots be observed.

P. *falciparum,* like *P. malariae*, does not produce hypnozoites in the liver, and relapses from the liver are not known to occur.

Epidemiology

P. falciparum occurs almost exclusively in tropical and subtropical regions.

Clinical Syndromes

The incubation period of *P. falciparum* is the shortest of the plasmodia, ranging from 7 to 10 days, and does not extend for months to years. Following the early flu-like symptoms, *P. falciparum* rapidly produces daily (quotidian) chills and fever, and severe nausea, vomiting, and diarrhea. The periodicity of the attacks then becomes tertian (36 to 48 hours), and fulminating disease develops. The term ***malignant tertian malaria*** is appropriate for this infection. Because it is similar to intestinal infections, the nausea, vomiting, and diarrhea have led to the observation that malaria is "the malignant mimic."

Although any malaria infection may be fatal, *P. falciparum* is the most likely to be so if left untreated. The increased numbers of erythrocytes infected and destroyed result in toxic cellular debris, adherence of red cells to vascular endothelium and to adjacent red cells, and formation of capillary plugging by masses of red cells, platelets, leukocytes, and malarial pigment.

Involvement of the brain (**cerebral malaria**) is most often seen in *P. falciparum* infection. Capillary plugging from an accumulation of malarial pigment and masses of cells can result in coma and death.

Kidney damage is also associated with *P. falciparum* malaria, resulting in so-called **blackwater fever.** Intravascular hemolysis with rapid destruction of red cells produces a marked hemoglobinuria and can result in acute renal failure, tubular necrosis, nephrotic syndrome, and death. Liver involvement is characterized by abdominal pain, vomiting of bile, severe diarrhea, and rapid dehydration.

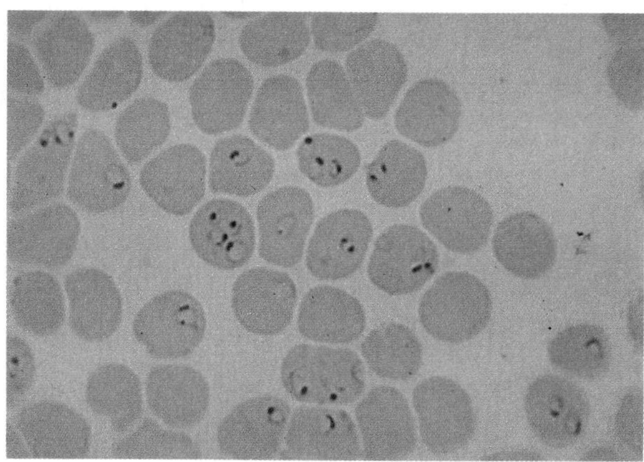

FIGURE 48-3 Ring forms of *Plasmodium falciparum.* Note the multiple ring forms within the individual erythrocytes, characteristic of *P. falciparum.*

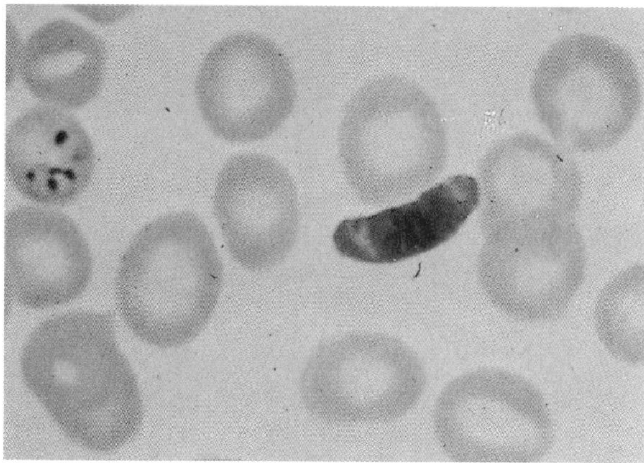

FIGURE 48-4 Mature gametocyte of *Plasmodium falciparum.* The presence of this sausage-shaped form is diagnostic of *P. falciparum* malaria.

Laboratory diagnosis

Thick and thin blood films are searched for the characteristic rings of *P. falciparum,* which can frequently occur in multiples within a single cell, as well as in the accolé position (Figure 48-3), and for the distinctive crescentic gametocytes (Figure 48-4).

Laboratory personnel must perform a thorough search of the blood films because mixed infections can occur with any combination of the four species, but most often the combination is *P. falciparum* and *P. vivax.* The detection and proper reporting of a mixed infection bears directly on the treatment modality chosen.

Treatment, Prevention, and Control

Treatment of malaria is based on the history regarding travel to endemic areas, prompt clinical review and differential diagnosis, accurate and rapid laboratory work, and correct usage of antimalarial drugs.

Because chloroquine-resistant strains of *P. falciparum* are present in many parts of the world, physicians must review all current protocols for proper treatment of *P. falciparum* infections, noting particularly where chloroquine resistance is known to occur. If the patient's history indicates the origin is not from a chloroquine-resistant area, the drug of choice is either chloroquine or parenteral quinine. Patients infected with chloroquine-resistant *P. falciparum* (or *P. vivax*) may be treated with other agents including mefloquine, quinine, quinidine, Fansidar (pyrimethamine-sulfadoxine), or doxycycline. Since quinine and Fansidar are potentially toxic, they are used more often for treatment than prophylaxis. Amodiaquine, an analogue of chloroquine, is effective against chloroquine-resistant *P. falciparum*; however, toxicity limits its use. When there is uncertainty whether the *P. falciparum* is chloroquine-resistant, it is advisable to assume the strain is resistant and treat accordingly. If the laboratory reports a mixed infection involving *P. falciparum* and *P. vivax,* the treatment must not only eradicate *P. falciparum* from the erythrocytes but also eradicate the liver stages of *P. vivax* to avoid relapses. Failure on the part of laboratory detection and reporting to establish such a mixed infection can result in inappropriate treatment and unnecessary delay in accomplishing a complete cure.

P. falciparum infection can be prevented and controlled exactly as for *P. vivax* and the other human malarias. The problem with chloroquine resistance complicates the management of these patients but can be overcome by the physician's awareness of appropriate regimens.

BABESIA

Babesia are intracellular sporozoan parasites that morphologically resemble plasmodia. Babesiosis is a zoonosis infecting a variety of animals such as deer, cattle, and rodents with humans as accidental hosts. Infection is transmitted by Ixodid ticks. *Babesia microti* is the usual cause of babesiosis in the United States.

Physiology and Structure

Human infection follows contact with an infected tick (Figure 48-5). The infectious pyriform bodies are introduced into the bloodstream and infect erythrocytes. The intraerythrocytic trophozoites multiply by binary fission, forming tetrads, and then lyse the erythrocyte, releasing the merozoites. These can reinfect other cells to maintain the infection. Infected cells can also be ingested by feeding ticks, in which additional replication can take place. Infection in the tick population can also be maintained by transovarian transmission. The infected cells in humans resemble the ring forms of *Plasmodium falciparum,* but malarial pigment or other stages of growth characteristically seen with plasmodial infections are not seen with careful examination of blood smears.

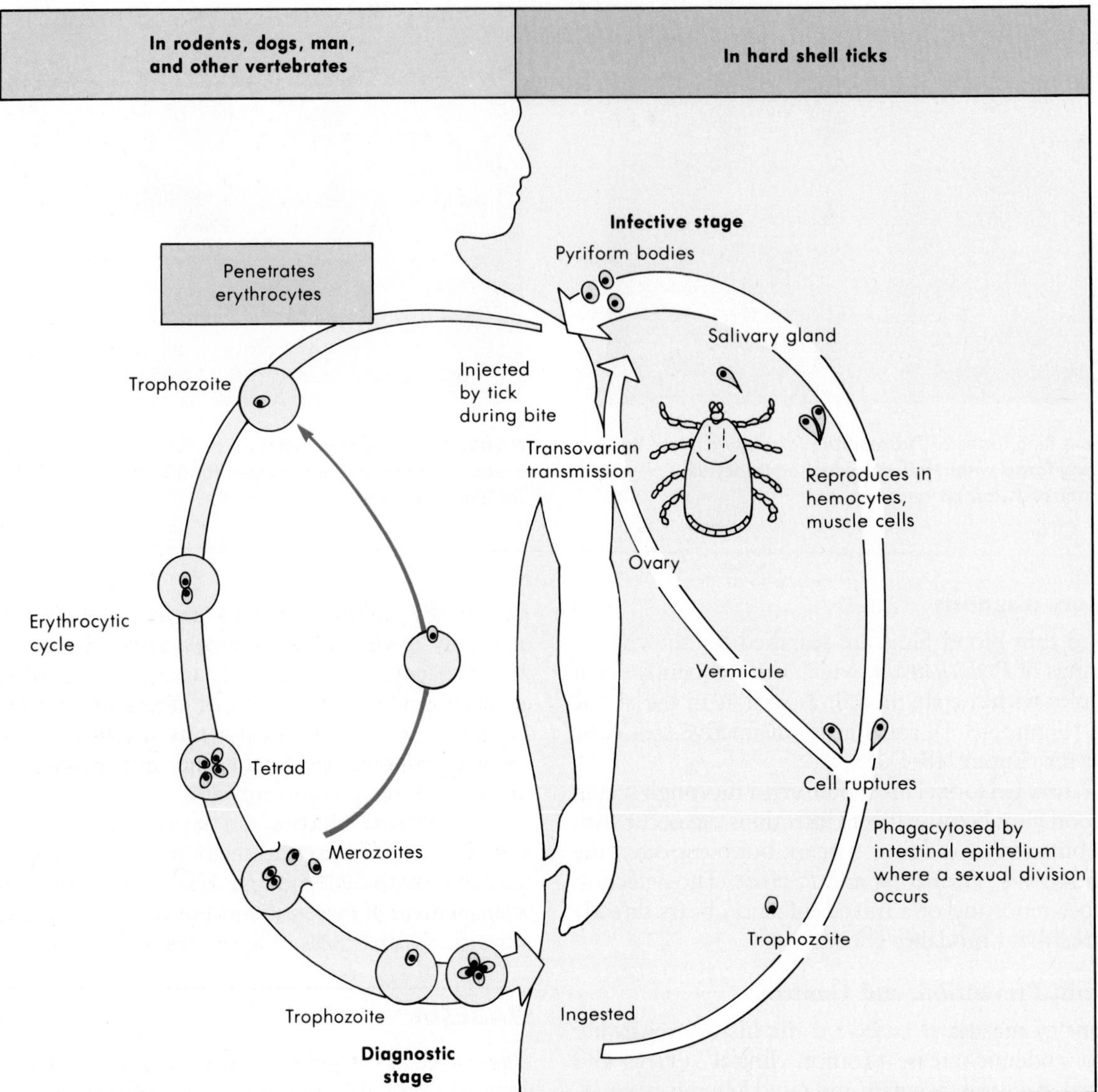

FIGURE 48-5 Life cycle of *Babesia*.

Epidemiology

More than 70 different species of *Babesia* are found in Africa, Asia, Europe, and North America, with *B. microti* responsible for disease along the northeastern seaboard of the United States (e.g., Nantucket Island, Martha's Vineyard, Shelter Island). *Ixodes dammini* is the tick vector responsible for transmitting babesiosis in this area, and the natural reservoir hosts are field mice, voles, and other small rodents. Serologic studies in endemic areas have demonstrated a high incidence of past exposure to *Babesia*. Presumably, most infections are asymptomatic or mild. *B. divergens*, which has been reported more frequently from Europe, causes severe, often fatal, infections in individuals who have undergone splenectomies. Although most infections follow tick bites, transfusion-related infections have been demonstrated.

Clinical Syndromes

After an incubation period of 1 to 4 weeks, symptomatic patients experience general malaise, fever without periodicity, headache, chills, sweating, fatigue, and weakness. As the infection progresses with increased destruction of erythrocytes, hemolytic anemia develops and the patient may experience renal failure. Hepatomegaly and splenomegaly can develop in advanced disease. Low-grade parasitemia may persist for weeks. Splenectomy or functional asplenia, immunosuppression, or advanced age increases individual susceptibility to infections, as well as more severe disease.

Laboratory Diagnosis

Examination of blood smears is the diagnostic method of choice. Laboratory personnel must be experienced in differentiating *Babesia* and *Plasmodium.* Infected patients may have negative smears because of the low-grade parasitemia. These infections can be diagnosed by inoculating samples of blood into hamsters, which are highly susceptible to infection. Serologic tests are also available for diagnosis.

Treatment, Prevention, and Control

The drugs of choice are clindamycin combined with quinine. Various other antiprotozoal regimens including chloroquine and pentamidine have been used with variable results. However, most patients with mild disease recover without specific therapy. Exchange blood transfusion has also been successful in splenectomized patients with severe infections caused by *B. microti* or *B. divergens.* The use of protective clothing and insect repellents can minimize tick exposure in endemic areas, which is critical for prevention of disease. Ticks must feed on humans for several hours before the organisms are transmitted, so prompt removal of ticks can be protective.

TOXOPLASMA GONDII

T. gondii is a typical coccidian parasite related to *Plasmodium*, *Isospora,* and other members of the phylum Apicomplexa. *T. gondii* is an intracellular parasite, and it is found in a wide variety of animals, including birds and humans. Only one species exists, and there appears to be little strain-to-strain variation. The essential reservoir host of *T. gondii* is the common house cat and other felines.

Physiology and Structure

Organisms develop in the intestinal cells of the cat, as well as during an extraintestinal cycle with passage to the tissues via the bloodstream (Figure 48-6). The organisms from the intestinal cycle are passed in cat feces and mature in the external environment within 3 to 4 days into infective oocysts. These oocysts, similar to those of *Isospora belli,* the human intestinal protozoan parasite, can be ingested by mice and other animals (including humans) and produce acute and chronic infection of various tissues, including brain. Infection in cats is established when the tissues of infected rodents are eaten.

Some infective forms or **trophozoites** from the oocyst develop as slender crescentic types called **tachyzoites.** These are rapidly multiplying forms that are responsible for both the initial infection and the tissue damage. Slow-growing, shorter forms called **bradyzoites** also develop and form cysts in chronic infections.

Epidemiology

Human infection with *T. gondii* is ubiquitous; however, it is increasingly apparent that certain immunocompromised individuals (AIDS patients) are more likely to have severe manifestations. The wide variety of animals – both carnivores and herbivores, as well as birds – harboring the organism accounts for the widespread transmission.

Humans become infected from two sources: (1) ingestion of improperly cooked meat from animals serving as intermediate hosts and (2) the ingestion of infective oocysts from cat fecal contamination. Transplacental infection from an infected mother can occur with devastating results for the fetus. Serologic studies show an increased prevalence in human populations where the consumption of uncooked meat or meat juices is popular. It is noteworthy that serologic tests of human and rodent populations are negative in the few geographical areas where cats have not existed. Outbreaks of toxoplasmosis in the United States are usually traced to poorly cooked meat (e.g., hamburgers), as well as contact with cat feces.

Transplacental infection can occur in pregnancy either from infection acquired from meat and meat juices or from contact with cat feces. Transfusion infection via contaminated blood can occur but is not common.

Although the rate of seroconversion is similar for individuals within a geographical location, the rate of severe infection is dramatically affected by the immune status of the individual. Patients with defects in cell-mediated immunity, especially those with HIV infection or following organ transplantation (or immunosuppressive therapy), are most likely to have disseminated or central nervous system disease. Illness in this setting is generally believed to be caused by reactivation of previously latent infection rather than new exposure to the organism.

Clinical Syndromes

Most *T. gondii* infections are benign and asymptomatic, with symptoms occurring as the parasite moves in the blood to tissues where it becomes an intracellular parasite. When symptomatic disease occurs, the infection is characterized by cell destruction, reproduction of more organisms, and eventual cyst formation. Many different tissues may be affected; however, the organism has a particular predilection for cells of the lung, heart, lymphoid organs, and the central nervous system including the eye.

Symptoms of acute disease include chills, fever, headaches, myalgia, lymphadenitis, and fatigue, occasionally resembling infectious mononucleosis. The chronic form symptoms are lymphadenitis, occasionally a rash, evidence of hepatitis, encephalomyelitis, and myocarditis. In some case chorioretinitis appears and may lead to blindness.

Congenital infection with *T. gondii* also occurs in infants born to mothers who are infected during pregnancy. If infected in the first trimester the result is spontaneous abortion, stillbirth, or severe disease. Manifestations in the infant infected after the first trimester include epilepsy, encephalitis, microcephaly, intracranial calcifications, hydrocephalus, psychomotor or mental retardation, chorioretinitis, blindness, anemia, jaundice, rash, pneumonia, diarrhea, and hypothermia. Infants may be asymptomatic at birth only to develop disease months to years later. Most often these children develop chorioretinitis with or without blindness, or other neurological

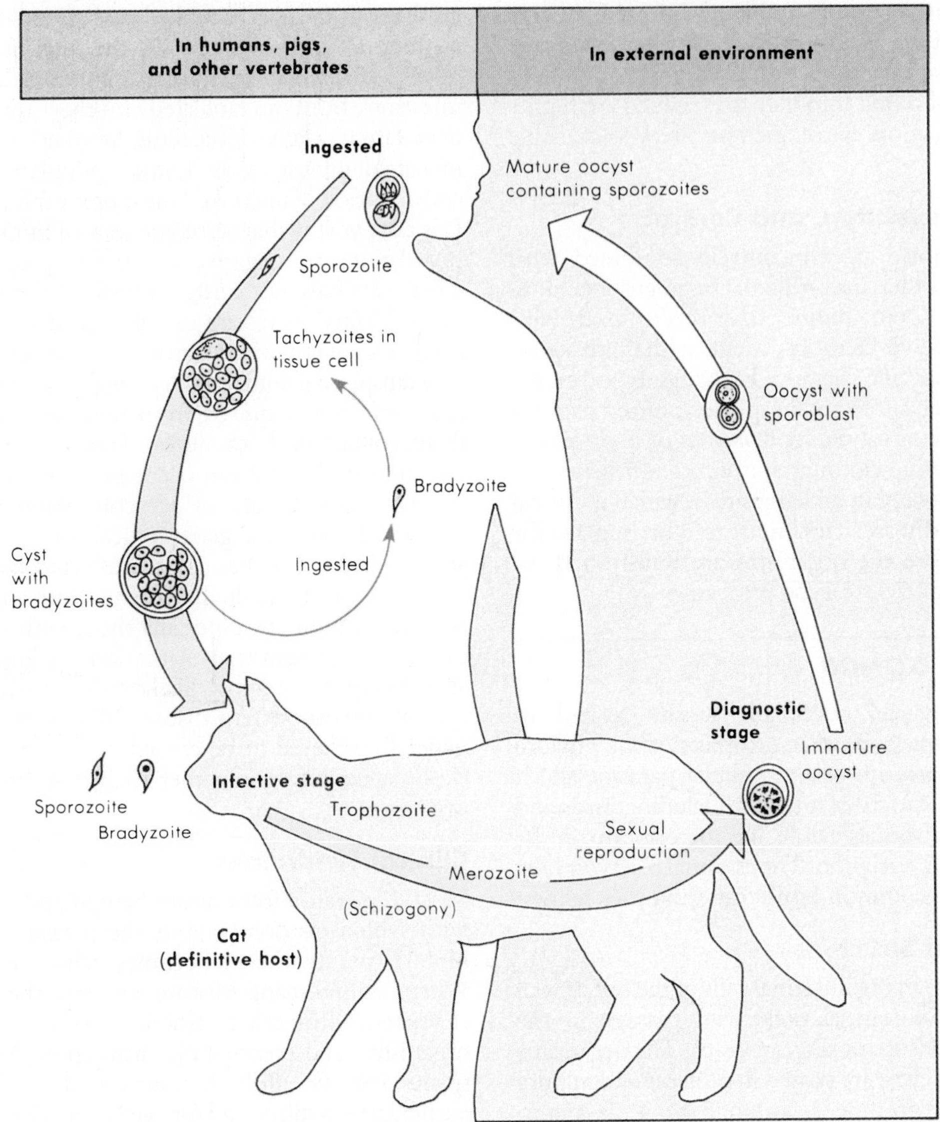

FIGURE 48-6 Life cycle of *Toxoplasma gondii.*

problems including retardation, seizures, microcephaly, or hearing loss.

In immunocompromised older individuals a different spectrum of disease is seen. Reactivation of latent toxoplasmosis is a special problem in these individuals. The presenting symptoms of *Toxoplasma* infection in immunocompromised patients are usually neurological, most frequently consistent with diffuse encephalopathy, meningoencephalitis, or cerebral mass lesions. Reactivation of cerebral toxoplasmosis has emerged as a major cause of encephalitis in patients with AIDS. The disease is usually multifocal with more than one mass lesion appearing in the brain at the same time. Symptoms are related to the location of the lesions and may include hemiparesis, seizures, visual impairment, confusion, and lethargy. Other sites of infection that have been reported include the eye, lung, and testes. Although disease is seen predominantly in patients with AIDS, it may also occur with similar manifestations in other immunocompromised patients, in particular those undergoing solid organ transplantation.

Laboratory Diagnosis

Serologic testing is required, and the diagnosis of acute active infection is established by increasing antibody titers documented in serially collected blood. Because contact with the organism is common, attention to increasing titers is essential to differentiate acute, active infection from previous asymptomatic or chronic infection. Currently the ELISA test for detecting IgM antibodies appears to be the most reliable procedure because of its simplicity and rapidity in documenting acute infections. The test is not generally satisfactory in AIDS patients with latent or reactivated infections because they fail to produce an IgM response or increasing IgG titer.

Demonstration of these organisms as trophozoites and cysts in tissue and body fluids is the definitive method of diagnosis (Figure 48-7). Biopsy specimens from lymph nodes, brain, myocardium, or other suspected tissue, or body fluids including cerebrospinal fluid, amniotic fluid, or bronchoalveolar lavage fluid can be examined directly for the organisms. Newer monoclonal antibody–based fluorescent stains may facilitate direct detection of *T. gondii* in tissue. Culture methods for *T. gondii* are largely experimental and not usually available in clinical laboratories. The two methods available are to inoculate potentially infected material into either mouse peritoneum or tissue culture.

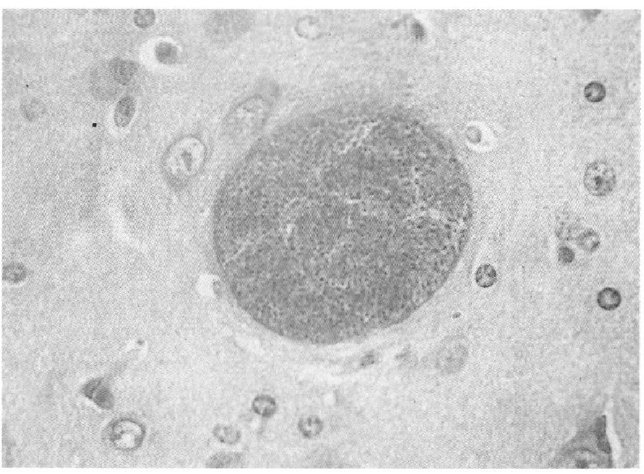

FIGURE 48-7 Cyst of *Toxoplasma gondii* in mouse brain. Hundreds of organisms may be present in the cyst, which may become active and initiate disease with decreased host immunity (e.g., immunosuppression in transplant patients, diseases such as AIDS).

Treatment, Prevention, and Control

Therapy of toxoplasmosis depends on the nature of both the infectious process and the immunocompetence of the host. Most mononucleosis-like infections in normal hosts resolve spontaneously and do not require specific therapy. In contrast, disseminated or central nervous system infection in immunocompromised individuals must be treated. Before its association with HIV infection, immunocompromised patients with toxoplasmosis were treated for 4 to 6 weeks. In the setting of HIV infection discontinuing therapy after 4 to 6 weeks is associated with a relapse rate of 25%. Such patients are currently treated with an initial high dose regimen of pyrimethamine plus sulfadiazine and then continued on lower doses of both drugs indefinitely. Although pyrimethamine plus sulfadiazine is the regimen of choice, toxicity (rash and bone marrow suppression) may necessitate changes to alternative agents. Clindamycin plus pyrimethamine is the best studied alternative. Atovaquone and azithromycin (each alone or with pyrimethamine) also have some activity, although their efficacy and safety compared to clindamycin-pyrimethamine need to be assessed. Trimethoprim-sulfamethoxazole is not an acceptable alternative to pyrimethamine-sulfadiazine for treatment of disseminated or central nervous system toxoplasmosis. The use of corticosteroids is indicated as part of therapy of cerebral edema and in ocular infections that involve or threaten the macula.

Infections in the first trimester of pregnancy are difficult to manage because of the teratogenicity of pyrimethamine in laboratory animals. Both clindamycin and spiramycin have been substituted with apparent success. Spiramycin does not appear to be effective therapy for toxoplasmosis in immunocompromised individuals.

As more immunocompromised patients at risk for disseminated infection are identified, greater emphasis is placed on preventive measures and specific prophylaxis. Routine serologic screening of patients before organ transplantation and early in the course of HIV infection is now being performed. Individuals with positive serologic tests are at much higher risk for development of disease and are now being considered for prophylaxis. Trimethoprim-sulfamethoxazole, which is also used as prophylaxis to prevent *Pneumocystis* infections, also appears to be effective at preventing infections with *T. gondii*. Additional preventive measures for pregnant women and immunocompromised hosts should include avoidance of consumption and handling of raw or undercooked meat and exposure to cat feces.

SARCOCYSTIS LINDEMANNI

S. lindemanni is a typical coccidian closely related to the intestinal forms, *S. suihominis*, *S. bovihominis*, and *Isospora belli*, and the blood and tissue parasite, *Toxoplasma gondii*. *S. lindemanni* occurs worldwide in various animals, especially sheep, cattle, and pigs. Humans are accidentally infected only as the result of eating meat from these animals. Most infections are asymptomatic, but occasionally an infection may cause myositis, swelling of muscle, dyspnea, and eosinophilia. Infection of the myocardium has been observed but is extremely rare. There is no specific treatment for the muscle infection.

PNEUMOCYSTIS CARINII

The taxonomic position of this extracellular opportunistic organism producing interstitial plasma cell pneumonia is not clear, although recent evidence indicates a relationship to fungi. However, because *Pneumocystis* has historically been placed with sporozoans in phylum Apicomplexa, it will be in this section.

Physiology and Structure

The life cycle of *P. carinii* appears to consist of a resistant cyst stage and sporozoites released from the cyst in an asexual reproductive process (sporogony). These become trophozoites and are capable of attaching to the surface of pulmonary epithelial cells. Asexual reproduction of trophozoites on cell surfaces eventually leads to the cyst stage and reproduction, producing additional sporozoites.

Epidemiology

This is a cosmopolitan organism in humans and other animals. Rodents especially have been suggested as reservoir hosts. Transmission from host to host is apparently by droplet inhalation and close contact. This opportunistic organism is present in many persons who are completely asymptomatic. Symptomatic disease, **pneumocystosis,** develops when some imbalance or debilitating illness (e.g., AIDS) is present, suggesting a long-term carrier state.

Pneumocystosis is seen primarily in premature and malnourished children in crowded institutions such as orphanages and hospitals. It is also seen in adults in chronic disease wards and is the most common opportunistic infection seen in patients with AIDS and other immune deficiencies. As many as 85% of individuals with AIDS will develop *Pneumocystis* pneumonia.

Clinical Syndromes

Pneumocystis most often causes an interstitial pneumonitis with plasma cell infiltrates. Subclinical infections in healthy individuals are probably frequent, and the organism may remain latent for long periods of time. Onset of the disease is insidious, but it can be suspected in patients who are malnourished or immunocompromised and who develop fever and pneumonitis not otherwise explainable.

As the disease progresses, the patient experiences weakness, dyspnea, and tachypnea, leading to cyanosis. Radiology of the lungs shows infiltrations spreading from hilar areas, giving the lungs a so-called "ground glass" appearance. In these cases the arterial oxygen tension is low, and carbon dioxide tension is normal or low. Death is the result of asphyxia.

In the past few years extrapulmonary infections with *P. carinii* have been described in patients with AIDS. Multiple sites of involvement have been observed, including ear, eye, liver, and bone marrow. Most such patients have received aerosolized pentamidine as prophylaxis to prevent *P. carinii* pneumonia.

Laboratory Diagnosis

Examination of stained slides of impression smears of lung tissue obtained by brush biopsy, aspirates of bronchial washings, or sputum reveals the typical *P. carinii* organisms, as well as material obtained by percutaneous transthoracic needle aspiration (Figure 48-8). Bronchoalveolar lavage fluid alone is adequate for demonstration of organisms in more than 90% of AIDS patients. Induced sputum specimens may also be useful in AIDS patients because of the tremendous organism burden. The parasites can be stained with silver or Giemsa stain, or with specific fluorescein-labeled antibodies. Radiology is of value in establishing the typical appearance of the lungs infected with *P. carinii*. Serologic tests are not available as a diagnostic procedure.

Treatment, Prevention, and Control

The drug of choice is trimethoprim-sulfamethoxazole, with pentamidine as an alternative. Supportive measures such as oxygen and antibiotics may also be indicated.

Education regarding transmission of the organism, avoidance of crowding of infected patients, and eliminating possible contact with droplet transmission are all critical, as are prompt diagnosis and treatment. The organism and its transmission are difficult to control because of the extended carrier state and its presence as an opportunistic pathogen. Prophylaxis with trimethoprim-sulfamethoxazole or aerosolized pentamidine may be useful in individuals with AIDS.

LEISHMANIA

The hemoflagellates are flagellated insect-transmitted protozoa that infect blood and tissues. Three species of *Leishmania*, a protozoan hemoflagellate, produce human disease: *L. donovani*, *L. tropica*, and *L. braziliensis* (Table 48-2). The diseases are distinguished by the ability of the organism to infect deep tissues **(visceral leishmaniasis)**

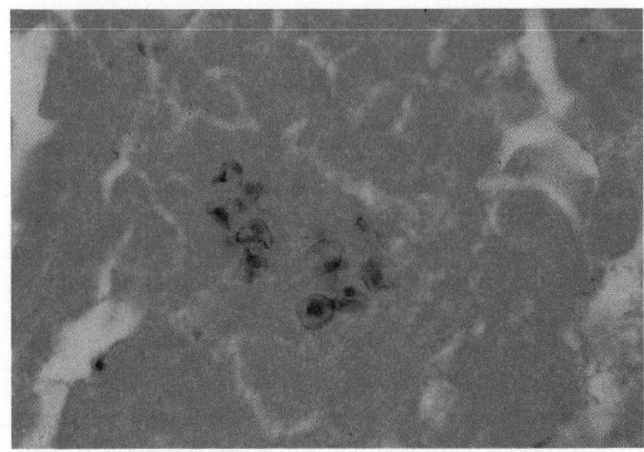

FIGURE 48-8 *Pneumocystis carinii* cysts stained with Gomori methenamine silver.

TABLE 48-2 Leishmaniasis in Humans

Parasite	Disease
L. donovani	Visceral leishmaniasis (kala-azar, dum dum fever)
L. tropica	Cutaneous leishmaniasis (Oriental sore, Delhi boil)
L. braziliensis	Mucocutaneous leishmaniasis (American leishmaniasis, espundia, chiclero ulcer)

or replicate only in cooler superficial tissues **(cutaneous** or **mucocutaneous leishmaniasis).** The reservoir hosts and geographical distribution differ for the three species, but transmission by sandflies (belonging to the genus *Phlebotomus* or *Lutzomyia*) is common to all leishmanial species.

Leishmania donovani

Physiology and Structure

The life cycles of all leishmania parasites differ in epidemiology, tissues affected, and clinical manifestations (Figure 48-9). The **promastigote** stage (long, slender form with a free flagellum) is present in the saliva of infected sandflies. Human infection is initiated by the bite of an infected sandfly, which injects the promastigotes into the skin where they lose their flagella, enter the amastigote stage, and invade reticuloendothelial cells. Reproduction occurs in the amastigote stage, and—as cells rupture—destruction of specific tissues develops (e.g., cutaneous tissues and visceral organs such as liver and spleen). The **amastigote** stage (Figure 48-10) is diagnostic for leishmaniasis, as well as the infectious stage for sandflies. Ingested amastigotes transform in the sandfly into the promastigote stage, which multiplies by binary fission in the fly midgut. After development, this stage will migrate to the fly proboscis where new human infection can be introduced during feeding.

Epidemiology

L. donovani of the classic **kala-azar** or **dum dum fever** type occurs in many parts of Asia, Africa, and Southeast Asia. Except for some rodents in Africa, there are few reservoir hosts. The vector is the *Phlebotomus* sandfly. Variants of *L. donovani* are also recognized. *L. donovani*

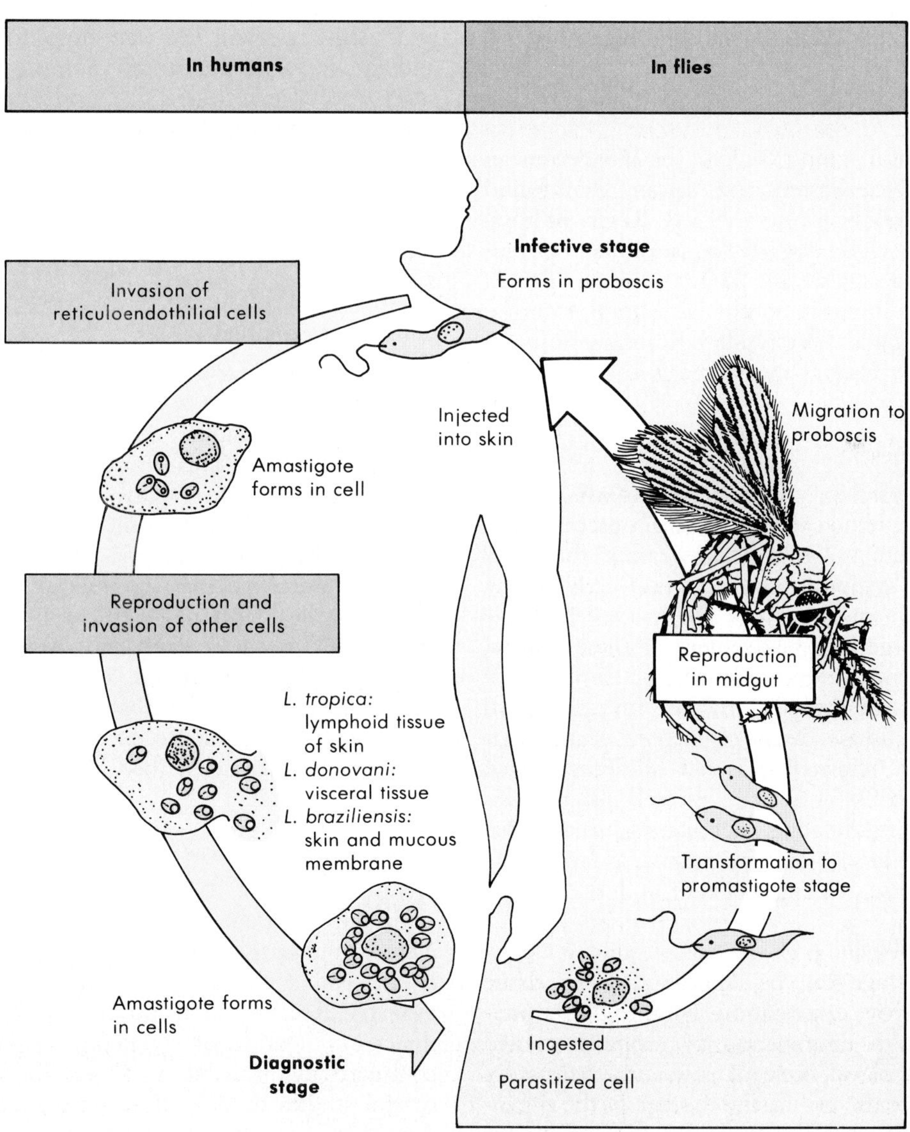

FIGURE 48-9 Life cycle of *Leishmania* species.

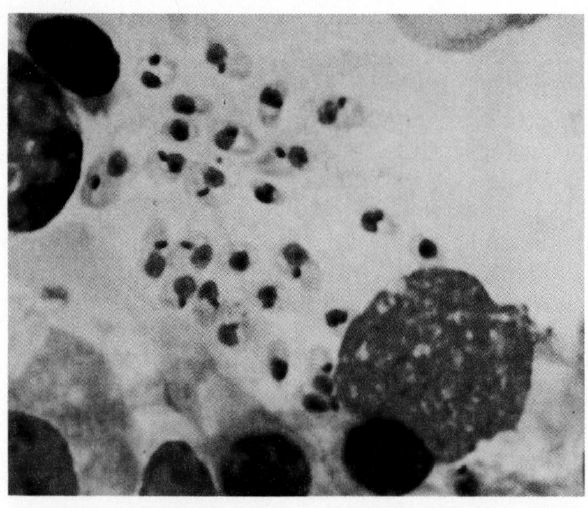

FIGURE 48-10 Giemsa-stained amastigotes (Leishman-Donovan bodies) of *Leishmania donovani* present in bone marrow. A small dark-staining kinetoplast can be seen next to the spherical nucleus in some parasites. (From Ash LR and Orihel TC: *Atlas of human parasitology*, ed 2, Chicago, 1984, American Society of Clinical Pathologists.)

infantum is present in countries along the Mediterranean basin (European, Near Eastern, and African) and is found in parts of China and the former U.S.S.R. Reservoir hosts of this organism include dogs, foxes, jackals, and porcupines. The vector is also the *Phlebotomus* sandfly. *L. donovani chagasi* is found in South and Central America, especially Mexico and the West Indies. Reservoir hosts are dogs, foxes, and cats, and the vector is the *Lutzomyia* sandfly.

Clinical Syndromes

The incubation period for **visceral leishmaniasis** may be from several weeks to a year, with gradual onset of fever, diarrhea, and anemia. Chills and sweating that may resemble malaria symptoms are common early in the infection. As organisms proliferate and invade cells of the liver and spleen, marked enlargement of these organs, weight loss, and emaciation occur. Kidney damage may also occur as cells of the glomeruli are invaded. With persistence of the disease, deeply pigmented, granulomatous areas of skin, referred to as *post–kala-azar dermal leishmaniasis,* occur. If untreated, visceral leishmaniasis develops into a fulminating, debilitating, and lethal disease in a few weeks or may persist as a chronic deteriorating disease, leading to death in 1 or 2 years.

Laboratory Diagnosis

The amastigote stage can be demonstrated in tissue biopsy, bone marrow examination, lymph node aspiration, and thorough examination of properly stained smears. Culture of blood, bone marrow, and other tissues often demonstrates the promastigote stage of the organisms. Serologic testing is also available.

Treatment, Prevention, and Control

Visceral leishmaniasis is treated with pentavalent antimonial compounds. The drug of choice is stibogluconate. Therapy is not uniformly successful, and relapse rates of 2% to 8% are seen. Alternative approaches include the addition of allopurinol or treatment with pentamidine or amphotericin B. Prompt treatment of human infections and control of reservoir hosts along with insect control help eliminate transmission of disease. Protection from sandflies by screening and insect repellents is also essential.

Leishmania tropica

Physiology and Structure

The life cycle of *L. tropica* is illustrated in Figure 48-9.

Epidemiology

Cutaneous leishmaniasis produced by *L. tropica* is present in many parts of Asia, Africa, Mediterranean Europe, and the southern region of the former U.S.S.R. In these regions the reservoir hosts are dogs, foxes, and rodents, and the vector is the sandfly *Phlebotomus.* Two related species are also recognized. *L. aethiopica* is endemic in Ethiopia, Kenya, and Yemen, with dogs and rodents as reservoir hosts and the vector the *Phlebotomus* sandfly. *L. mexicana* occurs in South and Central America, especially in the Amazon basin, with sloths, rodents, monkeys, and raccoons as reservoir hosts. The vector is the *Lutzomyia* sandfly.

Clinical Syndromes

The incubation period after a sandfly bite may be as short as 2 weeks, or 2 months may elapse before the first sign, a red papule, appears at the site of the fly's bite and feeding. This lesion becomes irritated, with intense itching, and begins to enlarge and ulcerate. Gradually, the ulcer becomes hard and crusted and exudes a thin serous material. At this stage secondary bacterial infection may complicate the disease. The lesion may heal without treatment in a matter of months but usually leaves a disfiguring scar. A disseminated nodular type of cutaneous leishmaniasis has been reported from Ethiopia, probably caused by an allergy to *L. aethiopica* antigens. Recently, a viscerotropic form of *L. tropica* has been described in persons returning from the Persian Gulf.

Laboratory Diagnosis

Demonstration of the amastigotes in properly stained smears from touch preparations or ulcer biopsy and culture of ulcer tissue are appropriate laboratory methods to determine the diagnosis. Serologic tests are also available. Recently, DNA probes have been developed for direct examination of cutaneous lesions. There are no commercially available products for these tests, and careful studies to determine accuracy of testing procedures have not yet been performed.

Treatment, Prevention, and Control

The drug of choice is stibogluconate, with an alternative treatment of applying heat directly to the lesion. Protection from sandfly bites using screening, protective clothing, and repellents is essential. Prompt treatment and eradication of the ulcers to prevent transmission, along with control of sandflies and reservoir hosts, will reduce the incidence of human infection.

Leishmania braziliensis

Physiology and Structure

The life cycle of *L. braziliensis* is illustrated in Figure 48-9.

Epidemiology

Mucocutaneous leishmaniasis produced by *L. braziliensis* is seen from the Yucatan peninsula into Central and South America, especially in those rain forests where chicle workers are exposed to sandfly bites while harvesting the chicle sap for chewing gum (thus the name **chiclero ulcer**). There are many jungle reservoir hosts, as well as domestic dogs. The vector is the *Lutzomyia* sandfly. The variant *L. braziliensis panamensis* is similar in all respects to *L. braziliensis* except for its more frequent occurrence in Panama and slight difference in growth in cultures. Reservoir hosts and the vector are similar to *L. braziliensis.*

Clinical Syndromes

The incubation period and appearance of ulcers for *L. braziliensis* are similar to *L. tropica,* requiring a few weeks to months for the papule to appear. The essential difference in clinical disease is the involvement and destruction of mucous membranes and related tissue structures. This is often combined with edema and secondary bacterial infection to produce severe and disfiguring facial mutilation.

Laboratory Diagnosis

The diagnostic tests are similar for all *Leishmania.* Organisms are demonstrated in ulcers or cultured tissue. Serologic testing is also available.

Treatment, Prevention, and Control

The drug of choice is stibogluconate; an alternative is amphotericin B. As with all the other leishmania complexes, screening, protective clothing, insect repellents, and prompt treatment are needed to prevent transmission and control disease. The protection of forest and construction workers in endemic areas is most difficult, and disease in those places may be effectively controlled only by vaccination. Work to develop a vaccine is currently under way.

TRYPANOSOMES

Trypanosoma, another hemoflagellate, causes two distinctly different forms of disease (Table 48-3). One is called **African trypanosomiasis,** or **sleeping sickness,** and is produced by *Trypanosoma brucei gambiense* and *T. brucei rhodesiense.* It is transmitted by tsetse flies. The second infection is called **American trypanosomiasis,** or **Chagas' disease,** produced by *T. cruzi.* It is transmitted by true bugs (triatomids, reduviids—so-called kissing bugs).

TABLE 48-3 *Trypanosoma* Species Responsible for Human Diseases

Parasite	Vector	Disease
T. brucei sspp. *gambiense* sspp. *rhodesiense*	Tsetse fly	African trypanosomiasis (sleeping sickness)
T. cruzi	Reduviids	American trypanosomiasis (Chagas' disease)

Trypanosoma brucei gambiense

Physiology and Structure

The life cycle of the African forms of trypanosomiasis is illustrated in Figure 48-11. The infective stage of the organism is the **trypomastigote,** present in the salivary glands of transmitting tsetse flies. This stage has a free flagellum and an undulating membrane running the full length of the body. The trypomastigotes enter the wound created by the fly bite and find their way into blood and lymph, eventually invading the central nervous system. Reproduction of the trypomastigotes in blood, lymph, and spinal fluid is by binary or longitudinal fission. These trypomastigotes in blood are then infective for biting tsetse flies, where further reproduction occurs in the midgut. The organisms then migrate to the salivary glands where an **epimastigote** form (having a free flagellum but only a partial undulating membrane) continues reproduction to the infective trypomastigote stage. Tsetse flies become infective 4 to 6 weeks after feeding on blood from a diseased patient.

Epidemiology

T. brucei gambiense is limited to tropical West and Central Africa, correlating to the range of the tsetse fly vector. The tsetse flies transmitting *T. brucei gambiense* prefer shaded stream banks for reproduction and proximity to human dwellings. Persons who work in such areas are at greatest risk of infection. An animal reservoir has not been proved, although several species of animals have been infected experimentally.

Clinical Syndromes

The incubation period of Gambian sleeping sickness varies from a few days to weeks. *T. brucei gambiense* produces chronic disease, often ending fatally, with central nervous system involvement after several years' duration. One of

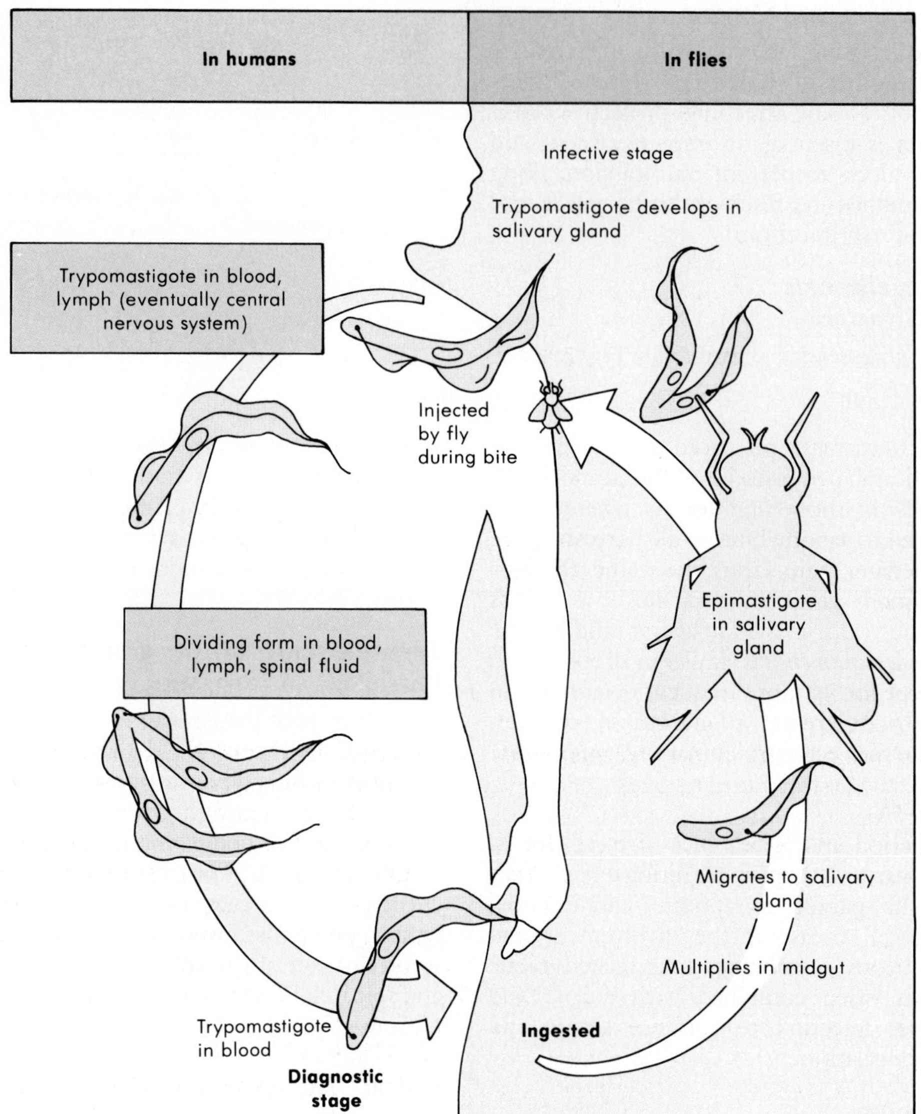

FIGURE 48-11 Life cycle of *Trypanosoma brucei*.

the earliest signs of disease is an occasional ulcer at the site of the fly bite. As reproduction of organisms continues, the lymph nodes are invaded and fever, myalgia, arthralgia, and lymph node enlargement result. Swelling of the posterior cervical lymph nodes is characteristic of Gambian disease and is called Winterbottom's sign. Patients in this acute phase often exhibit hyperactivity.

Chronic disease progresses to central nervous system involvement with lethargy, tremors, meningoencephalitis, mental retardation, and general deterioration. In the final stages of chronic disease, convulsions, hemiplegia, and incontinence occur, and the patient becomes difficult to arouse or respond, eventually progressing to a comatose state. Death is the result of central nervous system damage, combined with other infections such as malaria or pneumonia.

Laboratory Diagnosis

Organisms can be demonstrated in thick and thin blood films, in concentrated anticoagulated blood preparations, and in aspirations from lymph nodes and concentrated spinal fluid. Methods for concentrating parasites in blood may be helpful. Approaches include centrifugation of heparinized samples or anion-exchange chromatography. Levels of parasitemia vary widely, and several attempts to visualize the organism over a number of days may be necessary. Preparations should be fixed and stained immediately to avoid disintegration of the trypomastigotes. Serologic tests are also useful diagnostic techniques. Immunofluorescence, ELISA, precipitin, and agglutination methods have been used. Most reagents for such tests are not available commercially.

Treatment, Prevention, and Control

In the acute stages of the disease the drug of choice is suramin, with pentamidine as an alternative. In chronic disease with central nervous system involvement the drug of choice is melarsoprol, with alternatives of tryparsamide combined with suramin. DL-α-difluoromethylornithine (DFMO) has recently been introduced and holds promise for treatment of all stages of disease.

The most essential elements are control of breeding sites of the tsetse flies by clearing brush, using insecticides, and treating human cases to reduce transmission to flies. Persons going into known endemic areas should wear protective clothing and use screening, bed netting, and insect repellents.

Trypanosoma brucei rhodesiense

Physiology and Structure

The life cycle is similar to *T. brucei gambiense* (see Figure 48-11), with both trypomastigote and epimastigote stages and transmission by tsetse flies.

Epidemiology

The organism is found primarily in East Africa, especially the cattle-raising countries where tsetse flies breed in the brush rather than stream banks. *T. brucei rhodesiense* also differs from *T. brucei gambiense* in having domestic animal hosts (cattle and sheep) and wild game animals as reservoir hosts. This transmission and vector cycle makes the organism much more difficult to control than *T. brucei gambiense*.

Clinical Syndromes

The incubation period for *T. brucei rhodesiense* is shorter than for *T. brucei gambiense*. Acute disease (fever, rigors, and myalgia) occurs more rapidly and progresses to a fulminating, rapidly fatal illness. Infected persons are usually dead within 9 to 12 months if untreated.

This more virulent organism also develops in greater numbers in the blood, without lymphadenopathy, and CNS invasion occurs early in the infection, with lethargy, anorexia, and mental disturbance. The chronic stages described for *T. brucei gambiense* are not often seen because, in addition to rapid CNS disease, the organism produces kidney damage and myocarditis leading to death.

Laboratory Diagnosis

Examination of blood and spinal fluid is carried out as for *T. brucei gambiense* (Figure 48-12). Serologic tests are available; however, the marked variability of the surface antigens of trypanosomes limits the diagnostic usefulness of this approach.

Treatment, Prevention, and Control

The same treatment protocol applies as for *T. brucei gambiense*, with early treatment for the more rapid neurological manifestations. Similar prevention and control measures are needed: tsetse fly control and use of protective clothing, screens, netting, and insect repellent. In addition, early treatment is essential to control transmission, detect infection, and determine treatment in domestic animals. Control of infection in game animals is difficult, but infection can be reduced if tsetse fly control measures, specifically eradication of brush and grassland breeding sites, are applied.

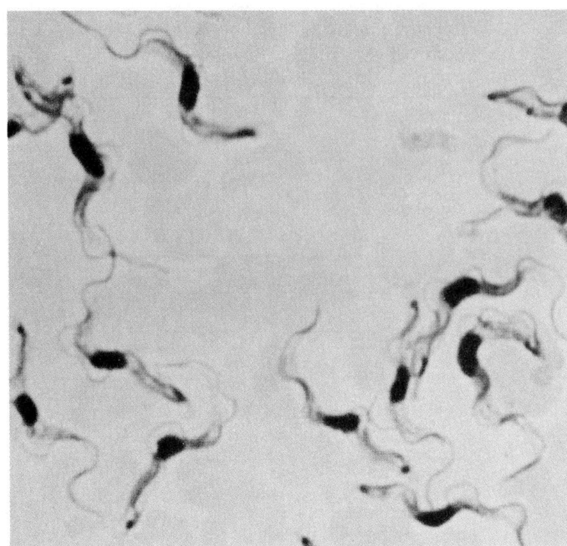

FIGURE 48-12 Trypomastigote stage of *Trypanosoma gambiense* in a blood smear. (From Ash LR and Orihel TC: *Atlas of human parasitology*, ed 2, Chicago, 1984, American Society of Clinical Pathologists.)

Trypanosoma cruzi

Physiology and Structure

The life cycle of *T. cruzi* (Figure 48-13) differs from *T. brucei* with the development of an additional form called an amastigote (Figure 48-14). The amastigote is an intracellular form with no flagellum and no undulating membrane. It is smaller than the trypomastigote, oval, and found in tissues. The infective trypomastigote, present in the feces of a reduviid bug ("kissing bug"), enters the wound created by the biting, feeding bug. The bugs have been called kissing bugs because they frequently bite people around the mouth and in other facial sites. They are notorious for biting, feeding on blood and tissue juices, and then defecating into the wound. The organisms in the feces of the bug enter the wound and are usually aided in penetration by the patient's rubbing or scratching the irritated site.

The trypomastigotes then migrate to other tissues (e.g., cardiac muscle, liver, brain), lose the flagellum and undulating membrane, and become the smaller, oval, intracellular amastigote form. These intracellular amastigotes multiply by binary fission and eventually destroy the host cells. Then they are liberated to enter new host tissue as intracellular amastigotes or to become trypomastigotes

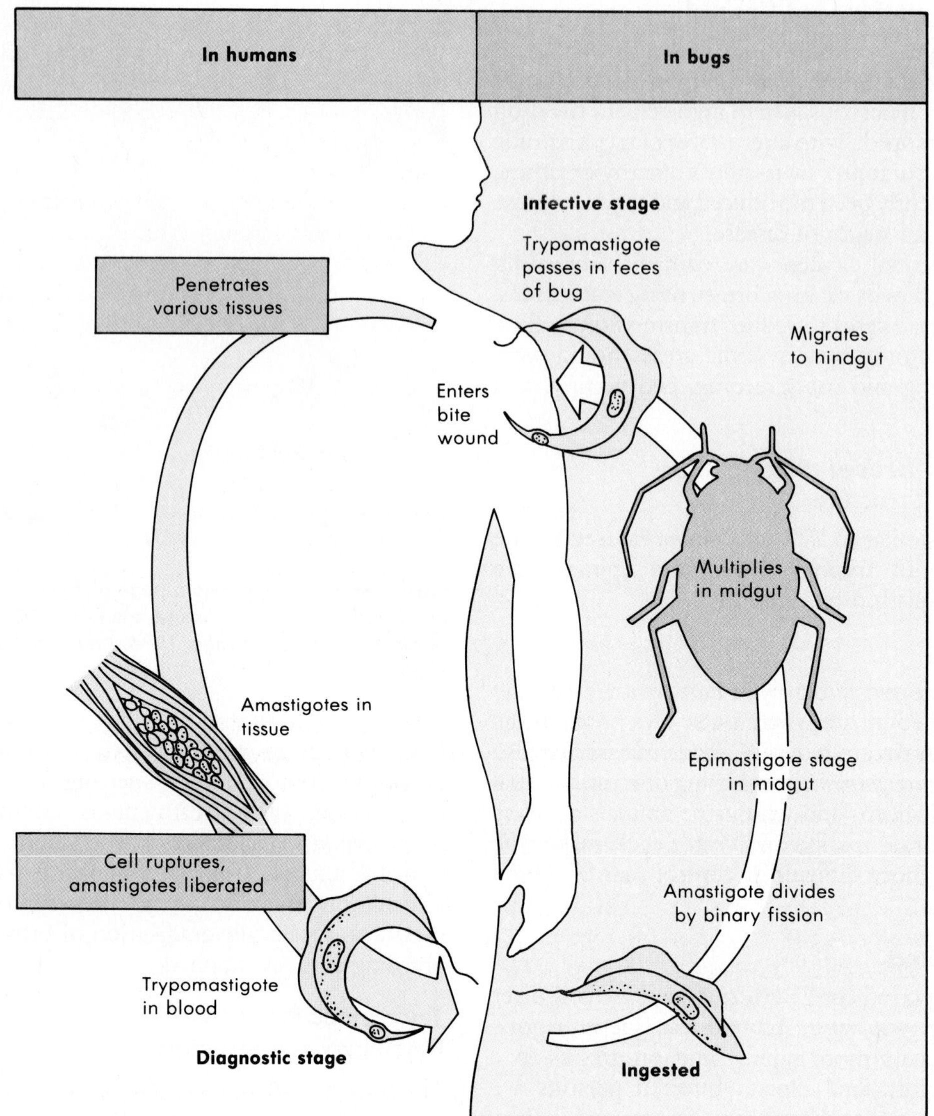

FIGURE 48-13 Life cycle of *Trypanosoma cruzi.*

infective for feeding reduviid bugs. Ingested trypomastigotes develop into epimastigotes in the midgut of the insect and reproduce by longitudinal binary fission. The organisms migrate to the hindgut of the bug, develop into metacyclic trypomastigotes, and then leave the bug in the feces after biting, feeding, and defecating, initiating a new human infection.

Epidemiology

T. cruzi occurs widely in both reduviid bugs and a broad spectrum of reservoir animals in North, Central, and South America. Human disease is found most often among children in South and Central America, where there is a direct correlation between infected wild animal reservoir hosts and the presence of infected bugs whose nests are found in human homes. Cases are rare in the United States because the bugs prefer nesting in animal burrows and because homes are not as open to nesting as those in South and Central America.

Clinical Syndromes

Chagas' disease may be asymptomatic, acute, or chronic. One of the earliest signs is development at the site of the bug bite of an erythematous and indurated area called a **chagoma.** This is often followed by a rash and edema around the eyes and face. The disease is most severe in children less than 5 years of age and frequently is seen as an acute process with central nervous system involvement. Acute infection is also characterized by fever, chills, malaise, myalgia, and fatigue. Parasites may be present in the blood during the acute phase; however, they are sparse in patients older than 1 year. Death may ensue a few weeks after an acute attack, the patient may recover, or the patient may enter the chronic phase as organisms

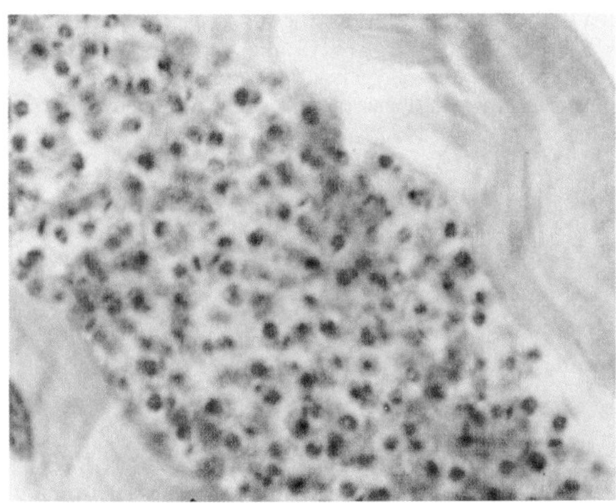

FIGURE 48-14 Amastigote stage of *Trypanosoma cruzi* in skeletal muscle. (From Ash LR and Orihel TC: *Atlas of human parasitology*, ed 2, Chicago, 1984, American Society of Clinical Pathologists.)

proliferate and enter the heart, liver, spleen, brain, and lymph nodes.

Chronic Chagas' disease is characterized by hepatosplenomegaly, myocarditis, and enlargement of the esophagus and colon as a result of destruction of nerve cells (e.g., Auerbach's plexus) and other tissues controlling the growth of these organs.

Megacardium and electrocardiographic changes are commonly seen in chronic disease. Involvement of the central nervous system may produce granulomas in the brain with cyst formation and a meningoencephalitis. Death from chronic Chagas' disease results from tissue destruction in the many areas invaded by the organisms, and sudden death results from complete heart block and brain damage.

Laboratory Diagnosis

T. cruzi can be demonstrated in thick and thin blood films or concentrated anticoagulated blood early in the acute stage. As the infection progresses, the organisms leave the bloodstream and become difficult to find. Biopsy of lymph nodes, liver, spleen, or bone marrow may demonstrate the organisms in the amastigote stage. Culture of blood or inoculation into laboratory animals may be useful when the parasitemia is low. Serologic tests are also available. In endemic areas, xenodiagnosis is widely used.

Treatment, Prevention, and Control

Treatment of Chagas' disease is limited by the lack of reliable agents. The drug of choice is nifurtimox. Although it has some activity against the acute phase of disease, it has little activity against tissue amastigotes and has a number of side effects. Alternative agents include allopurinol and benzimidazole, an imidazole compound. Education regarding the disease, its insect transmission, and the wild animal reservoirs is critical. Bug control, eradication of nests, and construction of homes to prevent nesting of bugs are also essential. The use of DDT in bug-infested homes has demonstrated a drop in both malaria and Chagas' disease transmission. Screening of blood by serologic means or excluding blood donors from endemic areas prevents some infections that would otherwise be associated with transfusion therapy.

Development of a vaccine is possible because *T. cruzi* does not have the wide antigenic variation observed with the African trypanosomes.

CASE STUDY AND QUESTIONS

The patient was a 44-year-old female heart transplant patient, approximately 1 year after transplant. The patient complains to her primary physician about headache, nausea, and vomiting. She has no skin lesions. A head CT scan demonstrates ring-enhancing lesions. A biopsy of the lesions is performed. All cultures (bacterial, fungal, viral) are negative. Special stains of the tissue revealed multiple cystlike structures of varying size.

1. What is the differential diagnosis of infectious agents in this patient? What is the most likely etiological agent?
2. What other tests would you do to confirm the diagnosis?
3. What aspects of the medical history might suggest a risk for infection with this agent?
4. What are the therapeutic options and the likelihood of successful therapy?

Bibliography

Beaver PC, Jung RC, and Cupp EW: *Clinical parasitology*, ed 9, Philadelphia, 1984, Lea & Febiger.

Benenson MW et al.: Oocyst-transmitted toxoplasmosis associated with ingestion of contaminated water, *N Engl J Med* 307:666-669, 1982.

Bittencourt AL et al.: Esophageal involvement in congenital Chagas' disease: report of a case with megaesophagus, *Am J Trop Med Hyg* 33:30-33, 1984.

Bruce-Chwatt LJ: The challenge of malaria vaccine: trials and tribulations, *Lancet* 1:371-373, 1987.

Corredor A et al.: Epidemiology of visceral leishmaniasis in Colombia, *Am J Trop Med Hyg* 40:480-486, 1989.

Cregan P, Yamamoto A, Lum A et al.: Comparison of four methods for rapid detection of *Pneumocystis carinii* in respiratory specimens, *J Clin Microbiol* 28:2432-2436, 1990.

Edman JC, Kovacs JA, Masur H et al.: Ribosomal RNA sequence shows *Pneumocystis carinii* to be a member of the fungi, *Nature* 334:19-22, 1988.

Gombert ME et al.: Human babesiosis: clinical and therapeutic considerations, *JAMA* 248:3005-3007, 1982.

Howard BJ et al.: *Clinical and pathogenic microbiology*, St. Louis, 1987, Mosby.

Kreutzer BD et al.: Identification of *Leishmania* sp. by multiple isozyme analysis, *Am J Trop Med Hyg* 32:703-715, 1983.

Luft BJ and Remington JS: Toxoplasmic encephalitis, *J Infect Dis* 157:1-6, 1988.

Markell EK, Voge M, and John DT; *Medical parasitology*, ed 7, Philadelphia, 1992, WB Saunders.

Northfelt D, Clement MJ, and Safrin S: Extrapulmonary pneumocystosis: clinical features in human immunodeficiency virus infection, *Medicine* 69:392-398, 1990.

Rieckmann KH et al.: *Plasmodium vivax* resistance to chloroquine? *Lancet* 2:1183-1184, 1989.

Sharma GK: Malaria: a critical review, *J Commun Dis* 19:187-290, 1987.

Wong B et al.: Central nervous system toxoplasmosis in homosexual men and parenteral drug abusers, *Ann Intern Med* 100:36-42, 1984.

bacterial infection. Worms that migrate into the vagina may produce genitourinary problems and granulomas.

There is evidence that worms attached to the bowel wall may produce inflammation and granuloma formation around the eggs. Although the adult worms may occasionally invade the appendix, there remains no proven relationship between pinworm invasion and appendicitis. Penetration through the bowel wall into the peritoneal cavity, liver, and lungs has been recorded infrequently.

Laboratory Diagnosis

The diagnosis of enterobiasis is usually suggested by the clinical manifestations and confirmed by detection of the characteristic eggs on the anal mucosa. Occasionally, the adult worms are seen by laboratory personnel in stool specimens, but the method of choice for diagnosis involves use of an anal swab with a sticky surface that picks up the eggs (Figure 49-2) for microscopic examination. Sampling can be done with clear tape or commercially available swabs. The sample should be collected when the child arises, before bathing or defecation, to pick up eggs laid by migrating worms during the night. Parents can collect the specimen and deliver it to the physician for immediate microscopic examination. Three swabbings, one per day for 3 consecutive days, may be required for detecting the diagnostic eggs. The eggs are rarely seen in fecal specimens. Systemic signs of infection such as eosinophilia are rare.

Treatment, Prevention, and Control

The drug of choice is pyrantel pamoate; as an alternative drug, mebendazole is used. To avoid reintroduction of the organism and reinfection in the family environment, it is customary to treat the entire family simultaneously. Although cure rates are high, reinfection is common. Repeat treatment after 2 weeks may be useful in preventing reinfection.

Personal hygiene, clipping of fingernails, thorough washing of bed clothes, and prompt treatment of infected individuals all contribute to control. When housecleaning is done in the home of an infected family, dusting under beds, on window sills, and over doors should be done with a damp mop to avoid inhalation of infectious eggs.

ASCARIS LUMBRICOIDES

Physiology and Structure

These large (20 to 35 cm in length) pink worms have a more complex life cycle than *Enterobius vermicularis* (Figure 49-3) but are otherwise typical of an intestinal roundworm.

The ingested infective egg releases a larval worm that penetrates the duodenal wall, enters the bloodstream, is carried to the liver and the heart, and then enters the pulmonary circulation. The larvae break free in the alveoli of the lungs, where they grow and molt. In about 3 weeks the larvae pass from the respiratory system to be coughed up, swallowed, and returned to the small intestine.

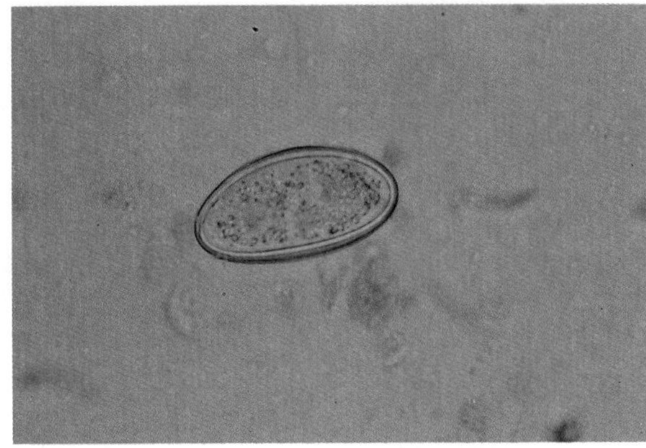

FIGURE 49-2 *Enterobius vermicularis* egg. The thin-walled eggs are 50 to 60 μm by 20 to 30 μm, ovoid, and flattened on one side (not because children sit on them—but this is an easy way to correlate the egg morphology with the epidemiology of the disease).

As the male and female worms mature in the small intestine (primarily jejunum), fertilization of the female by the male initiates egg production, which may amount to 200,000 eggs per day for as long as a year. Female worms can also produce unfertilized eggs in the absence of males. Eggs are found in the feces 60 to 75 days after the initial infection. Fertilized eggs become infectious after approximately 2 weeks in the soil.

Epidemiology

Ascaris lumbricoides is prevalent in areas of poor sanitation and where human feces are used as fertilizer. Because both food and water are contaminated with *Ascaris* eggs, this parasite more than any other affects the world's population. Although no animal reservoir is known for *A. lumbricoides,* an almost identical species from pigs, *Ascaris suum,* can infect humans. This species is seen in swine growers and is associated with the use of pig manure for gardening. *Ascaris* eggs are quite hardy and can survive extreme temperatures and persist for several months in feces and sewage. Ascariasis is the most common helminth worldwide, with an estimated 1 billion individuals infected.

Clinical Syndromes

Infections that are caused by the ingestion of only a few eggs may produce no symptoms; however, even a single adult ascaris may be dangerous because it can migrate into the bile duct and liver and create tissue damage. Furthermore, because the worm has a tough flexible body, it can occasionally perforate the intestine, creating peritonitis with secondary bacterial infection. The adult worms do not attach to the intestinal mucosa but depend on constant motion to maintain their position within the bowel lumen.

Following infection with many larvae, migration of worms to the lungs can produce pneumonitis resembling

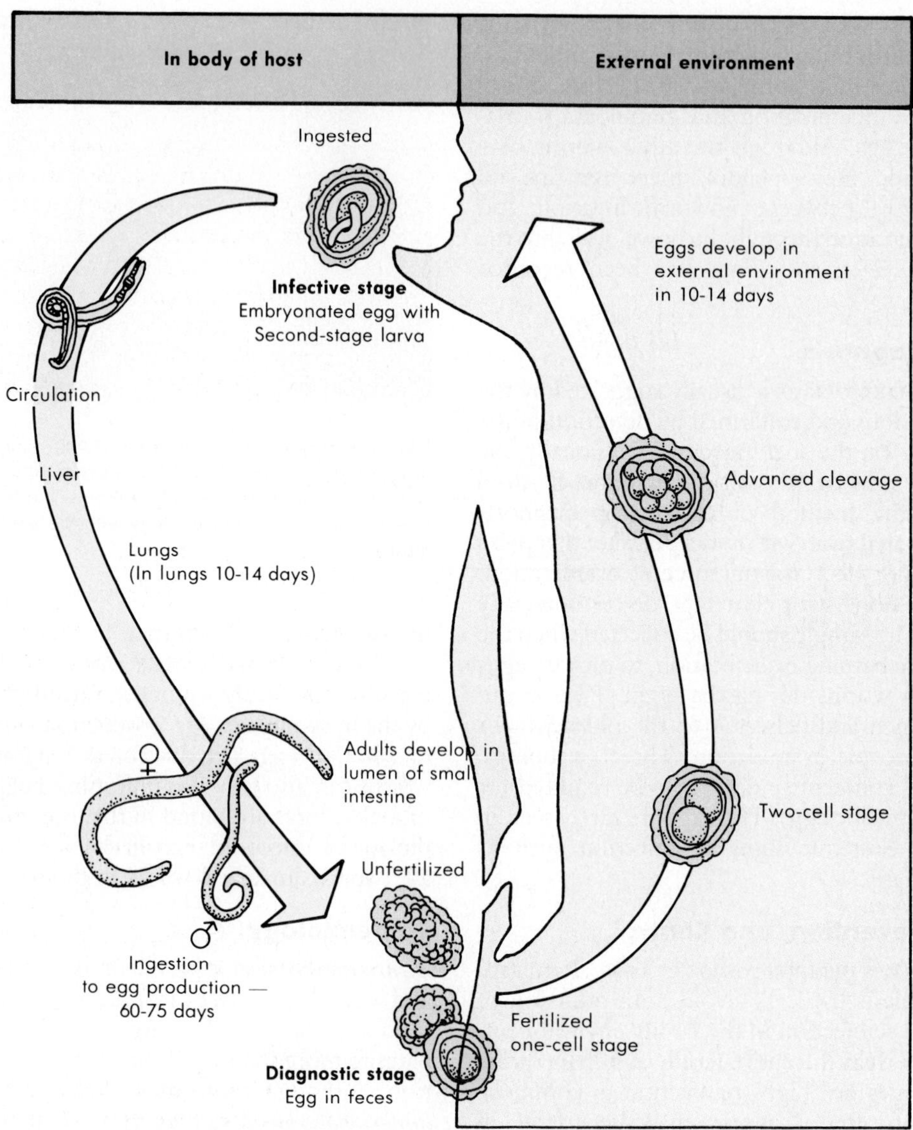

FIGURE 49-3 Life cycle of *Ascaris lumbricoides.*

an asthmatic attack. Pulmonary involvement is related to the degree of hypersensitivity induced by previous infections and the intensity of the current exposure and may be accompanied by eosinophilia and oxygen desaturation. Also, a tangled bolus of mature worms in the intestine can result in obstruction, perforation, and occlusion of the appendix. As mentioned previously, migration into the bile duct, gallbladder, and liver can produce severe tissue damage. This migration can occur in response to fever, drugs other than those used to treat ascariasis, and some anesthetics. Patients with many larvae may also experience abdominal tenderness, fever, distention, and vomiting.

Laboratory Diagnosis

Examination of the sediment of concentrated stool reveals the knobby-coated, bile-stained, fertilized and unfertilized eggs. Eggs are oval, 55 to 75 μm long and 50 μm wide. The thick-walled outer shell can be partially removed (decorticated egg). Occasionally, adult worms pass with the feces, which can be quite dramatic because of their large size (20 to 35 cm long). Roentgenologists may also visualize the worms in the intestine, and cholangiograms often disclose their presence in the biliary tract of the liver. The pulmonary phase of the disease may be diagnosed by the finding of larvae and eosinophils in sputum.

Treatment, Prevention, and Control

Treatment of symptomatic infection is highly effective. The drug of choice is mebendazole; pyrantel pamoate and piperazine are alternatives. Patients with mixed parasitic infections *(Ascaris lumbricoides* and other helminths, *Giardia lamblia,* and *Entamoeba histolytica)* in the stool should be treated for ascariasis first to avoid provoking worm migration and possible intestinal perforation.

Education, improved sanitation, and avoidance of human feces as fertilizer are critical. A program of mass treatment in highly endemic areas has been suggested, but this may not be economically feasible. Furthermore, eggs can persist in contaminated soil for 3 years or more. Certainly, improved personal hygiene among individuals who handle food is an important aspect of control.

TOXOCARA CANIS AND *T. CATI*

Physiology and Structure

Toxocara canis and *T. cati* are ascarid worms naturally parasitic in the intestines of dogs and cats that accidentally infect humans, producing a disease called **visceral larval migrans** or **toxocariasis.** When ingested by humans, the eggs of these worms can hatch into larval forms that cannot follow the normal developmental cycle as in the natural dog or cat host. They can penetrate the human gut and reach the bloodstream and then migrate as larvae to various human tissues. They do not develop beyond the migrating larval form.

Epidemiology

Wherever infected dogs and cats are present, the eggs are a threat to humans. This is especially true for children who are exposed more readily to contaminated soil and who tend to put objects in their mouth.

Clinical Syndromes

The clinical manifestations of toxocariasis in humans are related to the migration of the larvae through tissues. The larvae may invade any tissue of the body, where they can induce bleeding, the formation of eosinophilic granulomas, and necrosis. Patients may be asymptomatic and have only eosinophilia, but they can also have serious disease directly related to the number and location of the lesions caused by the migrating larvae and the degree to which the host is sensitized to the larval antigens. The organs most frequently involved include the lungs, heart, kidney, liver, skeletal muscles, eye, and central nervous system. Signs and symptoms include cough, wheezing, fever, rash, anorexia, seizures, fatigue, and abdominal discomfort. On examination, patients may have hepatosplenomegaly, as well as nodular pruritic skin lesions. Death may result from respiratory failure, cardiac arrhythmia, or brain damage. Ocular disease can also occur with the movement of larvae through the eye and may be mistaken for malignant retinoblastoma. Prompt diagnosis is required to avoid unnecessary enucleation.

Laboratory Diagnosis

Diagnosis of visceral larval migrans is based on clinical findings, the presence of eosinophilia, known exposure to dogs or cats, and serologic confirmation. ELISA assays are readily available and appear to offer the best serologic marker for disease. Examination of feces from infected patients is not useful because egg-laying adults are not present. However, examination of fecal material from infected pets often supports the diagnosis. Tissue examination for larvae may provide a definitive diagnosis but may be negative because of sampling error.

Treatment, Prevention, and Control

Treatment is primarily symptomatic since antiparasitic agents are not of proven benefit. The drug of choice is diethylcarbamazine or thiabendazole. Mebendazole is an acceptable alternative. Corticosteroid therapy may be lifesaving if the patient has serious pulmonary, myocardial, or central nervous system involvement since a major component of the infection is an inflammatory response to the organism. This zoonosis can be greatly reduced if pet owners conscientiously eradicate worms from their animals and clean up pet fecal material from yards and school playgrounds. Children's play areas and sandboxes should be carefully monitored.

TRICHURIS TRICHIURA

Physiology and Structure

Commonly called **"whipworm"** because it resembles the handle and lash of a whip, *T. trichiura* has a simple life cycle (Figure 49-4). Ingested eggs hatch into a larval worm in the small intestine and then migrate to the cecum, where they penetrate the mucosa and mature to adults. Three months after the initial infection, the fertilized female worm will start laying eggs and may produce 3000 to 10,000 eggs per day. Female worms can live for as long as 8 years. Eggs passed into the soil will mature and become infectious in 3 weeks. *T. trichiura* eggs are distinctive with dark bile staining, barrel shape, and the presence of polar plugs in the egg shell (Figure 49-5).

Epidemiology

Similar to *Ascaris lumbricoides,* distribution is worldwide and prevalence is directly correlated with poor sanitation and use of human feces as fertilizer. No animal reservoir is recognized.

Clinical Syndromes

The clinical manifestations of trichuriasis are generally related to the intensity of the worm burden. Most infections are with small numbers of *Trichuris* and are usually asymptomatic, although secondary bacterial infection may occur because the heads of the worms penetrate deep into the intestinal mucosa. Infections with many larvae may produce abdominal pain and distention, bloody diarrhea, weakness, and weight loss. Appendicitis may occur as worms fill the lumen, and prolapse of the rectum is seen in children because of the irritation and straining during defecation. Anemia and eosinophilia are also seen in severe infections.

Laboratory Diagnosis

Stool examination reveals the characteristic bile-stained eggs with polar plugs. Light infestations may be difficult to detect because of the paucity of eggs in the stool specimens.

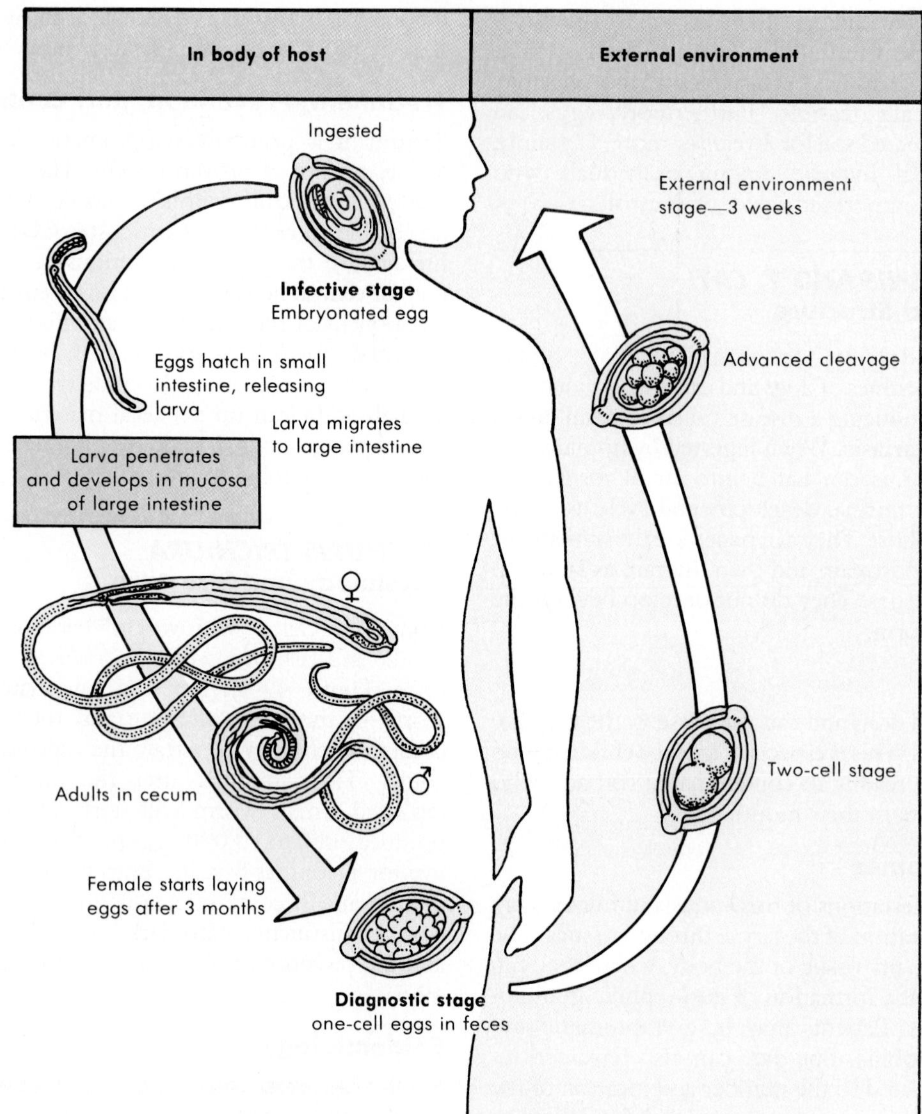

FIGURE 49-4 Life cycle of *Trichuris trichiura.*

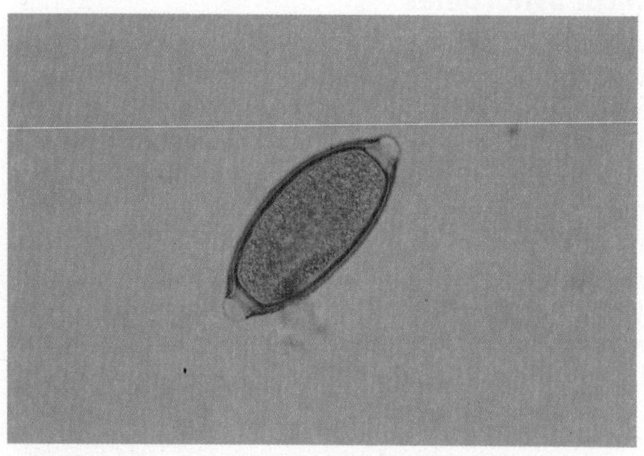

FIGURE 49-5 *Trichuris trichiura* egg. The eggs are barrel shaped, measuring 50 μm by 24 μm, with a thick wall and two prominent plugs at the ends. Internally, an unsegmented ovum is present.

Treatment, Prevention, and Control

The drug of choice is mebendazole. As for *Ascaris lumbricoides,* prevention depends on education, good personal hygiene, adequate sanitation, and avoiding the use of human feces as fertilizer.

HOOKWORMS

Ancylostoma duodenale and *Necator americanus*

Physiology and Structure

The two human hookworms are *Ancylostoma duodenale* (Old World hookworm) and *Necator americanus* (New World hookworm). Differing only in geographical distribution, structure of mouthparts, and relative size, these two species will be discussed together as agents of hookworm infection. The human phase of the hookworm

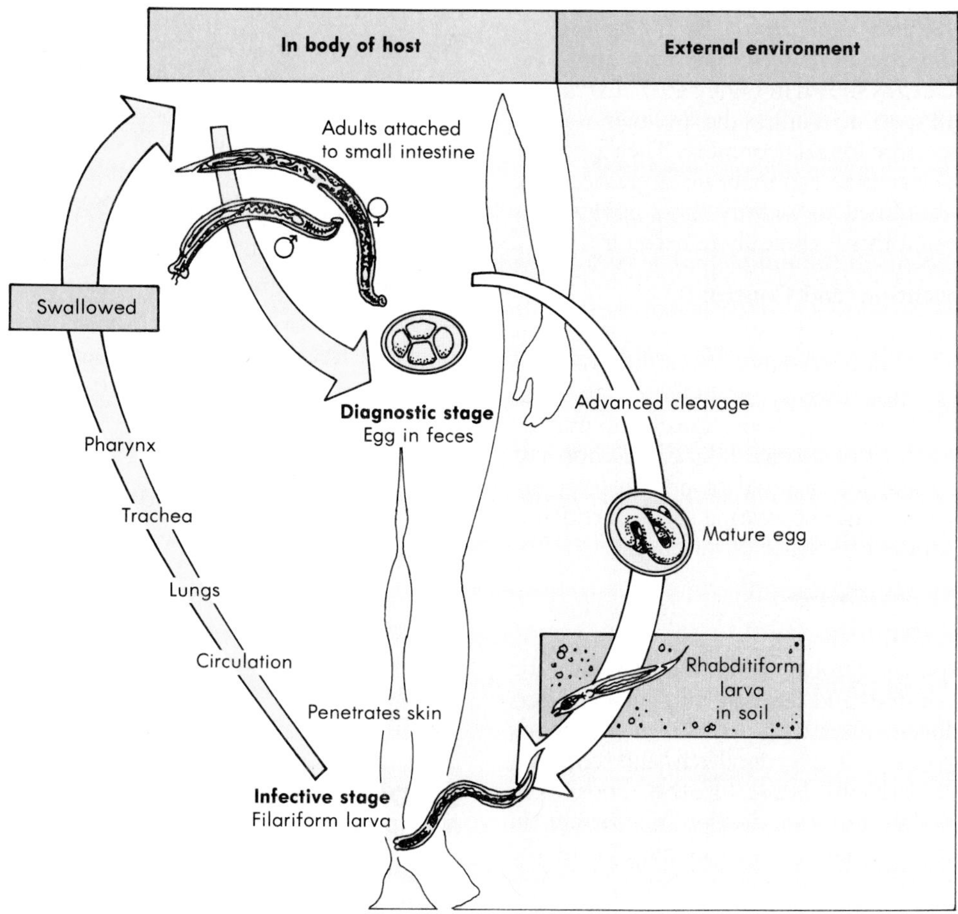

FIGURE 49-6 Life cycle of human hookworms.

life cycle is initiated when a **filariform** (infective form) larva penetrates intact skin (Figure 49-6). The larva then enters the circulation, is carried to the lungs and, like *Ascaris lumbricoides,* is coughed up, swallowed, and develops to adulthood in the small intestine. The adult *N. americanus* has a hooklike head, which accounts for the name commonly used. Adult worms lay as many as 10,000 to 20,000 eggs per day, which are released into feces. Egg laying is initiated 4 to 8 weeks after the initial exposure and can persist for as long as 5 years. On contact with soil, the **rhabditiform** (noninfective) larvae are released from the eggs and within 2 weeks develop into filariform larvae. The filariform larvae can then penetrate exposed skin (e.g., bare feet) and initiate a new cycle of human infection.

Both species have mouthparts designed for sucking blood from injured intestinal tissue; *A. duodenale* has chitinous teeth, and *N. americanus* has shearing chitinous plates.

Epidemiology

Transmission of hookworm infection requires deposition of egg-containing feces on shady, well-drained soil and is favored by warm, humid (tropical) conditions. Hookworm infections are reported worldwide where direct contact with contaminated soil can lead to human disease, but occur primarily in warm subtropical and tropical regions, and in southern parts of the United States. It is estimated that more than 900 million individuals worldwide are infected with hookworms, including 700,000 in the United States.

Clinical Syndromes

Skin-penetrating larvae may produce an allergic reaction and rash at sites of entry, and larvae migrating in the lungs can cause pneumonitis. Adult worms produce the gastrointestinal symptoms of nausea, vomiting, and diarrhea. As blood is lost from feeding worms, a microcytic hypochromic anemia develops. Daily blood loss is estimated at 0.15 to 0.25 ml for each adult *A. duodenale* and 0.03 ml for each adult *N. americanus*. In severe chronic infections, emaciation and mental and physical retardation may occur related to anemia from blood loss and nutritional deficiencies. Also, intestinal sites may be secondarily infected by bacteria when the worms migrate along the intestinal mucosa.

Laboratory Diagnosis

Stool examination reveals the characteristic non–bile-stained segmented eggs shown in Figure 49-7. Larvae are not found in stool specimens unless the specimen was left at ambient temperature for a day or more. The eggs of *A. duodenale* and *N. americanus* cannot be distinguished. The larvae must be examined to identify these hookworms specifically, although this is clinically unnecessary.

Treatment, Prevention, and Control

The drug of choice is mebendazole; pyrantel pamoate is an alternative. In addition to eradication of the worms to stop blood loss, iron therapy is indicated to raise hemoglobin levels to normal. Blood transfusion may be necessary in severe cases of anemia. Education, improved sanitation, and controlled disposal of human feces are critical. The simple practice of wearing shoes in endemic areas helps reduce the prevalence of infection.

Ancylostoma braziliense

Physiology and Structure

A. braziliense, a species of hookworm, is naturally parasitic in the intestines of dogs and cats and accidentally infects humans. It produces a disease properly called **cutaneous larva migrans** but also called "ground itch" and "creeping eruption." The filariform larvae of this hookworm penetrate intact skin but can develop no further in humans. The larvae remain trapped in the skin of the wrong host for weeks or months, wandering through subcutaneous tissue and creating serpentine tunnels.

Epidemiology

Similar to the situation with *Ascaris* worms, the threat of infection is greatest among children coming into contact with soil or sandboxes contaminated with animal feces containing hookworm eggs. Infections are prevalent throughout the year on beaches in subtropical and tropical regions; in summer, infection is reported as far north as the Canadian-U.S. border.

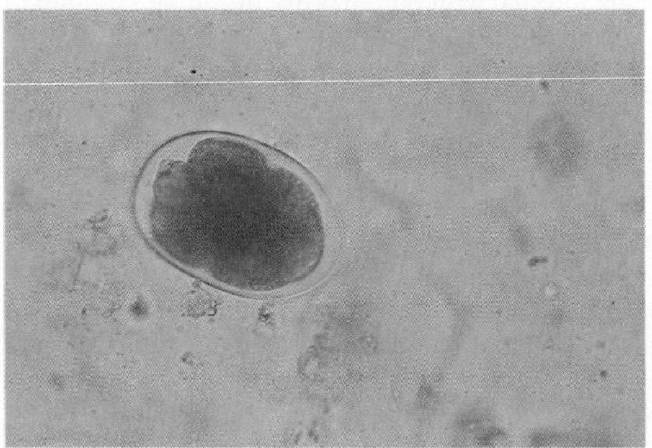

FIGURE 49-7 Human hookworm egg. The eggs are 60 to 75 μm long and 35 to 40 μm wide, thin shelled, and enclose a developing larva.

Clinical Syndromes

The migrating larvae may provoke a severe erythematous and vesicular reaction. The pruritus and scratching of the irritated skin may lead to secondary bacterial infection. About half of the patients will develop transient pulmonary infiltrates with peripheral eosinophilia (Löffler's syndrome), presumably due to pulmonary migration of the larvae.

Laboratory Diagnosis

Occasionally, larvae are recovered in skin biopsy or following freezing of the skin, but most diagnoses are based on the clinical appearance of the tunnels and a history of contact with dog and cat feces. The larvae are rarely found in sputum.

Treatment, Prevention, and Control

The drug of choice is thiabendazole. Antihistamines may be helpful in controlling the pruritus. This zoonosis, as with animal *Ascaris*, can be reduced by educating pet owners to treat their animals for worm infections and to pick up pet feces from yards, beaches, and sandboxes. In endemic areas shoes or sandals should be worn to prevent infection.

STRONGYLOIDES STERCORALIS

Physiology and Structure

Although the morphology of these worms and epidemiology of their infections are similar to the hookworm, the life cycle of *S. stercoralis* (Figure 49-8) differs in three aspects: (1) eggs hatch into larvae in the intestine and before they are passed in feces; (2) larvae can mature into filariforms and cause autoinfections; and (3) a free-living, nonparasitic cycle can be established outside the human host.

In direct development, like the hookworm, a skin-penetrating larva enters the circulation and follows the pulmonary course. It is coughed up and swallowed, and adults develop in the small intestine. Adult females burrow into the mucosa of the duodenum and reproduce parthenogenetically. Each female produces about one dozen eggs per day, which hatch within the mucosa and release rhabditiform larvae into the lumen of the bowel. The rhabditiform larvae are distinguished from the larvae of hookworms by their short buccal capsule and large genital primordium. The rhabditiform larvae are passed in the stool and may either continue the direct cycle by developing into infective filariform larvae or develop into free-living adult worms and initiate the indirect cycle.

In indirect development the larvae in the soil develop into free-living adults that produce eggs and larvae. Several generations of this nonparasitic existence may occur before new larvae again become skin-penetrating parasites.

Finally, in **autoinfection**, rhabditiform larvae in the intestine do not pass with feces but become filariform larvae. These penetrate the intestinal or perianal skin and follow the circulation-pulmonary-cough-and-swallow course to become adults, producing more larvae in the intestine. This cycle can persist for years and can lead to hyperinfection and massive or disseminated—often fatal—infection.

Epidemiology

Similar to hookworms in its requirements for warm temperatures and moisture, *S. stercoralis* demonstrates low prevalence but a somewhat broader geographical distribution, including parts of the northern United States and Canada. Sexual transmission also occurs. Animal reservoirs such as domestic pets are recognized.

Clinical Syndromes

Individuals with strongyloidiasis frequently are afflicted with pneumonitis from migrating larvae similar to that seen in both ascariasis and hookworm infection. The intestinal infection is usually asymptomatic. However, heavy worm loads may involve the biliary and pancreatic ducts, the entire small bowel, and the colon, causing inflammation and ulceration leading to epigastric pain and tenderness, vomiting, diarrhea (occasionally bloody), and malabsorption. Symptoms mimicking peptic ulcer disease coupled with peripheral eosinophilia should strongly suggest the diagnosis of strongyloidiasis.

Autoinfection may lead to chronic strongyloidiasis that can last for years even in nonendemic areas. Although many of these chronic infections may be asymptomatic, as many as two thirds of the patients have recurring episodic symptoms referable to the involved skin, lungs, and intestinal tract. Individuals with chronic strongyloidiasis are at risk of developing severe, life-threatening **hyperinfection syndrome** if the host-parasite balance is disturbed by any drug or illness that compromises the host's immune status. Hyperinfection syndrome is seen most commonly in individuals immunocompromised by malignancies (especially hematological malignancies) and/or corticosteroid therapy. Hyperinfection syndrome has also been observed following solid organ transplantation and in malnourished individuals. It appears that loss of cellular immune function is associated with the conversion of rhabditiform larvae to filariform larvae followed by dissemination of the larvae via the circulation to virtually any organ. Most commonly, extraintestinal infection involves the lung and includes bronchospasm, diffuse infiltrates, and occasionally cavitation. Widespread dis-

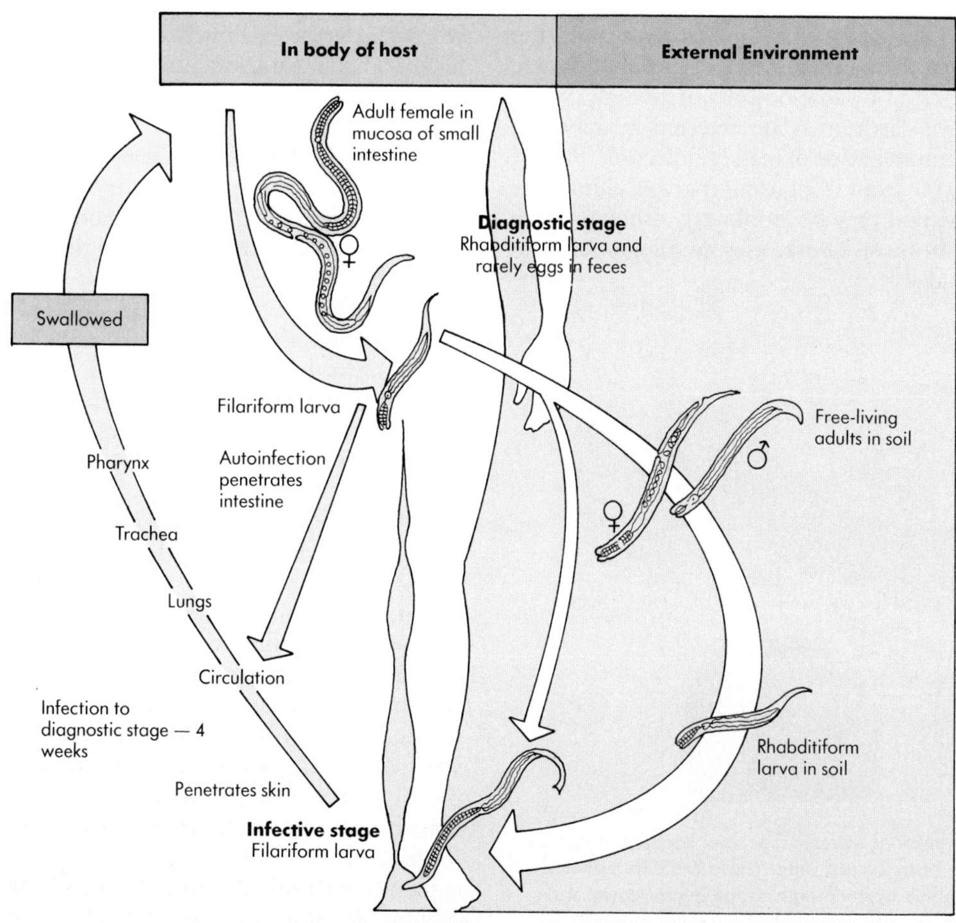

FIGURE 49-8 Life cycle of *Strongyloides stercoralis.*

semination involving abdominal lymph nodes, liver, spleen, kidneys, pancreas, thyroid, heart, brain, and meninges is not uncommon. Intestinal symptoms of hyperinfection syndrome include profound diarrhea, malabsorption, and electrolyte abnormalities. Notably, hyperinfection syndrome is associated with a high mortality of approximately 86%. Bacterial sepsis, meningitis, peritonitis, or endocarditis secondary to larval spread from the intestine are frequent and often fatal complications of hyperinfection syndrome.

Laboratory Diagnosis

Diagnosis of strongyloidiasis may be difficult because of intermittent passage of low numbers of first-stage larvae in stool. Examination of concentrated stool sediment reveals the larval worms (Figure 49-9) but, in contrast with hookworm infections, eggs are generally not seen. Collecting samples from three stools, one per day for 3 days, as for *Giardia lamblia*, is recommended because *S. stercoralis* larvae may occur in "showers," with many present one day and few or none the next. Several authors favor the Baermann funnel gauze method of concentrating living *S. stercoralis* larvae from fecal specimens. This method employs a funnel with a stopcock and a gauze insert. The funnel is filled with lukewarm water to a level just covering the gauze, and a specimen of stool is placed on the gauze, partially in contact with the water. The larvae in the stool migrate through the gauze into the water and then sediment into the neck of the funnel where they may be detected by low-power microscopy. When absent from stool, larvae may be detected in duodenal aspirates or in sputum in case of massive infection. Finally, culture of the larvae from stool using charcoal cultures or an agar plate method may be employed, although these are not routine in most laboratories. Serologic tests are generally not available.

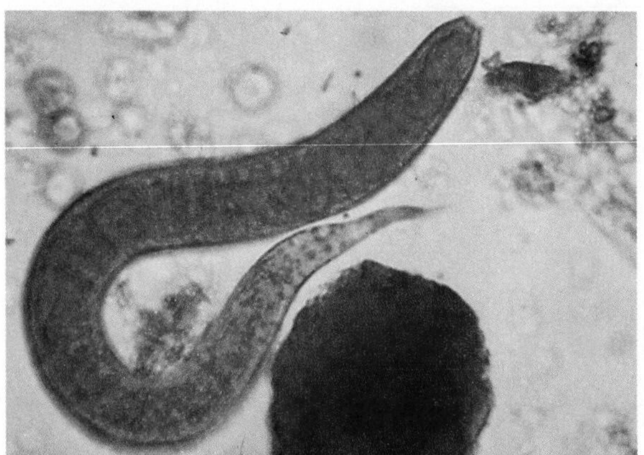

FIGURE 49-9 *Strongyloides stercoralis* larvae. Larvae are 180 to 380 μm long and 14 to 24 μm wide. These are differentiated from hookworm larvae by the length of the buccal cavity and esophagus, as well as the structure of the genital primordium.

Treatment, Prevention, and Control

All infected patients should be treated to prevent autoinfection and potential dissemination (hyperinfection) of the parasite. The drug of choice is thiabendazole, with mebendazole as an alternative. Patients in endemic areas who are about to undergo immunosuppressive therapy should have at least three stool examinations to rule out *S. stercoralis* infection and avoid the risks of autoinfection. Strict infection control measures should be enforced when caring for individuals with hyperinfection syndrome since stool, saliva, vomitus, and body fluids may contain infectious filariform larvae. Similar to hookworm, *Strongyloides* control requires education, proper sanitation, and prompt treatment of existing infections.

TRICHINELLA SPIRALIS

Physiology and Structure

Trichinella spiralis is the etiological agent of trichinosis. The adult form of this organism lives in the duodenal and jejunal mucosa of flesh-eating mammals worldwide. The infectious larval form is present in the striated muscles of both carnivorous and omnivorous mammals. Among domestic animals, swine are most frequently involved. Figure 49-10 illustrates the simple, direct life cycle, which terminates in the musculature of humans where the larvae eventually die and calcify. The infection begins when meat containing encysted larvae is digested. The larvae leave the meat in the small intestine and within 2 days develop into adult worms. A single fertilized female worm produces more than 1500 larvae in 1 to 3 months. These larvae move from the intestinal mucosa into the bloodstream and are carried in the circulation to various muscle sites throughout the body, where they coil in striated muscle fibers and become encysted (Figure 49-11). The muscles invaded most frequently include the extraocular muscles of the eye, the tongue, the deltoid, pectoral, and intercostal muscles, the diaphragm, and the gastrocnemius. The encysted larvae remain viable for many years and would be infectious if ingested by a new animal host.

Epidemiology

Trichinosis occurs worldwide in humans, and its greatest prevalence is associated with consumption of pork products. In addition to its transmission from pigs, many carnivorous and omnivorous animals harbor the organism and are potential sources of human infection. Notably, polar bears and walruses in the Arctic account for outbreaks in human populations—especially with a strain of *T. spiralis* that is more resistant to freezing than the *T. spiralis* strains found in the continental United States and other temperate regions. It is estimated that more than 1.5 million Americans carry live *Trichinella* cysts in their musculature and that 150,000 to 300,000 acquire new infection annually.

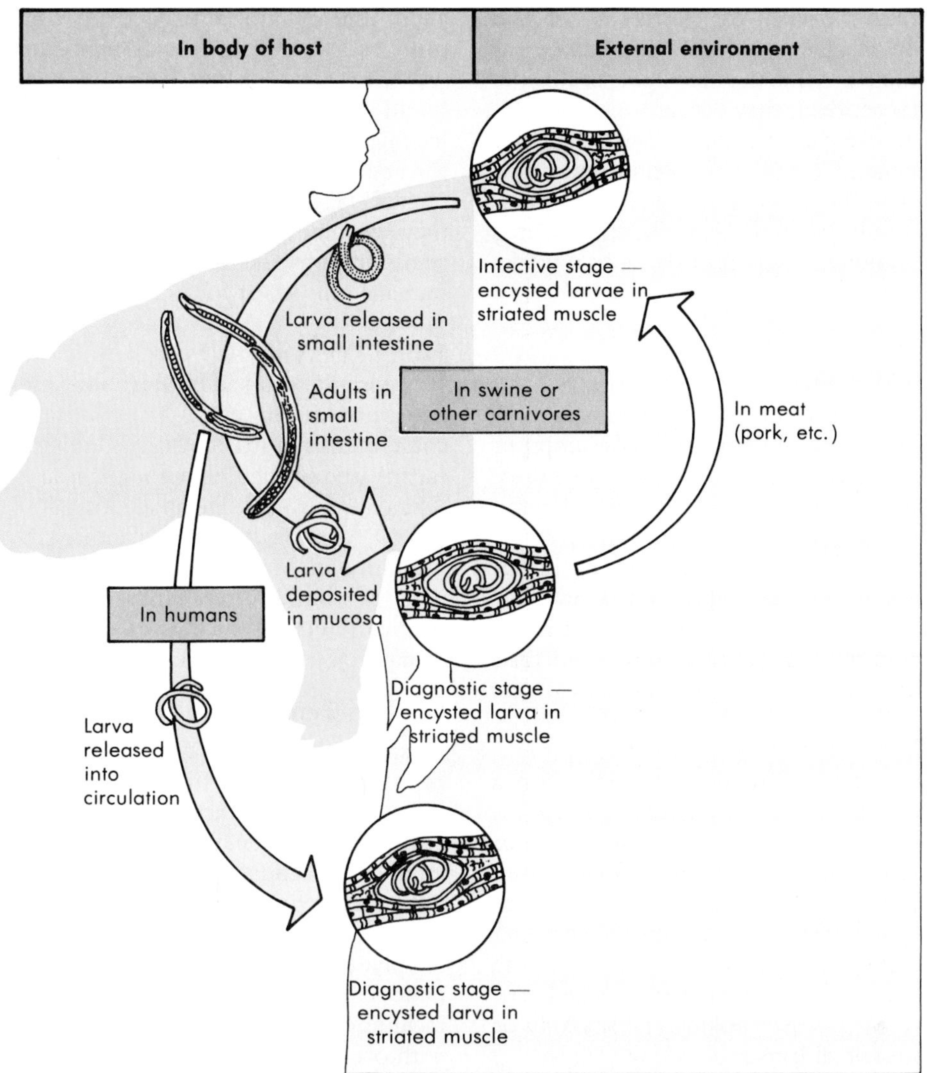

FIGURE 49-10 Life cycle of *Trichinella spiralis.*

Clinical Syndromes

Trichinosis is one of the few tissue parasitic diseases still seen in the United States. As with other parasitic infections most patients have minimal or no symptoms. The clinical presentation depends largely on the tissue burden of organisms and the location of the migrating larvae. Patients in whom 10 or fewer larvae are deposited per gram of tissue are usually asymptomatic; those with 100 or more generally have significant disease; and those with 1000 to 5000 have a very serious course that occasionally ends in death. In mild infections with few migrating larvae, patients may experience only a flu-like syndrome with slight fever and mild diarrhea. With more extensive larval migration, persistent fever, gastrointestinal distress, marked eosinophilia, muscle pain, and periorbital edema occur. "Splinter" hemorrhages beneath the nails are also a common finding, thought to be caused

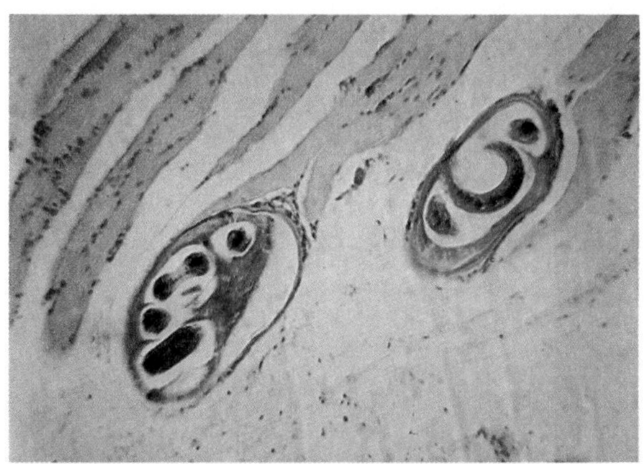

FIGURE 49-11 Encysted larva of *Trichinella spiralis* in biopsied muscle. (From Finegold SM and Baron EJ, editors: *Bailey and Scott's diagnostic microbiology*, ed 7, St. Louis, 1986, Mosby.)

by vasculitis resulting from toxic secretions of the migrating larvae. In heavy infections severe neurological symptoms, including psychosis, meningoencephalitis, and cerebrovascular accident, may occur.

Patients who survive the migration, muscle destruction, and encystment of larvae in moderate infections experience a decline in clinical symptoms in 5 or 6 weeks. Lethal trichinosis results when myocarditis, encephalitis, and pneumonitis combine; the patient dies 4 to 6 weeks after infection. Respiratory arrest often follows heavy invasion and muscle destruction in the diaphragm.

Laboratory Diagnosis

Diagnosis is usually established with clinical observations, especially when an outbreak can be traced to consumption of improperly cooked pork or bear meat. The laboratory may confirm this if the encysted larvae are detected in the implicated meat or biopsied muscle from the patient. Marked eosinophilia is characteristically present in patients with trichinosis. Serologic procedures are also available for confirmation. Significant antibody titers are usually absent before the third week of illness but then may persist for years.

Treatment, Prevention, and Control

Treatment of trichinosis is primarily symptomatic since there are no good antiparasitic agents for tissue larvae. Treatment of the adult worms in the intestine with mebendazole may halt the production of new larvae. Steroids are recommended for severe symptoms, along with thiabendazole or mebendazole. Education regarding pork and bear meat transmission is essential, especially the recommendation that pork and bear meat be cooked until the interior is gray. Microwave cooking and smoking or drying meat do not kill all larvae.

Laws regulating the feeding of garbage to pigs help control transmission, as may regulations controlling the foraging of bears in garbage pits and public parks. Freezing pork, as conducted in federally inspected meat packing plants, has reduced transmission. Quick freezing of pork at − 40° C effectively destroys the organisms, as does low-temperature storage at − 15° C for 20 days or more.

WUCHERERIA BANCROFTI AND *BRUGIA MALAYI*

Physiology and Structure

Because of their many similarities, *Wuchereria bancrofti* and *Brugia malayi* will be discussed together. Human infection is initiated by introduction of infective larvae, present in the saliva of a biting mosquito, into a bite wound (Figure 49-12). Various species of *Anopheles*, *Aedes* and *Culex* mosquitoes are known to be vectors of Bancroft's and Malayan filariasis. The larvae migrate from the location of the bite to the lymphatics, primarily in the arms, legs, or groin, where growth to adulthood occurs. From three to 12 months after the initial infection, the adult male worm fertilizes the female, who in turn produces the sheathed larval microfilariae that find their way into the circulation. The presence of microfilariae in blood is diagnostic for human disease and is infective for feeding mosquitoes. In the mosquito the larvae move through the stomach and thoracic muscles in developmental stages and finally migrate to the proboscis. There they become an infective third-stage larva and are transmitted by the feeding mosquito. The adult form in humans can persist for as long as 10 years.

Epidemiology

W. bancrofti occurs in both tropical and subtropical areas and is endemic in central Africa, along the Mediterranean coast, in many parts of Asia (including China, Korea, and Japan), and in the Philippines. It is also present in Haiti, Trinidad, Surinam, Panama, Costa Rica, and Brazil. No animal reservoir has been identified. *B. malayi* is found primarily in Malaysia, India, Thailand, Vietnam, and parts of China, Korea, Japan, and many Pacific islands. Animal reservoirs such as cats and monkeys are recognized.

Clinical Syndromes

In some patients there is no sign of disease, even though blood specimens may show many microfilariae present. In other patients early acute symptoms are fever, lymphangitis and lymphadenitis with chills, and recurrent febrile attacks. The acute presentation is thought to be due to the inflammatory response to the presence of molting adolescent worms and dead or dying adults within the lymphatic vessels. As the infection progresses, the lymph nodes enlarge, possibly involving many parts of the body, including the extremities, the scrotum, and the testes, with occasional abscess formation. This results from the physical obstruction of lymph in the vessels caused by the presence of adult worms and host reactivity in the lymphatics. This process may be complicated by recurrent bacterial infections, which contribute to the tissue damage. The thickening and hypertrophy of tissues infected with the worms may lead to the enlargement of tissues, especially the extremities, progressing to **filarial elephantiasis**. Filariasis of this type is thus a chronic, debilitating, and disfiguring disease requiring prompt diagnosis and treatment. Occasionally, ascites and pleural effusions secondary to rupture of enlarged lymphatics into the peritoneal or pleural cavities may be observed.

Laboratory Diagnosis

Eosinophilia is usually present during acute inflammation episodes; however, demonstration of microfilariae in blood is required for definitive diagnosis. Microfilariae can be demonstrated in Giemsa-stained blood films as for malaria (Figure 49-13). Concentrations of anticoagulated blood specimens and urine specimens are also valuable procedures. Buffy coat films serve to concentrate the white blood cells and are useful for detection of microfilariae. The presence of small numbers of microfilariae in

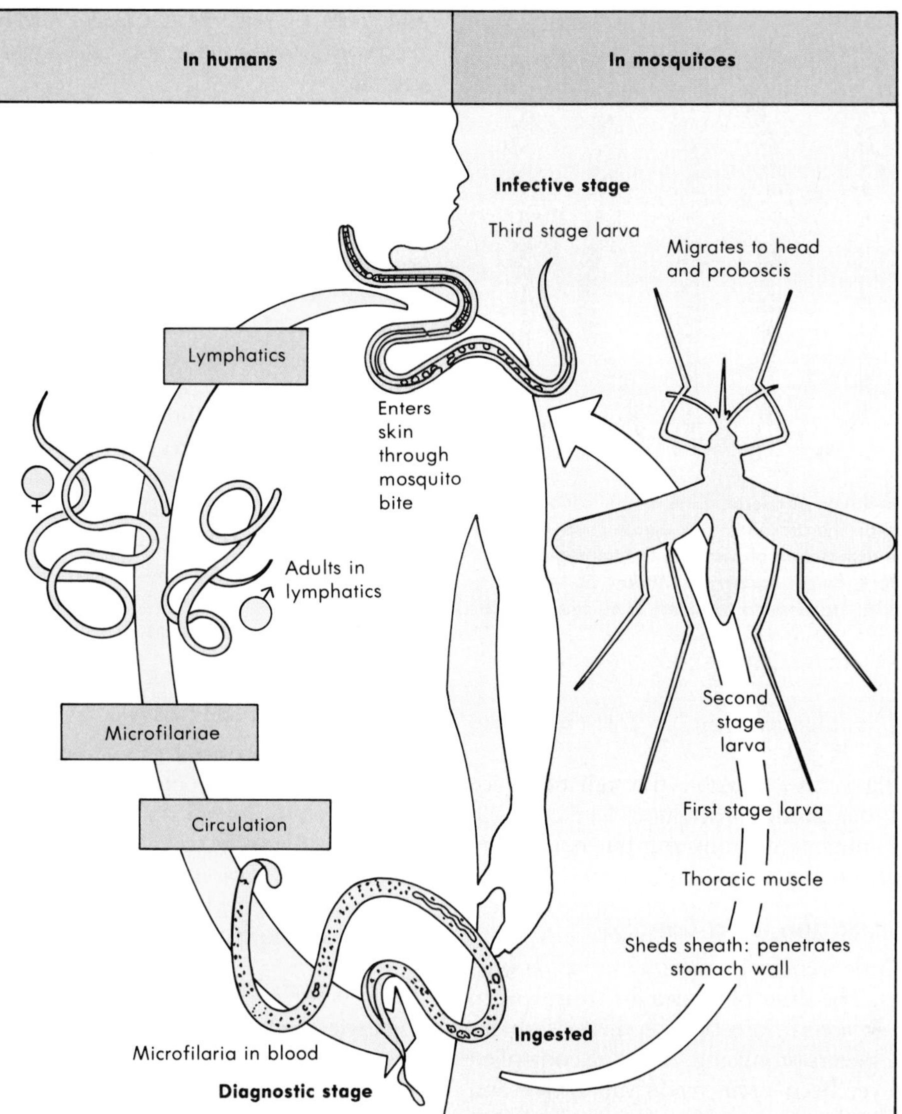

FIGURE 49-12 Life cycle of *Wuchereria bancrofti.*

blood can be detected by means of a membrane filtration technique in which anticoagulated blood is mixed with saline and forced through a 5 μm membrane filter. Following several washes with saline or distilled water the filter may be examined microscopically for living microfilariae or dried, fixed, and stained as for a thin blood film.

Both *W. bancrofti* and *B. malayi* have a periodicity in production of microfilariae—**"nocturnal periodicity."** This results in greater numbers of microfilariae in blood at night. It is recommended that blood specimens be taken between 10 PM and 4 AM to detect infection.

W. bancrofti, as well as *B. malayi* and *Loa loa,* demonstrate a sheath on their microfilariae. This can be the first step in identifying the specific types of filariasis. Further identification is based on study of head and tail structures (Figure 49-14). Clinically, an exact species identification is not critical, because treatment for all the

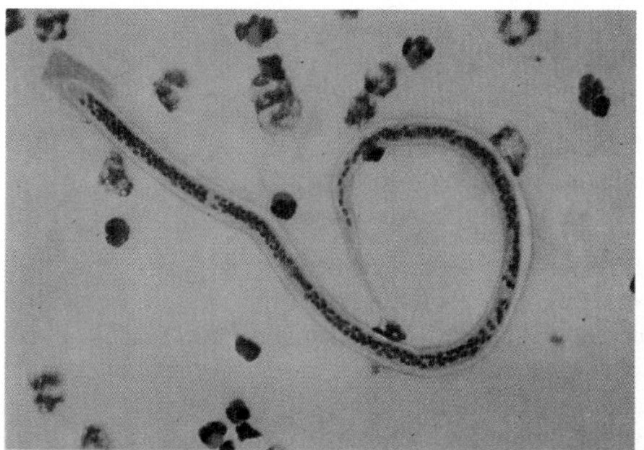

FIGURE 49-13 *Wuchereria bancrofti* microfilaria in blood smear. (From Finegold SM and Baron EJ, editors: *Bailey and Scott's diagnostic microbiology,* ed 7, St. Louis, 1986, Mosby.)

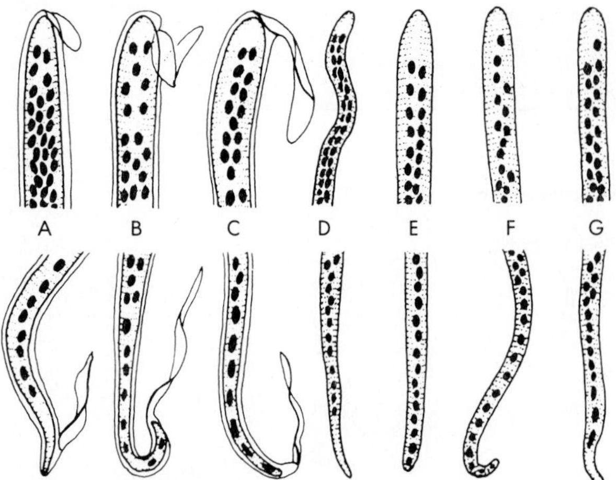

FIGURE 49-14 Differentiation of microfilariae. Identification of microfilariae is based on the presence of a sheath covering the larvae, as well as the distribution of nuclei in the tail region. *A, Wuchereria bancrofti; B, Brugia malayi; C, Loa loa; D, Onchocerca volvulus; E, Mansonella perstans; F, M. streptocerca;* and *G, M. ozzardi.*

filarial infections is identical, except for *Onchocerca volvulus.*

Serologic testing is also available through reference laboratories as a diagnostic procedure. Detection of circulating filarial antigens is promising but not widely available as a diagnostic test.

Treatment, Prevention, and Control

Treatment is of little benefit in most cases of chronic lymphatic filariasis. The drug of choice for treatment of *W. bancrofti* and *B. malayi* infections is diethylcarbamazine. Ivermectin appears promising, although controlled studies have not yet been performed. Supportive and surgical therapy for lymphatic obstruction may be of some cosmetic help. Education regarding filarial infections, mosquito control, use of protective clothing and insect repellents, and treatment of infections to prevent further transmission is essential. Control of *B. malayi* infections is more difficult because of the presence of disease in animal reservoirs.

LOA LOA

Physiology and Structure

The life cycle of *Loa loa* is similar to that illustrated in Figure 49-12, except the vector is a biting fly called *Chrysops*, the mango fly. Approximately 6 months after infection, production of microfilariae will start and can persist for 17 years or more. Adult worms can migrate through subcutaneous tissues, muscle, and in front of the eyeball.

Epidemiology

Loa loa is confined to the equatorial rain forests of Africa and is endemic in tropical West Africa, the Congo basin, and parts of Nigeria. Monkeys in these areas serve as reservoir hosts in the life cycle, with mango flies as vectors.

Clinical Syndromes

Symptoms usually do not appear until a year or so after the fly bite, because the worms are slow in reaching adulthood. One of the first signs of infection is the so-called fugitive or **Calabar swellings.** These swellings are transient and usually appear on the extremities, produced as the worms migrate through subcutaneous tissues, creating large nodular areas that are painful and pruritic. Because eosinophilia (50% to 70%) is observed, Calabar swellings are believed to be the result of allergic reactions to the worms or their metabolic products.

Adult *Loa loa* worms can also migrate under the conjunctiva, producing irritation, painful congestion, edema of the eyelids, and impaired vision. The presence of a worm in the eye can obviously cause anxiety in the patient. The infection may be long-lived and in some cases asymptomatic.

Laboratory Diagnosis

The clinical observation of Calabar swellings or migration of worms in the eye, combined with eosinophilia, should alert the physician to consider infection with *Loa loa*. The microfilariae can be found in blood. In contrast with the other filariae, *Loa loa* is primarily present during the daytime. Serologic testing can also be useful for confirming the diagnosis but is not readily available.

Treatment, Prevention, and Control

Diethylcarbamazine is effective against both adults and microfilariae; however, destruction of the parasites may induce severe allergic reactions that require treatment with corticosteroids. The role of ivermectin remains undefined for this infection. Surgical removal of worms migrating across the eye or bridge of the nose can be accomplished by immobilizing the worm with instillation of a few drops of 10% cocaine. Education regarding the infection and its vector, especially for persons entering the known endemic areas, is essential. Protection from fly bites by using screening, appropriate clothing, and insect repellents, along with treatment of cases, is also critical in reducing the incidence of infection. However, the presence of disease in animal reservoirs (e.g., monkeys) limits the feasibility of controlling this disease.

MANSONELLA SPECIES

Filarial infections caused by *Mansonella* species are less important than those previously discussed, but physicians should be aware of the names because they may encounter patients with these infections. Infections caused by these organisms are generally asymptomatic but may cause dermatitis, lymphadenitis, hydrocele, and, rarely, lymphatic obstruction resulting in elephantiasis.

All of the *Mansonella* species produce nonsheathed microfilariae in blood and subcutaneous tissues, and all are transmitted by biting midges (*Culicoides*) or black flies (*Simulium*). All of these species are treatable with diethylcarbamazine as for previous filarial infections. Species identification, if desired, can be accomplished with blood smears, noting the structure of the microfilariae. Serologic tests are also available.

Prevention and control require measures involving insect repellents, screening, and other precautions as for all insect-transmitted diseases.

Mansonella perstans

Mansonella perstans occurs primarily in parts of tropical Africa and Central and South America. It may produce allergic skin reactions, edema, and Calabar swellings similar to *Loa loa*. Reservoir hosts are chimpanzees and gorillas.

Mansonella ozzardi

Mansonella ozzardi is found primarily in Central and South America and the West Indies. It may produce swelling of the lymph nodes and occasional hydrocele. There are no known reservoir hosts.

Mansonella streptocerca

M. streptocerca occurs primarily in Africa, especially in the Congo basin. It may produce edema in the skin and, rarely, a form of elephantiasis. Monkeys serve as reservoir hosts.

ONCHOCERCA VOLVULUS

Physiology and Structure

Infection occurs following introduction of larvae of *O. volvulus* through the skin during the biting and feeding of the *Simulian* or blackfly vector (Figure 49-15). The larval worms migrate from skin to subcutaneous tissue and develop into adult male and female worms. The adults become encased in fibrous subcutaneous nodules within which they may remain viable for as long as 15 years. The female worm, after fertilization by the male, begins producing as many as 2000 nonsheathed microfilariae each day. The microfilariae exit the capsule and migrate to the skin, eye, and other body tissues. These nonsheathed microfilariae appearing in skin tissue are infective for feeding black flies.

Epidemiology

Onchocerca volvulus is endemic in many parts of Africa, especially in the Congo basin and the Volta River basin. In the Americas it occurs in many Central and South American countries. Onchocerciasis affects more than 50 million people worldwide and causes blindness in approximately 5% of infected individuals.

Several species of the black fly genus *Simulium* serve as vectors, but none so appropriately named as the principal vector, *Simulium damnosum* ("the damned black fly"). These black flies, or buffalo gnats, breed in fast-flowing streams, which makes control or eradication by insecticides almost impossible because the chemicals are rapidly washed away from the eggs and larval flies.

There is a greater prevalence of infection in men than women in endemic areas because of their work in or near the streams where the black flies are breeding. Studies in endemic areas in Africa have shown that 50% of men will be totally blind before they are 50 years of age. This accounts for the common term, **"river blindness,"** applied to the disease onchocerciasis. This fear of blindness has created an additional problem in many parts of Africa, because whole villages leave the area near streams and farmland that could produce food. The migrating populations then find themselves in areas where starvation faces them.

Clinical Syndromes

Clinical onchocerciasis is characterized by infection involving the skin, subcutaneous tissue, lymph nodes, and eyes. The clinical manifestations of the infection are due to the acute and chronic inflammatory reaction to antigens released by the microfilariae as they migrate through the tissues. The incubation period from infectious larvae to adult worms is from several months to a year. Disease initially is seen with fever, eosinophilia, and urticaria. As the worms mature, copulate, and begin producing microfilariae, subcutaneous nodules begin to appear and can occur on any part of the body. These nodules are most dangerous when they are present on the head and neck because the microfilariae may migrate to the eyes and cause serious tissue damage, leading to blindness. The mechanisms for development of eye disease are thought to be a combination of both direct invasion by the microfilaria and antigen-antibody complex deposition within the ocular tissues. Patients progress from conjunctivitis with photophobia to punctate and sclerosing keratitis. Internal eye disease with anterior uveitis, chorioretinitis, and optic neuritis may also occur.

Within the skin the inflammatory process results in loss of elasticity and areas of depigmentation, thickening, and atrophy. A number of skin conditions are related to the presence of this parasite, including pruritus, hyperkeratosis, myxedematous thickening, and a form of elephantiasis called "hanging groin" when the nodules are located near the genitalia.

Laboratory Diagnosis

Diagnosis of onchocerciasis is made by demonstration of microfilaria in skin snip preparations from the infrascapular or gluteal region. A sample is obtained by raising the skin with a needle and shaving the epidermal layer with a razor. The specimen is incubated in saline for several hours, then inspected with a dissecting microscope for the presence of nonsheathed microfilaria. In patients with ocular disease, the organism may also be seen in the anterior chamber with the aid of a slit lamp. Serologic and

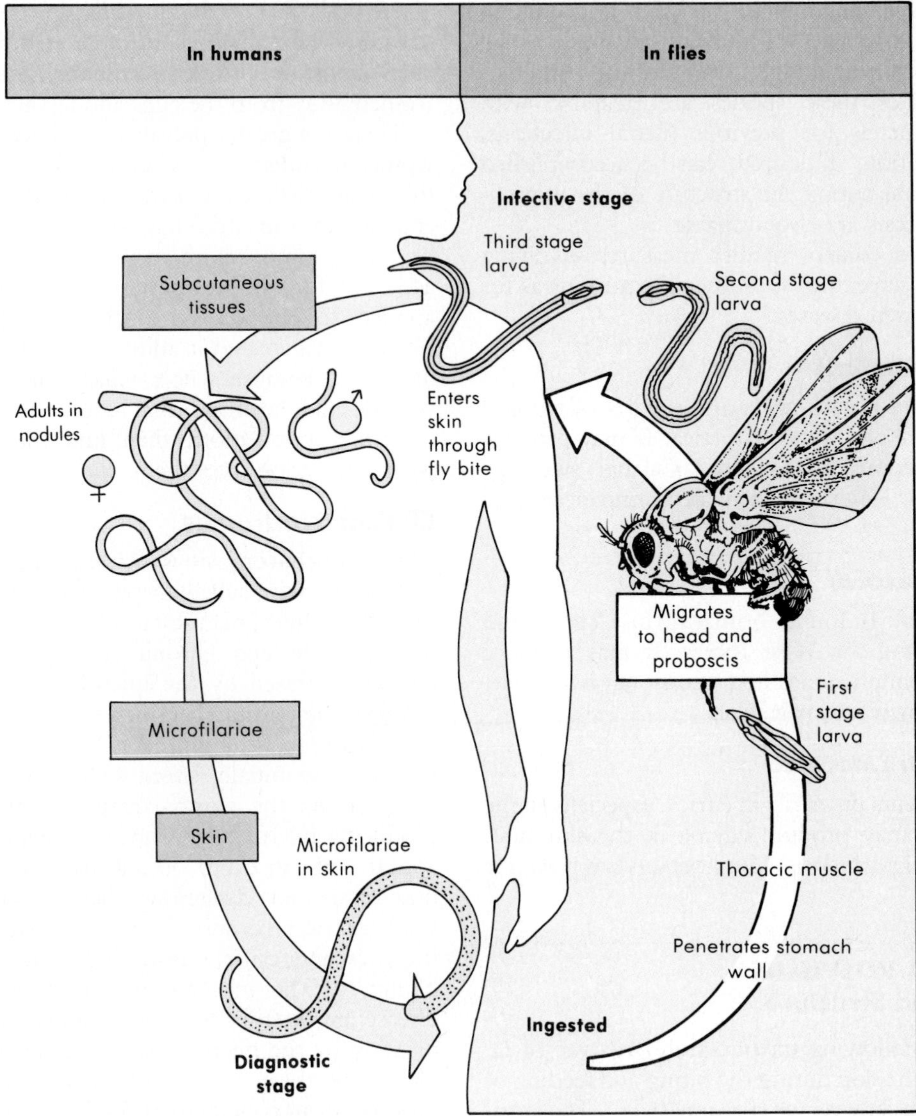

FIGURE 49-15 Life cycle of *Onchocerca volvulus.*

culture methods are not helpful, although efforts to develop serologic detection methods are ongoing.

Treatment, Prevention, and Control

Surgical removal of the encapsulated nodule is often performed to remove the adult worms and stop production of microfilariae. In addition, treatment with diethylcarbamazine followed by suramin is recommended; an alternative drug is mebendazole. The drug ivermectin also holds promise for eradication of migrating microfilariae.

Education regarding the disease and its black fly transmission is essential. Protection from black fly bites by use of protective clothing, screening, and insect repellents, as well as prompt diagnosis and treatment of infections to prevent further transmission, is critical.

Although control of black fly breeding is difficult because insecticides wash away in the streams, some form of biological control of this vector may reduce fly reproduction and disease transmission.

DIROFILARIA IMMITIS

Several mosquito-transmitted filaria infect dogs, cats, raccoons, and bobcats in nature and occasionally are found in humans. *Dirofilaria immitis*, the dog heartworm, is notorious for forming a lethal worm bolus in the dog's heart. This nematode may also infect humans, producing a subcutaneous nodule or a so-called "coin lesion" in the lung. Only very rarely have these worms been found in human hearts.

The "coin lesion" in the lung presents a problem to both the radiologist and the surgeon because it resembles a malignancy requiring surgical removal. Unfortunately, no laboratory test currently available can provide an

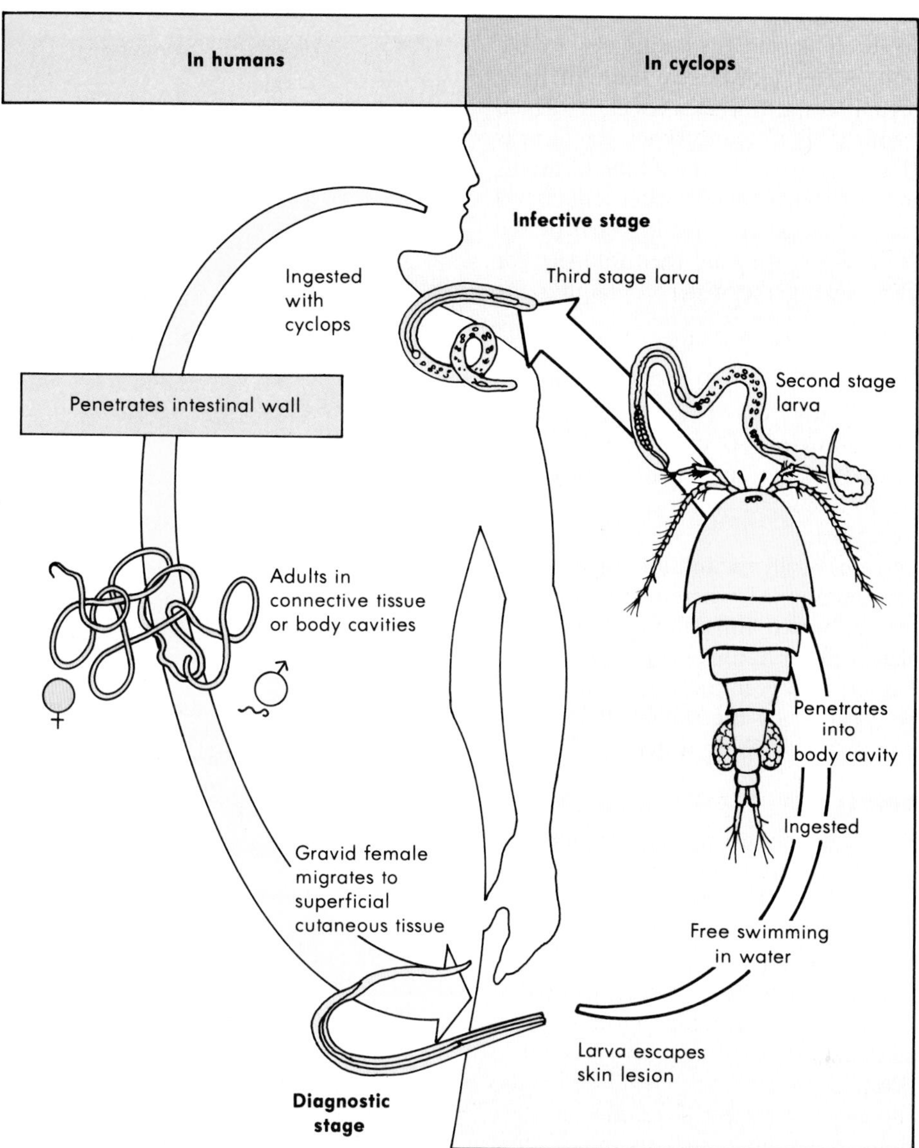

FIGURE 49-16 Life cycle of *Dracunculus medinensis.*

accurate diagnosis of dirofilariasis. Peripheral eosinophilia is rare, and the radiographic features are insufficient to allow one to distinguish pulmonary dirofilariasis from bronchogenic carcinoma. Serologic tests are not sufficiently sensitive or specific to preclude the surgical intervention. A definitive diagnosis is made when a thoracotomy specimen is examined microscopically, revealing the typical cross-sections of the parasite.

Transmission of the filarial infections can be controlled by mosquito control and a prophylactic use of the drug ivermectin in dogs.

DRACUNCULUS MEDINENSIS

The name *Dracunculus medinensis* means "little dragon of Medina." This is a very ancient worm infection thought by some scholars to be the "fiery serpent" noted by Moses with the Israelites at the Red Sea.

Physiology and Structure

D. medinensis is not a filarial worm but is a tissue-invading nematode of medical importance in many parts of the world. The worms have a very simple life cycle, depending on fresh water and a microcrustacean (copepod) of the genus *Cyclops* (Figure 49-16). When *Cyclops* harboring larval *D. medinensis* are ingested in drinking water by humans and other mammals, the infection is initiated with liberation of the larvae in the stomach. These larvae penetrate the wall of the digestive tract and migrate to the retroperitoneal space where they mature. These larvae are not microfilariae and do not appear in blood or other tissues. Male and female worms mate in the retroperitoneum, and the fertilized female then migrates to the subcutaneous tissues, usually in the extremities. When the fertilized female worm becomes gravid, a vesicle is formed in the host tissue, which will ulcerate. When the ulcer is completely formed, the worm protrudes a loop of uterus through the ulcer. On contact with water, the larval worms are released. The larvae are then ingested by the *Cyclops* in fresh water, where they are then infective for humans or animals drinking the water containing the *Cyclops*.

Epidemiology

D. medinensis occurs in many parts of Asia and equatorial Africa, infecting an estimated 10 million individuals. Reservoir hosts include dogs and many fur-bearing animals that come into contact with drinking water containing infective *Cyclops*.

Human infections are usually the result of ingestion of water from so-called "step wells" where people stand or bathe in the water—at which time the gravid female worm discharges larvae from lesions on the arms, legs, feet, and ankles to infect *Cyclops* in the water. Ponds and standing water are occasionally the source of infection when humans use these for drinking water.

Clinical Syndromes

Symptoms of infection usually do not appear until the gravid female creates the vesicle and the ulcer in the skin for liberation of larval worms. This occurs usually 1 year after the initial exposure. At the site of the ulcer there is erythema and pain, as well as an allergic reaction to the worm. There is also the possibility of abscess formation and secondary bacterial infection, leading to further tissue destruction and inflammatory reaction, with intense pain and sloughing of skin.

If the worm is broken in attempts to remove it, there may be toxic reactions, and if the worm dies and calcifies, there may be nodule formation and some allergic reaction. Once the gravid female has discharged all the larvae, it may retreat into deeper tissue where it is gradually absorbed or may simply be expelled from the site.

Laboratory Diagnosis

Diagnosis is established by observation of the typical ulcer and flooding the ulcer with water to recover the discharge of larval worms. Occasionally, x-ray examination reveals worms in various parts of the body.

Treatment, Prevention, and Control

The ancient method of slowly wrapping the worm on a twig is still used in many endemic areas (Figure 49-17). Surgical removal is also a practical and reliable procedure for the patient. The drug of choice for treatment is niridazole; alternative drugs are metronidazole and thiabendazole. These drugs have an antiinflammatory effect and will either eliminate the worm or make surgical removal easier.

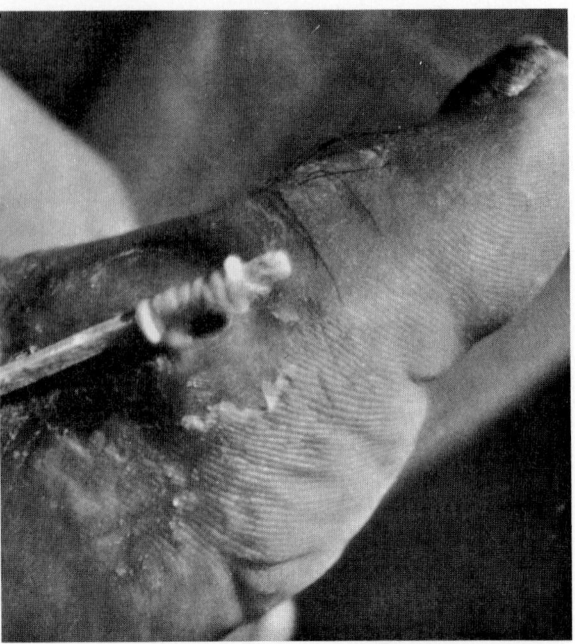

FIGURE 49-17 Removal of a *Dracunculus medinensis* adult from an exposed ulcer by winding the worm slowly around a stick. (From Binford CH and Conner DH: *Pathology of tropical and extraordinary diseases*, Washington DC, 1976, Armed Forces Institute of Pathology.)

Education regarding the life cycle of the worm and avoidance of water contaminated with *Cyclops* are critical. Protection of drinking water by prohibiting bathing and washing of clothing in wells is essential. Persons who live in or travel to endemic areas should boil water before consuming it. Treatment of water with chemicals and the use of fish that consume *Cyclops* as food are also helpful. Prompt diagnosis and treatment of cases also limit further transmission. These preventive measures have been incorporated into an ongoing global effort to eliminate dracunculiasis.

CASE STUDY AND QUESTIONS

A 10-year-old boy was brought in by his father for evaluation of crampy abdominal pain, nausea, and mild diarrhea for approximately 2 weeks. On the day before evaluation the boy reported to his parents that he passed a large worm into the toilet during a bowel movement. He flushed the worm before the parents could see it. Physical examination was completely unremarkable. He had no fever, cough or rash and did not complain of anal pruritus. His travel history was unremarkable. An examination of a stool specimen revealed the diagnosis.

1. Which intestinal parasites of humans are nematodes?
2. Which nematode is likely in this case, and what diagnostic forms may be found in stool?

3. What is the most likely means of acquisition of this parasite?
4. Is this patient at risk of autoinfection?
5. Describe the life cycle of this parasite.
6. Can this parasite cause extraintestinal symptoms? What other organs may be invaded, and what might stimulate extraintestinal invasion?

Bibliography

Chandrasoma PT and Mendis KN: *Enterobius vermicularis* in ectopic sites, *Am J Trop Med Hyg* 26:644-649, 1977.

Davidson RA et al.: Risk factors for strongyloidiasis: a case control study, *Arch Intern Med* 144:321-324, 1984.

Gilman RH et al.: The adverse effects of heavy *Trichuris* infection, *Trans R Soc Trop Med Hyg* 77:432-438, 1983.

Irga-Siegman Y et al.: Syndrome of hyperinfection with *Strongyloides stercoralis*, *Rev Infect Dis* 3:397-407, 1981.

Lynch NR et al.: Seroprevalence of *Toxocara canis* infection in tropical Venezuela, *Trans R Soc Trop Med Hyg* 82:275-281, 1988.

MacKenzie CD et al.: Variations in host responses and the pathogenesis of human onchocerciasis, *Rev Infect Dis* 7:802-808, 1985.

Markell EK, Voge M, and John DT: *Medical parasitology*, ed 7, Philadelphia, 1992, WB Saunders.

Nanduri J and Kuzura JW: Clinical and laboratory aspects of filariasis, *Clin Microbiol Rev* 2:39-50, 1989.

Ro JY et al.: Pulmonary dirofilariasis: the great imitator of primary or metastatic lung tumor, *Hum Pathol* 30:69-76, 1989.

Warren KS: Hookworm control, *Lancet* II 897-898 (Oct. 15), 1988.

CHAPTER 50

Trematodes

THE trematodes **(flukes)** are members of the Platyhelminthes and are generally flat, fleshy, leaf-shaped worms. In general, they are equipped with two muscular suckers: an oral type, which is the beginning of an incomplete digestive system, and a ventral sucker, which is simply an organ of attachment. The digestive system consists of lateral tubes that do not join to form an excretory opening. Most flukes are hermaphroditic, with both male and female reproductive organs in a single body. Schistosomes are the only exception—they have cylindrical bodies (like the nematodes), and separate male and female worms exist.

All flukes require intermediate hosts for completion of their life cycles, and without exception the first intermediate hosts are mollusks (snails and clams). In these hosts an asexual reproductive cycle occurs that is a type of germ cell propagation. Some flukes require various second intermediate hosts before reaching the final host and developing into adult worms. This variation is discussed with the individual species.

Fluke eggs are equipped with a lid at the top of the shell, called an **operculum,** that opens to allow the larval worm to find its appropriate snail host. The schistosomes do not have an operculum, but rather the egg shell splits open to liberate the larva. The primary medically significant trematodes are summarized in Table 50-1.

FASCIOLOPSIS BUSKI

A number of intestinal flukes are recognized, including *Fasciolopsis buski, Heterophyes heterophyes*, *Metagonimus yokogawai*, *Echinostoma ilocanum*, and *Gastrodiscoides hominis. F. buski* is the largest, most prevalent, and most important intestinal fluke. The other flukes are similar to *F. buski* in many respects (epidemiology, clinical syndromes, treatment) and are not discussed further. It is important only that physicians recognize the relationship among these different flukes.

Physiology and Structure

This large intestinal fluke demonstrates a typical life cycle (Figure 50-1). Humans ingest the encysted larval stage **(metacercaria)** when they peel the husks from aquatic vegetation (e.g., water chestnuts) with the teeth. The metacercariae are scraped from the husk, swallowed, and develop into immature flukes in the duodenum. The fluke attaches to the mucosa of the small intestine with two muscular suckers, develops into an adult form, and

TABLE 50-1 Medically Significant Trematodes

Trematode	Common name	Intermediate host	Biological vector	Reservoir host
Fasciolopsis buski	Giant intestinal fluke	Snail	Water plants (e.g., water chestnuts)	Pigs, dogs, rabbits, humans
Fasciola hepatica	Sheep liver fluke	Snail	Water plants (e.g., watercress)	Sheep, cattle, humans
Opisthorchis (Clonorchis) sinensis	Chinese liver fluke	Snail, freshwater fish	Uncooked fish	Dogs, cats, humans
Paragonimus westermani	Lung fluke	Snail, freshwater crabs, or crayfish	Uncooked crabs, crayfish	Pigs, monkeys, humans
Schistosome species	Blood fluke	Snail	None	Primates, rodents, domestic pets, livestock, humans

undergoes self-fertilization. Egg production is initiated 3 months after the initial infection with the metacercariae. The operculated eggs pass in feces to water, where the operculum at the top of the egg shell pops open, liberating a free-swimming larval stage **(miracidium).** Glands at the pointed anterior end of the miracidium produce lytic substances that allow the penetration of the soft tissues of snails. In the snail tissue the miracidium develops through a series of stages by asexual germ cell propagation. The final stage **(cercaria)** in the snail is a free-swimming form that, after release from the snail, encysts on the aquatic vegetation, becoming the metacercariae, or infective stage.

Epidemiology

Because it depends on the distribution of its appropriate snail host, *F. buski* is found only in China, Vietnam, Thailand, parts of Indonesia, Malaysia, and India. Pigs, dogs, and rabbits serve as reservoir hosts in these endemic areas.

Clinical Syndromes

The symptomatology of *F. buski* infection relates directly to the worm burden in the small intestine. The attachment of the flukes in the small intestine can produce inflammation, ulceration, and hemorrhage. Severe infections produce abdominal discomfort similar to that of duodenal ulcer, as well as diarrhea. Stools may be profuse, a malabsorption syndrome that is similar to giardiasis is common, and intestinal obstruction can occur. Marked eosinophilia is also present. Although death can occur, it is rare.

Laboratory Diagnosis

Stool examination reveals the large, golden, bile-stained eggs with an operculum on the top (Figure 50-2). The

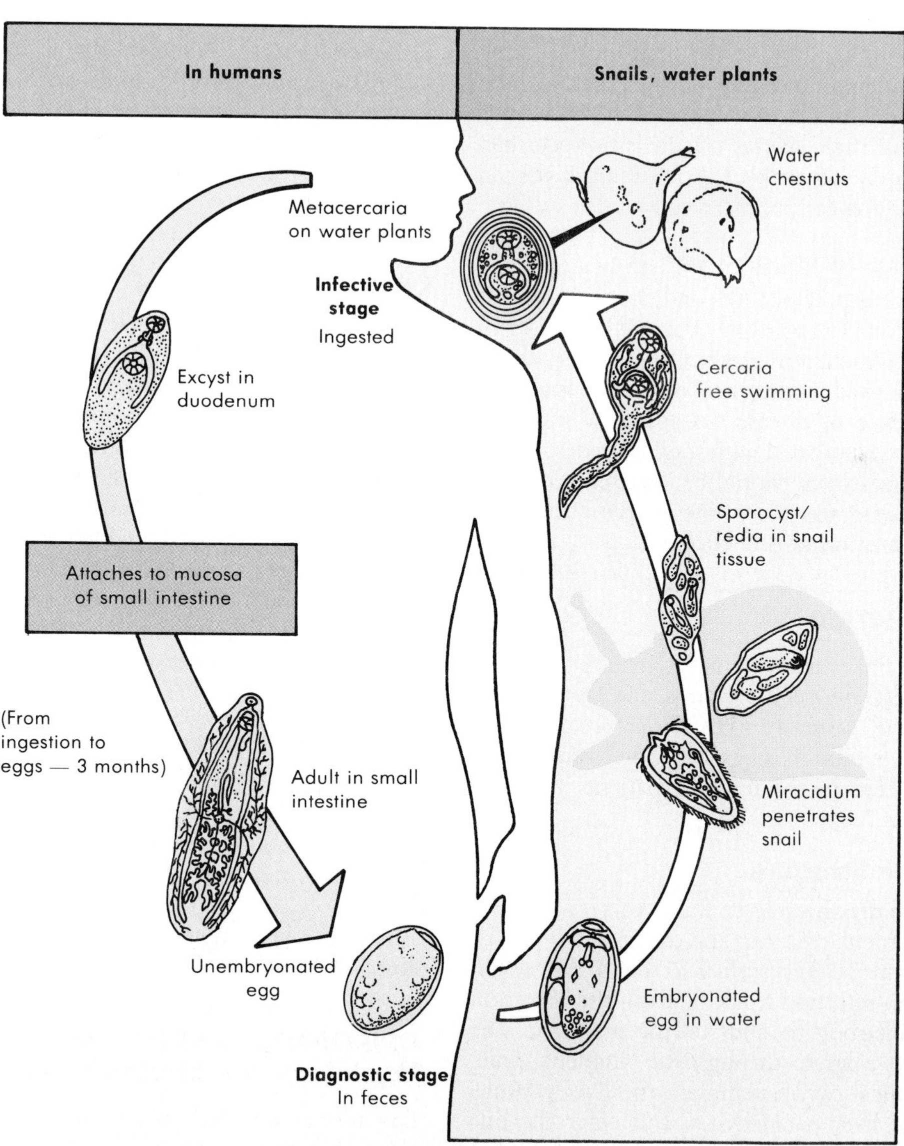

FIGURE 50-1 Life cycle of *Fasciolopsis buski* ("giant intestinal fluke").

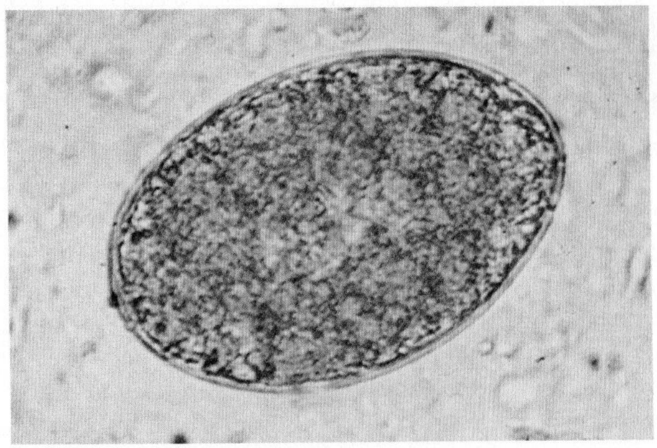

FIGURE 50-2 *Fasciolopsis buski* egg. The eggs are oval, large (75 to 100 μm by 130 to 150 μm), and surrounded by a thin shell. Although an operculum is present, it is rarely seen. (From Koneman EW, Allen SD, Dowell VR, and Sommers HM: *Color atlas and textbook of diagnostic microbiology*, ed 2, Philadelphia, 1979, JB Lippincott.)

measurements and appearance of *F. buski* eggs are similar to that of the liver fluke *Fasciola hepatica*, and differentiation of the eggs of these species usually is not possible. Large (approximately 1.5 cm by 3.0 cm) adult flukes can rarely be found in feces or specimens collected at surgery.

Treatment, Prevention, and Control

The drug of choice is praziquantel, and the alternative is niclosamide. Education regarding safe consumption of infective aquatic vegetation (particularly water chestnuts), proper sanitation, and control of human feces will reduce the incidence of disease. In addition, the snail population may be eliminated with molluscacides. When infection occurs, treatment should be initiated promptly to minimize its spread. Control of the reservoir hosts will also reduce transmission of the worm.

FASCIOLA HEPATICA

A number of liver flukes are recognized, including *Fasciola hepatica*, *Opisthorchis sinensis*, *O. felineus*, and *Dicrocoelium dendriticum*. Only *F. hepatica* and *O. sinensis* are discussed in this chapter, although eggs of other flukes are occasionally detected in the feces of patients in other geographical areas.

Physiology and Structure

Commonly called the **sheep liver fluke,** this is a parasite of herbivores (particularly sheep and cattle) and humans. Its life cycle (Figure 50-3) is similar to that of *Fasciolopsis buski,* with human infection resulting from the ingestion of watercress that harbors the encysted metacercariae. The larval flukes then migrate through the duodenal wall, across the peritoneal cavity, penetrate the liver capsule, pass through the liver parenchyma, and enter the bile ducts to become adult worms. Approximately 3 to 4 months after the initial infection the adult flukes start producing operculated eggs identical to those of *F. buski* as seen in stool examination.

Epidemiology

Infections have been reported worldwide in sheep-raising areas, with the appropriate snail as an intermediate host, including the former Soviet Union, Japan, Egypt, and many Latin American countries. Outbreaks are directly related to human consumption of contaminated watercress in areas where infected herbivores are present. Human infection is rare in the United States, but several well-documented cases have been reported in travelers from endemic areas.

Clinical Syndromes

Migration of the larval worm through the liver produces irritation of this tissue, tenderness, and hepatomegaly. Right upper quadrant pain, chills, and fever with marked eosinophilia are commonly observed. As the worms take up residence in the bile ducts, their mechanical irritation and toxic secretions produce hepatitis, hyperplasia of the epithelium, and biliary obstruction. Some worms penetrate eroded areas in the ducts and invade the liver to produce necrotic foci referred to as "liver rot." In severe infections secondary bacterial infection can occur, and portal cirrhosis is common.

Laboratory Diagnosis

Stool examination reveals operculated eggs indistinguishable from the eggs of *F. buski.* Exact identification is a therapeutic problem because treatment is not the same for both. Whereas *F. buski* responds favorably to praziquantel, *F. hepatica* does not. Where exact identification is desired, a sample of the patient's bile differentiates the species; if the eggs are present in bile, they are *Fasciola hepatica* and not *F. buski,* which is limited to the small intestine. Eggs may appear in stool samples from persons who have eaten infected sheep or cattle liver. The spurious nature of this finding can be confirmed by having the patient refrain from eating liver and then rechecking the stool.

Treatment, Prevention, and Control

In contrast to *F. buski*, *F. hepatica* responds poorly to praziquantel. Treatment with bithionol or the benzimidazole compound, triclabendazole, has been effective. Preventive measures are similar to those for *F. buski* control—especially avoiding ingestion of watercress and other uncooked aquatic vegetation in areas frequented by sheep and cattle.

OPISTHORCHIS SINENSIS

Physiology and Structure

This trematode, also referred to as *Clonorchis sinensis* in older literature, is commonly called the **Chinese liver**

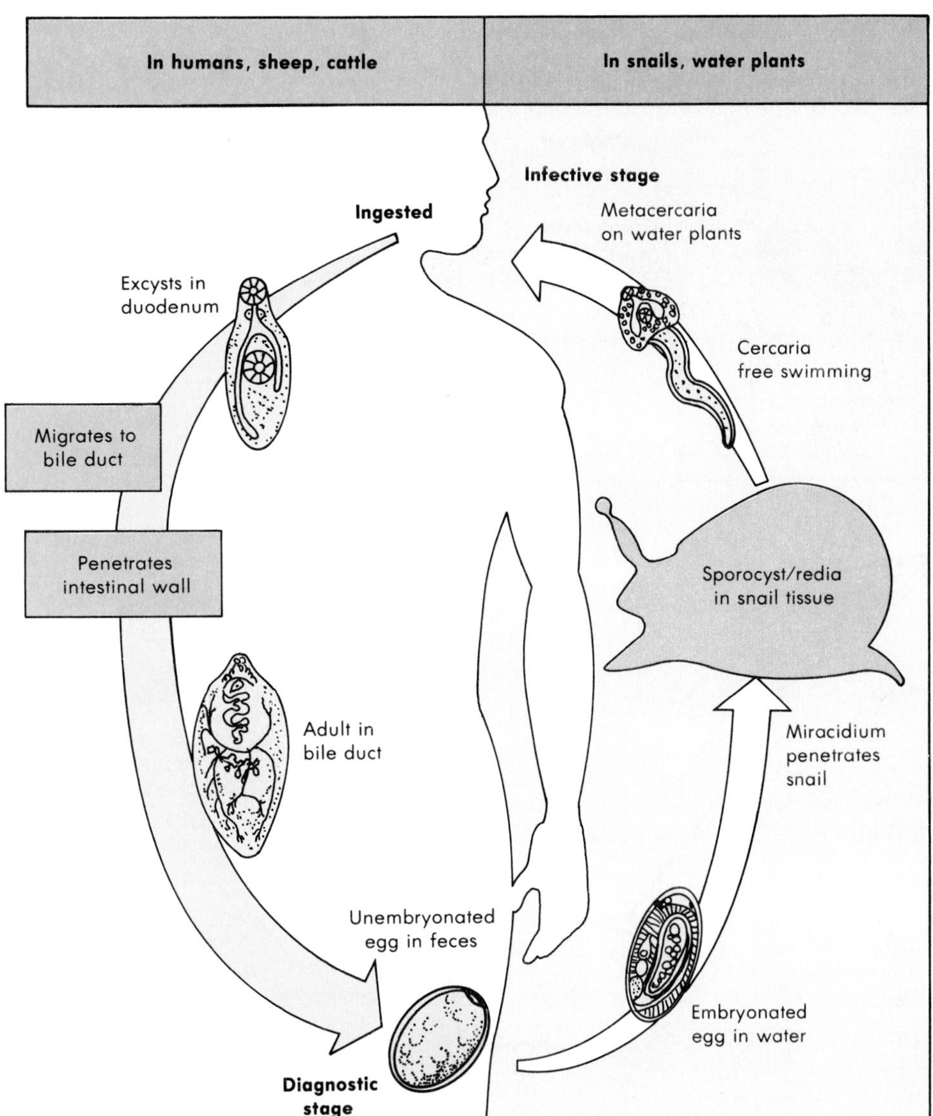

FIGURE 50-3 Life cycle of *Fasciola hepatica* ("sheep liver fluke").

fluke. Figure 50-4 illustrates this fluke's life cycle, which involves two intermediate hosts. *O. sinensis* differs from other fluke cycles because the eggs are eaten by the snail and then reproduction begins in the soft tissues of the snail. *O. sinensis* also requires a second intermediate host, freshwater fish, where the cercariae encyst and develop into infective metacercariae. When uncooked freshwater fish harboring metacercariae are eaten, flukes develop first in the duodenum and then migrate to the bile ducts where they become adults. The adult fluke undergoes self-fertilization and begins producing eggs. *O. sinensis* may survive in the biliary tract for as long as 50 years, producing approximately 2000 eggs per day. These eggs pass with feces and are once again eaten by snails, reinitiating the cycle.

Epidemiology

O. sinensis is found in China, Japan, Korea, and Vietnam, where it is estimated to infect approximately 19 million individuals. It is one of the most frequent infections seen among Asian refugees and can be traced to the consumption of raw, pickled, smoked, or dried freshwater fish harboring viable metacercariae. Dogs, cats, and fish-eating mammals also serve as reservoir hosts.

Clinical Syndromes

Infection in humans is usually mild and asymptomatic. Severe infections with many flukes in the bile ducts produce fever, diarrhea, epigastric pain, hepatomegaly, anorexia, and occasionally jaundice. Biliary obstruction may occur, and chronic infection can result in adenocar-

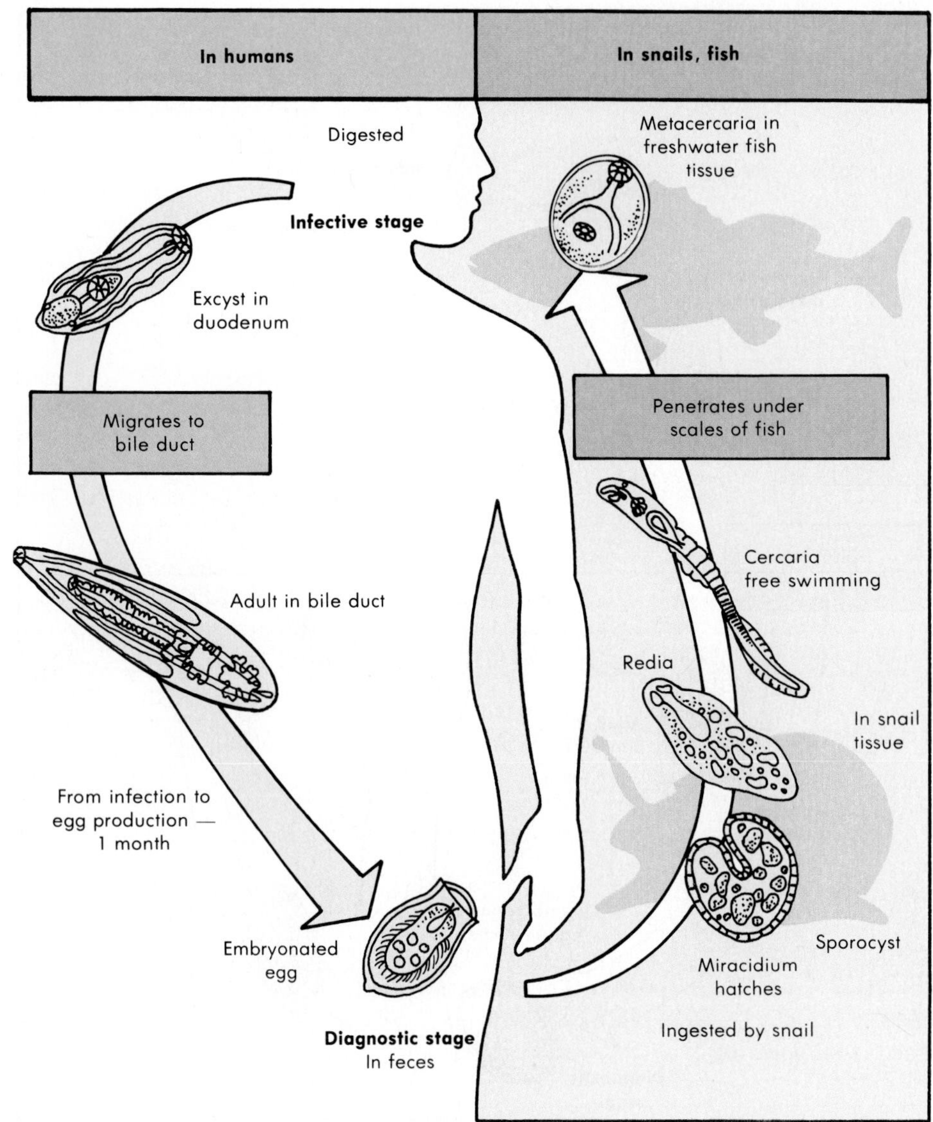

FIGURE 50-4 Life cycle of *Opisthorchis sinensis* ("Chinese liver fluke").

cinoma of the bile ducts. Invasion of the gallbladder may produce cholecystitis, cholelithiasis, and impaired liver function, as well as liver abscesses.

Laboratory Diagnosis

The diagnosis is made by recovering the distinctive eggs from stools. The eggs measure 27 to 35 μm by 12 to 19 μm and are characterized by a distinct operculum with prominent shoulders and a tiny knob at the posterior (abopercular) pole (Figure 50-5). In mild infections repeated examinations of stool or duodenal aspirates may be necessary. In acute symptomatic infection there is usually an eosinophilia and elevation of serum alkaline phosphatase levels. Radiographic imaging procedures may detect abnormalities of the biliary tract.

Treatment, Prevention, and Control

The drug of choice is praziquantel. Prevention of infection is accomplished by not eating uncooked fish and by implementing proper sanitation policies, including disposal of human, dog, and cat feces in adequately protected sites so that they cannot contaminate water supplies with the intermediate snail and fish hosts.

PARAGONIMUS WESTERMANI

Physiology and Structure

Paragonimus westermani, commonly called the **lung fluke,** is one of several species of *Paragonimus* that infect humans and many other animals. Figure 50-6 shows a familiar fluke life cycle from egg to snail to infective metacercaria. The infective stage occurs in a second intermediate

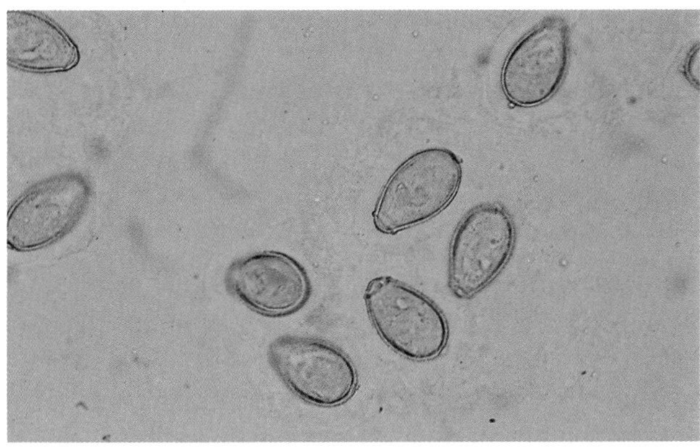

FIGURE 50-5 *Opisthorchis sinensis* egg. These ovoid eggs are small (22 to 30 μm long by 12 to 19 μm wide) and have a yellowish-brown thick shell with a prominent operculum at one end and a small knob at the other end.

host—the muscles and gills of freshwater crabs and crayfish. In humans who ingest infected meat, the larval worm hatches in the stomach and follows an extensive migration through the intestinal wall to the abdominal cavity, then through the diaphragm, and finally to the pleural cavity. Adult worms reside in the lungs and produce eggs that are liberated from ruptured bronchioles and appear in sputum or, when swallowed, in feces.

Epidemiology

Paragonimiasis occurs in many countries in Asia, Africa, India, and Latin America. It can be seen in refugees from Southeast Asia. Its prevalence is directly related to the consumption of uncooked freshwater crabs and crayfish. It is estimated that approximately 3 million individuals are infected with this lung fluke. As many as 1% of all Indochinese immigrants to the United States are infected

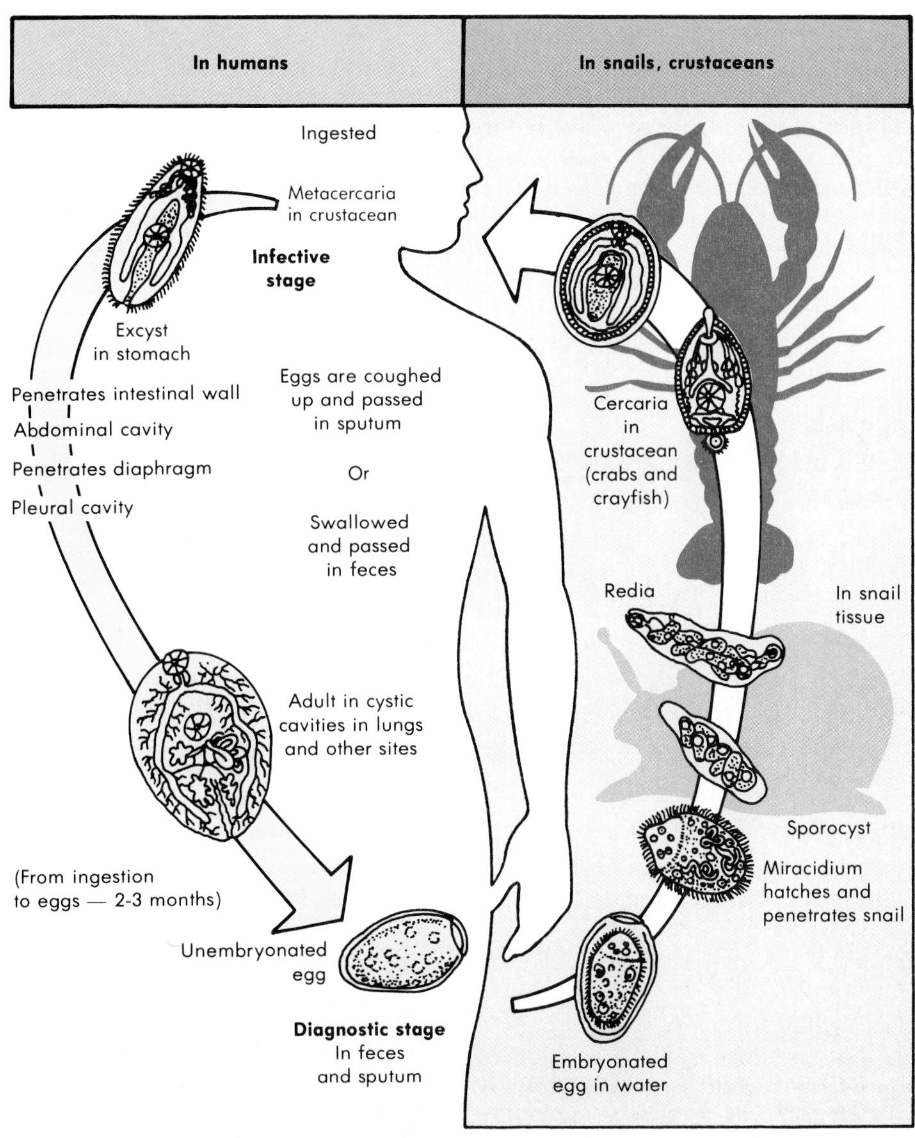

FIGURE 50-6 Life cycle of *Paragonimus westermani* ("Oriental lung fluke").

with *P. westermani*. A wide variety of shore-feeding animals (e.g., wild boars, pigs, and monkeys) serve as reservoir hosts, and some human infections result from ingestion of meat containing migrating larval worms from these reservoir hosts. Human infections endemic to the United States are usually caused by a related species, *Paragonimus kellicotti*, which is found in crabs and crayfish in eastern and midwestern waters.

Clinical Syndromes

The clinical manifestations of paragonimiasis may be due to larvae migrating through tissues or to adults established in the lungs or other ectopic sites. The onset of disease coincides with larval migration and is associated with fever, chills, and high eosinophilia. The adult flukes in the lungs first produce an inflammatory reaction that results in fever, cough, and increased sputum. As destruction of lung tissue progresses, cavitation occurs around the worms, sputum is blood tinged and dark with eggs (so-called rusty sputum), and patients experience severe chest pain. The resulting cavity may become secondarily infected with bacteria. Dyspnea, chronic bronchitis, bronchiectasis, and pleural effusion may be seen. Chronic infections lead to fibrosis in the lung tissue. Location of larvae, adults, and eggs in ectopic sites may produce severe clinical symptoms depending on the site involved. The migration of larval worms may result in invasion of the spinal cord and brain, producing severe neurological disease (visual problems, motor weakness, and convulsive seizures) referred to as **cerebral paragonimiasis.** Migration and infection may also occur in subcutaneous sites, in the abdominal cavity, and in the liver.

Laboratory Diagnosis

Examination of sputum and feces will reveal the golden-brown, operculated eggs (Figure 50-7). Pleural effusions, when present, should also be examined for eggs. Chest x-ray films often show infiltrates, nodular cysts, and pleural effusion. Marked eosinophilia is common. Serologic procedures are available through reference laboratories and can be helpful, particularly in cases with extrapulmonary (e.g., central nervous system) involvement.

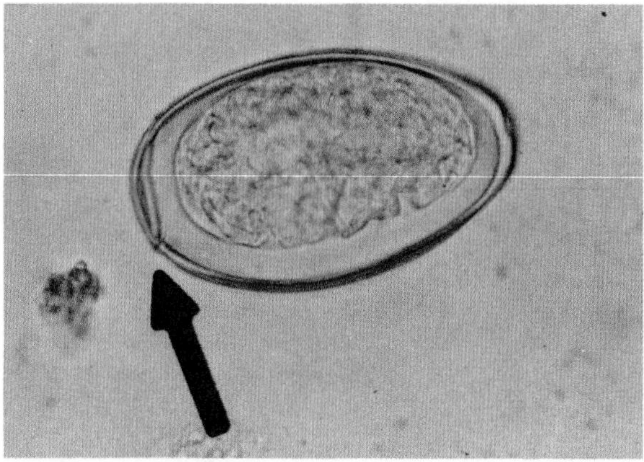

FIGURE 50-7 *Paragonimus westermani* egg. These large ovoid eggs (80 to 120 μm long and 45 to 70 μm wide) have a thick yellowish-brown shell and a distinct operculum (*arrow*). (From Koneman EW, Allen SD, Dowell VR, and Sommers HM: *Color atlas and textbook of diagnostic microbiology*, ed 2, Philadelphia, 1979, JB Lippincott.)

Treatment, Prevention, and Control

The drug of choice is praziquantel, with bithionol as an alternative. Education regarding the consumption of uncooked freshwater crabs and crayfish, as well as the flesh of animals found in endemic areas, is critical. Pickling and wine-soaking of crabs and crayfish will not kill the infective metacercarial stage. Proper sanitation and control of the disposal of human feces are essential.

SCHISTOSOMES

Schistosomiasis is a major parasitic infection of tropical areas, with some 200 million infections worldwide. The three schistosomes most frequently associated with human disease are *Schistosoma mansoni*, *S. japonicum*, and *S. haematobium*. They collectively produce the disease called **schistosomiasis,** also known as **bilharziasis** or "**snail fever.**" As discussed earlier, the schistosomes differ from other flukes: they are male and female rather than hermaphroditic, and their eggs do not have an operculum. They also are obligate intravascular parasites and are not found in cavities, ducts, and other tissues. The infective forms are skin-penetrating cercariae liberated from snails, and these differ from other flukes in that they are not eaten on vegetation, in fish, or in crustaceans.

Figure 50-8 illustrates the life cycle of the different schistosomes. It is initiated by ciliated, free-swimming cercaria in fresh water that penetrate intact skin, enter the circulation, and develop in the intrahepatic portal circulation (*S. mansoni* and *S. japonicum*) or in the vessicle, prostate, rectal and uterine plexuses and veins (*S. haematobium*). The female has a long, slender, cylindrical body, whereas the shorter male, which appears cylindrical, is actually flat. The cylindrical appearance derives from folding the sides of the body to produce a groove, the gynecophoral canal, in which the female resides for fertilization. Both sexes have oral and ventral suckers and an incomplete digestive system, typical of a fluke.

As the worms develop in the portal circulation, they elaborate a remarkable defense against host resistance. They coat themselves with substances that the host recognizes as itself; consequently, there is little protective response directed against their presence in blood vessels. This protective mechanism accounts for chronic infections that may last 20 to 30 years or longer.

After developing in the portal vein, the male and female adult worms pair up and migrate to their final locations, where fertilization and egg production begins. *S. mansoni* and *S. japonicum* are found in mesenteric veins and produce **intestinal schistosomiasis;** *S. haematobium* occurs in veins around the urinary bladder and causes **vesicular schistosomiasis**. On reaching the submucosal venules of their respective locations, the worms initiate oviposition, which may continue at the rate of 300 to 3000 eggs daily for 4 to 35 years. Although the host inflammatory response to the adult worms is minimal, the eggs elicit an intense inflammatory reaction with both mononuclear and polymorphonuclear cellular infiltrates and the formation of microabscesses. In addition, the larvae inside the eggs produce enzymes that aid in tissue destruction and allow the eggs to pass through the mucosa and into the lumen of the bowel and bladder, where they are passed to the external environment in the feces and urine, respectively.

The eggs hatch quickly upon reaching fresh water to release motile miracidia. The miracidia then invade the appropriate snail host where they develop into thousands of infectious cercariae. The free-swimming cercariae are released into the water where they are immediately infectious for humans and other mammals.

The infection is similar in all three species of human schistosomes in that disease results primarily from the host's immune response to the eggs. The very earliest signs and symptoms are due to the penetration of the cercariae through the skin. Immediate and delayed hypersensitivity to parasite antigens results in an intensely pruritic papular skin rash.

The onset of oviposition results in a symptom complex known as **Katayama syndrome**, which is marked by fever, chills, cough, urticaria, arthralgias, lymphadenopathy, splenomegaly, and abdominal pain. This syndrome is typically seen 1 to 2 months after primary exposure and may persist for 3 months or more. It is thought to be due to the massive release of parasite antigens with subsequent

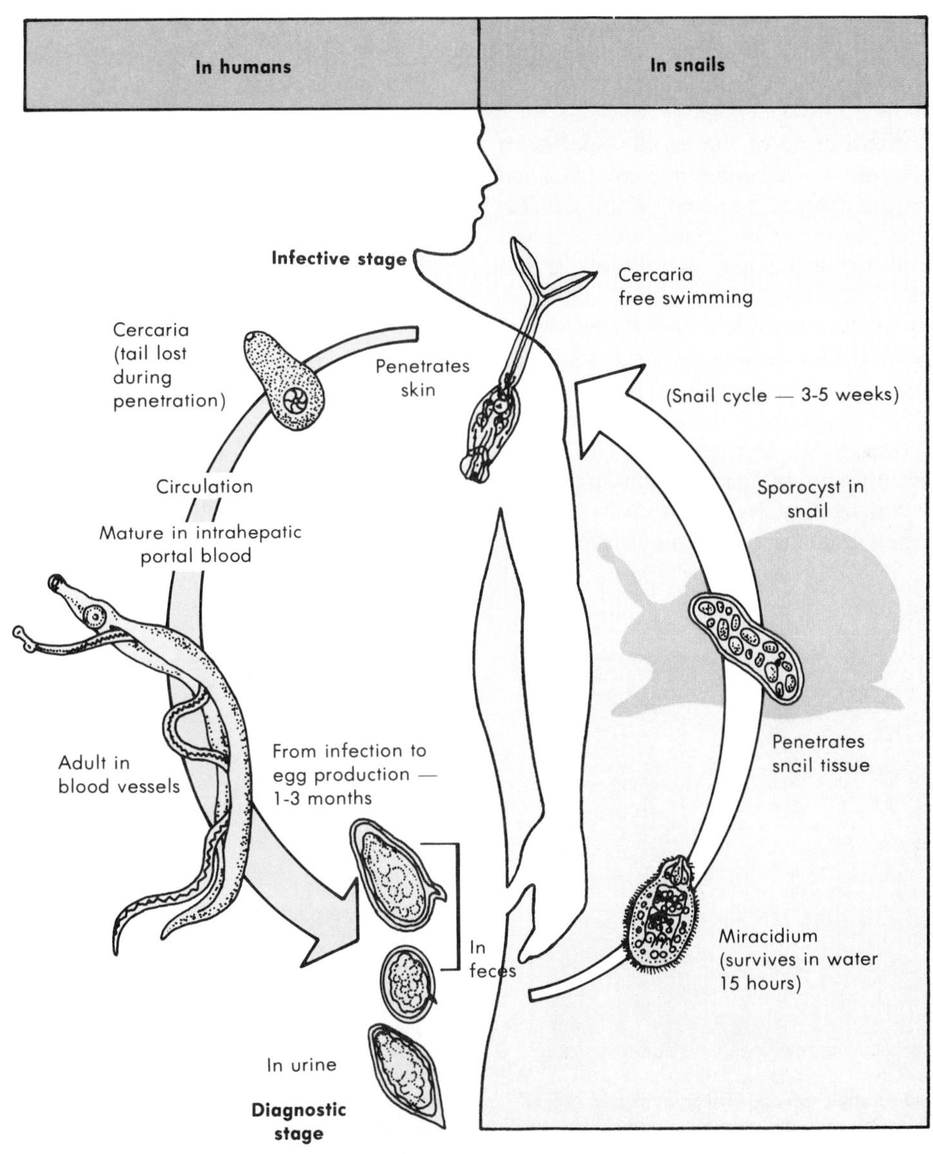

FIGURE 50-8 Life cycle of schistosomes.

immune complex formation. Associated laboratory abnormalities include leukocytosis, eosinophilia, and a polyclonal gammopathy.

The more chronic and significant phase of schistosomiasis is due to the presence of the eggs in various tissues and the resulting formation of granulomas and fibrosis. The retained eggs induce extensive inflammation and scarring, the clinical significance of which is directly related to the location and number of eggs.

Because of differences in some aspects of disease and epidemiology, these worms are discussed as separate species.

Schistosoma Mansoni

Physiology and Structure

S. mansoni usually resides in the small branches of the inferior mesenteric vein near the lower colon. The species of *Schistosoma* can be differentiated by their characteristic egg morphology (Figures 50-9 to 50-11). The eggs of *S. mansoni* are oval, possess a sharp lateral spine, and measure 115 to 175 μm by 45-70 μm (see Figure 50-9).

Epidemiology

The geographical distribution of the various species of *Schistosoma* depends on the availability of a suitable snail host. *S. mansoni* is the most widespread of the schistosomes and is endemic in Africa, Saudi Arabia, and Malagasy. It has also become well established in the Western Hemisphere, particularly in Brazil, Surinam, Venezuela, parts of the West Indies, and Puerto Rico. Cases originating in these areas occur in the United States. In all of these areas there are also reservoir hosts, specifically primates, marsupials, and rodents. Schistosomiasis may be considered a disease of economic progress—the development of massive land irrigation projects in desert and tropical areas has resulted in the dispersion of infected humans and snails to previously uninvolved areas.

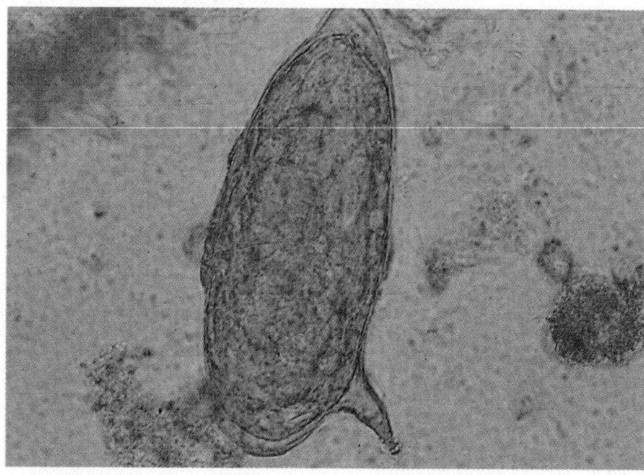

FIGURE 50-9 *Schistosoma mansoni* egg. These eggs are 115 to 175 μm long and 45 to 70 μm wide, contain a miracidium, and are enclosed in a thin shell with a prominent lateral spine.

Clinical Syndromes

As noted previously, cercarial penetration of the intact skin may be seen as a dermatitis with allergic reactions, pruritus, and edema. Migrating worms in the lungs may produce cough, and as they reach the liver, hepatitis may appear.

Infections with *S. mansoni* may produce hepatic and intestinal abnormalities. As the flukes take residence in the mesenteric vessels and egg laying begins, fever, malaise, abdominal pain, and tenderness of the liver may be observed. Deposition of eggs in the bowel mucosa results in inflammation and thickening of the bowel wall with associated abdominal pain, diarrhea, and blood in the stool. Importantly, eggs may be carried by the portal vein

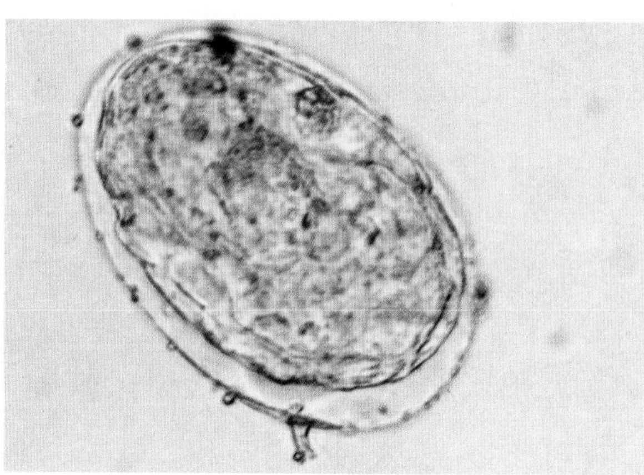

FIGURE 50-10 *Schistosoma japonicum* egg. These eggs are smaller than those of *S. mansoni* (70 to 100 μm long by 55 to 65 μm wide) and have a spine that is inconspicuous. (From Ash LR, Orihel TC: *Atlas of human parasitology*, ed 2, Chicago, 1984, *American Society of Clinical Pathologists.*)

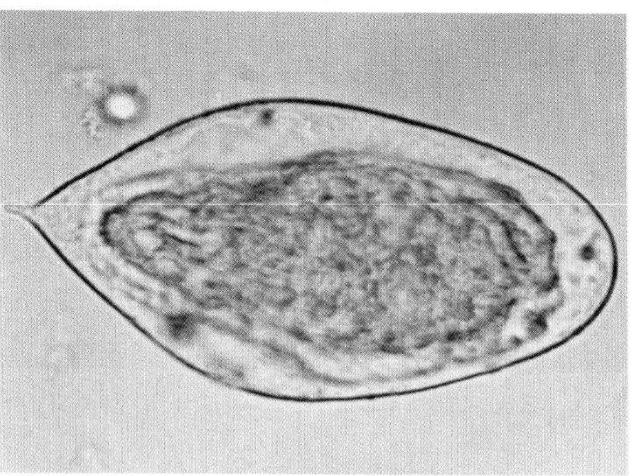

FIGURE 50-11 *Schistosoma haematobium* egg. These eggs are similar in size to those of *S. mansoni* but can be differentiated by the presence of a terminal spine. (From Ash LR, Orihel TC: *Atlas of human parasitology*, ed 2, Chicago, 1984, American Society of Clinical Pathologists.)

to the liver, where inflammation can lead to periportal fibrosis and eventually to portal hypertension and its associated manifestations.

Chronic infection with *S. mansoni* shows a dramatic hepatosplenomegaly with large accumulations of ascitic fluid in the peritoneal cavity. On gross examination, the liver is studded with white granulomas **(pseudotubercles)**. Although *S. mansoni* eggs are primarily deposited in the intestine, eggs may appear in the spinal cord, lungs, and other sites. A similar fibrotic process occurs at each site. Severe neurological problems may follow when eggs are deposited in the spinal cord and brain. In fatal schistosomiasis caused by *S. mansoni*, fibrous tissue reaction to the eggs in the liver surrounds the portal vein in a thick, grossly visible layer ("clay pipestem fibrosis").

Laboratory Diagnosis

The diagnosis of schistosomiasis is usually established by the demonstration of characteristic eggs in feces. Stool examination reveals the large golden eggs with a sharp lateral spine (see Figure 50-9). Concentration techniques may be necessary in light infections. Rectal biopsy is also helpful to see the egg tracks laid by the worms in rectal vessels. Quantitation of egg output in stool is useful in estimating the severity of infection and in following response to therapy. Serologic tests are also available but are largely of epidemiological interest only. The development of newer tests using stage-specific antigens may allow the distinction of active from inactive disease and thus have greater clinical utility.

Treatment, Prevention, and Control

The drug of choice is praziquantel, and the alternative is oxamniquine. Antihelminthic therapy may terminate oviposition but will not affect lesions caused by eggs already deposited in tissues. Schistosomal dermatitis and the Katayama syndrome may be treated with the administration of antihistamines and corticosteroids. Education regarding the life cycles of these worms is essential, as well as control of snails using molluscacides. Improved sanitation and control of human fecal deposits are critical. Mass treatment may one day be practical, and the development of a vaccine may be forthcoming.

Schistosoma Japonicum

Physiology and Structure

S. japonicum resides in branches of the superior mesenteric vein around the small intestine and in the inferior mesenteric vessels. *S. japonicum* eggs (Figure 50-10) are smaller, almost spherical, and possess a tiny spine. These eggs are produced in greater numbers than those of *S. mansoni* and *S. haematobium*. Because of the size, shape, and numbers of these eggs, they are carried to more sites in the body (liver, lungs, brain), and infection with a few *S. japonicum* adults can be more severe than infections involving similar numbers of *S. mansoni* or *S. haematobium*.

Epidemiology

This **Oriental blood fluke** is found only in China, Japan, the Philippines, and on the island of Sulawesi, Indonesia. Epidemiological problems correlate directly with a broad range of reservoir hosts, many of which are domestic (cats, dogs, cattle, horses, and pigs).

Clinical Syndromes

The initial stages of infection with *S. japonicum* are similar to those of *S. mansoni*, with dermatitis, allergic reactions, fever, malaise followed by abdominal discomfort, and diarrhea. The Katayama syndrome associated with the onset of oviposition is observed more commonly with *S. japonicum* than with *S. mansoni*. In chronic *S. japonicum* infection, hepatosplenic disease, portal hypertension, bleeding esophageal varices, and accumulation of ascitic fluid are commonly seen. Granulomas that appear as pseudotubercles in and on the liver are common, along with the "clay pipestem fibrosis" as described for *S. mansoni*.

S. japonicum frequently involves cerebral structures when eggs reach the brain and granulomas develop around them. The neurological manifestations include lethargy, speech impairment, visual defects, and seizures.

Laboratory Diagnosis

Stool examination demonstrates the small golden eggs with tiny spines; usually, rectal biopsy is similarly revealing. Serologic tests are available.

Treatment, Prevention, and Control

The drug of choice is praziquantel. Prevention and control may be achieved by measures similar to those for *S. mansoni*, especially education of populations in endemic areas regarding proper water purification, sanitation, and control of human fecal deposits. Control of *S. japonicum* must also involve the broad range of reservoir hosts and consider the fact that people work in rice paddies and on irrigation projects where infected snails are present. Mass treatment may offer help, and a vaccine may be developed someday.

Schistosoma Haematobium

Physiology and Structure

Following development in the liver, these blood flukes migrate to the vesicular, prostatic, and uterine plexuses of the venous circulation, occasionally the portal bloodstream, and only rarely in other venules.

Large eggs with a sharp terminal spine (Figure 50-11) are deposited in the wall of the bladder and occasionally in the uterine and prostatic tissues. Those deposited in the bladder wall can break free and are found in urine.

Epidemiology

S. haematobium occurs throughout the Nile Valley and in many other parts of Africa, including islands off the eastern coast. It also appears in Asia Minor, Cyprus, southern Portugal, and India. Reservoir hosts include monkeys, baboons, and chimpanzees.

Clinical Syndromes

Early stages of infection with *S. haematobium* are similar to those of infections involving *S. mansoni* and *S. japonicum,* with dermatitis, allergic reactions, fever, and malaise. Unlike the other two schistosomes, *S. haematobium* produces hematuria, dysuria, and urinary frequency as early symptoms. Associated with hematuria, bacteriuria is frequently a chronic condition. Egg deposition in the walls of the bladder eventually may result in scarring with loss of bladder capacity and the development of obstructive uropathy.

Patients with *S. haematobium* infections involving many flukes frequently demonstrate a squamous cell carcinoma of the bladder. It is commonly stated that the leading cause of cancer of the bladder in Egypt and other parts of Africa is *S. haematobium.* The granulomas and pseudotubercles of *S. haematobium* seen in the bladder may also be present in the lungs. Fibrosis of the pulmonary bed from egg deposition leads to dyspnea, cough, and hemoptysis.

Laboratory Diagnosis

Examination of urine specimens reveals the large, terminally spined eggs. Occasionally bladder biopsy is helpful in establishing the diagnosis. *S. haematobium* eggs may appear in stool examination if worms have migrated to mesenteric vessels. Serologic tests are also available.

Treatment, Prevention, and Control

The drug of choice is praziquantel. At present, education, possible mass treatment, and development of a vaccine are the best approaches to control of *S. haematobium* disease. The basic problems of irrigation projects (e.g., dam building), migratory human populations, and multiple reservoir hosts make prevention and control extremely difficult.

CERCARIAL DERMATITIS ("SWIMMER'S ITCH")

Several nonhuman schistosomes have cercariae that penetrate human skin, producing a severe dermatitis, but these cannot develop into adult worms. The natural hosts of these schistosomes are birds and other shore-feeding animals from freshwater lakes throughout the world and a few marine beaches. The intense pruritus and urticaria from this skin penetration may lead to secondary bacterial infection from scratching the sites of infection.

Treatment consists of oral trimeprazine and topical applications of palliatives. When indicated, sedatives may be given. Control is difficult because of bird migration and transfer of live snails from lake to lake. Molluscicides such as copper sulfate have produced some reduction in snail populations. Immediate drying of the skin when leaving such waters offers some protection.

CASE STUDY AND QUESTIONS

A 45-year-old Egyptian male is referred for evaluation of hematuria and urinary frequency of 2 months' duration. This individual lived in the Middle East for most of his life but for the past year has lived in the United States. He denies previous renal or urological problems. His physical examination is unremarkable. A midstream urine specimen is grossly bloody.

1. What is the differential diagnosis of hematuria in this patient?
2. What was the etiological agent of this patient's urological process?
3. What exposures might put an individual at risk for this infection?
4. What are the major complications of this infection?
5. How is this disease treated?

Bibliography

Beaver PC, Jung RC, and Cupp EW: *Clinical parasitology*, ed 9, Philadelphia, 1984, Lea & Febiger.

Burton K et al.: Pulmonary paragonimiasis in Laotian refugee children, *Pediatrics* 70:246-248, 1982.

James SL: *Schistosoma* spp: progress toward a defined vaccine, *Exp Parasitol* 63:247-252, 1987.

Johnson RJ et al.: Paragonimiasis, diagnosis and use of praziquantel in treatment, *Rev Infect Dis* 7:200-206, 1985.

Markell EK, Voge M, and John DT: *Medical parasitology*, ed 7, Philadelphia, 1992, WB Saunders.

Nash TE, Cheever AW, Ottesen EA, Cook JA: Schistosoma infection in humans: perspectives and recent findings, *Ann Intern Med* 97:740-754, 1982.

Warren KS: Selective primary health care: Strategies for control of disease in the developing world. I. Schistosomiasis, *Rev Infect Dis* 4:715-726, 1982.

Wongratanacheewin S, Bunnag D, Vaeusorn N, and Sirisinba S: Characterization of humoral immune response in the serum and bile of patients with opisthorchiasis and its application in immunodiagnosis, *Am J Trop Med Hyg* 38:356-362, 1988.

CHAPTER 51

Cestodes

THE bodies of cestodes, **tapeworms,** are flat and ribbonlike, and the heads are equipped with organs of attachment. The head, or **scolex,** of the worm usually has four muscular cup-shaped suckers, and a crown of hooklets. An exception is seen with *Diphyllobothrium latum,* the fish tapeworm, whose scolex is equipped with a pair of long, lateral muscular grooves and lacks hooklets.

The individual segments of tapeworms are called **proglottids,** and the chain of proglottids is called a **strobila.**

All tapeworms are hermaphroditic, with male and female reproductive organs present in each mature proglottid. The eggs of most tapeworms are nonoperculated and contain a six-hooked hexacanth embryo; the one exception, *Diphyllobothrium latum,* has an unembryonated operculated egg similar to fluke eggs. Tapeworms have no digestive system, and food is absorbed from the host intestine through the soft body wall of the worm. Most tapeworms found in the human intestine have complex life cycles involving intermediate hosts, and in some instances (cysticercosis, echinococcosis, sparganosis) humans serve as a form of intermediate host that harbors larval stages. These extraintestinal larval infections are at times more serious than the presence of adult worms in the intestine. The most common cestodes of medical importance are listed in Table 51-1.

TAENIA SOLIUM

Physiology and Structure

After a person ingests pork muscle containing a larval worm called a **cysticercus** ("bladder worm"), attachment of the scolex with its four muscular suckers and crown of hooklets initiates infection in the small intestine (Figure 51-1). The worm then produces proglottids until a strobila of proglottids is developed, which may be several meters in length. The sexually mature proglottids contain eggs, and as these proglottids leave the host in feces they can contaminate water and vegetation ingested by swine. The eggs in swine become a six-hooked larval form called an **oncosphere** that penetrates the pig's intestinal wall, migrates in the circulation to the tissues, and becomes a cysticercus to complete the cycle.

Epidemiology

T. solium infection is directly correlated with eating insufficiently cooked pork and is prevalent in Africa, India, Southeast Asia, China, Mexico, Latin American countries, and Slavic countries. It is seen infrequently in the United States.

Clinical Syndromes

Adult *Taenia solium* in the intestine seldom causes appreciable symptoms. The intestine may be irritated

TABLE 51-1 Medically Important Cestodes

Cestode	Common name	Reservoir for larvae	Reservoir for adults
Taenia solium	Pork tapeworm	Hogs	Humans
	Cysticercosis	Humans	—
Taenia saginata	Beef tapeworm	Cattle	Humans
Diphyllobothrium latum	Fish tapeworm	Freshwater crustaceans Freshwater fish	Humans, dogs, cats, bears
Echinococcus granulosus	Unilocular hydatid cyst	Herbivores, humans	Canines
Echinococcus multilocularis	Alveolar hydatid cyst	Herbivores, humans	Foxes, wolves, dogs, cats
Hymenolepsis nana	Dwarf tapeworm	Rodents, humans	Rodents, humans
Hymenolepsis diminuta	Dwarf tapeworm	Insects	Rodents, humans
Dipylidium caninum	Pumpkin seed tapeworm	Fleas	Dogs, cats

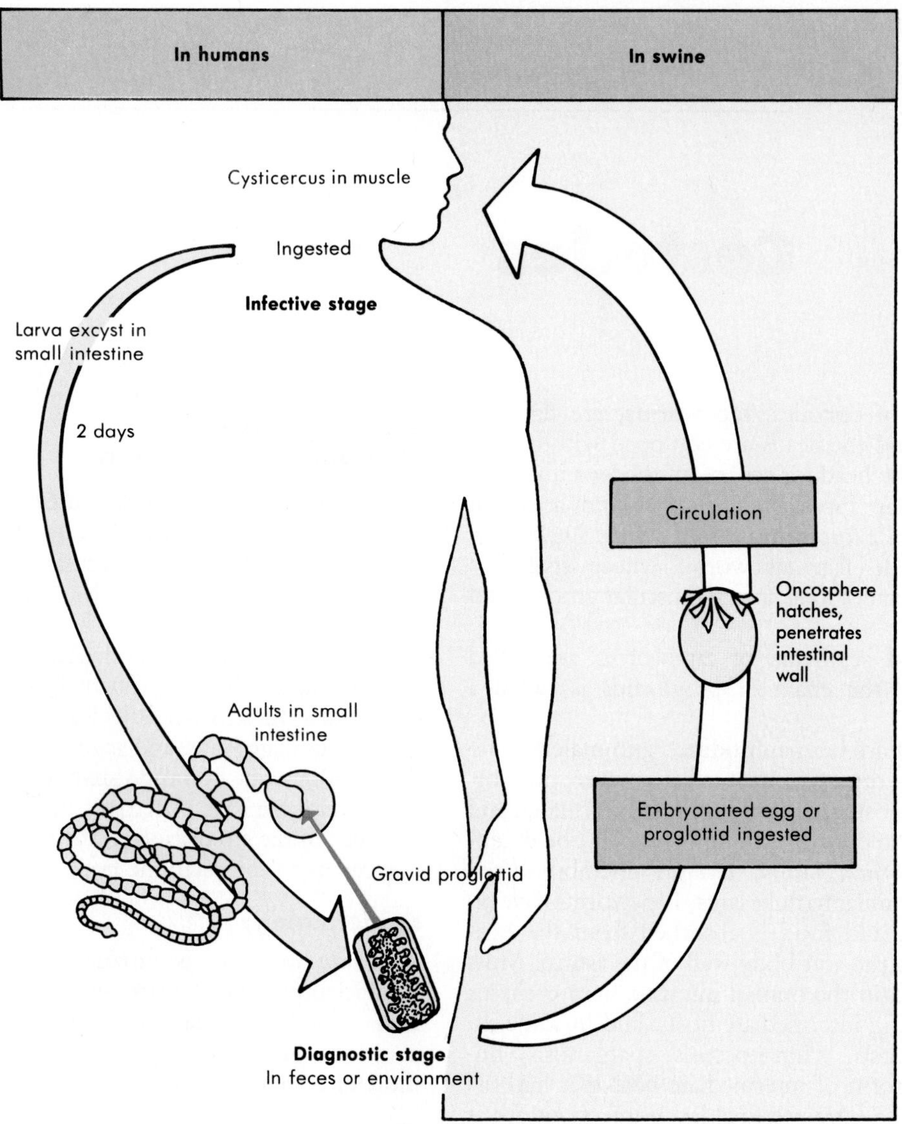

FIGURE 51-1 Life cycle of *Taenia solium* ("pork tapeworm").

at sites of attachment, and abdominal discomfort, chronic indigestion, and diarrhea may occur. Most patients become aware of the infection only when they see proglottids or a strobila of proglottids in their feces.

Laboratory Diagnosis

Stool examination may reveal proglottids and eggs, and treatment may produce the entire worm for identification. The eggs are spherical, 30 to 40 μm in diameter, and possess a thick, radially striated shell containing a 6-hooked hexacanth embryo (Figure 51-2). The eggs are identical to those of *Taenia saginata* (beef tapeworm), so eggs alone are not sufficient for species identification. Critical examination of the proglottids reveals their internal structure, which is important for differentiation of *T. solium* and *T. saginata*. Gravid proglottids of *T. solium* are smaller than those of *T. saginata* and contain

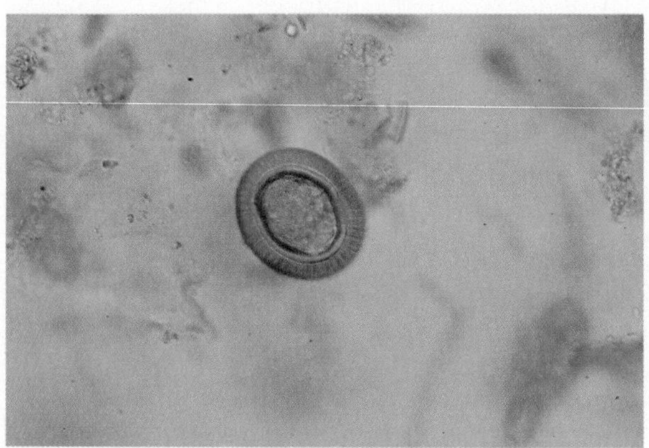

FIGURE 51-2 *Taenia* egg. The eggs are spherical, 40 μm in diameter, and contain 3 pairs of hooklets internally. The eggs of the different *Taenia* species cannot be differentiated.

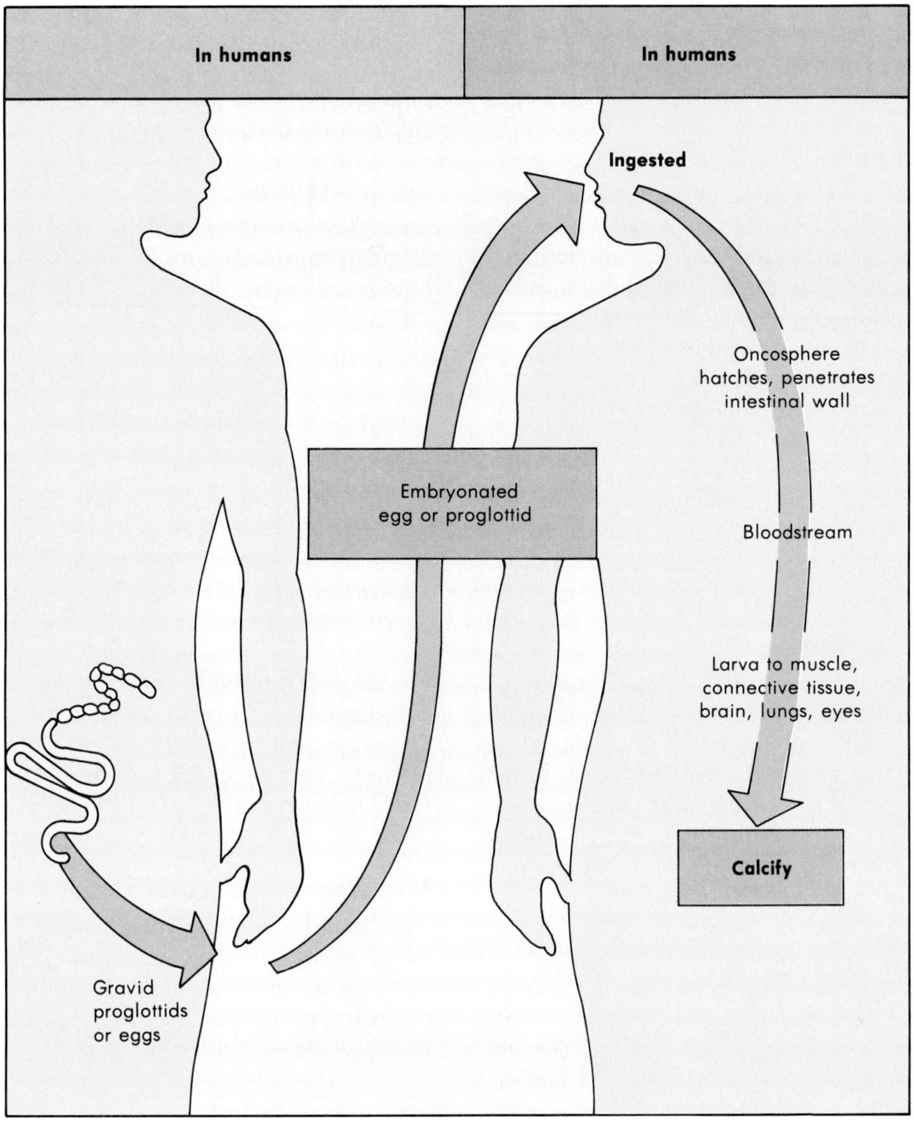

FIGURE 51-3 Development of human cysticercosis.

only 7 to 13 lateral uterine branches versus 15 to 30 for the beef tapeworm.

Treatment, Prevention, and Control

The drug of choice is niclosamide; praziquantel, paromomycin, or quinacrine are effective alternatives. Prevention of pork tapeworm infections requires that pork either be cooked until the interior of the meat is gray or be frozen at −20° C for at least 12 hours. Sanitation is critical; every effort must be made to keep human feces containing *T. solium* eggs out of water and vegetation ingested by pigs.

CYSTICERCOSIS

Physiology and Structure

Cysticercosis involves infection of individuals with the larval stage of *T. solium,* the cysticerci, which normally infects pigs (Figure 51-3). Human ingestion of water or vegetation contaminated with *T. solium* eggs from human feces initiates the infection. Autoinfection may occur when eggs from an individual infected with the adult worm are transferred from the perianal area to the mouth on contaminated fingers. Once ingested, the eggs hatch in the stomach of the intermediate host, releasing the hexacanth embryo or oncosphere. The oncosphere penetrates the intestinal wall and migrates in the circulation to the tissues, where it develops into a cysticercus over 3 to 4 months. The cysticerci may develop in muscle, connective tissue, brain, lung, and eyes and remain viable for as long as 5 years.

Epidemiology

Cysticercosis is found in the areas where *Taenia solium* is prevalent and is directly correlated with human fecal contamination. In addition to fecal-oral transmission, autoinfection may occur when a proglottid containing eggs is regurgitated from the small intestine into the stomach, allowing the eggs to hatch and release the infectious oncosphere.

Clinical Syndromes

A few cysticerci in nonvital areas (subcutaneous tissues, among others) may not provoke symptoms, but serious disease may follow as the cysticerci lodge in vital areas such as the brain or eyes. In the brain they may produce hydrocephalus, meningitis, cranial nerve damage, seizures, hyperactive reflexes, and visual defects. In the eye, loss of visual acuity may occur, and if the larvae lodge along the optic tract, visual field defects result. Tissue reaction to viable larvae may be only moderate, thus minimizing symptoms. However, the death of the larvae results in the release of antigenic material that stimulates a marked inflammatory reaction with exacerbation of symptoms and resulting fever, muscle pains, and eosinophilia.

Laboratory Diagnosis

The presence of cysticerci is usually established by the appearance of calcified cysticerci in soft tissue roentgenograms, surgical removal of subcutaneous nodules, and visualization of cysts in the eye. Central nervous system lesions may be detected by computed tomography, radioisotope scanning, or ultrasonography. Serologic studies may be useful, but false positives may occur in individuals with other helminthic infections.

Treatment, Prevention, and Control

The drug of choice for cysticercosis is praziquantel. Albendazole has also been used successfully in the treatment of parenchymal neurocysticercosis. Concomitant steroid administration may be necessary in minimizing the inflammatory response to dying larvae. Surgical removal of cerebral and ocular cysts may be necessary. Critical to prevention and control of human infection are the treatment of human cases harboring adult *T. solium* to reduce egg transmission and the controlled disposal of human feces. These measures will also reduce infection in pigs.

TAENIA SAGINATA

Physiology and Structure

The life cycle of *T. saginata*, the **beef tapeworm,** is similar to that of *T. solium* (Figure 51-4), with infection resulting after cysticerci are ingested in insufficiently cooked beef. Following excystment, the larvae develop into adults in the small intestine and initiate egg production in maturing proglottids. The adult worm may parasitize the jejunum and small intestine of humans for as long as 25 years, attaining a length of 10 m. A major difference, in contrast with *T. solium* infections, is that cysticercosis produced by *T. saginata* does not occur in humans. The adult *T. saginata* worm also differs from *T. solium* because it lacks a crown of hooklets on the scolex and has a different proglottid uterine branch structure. These facts are important in differentiating between the two tapeworms but do not affect the selection of therapy.

Epidemiology

T. saginata occurs worldwide and is one of the most frequent causes of cestode infection seen in the United States. Humans and cattle perpetuate the life cycle: human feces contaminate water and vegetation with eggs, which are then ingested by cattle. The cysticerci in cattle produce adult tapeworms in humans when rare or insufficiently cooked beef is eaten.

Clinical Syndromes

The syndrome that results from *T. saginata* infection is similar to intestinal infection with *T. solium*. Patients are generally asymptomatic or may complain of vague abdominal pains, chronic indigestion, and hunger pains. Proglottids may pass out of the anus directly.

Laboratory Diagnosis

The diagnosis of *T. saginata* infection is similar to that of *T. solium,* with recovery of proglottids and eggs, or recovery of the entire worm with a scolex lacking hooklets. Study of the uterine branches in the proglottids differentiates *T. saginata* from *T. solium*.

Treatment, Prevention, and Control

Treatment is identical to treatment for the intestinal phase of *T. solium*. A single dose of niclosamide is highly effective in elimination of the adult worm. Education regarding cooking of beef and control of the disposal of human feces are critical measures.

DIPHYLLOBOTHRIUM LATUM

Physiology and Structure

One of the largest tapeworms (20 to 30 feet long), *Diphyllobothrium latum* (the **fish tapeworm**) has a complex life cycle involving two intermediate hosts—freshwater crustaceans and freshwater fish (Figure 51-5). The ribbonlike larval worm in the flesh of freshwater fish is called a **sparganum.** Ingestion of this sparganum in raw or insufficiently cooked fish initiates infection. The scolex of *D. latum* is lance shaped and has long, lateral grooves (bothria), which serve as organs of attachment. The proglottids of *D. latum* are broad, have a central uterine structure resembling a rosette, and produce eggs having an operculum, like fluke eggs, and a knob on the shell at the bottom of the egg. The adult worms may produce eggs for months or years. More than 1 million eggs per day are released into the fecal stream. Upon reaching fresh water, the unembryonated operculate eggs require a period of 2 to 4 weeks to develop a ciliated, free-swimming larval form called a **coracidium**. The fully developed coracidium leaves the egg via the operculum

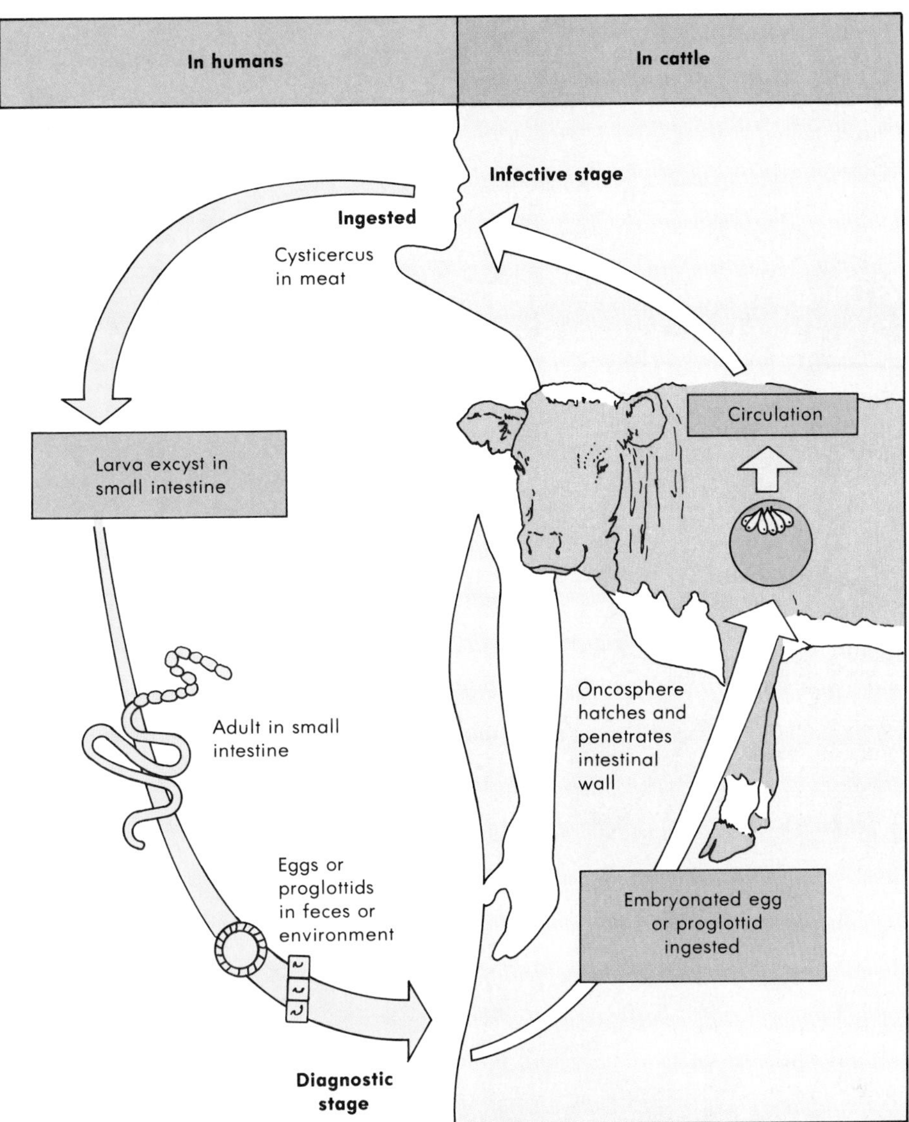

FIGURE 51-4 Life cycle of *Taenia saginata* ("beef tapeworm").

and is ingested by tiny crustaceans called **copepods** (e.g., *Cyclops* and *Diaptomus*) where it develops into a procercoid larval form. The crustacean harboring the larval stage is then eaten by a fish, and the infectious plerocercoid or sparganum larvae develop in the musculature of the fish. If the fish is in turn eaten by another fish, the sparganum simply migrates into the muscles of the second fish. Humans are infected when they eat raw or undercooked fish containing the larval forms.

Epidemiology

D. latum occurs worldwide, most prevalently in cool lake regions where raw or pickled fish is popular. Insufficient cooking over campfires and tasting and seasoning "gefilte fish" account for many infections. A reservoir of infected wild animals, such as bears, minks, walruses, and members of the canine and feline families that eat fish, are also sources for human infections. The practice of dumping raw sewage into freshwater lakes contributes to the propagation of this tapeworm.

Clinical Syndromes

Clinically, as is the case with most adult tapeworm infections, most *D. latum* infections are asymptomatic. Occasionally individuals complain of epigastric pain, abdominal cramping, nausea, vomiting, and weight loss. As many as 40% of *D. latum* carriers may have low serum levels of vitamin B_{12}, presumably as a result of the competition between the host and the worm for dietary vitamin B_{12}. A small percentage (0.1% to 2%) of individuals infected with *D. latum* develop clinical signs of vitamin B_{12} deficiency, including megaloblastic anemia and neurological manifestations such as numbness, paresthesia, and loss of vibration sense.

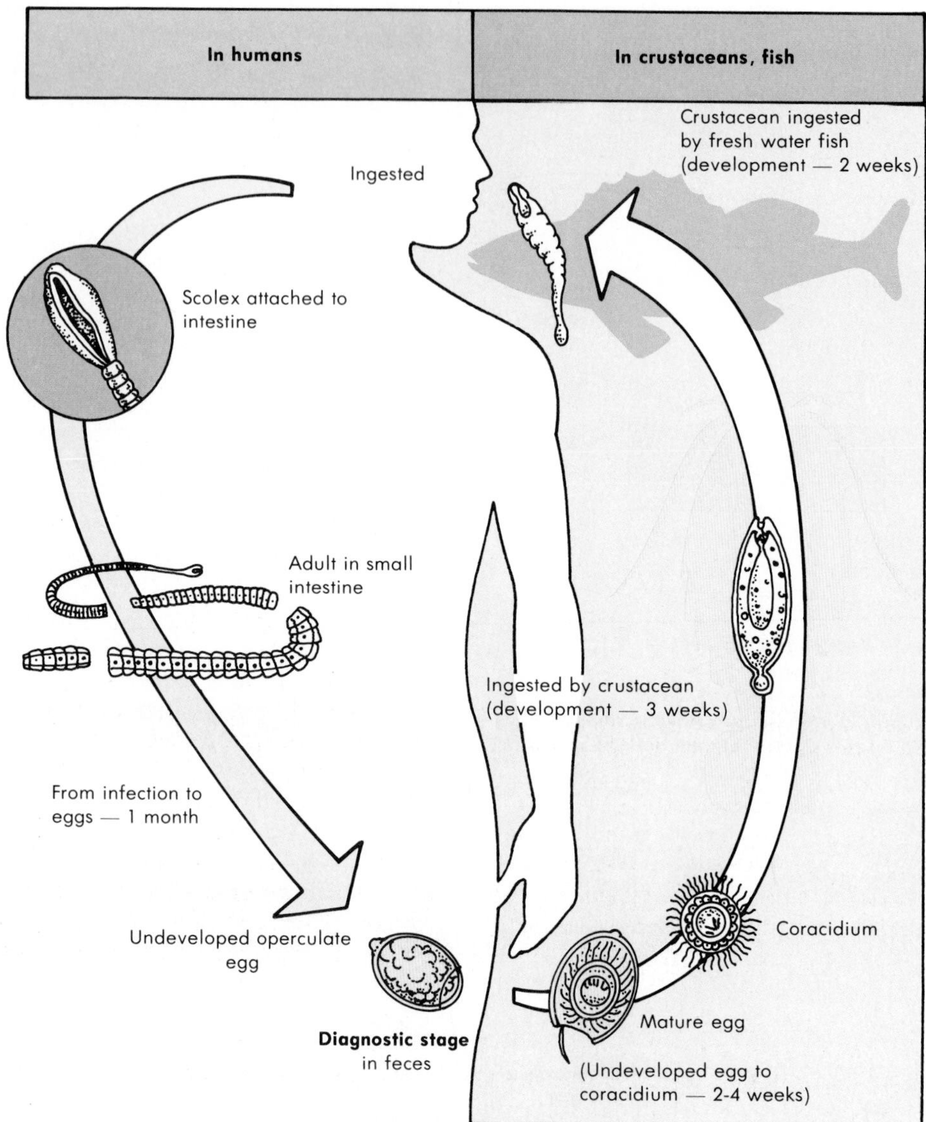

FIGURE 51-5 Life cycle of *Diphyllobothrium latum* ("fish tapeworm").

Laboratory Diagnosis

Stool examination reveals the bile-stained, operculated egg with its knob at the bottom of the shell (Figure 51-6). Typical proglottids with the rosette uterine structure may also be found in stool specimens. Concentration techniques are usually not necessary since the worms produce large numbers of ova.

Treatment, Prevention, and Control

The drug of choice is niclosamide; praziquantel and paromomycin are acceptable alternatives. Vitamin B_{12} supplementation may be necessary in those individuals with evidence of clinical vitamin B_{12} deficiency. The prevalence of this infection is reduced by avoiding the ingestion of insufficiently cooked fish, controlling the disposal of human feces, especially the proper treatment of sewage before disposal in lakes, and promptly treating infections.

SPARGANOSIS

Physiology and Structure

The larval forms of several tapeworms closely related to *D. latum* (most often *Spirometra* spp.) can produce human disease in subcutaneous sites and in the eye. In these cases humans act as the end-stage host for the larval stage, or sparganum. Infections are acquired primarily by drinking pond water and ditch water that contains crustaceans (copepods) that carry a larval tapeworm. This larval form penetrates the intestinal wall and migrates to various sites in the body, where it develops into a

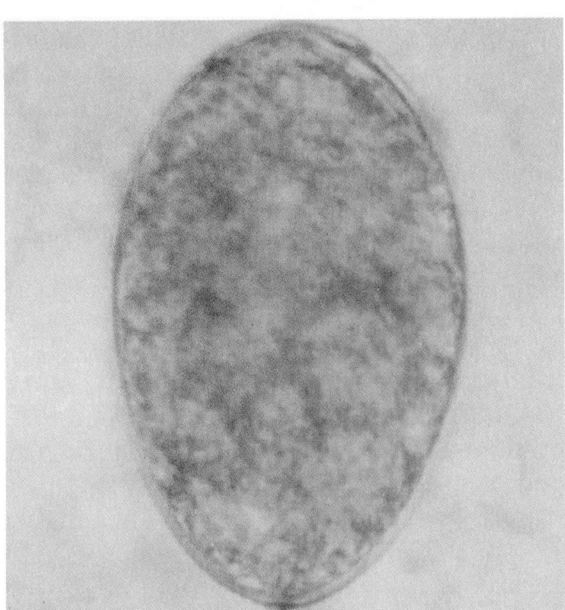

FIGURE 51-6 *Diphyllobothrium latum* egg. Unlike other tapeworm eggs, *D. latum* eggs are operculated. The eggs are 45 μm × 70 μm in size. (From Lennette EH, Balows A, Hausler WJ, and Shadomy HJ: *Manual of clinical microbiology*, ed 4, Washington, DC, 1985, American Society for Microbiology.)

sparganum. Infections may also occur if tadpoles, frogs, and snakes are ingested raw, or if the flesh of these animals is applied to wounds as a poultice. The larval worm leaves the relatively cold flesh of the dead animal and migrates into the warm human flesh.

Epidemiology

Cases have been reported from various parts of the world, including the United States, but the infection is most prevalent in the Orient. Regardless of location, drinking contaminated water and eating raw tadpole, frog, and snake flesh lead to infection.

Clinical Syndromes

In subcutaneous sites sparganosis can produce painful inflammatory tissue reactions and nodules. In the eye the tissue reaction is intensely painful, and periorbital edema is common. Corneal ulcers may develop with ocular involvement. Ocular disease is frequently associated with the use of frog or snake flesh as a poultice over a wound near the eye.

Laboratory Diagnosis

Sections of tissue removed surgically show characteristic tapeworm features: highly convoluted parenchyma and dark staining calcareous corpuscles.

Treatment, Prevention, and Control

Surgical removal is the customary approach. The drug praziquantel may be used; however, there is no clinical data to support its efficacy. Education regarding possible contamination of drinking water with crustaceans harboring larval worms is essential. This is most likely to occur in pond water and ditch water. Ingestion of raw frog and snake flesh or their use as poultices over wounds also should be avoided.

ECHINOCOCCUS GRANULOSUS

Physiology and Structure

Infection with *Echinococcus granulosus* is another example of accidental human infection, with humans serving as dead-end intermediate hosts in a life cycle naturally occurring in other animals. *E. granulosus* adult tapeworms are found in nature in the intestines of canines (dog, fox, wolf, coyote, jackal, dingo); the larval cyst stage is present in the viscera of herbivores (sheep, cattle, swine, deer, moose, elk; Figure 51-7). The worm consists of a *Taenia*-like scolex with four sucking disks and a double row of hooklets, and a strobila containing three proglottids – one immature, one mature, and one gravid. Adult tapeworms in the canine intestine produce infective eggs that pass in feces. The eggs are identical in appearance to those of *Taenia* species. When these eggs are ingested by humans, a six-hooked larval stage called an oncosphere hatches. The oncosphere penetrates the human intestinal wall and enters the circulation to be carried to various tissue sites, primarily the liver and lungs but also the central nervous system and bone. This same cycle occurs in the viscera of herbivores. When the herbivore is killed by a canine predator or viscera is fed to canines, the ingestion of cysts produces adult tapeworms in the canine intestine to complete the cycle and initiate new egg production. Adult tapeworms do not develop in the intestines of either herbivores or humans.

In humans the larvae form a **unilocular hydatid cyst,** which is a slow-growing, tumor-like, and space-occupying structure enclosed by a laminated germinative membrane. This membrane produces structures on its wall called **brood capsules,** where tapeworm heads **(protoscolices)** develop. **Daughter cysts** may develop in the original mother cyst, and these also produce brood capsules and protoscolices. The cysts and daughter cysts also accumulate fluid as they grow. This fluid is potentially toxic; if spilled into body cavities, anaphylactic shock and death can result. Spillage and the escape of protoscolices can lead to the development of cysts in other sites, because the protoscolices have the germinative potential to form new cysts. Eventually, the brood capsules and daughter cysts disintegrate within the mother cyst, liberating the accumulated protoscolices. These become known as **"hydatid sand."** This type of echinococcus cyst is called a unilocular cyst to differentiate it from related cysts that grow differently. The unilocular cyst is generally about 5 cm in diameter, but some as large as 20 cm, containing almost 2 liters of cyst fluid, have been reported. Over long periods the cyst may die and become calcified.

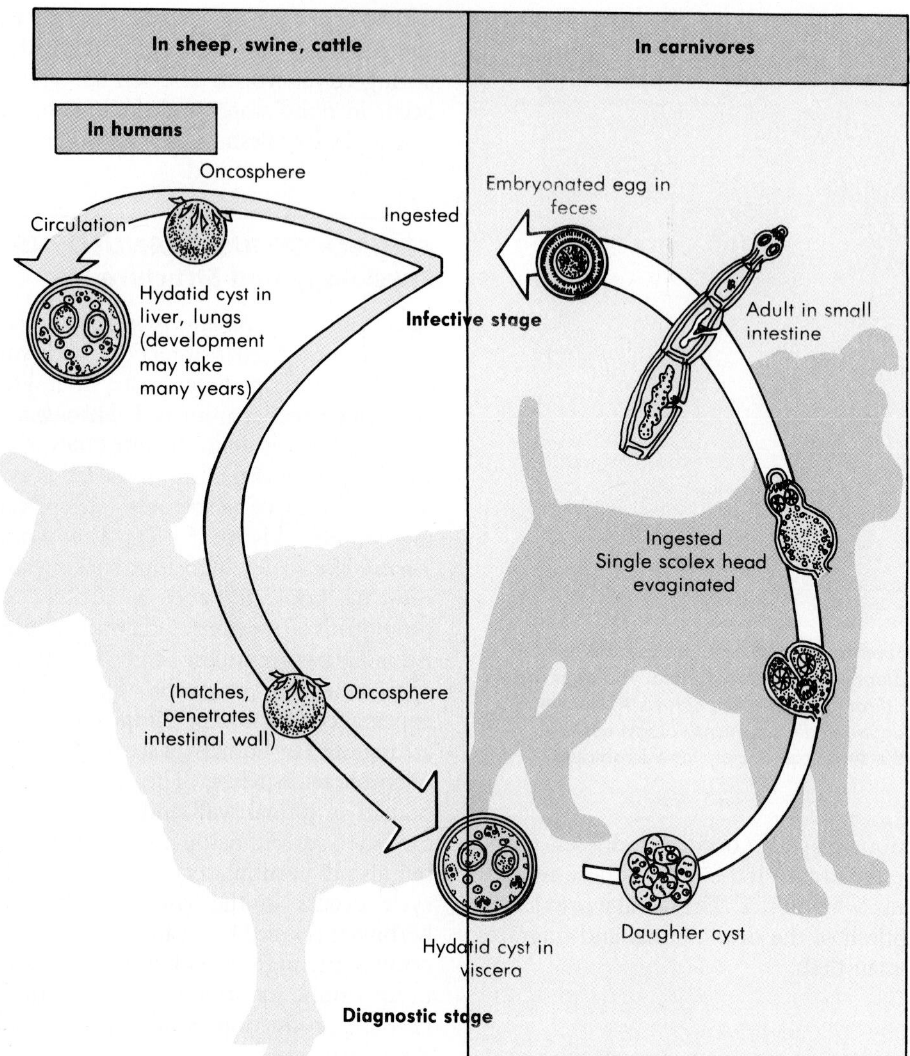

FIGURE 51-7 Life cycle of *Echinococcus granulosus.*

Epidemiology

Human infection with *E. granulosus* unilocular cyst is directly correlated with raising sheep in many countries in Europe, South America, Africa, Asia, Australia, and New Zealand. It occurs in Canada and in the United States, with cases reported from Alaska, Utah, New Mexico, Arizona, California, and the lower Mississippi valley. Human infection follows ingestion of contaminated water or vegetation, as well as hand-to-mouth transmission of canine feces carrying the infective eggs.

Clinical Syndromes

Because the unilocular cyst grows slowly, 5 to 20 years may pass before any symptoms appear. In many instances it appears that the cyst is as old as its host. The pressure of the expanding cyst in an organ is usually the first sign of infection. In the majority of cases the cysts are located in the liver or lung. In the liver the cyst may exert pressure on both bile ducts and blood vessels and create pain and biliary rupture. In the lungs cysts may produce cough, dyspnea, and chest pains. Rupture of the cysts may occur in 20% of cases, producing fever, urticaria, and occasionally anaphylactic shock and death caused by the release of antigenic cyst contents. Cyst rupture may also lead to dissemination of infection resulting from the release of thousands of protoscolices. In bone the cyst is responsible for erosion of the marrow cavity, as well as the bone itself. In the brain severe damage may occur as a result of the cyst's tumor-like growth into brain tissue.

Laboratory Diagnosis

Diagnosis of hydatid disease is difficult and depends primarily on clinical, radiographic, and serologic findings. Radiologic examination, scanning procedures, tomography, and ultrasound techniques are all valuable and may provide the first evidence of the cyst's presence. Aspiration of cyst contents may demonstrate the protoscolices ("hydatid sand"); however, it is contraindicated because

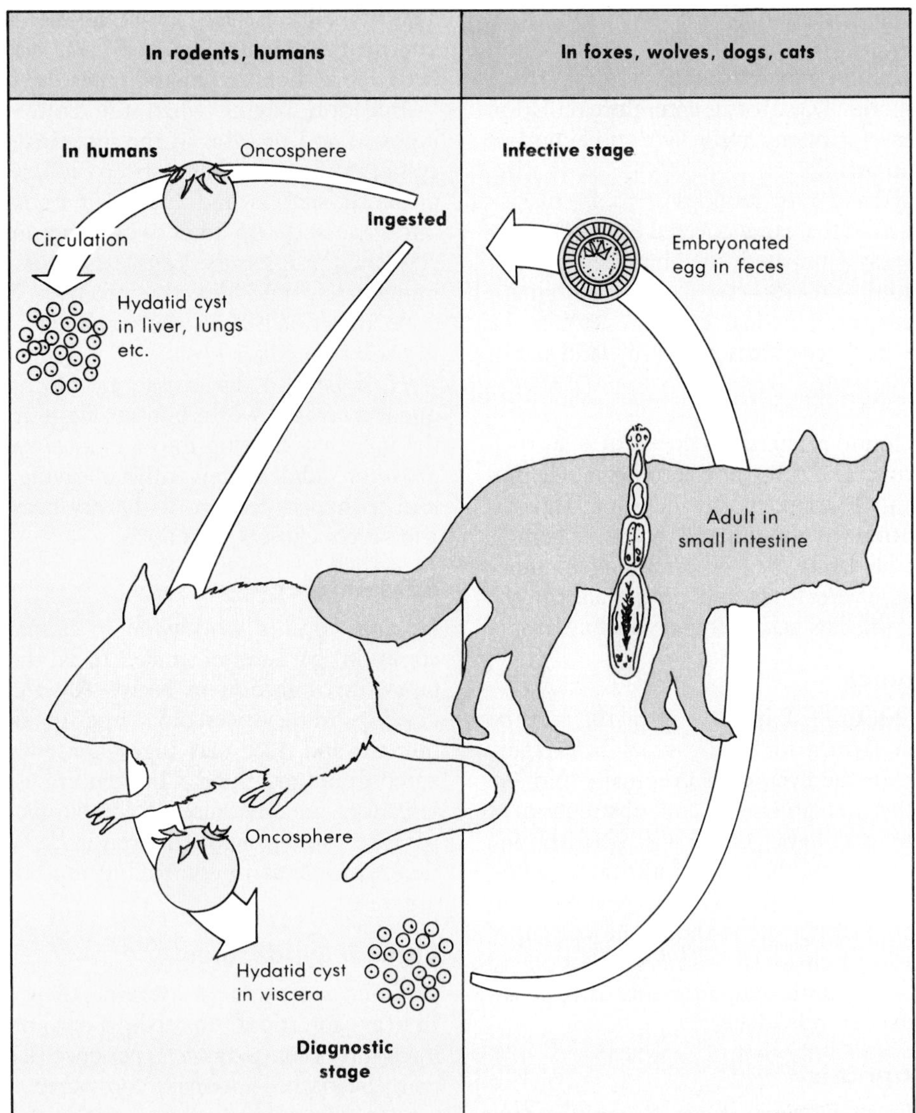

FIGURE 51-8 Life cycle of Echinococcus multilocularis.

of the risk of anaphylaxis and dissemination of the infection. Serologic testing may be useful but is negative in 10% to 40% of infections.

Treatment, Prevention, and Control

Surgical resection of the cyst is the treatment of choice. In some instances the cyst is first aspirated to remove the fluid and hydatid sand, then instilled with formalin to kill and detoxify remaining fluid, and finally rolled into a marsupial pouch and sewn shut. If the condition is inoperable because of the cyst's location, medical therapy with high-dose albendazole, mebendazole, or praziquantel may be considered. The most important factor in preventing and controlling echinococcosis is education regarding the transmission of infection and the role of canines in the life cycle. Proper personal hygiene and washing of hands and cooking utensils in environments inhabited by dogs are critical. Dogs should not be allowed in the vicinity of animal slaughter and should never be fed the viscera of slain animals. In some areas the killing of stray dogs has reduced the incidence of infection.

ECHINOCOCCUS MULTILOCULARIS

Physiology and Structure

Like infection with *E. granulosus,* human infection with *E. multilocularis* is accidental (Figure 51-8). Adult *E. multilocularis* tapeworms are primarily found in foxes and wolves, although farm dogs and cats harbor them in some rural environments. The intermediate hosts that harbor the cyst stage are rodents (mice, voles, shrews, and lemmings). Humans become infected with the cyst stage as a result of contact with fox, dog, or cat feces contaminated with eggs. Trappers and workers who handle fur pelts may become infected by inhaling fecal dust carrying eggs.

Infective eggs hatch in and penetrate the intestinal tract to become oncospheres. These forms enter the circulation and take up residence primarily in the liver and lungs but also possibly in the brain.

The **alveolar hydatid cyst** develops as an alveolar or honeycombed structure that is *not* covered by a unilocular limiting mother cyst–laminated membrane. The cyst grows via exogenous budding, eventually resembling a carcinoma. In humans individual cysts are said to be "sterile" and rarely produce protoscolices (hydatid sand).

Epidemiology

E. multilocularis is found primarily in northern areas such as Canada, the former U.S.S.R., northern Japan, Central Europe, and Alaska, Montana, North and South Dakota, Minnesota, and Iowa in the United States. There is evidence that the life cycle may be extending to other midwestern states, where foxes and mice transmit the organism to dogs and cats and eventually to humans.

Clinical Syndromes

E. multilocularis, because of its slow growth, may be present in human tissues for many years before any symptoms appear. In the liver, cysts eventually mimic a carcinoma, with liver enlargement and obstruction of biliary and portal pathways. Often the growth will metastasize to the lungs and brain. Malnutrition, ascites, and portal hypertension produced by *E. multilocularis* create the appearance of hepatic cirrhosis. Among all of the worm infections of humans, *E. multilocularis* is one of the most lethal. If left untreated, mortality is approximately 70% of infected individuals.

Laboratory Diagnosis

Unlike *E. granulosus,* the tissue form *E. multilocularis* presents no protoscolices, and the material so resembles a neoplasm that even pathologists mistake it for carcinoma. Radiologic procedures and scanning techniques are helpful, and serologic methods are available.

Treatment, Prevention, and Control

Surgical removal of the cyst is indicated, especially if an entire hepatic area can be resected. The same surgical approach applies to lesions in the lung, wherein a lobe can be resected. Mebendazole and albendazole, as used for treatment of *E. granulosus*, have shown clinical cures. As with *E. granulosus*, education, proper personal hygiene, and deworming of farm dogs and cats are critical. It is extremely important to treat these animals if they have contact with children.

HYMENOLEPIS NANA

Physiology and Structure

Hymenolepis nana, the **dwarf tapeworm,** is only 2 to 4 cm in length, unlike *Taenia*, which measures several meters. The life cycle is also simple and does not require an intermediate host (Figure 51-9), although mice and beetles may be infected and enter the cycle.

Infection begins when the embryonated eggs are ingested and develop in the intestinal villi into a larval cysticercoid stage. This cysticercoid larva attaches its four muscular suckers and crown of hooklets to the small intestine, and the adult worm produces a strobila of egg-laden proglottids. Eggs passing in the feces are then immediately and directly infective, initiating another cycle. Infection may also be acquired by ingesting infected insect intermediate hosts.

H. nana also can cause autoinfection, with a subsequent increased worm burden. Eggs are able to hatch in the intestine, develop into a cysticercoid larva, and then grow into adult worms without leaving the host. This can lead to hyperinfection, with very heavy worm burdens and severe clinical symptoms.

Epidemiology

H. nana occurs worldwide in humans and is also a common parasite of mice. It is the most common tapeworm infection in North America. It occasionally develops its cysticercoid stage in beetles, and both humans and mice may ingest these beetles in contaminated grain and flour. Children are especially at risk of infection, and, because of the simple life cycle of the parasite, families with children in day-care centers experience problems in controlling the transmission of this organism.

Clinical Syndromes

With few worms in the intestine, there are no symptoms. In heavy infections, especially if autoinfection and hyperinfection occur, patients experience diarrhea, abdominal pain, headache, anorexia, and other vague complaints.

Laboratory Diagnosis

Stool examination reveals the characteristic *H. nana* egg with its six-hooked embryo and polar filaments (Figure 51-10).

Treatment, Prevention, and Control

The drug of choice is praziquantel; an alternative is niclosamide. Treatment of cases, improved sanitation, and proper personal hygiene are essential, especially in the family and institutional environments.

HYMENOLEPIS DIMINUTA

Physiology and Structure

H. diminuta, closely related to *H. nana,* is primarily a tapeworm of rats and mice, but it is also found in humans. It differs from *H. nana* in size, measuring 20 to 60 cm, the scolex lacks hooklets, and the egg is larger, bile stained, and has no polar filaments. The life cycle of *H. diminuta* is more complex and requires larval insects ("meal worms") to reach the infective cysticercoid stage.

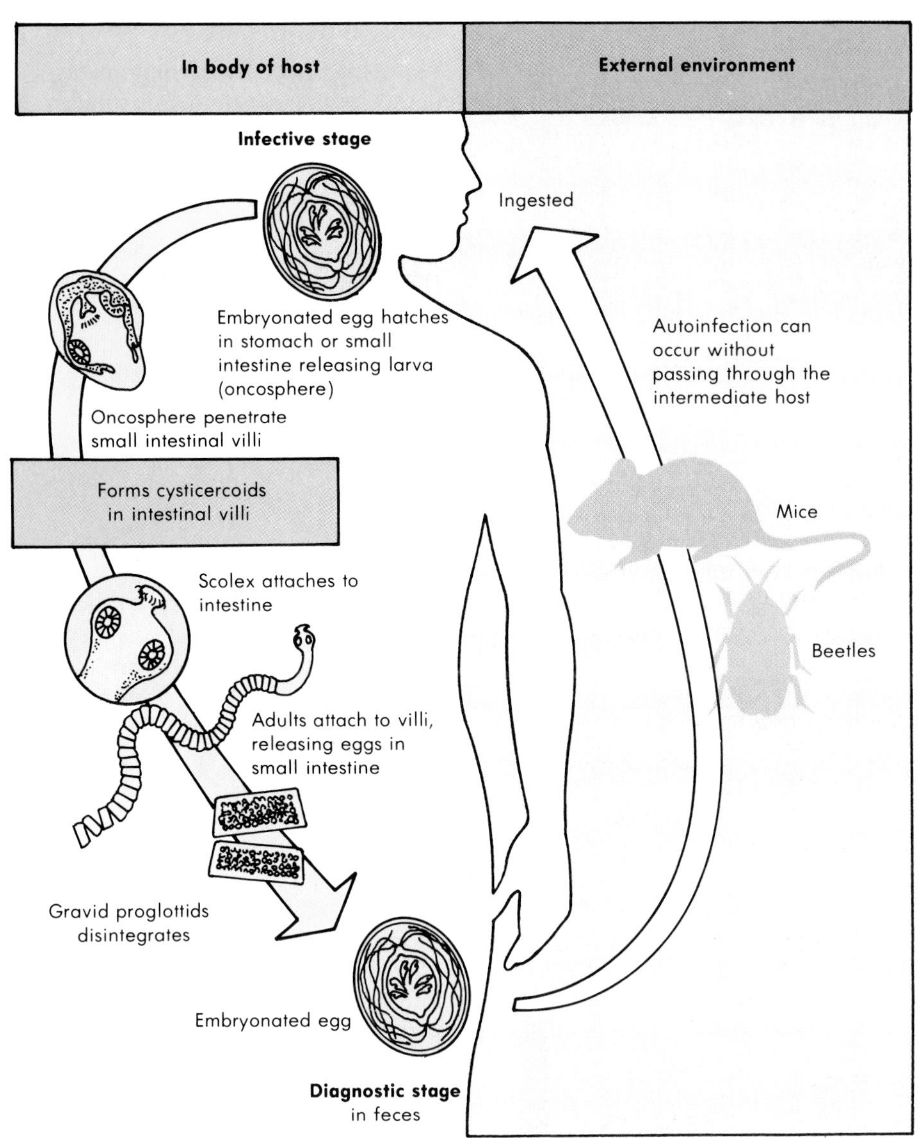

FIGURE 51-9 Life cycle of Hymenolepis nana ("dwarf tapeworm").

Epidemiology

Infections have been found all over the world, including in the United States. Larval beetles and other larval insects become infected when they feed on rat feces carrying *H. diminuta* eggs. Humans are infected by ingesting the larval insects ("meal worms") in contaminated grain products (e.g., flour, cereals).

Clinical Syndromes

Mild infections show no symptoms, but heavier worm burdens produce nausea, abdominal discomfort, anorexia, and diarrhea.

Laboratory Diagnosis

Stool examination demonstrates the characteristic bile-stained egg that lacks polar filaments.

Treatment, Prevention, and Control

The drug of choice is niclosamide, with praziquantel an alternative. Rodent control in areas where grain products are produced or stored is essential. Thorough inspection of uncooked grain products to detect meal worms is also important.

DIPYLIDIUM CANINUM

Physiology and Structure

This small tapeworm, averaging about 15 cm in length, is primarily a parasite of dogs and cats, but it can infect humans – especially children whose mouths are licked by infected pets. The life cycle involves development of larval worms in dog and cat fleas. These fleas, when crushed by the teeth of the infected pet, are carried on the tongue to

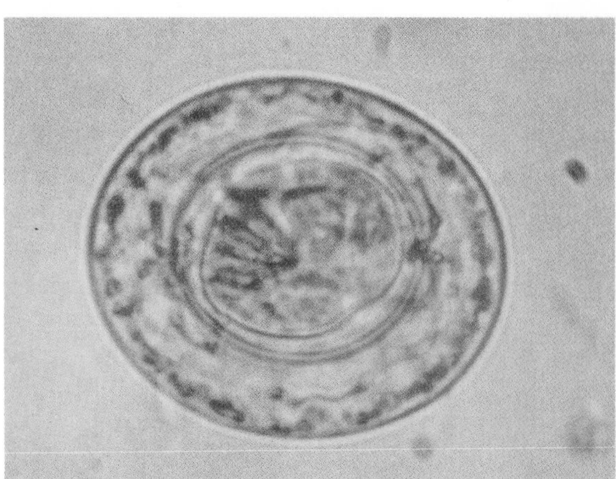

FIGURE 51-10 *Hymenolepis nana* egg. The eggs are 30 to 45 μm in diameter, with a thin shell, containing a six-hooked embryo. (From Lennette EH, Balows A, Hausler WJ, and Shadomy HJ: *Manual of clinical microbiology*, ed 4, Washington, DC, 1985, American Society for Microbiology.)

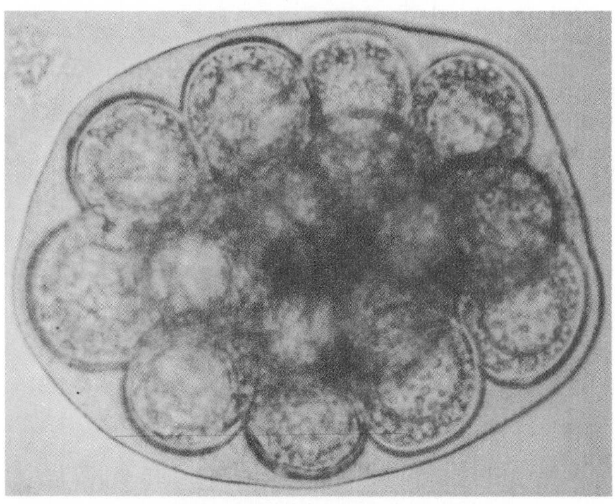

FIGURE 51-11 *Dipylidium caninum* eggs. Free eggs are rarely seen. Instead, egg packets containing 8 to 15 six-hooked oncospheres enclosed in a thin membrane are most commonly found in fecal specimens. (From Lennette EH, Balows A, Hausler WJ, and Shadomy HJ: *Manual of clinical microbiology*, ed 4, Washington, DC, 1985, American Society for Microbiology.)

the child's mouth in kissing or licking. Swallowing the infected flea leads to intestinal infection.

Because of the size and shape of the mature and terminal proglottids, *D. caninum* is often called the **"pumpkin seed tapeworm."** The eggs are distinctive because they occur in packets covered with a tough clear membrane. There may be as many as 25 eggs in a packet, and a single egg free of the packet is seldom seen.

Epidemiology

D. caninum occurs worldwide, especially in children. Its distribution and transmission are directly correlated with dogs and cats infected with fleas.

Clinical Syndromes

Light infections are asymptomatic; heavier worm burdens produce abdominal discomfort, anal pruritus, and diarrhea. Anal pruritus results from the active migration of the motile proglottid.

Laboratory Diagnosis

Stool examination reveals the colorless egg packets (Figure 51-11), and proglottids may be in feces brought to physicians by patients.

Treatment, Prevention, and Control

The drug of choice is niclosamide; praziquantel or paromomycin are alternatives. Dogs and cats should be dewormed and not be allowed to lick the mouths of children. Pets should be treated to the eradicate fleas.

CASE STUDY AND QUESTIONS

A 30-year-old Hispanic male enters the emergency department following a focal neurological seizure. The patient had recently emigrated from Mexico and was in his usual state of good health before the seizure. Neurological examination revealed no focal findings. A head CT scan was remarkable for multiple small cystic lesions in both cerebral hemispheres. Punctate calcification was noted in several of the lesions. A lumbar puncture revealed a CSF glucose level of 65 mg/dl (normal) and a protein of 38 mg/dl (normal). There were 20 white blood cells per mm^3 (abnormal) with a differential of 5% neutrophils, 90% lymphocytes, and 5% monocytes. A PPD skin test was negative with positive controls. Serologic test for HIV was negative.

1. What is the differential diagnosis of this patient's neurological process?
2. Which parasite or parasites may cause this condition?
3. What diagnostic tests are available for this infection?
4. What are your therapeutic options?
5. How do people become infected with this parasite?
6. What other tissue sites may be involved outside of the central nervous system? How would you document these additional foci of infection?

Bibliography

Beaver PC, Jung RC, and Cupp EW: *Clinical parasitology*, ed 9, Philadelphia, 1984, Lea & Febiger.

Blenkharn JI, Benjamin IS, and Blumgart LH: Bacterial infection of hepatic hydatid cysts with *Haemophilus influenzae*, *J Infect* 15:169-171, 1987.

Coltorti E et al.: Field evaluation of an enzyme immunoassay for detection of asymptomatic patients in a hydatid control program, *Am J Trop Med Hyg* 38:603-607, 1988.

Cook GC: Neurocysticercosis: parasitology, clinical presentation, diagnosis, and recent advances in management, *Q J Med* 68:575-583, 1988.

Desowitz RS: *New Guinea tapeworms and Jewish grandmothers*, New York, 1983, Avon/Discus.
Groll E: Praziquantel for cestode infections in man, *Acta Trop* 37:293-296, 1980.
Kammerer WS and Schantz PM: Long-term follow-up of human hydatid disease (*Echinococcus granulosus*) treated with a high dose mebendazole regimen, *Am J Trop Med Hyg* 33:132-137, 1984.
Leiby PD and Kritsky DC: *Echinococcus multilocularis*: a possible domestic life cycle in Central North America and its public health importance, *J Parasitol* 58:1213-1215, 1972.
Markell EK, Voge M, and John DT: *Medical parasitology*, ed 7, Philadelphia, 1992, WB Saunders.
Saimot AG et al.: Albendazole as a potential treatment for human hydatidosis, *Lancet* 2:652-656, 1983.
Schmidt GD and Roberts LS: *Foundations of parasitology*, ed 4, St. Louis, 1989, Mosby.

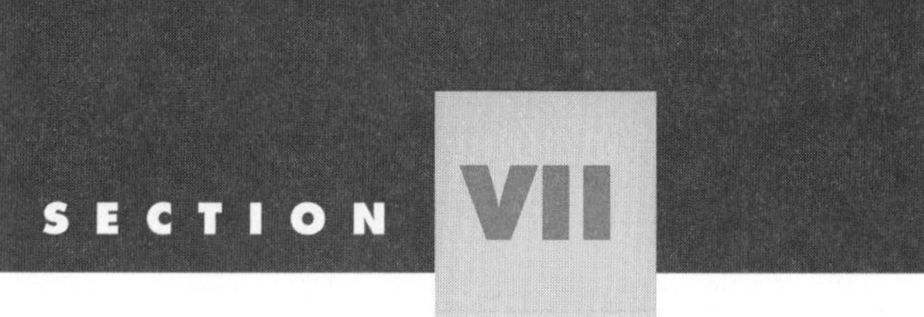

VIROLOGY

CHAPTER 52

Introduction to Viral Disease

VIRUSES cause disease after they break through the natural protective barriers of the body, evade immune control, and either kill cells of an important tissue (e.g., brain) or trigger a destructive immune/inflammatory response. The outcome of a viral infection is determined by the nature of the virus-host interaction and the host's response to the infection (Box 52-1). The immune response is the best treatment, but it is also a major factor in the pathogenesis of a viral infection. The nature of the disease and its symptoms are determined by the target tissue. The severity of disease may be determined by many viral and host parameters, including the strain of virus, the inoculum size, and the general health of the infected individual. The effectiveness of the immune response in resolving the infection generally determines the severity and length of disease.

A particular disease may be caused by several viruses that have a common tissue **tropism** (preference) (e.g., hepatitis: liver; common cold: upper respiratory tract; encephalitis: central nervous system). A particular virus may cause several different diseases or no observable symptoms. For example, herpes simplex virus type 1 can cause gingivostomatitis, pharyngitis, herpes labialis (cold sores), genital herpes, encephalitis or keratoconjunctivitis, depending on the affected cell type, or it can cause no disease at all. Although normally benign, this virus can be life threatening in a newborn or immunocompromised individual.

Many viruses encode activities **(virulence factors)** that promote the efficiency of virus replication, transmission, access and binding to target tissue, or escape from immune recognition and resolution (see Chapter 11). These activities may not be essential for viral growth in tissue culture but are required for pathogenicity or survival in the host. Loss of these virulence factors results in **attenuation** of the virus. Many live virus vaccines are attenuated virus strains.

This chapter will discuss viral disease at the cellular level (cytopathogenesis), the host level (mechanisms of disease and the immune response), and the population level (epidemiology and control). The properties of the virus responsible for these actions will be stressed in each case.

BOX 52-1 Determinants of Viral Disease

NATURE OF THE DISEASE

- Target tissue
  - Portal of entry of virus
  - Access of virus to target tissue
  - Tissue tropism of virus (viral attachment protein)
  - Permissiveness of cells for virus replication
- Viral pathogen (strain)

IMMUNE STATUS

- Competence of the immune system
- Prior immunity to the virus

SEVERITY OF DISEASE

- Cytopathic ability of virus
- Immunopathology
- Virus inoculum size
- Length of time before resolution of infection
- General health of the individual
  - Nutrition
  - Other diseases influencing immune status
- Genetic makeup of the individual
- Age

INFECTION OF THE TARGET TISSUE

The virus gains entry into the body through breaks in the skin and through the mucoepithelial membranes at the orifices of the body (eyes, respiratory tract, mouth, genitalia, and gastrointestinal tract). The skin is an excellent barrier to infection, and the orifices are protected by tears, mucus, ciliated epithelium, stomach acid, bile, and IgA. *Inhalation is probably the most common route of viral infection.*

Upon entry into the body, the virus replicates in cells that express viral receptors and that have the appropriate biosynthetic machinery. Symptoms may or may not accompany virus replication at the primary site. The virus may replicate and remain at the primary site or may disseminate to other tissues by way of the bloodstream, the mononuclear phagocyte and lymphatic system, or through neurons (Figure 52-1). The mononuclear phagocyte system (reticuloendothelial system) consists of blood and tissue macrophages (e.g., dendritic cells of skin, Kupffer's cells of the liver, and microglial cells of the brain).

The bloodstream and the lymphatic system are the predominant means of viral transfer in the body. The virus may gain access to the bloodstream and lymphatic system following cell damage, by phagocytosis, or by active transport mechanisms. Many viruses infect and are transported across the mucoepithelial cells of the oropharynx, gastrointestinal, vaginal, and anal tracts. Several enteric viruses (picornaviruses and reoviruses) bind to receptors on M cells, which translocate the virus to the underlying Peyer's patches of the lymphatic system.

Transport of virus in the blood is termed a **viremia**. The virus may be free in the plasma or associated in lymphocytes or macrophages. Viruses taken up by phagocytic macrophages may be inactivated, replicate, or be delivered to other tissues by way of the mononuclear phagocyte system (e.g., lymph nodes, spleen, liver, and other tissues). Replication of virus in macrophages, the endothelial lining of blood vessels, or the liver can amplify the infection and initiate a secondary viremia. For many virus infections, a secondary viremia precedes delivery of virus to the target tissue (liver, skin, etc.) and symptoms.

Viruses may gain access to the central nervous system or brain from the bloodstream, from infected meninges or cerebral spinal fluid, by migration of infected macrophages, or by infection of peripheral and sensory neurons (olfactory). Viruses in the blood may infect and disrupt the endothelial cell lining and exit the blood vessels or traverse the blood-brain barrier to infect the central nervous system. The meninges are accessible to many viruses spread by viremia and may provide access to neurons. Herpes simplex, varicella-zoster, and rabies initially infect mucoepithelium, skin, or muscle, then the peripheral innervating neuron, which transports the virus to the central nervous system or brain.

VIRAL PATHOGENESIS

Cytopathogenesis

There are three potential outcomes following the viral infection of a cell: failed infection **(abortive infection)**, cell death **(lytic infection)**, or virus production without cell death (nonlytic) **(persistent infection)** (Box 52-2; Table 52-1). Persistent infections include chronic, latent-

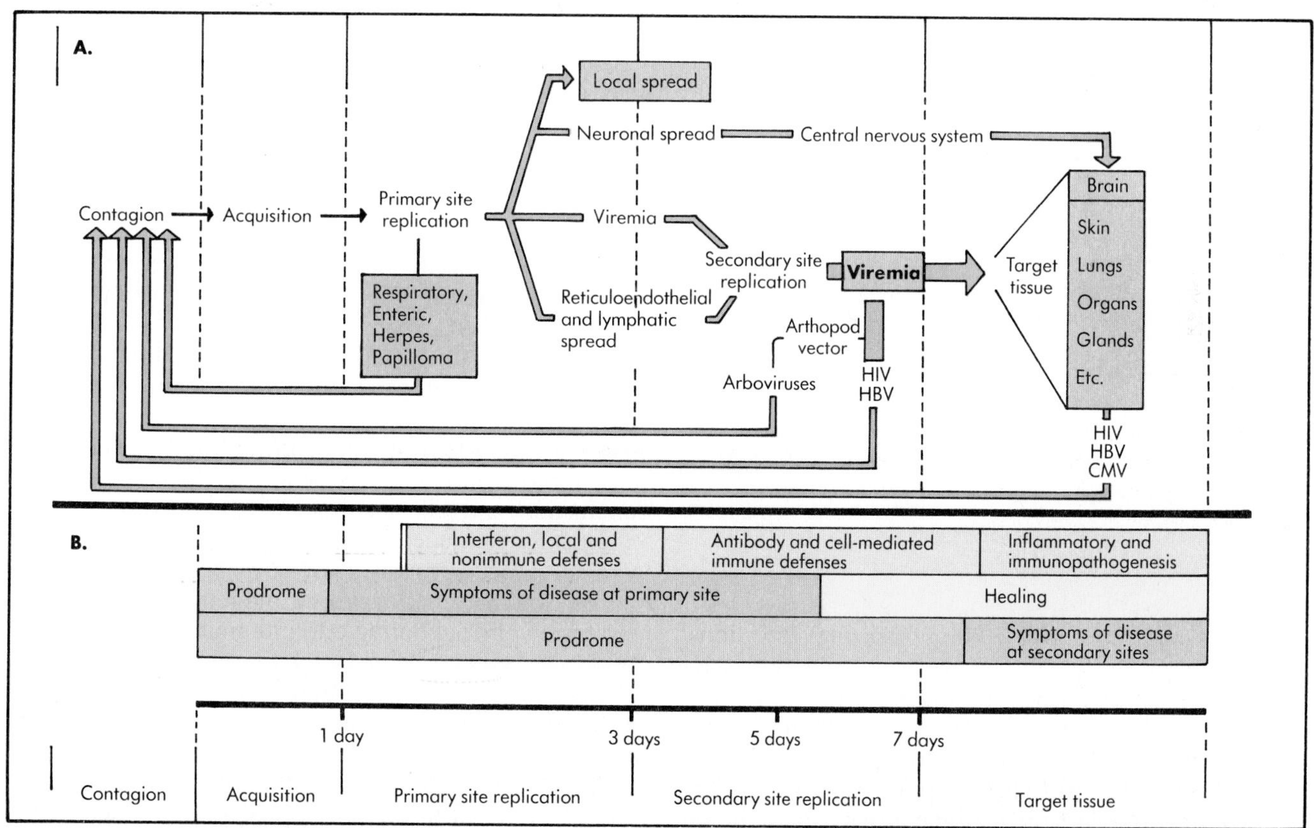

FIGURE 52-1 **A,** The stages of viral infection. The virus is released from one individual, acquired by another, replicates, and initiates a primary infection at the site of acquisition. Depending on the virus, it may spread to other body sites and finally to a target tissue characteristic of the disease. The cycle is continued by release of new virus. The thickness of the arrow denotes amplification of the original virus inoculum upon replication. The boxes indicate a site or cause of symptoms. **B,** Time course of viral infection. The time course of symptoms and immune response correlate with the stage of virus infection and whether the virus causes symptoms at the primary site or only after dissemination to another site (secondary site).

BOX 52-2 Determinants of Viral Pathogenesis

INTERACTION OF VIRUS WITH TARGET TISSUE

Access to target tissue
- Stability of virus in the body
  - Temperature
  - Acid and bile of the gastrointestinal tract
- Ability to cross skin or mucous epithelial cells (e.g., cross the gastrointestinal tract into the bloodstream)
- Ability to establish viremia
- Ability to spread through the reticuloendothelial system

Recognition of target tissue
- Specificity of viral attachment proteins
- Tissue-specific expression of receptors

CYTOPATHOLOGICAL ACTIVITY OF THE VIRUS

Efficiency of virus replication in the cell
- Optimum temperature for replication
- Permissivity of host

Cytotoxic viral proteins

Degradative viral enzymes

Accumulation of viral proteins and structures (inclusion bodies)

Altered cell metabolism (e.g., cell immortalization)

IMMUNE RESPONSE

Nonspecific antiviral immune responses
- Interferon
- Natural killer cells and macrophages

Antigen specific immune responses
- T-lymphocyte responses
- Antibody responses

Viral mechanisms of escape of immune responses

IMMUNE ESCAPE MECHANISMS (SEE TABLE 52-6)

IMMUNOPATHOLOGY

Interferon: Flu-like symptoms

T-cell responses: Delayed type hypersensitivity

Antibody: Complement, antibody dependent cellular cytotoxicity, immune complexes

Other inflammatory responses

recurrent and transforming (immortalizing) infections. The nature of the infection is determined by both viral and cellular characteristics. A **nonpermissive** cell will not allow replication of a particular type or strain of virus. Viral mutants, which cause abortive infections do not multiply and therefore will disappear. A **permissive** cell provides the biosynthetic machinery (e.g., transcription factors, posttranslational processing enzymes) to support the complete replicative cycle of the virus. A **semipermissive** cell may be very inefficient or support some but not all steps in virus replication.

Replication of the virus can initiate changes in cells leading to cytolysis or alterations in the cell's appearance, functional properties, or antigenicity. The effects on the cell may result from virus takeover of macromolecular synthesis, accumulation of viral proteins or particles, or modification of cellular structures, such as incorporation of glycoproteins in cell membranes (Table 52-2).

TABLE 52-1 Types of Viral Infections at the Cellular Level

Type	Virus production	Fate of cell
Abortive	–	No effect
Cytolytic	+	Death
Persistent		
Productive	+	Senescence
Latent	–	No effect
Transforming		
DNA viruses	–	Immortalization
RNA viruses	+	Immortalization

Lytic Infections

Virus replication is often incompatible with essential cell functions and viability. Some viruses prevent the synthesis of cellular macromolecules or produce degradative enzymes and toxic proteins. This prevents growth and repair and leads to the death of the cell. Herpes simplex and other viruses produce proteins that inhibit cellular DNA and mRNA synthesis and other proteins that degrade host DNA to provide substrates for genome replication. Cellular protein synthesis may be actively blocked (e.g., polio virus inhibits translation of 5′capped cellular mRNA) or passively blocked (e.g., production of large numbers of viral mRNA that successfully compete for ribosomes) (see Chapter 7).

Replication of the virus and accumulation of viral components and progeny within the cell can disrupt cell structure and function or can disrupt lysosomes, causing autolysis. Expression of viral antigens on the cell surface and disruption of the cytoskeleton can change cell-to-cell interactions and cellular appearance and can make the cell a target for immune cytolysis.

Cell-surface expression of glycoproteins of some paramyxoviruses, herpesviruses, and retroviruses initiates the fusion of neighboring cells into multinucleated giant cells called **syncytia**. Cell-to-cell fusion may occur in the absence of new protein synthesis (fusion from without), as for Sendai and other paramyxoviruses, or may require new protein synthesis (fusion from within), as for herpes simplex virus. Syncytia formation allows the virus to spread from cell to cell and escape antibody detection. Syncytia formation by human immunodeficiency virus (HIV) also causes death of the cells.

Some viral infections cause characteristic changes in the appearance and properties of the target cells. These changes are especially apparent after infection of cells grown in tissue culture. Chromosomal aberrations and degradation can be detected by histological staining (e.g.,

TABLE 52-2 Mechanisms of Viral Cytopathogenesis

Mechanism	Representative viruses
Inhibition of cellular protein synthesis	Polioviruses, herpes simplex virus, togaviruses, poxviruses
Inhibition and degradation of cellular DNA	Herpesviruses
Alteration of cell membrane structure	
Glycoprotein insertion	All enveloped viruses
Syncytia formation	Herpes simplex virus, varicella-zoster virus, paramyxoviruses, human immunodeficiency virus
Disruption of cytoskeleton	Nonenveloped viruses (accumulation), herpes simplex virus
Permeability changes	Togaviruses, herpesviruses
Inclusion bodies	
Negri bodies (intracytoplasmic)	Rabies
Owl's eye (intranuclear)	Cytomegalovirus
Cowdry's type A (intranuclear)	Herpes simplex virus, subacute sclerosing panencephalitis (measles) virus
Intranuclear basophilic	Adenoviruses
Intracytoplasmic acidophilic	Poxviruses
Perinuclear cytoplasmic acidophilic	Reoviruses
Toxicity of virion components	Adenovirus fibers

marginated chromatin ringing the nuclear membrane in HSV- and adenovirus-infected cells). The presence of new, stainable structures within the nucleus or cytoplasm, called **inclusion bodies,** may result from virus-induced changes in the membrane or chromosomal structure or may represent the sites of virus replication or accumulations of viral capsids. The nature and location of these inclusion bodies are characteristic of particular viral infections and facilitate laboratory diagnosis (Table 52-2). Vacuolization, rounding of the cells, and other nonspecific histological changes indicative of sick cells may also result from viral infection.

Nonlytic Infections

A **persistent** infection occurs in an infected cell that is not killed by the virus. A persistent productive infection occurs for some viruses that are released gently from the cell by exocytosis or by budding from the plasma membrane. A **latent** infection occurs for DNA virus infections of cells that restrict or lack the machinery for transcription of all the viral genes. The specific transcription factors required by a virus may be expressed only in specific tissues, in growing but not resting cells, or following hormone or cytokine induction. For example, HIV establishes a latent infection of T lymphocytes, but replication is activated by T-cell mitogens. Herpes simplex virus establishes latent infection of neurons that lack the nuclear factors required to transcribe the immediate early viral genes, but stress and other stimuli activate virus replication.

Oncogenic Viruses

Some DNA viruses and retroviruses establish persistent infections that can also stimulate uncontrolled cell growth, causing **transformation** or **immortalization** of the cell (Figure 52-2). Characteristics of transformed cells include continued growth without senescence, alterations in cell morphology and metabolism, increased cell growth rate and sugar transport, loss of cell-contact–inhibition of growth, and ability to grow in suspension or semisolid agar.

Different oncogenic viruses have different mechanisms for immortalizing cells. Viruses immortalize cells either by promoting or providing growth stimulating genes or by removing the inherent braking mechanisms, which limit DNA synthesis and cell growth. Immortalization by DNA viruses occurs in semipermissive cells, which express only the early viral genes. Synthesis of viral DNA and progression into the late phase of mRNA and protein synthesis usually causes cell death, which precludes immortalization. Papillomavirus, SV40 virus, and adenovirus encode proteins that bind and inactivate cell growth regulatory proteins, such as p53 or the retinoblastoma gene product. This releases the brakes on cell growth. Epstein-Barr virus immortalizes B lymphocytes by stimulating cell growth (as a B-cell mitogen) and by inducing expression of the cell's bcl oncogene, which prevents programmed cell death (**apoptosis**).

Retroviruses have several potential mechanisms of immortalization. Some oncoviruses encode oncogene proteins (e.g., sis, ras, src, mos, myc, jun, fos), which are almost identical to the cellular proteins involved in cellular growth control (e.g., components of a growth factor signal cascade or growth regulating transcription factors). Overproduction or altered function of these oncogene products stimulates cell growth. These oncogenic viruses rapidly cause tumors. Human T-cell lymphotropic virus (HTLV-1) (the only identified human oncogenic retrovi-

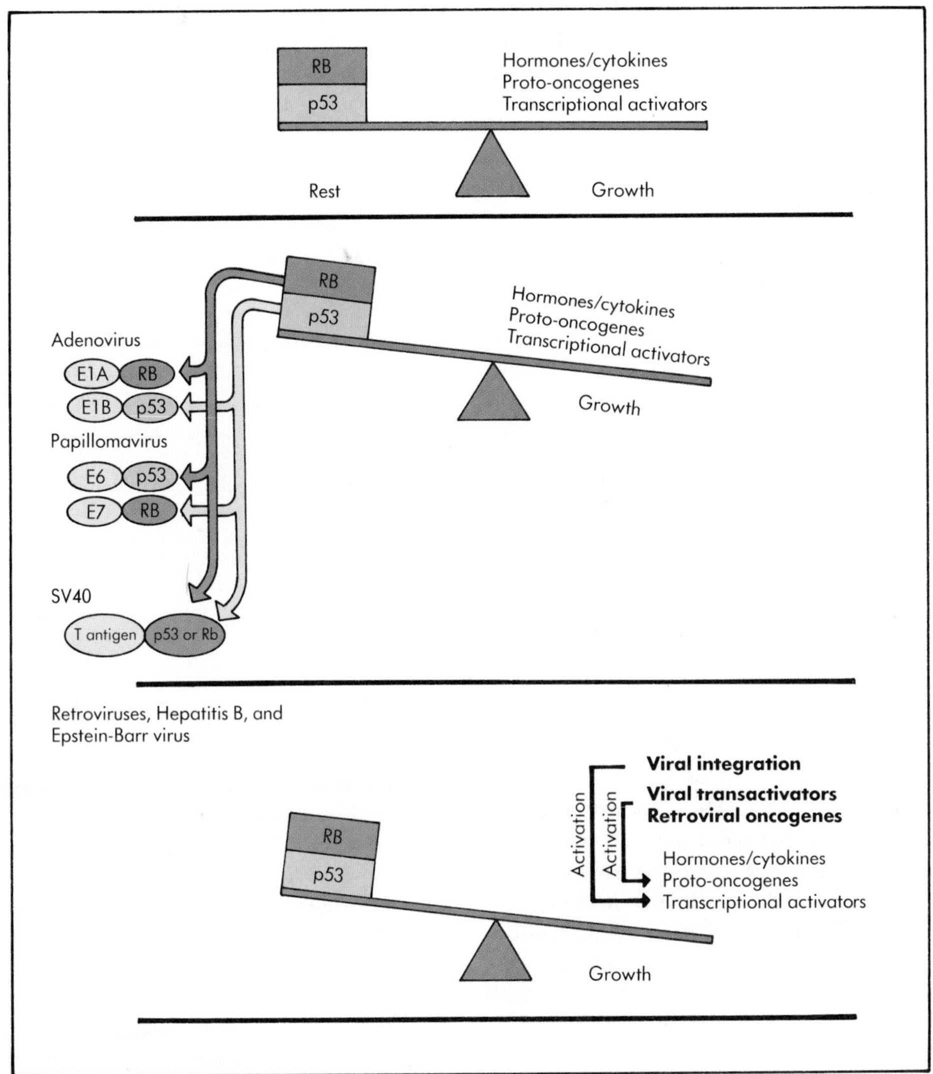

FIGURE 52-2 Mechanisms of viral transformation/immortalization. Cell growth is controlled by the balance of external and internal growth activators (accelerators) and growth suppressors such as p53 and the retinoblastoma gene product (RB) (brakes). Oncogenic viruses alter the balance by removing the brakes or enhancing the accelerators.

rus) has two potential mechanisms of leukemogenesis. HTLV-1 encodes a protein (tax) that transactivates gene expression, including genes for growth stimulating lymphokines. Integration of HTLV-1 near a cellular growth stimulating gene can cause the gene to be activated by the strong viral enhancer and promoter sequences encoded at each end of the viral genome (LTR sequences). HTLV-1 associated leukemias occur after 20 to 30 years. Retroviruses continue to produce virus in immortalized/transformed cells.

Viral transformation is the first step but is generally not sufficient for oncogenesis and tumor formation. Immortalized cells are more likely than normal cells to accumulate other mutations or chromosomal rearrangements after time to promote tumor cell development. Immortalized cells may also be more susceptible to cofactors and tumor promoters (e.g., phorbol esters and butyrate), which enhance tumor formation. Approximately 15% of human cancers can be related to oncogenic viruses such as HTLV-1, hepatitis B virus, papillomaviruses 16 and 18, and Epstein-Barr virus. Herpes simplex virus type 2 may be a cofactor for human cervical cancer.

HOST DEFENSES AGAINST VIRAL INFECTION

Humans are protected from viral infection by **natural barriers** (e.g., skin, mucus, ciliated epithelium, gastric acid, and bile), **nonspecific immune defenses** (e.g., fever, interferon, macrophages, natural killer cells), and **antigen-specific immune responses** (e.g., antibody and T cells). Skin is the best barrier to infection. Abrasions or breaks in the skin allow access to cells permissive to infection. On penetration of the natural barriers, the virus activates the nonspecific defenses, which attempt to limit

TABLE 52-3 Physicochemical Properties of Human Interferons

Property	Interferon		
	Alpha	Beta	Gamma
Previous designations	Leukocyte-IFN Type I	Fibroblast-IFN Type I	Immune IFN Type II
Genes	>20	One	One
Molecular weight (daltons)*			
Major subtypes	16,000-23,000	23,000	20,000-25,000
Cloned†	19,000	19,000	16,000
Glycosylation	No‡	Yes	Yes
pH 2 stability	Stable‡	Stable	Labile
Induction	Viruses	Viruses	Mitogens
Principal source	Epithelium, leukocytes	Fibroblast	Lymphocyte
Introns in gene	No	No	Yes
Homology with Hu-IFN-α	100%	30%-50%	<10%

From White DO: *Antiviral chemotherapy, interferons and vaccines,* Basel, 1984, Karger; and Samuel CE: *Virol* 183:1-11, 1991.
*Molecular weight of monomeric form. Interferons often occur as polymers.
†Nonglycosylated form, as produced in bacteria by recombinant DNA technology.
‡Most subtypes, but not all.

and control local viral replication and spread. Antigen-specific immune responses are the last to be activated and are generally systemic. The ultimate goal of the immune response is to eliminate the virus and the cells harboring or replicating the virus. The immune response is the best and in most cases the only means of controlling a virus infection. Both the humoral and the cellular immune responses are important for antiviral immunity. Failure to resolve the infection may lead to persistent or chronic infections or death.

Nonspecific Immune Defenses

Body temperature, fever, interferons and other cytokines, the mononuclear phagocyte system, and natural killer cells provide a local rapid response to viral infection and activate the specific immune defenses. Oftentimes the nonspecific defenses are sufficient to control a viral infection, thus preventing the occurrence of symptoms.

Virus infection can induce the release of cytokines (tumor necrosis factor, interleukin 1, etc.) and interferon (discussed later) from infected cells and macrophages. These soluble protein factors trigger local and systemic responses. Induction of fever and stimulation of the immune system are two of these systemic effects.

Body temperature and fever can limit the replication or destabilize some viruses. Many viruses are less stable (e.g., herpes simplex virus) or cannot replicate (rhinoviruses) as well at 37° C or higher.

Cells of the mononuclear phagocyte system phagocytize virus and cell debris from viral infected cells. Macrophages in the liver (Kupffer's cells) and spleen rapidly clear many viruses from the blood. Antibody and complement bound to a virus facilitate its uptake by macrophage (**opsonization**). Macrophages also present antigen to T lymphocytes and release interleukin 1 and interferon to initiate the antigen-specific immune response. Activated macrophage can also distinguish and kill infected target cells.

Natural killer (NK) cells are large granular lymphocytes. Interferon and specific lymphokines stimulate the differentiation of pre-NK cells to NK cells and activate NK cells to kill viral-infected cells. It is not known how NK cells distinguish viral-infected cells.

Interferon

Interferon was first described by Isaacs and Lindemann as a factor that "interferes" with the replication of many different viruses. Interferon is the body's first active defense against a viral infection. In addition to preventing viral replication, interferons activate the immune response and also enhance T-cell recognition of the infected cell. Interferon is a very important defense against infection but is also a cause of the malaise, myalgia, chills, and fever (nonspecific flu-like symptoms) associated with many viral infections.

Interferon comprises a family of proteins that can be subdivided by several properties, including size, stability, cell of origin, and mode of action (Table 52-3). The alpha- and beta-interferons share many properties including structural homology and mode of action. Alpha-interferon is made by B lymphocytes, monocytes, and macrophages. Beta-interferon is made by fibroblasts and other cells in response to virus infection and other stimuli. Gamma-interferon is produced later in infection by activated T cells. Although gamma-interferon inhibits virus replication, its structure and mode of action differ from the other interferons. Gamma-interferon is also known as macrophage activation factor.

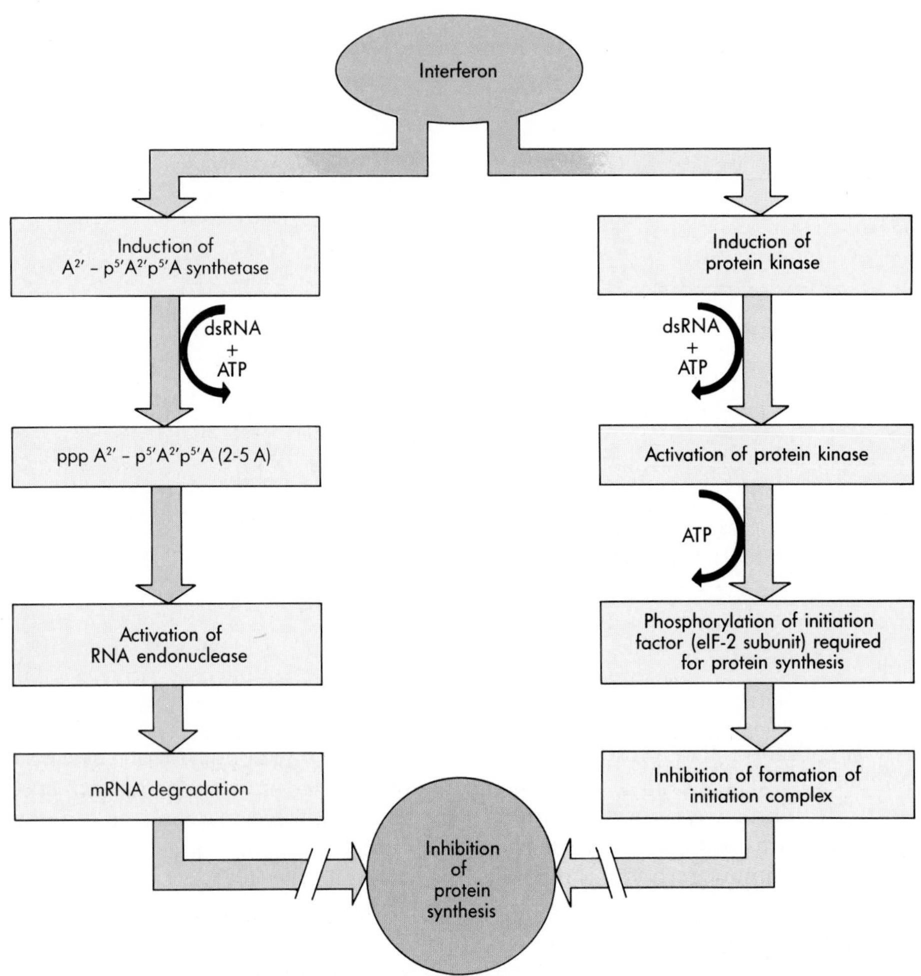

FIGURE 52-3 The two major routes for interferon inhibition of viral protein synthesis. One mechanism involves induction of an unusual polymerase (2-5A synthetase) that is activated by double-stranded RNA. The activated enzyme synthesizes an unusual adenine trinucleotide with a 2′, 5′-phosphodiester linkage. The trinucleotide activates an endonuclease that degrades mRNA. The other mechanism involves induction of a protein kinase that inactivates the eIF-2 initiation factor by phosphorylating one of the subunits to prevent initiation of protein synthesis.

One of the best inducers of alpha- and beta-interferon production is double-stranded RNA, such as the replicative intermediates of RNA viruses. One double-stranded RNA molecule per cell is sufficient to induce the production of interferon. Many of the other substances that promote interferon production reduce protein synthesis in the cell. This decreases the concentration of a repressor protein of the interferon gene, which allows expression of the interferon gene. Nonviral interferon inducers include intracellular microorganisms (e.g., mycobacteria, fungi, protozoa), immune stimulators or mitogens (e.g., endotoxins, phytohemagglutinin), double-stranded polynucleotides (e.g., poly I:C, poly dA:dT), synthetic polyanion polymers (e.g., polysulfates, polyphosphates, pyran), antibiotics (e.g., kanamycin, cyclohexamide), and low molecular weight synthetic compounds (e.g., tilorone, acridine dyes).

Alpha- and beta-interferon can be induced and released within hours of infection. The interferon binds to specific receptors on neighboring cells and induces the production of antiviral proteins. The major antiviral effects of interferon are produced by two enzymes, 2'-5' oligoadenylate (2-5A) synthetase (an unusual polymerase) and a protein kinase specific for ribosomal initiating factor eIF-2. Both of these enzymes must bind double-stranded RNA to be activated. Viral infection of the cell and production of double-stranded RNA activates these enzymes and triggers a cascade of biochemical events that leads to inhibition of protein synthesis, the degradation of mRNA (preferentially viral mRNA), and other activities. This essentially puts the cellular factory on strike and prevents viral replication (Figure 52-3). It must be stressed that interferon induces an **antiviral state** but does not directly block virus replication. The antiviral state lasts for 2 to 3 days, which may be sufficient for the cell to degrade and eliminate the virus without being killed.

TABLE 52-4 Some Biological Effects of Interferons

Effect	Comment
Inhibition of multiplication of viruses	
Inhibition of cell division	
Immunomodulation	
All cells	Increased expression of major histocompatibility antigens and Fc receptors
Natural killer cell	Activation and maturation
T cell	Proliferation suppressed; lymphokine release enhanced
DTH (CD4)	Modulation of delayed hypersensitivity
CTL (CD8)	Cytotoxicity increased
Macrophage	Activation

Interferons stimulate cell-mediated immunity by activating effector cells and by enhancing recognition of the viral-infected target cell. Interferons stimulate pre-natural killer cells to differentiate to natural killer cells to activate an *early, local* natural defense against infection. Activation of macrophages by gamma-interferon promotes the production of more interferon and secretion of other biological response modifiers, phagocytosis, recruitment, and inflammatory responses.

All interferon types stimulate the expression of major histocompatability (MHC) class I (HLA) and II antigens on the cell surface. Gamma-interferon increases the expression of MHC class II antigens on the macrophage to help promote antigen presentation to T cells. Alpha- and beta-interferon increases expression of MHC Class I antigens, which enhances the cell's ability to present antigen, making the cell a better target for cytotoxic T cells.

Interferon also has widespread regulatory effects on cell growth, protein synthesis, and the immune response (Table 52-4). All three interferon types block cell proliferation at appropriate doses.

Genetically engineered recombinant interferon is being used as an antiviral therapy for some viral infections (e.g., condyloma acuminata and hepatitis C virus). Effective treatment requires use of the correct interferon subtype, delivered promptly and at the appropriate concentration. Interferons have also been used in clinical trials for the treatment of certain cancers. Interferon treatment is accompanied by flu-like side effects such as chills, fever, and fatigue.

Antigen-Specific Immunity

Humoral and cell-mediated immunity play different roles in resolving viral infections. Humoral immunity (antibody) acts mainly on extracellular virions, whereas cell-mediated immunity (T cells) is directed at the virus-producing cell (Figure 52-4).

Humoral Immunity

Practically all viral proteins are foreign to the host and are **immunogenic** (capable of eliciting an antibody response). However, not all immunogens elicit protective immunity. **Protective humoral immunity** is developed against the structural antigens located at the surface of the virus. These antigens include the viral capsid proteins of naked viruses and the glycoproteins of enveloped viruses. An antibody response to other viral antigens may be useful for serologic analysis of the viral infection.

Antibody blocks the progression of disease by **neutralization** and **opsonization** of cell-free virus. Antibody can neutralize the virus by binding to the viral attachment proteins, preventing their interaction with target cells, or by destabilizing the virus, initiating its degradation. Binding of antibody to the virus also opsonizes the virus, promoting its uptake and clearance by macrophages. Antibody recognition of infected cells can also promote antibody-dependent cellular cytotoxicity.

The major antiviral role of antibody is to prevent the spread of extracellular virus to other cells and is especially important in preventing a viremia. Antibody is most effective at resolving cytolytic infections. Resolution occurs because the virus kills the cell factory and the antibody eliminates the extracellular virus. Antibody is the primary defense initiated by vaccination.

T-Cell Immunity

T-cell–mediated immunity promotes antibody and inflammatory responses (CD4 helper and delayed type hypersensitivity T lymphocytes) and kills infected cells (CD8 cytotoxic T lymphocytes). The T-cell immune response is directed against viral peptides bound to the hydrophobic cleft of an MHC antigen on the target cell surface. Macrophages and other antigen presenting cells initiate the immune response by processing and presenting the virus, viral protein, or vaccine to CD4 T cells. CD4 T cells recognize viral peptide antigens bound to MHC class II molecules. The peptides expressed on MHC class II antigens are obtained from viral proteins that were endocytosed or phagocytosed (exogenous route) and proteolytically degraded by the cell. The CD4 T cells release lymphokines and interferon γ, which activate (help) B cells, macrophages, and other T cells and initiate the delayed type hypersensitivity response.

Cytotoxic T (CD8) lymphocytes (CTL) kill infected cells and, as a result, eliminate the source of new virus. CTL are activated by lymphokines produced by helper T cells and kill cells expressing the appropriate complex of viral peptide with MHC class I protein. The peptides expressed on MHC class I antigens are obtained from viral proteins synthesized within the infected cell (endogenous route). CTL antigen targets include peptides derived from viral proteins that would not elicit protec-

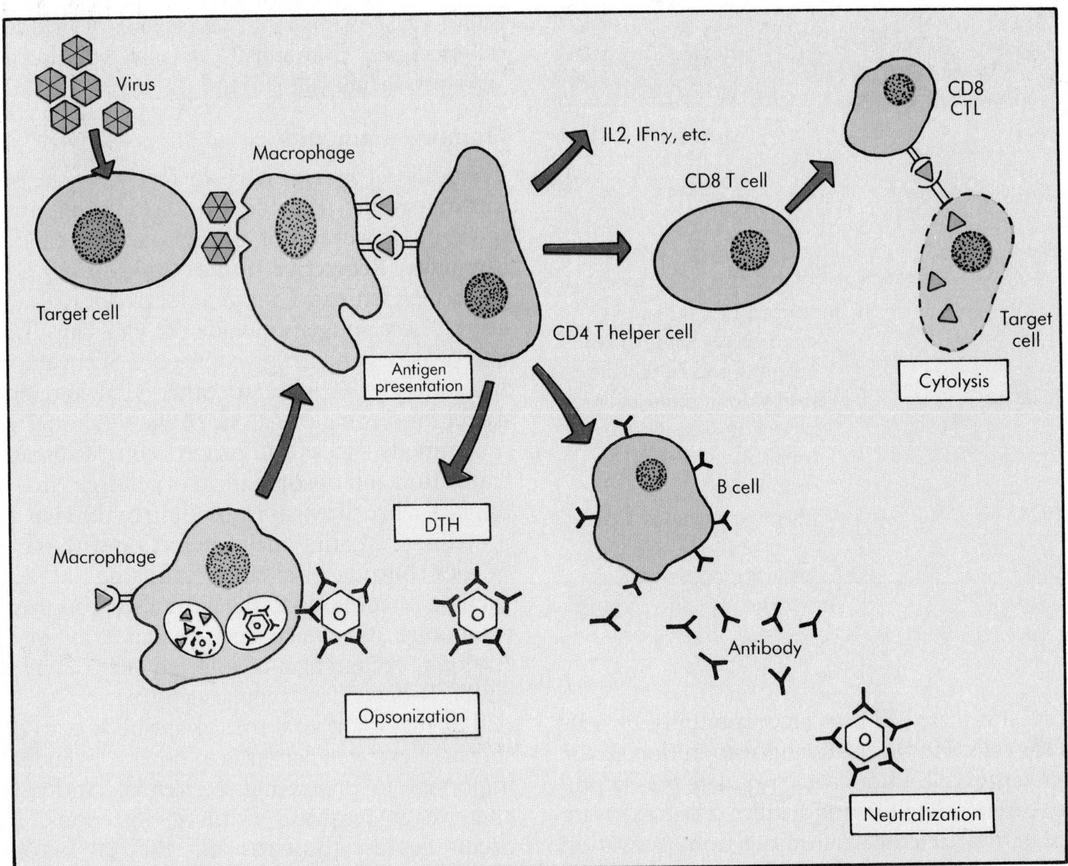

FIGURE 52-4 Antigen-specific antiviral immunity. The immune response is initiated by phagocytosis, proteolysis, and antigen presentation on macrophage-lineage cells. Antigen-specific T-helper and delayed type hypersensitivity *(DTH)* cells are activated and release lymphokines, which activate cytolytic T cells and B cells. Antibody binds to virus and neutralizes or opsonizes free virus. Macrophages phagocytose virus particles and restart the cycle.

tive antibody (e.g., intracellular or internal virion proteins, nuclear proteins, improperly folded or processed proteins [cell trash]) in addition to viral glycoproteins. For example, the matrix and nucleoproteins of influenza and the ICP4 (nuclear) protein of herpes simplex virus are targets for CTL lysis but do not elicit protective antibody.

Cell-mediated immunity is especially important for resolving infections by syncytia-forming viruses, which can spread from cell to cell without exposure to antibody (e.g., measles virus, herpes simplex virus, varicella-zoster virus); noncytolytic viruses (e.g., hepatitis A virus, measles virus); and controlling latent viruses (herpesviruses and papovaviruses).

Immune Response to Viral Challenge

The nature of the immune response to a viral infection is determined by host, viral, and other factors. Host factors include genetic background, immune status, age, and the general health of the individual. Viral factors include viral strain, infectious dose, and route of entry. The time required to initiate immune protection, the extent of the response, the level of control of the infection, and the potential for immunopathology resulting from the infection differ following a primary infection and a rechallenge.

Primary Viral Challenge

The nonspecific immune responses are the earliest antiviral responses to viral challenge and are often sufficient to limit virus spread. Interferon produced in response to most virus infections initiates protection of adjacent cells, enhances antigen presentation by promoting expression of MHC antigens, and initiates clearance of infected cells by activating natural killer cells. Virus and viral components released from the infected cells are phagocytosed by resident macrophages that mobilize and move to the lymph nodes. Macrophages in the liver and spleen are especially important for clearing virus from the bloodstream. The macrophages degrade and process the viral antigens and express appropriate peptide fragments on their cell surface bound to MHC class II antigens. Macrophages also release interleukin 1 and tumor necrosis factor (TNF) to promote helper T-cell activation and fever.

Antigen-specific responses are initiated later in the

TABLE 52-5 Human Viruses Infecting Cells of the Lymphocyte-Macrophage Lineage

Representative viruses	Comment
B cells	
Epstein-Barr virus	Immortalization and polyclonal B-cell activation
T cells	
Measles	Infects T cells and proliferates in activated cell
Human T lymphotropic virus 1 and 2	Retroviruses associated with T-cell lymphoma/leukemia
Human immunodeficiency virus 1 and 2	Kills helper cells, induces acquired immunodeficiency syndrome (AIDS)
Macrophages	
Yellow fever, dengue	Viral hemorrhagic fever
Rubella	Facilitates spread of virus
Human immunodeficiency virus	Persistence and infection in various tissues, including brain

course of infection. IgM-producing B lymphocytes and CD4 T cells respond to antigen at approximately the same time. IgM is the first antiviral antibody. CD4 T cells specific for viral antigens interact with macrophages, become activated, secrete interleukin 2, gamma-interferon, and other lymphokines, and proliferate. The lymphokines secreted by the CD4 T cells promote the development of B and T cells to activate IgG and IgA production and cytotoxic CD8 T cells. Swollen lymph nodes can result from activation and growth of lymphocytes in response to the viral challenge. IgG and IgA are produced 2 to 3 days after IgM. Secretory IgA is made in response to a viral challenge through the natural openings of the body: the eyes, mouth, and respiratory and gastrointestinal systems. CD8+ killer/suppressor T cells are present at approximately the same time as IgG. Resolution of the infection occurs later, when sufficient antibody is available to neutralize all virus progeny or when cellular immunity has been able to reach and eliminate the infected cells. DTH and CTL responses are required for resolution of most enveloped virus infections. In many cases, IgG and cytotoxic T cells in the blood are detected after virus replication has been controlled.

Infections of lymphocytes or macrophages are special cases for the immune response (Table 52-5). The virus may alter the function of the cell, or it may inactivate or target the cell for immune clearance. Measles and influenza virus infection of lymphocytes depress their function. HIV infection and cytolysis of CD4 T cells debilitate the immune system by eliminating these very important cells. The hyperactive T-cell responses to EBV, CMV, and HIV infection of lymphocytes cause the mononucleosis-like symptoms (lymphocytosis, swollen glands, malaise) associated with their infections. Viruses that can replicate in the macrophage are often hidden from immune clearance, which promotes their transport throughout the body. Lymphocytes and macrophages are long-lived cells, and many viruses establish persistent and latent infections of these cells.

Secondary Viral Challenge

In any war it is easier to eliminate an enemy if its identity and origin are known and if establishment of its foothold can be prevented. Similarly, prior immunity allows rapid, specific mobilization of defenses to prevent disease symptoms, promote rapid clearance of the virus, and prevent viral access to the target tissue. As a result, most secondary viral challenges are asymptomatic. Antibody and memory B and T cells are present in an immune individual to act on the virus infection and generate a more rapid and extensive anamnestic response. Secretory IgA provides an important defense to reinfection through the natural openings of the body but is produced only transiently. IgG antibody prevents viremic spread from the primary site of infection.

Viral Mechanisms for Escaping the Immune Response

A major factor in the virulence of a virus is its ability to escape immune resolution. Viruses may escape immune resolution by evading detection, preventing activation, or blocking the delivery of the immune response. Specific examples are presented in Table 52-6. Some viruses actually encode special proteins that suppress the immune response.

Immunopathology

Hypersensitivity and inflammatory reactions initiated by antiviral immunity can be the major cause of disease-related pathology (Table 52-7). Inflammatory responses can be initiated early in the infection by cell damage, interferon and lymphokines, and activation of the C3 component of complement by the alternative pathway. Later, inflammatory responses may be induced by immune complexes and complement activation (classical pathway), CD4 T-cell induced delayed type hypersensitivity, and immune cytolysis. Interferon and lymphokines initiate effects on multiple body systems to produce the symptoms usually associated with mild viral infections (e.g., fever, runny nose, malaise, headache). Cell damage,

TABLE 52-6 Viral Evasion of Immune Responses

Mechanism	Viral examples	Action
HUMORAL RESPONSE		
Hidden from antibody	Herpesviruses, retroviruses	Latent infection
Hidden from antibody	Herpes simplex virus, varicella-zoster virus, paramyxoviruses	Syncytia formation (cell-to-cell infection)
Antigenic variation	Lentiviruses (HIV)	Genetic change after infection
	Influenza virus	Annual genetic changes
Secretion of blocking antigen	Hepatitis B virus	Hepatitis B surface antigen
Decay of complement	Herpes simplex virus	Glycoprotein C binds and promotes C3 decay
INTERFERON		
Block production	Hepatitis B virus	Inhibits interferon transcription
	Epstein-Barr virus	Interleukin 10 analogue (BCRF1) blocks gamma-interferon production
Block action	Adenovirus	Inhibits up-regulation of MHC expression
	Adenovirus	VA1 RNA blocks double-stranded RNA activation of interferon-induced protein kinase
IMMUNE CELL FUNCTION		
Cytolysis of lymphoid cells	HIV	CD4 T cells
	Epstein-Barr virus	B cells
Impairment of function	HIV	Reduces cell surface expression of CD4 on T cell
	Measles virus	Suppresses natural killer, T, and B cells
Immunosuppressive factors	Epstein-Barr virus	BCRF (similar to interleukin-10) suppresses helper T cell responses
	HIV, cytomegalovirus	
DECREASED ANTIGEN PRESENTATION		
Reduced human leukocyte antigen expression	Adenovirus 12	Inhibits MHC class I transcription
		19 kd protein (E3 gene) binds MHC I heavy chain, blocks translocation to surface
	Cytomegalovirus	H301 protein binds beta-2-microglobulin, blocks surface expression
	Herpes simplex virus	Inhibits cell protein synthesis
INHIBITION OF INFLAMMATION		
	Poxvirus, adenovirus	Blocks interleukin 1 or tumor necrosis factor action

complement activation, and DTH usually initiate local responses characterized by neutrophil infiltration and more cell damage.

The inflammatory response initiated by cell-mediated immunity is difficult to control and will damage tissue. Enveloped virus infections are usually associated with more extensive immunopathology. For example, the classical symptoms of measles and mumps are due to the T cell–induced inflammatory and hypersensitivity responses rather than viral cytopathology. T cell–deficient individuals suffer atypical disease presentations.

The presence of large amounts of antigen in blood during viremias or chronic infections (e.g., hepatitis B virus) can initiate classic immune-complex hypersensitivity reactions. Immune complexes containing virus or viral antigen can activate the complement system, promoting inflammatory responses and tissue destruction. These immune complexes often accumulate in the kidney and cause renal problems.

For dengue and measles viruses, partial immunity to a related strain can initiate a more severe host response and disease upon challenge with a new strain. Antigen-specific T-cell and antibody responses are enhanced and induce significant inflammatory and hypersensitivity damage to infected endothelial cells (dengue hemorrhagic fever) or skin and the lung (atypical measles). In addition, a

TABLE 52-7 Viral Immunopathogenesis

Immunopathogenesis	Immune mediators	Examples
"Flu-like symptoms"	Interferon/lymphokines	Respiratory viruses, arboviruses (viremia-inducing viruses)
DTH and inflammation	T cells, PMNs, etc.	Enveloped viruses
Immune-complex disease	Antibody, complement, PMNs	Hepatitis B virus
Hemorrhagic disease	T cells antibody/complement	Dengue virus
Post infection cytolysis	T cells	Enveloped viruses (e.g., post measles encephalitis)
Immunosuppression	(see Table 52-6)	HIV, cytomegalovirus, measles virus, influenza virus

DTH, Delayed type hypersensitivity; *PMNs*, polymorphonuclear leukocytes.

non-neutralizing antibody can facilitate the uptake of dengue and yellow fever viruses into macrophages through Fc receptors, where they can replicate.

Children generally have a less active cell-mediated immune response than adults and generally have milder disease symptoms with several viral diseases (e.g., measles, mumps, Epstein-Barr virus, varicella-zoster virus). However, for hepatitis B virus, mild or no symptoms correlate with an inability to resolve the infection and results in chronic disease.

Viral Disease

The stages of viral infection are shown in Figure 52-1. The initial period before detection of characteristic disease symptoms is termed the **prodrome** or **incubation period.** During this period, the virus is replicating but has not reached the target tissue or induced sufficient damage to cause symptoms. The incubation period is relatively short if infection of the primary site produces the characteristic symptoms of the disease. Nonspecific flu-like symptoms may precede the characteristic disease symptoms. The incubation periods for many common viral infections are given in Table 52-8.

Viral infections may be apparent or inapparent and may cause acute or chronic disease. The symptoms of a viral disease are related to the function of the infected target tissue and the immunopathology induced by the infection. Clinical syndromes for specific viruses will be discussed in subsequent chapters and reviewed in Chapter 70. The ability of an individual's immune system to control and resolve a viral infection usually determines whether acute or chronic disease will result (Figure 52-5).

Inapparent infections result if no damage occurs to the infected tissue, if the infection is controlled before the virus reaches its target tissue, if the target tissue is expendable, if the damage is rapidly repaired, or if the level of damage is below a functional threshold for that particular tissue. Many infections of the brain are either inapparent or below the threshold of severe loss of function, but encephalitis results when loss of function becomes significant. Inapparent infections are frequently detected by the presence of virus-specific antibody in an individual. For example, although 97% of adults have antibody (seropositive) to varicella-zoster virus, less than half will remember having had chickenpox.

The susceptibility of an individual and the severity of the disease differ depending on factors such as exposure, immune status, age, general health of the individual, viral dose, and the genetics of both the virus and the host. Once infected, the host's immune status is probably the major factor in whether a viral infection causes a life-threatening disease, a benign lesion, or no symptoms at all.

TABLE 52-8 Incubation Periods of Common Viral Infections

Disease	Incubation period* (days)
Influenza	1-2
Common cold	1-3
Bronchiolitis, croup	3-5
Acute respiratory disease (adenoviruses)	5-7
Dengue	5-8
Herpes simplex	5-8
Enteroviruses	6-12
Poliomyelitis	5-20
Measles	9-12
Smallpox	12-14
Chickenpox	13-17
Mumps	16-20
Rubella	17-20
Mononucleosis	30-50
Hepatitis A	15-40
Hepatitis B	50-150
Rabies	30-100
Warts	50-150
AIDS	1-10 years

Modified from White DO and Fenner F: *Medical virology*, ed 3, New York, 1986, Academic Press.

*Until first appearance of prodromal symptoms. Diagnostic signs (e.g., rash, paralysis) may not appear until 2 to 4 days later.

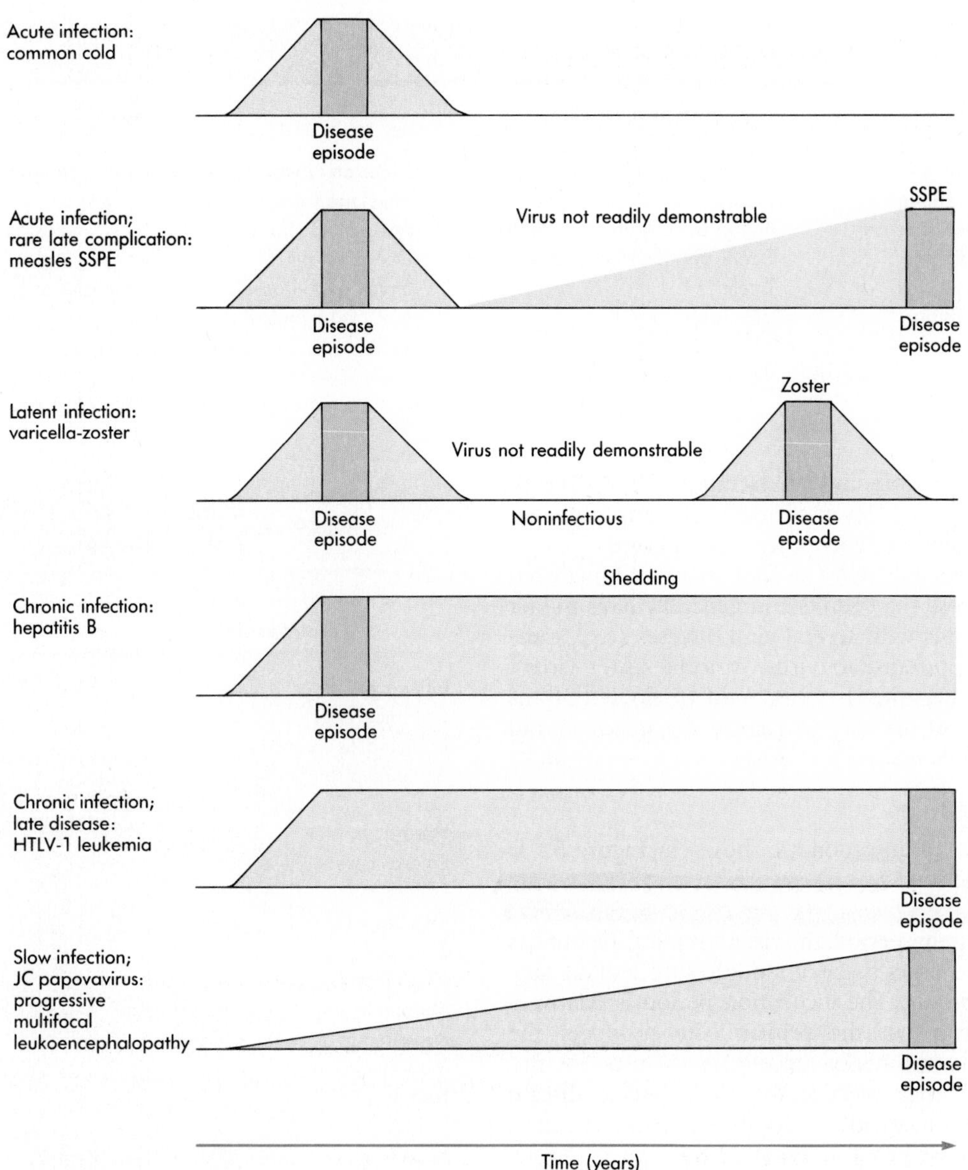

FIGURE 52-5 Diagram depicting acute infection and various types of persistent infection, as illustrated by the diseases indicated in the column at the left. *Vertical box* (green) illustrates disease episode. *SSPE*, subacute sclerosing panencephalitis. (Redrawn from White DO, Fenner F: *Medical virology*, ed 3, New York, 1986, Academic Press.)

Exposure

People are exposed to viruses throughout their lives. However, some situations, vocations, life-styles, or living arrangements increase the chance of contact with certain viruses. Many viruses are ubiquitous, and evidence of exposure (antibodies to the virus) can be detected in most young children (herpes simplex virus type 1, human herpesvirus 6, varicella-zoster virus, parvovirus B19) or by early adulthood (Epstein-Barr virus and many respiratory and enteric viruses). Poor hygiene and crowded living, school, and job conditions promote exposure to respiratory and enteric viruses. Day-care centers are consistent sources of viral infections, especially viruses spread by respiratory and fecal-oral routes. Travel, summer camp, and vocations that bring us in contact with a virus vector, such as mosquitos, put us at risk for infection by arboviruses and other zoonoses. Sexual promiscuity also promotes spread and acquisition of several viruses. Health care workers such as physicians, dentists, nurses, and technicians are frequently exposed to respiratory and other viruses but are especially at risk for acquiring viruses from contaminated blood (hepatitis B virus, human immunodeficiency virus) or vesicle fluid (herpes simplex virus).

Immune Status

The immune status of an individual is a crucial determinant for susceptibility, symptoms, and severity. The competence of the immune response determines how quickly and efficiently the infection is resolved, but it can also determine the severity of the symptoms related to the extent of immunopathogenesis. Rechallenge of an individual with prior immunity usually results in asymptomatic or mild disease. Immunosuppression by AIDS, cancer, or immunosuppressive therapy increases the risk to more serious disease upon primary infection (measles, vaccinia) and to recurrences of latent viruses (e.g., herpesviruses, papovaviruses).

Age

The age of the individual is an important factor in viral infections. Infants, children, adults, and the elderly are susceptible to different viruses and have different symptomatic responses to the infection. This may be due to differences in body size, tissue characteristics, recuperative abilities, and, most important, immune status. Differences in life-style, habits, school, and jobs at different ages in life determine when we are exposed to viruses.

Infants and children acquire a series of respiratory and exanthematous viral diseases because they have never been exposed and are immunologically naive. Infants are especially susceptible to more serious presentations of paramyxovirus respiratory infections and gastroenteritis because of the child's small size and physiological requirements (e.g., nutrients, water, and electrolytes). However, children generally do not develop as severe an immunopathologic response as adults, and some diseases (herpesviruses) are more benign in children.

The elderly are especially susceptible to new virus infections and reactivation of latent viruses. They are less able to initiate a new immune response, repair tissue damage, and recover, and are therefore more susceptible to outbreaks of influenza A and B. The elderly are more prone to zoster (shingles), a recurrence of varicella-zoster virus.

Other Host Factors

The general health and genetic makeup of an individual play important roles in determining the competence and nature of the immune response. Poor nutrition compromises the immune system and decreases tissue regenerative capacity. Immunosuppressive diseases and therapies allow virus replication or recurrence to proceed unchecked. Genetic differences in immune-response genes, genes for virus receptors, and other genetic loci can also affect the susceptibility of an individual and the severity of a virus infection.

EPIDEMIOLOGY

Infection of a population is similar to infection of an individual in that the virus must spread through the population and is controlled by immunization of the population (Box 52-3). To endure, viruses must continue to infect new, immunologically naive, susceptible hosts.

BOX 52-3 Viral Epidemiology

(Infection of a population instead of a person)

MECHANISMS OF VIRUS TRANSMISSION

Aerosols
Fomites (e.g., tissues, clothes)
Direct contact with secretions (e.g., saliva, semen)
Sexual contact
Blood transfusion or organ transplant
Zoonoses (animals, insects [arboviruses])

DISEASE/VIRUS FACTORS THAT PROMOTE TRANSMISSION

Stability of virion to the environment (e.g., drying, drinking water, detergents, temperature)
Replication and secretion of virus into transmittable aerosols/secretions (e.g., saliva, semen)
Ability to spread before symptoms
Transience or ineffectiveness of immune response to control reinfection or recurrence

RISK FACTORS

Age
Health
Immune status
Occupation: contact with agent or vector
Travel history
Life-style
Children in day care

CRITICAL COMMUNITY SIZE

GEOGRAPHY/SEASON

Presence of cofactors or vectors in the environment
Habitat and season for arthropod vectors (mosquitos)
School session: close proximity and crowding
Home heating season

MODES OF CONTROL

Quarantine
Elimination of the vector
Immunization
- Natural infection
- Vaccination

Maintenance of a Virus in the Population

Persistence of a virus in a community depends on the availability of a critical number of immunologically naive (seronegative), susceptible individuals. The efficiency of the route of transmission determines the size of the susceptible population required for continuation. Immunization, by natural or vaccination routes, is the best means of reducing the number of susceptible individuals.

Transmission of Viruses

Viruses are transmitted by direct contact (including sexual contact), injection or transplantation with contaminated fluids, blood, or organs, and the respiratory and fecal-oral routes (Figure 52-1). The route of transmission depends on the source of virus (tissue site of virus replication and secretion) and the ability of the virus to endure the hazards and barriers of the environment and the body en route to the target tissue. For example, viruses that replicate in the respiratory tract (e.g., influenza A) are released in aerosol droplets, whereas enteric viruses (e.g., picornaviruses and reoviruses) are passed by the fecal-oral route. Cytomegalovirus is transmitted in most bodily secretions because it infects epithelial and other cells found in skin, secretory glands, the lungs, liver, and other organs. Arthropods or animal bites can also introduce togaviruses and rhabdoviruses to human hosts.

The presence or absence of an envelope is the major structural determinant for the mode of viral transmission. Nonenveloped viruses can withstand drying, detergents, and extremes of pH and temperature, whereas enveloped viruses generally cannot. Most nonenveloped viruses can withstand the acidic environment of the stomach and the detergent-like bile of the intestines, as well as mild disinfection and insufficient sewage treatment procedures. Nonenveloped viruses are generally transmitted by respiratory and fecal-oral routes and can often be acquired from contaminated objects, termed **fomites**. Hepatitis A virus, a picornavirus, is transmitted by the fecal-oral route and acquired from contaminated water, shellfish, and food. Rhinoviruses and many other nonenveloped viruses can be spread by contact with fomites such as handkerchiefs or toys.

Unlike the sturdy naked capsid viruses, enveloped viruses are more fragile. They require an intact envelope for infectivity. Enveloped viruses must remain wet and are spread in respiratory droplets, blood, by injection, organ transplants, mucus, saliva, and semen. Most enveloped viruses are also labile to acid and detergents, which precludes fecal-oral transmission.

Animals can also act as **vectors** to spread viral disease to other animals and humans and even to other locales. They can also be **reservoirs** for the virus to maintain and amplify the virus in the environment. Viral diseases that are shared by animals or insects and man are a **zoonosis**. Arthropods, including mosquitos, ticks, and sandflies, can act as vectors for togaviruses, flaviviruses, bunyaviruses, and reoviruses. These viruses are often referred to as **arboviruses** because they are *ar*thropod *bo*rne. Most arboviruses have a very broad host range, which may include specific insects, birds, reptiles, and mammals in addition to humans. Raccoons, foxes, dogs, and cats are vectors for rabies virus.

Other factors that can promote the transmission of viruses include the potential for asymptomatic infection, crowding, occupation, life-style, day-care centers, and travel. Many viruses are released before symptoms appear, making it difficult to restrict transmission (e.g., HIV, varicella-zoster virus). Viruses that cause persistent productive infections (e.g., cytomegalovirus, HIV) are a continual source of virus that may result in spread to immunologically naive individuals. Viruses with many different serotypes (rhinoviruses) or viruses capable of changing their antigenicity (influenza and HIV) readily find immunologically naive populations.

Geographical and Seasonal Considerations

The geographical distribution of a virus is usually determined by the presence of cofactors, vectors, or an immunologically naive, susceptible population. Many of the arboviruses are limited to the ecological niche of their arthropod vectors. Extensive global transportation is eliminating many of the geographical restrictions to virus distribution.

Seasonal differences in the occurence of viral disease correspond with behaviors that promote the spread of the virus. Respiratory viruses are more prevalent in the winter because of crowding and temperature and humidity conditions that facilitate the spread or stabilize the extracorporal virus. Enteric viruses are more prevalent during the summer, possibly because of less effective hygiene. The seasonal differences in arboviral diseases reflect the life cycle of the arthropod vector or its reservoir (e.g., birds).

Outbreaks, Epidemics, and Pandemics

Outbreaks of a virus infection often result from introduction of a virus (such as hepatitis A) into a new location. The outbreak is initiated from a common source (e.g., food preparation), and identification of the source can often stop the outbreak. **Epidemics** occur over a larger geographical area and generally result from introduction of a new strain of virus to an immunologically naive population. **Pandemics** are worldwide epidemics, usually resulting from introduction of a new virus (e.g., HIV). Pandemics of influenza A have occurred approximately every 10 years caused by the introduction of new strains of virus.

CONTROL OF VIRUS SPREAD

The spread of a virus can be controlled by quarantine, good hygiene, change in life-style, elimination of the vector, and immunization of the population. Quarantine was once the only means of limiting virus epidemics and is most effective for viruses that are always symptomatic (e.g., measles, smallpox). Quarantine is used in the hospital to limit nosocomial spread of viruses, especially to high-risk patients (e.g., immunosuppressed individuals). Proper sanitation of contaminated items and disinfection of the water supply can limit the spread of enteric viruses. Changes in life-styles have made a difference in the spread of sexually transmitted viruses such as HIV, hepatitis B virus, and herpes simplex virus. Elimination of the arthropod or its ecological niche (drain the swamps) has proved effective for controlling arboviruses.

The best way to limit virus spread is to immunize the population. Natural infection or vaccination protects the individual and reduces the size of the immunologically naive, susceptible population necessary to continue the spread of the virus.

QUESTIONS

1. List the routes by which a virus gains entry into the body, the barriers to infection at each route, and a virus that infects by that route.
2. Describe or draw the path of a virus that is transmitted by an aerosol and causes lesions on the skin (similar to varicella).
3. Identify the structures that elicit a protective antibody response for adenovirus, influenza A virus, polio virus, and rabies virus.
4. Describe the major roles of each of the following in promoting resolution of a virus infection: interferon, macrophage, natural killer cells, CD4 T cells, CD8 T cells, and antibody.
5. Why are alpha- and beta-interferons produced before gamma-interferon?
6. How does the nucleoprotein of influenza virus become an antigen for cytolytic CD8 T cells?
7. Herpes simplex virus causes primary and recurrent disease. Describe and compare the nature and time course of the immune response to these infections.
8. Describe the immune escape mechanisms used by herpes simplex virus, adenovirus, influenza A virus, hepatitis B virus, and rabies.
9. What events occur during the prodrome periods of a respiratory viral disease (e.g., parainfluenza virus) and encephalitis (e.g., St. Louis encephalitis virus)?
10. List the viral characteristics (structure, replication, target tissue) that would promote transmission by the fecal-oral route, by arthropods, by fomites, in mother's milk, and by sexual activity.
11. Describe the different mechanisms by which oncogenic viruses immortalize cells.

References

Belshe RB: *Textbook of human virology,* ed 2, St. Louis, 1991, Mosby.

Ellner PD, Neu HC: *Understanding infectious disease*, St. Louis, 1992, Mosby.

Emond RTD and Rowland HAK: *Color atlas of infectious diseases*, ed 2, St. Louis, 1987, Mosby.

Gorbach SL, Bartlett, JG, and Blacklow NR: *Infectious diseases*, Philadelphia, 1992, WB Saunders.

Hart CA, Broadhead RL: *Color atlas of pediatric infectious diseases*, St. Louis, 1992, Mosby.

Haukenes G, Haaheim LR, and Pattison JR: *A practical guide to clinical virology*, New York, 1989, John Wiley & Sons.

Krugman S, Katz SL, Gerson AA, and Wilfert CM: *Infectious diseases of children*, ed 9, St. Louis, 1992, Mosby.

Mandell GL, Douglas RG Jr., and Bennett JE: *Principles and practice of infectious disease*, ed 3, New York, 1990, Churchill Livingstone.

Mims CA, White DO: *Viral pathogenesis and immunology*, Oxford, 1984, Blackwell Scientific Publications.

Shulman ST, Phair JP, and Sommers HM: *The biologic and clinical basis of infectious diseases*, ed 4, Philadelphia, 1992, WB Saunders.

White DO, Fenner FJ: *Medical virology*, ed 3, Orlando, Fla, 1986, Academic Press.

CHAPTER 53

Laboratory Diagnosis of Viral Disease

THE first clues for making the diagnosis of a viral infection are obtained from the patient's history and symptoms and by exclusion of other types of infection (e.g., bacterial, fungal). Viral laboratory studies can confirm the diagnosis and identify the viral agent of infection. Identification of a viral agent can direct the choice of appropriate therapy and is useful for defining the disease process, epidemiological monitoring, and educating physicians and patients.

Laboratory confirmation of a viral diagnosis can be made by observation of virus-induced **cytopathological effects (CPE)** on cells, electron microscopic detection of viral particles, isolation and growth of the virus, detection of viral components (e.g., proteins, enzymes, and nucleic acids) or evaluation of the patient's immune response to the virus (**serology**). Virus, viral antigens, or CPE can be detected by cytologic examination of clinical specimens or in tissue culture cells grown and infected in the laboratory (Box 53-1).

CYTOLOGY

Cytologic examination of specimens can provide a rapid initial diagnosis for those viruses that produce a characteristic cytopathologic effect. Characteristic CPE include changes in cell morphology, cell lysis, vacuolation, syncytia formation (Figure 53-1), and presence of inclusion bodies. **Inclusion bodies** are histological changes in cells caused by the presence of viral components, or virus-induced changes in cell structures. **Cowdry Type A** inclusions in single cells or in large **syncytia** (multiple cells fused together) are characteristic for herpes simplex virus (HSV) and varicella-zoster virus (VZV) infections (Figure 53-2). Cytomegalovirus infection is indicated by nuclear, **owl-eye inclusion bodies** in cells of tissues or in urine sediment. Rabies infection may be detected by finding **Negri bodies** (rabies virus inclusions) in brain tissue (Figure 53-3).

BOX 53-1 Laboratory Procedures for Diagnosis of Viral Infections

- Cytologic examination
- Electron microscopy
- Virus isolation and growth
- Detection of viral proteins (antigens and enzymes)
- Detection of viral genetic material
- Serology

ELECTRON MICROSCOPY

Electron microscopy is not a standard clinical laboratory technique, but it can be used to detect and identify some viruses. Sufficient numbers of virus particles must be present to allow detection by electron microscopy. Addition of virus-specific antibody to a sample can facilitate detection and simultaneous identification of virus (**immunoelectron microscopy**) by clumping the viral particles. This approach is useful for enteric viruses, such as rotavirus, which are produced in large quantity

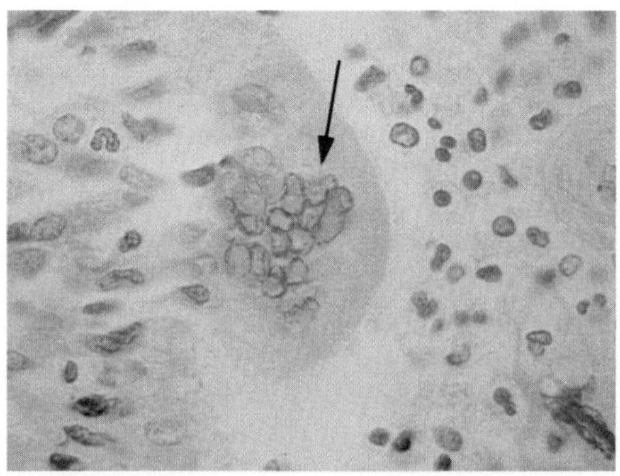

FIGURE 53-1 Syncytium formation by measles virus. Multinucleated giant cell visible in a histological section of lung biopsy from a measles virus–induced giant-cell pneumonia in an immunocompromised child. (From Hart CA, Broadhead RL: *A color atlas of pediatric infectious diseases*, London, 1992, Wolfe.)

and have a characteristic morphology. Appropriately processed tissue from a biopsy or clinical specimen can also be examined for viral structures.

VIRAL ISOLATION AND GROWTH

The "gold standard" for proving the viral etiology of a syndrome is recovery and growth of the agent. The patient's symptoms, travel history, season of the year, and a presumptive diagnosis help in choosing the appropriate procedures for isolating a viral agent (Table 53-1). For example, symptoms of central nervous system disease following parotitis suggest collection of cerebrospinal fluid and urine for the isolation of mumps virus. A focal encephalitis with a temporal lobe–localization preceded by headaches and disorientation suggests herpes simplex virus and the need for biopsy of brain tissue for cytology and viral isolation. Meningitis symptoms during the summer suggest an enterovirus etiology for which cerebrospinal fluid, throat swab, and stool would be appropriate specimens.

The selection of the appropriate specimen for viral culture is often complicated because several viruses may cause the same clinical disease. For example, aseptic meningitis can be caused by many agents, and several types of specimens may be required to identify the causal virus.

Specimens should be collected early in the acute phase of infection before viral shedding ceases. Viral shedding for respiratory viruses may last only 3 to 7 days and lapse before the end of the symptoms. Herpes simplex virus and varicella-zoster virus may not be recoverable from lesions more than 5 days after onset. Isolation of an enterovirus from the cerebrospinal fluid may be possible for only 2 to 3 days after onset of the central nervous system manifestations. In addition, antibody produced in response to the infection may block detection of virus.

The shorter the interval between collection of a specimen and its delivery to the laboratory, the greater the potential for isolating a virus. Many viruses are labile, and the samples are susceptible to bacterial and fungal overgrowth. Viruses are best transported and stored on ice and in special media that contain antibiotics and proteins such as serum albumin or gelatin. Significant losses in infectious titer occur when enveloped viruses (e.g., herpes simplex virus, varicella-zoster virus, influenza virus) are kept at room temperature or frozen at −20° C. This is not observed with nonenveloped viruses (e.g., adenoviruses, enteroviruses).

Virus Growth

Virus can be grown in tissue culture, embryonated eggs, or experimental animals (Box 53-2). Embryonated eggs are still used for the growth of virus for some vaccines but have been replaced by cell cultures for routine virus isolation in clinical laboratories. Experimental animals are rarely used in clinical laboratories.

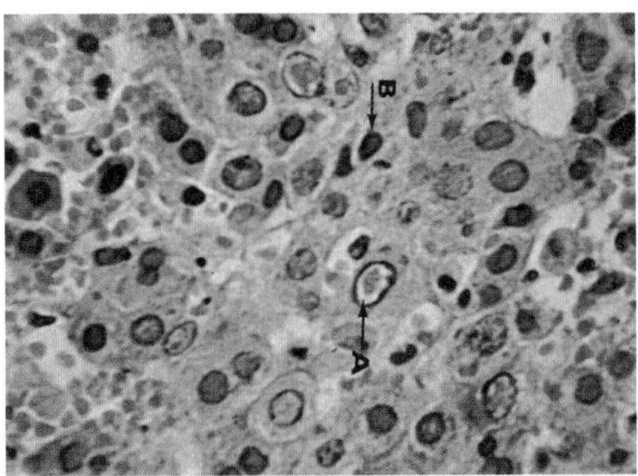

FIGURE 53-2 Herpes simplex virus–induced cytopathological effects. **A,** A biopsy of an HSV-infected liver shows an eosinophilic Cowdry Type A intranuclear inclusion body surrounded by a halo and a ring of marginated chromatin at the nuclear membrane. **B,** An infected cell exhibits a smaller condensed nucleus (pyknotic). (From Emond RTD, Rowland HAK: *A color atlas of infectious diseases,* ed 2, London, 1987, Wolfe.)

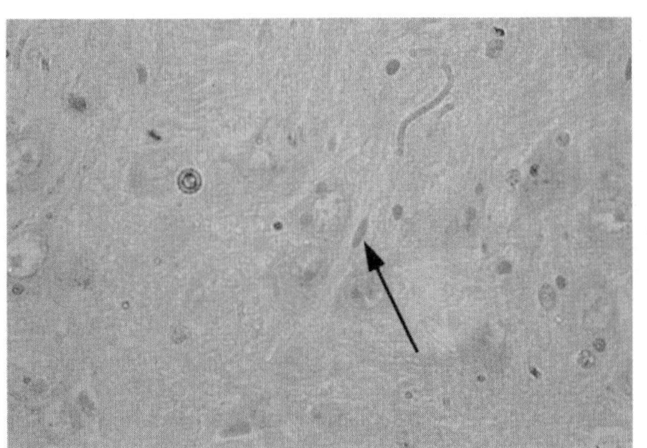

A

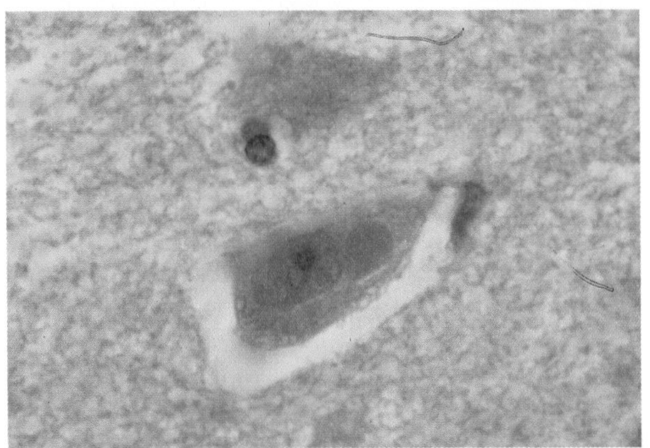

B

FIGURE 53-3 Negri bodies caused by rabies. **A,** A section of brain from a patient with rabies demonstrates Negri bodies. **B,** Higher magnification from another biopsy. (*A,* From Hart CA, Broadhead RL: *A color atlas of pediatric infectious diseases,* London, 1992, Wolfe.)

TABLE 53-1 Specimens for Viral Diagnosis

Common pathogenic viruses	Specimens for culture	Comments
RESPIRATORY		
Adenovirus, influenza, enterovirus (picornavirus)*, rhinovirus, paramyxovirus†, rubella virus, herpes simplex virus	Nasal washing, throat swab, nasal swab, sputum	Virus is also shed in stool*; measles and mumps may also be in urine†
GASTROINTESTINAL		
Reovirus, rotavirus, adenovirus, Norwalk virus, and calicivirus	Stool, rectal swab	Samples are analyzed by electron microscopy and antigen detection; viruses are not cultured
MACULOPAPULAR RASH		
Adenovirus, enterovirus (picornavirus)	Throat swab and rectal swab	
Rubella virus and measles virus		
VESICULAR RASH		
Coxsackievirus, echovirus, herpes simplex virus, and varicella-zoster virus	Vesicle fluid, scraping or swab	Initial diagnosis of HSV and VZV can be obtained from vesicle scraping (Tzanck smear)
CENTRAL NERVOUS SYSTEM (ASEPTIC MENINGITIS, ENCEPHALITIS)		
Enterovirus (picornavirus)	Stool	
Arboviruses (togaviruses, bunyaviruses, etc.)	Viruses rarely cultured	Diagnosis by serologic test
Rabies virus	Tissue, saliva, brain biopsy	Diagnosis by immunofluorescence analysis for antigen
Herpes simplex virus, cytomegalovirus, mumps virus, measles virus	Cerebrospinal fluid, brain biopsy	Virus isolation and immunofluorescence analysis for antigen
URINARY		
Adenovirus, cytomegalovirus	Urine	Cytomegalovirus may be shed without apparent disease
EYE		
Adenovirus, herpes simplex virus, enterovirus (picornavirus)	Conjunctival swab or scraping, throat swab	

Data from Cherneskey MA, Ray CG, Smith TF: *Laboratory diagnosis of viral infections*, Washington, DC, 1982, Cumitech 15. American Society of Microbiology; and Hsiung GD: *Diagnostic virology*, New Haven, 1982, Yale University Press.

Cell Culture

Different types of tissue culture cells are used for virus growth. **Primary cell cultures** are obtained by dissociating specific animal organs with trypsin or collagenase. The cells are grown as monolayers (fibroblast or epithelial) or in suspension (lymphocyte) in artificial media supplemented with bovine serum or another source of growth factors. Primary cells can be dissociated with trypsin and passed or transferred to become **secondary cell cultures**. **Diploid cell strains** are cultures of a single cell type capable of being passed a large but finite number of times before they will senesce or undergo a significant change in their characteristics. Tumor cells and cells immortalized by viruses or chemicals can be grown as **cell lines** and consist of a single cell type that can be passed continuously without senescing.

Primary monkey kidney cells are excellent for recovery of myxoviruses, paramyxoviruses, many enteroviruses, and some adenoviruses. Human fetal diploid cells, generally fibroblastic cells, support the growth of a broad spectrum of viruses (e.g., herpes simplex virus, varicella-zoster virus, adenoviruses, picornaviruses) and are the only cells in which cytomegalovirus is recovered. HEp-2 cells, a continuous line of epithelial cells derived from a human cancer, are particularly excellent for recovering respiratory syncytial virus, adenoviruses, and herpes simplex virus. Many clinically significant viruses can be recovered in at least one of these cell cultures.

Virus Detection

Detection and initial identification of the virus can be made by observation of the virus-induced CPE in the cell monolayer (Box 53-3 and Figure 53-4). A single virus may cause a focus of cytopathology (**plaque**). The type of cell culture, the characteristics of the CPE, and the rapidity of viral growth can be used for an initial identification of many clinically important viruses. This approach for identifying viruses is similar to bacterial identification based on growth and morphology of colonies on selective differential media.

Some viruses grow slowly or not at all or do not readily cause CPE in cell lines typically used in clinical virology laboratories. Specimens submitted for the isolation of viruses such as human immunodeficiency virus, coxsackie A virus, and togaviruses require, respectively, co-cultivation with normal human peripheral blood mononuclear cells, inoculation of suckling mice, or the use of special cell cultures, which are not available except in highly specialized virology laboratories. These viruses are most frequently diagnosed serologically or by detection of viral genomes or antigens.

Characteristic viral properties can also be used to identify viruses that do not cause classic CPE. Rubella virus infection may not cause CPE but will prevent (interfere with) the replication of picornaviruses in a process known as **heterologous interference**. Influenza virus, parainfluenza virus, mumps virus, and togavirus infected cells express a viral glycoprotein (hemagglutinin) that binds erythrocytes of defined animal species to the infected cell surface **(hemadsorption)** (Figure 53-5). Virus released into the cell culture medium can be detected by agglutination of erythrocytes, a process termed **hemagglutination.**

The amount of virus can be quantitated by the titer of virus that causes cytopathology in tissue culture (tissue culture dose: $\mathbf{TCD_{50}}$), kills 50% of a set of test animals (lethal dose: $\mathbf{LD_{50}}$), or initiates a detectable symptom,

BOX 53-2 Systems for Propagation of Viruses

People
Animals
- Cows (e.g., Jenner's cowpox vaccine), chickens, mice, rats, suckling mice, etc.

Embryonated eggs
Organ and tissue culture
- Organ culture
- Primary tissue culture
- Cell lines: diploid
- Tumor or immortalized cell lines

BOX 53-3 Viral Cytopathologic Effects

Cell death
- Cell rounding
- Degeneration
- Aggregation
- Loss of attachment to substratum

Characteristic histological changes: inclusion bodies in the nucleus or cytoplasm, margination of chromatin
Syncytia: multinucleated giant cells caused by virus-induced cell-cell fusion.
Cell surface changes
- Viral antigen expression
- Hemadsorption (hemagglutinin expression)

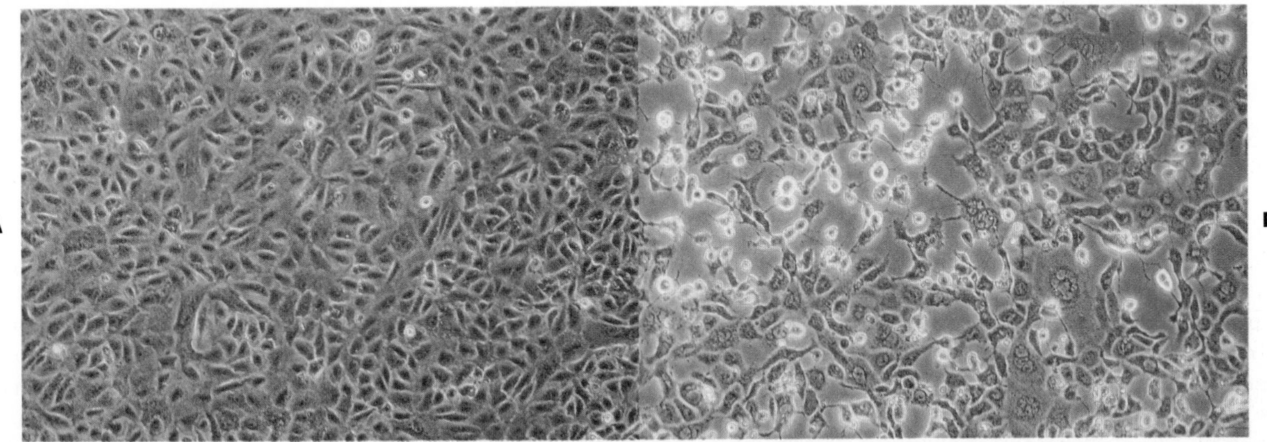

FIGURE 53-4 Cytopathological effects of herpes simplex virus infection. **A,** Uninfected Vero cells, an African green monkey kidney cell line. **B,** HSV-1-infected Vero cells showing rounded cells, multinucleated cells, and loss of the monolayer.

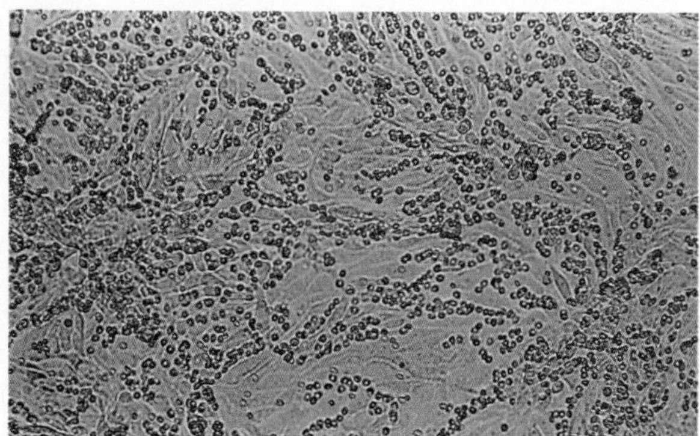

FIGURE 53-5 Hemadsorption of erythrocytes to influenza-infected cells. Influenza, mumps, and parainfluenza viruses and many togaviruses express a hemagglutinin that will bind erythrocytes of selected animal species.

BOX 53-4	Assays for Viral Proteins and Nucleic Acids

PROTEIN

Protein patterns (electrophoresis)
Enzyme activities
Antigen detection (IF, ELISA, western blot, etc.)

NUCLEIC ACIDS

Restriction endonuclease cleavage patterns
Electrophoretic mobilities of RNA for segmented RNA viruses (electrophoresis)
DNA genome hybridization in situ (cytochemistry)
Southern, Northern, and dot blots
Polymerase chain reaction (PCR)

antibody, or other response in 50% of a set of test animals (infectious dose: $\mathbf{ID_{50}}$). The number of infectious viruses can also be evaluated by a count of the plaques produced by tenfold dilutions of sample (**plaque forming units [pfu]**). The ratio of viral particles to pfu is always greater than 1 because a large number of defective viral particles are produced during virus replication.

Interpretation of Culture Results

In general the detection of any virus in host tissues, cerebrospinal fluid, blood, or vesicular fluid can be considered highly significant. However, virus shedding may be induced by an underlying condition (e.g., another infection, immune suppression, or stress) and unrelated to the disease symptoms. Certain viruses can be intermittently shed without symptoms for periods ranging from weeks (enteroviruses in feces) to many months or years (herpes simplex virus or cytomegalovirus in the oropharynx and vagina; adenoviruses in the oropharynx and intestinal tract). Failure to isolate a virus when a viral infection is present is usually due to problems with the clinical sample (e.g., improper handling, the time the sample is taken, or presence of neutralizing antibody).

DETECTION OF VIRAL PROTEINS

Viral replication produces enzymes and other proteins that can be detected by biochemical, immunological, and molecular biological means (Box 53-4). The viral proteins can be separated by electrophoresis and their patterns used to identify and distinguish different viruses. For example, electrophoretically separated herpes simplex virus–infected cell proteins and virion proteins have different patterns for different types and strains of HSV-1 and HSV-2.

Detection and assay of characteristic enzymes can identify and quantitate specific viruses. For example, the presence of reverse transcriptase in serum or cell culture indicates the presence of a retrovirus.

Antibodies can be used as sensitive and specific tools to detect, identify, and quantitate the presence of virus and viral antigen in clinical specimens or cell culture **(immunohistochemistry)**. Antigen is detected with antiviral antibodies that have been covalently modified with fluorescent, enzymatic, or radioactive labels. Antiviral antibodies may be obtained from convalescent patients or may be prepared in animals. Monoclonal antibodies are also available that can recognize individual epitopes on viral antigens. Monoclonal antibodies have the specificity to distinguish viral mutants and strains that differ in these proteins.

Viral antigens on the cell surface or within the cell can be detected by **immunofluorescence** and **enzyme immunoassay (EIA)**. Direct immunofluorescence (DFA) uses a fluorescent primary antiviral antibody (e.g., fluorescein isothiocyanate labeled rabbit antiviral antibody), whereas indirect immunofluorescence (IFA) uses a fluorescent second antibody (e.g., fluorescein isothiocyanate labeled goat antirabbit [FITC-GAR] antibody to recognize the primary antiviral antibody and to locate the antigen (Figure 53-6 and Figure 53-7). For EIA, an enzyme such as horseradish peroxidase or alkaline phosphatase is conjugated to the antibody and converts a substrate into a chromophore to mark the antigen. Virus or antigen released from infected cells can be detected by **enzyme linked immunosorbentassay (ELISA), radioimmunoassay (RIA),** and **latex agglutination (LA)** (see section on Serology).

Cytomegalovirus detection can be enhanced by using a combination of cell culture and immunological methods. The clinical sample is centrifuged onto cells grown on a coverslip or the bottom of a shell vial. This increases the efficiency and accelerates the process of virus entry into the cells on the coverslip. The cells can then be analyzed by IF or EIA for early viral antigens, which are detectable within 24 hours instead of after 7 to 14 days for CPE.

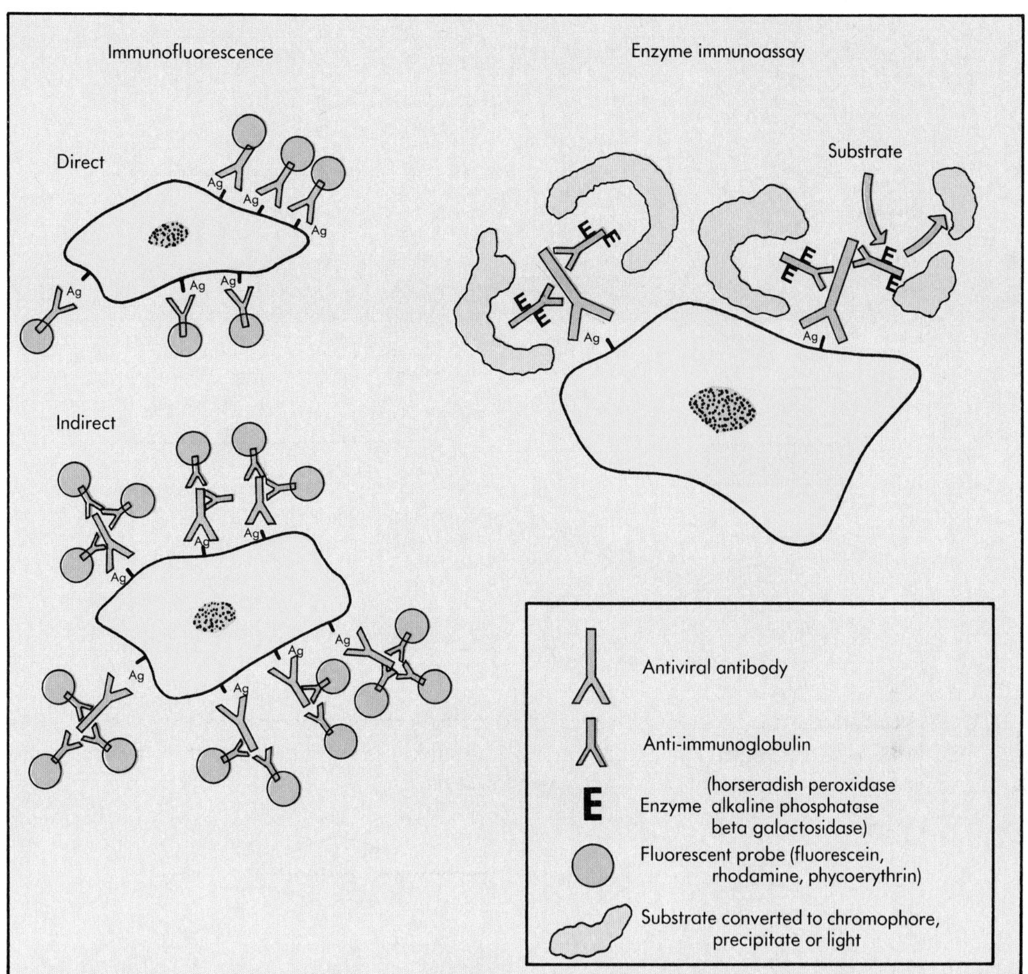

FIGURE 53-6 Immunofluorescence and enzyme immunoassays (EIA) for antigen localization in cells. Antigen can be detected by **direct** assay with antiviral antibody modified covalently with a fluorescent or enzyme probe or by **indirect** assay using antiviral antibody and chemically modified anti-immunoglobulin. The enzyme converts substrate to a precipitate, chromophore or light.

DETECTION OF VIRAL GENETIC MATERIAL

The genome structure and genetic sequence is a major distinguishing characteristic of the family, type, and strain of virus (see Box 53-4). Electrophoretic separation of RNA genome segments (influenza and reoviruses) or restriction endonuclease cleavage products of DNA virus genomes distinguish different types and strains of virus. The patterns of RNA or DNA are like genetic fingerprints for these viruses. Different strains of herpes simplex virus types 1 and 2 can also be distinguished in this manner.

DNA probes with sequences complementary to specific regions of a viral genome can be used to detect, locate, and quantitate viral nucleic acids in clinical specimens (Figure 53-8). DNA probes can be used like antibodies as sensitive and specific tools for detecting the presence of virus. However, DNA probes can detect the virus even in the absence of virus replication. DNA probe analysis is especially useful for slowly replicating or

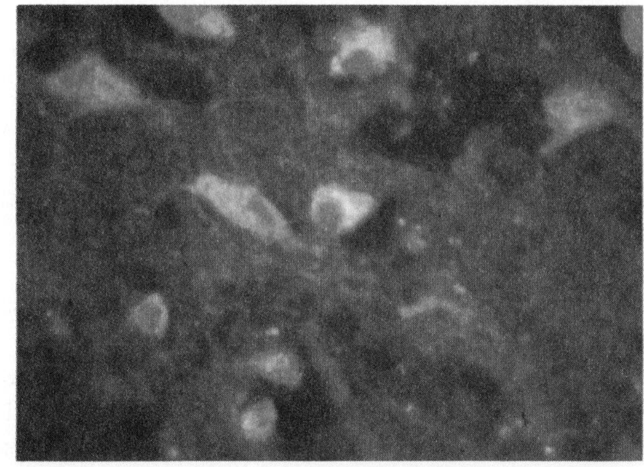

FIGURE 53-7 Immunofluorescence localization of herpes simplex virus–infected nerve cells in a brain section from a case of herpes encephalitis. (From Emond RTD, Rowland HAK: *A color atlas of infectious diseases*, ed 2, London, 1987, Wolfe.)

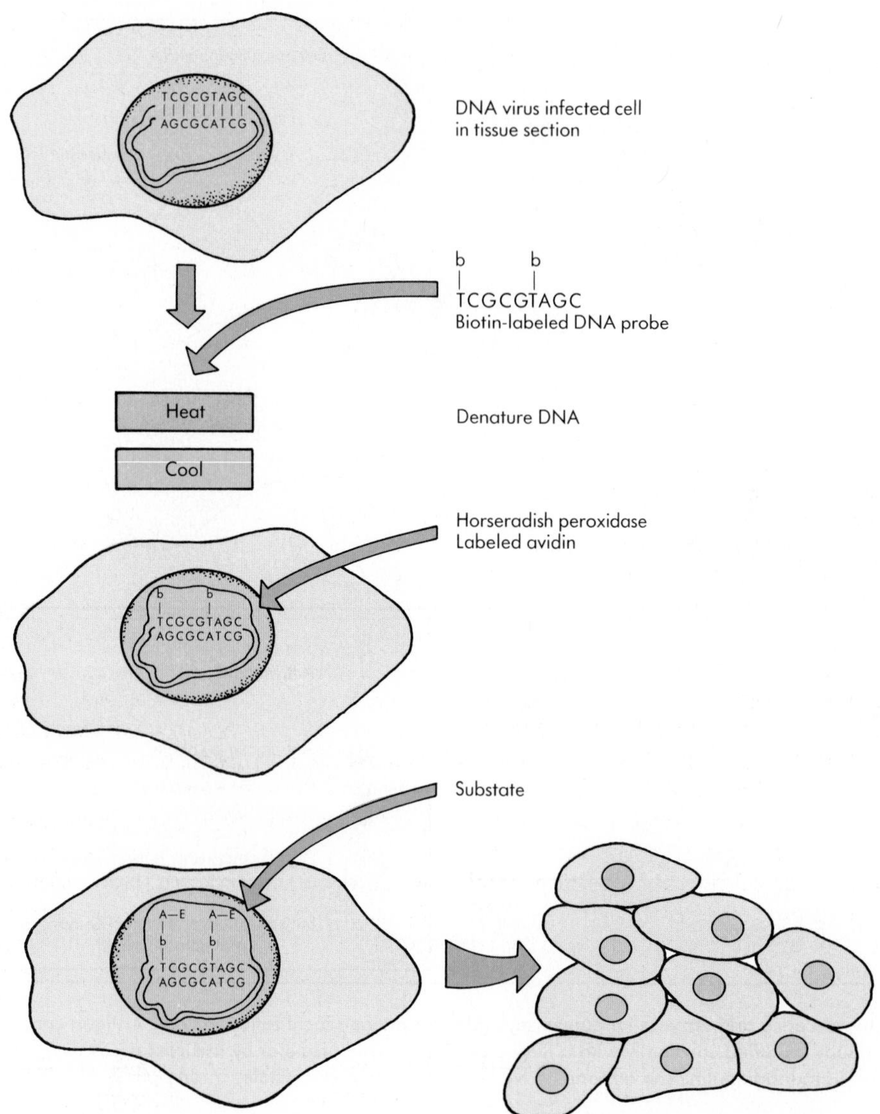

FIGURE 53-8 DNA probe analysis of virus-infected cells. Virus-infected cells can be localized in histologically prepared tissue sections using DNA probes as small as 9 nucleotides or bacterial plasmids containing the viral gene. A tagged DNA probe is added to the sample. In this case the DNA probe is labeled with biotin-modified thymidine, but radioactivity can also be used. The sample is heated to denature the DNA and cooled to allow the probe to hybridize to the complementary sequence. Enzyme-labeled avidin is added to bind to the biotin on the probe. Addition of the appropriate substrate will color the nuclei of virally infected cells.

nonproductive virus infections such as cytomegalovirus and human papillomavirus.

DNA probes are chemically synthesized or are obtained by cloning fragments or an entire viral genome into bacterial vectors (plasmids, cosmids). DNA copies of RNA viruses are made with the retrovirus reverse transcriptase and then cloned into vectors. The DNA probes are labeled with radioactive or chemically modified nucleotides (e.g., biotinylated uridine, bromodeoxyuridine) to allow their detection and quantitation.

The DNA probes can detect specific viral genetic sequences in fixed, permeabilized tissue biopsies by **in situ hybridization**. Viral nucleic acids in extracts from a clinical sample can be detected by fixing a small volume of the extract onto a nitrocellulose filter (**dot blot**) and then probing the filter with labeled, specific viral DNA. Alternatively, viral DNA or restriction endonuclease cleavage products of viral DNA can be separated electrophoretically, transferred onto a nitrocellulose filter (**Southern blot**—DNA:DNA probe hybridization), and then identified by their characteristic electrophoretic mobility and by hybridization with a specific genetic probe. Electrophoretically separated viral RNA (**Northern blot**—RNA:DNA probe hybridization) blotted onto a nitrocellulose filter can be detected in a similar manner.

Hybridization of the probe to the viral nucleic acids is detected by autoradiography, fluorescent, or EIA-like methods. For example, a biotin-labeled DNA probe can

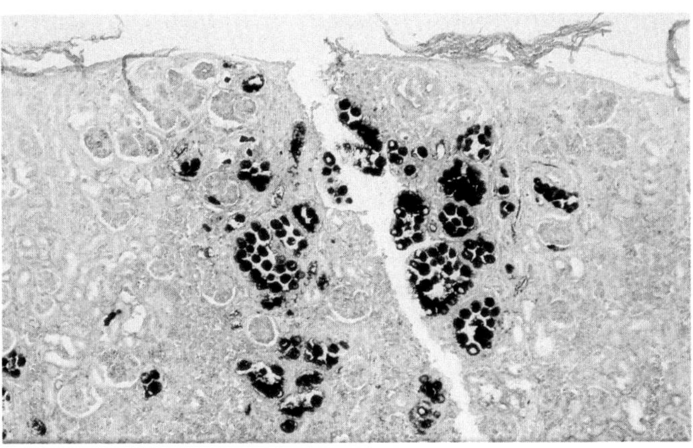

FIGURE 53-9 In situ localization of cytomegalovirus infection using a genetic probe. CMV infection of the renal tubules of a kidney is localized with a biotin-labeled, CMV-specific DNA probe and visualized with horseradish peroxidase–conjugated avidin conversion of substrate in a manner similar to enzyme immunoassay. (Courtesy Donna Zabel, Akron Children's Hospital Medical Center.)

be used with fluorescent- or enzyme- (horseradish peroxidase) labeled avidin (a protein that binds tightly to biotin) to detect viral nucleic acids in a cell in a manner similar to indirect immunofluorescence or EIA localization of antigen. Many viral probes and kits for detecting viruses are now commercially available. This approach is useful for detecting and locating viral genomes in patient samples even in the absence of CPE or significant amounts of viral antigen, and for studying the expression of specific viral genes in different cell types (Figure 53-9).

The **polymerase chain reaction (PCR)** can detect single copies of viral DNA and is one of the newest genetic analysis techniques (Figure 53-10). A sample is incubated with two short DNA oligomers that are complementary to the ends of a known genetic sequence of the viral DNA, a heat-stable DNA polymerase, nucleotides, and buffers. The oligomers hybridize to the viral DNA and act as primers for the polymerase, which copies a segment of the DNA. The sample is heated to denature the DNA (separating the strands of the double helix) and cooled to allow hybridization of primers to the new DNA. Each copy of DNA becomes a new template. The process is repeated many (20 to 40) times to amplify the original DNA sequence in an exponential manner. A millionfold amplification of a target sequence can be accomplished in a few hours. This technique is especially useful for detecting latent and integrated virus sequences, such as for retroviruses, herpesviruses, papillomaviruses and other papovaviruses.

VIRAL SEROLOGY

The humoral immune response provides a history of a patient's infections. Serology can be used to identify the virus and its strain or serotype, evaluate the course of an infection, or determine if it is a primary or a reinfection and if acute or chronic. Serologic data on a virus infection are provided by the antibody type and titer and the identity of the antigenic targets. Serologic diagnosis is used for viruses that are difficult to isolate and grow in cell culture and viruses with a slower course of disease (Box 53-5).

The relative antibody concentration is reported as a **titer.** A titer is the inverse of the greatest dilution (lowest concentration) (e.g., dilution of 1:64 = titer of 64) of patient serum that retains activity (e.g., binds to viral antigen, inhibits a specific viral activity, or competes with and blocks the binding and detection of a radioactive or otherwise labeled antibody).

Production of antibody in response to a primary infection results in **seroconversion**. Detection of virus-specific IgM antibody generally indicates recent primary infection and is present during the first 2 to 3 weeks of a primary infection. Seroconversion is indicated by a *fourfold or greater increase in antibody titer* between serum taken during the **acute phase** of disease and that taken at least 2 to 3 weeks later during the **convalescent phase**. Reinfection or recurrence later in life causes an anamnestic (secondary or booster) response. Antibody titers may remain high for frequent recurrent disease (e.g., herpesviruses).

A fourfold increase in antibody titer between acute and convalescent sera is required to indicate seroconversion because of the inherent imprecision of serologic assays based on twofold serial dilutions. For example, samples with 512 units and 1023 units of antibody would both give a signal upon a 512-fold dilution but not a 1024-fold dilution and would be reported as 512. Samples with 1020 units and 1030 units are not significantly different but would be reported as titers of 512 and 1024, respectively.

The course of a chronic infection can also be determined by a **serologic profile**. The presence and titers of antibody to several key viral antigens can describe the stage of disease for certain viruses. This is especially useful for viruses with a slower course of disease (e.g., hepatitis B and Epstein-Barr virus infectious mononucleosis). In general, the first antibodies to be detected are directed against antigens most available to the immune system (e.g., on the virion or infected-cell surfaces). Later in the infection, when cells have been lysed by the infecting virus or the cellular immune response, antibodies directed against the intracellular viral proteins and enzymes are detected. For example, antibodies to the envelope and capsid antigens of Epstein-Barr virus are detected first. Then during convalesence, antibodies are detected to nuclear antigens, such as the Epstein-Barr virus nuclear antigen (EBNA).

A serologic **battery** or **panel** consisting of assays for several viruses may be used for the diagnosis of certain disease syndromes. Local epidemiological factors, time of year, patient factors (immunocompetency), travel history, and patient age influence the choice of virus assays to be

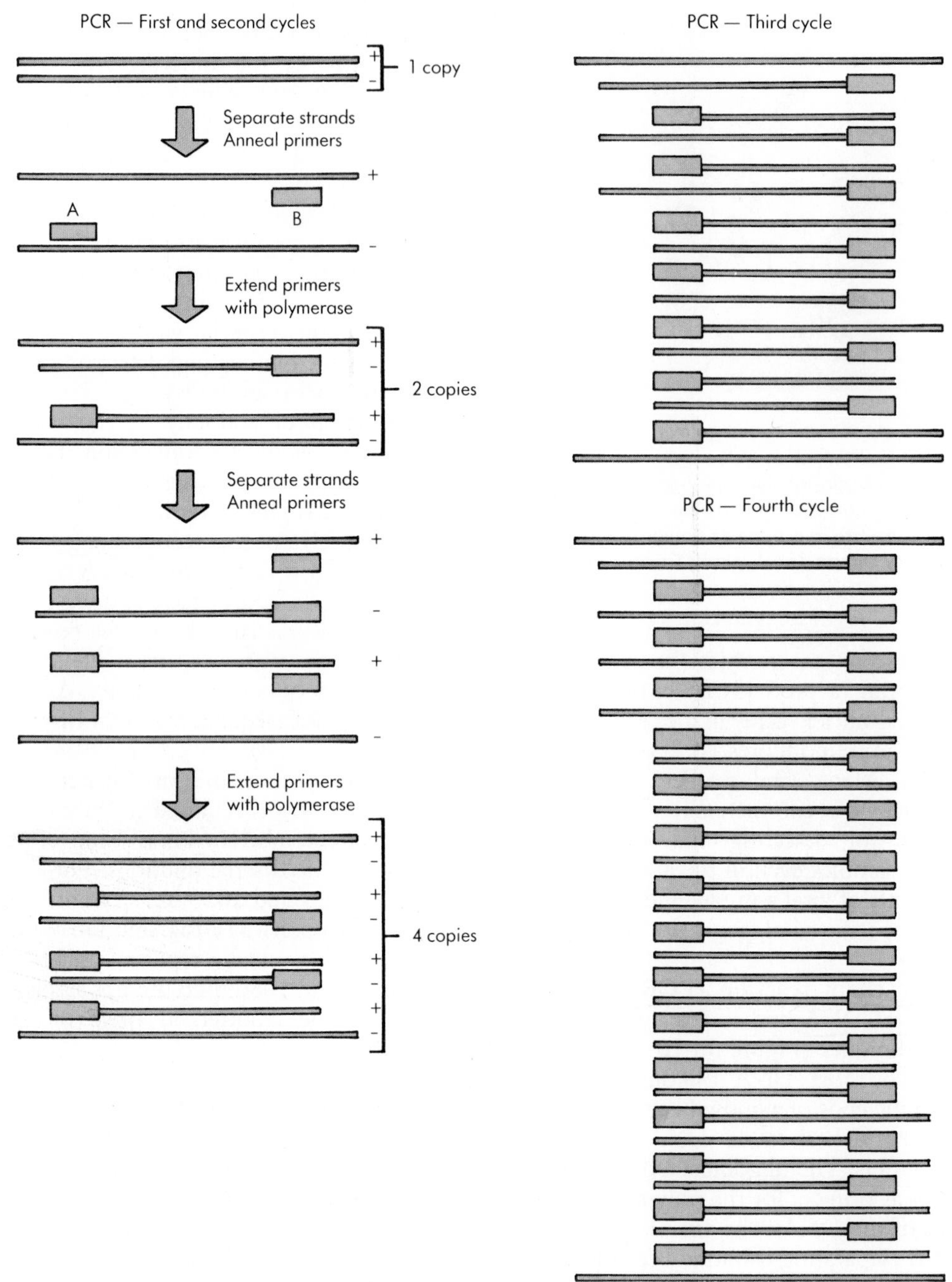

FIGURE 53-10 Polymerase chain reaction (PCR). The polymerase chain reaction is a rapid means of amplifying a known sequence of DNA. A sample is mixed with a heat-stable DNA polymerase, excess deoxyribonucleotide triphosphates, and two DNA oligomers (primers), which complement the ends of the target sequence to be amplified. The mixture is heated to denature the DNA and then cooled to allow binding of the primers to the target DNA and extension of the primers by the polymerase. The cycle is repeated 20 to 30 times. After the first cycle, only the sequence bracketed by the primers will be amplified. (Modified from Blair GE, Blair Zajdel ME: *Biochem Educ* 20:87-90, 1992.)

included on a panel. For example, herpes simplex virus, mumps, western equine encephalitis, eastern equine encephalitis, St. Louis encephalitis, and California encephalitis viruses may be included in a panel of tests for central nervous system diseases.

Serologic Test Methods

Complement fixation is a standard but technically difficult serologic test (Box 53-6). The patient's serum sample is reacted with lab-derived antigen and extra complement. Antibody-antigen complexes will activate

BOX 53-5 Viruses Diagnosed by Serology*

Epstein-Barr virus
Rubella virus
Hepatitis A, B, C, D, E
Human immunodeficiency virus
Arboviruses (encephalitis viruses)

*Serology is also used to determine the immune status for other viruses.

BOX 53-6 Serologic Assays

Complement fixation
Hemagglutination inhibition (HI)*
Neutralization*
Immunofluorescence (direct and indirect)
Latex agglutination
In situ enzyme immunoassay (EIA)
Enzyme linked immunosorbent assay (ELISA)
Radioimmunoassay (RIA)

*For detection of antibody and not antigen.

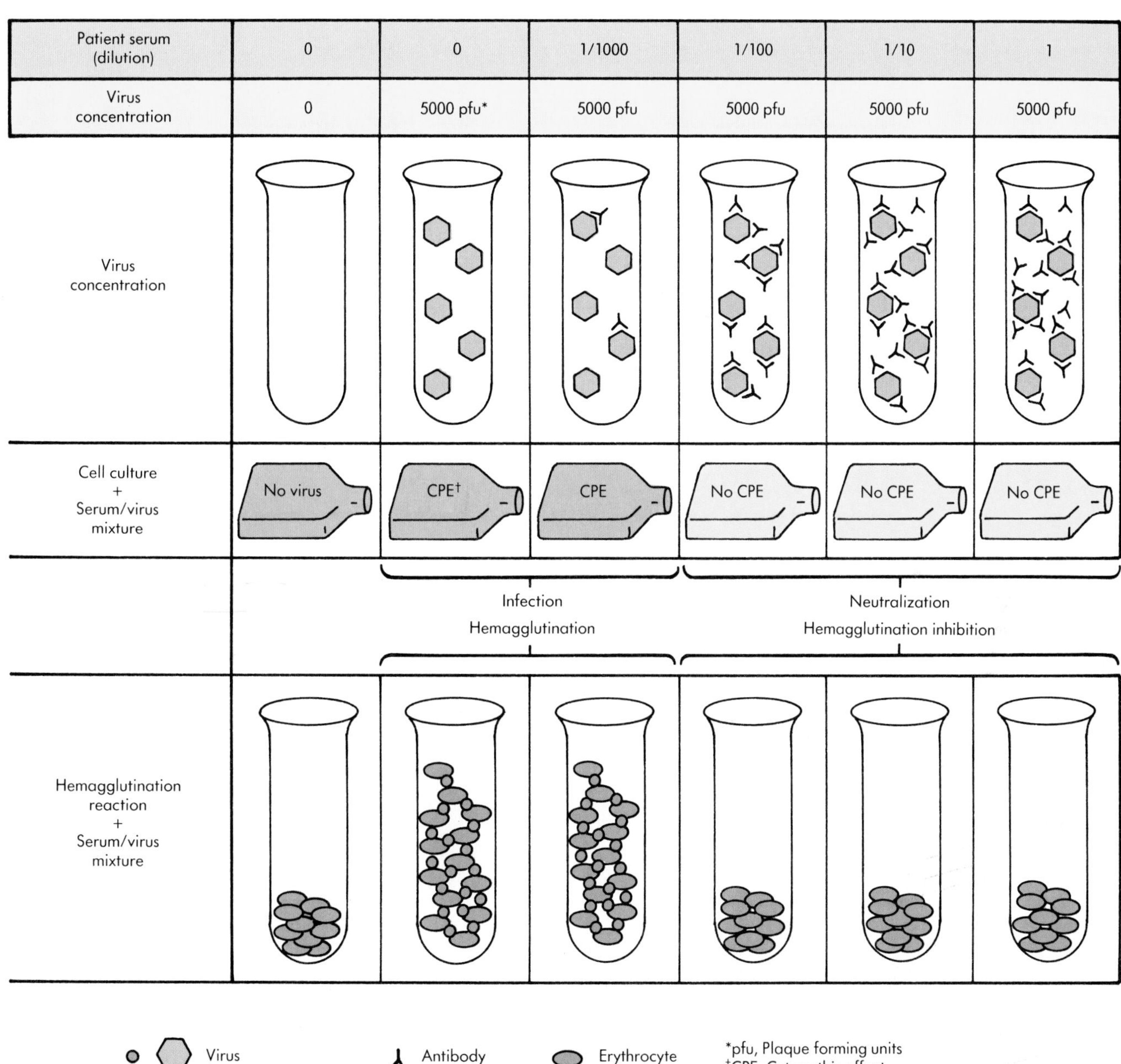

FIGURE 53-11 Neutralization, hemagglutination, and hemagglutination inhibition assays. In the assay shown, tenfold dilutions of serum were incubated with virus. Aliquots of the mixture were then added to either cell cultures or erythrocytes. In the absence of antibody, the virus infected the monolayer (indicated by CPE) and caused hemagglutination (formed a gel-like suspension of erythrocytes). In the presence of the antibody, infection was blocked (neutralization) and hemagglutination was inhibited (HI), allowing the erythrocytes to pellet. The titer of antibody in the serum was 100.

and fix (use up) the complement. The residual complement is assayed by lysis of red blood cells coated with antibody. Antibodies measured by this system generally develop slightly later in the course of an illness than those measured by other techniques.

Neutralization and **hemagglutination inhibition (HI)** are tests that assay antibody recognition and binding to virus. Antibody coating of the virus blocks its binding to indicator cells (Figure 53-11). For neutralization, antibody inhibits infection and cytopathology in tissue culture cells. A neutralization antibody response is virus-type specific and often develops with the onset of symptoms and persists for long periods. HI is used for those viruses that can selectively agglutinate erythrocytes of various animal species (e.g., chicken, guinea pig, human). Antibody present in serum will prevent a standardized amount of virus from binding to and agglutinating erythrocytes.

The indirect fluorescent antibody test and solid phase immunoassays (SPIA) such as latex agglutination (LA),

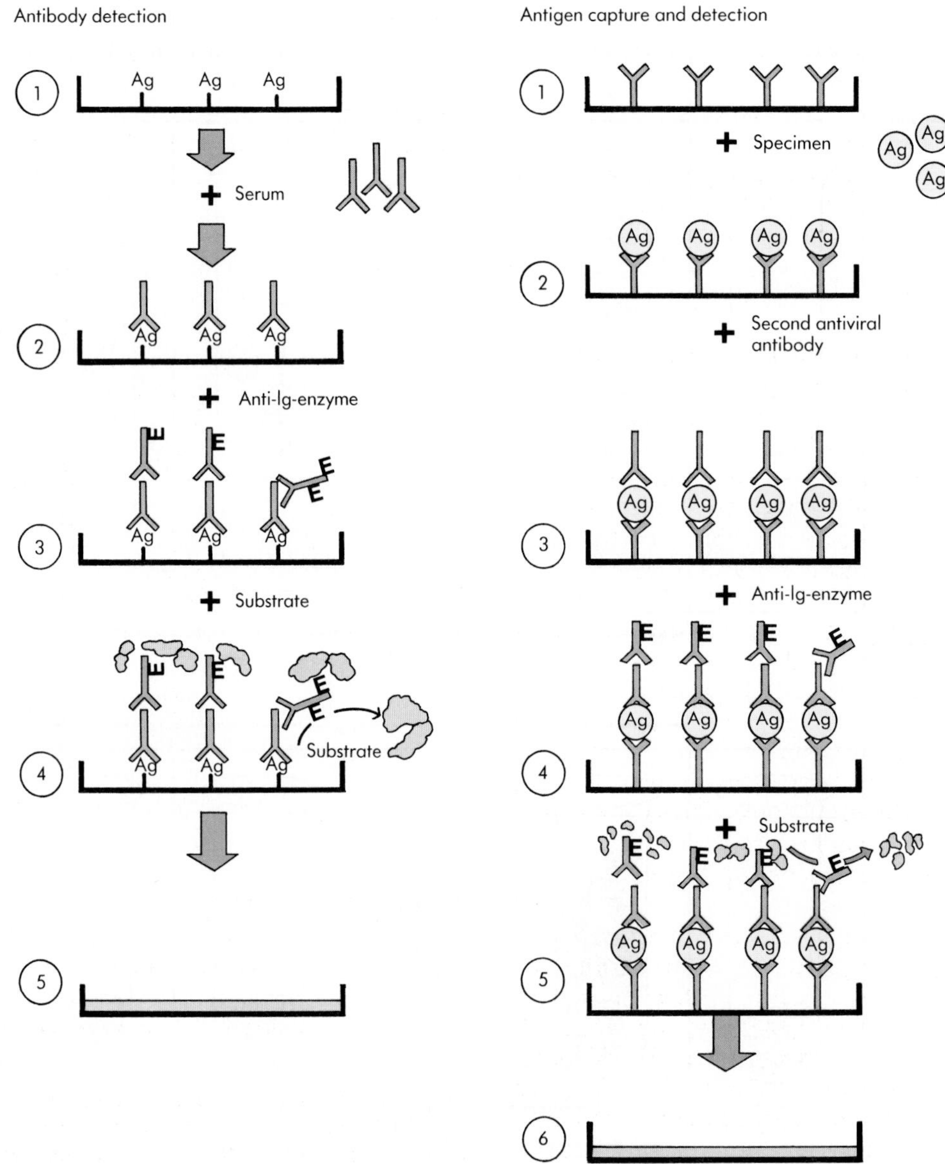

FIGURE 53-12 Enzyme immunoassays for quantitation of antibody or antigen. Antibody detection: *1,* Viral antigen, obtained from infected cells, virions, or genetic engineering, is affixed to a surface. *2,* Patient serum is added and allowed to bind to the antigen. Unbound antibody is washed away. *3,* Enzyme-conjugated antihuman antibody is added, and unbound antibody is washed away. *4,* Substrate is added and *5,* converted into chromophore, precipitate, or light. Antigen capture and detection: *1,* Antiviral antibody is affixed to a surface. *2,* Specimen containing antigen is added, and unbound antigen is washed away. *3,* A second, antiviral antibody is added to detect the captured antigen. *4,* Enzyme-conjugated anti-antibody is added, washed, and followed by *5,* substrate, which is, *6,* converted into chromophore, precipitate, or light.

enzyme linked immunosorbent test (ELISA), and radioimmunoassay (RIA) are used to detect and quantitate specific antibody-virus antigen immune complexes. In these assays virus-specific antibody is separated from other antibodies in patient serum by binding to an immobilized antigen or by precipitation of the appropriate immune complexes. The patient's IgG or IgM can then be detected using a second antihuman antibody that has been chemically modified with a fluorescent, radioactive, or enzyme probe.

The **indirect fluorescent antibody** test (see Figures 53-6 and 53-7) can be used to detect virus-specific antibody in the patient's serum using virus-infected cells fixed onto wells of a microscope slide. The titer of this antibody is the reciprocal of the highest dilution that still exhibits fluorescent staining.

Latex agglutination (LA) is a rapid, technically simple assay for determination of antibody or soluble antigen. Virus-specific antibody causes clumping of latex particles coated with viral antigens. Conversely, antibody-coated latex particles are used to detect soluble viral antigen. **Passive hemagglutination** utilizes antigen-modified erythrocytes as indicators instead of latex particles.

The **enzyme linked immunosorbent assay (ELISA)** uses antigen immobilized on a plastic surface, bead, or filter to capture and separate the virus-specific antibody from other antibodies in a patient's serum (Figure 53-12). The affixed patient antibody is then detected by an antihuman antibody with a covalently linked enzyme (e.g., horseradish peroxidase, alkaline phosphatase or beta-galactosidase). It is quantitated spectrophotometrically by the intensity of color produced on enzyme conversion of an appropriate substrate. The many variations of ELISA assays differ in their means of antibody or antigen capture or detection. An example of a commonly used ELISA test is the home pregnancy test for human choriogonadotrophin hormone.

ELISA assays can also be used to quantitate soluble antigen in a patient sample. Soluble antigen is captured and concentrated by immobilized antibody and then detected with a different antibody labeled with the enzyme.

Western blot analysis is a newer variation of an ELISA. Viral proteins separated by electrophoresis according to their molecular weight or charge are transferred (blotted) onto a filter paper (e.g., nitrocellulose, nylon). When exposed to patient's serum, the immobilized proteins capture virus-specific antibody and are visualized with an enzyme-conjugated antihuman antibody. Western blot analysis is used to confirm ELISA results for human immunodeficiency virus infection (Figure 53-13).

Radioimmunoassay uses radiolabeled (e.g., ^{125}I) antibody or antigen to quantitate antigen-antibody complexes. RIA can be performed as a capture assay, as described previously for ELISA, or a competition assay. In a competition assay, antibody in a patient's serum is quantitated by its ability to compete with and replace a laboratory-prepared radiolabeled antibody from antigen-antibody complexes. The antigen-antibody complexes are precipitated and separated from free antibody, and the radioactivity is measured for both fractions. The amount of patient antibody is then quantitated from standard curves prepared using known quantities of competing antibody.

Limitations to the Use of Serology

There are limitations to the use and interpretation of serology. The presence of antiviral antibody indicates previous infection but is not sufficient to indicate when the infection occurred. Virus-specific IgM, a fourfold increase in titer between acute and convalescent serum or specific antibody profiles, will indicate recent infection. False-positive or false-negative tests may confuse t ie diagnosis. Interfering antibody may be present, ; d

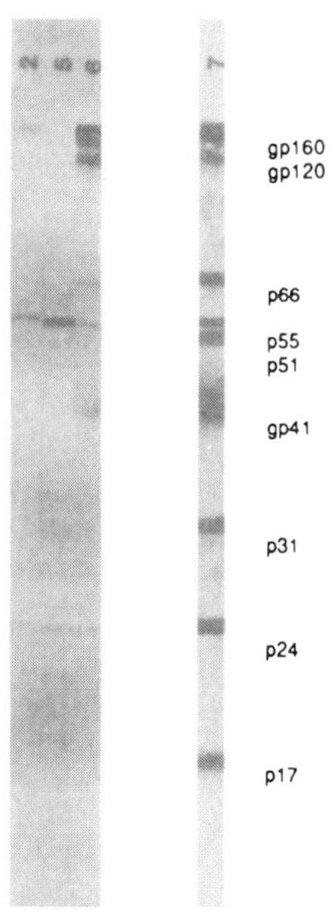

Strip	Interpretation	Bands Present
2	INDETERMINATE	p24, p55, gp160
5	INDETERMINATE	p24, p55
6	INDETERMINATE	p24, gp41, p55, p66, gp120, gp160
7	POSITIVE	p17, p24, p31, gp41, p51, p55, p66, gp120, gp160

FIGURE 53-13 Western blot analysis of human immunodeficiency virus (HIV) antigens and antibody. HIV protein antigens are separated by electrophoresis and blotted onto nitrocellulose paper strips. The strip is incubated with patient antibody, washed to remove unbound antibody, and then reacted with enzyme conjugated antihuman antibody and chromophoric substrate. Serum from an HIV-infected individual will bind and identify the major antigenic proteins of HIV. Of the four sera shown, only serum 7 recognizes all the antigens and is definitively positive. (From Belshe RB, editor: *Textbook of human virology*, ed 2, St. Louis, 1991, Mosby.)

serologic cross-reactions between different viruses may confuse the identity of the infecting agent (e.g., parainfluenza and mumps express related antigens). Conversely, the antibody used in the assay may be too specific and may not recognize other viruses from the same family, giving a false-negative result (e.g., rhinovirus). A good understanding of the clinical symptoms and a knowledge of the limitations and potential problems with serologic assays will aid in making the diagnosis.

QUESTIONS

1. Brain tissue was obtained at autopsy from an individual who died of rabies. What procedures could be used to confirm the presence of rabies virus–infected cells in the brain tissue?
2. A cervical Pap smear was taken from a woman with a vaginal papilloma (wart). Certain types of papilloma have been associated with cervical carcinoma. What method(s) would be appropriate to detect and identify the type of papilloma in the cervical smear?
3. A legal case would be settled by identification of the source of an HSV infection. Serum and viral isolates were obtained from the individual and two contacts. What methods could be used to determine whether the individual was infected with HSV-1 or HSV-2? What methods could be used to allow comparison of the type and strain of HSV obtained from all three individuals?
4. Serum was taken from a 50-year-old man with "flu-like" symptoms during the disease and 3 weeks later. The hemagglutination inhibition data for the current strain of influenza A (H3N2) are presented at top, right. Hemagglutination is indicated by the filled circle. Was the individual infected with the current strain of influenza A?

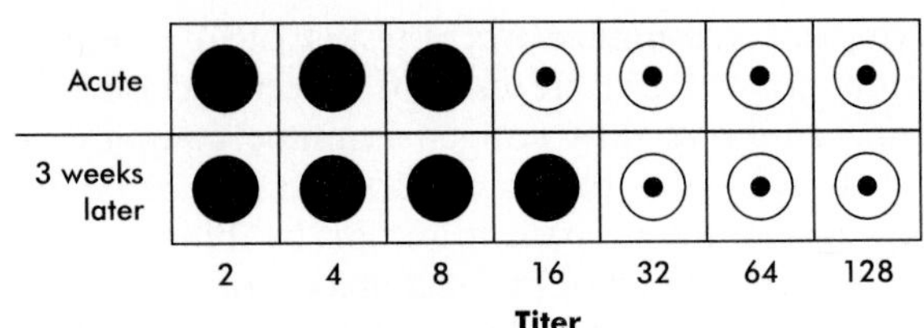

5. A policeman stuck his finger with a drug addict's syringe needle by accident. He is concerned that he may be infected with human immunodeficiency virus. Samples were taken from the policeman 1 month later for analysis. What assays would be appropriate to determine whether the individual was infected with HIV? In this case, it may be too early to detect an antibody response to the virus. What procedures would be appropriate to assay for virus or viral components?

Bibliography

Chernesky MA, Ray CG, and Smith TF: *Laboratory diagnosis of viral infections*, Washington DC, 1982, American Society for Microbiology.

Hsiung GD: *Diagnostic virology*, ed 3, New Haven, Conn., 1982, Yale University Press.

Lennette DA, Specter S, and Thompson KD, editors: *Infections: the role of the clinical laboratory*, Baltimore, 1979, University Park Press.

Lennette EH, editor: *Laboratory diagnosis of viral infections*, New York, 1985, Marcel Dekker.

Menegus MA: Diagnostic virology. In Belshe RB, editor: *Textbook of human virology*, ed 2, St. Louis, 1991, Mosby.

Specter S, Lancz G, editors: *Clinical virology manual*, ed 2, New York, 1992, Elsevier.

CHAPTER 54

Papovaviruses

THE papovavirus group (Papovaviridae) includes the papillomaviruses and polyomaviruses (Table 54-1). Many viruses in both genera infect animals other than humans, and papovaviruses are known to cause chronic latent infections in their natural hosts. Human papillomaviruses cause warts. BK and JC viruses, members of the *Polyomavirus* genus, are associated with renal disease and progressive multifocal leukoencephalopathy, respectively, in immunosuppressed individuals. SV-40 (simian virus-40) is the prototype polyomavirus. Although these two genera are in the same family, they differ in size, antigenic determinants, and biological properties.

The papovaviruses are small, nonenveloped icosahedral capsid viruses with double-strand circular DNA genomes (Box 54-1). They encode proteins that promote cell growth. In a permissive cell type this facilitates lytic virus replication. However, these proteins may oncogenically transform a cell that is nonpermissive. The polyoma viruses and especially SV-40 have been studied extensively as model oncogenic viruses. Certain genotypes of human papillomaviruses (HPV) are closely associated with human cancers such as cervical carcinoma.

HUMAN PAPILLOMAVIRUSES
Structure and Replication

The icosahedral capsid of human papillomaviruses (HPV) is 50 to 55 nm in diameter and consists of two structural proteins forming 72 capsomeres (Figure 54-1). The HPV genome is circular and has approximately 8000 base pairs. The HPV DNA encodes seven or eight early (depending on the virus) (E1-E8) and two late (structural) (L1, L2) genes, all located on one strand (the plus strand) (Figure 54-2).

Classification of HPV is based on DNA relatedness because these viruses cannot be grown readily in tissue culture. Based on DNA sequence homology, at least 58 HPV types have been identified and classified in 1 of 16 (A through P) groups. HPV can be distinguished further as cutaneous HPV or mucosal HPV based on the site of infection and replication. Viruses in similar groups frequently cause similar types of warts.

Individual HPV types have very limited host and tissue tropisms. The papillomaviruses require specific nuclear factors for transcription and replication that are characteristic of the different layers and types of skin and mucosa. A model skin organ culture system (raft) has recently been developed that supports virus replication. In this model, keratinocytes differentiate as if in skin and express the transcription factors that are required for HPV replication at the appropriate differentiation stage correlating with the expression of specific keratins. HPV

TABLE 54-1 Human Papovaviridae and Their Diseases

Virus	Disease
Papillomavirus	Warts
Polyomavirus	
BK virus	Renal disease*
JC virus	Progressive multifocal leukoencephalopathy*

*Disease occurs in immunosuppressed patients.

BOX 54-1 Unique Properties of Papovaviruses

Small icosahedral capsid virion
Double-stranded circular DNA genome, replicated and assembled in the nucleus
Two major genera:
- Papilloma HPV types 1-58+ (as determined by genotype; types defined by DNA homology, tissue tropism, and association with oncogenesis)
- Polyoma: SV-40, JC, and BK viruses

Viruses have defined tissue tropisms determined by receptor interactions and the transcriptional machinery of the cell
Viruses encode proteins that promote cell growth by binding to the cellular growth suppressor proteins p53 and RB. Polyoma T antigen binds to both RB and p53. Papillomavirus E6 binds p53 and E7 binds RB
Viruses can cause lytic infections in permissive cells but cause abortive, persistent, or latent infections or immortalize (transform) nonpermissive cells

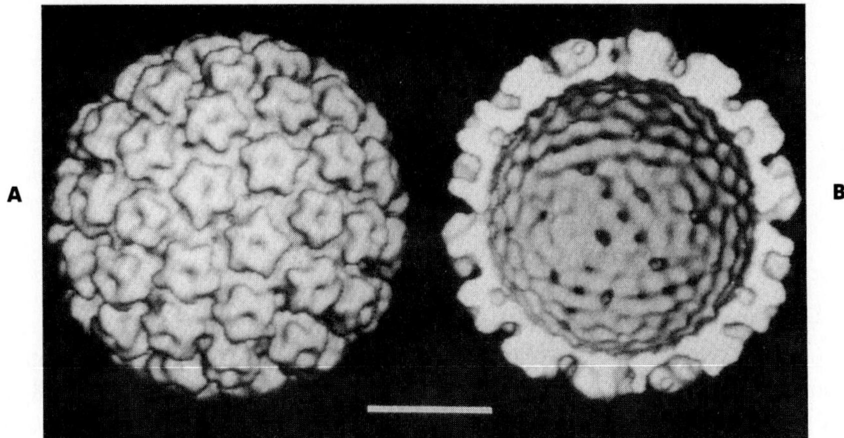

FIGURE 54-1 Computer reconstruction of cryoelectron micrographs of the human *papillomavirus*. **A,** View of the surface of HPV shows the presence of 72 capsomeres arranged in an icosahedron. All the capsomeres (pentons and hexons) appear to form a regular five-pointed, star-shaped head. **B,** A computer cross-section of the capsid shows the interaction of the capsomeres and channels in the capsid. (From Baker TS, Newcomb WW, Olson NH, et al.: *Biophysical J* 60:1445-1456, 1991.)

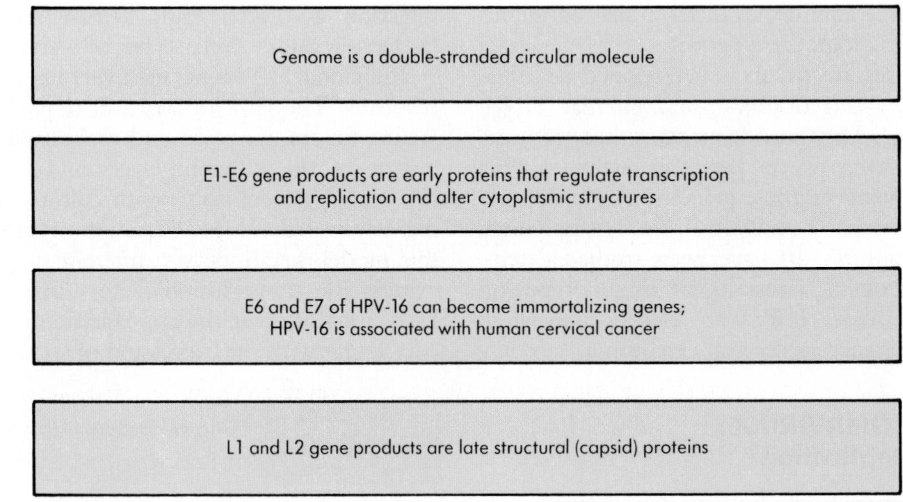

Genome is a double-stranded circular molecule
E1-E6 gene products are early proteins that regulate transcription and replication and alter cytoplasmic structures
E6 and E7 of HPV-16 can become immortalizing genes; HPV-16 is associated with human cervical cancer
L1 and L2 gene products are late structural (capsid) proteins

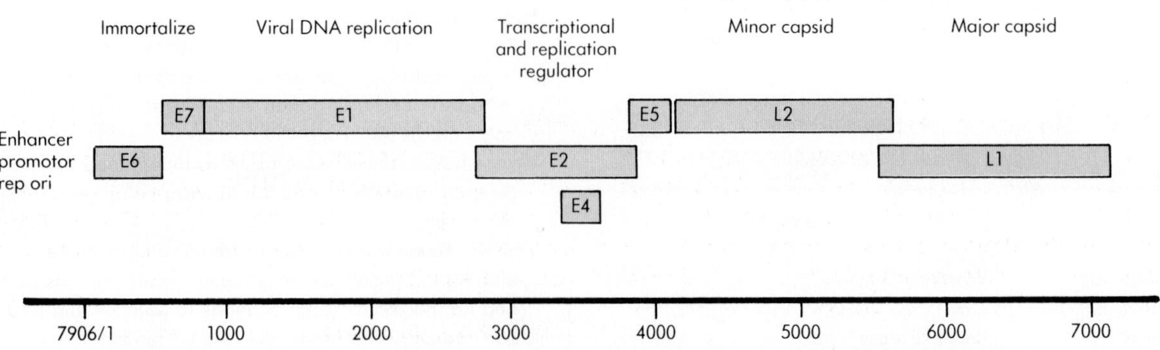

FIGURE 54-2 Genome of human papillomavirus (HPV-16). DNA is normally a double-stranded circular molecule but is shown in its linear, integrated form. *E6,* oncogene protein that binds p53; *E7,* oncogene protein that binds RB105; *rep ori,* origin of replication; L1, major capsid protein; *L2,* minor capsid protein. (Courtesy Tom Broker, M.D.)

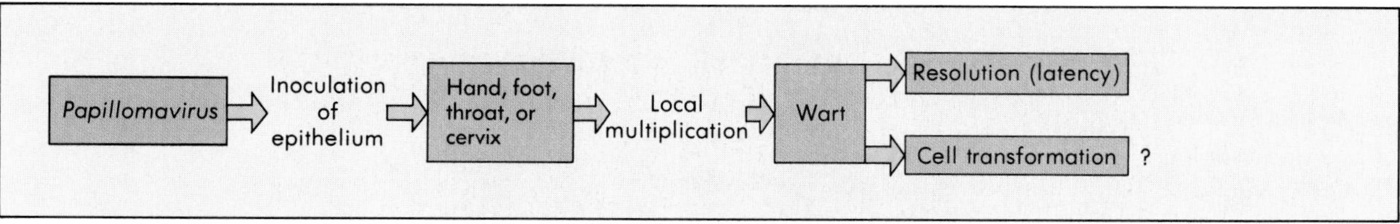

FIGURE 54-3 Progression of papillomavirus infection.

will replicate in the differentiating epithelial cells of either skin or mucosa. The virus remains latent in the basal layer of cells.

Pathogenesis

Papillomaviruses infect and replicate in the squamous epithelium of skin and mucous membranes to induce epithelial proliferation, a **wart**. Viral infection remains local and generally regresses spontaneously (Figure 54-3; see also Figure 54-6, A). The papillomavirus remains in the basal layer of the epithelium, and expression of its genes correlates with the differentiation stage of the skin. The papillomavirus genome can persist in the cells and may cause recurrences. A summary of HPV pathogenic mechanisms is given in Box 54-2.

HPV has been studied extensively for its oncogenic potential. Viral DNA has been found in both benign and malignant tumors, especially mucosal papillomas. HPV 16 and 18 cause cervical papillomas and dysplasia, and at least 85% of cervical carcinomas contain integrated HPV DNA. The E6 and E7 proteins of HPV 16 and 18 have been identified as oncogenes, which bind and inactivate the cellular growth (transformation) suppressor proteins, p53 and p105 retinoblastoma gene product (RB). The E6 binds the p53 protein, and E7 binds to RB. Without these brakes on cell growth, the cell is more susceptible to mutation, chromosomal aberrations or the action of a cofactor, and become cancerous.

The mechanism by which papillomas resolve is not known. The importance of cell-mediated immunity is suggested since immunosuppressed individuals have recurrences and more severe presentations of papovavirus infections, including papillomaviruses.

BOX 54-2 Disease Mechanisms of Papovaviruses

PAPILLOMAVIRUSES

- Virus is acquired by close contact and infects epithelial cells of either the skin or mucous membranes
- Tissue tropism and disease presentation is dependent on the papillomavirus type
- Virus replication is dependent on the epithelial cell differentiation stage: persistent in the basal layer and active in differentiated keratinocytes
- Causes benign outgrowth of cells into warts
- Warts resolve spontaneously: Immune response?????
- Certain types are associated with dysplasia that may become cancerous with the action of cofactors
- DNA of specific HPV types is present (integrated) in the tumor cell chromosome

POLYOMAVIRUSES (JC AND BK)

- Virus is probably acquired through the respiratory route and spread by viremia to the kidney early in life
- Infections are asymptomatic
- Virus establishes persistent/latent infection in kidney, lungs, etc.
- In immunocompromised individuals, JC is activated, spreads to the brain, and causes progressive multifocal leukoencephalopathy (PML), a conventional slow virus disease
- In PML, JC partially transforms astrocytes and kills oligodendrocytes, yielding characteristic lesions and sites of demyelination

Epidemiology

HPV is relatively stable to inactivation and can be transmitted by fomites, such as contaminated surfaces, bathroom floors, or towels (Box 54-3). HPV infections are transmitted by direct contact and acquired through small breaks in the skin or mucosa. Inoculation during sexual intercourse, while passing through an infected birth canal, or by the childhood habit of chewing warts is known to occur.

Plantar, common, and flat warts are most common in children and young adults. The lower incidence of these warts in adults may result from acquired immunity. Genital warts are most common among sexually active individuals, underscoring their status as a sexually transmitted disease. Recent studies suggest that genital HPV infections may occur in 10% to 20% of females. Asymptomatic shedding may promote transmission. Laryngeal papillomas occur in young children and middle-age adults.

Clinical Syndromes

Skin Warts

Most persons with infection have the common HPV types (1 through 4), which infect keratinized surfaces usually on the hands and feet (Figure 54-4). Initial

BOX 54-3 Epidemiology of Papovaviruses

DISEASE/VIRAL FACTORS

Capsid virus is resistant to inactivation
Virus persists in host
Asymptomatic shedding is likely

TRANSMISSION

Papilloma: direct contact, sexual contact for certain virus types, or passage through infected birth canal for laryngeal papillomas (types 6 and 11)
Polyoma: inhalation of infectious aerosols

WHO IS AT RISK?

Papilloma: warts are common; sexually active individuals are at risk for infection with HPV types correlated with oral and genital cancers
Polyoma: immunocompromised-PML

GEOGRAPHY/SEASON

Worldwide
No seasonal incidence

MODES OF CONTROL

None

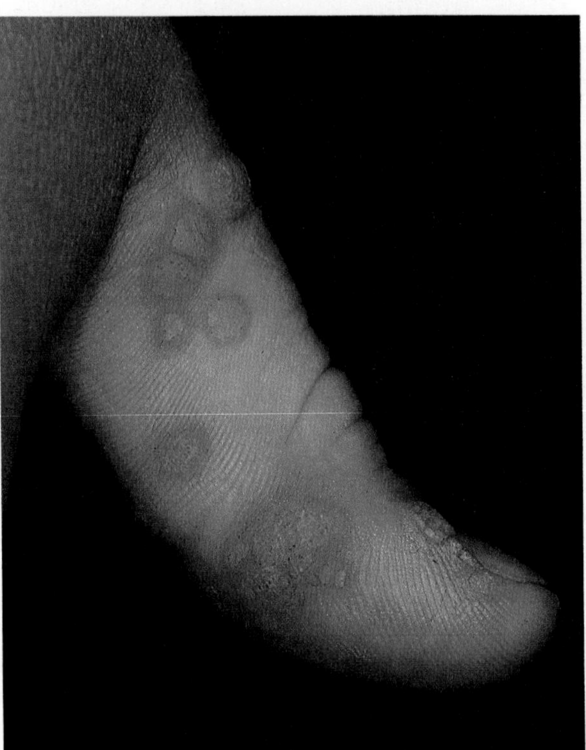

FIGURE 54-4 Common warts with thrombosed vessels (black dots) on the surface. (From Habif TP: *Clinical dermatology: a color guide to diagnosis and therapy*, St. Louis, 1985, Mosby.)

infection occurs in childhood or early adolescence (Table 54-2).

Benign Head and Neck Tumors

Single oral papillomas are the most benign epithelial tumors of the oral cavity. They are pedunculated with a fibrovascular stalk and usually have a rough papillary appearance to their surface. They can occur in any age-group, are usually solitary, and rarely recur after surgical excision. **Laryngeal papillomas** are commonly associated with HPV-6 and HPV-11 and are the most common benign epithelial tumors of the larynx. Laryngeal papillomatosis is usually considered a life-threatening condition in children because of the danger of airway obstruction. Occasionally, papillomas may extend down the trachea and into the bronchi.

Anogenital Warts

Genital warts (**condyloma acuminatum**) occur almost exclusively on the squamous epithelium of the external genitalia and perianal areas. Approximately 90% are caused by HPV types 6 and 11. Anogenital lesions infected with these HPV types rarely progress to malignancy in otherwise healthy individuals.

Cervical Dysplasia, Neoplasia

HPV infection of the genital tract is now recognized as a common sexually transmitted disease. Cytologic changes characteristic of this viral infection (**koilocytotic cells**) are detected in approximately 5% of all Papanicolaou stained cervical smears (Figure 54-5). Infection of the female genital tract by HPV types 16 and 18 and, rarely, by other types of HPV is associated with intraepithelial cervical neoplasia and cancer. The first neoplastic changes noted by light microscopy are termed *dysplasia*. Approximately 40% to 70% of the mild dysplasias undergo spontaneous regression.

The development of cervical cancer is thought to proceed through a continuum of progressive cellular changes from mild (cervical intraepithelial neoplasia, CIN I) to moderate (CIN II), to severe dysplasia and/or carcinoma in situ. This sequence of events has been documented by a number of studies to progress over a period of 1 to 4 years.

Laboratory Diagnosis

A wart can be confirmed microscopically by its characteristic histological appearance, consisting of hyperplasia of **prickle cells** and the production of excess keratin (hyperkeratosis) (Figure 54-6). Papillomavirus infection can be detected by the presence of koilocytotic (vacuolated cytoplasm) squamous epithelial cells, which are rounded and occur in clumps (see Figure 54-5 and Table 54-3). DNA molecular probes are the method of choice for establishing the presence of HPV infection in cervical

TABLE 54-2 Clinical Syndromes Associated With Papillomaviruses

Syndrome	HPV types	
	Common	Uncommon
SKIN WARTS		
Plantar wart	1	2, 4
Common wart	2, 4	1, 7, 26, 29
Flat wart	3, 10	27, 28, 41
Epidermodysplasia verruciformis	5, 8, 17, 20, 36	9, 12, 14, 15, 19, 21-25, 38, 46
BENIGN HEAD AND NECK TUMORS		
Laryngeal papilloma	6, 11	
Oral papilloma	6, 11	2, 16
Conjunctival papilloma	11	
ANOGENITAL WART		
Condyloma acuminatum	6, 11	1, 2, 10, 16, 30, 44, 45
Cervical intraepithelial neoplasia, cancer	16, 18	11, 31, 33, 35, 42, 43, 44

Modified from Balows A et al., editors: *Laboratory diagnosis of infectious diseases: principles and practice*, vol 2, New York, 1988, Springer-Verlag.

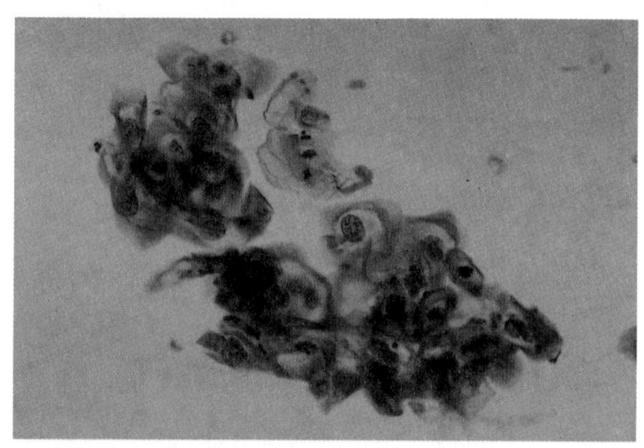

FIGURE 54-5 Papanicolaou stain of the exfoliated cervical-vaginal squamous epithelial cells showing perinuclear cytoplasmic vacuolization and nuclear enlargement ("koilocytosis") characteristic of HPV infection (×400).

swabs and in tissue. Human papillomavirus virions can be seen by electron microscopy in lesions as can HPV antigens by immunofluorescent and immunoperoxidase techniques. Papillomaviruses do not grow in cell cultures, and tests for HPV antibodies are rarely used except in research surveys.

Treatment, Prevention, and Control

Spontaneous disappearance of warts is the rule, but this may take many months to years. Painful or bulky lesions are removed by surgical cryotherapy, electrocautery, or chemical means, although recurrences are common. Injection of interferon is also beneficial. Surgery may be necessary for laryngeal papillomas.

At present the best means of prevention is avoidance of direct contact with infected tissue.

POLYOMAVIRUSES

Relatively little is known of the human polyomaviruses (BK and JC viruses) because they do not usually cause disease and are difficult to grow in cell cultures. SV-40 and murine polyomaviruses have been studied extensively as tumor-causing viruses.

Structure and Replication

The polyomaviruses are slightly smaller (45 nm in diameter) and contain less nucleic acid (5000 base pairs) than the papillomaviruses (see Box 54-1). The genomes of BK virus, JC virus, and SV-40 are closely related and divided into early, late, and noncoding regions (Figure 54-7). The early region on one strand codes for nonstructural T (transformation) proteins (including large T antigen), and the late region, on the other strand, codes for three viral capsid proteins (VP1, VP2, VP3) (Box 54-4). The noncoding region is the origin of DNA replication and the site of the transcriptional control sequences for both early and late genes.

The replicative cycle includes penetration by pinocytosis, followed by uncoating and viral multiplication in the nucleus. As with the papillomaviruses, polyomavirus replication is very dependent on host cell factors. Permissive cells allow late transcription of late viral mRNA and virus replication, which results in cell death. Some nonpermissive cells allow expression of only the early genes including T antigen, potentially leading to oncogenic transformation of the cell.

The large T antigen of SV-40 (and possibly JC and

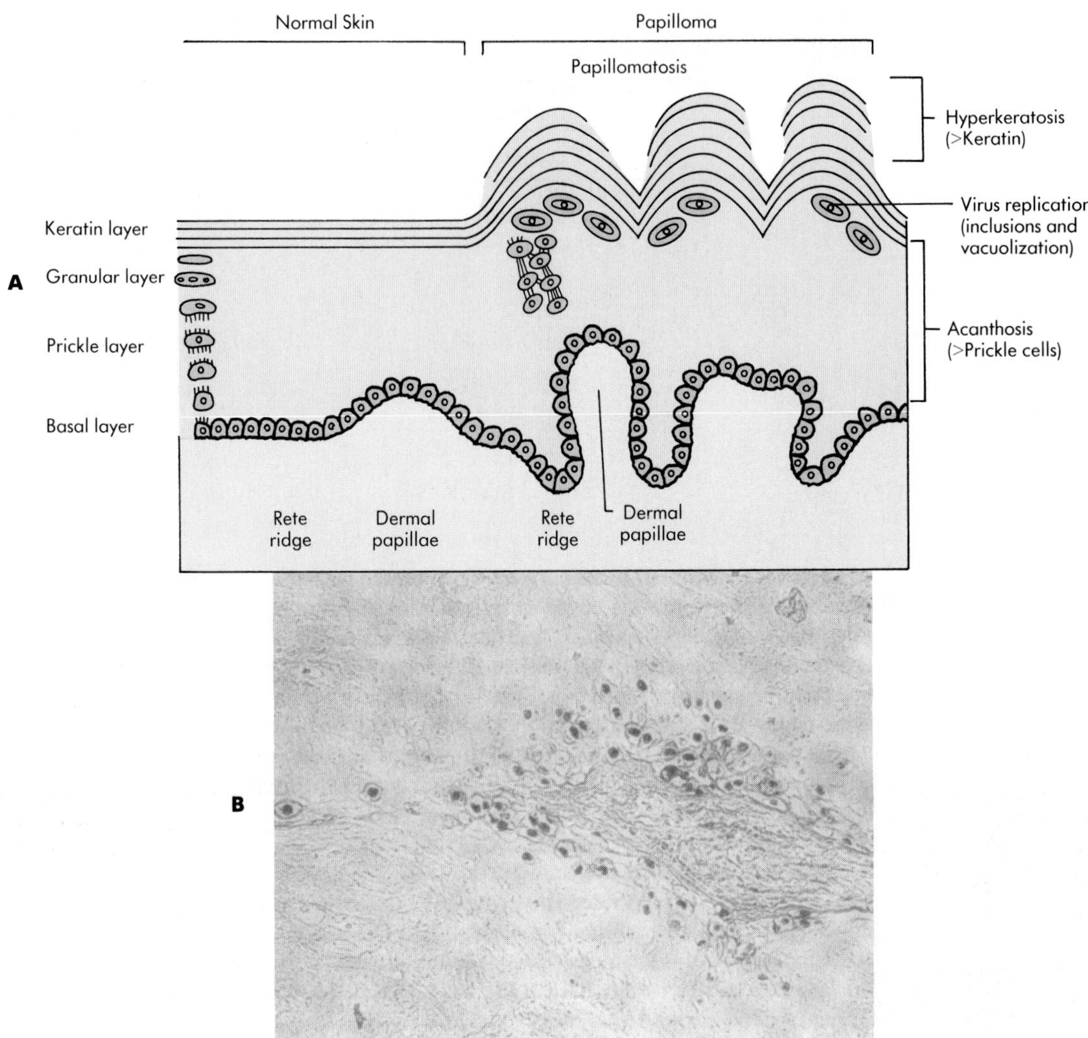

FIGURE 54-6 A, Comparison of normal skin and a papilloma (wart). *Papillomavirus* infection promotes the outgrowth of prickle cells (acanthosis), which thickens the skin and promotes the production of keratin (hyperkeratosis) forming epithelial spikes (papillomatosis). Virus replication occurs in the granular cells close to the final keratin layer. (Modified from Jenson AB et al. In Hooks J, Jordan W, editors: *Viral infections in oral medicine*, New York, 1982, North-Holland Elsevier.) **B,** DNA probe analysis of an HPV-6-induced anogenital condyloma. A biotin-labeled DNA probe was localized by horseradish peroxidase–conjugated avidin conversion of substrate to a chromogen precipitate. Dark staining is seen over nucleii of koilocytotic cells. (From Belshe RB, editor: *Textbook of human virology*, ed 2, St. Louis, 1991, Mosby.)

BK) has several functions. T antigen of SV-40 binds to DNA and controls both early and late gene transcription, as well as viral DNA replication. In addition, the T antigen binds to the two major cellular growth suppressor proteins, p53 and p105RB, and as a result promotes cell growth.

The polyomavirus genome is used very efficiently. The noncoding region of the genome contains the initiation sites for both the early and late mRNAs, as well as the origin for DNA replication. The three late proteins are produced from mRNAs, which have the same initiation site, and then are processed into three unique mRNAs.

The viral DNA is maintained and replicated bidirectionally similar to a bacterial plasmid. DNA replication precedes late mRNA transcription and protein synthesis.

TABLE 54-3 Laboratory Diagnosis of *Papillomavirus* Infections

Test	Detects
Cytology	Koilocytotic cells
Electron microscopy	Virus
In situ DNA probe analysis*	Viral nucleic acid
Immunofluorescent and immunoperoxidase staining	Viral structural antigens
Southern blot hybridization	Viral nucleic acid
Culture	Not useful

*Method of choice.

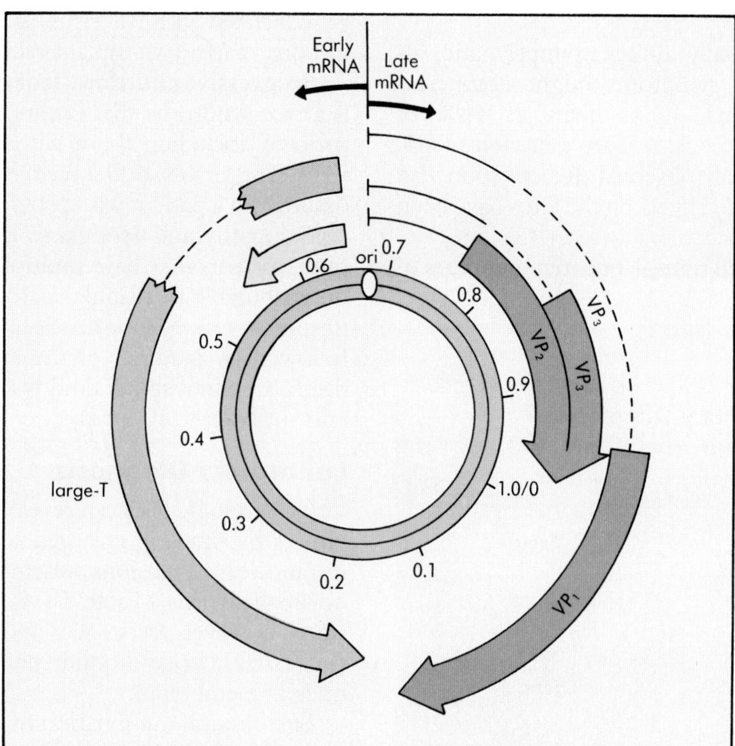

FIGURE 54-7 Genome of SV-40 virus. The SV-40 genome is a prototype of other polyomaviruses and contains an early, late, and noncoding region. The noncoding region contains the start sequences for both the early and late genes and for DNA replication (*ori*). The individual early mRNAs and late mRNAs are processed from larger nested transcripts. (Redrawn from Butel JS, Jarvis DL: *Biochem Biophys Acta* 865:171, 1986.)

Assembly of the virus occurs in the nucleus, and virus is released by cell lysis.

Pathogenesis

Polyomavirus infection is limited to specific hosts and cell types within that host. JC and BK viruses probably enter the respiratory tract, infect lymphocytes, and then the kidney with minimum cytopathology. BK establishes latent infection in the kidney, and JC establishes in the kidney, lungs, and reticuloendothelial system. Replication is blocked in immunocompetent individuals.

In immunocompromised patients, reactivation of virus in the kidney leads to virus shedding in the urine and potentially severe urinary tract infection (BK) or viremia and central nervous system infection (JC) (Figure 54-8). JC crosses the blood-brain barrier by replicating in the endothelial cells of capillaries. An abortive infection of astrocytes results in partial transformation, yielding enlarged cells with abnormal nucleii resembling glioblastomas. Productive lytic infections of oligodendrocytes cause demyelination (see Box 54-3). Like SV-40 virus, BK and JC cause tumors when injected into hamsters; however, they are not associated with any human tumors.

Epidemiology

Polyomavirus infections are ubiquitous, and most humans are infected with both JC and BK by the age of 15 years (see Box 54-3). Respiratory transmission is the probable mode of spread. Immune suppression after organ transplantation or during pregnancy will allow reactivation of latent infections.

Early batches of poliomyelitis vaccine were contaminated with SV-40, a simian polyomavirus, that was undetected in the primary monkey cell cultures used to prepare the vaccine. Although many people were vaccinated with the contaminated vaccines, no SV-40–related tumors have been reported during 25 years of follow-up.

BOX 54-4 *Polyomavirus* **Proteins**

EARLY

Large T	Regulation of early and late mRNA transcription; DNA replication; cell growth promotion/transformation
Small T	Viral DNA replication

LATE

VP1	Major capsid protein and viral attachment protein
VP2	Minor capsid protein
VP3	Minor capsid protein

Clinical Syndromes

Primary infection is virtually always asymptomatic, although mild respiratory symptoms might occur and cystitis has been reported. In as many as 40% of immunocompromised patients, urinary excretion of BK and JC viruses is commonly observed. Reactivation also occurs in pregnancy, but no effects on the fetus have been established.

Ureteral stenosis in renal transplant patients appears to be associated with BK virus, as does hemorrhagic cystitis in bone marrow transplant recipients.

Progressive multifocal leukoencephalopathy (PML) is a rare syndrome that occurs in immunocompromised patients, including those with AIDS, and is due to JC virus. The virus was first recovered by co-culture of brain tissue from a patient with progressive multifocal leukoencephalopathy and Hodgkin's disease. As the name implies, patients may have multiple neurological symptoms unattributable to a single anatomical lesion. Impairment of speech, vision, coordination, and/or mentation occurs, followed by paralysis of the arms and legs, and finally death. Cerebral spinal fluid is normal and does not contain antibody to JC virus.

TABLE 54-4 Laboratory Diagnosis of *Polyomavirus* (JC and BK) Infections

Test	Detects
Pap smear of urinary epithelial cells	Viral inclusions
Electron microscopy	Virions
Immunofluorescence and immunoperoxidase staining	Viral antigens
DNA probe analysis	Viral nucleic acid
Nucleic acid hybridization in clinical specimens	BK and JC viruses nucleic acids
Cell culture	
Human diploid lung fibroblasts	Virus isolation—BK
Primary human fetal glial cells	Virus isolation—JC*

*Not useful.

Laboratory Diagnosis

Urine cytologic tests can reveal the presence of JC or BK viruses by showing enlarged cells with dense basophilic intranuclear inclusions resembling those induced by cytomegalovirus (Table 54-4). Cytomegalovirus inclusions, however, are smaller and have a larger halo effect (i.e., a clear zone around the inclusion but within the nuclear membrane).

Histological examination of brain tissue from cases of progressive multifocal leukoencephalopathy reveals foci of demyelination surrounded by oligodendrocytes with inclusions. These cells are adjacent to areas of demyelination. The term *leukoencephalopathy* refers to the restriction of lesions to the white matter. There is little if any inflammatory cell response. Electron microscopy or DNA probe analysis can be used to detect viral particles in brain tissue.

BK virus can be cultured in diploid fibroblast cells or Vero monkey kidney cells, both of which are available for

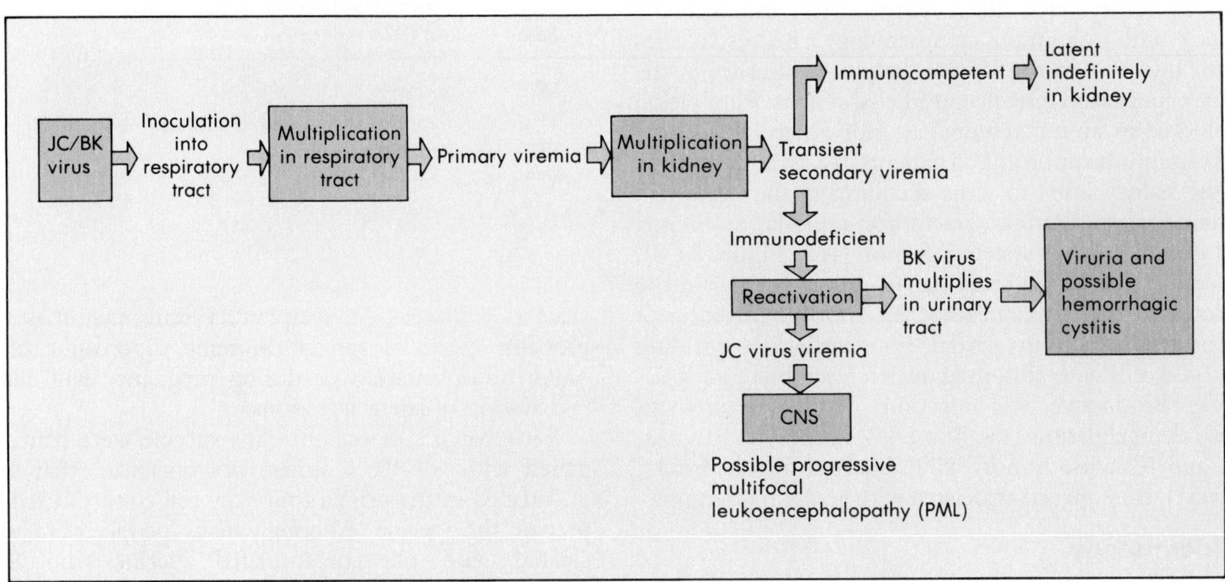

FIGURE 54-8 Mechanisms of spread of polyomaviruses within the body.

use in clinical laboratories. JC virus grows best in primary human fetal glial cells, which are not readily available. Culture of JC virus is therefore performed only in a few research laboratories.

Quicker methods of analysis now include in situ immunofluorescence, immunoperoxidase, DNA probe analysis, and polymerase chain reaction (PCR) analysis for genetic sequences.

Treatment, Prevention, and Control

No specific treatment is available, other than decreasing the immune suppression responsible for allowing the polyomavirus reactivation and symptoms. The ubiquitous nature of polyomaviruses and the lack of understanding of their modes of transmission make preventing primary infection unlikely.

CASE STUDY AND QUESTIONS

A 25-year-old carpenter noticed the appearance of several hyperkeratotic papules (warts) on the palm side of his index finger. They did not change in size and caused him only minimal discomfort. After a year, they spontaneously disappeared.

1. Will this virus infection spread to other body sites?
2. After disappearance, is the infection likely to be completely resolved or persist in the host?
3. What viral/cellular/host conditions regulate the replication of this virus and other papovaviruses?
4. How would the papillomavirus type causing this infection be identified?
5. Is it likely that this papillomavirus type is associated with human cancer? If not, which HPV types are associated with cancer and which cancers?

Bibliography

Arthur RR, Keerti VS, Baust SJ, Santos GW, and Saral R: Association of BK viruria with hemorrhagic cystitis in recipients of bone marrow transplants, *N Engl J Med* 315:230-234, 1986.

Crum CP, Barber S, Roche JK: Pathobiology of papillomavirus-related cervical diseases. *Clin Microbiol Rev* 4:270-285, 1991.

Fields BN and Knipe DM, editors: *Virology*, ed 2, New York, 1990, Raven Press.

Houff SA et al.: Involvement of JC virus-infected mononuclear cells from the bone marrow and spleen in the pathogenesis of progressive multifocal leukoencephalopathy, *N Engl J Med* 318:301, 1988.

Howley PM: Role of the human papillomaviruses in human cancer, *Cancer Res* 51(18 suppl): 5019S-5022S, 1991.

Hseuh C, Reyes CV: Progressive multifocal leukoencephalopathy, *Am Fam Physician* 37:129-132, 1988.

Human papilloma viruses, *Obstet Gynecol Clin North Am* June 1987 (this monograph contains a series of reviews).

Major EO, Amemiya K, Tornatore CS, Houff SA, Berger JR: Pathogenesis and molecular biology of progressive multifocal leukoencephalopathy, *Clin Microb Rev* 5:49-73, 1992.

zur-Hausen H: Viruses in human cancers, *Science* 254: 1167-1173, 1991.

CHAPTER 55

Adenoviruses

Adenoviruses were first isolated in 1953 in human adenoid cell culture. Since then approximately 100 serotypes, at least 42 of which infect humans, have been recognized. All human serotypes are included in a single genus within the family Adenoviridae. Based on DNA homology studies and hemagglutination patterns, the 42 serotypes belong to one of six subgroups (A-F) (Table 55-1). The viruses in each subgroup share many properties.

The first human adenoviruses to be identified were numbered 1 to 7 and are the most common. Common disorders caused by the adenoviruses include respiratory tract infection, conjunctivitis, hemorrhagic cystitis, and gastroenteritis. Several adenoviruses have oncogenic potential in animals and have been extensively studied by molecular biologists. These studies have elucidated many viral and eukaryotic intracellular processes. For example, analysis of the gene for the adenovirus hexon led to the discovery of introns and splicing of eukaryotic mRNAs. Adenovirus is also being used for gene replacement therapy (e.g., cystic fibrosis).

TABLE 55-1 Illnesses Associated With Adenoviruses

Illness category	Most common serotypes
Endemic respiratory disease	1, 2, 5
Acute respiratory disease of military recruits	3, 4, 7, 14, 21
Adenoviral pneumonias	3, 4, 7b, 14, 21
Epidemic keratoconjunctivitis	8, 19
Pharyngoconjunctival fever	3, 7
Less common syndromes	
Pertussis syndrome	1, 2, 3, 5
Acute hemorrhagic cystitis	1, 4, 7, 11, 21
Hepatic disorders	3, 7
Gastroenteritis	9, 12, 13, 18, 25, 26, 27, 28, 40, 41, 42
Intussusception	1, 2, 5
Musculoskeletal disorders	7
Genital infections	19
Skin infections	2, 4, 7, 21
Infections in immunocompromised hosts	32, 34, 35, 36

From Liu C: Adenoviruses. In Belshe RB, editor: *Textbook of human virology*, ed 2, St. Louis, 1991, Mosby.

STRUCTURE AND REPLICATION

Adenoviruses are double-stranded DNA viruses with a genome molecular weight of 20 to 25 $\times$ 10^6 daltons. The adenovirus genome is a linear double-stranded DNA with a terminal protein (TP, 55,000 d) covalently attached at each 5′end. The virions are nonenveloped icosadeltahedrons with a diameter of 70 to 90 nm (Figure 55-1 and Box 55-1). The capsid comprises 240 capsomeres, which consist of **hexons** and **pentons**. The 12 pentons, located at each of the vertices, contain a penton base and a fiber. The fiber contains the **viral attachment proteins** and will act as a hemagglutinin. The penton base and fiber are toxic to cells. The penton base will cause cells to become round, and the fibers inhibit cellular macromolecular synthesis. The pentons and fibers also contain type-specific antigens.

The core complex, within the capsid, includes viral DNA and at least two major proteins. At least 11 polypeptides are contained in the adenovirus virion, 9 of which have an identified structural function (Table 55-2).

A map of the adenovirus genome (Figure 55-2) shows the locations of the viral genes. The genes are transcribed from both DNA strands and in both directions at different times during the replication cycle. Most of the RNA transcribed from the adenovirus genome are processed into several individual mRNA in the nucleus. Early proteins promote cell growth and DNA replication. Late proteins, synthesized after the onset of viral DNA replication, are primarily structural.

Replication of adenoviruses has been studied extensively in HeLa cell culture. One virus cycle takes approximately 32 to 36 hours and produces 10,000 virions. The viral fiber proteins interact with cell surface receptors (approximately 100,000 fiber receptors are present on each cell) and then enter the cell by endocytosis. The virus lyses the endosomal vesicle, and the capsid delivers the DNA genome to the nucleus. Release of the capsid also allows inhibition of macromolecular synthesis by the toxic effects of the penton and fiber proteins. This entire process requires 2 hours.

A

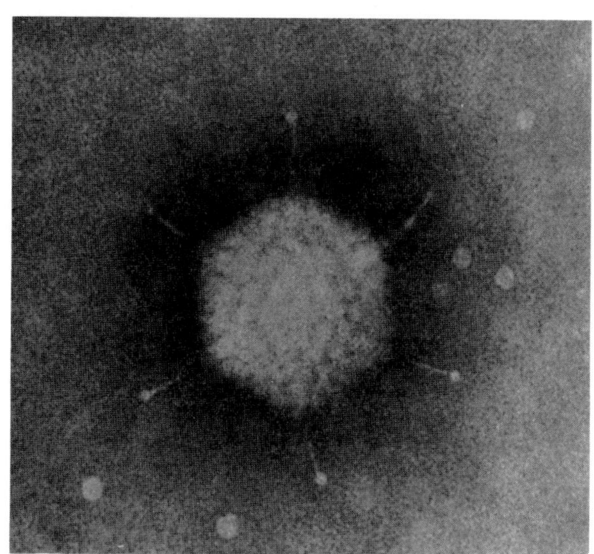

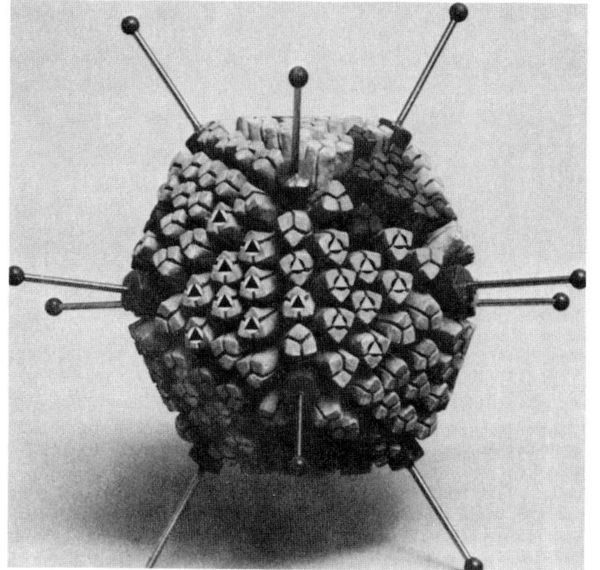

B

FIGURE 55-1 A, Electron micrograph of adenovirus virion with fibers. **B,** Model of adenovirus virion with fibers. (**A** from *J Molecular Biol* 13:13, 1965; **B** from Ginsberg HS: *The adenoviruses*, New York, 1984, Plenum Publishers.)

BOX 55-1 Unique Features of Adenoviruses

Naked icosadeltahedral capsid with fibers (viral attachment proteins) at vertices
Linear double-stranded genome with 5′ terminal proteins
Encodes proteins to promote mRNA and DNA synthesis including its own DNA polymerase
Human adenoviruses are grouped A through F by DNA homologies and by serotype (>42 types)
Serotype is mainly due to differences in the penton base and fiber protein, which determine the tissue tropism and disease
Causes lytic, persistent, and latent infections of humans and some strains can immortalize certain animal cells

Early transcriptional events, following shutdown of host cell macromolecular synthesis, lead to gene products that stimulate cell growth and promote viral DNA replication. Transcription of the E1A gene, processing of the primary transcript (splicing out introns to yield three mRNAs), and translation produce transactivator proteins required for transcription of the other early proteins. Other early proteins include more DNA-binding proteins, the DNA polymerase, and a protein to assist in escaping the immune response. The E1A and E1B proteins stimulate cell growth by binding to the cellular growth suppressor proteins p53 (E1A) and RB (retinoblastoma gene product) (E1B). In permissive cells, activities in the growing cells facilitate transcription and replication of the genome, which ultimately causes cell death. In nonpermissive cells, E1A and E1B promote cell growth without cell death and contribute to the oncogenic activity of the virus in rodent cells.

Viral DNA replication occurs in the nucleus by a viral DNA polymerase from both strands of the DNA. The polymerase uses a primer consisting of a 55,000 d viral protein (terminal protein "TP")–cytosine monophosphate primer.

Late gene transcription starts after DNA replication. Most of the individual late mRNAs are generated from a large (83% of the genome) primary transcript encoded by the right strand of the genome that is processed into individual mRNAs.

Capsid proteins are produced in the cytoplasm and then transported to the nucleus for viral assembly. Empty capsids assemble, and then the viral DNA and core proteins enter the capsid through an opening at one of the vertices. Cleavage of several of the capsid proteins and the terminal protein attached to the DNA lead to maturation of the particle into a stable and infectious virion. The replication and assembly process is inefficient and error prone (11 to 2300 particles produced per plaque forming unit). This results in accumulations of DNA, protein, and large numbers of defective particles in nuclear inclusion bodies. The virus remains in the cell until the cell degenerates and lyses.

PATHOGENESIS AND IMMUNITY

Adenoviruses infect epithelial cells lining respiratory and enteric organs (Box 55-2). Following local replication, viremia may occur with spread to visceral organs (Figure 55-3). This dissemination is more likely to occur in

TABLE 55-2 Major Adenovirus Structural Proteins

Location	Number	Molecular weight	Name	Comment
Capsid				
	II	120 Kd	Hexon protein	Contains family antigen and some serotyping antigens
	III	85 Kd	Penton base protein	Toxic to tissue culture cells
	IV	62 Kd	Fiber	Responsible for attachment and hemagglutination; contains some serotyping antigens
	VI	24 Kd	Hexon-associated proteins	
	VIII	13 Kd		
	IX	12 Kd	Penton-associated proteins	
	IIIa	66 Kd		
Core				
	V	48 Kd	Core protein 1 DNA-binding protein	
	VII	18 Kd	Core protein 2 DNA-binding protein	

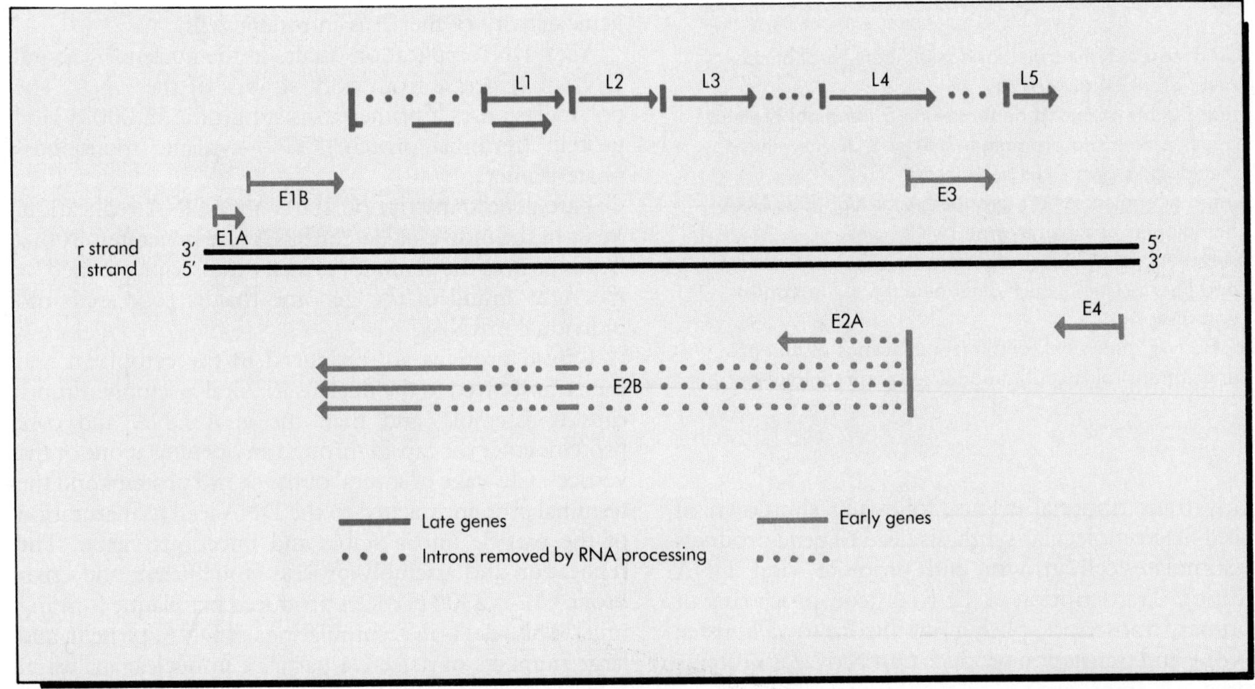

FIGURE 55-2 Genome map of adenovirus type 2. Genes are transcribed from both strands (*l* and *r*) in opposite directions. The early genes are transcribed from four promoter sequences. All of the late genes are transcribed from one promoter sequence. Alternative splicing patterns of primary RNA transcripts produce the full repertoire of viral proteins. The splicing pattern for the E2 transcript is shown as an example. *E*, Early protein; *L*, Late protein. (Modified from Jawetz E, Melnick JL, Adelberg EA, editors: *Review of medical microbiology*, ed 17, Norwalk, Conn, 1987, Appleton & Lange.)

immunocompromised patients. Differences in viral fiber proteins result in different target cell specificity among adenovirus serotypes. The virus has a propensity to become latent in lymphoid tissue, such as adenoids, tonsils, or Peyer's patches, and can be reactivated by immunosuppression or infection with other agents. Although certain adenoviruses (groups A and B) can transform and are oncogenic in rodent cells, adenovirus transformation of human cells has not been observed. The time course of adenovirus infection is shown in Figure 55-4.

The histological hallmark of adenovirus infection is a dense central intranuclear inclusion within an infected epithelial cell consisting of viral DNA and protein (Figure 55-5). These may resemble inclusions seen with cytomegalovirus, but adenovirus does not cause cellular enlargement (cytomegaly). Mononuclear cell infiltrates and epithelial cell necrosis accompany the characteristic inclusions.

BOX 55-2 Disease Mechanisms of Adenoviruses

- Virus spread by aerosol, close contact, or fecal-oral means to establish pharyngeal infection. Fingers spread virus to eyes
- Virus infects epithelial cells of mucous membranes in the respiratory tract, gastrointestinal tract, and conjunctiva/cornea causing cell damage directly
- Persists in lymphoid tissue (e.g., tonsils, adenoids, Peyer's patches)
- Antibody is important for prophylaxis and resolution
- Disease is determined by the tissue tropism of the specific group/serotype of the virus strain

Antibody is important for resolving lytic adenovirus infections and is associated with protection from reinfection by the same serotype. Cell-mediated immunity is important in limiting virus outgrowth since immunosuppressed individuals suffer recurrent disease.

Adenovirus encodes several early proteins that help the virus avoid immune defenses. During virus replication, a short RNA segment is produced that forms a double-stranded duplex and blocks initiation of the antiviral state by interferon. A 19,000 d early protein binds to the heavy chain of class I major histocompatability antigen and prevents it from reaching the cell membrane, thus preventing the cell from presenting antigenic targets to cytotoxic T cells. Several proteins inhibit tumor necrosis factor (TNF) induction of inflammation, which limits immunopathology and the severity of the disease symptoms.

EPIDEMIOLOGY

Adenovirus virions are stable to drying, detergents, the gastrointestinal tract (acid, protease, and bile) and even mild chlorine treatment (Box 55-3). This allows their spread by the fecal-oral route and by fingers and fomites, including towels and medical instruments and in poorly chlorinated swimming pools.

Adenovirus is spread exclusively by human-to-human transmission with no apparent animal reservoirs for the virus. Adenoviruses are spread mainly by respiratory or fecal-oral contact. Virus spread is promoted by close interaction, as in classrooms and military barracks. Adenoviruses may be shed intermittently and over long periods from the pharynx and especially in feces. Most infections are asymptomatic, which greatly facilitates their spread in the community.

Adenoviruses 1 through 7 are the most prevalent serotypes. From 5% to 10% of pediatric respiratory disease can be attributed to adenoviruses types 1, 2, and

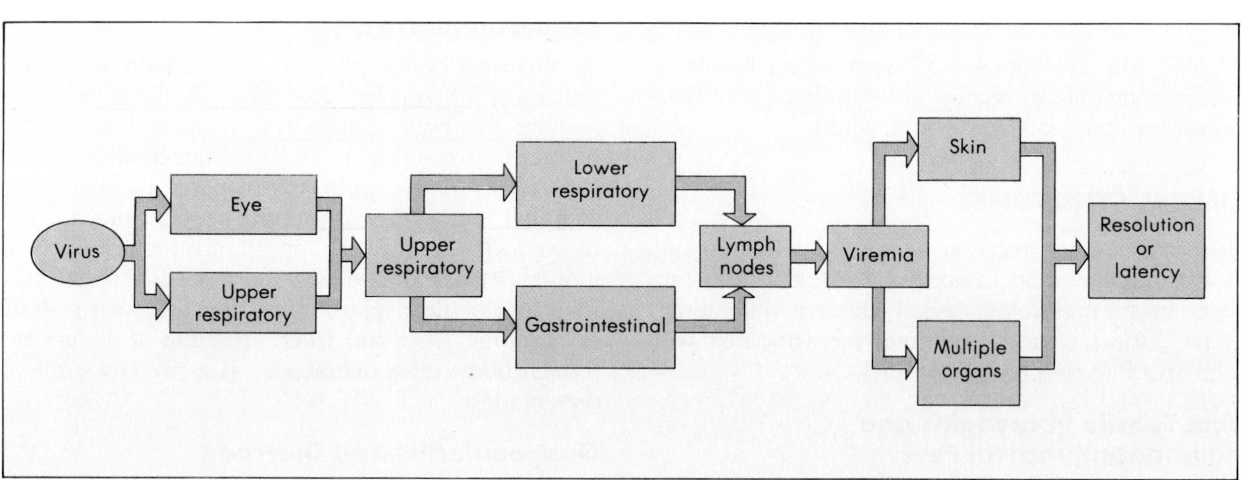

FIGURE 55-3 Mechanisms of adenovirus spread within the body.

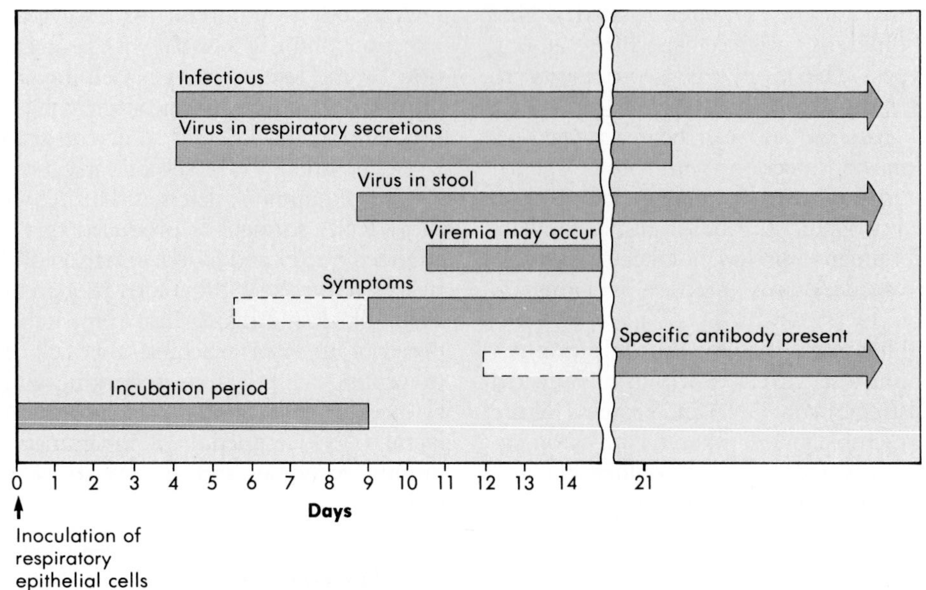

FIGURE 55-4 Time course of adenovirus respiratory tract infection.

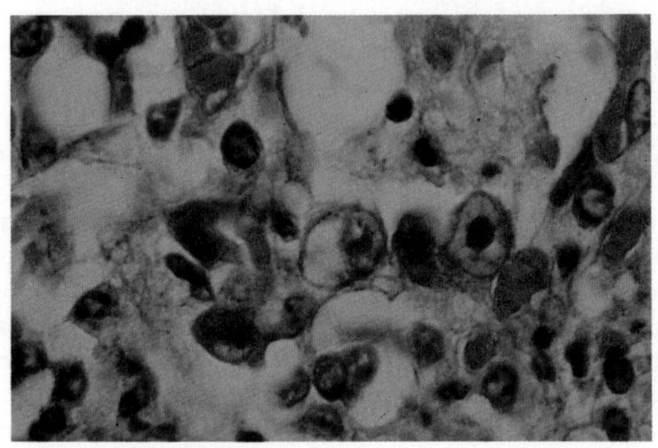

FIGURE 55-5 Histology of adenovirus infection. Inefficient assembly of virions yields basophilic nuclear inclusion bodies containing DNA, protein, and virions.

5. Adenovirus serotypes 4 and 7 seem especially able to spread among military recruits, since antibody prevalence to these serotypes is low in young adults.

CLINICAL SYNDROMES

Adenoviruses cause infection primarily in children and, less commonly, adults. Infection by reactivated virus occurs in immunocompromised children and adults. Several distinct clinical syndromes are associated with adenovirus infection (see Table 55-1).

Acute Febrile Pharyngitis and Pharyngoconjunctival Fever

Adenovirus causes pharyngitis, which is often accompanied by conjunctivitis (**pharyngoconjunctival fever**). Pharyngitis alone occurs in young children, particularly those younger than 3 years of age, and may mimic streptococcal infection. Pharyngoconjunctival fever occurs more often in outbreaks involving older children.

Acute Respiratory Disease

Acute respiratory disease is a syndrome of fever, cough, pharyngitis, and cervical adenitis seen primarily in outbreaks among military recruits because of serotypes 4 and 7.

Other Respiratory Diseases

Adenoviruses are definite but infrequent causes of true viral pneumonia in both children and adults (Figure 55-6). Laryngitis, croup, and bronchiolitis may also occur. Pertussis-like illness with a prolonged clinical course has been associated with adenoviruses.

Conjunctivitis and Epidemic Keratoconjunctivitis

Adenoviruses cause a follicular conjunctivitis in which the mucosa of the palpebral conjunctiva becomes pebbled or nodular and both conjunctivae (palpebral and bulbar) become inflamed (Figure 55-7). Conjunctivitis may occur sporadically or in outbreaks that can be traced to a common source (e.g., swimming pools). Epidemic keratoconjunctivitis may be an occupational hazard for industrial workers and was most striking in the naval shipyards of Pearl Harbor, causing more than 10,000 cases during 1941 and 1942. Irritation of the eye by a foreign body, dust, debris, etc., is a risk factor for this presentation.

Gastroenteritis and Diarrhea

Adenovirus is a major cause of acute viral gastroenteritis, accounting for 15% of hospitalized cases. Adenovirus serotypes 40, 41, and 42 have been grouped as enteric

BOX 55-3 Epidemiology of Adenoviruses

DISEASE/VIRAL FACTORS

Capsid virus is resistant to inactivation by the gastrointestinal tract and drying

Disease symptoms may resemble other respiratory virus infections

May cause asymptomatic shedding

TRANSMISSION

Direct contact via respiratory droplets and fecal material, on hands, on fomites (e.g., towels, contaminated medical instruments), close contact, and in inadequately chlorinated swimming pools

WHO IS AT RISK?

Persons in day-care centers, military training camps, and swimming clubs

GEOGRAPHY/SEASON

Worldwide

No seasonal incidence

MODES OF CONTROL

A live vaccine is available for serotypes 4 and 7 for military use

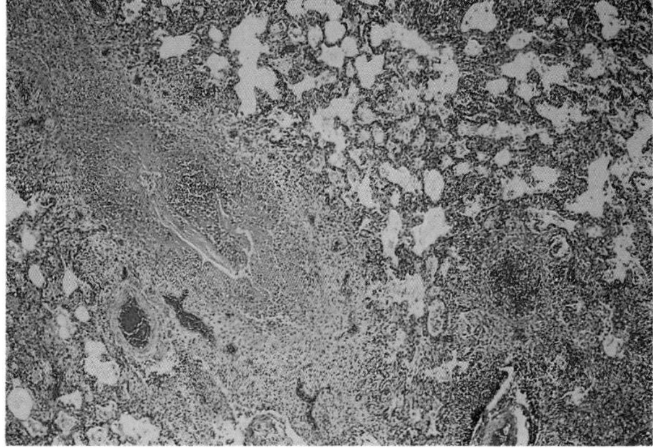

FIGURE 55-6 Hematoxylin and eosin-stained sample of adenovirus pneumonia, showing inflammation, necrosis, and exudate.

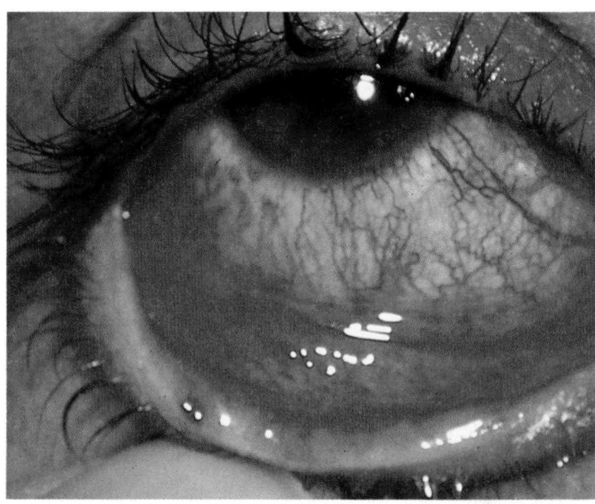

FIGURE 55-7 Conjunctivitis due to adenovirus.

adenoviruses (group F) and appear to be responsible for episodes of diarrhea in infants. These enteric adenoviruses will not replicate in the same tissue culture cells as other adenoviruses and rarely cause fever or respiratory symptoms.

Other Presentations

Adenovirus has also been associated with a pertussis-like illness, intussusception in young children, acute hemorrhagic cystitis with dysuria and hematuria in young boys, musculoskeletal disorders, and genital and skin infections.

Systemic Infection in Immunocompromised Patients

Immunocompromised patients are at risk of serious adenovirus infections, although not as often as from infections caused by the herpesviruses. Diseases include pneumonia and hepatitis. Infection can be from exogenous or endogenous (reactivation) sources.

LABORATORY DIAGNOSIS

Isolation of most adenovirus types is best accomplished in cell cultures derived from epithelial cells (e.g., primary human embryonic kidney (HEK) cells or continuous (transformed) lines such as HeLa or human epidermal carcinoma (HEp-2) cells. The virus causes a lytic infection with characteristic inclusion bodies within 2 to 20 days. Recovery in cell culture requires an average of 6 days.

Isolation of virus may not always be relevant to the actual disease, since adenovirus may be shed into feces for weeks to months after infection. For the results to be significant, the isolate should be obtained from a site or secretion relevant to the disease symptoms. Isolation of adenovirus from the throat of a patient with pharyngitis is usually diagnostic if laboratory findings eliminate other common etiologies such as *Streptococcus pyogenes*.

Immunoassays, including fluorescent antibody and enzyme linked immunosorbent assays, and DNA probe analysis can be used to detect and type/group the virus in clinical samples and after tissue culture growth. Enzyme immunoassay, DNA probe analysis, and immune electron microscopy are used to identify enteric adenovirus serotypes 40, 41, and 42, which do not grow in readily available cell cultures but may be responsible for infant diarrhea. Characteristic intranuclear inclusions can be seen in infected tissue during histological examination. Inclusions, however, are rare and must be distinguished from those resulting from cytomegalovirus.

Serologic assays such as complement fixation, hemagglutination inhibition, enzyme immunoassay, and neutralization techniques have been used to detect type-specific antibodies following adenovirus infection. A fourfold rise in antibody level or seroconversion between acute and convalescent serum specimens is necessary before the result can be considered diagnostic of active infection. Serologic diagnosis is rarely used except to confirm the significance of a fecal or upper respiratory isolate by its serotype.

TREATMENT, PREVENTION, AND CONTROL

There is no known treatment for adenovirus infection. Live oral vaccines have been used to prevent adenovirus 4 and 7 infections in military recruits, but they are not used in civilian populations. The widespread use of live adenovirus vaccines is unlikely since members of the adenovirus family are oncogenic in some species. However, genetically engineered subunit vaccines could be prepared and used in the future.

CASE STUDY AND QUESTIONS

A 7-year-old boy attending summer camp complained of sore throat, headache, cough, red eyes, and tiredness, and was sent to the infirmary. His temperature was 40° C. Within hours, other campers and counselors visited the infirmary with similar symptoms. Symptoms lasted for 5 to 7 days. All the patients went swimming in the camp pond. More than 50% of the camp complained of symptoms similar to the initial case. The public health department identified the agent as adenovirus serotype 3.*

1. Which adenovirus syndrome does the symptoms describe?
2. An outbreak as large as this suggests a common source of infection. What was the most likely source(s)? What were the most likely routes of transmission that spread the virus?
3. What physical properties of the virus facilitate its transmission?
4. What precautions or actions should the camp owners take to prevent other outbreaks?
5. What sample(s) would have been used by the public health department, and what tests would be required to obtain the diagnosis?

Bibliography

Balows A, Hausler WJ Jr, and Lennette EH, editors: *Laboratory diagnosis of infectious diseases: principles and practice*, vol II, New York, 1988, Springer-Verlag.

Ginsberg HS: *The adenoviruses*, New York, 1984, Plenum Publishers.

Horowitz, M: Adenoviruses and their replication. In Fields BN and Knipe DM: *Virology*, ed 2, New York, 1990, Raven Press.

Liu C: Adenoviruses. In Belshe RB, editor: *Textbook on human virology*, ed 2, St. Louis, 1991, Mosby.

Yolken RH and Eiden JJ: Rotavirus, Enteric Adenoviruses. In Belshe RB, editor: *Textbook on human virology*, ed 2, St. Louis, 1991, Mosby

*Modified from Outbreak of pharyngoconjunctival fever at a summer camp—North Carolina, *MMWR* 41:342-344, 1991.

CHAPTER 56

Human Herpesviruses

THE human herpesviruses are grouped into three subfamilies based on differences in viral characteristics (genome structure, tissue tropism, cytopathology, and site of latent infection), as well as pathogenesis and disease presentation. The human herpesviruses include herpes simplex (HSV) type 1 and type 2 and varicella zoster (VZV) viruses, cytomegalovirus (CMV), human herpesvirus 6 (HHV6) and human herpesvirus 7 (HHV7), and Epstein-Barr (EBV) (Table 56-1).

The herpesviruses are a diverse group of large DNA viruses that share a common virion morphology, basic mode of replication, the capacity to establish latent/recurrent infections, and the importance of cell-mediated immunity for controlling infection and causing symptoms. The herpesviruses can cause lytic, persistent, latent/recurrent, and (for Epstein-Barr virus) immortalizing infections (Box 56-1).

Herpesvirus infections are common, and the viruses are ubiquitous. Although they usually cause benign disease, the herpesviruses can cause significant morbidity and mortality, especially in immunosuppressed individuals. Fortunately, the herpesviruses encode enzymes that are targets for antiviral agents, and several of these compounds are therapeutically useful.

STRUCTURE OF THE HERPESVIRUSES

The herpesviruses are large enveloped viruses containing double-stranded deoxyribonucleic acid (DNA). The virion is approximately 150 nm in diameter and has the

TABLE 56-1 Properties Distinguishing the Herpesviruses

Subfamily	Virus	Primary target cell	Site of latency	Means of spread
ALPHA-HERPESVIRINAE				
Human herpesvirus 1	Herpes simplex type 1 (HSV-1)	Mucoepithelial	Neuron	Close contact
Human herpesvirus 2	Herpes simplex type 2 (HSV-2)	Mucoepithelial	Neuron	Close contact
Human herpesvirus 3	Varicella zoster virus (VZV)	Mucoepithelial	Neuron	Respiratory and close contact
GAMMA-HERPESVIRINAE				
Human herpesvirus 4	Epstein-Barr virus (EBV)	B lymphocyte and epithelial cells	B lymphocyte	Close contact (kissing disease)
BETA-HERPESVIRINAE				
Human herpesvirus 5	Cytomegalovirus (CMV)	Monocyte, lymphocyte, and epithelial cells	Monocyte, lymphocyte, and ?	Close contact, transfusions, tissue transplant, and congenital
Human herpesvirus 6	Herpes lymphotropic virus (HHV6)	T lymphocytes and ?	T lymphocytes and ?	Respiratory and close contact?
Human herpesvirus 7	Human herpesvirus 7 (HHV7)	T lymphocytes and ?	T lymphocytes and ?	?

? indicates that other cells may also be the primary target or site of latency.

BOX 56-1 Unique Features of Herpesviruses

- Large enveloped icosadeltahedral capsid containing a double-stranded DNA genome
- Encodes many proteins that regulate mRNA/DNA synthesis and the shutoff of host cell DNA, RNA, and protein synthesis
- Encodes enzymes (thymidine kinase, DNA polymerase) that promote viral DNA replication and are good targets for **antiviral drugs**
- DNA replication and assembly occurs in nucleus, virus buds from nuclear membrane, and is released by exocytosis and cell lysis
- Can cause lytic, persistent, latent, and for EBV, immortalizing infections

characteristic morphology shown in Figure 56-1. The DNA core is surrounded by an icosadeltahedral capsid containing 162 capsomeres. This is enclosed by a glycoprotein-containing envelope. Herpesviruses encode several glycoproteins for viral attachment, fusion, and immune escape. The space between the envelope and the capsid is called the **tegument** and contains viral proteins and enzymes. As enveloped viruses, the herpesviruses are sensitive to acid, solvents, detergents, and drying.

Herpesvirus genomes are linear double-stranded DNA but differ in size and gene orientation (Figure 56-2). Direct or inverted repeat sequences bracket unique regions of the genome (U_L [unique-long], U_S [unique-short]), allowing circularization and recombination within the genome. Recombination between inverted repeats of HSV, CMV, and VZV allows large portions of the genome to switch the orientation of their U_L and U_S gene segments with respect to each other.

REPLICATION OF THE HERPESVIRUSES

Herpesvirus replication is initiated by the interaction of viral glycoproteins with cell surface receptors. The tropism of some herpesviruses (e.g., EBV) is restricted by the tissue-specific expression of receptors. The nucleocapsid is then released into the cytoplasm by fusion of the envelope with either the plasma membrane or vesicle membranes, depending on the virion strain and cell type. Enzymes and transcription factors are carried into the cell in the tegument of the virion. The nucleocapsid docks with the nuclear membrane and delivers the genome into the nucleus, where transcription and replication of the genome occur.

Transcription of the viral genome and viral protein synthesis proceed in a coordinated and regulated manner in three phases: (1) **Immediate early proteins** (α) consisting of DNA-binding proteins important for regulation of gene transcription; (2) **Early proteins** (β) consisting of more transcription factors and enzymes, including the DNA polymerase; and (3) **Late proteins** (γ) consisting mainly of structural proteins.

The viral genome is transcribed by cellular DNA-dependent RNA polymerases and regulated by viral-encoded and cellular nuclear factors. The interplay of these factors determines whether the infection will be lytic, persistent, or latent. Cells that promote latent infection restrict transcription to specific immediate early genes. Progression to early and late gene expression results in cell death and lytic infection.

Replication of the viral genome is performed by the viral-encoded DNA polymerase. Viral-encoded scavenging enzymes provide deoxyribonucleotide substrates for the polymerase and are targets of antiviral drugs. These enzymes facilitate replication of the virus in nongrowing cells that lack sufficient substrates for viral DNA synthesis.

Empty procapsids assemble in the nucleus, are filled with DNA, acquire an envelope at the nuclear membrane and exit the cell by exocytosis or by lysis of the cell. Transcription, protein synthesis, glycoprotein processing, and exocytic release from the cell are performed by cellular machinery. The replication of HSV will be discussed in more detail later.

HERPES SIMPLEX VIRUS

Herpes simplex virus was the first of the human herpesviruses to be recognized. The name *herpes* is derived from a Greek word meaning to creep. "Cold sores" were described in antiquity, and their viral etiology was established in 1919.

The two types of HSV, 1 and 2, share many characteristics including DNA homology, antigenic determinants, tissue tropism, and disease symptoms. However, they can still be distinguished by differences in these properties.

Structure

The HSV genome is large enough to encode approximately 80 proteins. Among these are DNA-binding proteins that coordinate and promote the transcription and replication of the DNA. The HSV genome also encodes enzymes, including a DNA-dependent DNA polymerase and scavenging enzymes such as deoxyribonuclease, thymidine kinase, and ribonucleotide reductase, as well as other enzymes. Ribonucleotide reductase converts ribonucleotides to deoxyribonucleotides, and thymidine kinase phosphorylates the deoxyribonucleotides to provide substrates for replication of the viral genome. The substrate specificities of these enzymes and the DNA polymerase differ significantly from their cellular analogue and thus represent good targets for the development of antiviral chemotherapy.

HSV encodes at least 11 glycoproteins that serve as viral attachment (gB,gC,gD,gH), fusion (gB), structural, immune escape proteins (gC,gE,gI), and other functions. For example, the C3 component of the complement system binds to gC and is depleted from serum. The Fc

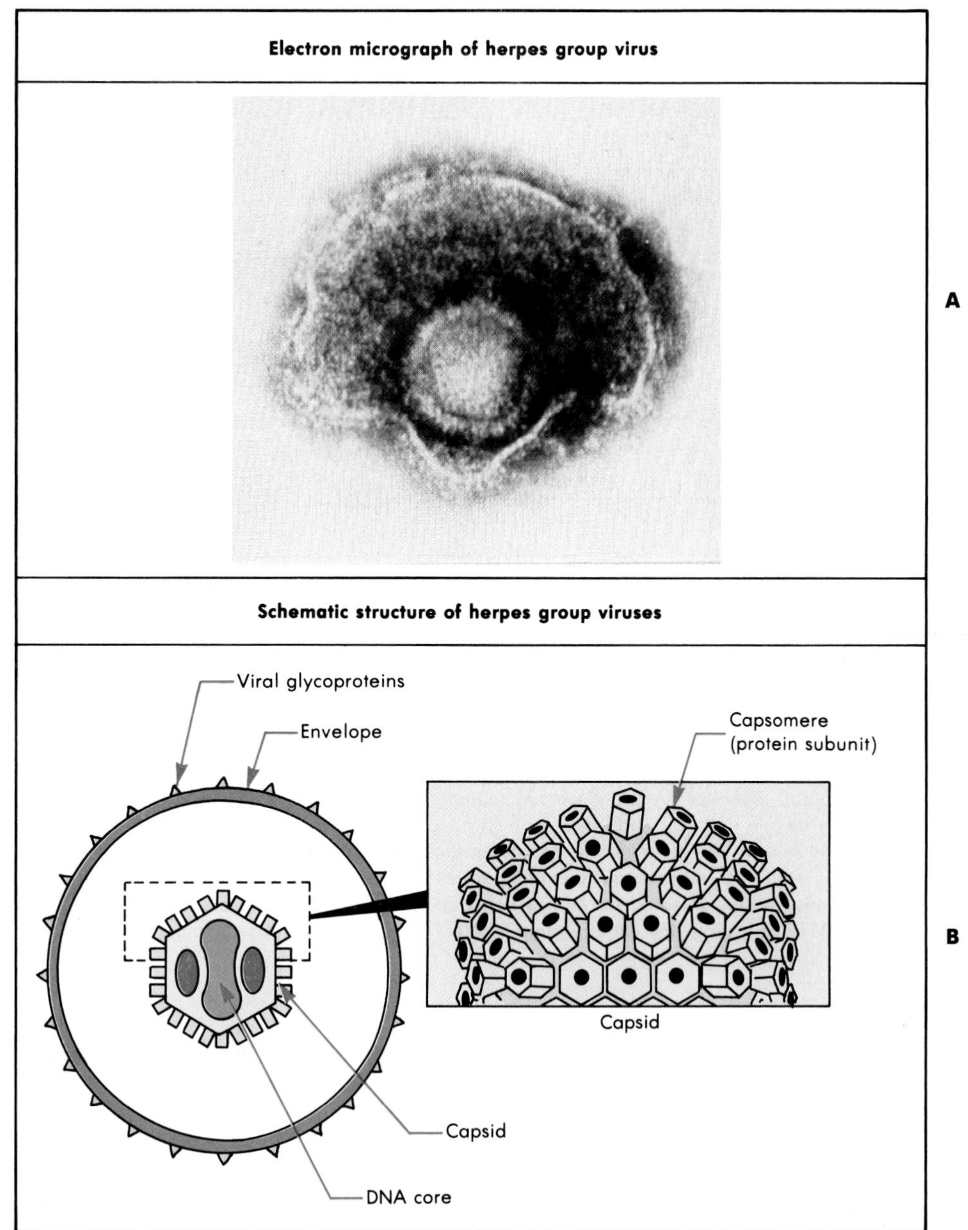

FIGURE 56-1. Electron micrograph **(A)** and general schematic structure **(B)** of the herpesviruses. The DNA genome of the herpesvirus in the core is surrounded by an icosahedral capsid and a membrane envelope. Glycoproteins are inserted into the envelope.

portion of IgG binds to a gE/gI complex, camouflaging the virus and virus- infected cells. These actions reduce the antiviral effectiveness of antibody.

Replication

HSV can infect most types of human cells and even cells of other species. The virus generally causes lytic infections of fibroblast and epithelial cells and latent infections of neurons (see Figure 7-10).

HSV-1 binds initially to heparan sulfate, a proteoglycan found on the outside of many cell types and then interacts with a protein closer to the cell surface. Although receptors for both types of HSV are expressed on similar cells, the two viruses bind to different structures.

The major route of HSV penetration is fusion at the cell surface membrane. The virion releases a protein that promotes the initiation of viral gene transcription, a viral-encoded protein kinase, and cytotoxic proteins into the cytoplasm upon fusion.

The immediate early gene products are transcribed first. These DNA-binding proteins stimulate DNA synthesis and promote the transcription of the early viral genes. During a latent infection, a specific RNA is the only detectable viral product synthesized in these cells

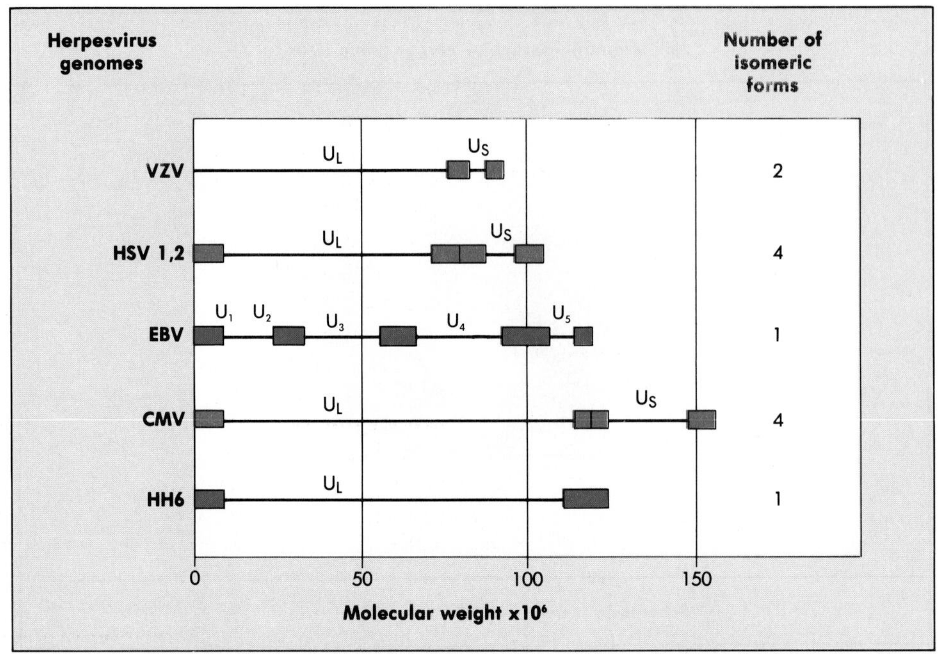

FIGURE 56-2 Herpesvirus genomes. The genomes of the herpesvirus are double-stranded DNA. The length and complexity of the genome differ for each of the viruses. Inverted repeats in HSV, VZV, and CMV allow the genome to recombine with itself to form isomers. Large genetic repeat sequences are boxed. Direct repeat DNA sequences: blue; indirect repeat DNA sequences: red; U_L: large unique sequence; U_S: small unique sequence. The genome of HSV and CMV have two sections, the unique long (U_L) and the unique short (U_S), each of which is bracketed by two sets of inverted repeats of DNA. The inverted repeats facilitate the replication of the genome but also allow the U_L and the U_S regions to invert independently of each other to give four different genome configurations or isomers. VZV has only one set of inverted repeats and can form two isomers. EBV exists in only one configuration with several unique regions surrounded by direct repeats.

(latency associated transcript [LAT]) and virus replication does not procede further.

The early proteins consist of mostly enzymes including the DNA-dependent polymerase. As catalytic proteins, relatively few copies of these enzymes are required to promote replication. Other early proteins inhibit the production and initiate the degradation of cellular messenger ribonucleic acid (mRNA) and DNA. Expression of the early and late genes generally leads to cell death.

Replication of the genome starts as soon as the polymerase is synthesized. This also triggers late gene transcription. Circular, end-to-end concatameric forms of the genome are made initially. Later in the infection, the DNA is replicated by a rolling-circle mechanism to produce a linear string of genomes in a fashion resembling a roll of toilet paper. Cleavage of the concatamers into individual genomes may occur before or as the DNA is sucked into a procapsid.

The late genes encode structural and other proteins. Many copies of these proteins are required. The capsid proteins are transported to the nucleus, where they are assembled into empty procapsids and filled with DNA. The glycoproteins are synthesized and then receive the high mannose N-linked glycan precursor at the endoplasmic reticulum. The glycoproteins then diffuse to the contiguous nuclear membrane. DNA-containing capsids associate and bud from viral glycoprotein-modified portions of the nuclear membrane. The virus buds into the endoplasmic reticulum and is transferred in a vesicle to the Golgi apparatus, where the glycoproteins are processed. The virus is released by exocytosis or cell lysis. The virus is also spread by cell-cell fusion and through intracellular bridges.

Pathogenesis and Immunity

The mechanisms of pathogenesis of HSV-1 and HSV-2 are very similar (Box 56-2). Both viruses initially infect and replicate in mucoepithelial cells and then establish latent infection of the innervating neurons. The site of infection and the subsequent disease is predominantly dependent on the means of acquisition of the virus. HSV-1 is usually associated with infections above the waist and HSV-2 with infections below the waist (Figure 56-3). Other differences between the two types include receptor specificity, growth characteristics, and antigenicity. HSV-2 has a greater potential to cause viremia and associated systemic flu-like symptoms.

HSV can cause lytic infections of most cells, persistent

BOX 56-2 Disease Mechanisms for Herpes Simplex Virus

HSV: Disease initiated by direct contact and is dependent on infected tissue (e.g., oral, genital, encephalitis)
Causes direct cytopathology
Avoids antibody by cell-cell spread (syncytia)
Establishes latency in neurons (hides from immune response)
Reactivates from latency by stress or immune suppression
CMI **required** for resolution with limited role for antibody
CMI-induced immunopathology contributes to symptoms

infections of lymphocytes and macrophages, and latent infection of neurons. Cytolysis generally results from virus-induced inhibition of cellular macromolecular synthesis, degradation of host cell DNA, membrane permeation, cytoskeletal disruption, and senescence of the cell. Changes in nuclear structure and margination of the chromatin occur, along with the production of *Cowdry's type A acidophilic intranuclear inclusion bodies*. Many strains of HSV also initiate syncytia formation. In tissue culture, HSV rapidly infects and kills cells. The cells become rounder and fall off the monolayer, producing plaques.

The virus initiates infection of mucosal membranes or enters through breaks in the skin. HSV usually causes a localized infection that may be inapparent or produce vesicular lesions. The virus replicates in the cells at the base of the lesion, and the vesicular fluid contains infectious virions. The lesion is caused by a combination of viral pathology and immunopathology. The lesion generally heals without producing a scar. The virus spreads to adjacent cells and to the innervating neuron. After infection of the neuron, the nucleocapsid is transported to the cell nucleus and initiates a latent infection.

Latent infection occurs in neurons and results in no detectable damage. Virus replication can be activated by various stimuli (e.g., stress, trauma, fever, or sunlight), and then the virus travels back down the nerve, causing lesions at the dermatome. Recurrences will therefore occur at the same spot each time.

Control and resolution of the HSV infection requires both humoral and cellular immunity. Antibody directed against the glycoproteins of the virus neutralize extracellular virus, limiting its spread. Antibody to HSV-1 also protects against future challenge by other strains of HSV-1 and to some extent against infections by HSV-2, and vice versa. However, the virus can escape antibody neutralization and clearance by direct cell-to-cell spread and latent infection of the neuron. Also, the virion and virus-infected cells express antibody (Fc) and complement receptors that weaken these humoral defenses. As a result, the *cell-mediated immune response is essential for controlling and resolving HSV infections*. In the absence of functional cell-mediated immunity, HSV infection disseminates to the vital organs and brain.

During primary infection, interferon and natural killer cells limit the progression of the infection. Delayed type hypersensitivity and cytotoxic T killer cell responses and activated macrophages kill infected cells and resolve the current disease. However, the immunopathology caused by the cell-mediated and inflammatory responses is a major cause of the symptoms.

Recurrent infections are generally less severe, more localized, and of shorter duration than primary episodes. Reactivation of the virus occurs despite the presence of antibody. The trigger for reactivation is stress, which may have a dual effect: (1) to promote the replication of the virus in the nerve and (2) to depress cell-mediated immunity transiently. Activation of memory cells, antibody responses, and the presence of local immunity resolve the infection more quickly than for a primary infection.

Epidemiology

The ability of HSV to establish latency with the potential for asymptomatic recurrence allows an individual to be a lifelong source of contagion (Box 56-3). As an enveloped virus, HSV is very labile and is readily inactivated by drying, detergents, and conditions of the G.I. tract. Although HSV can infect animal cells, HSV is exclusively a human disease.

HSV is transmitted in vesicle fluid, saliva, and vaginal secretions. Both HSV types can cause oral and genital lesions. HSV-1 is usually spread by oral contact (kissing) or by sharing glasses, toothbrushes, and other saliva-contaminated items. HSV-1 infection of fingers or body can result from mouth-to-skin contact and enters through a break in the skin. Autoinoculation may also cause infection of the eyes.

HSV-1 infection is common. In underdeveloped areas the prevalence of antibody to HSV-1 is greater than 90% by 2 years of age. This may reflect crowded living conditions or poor hygiene.

HSV-2 is spread mainly by sexual contact, autoinoculation, or from the mother at birth. Depending on sexual practices, HSV-2 may infect the genitalia, anorectal tissues, or oropharynx. The virus may then cause symptomatic or asymptomatic primary infection or recurrences. Infection of the neonate may occur during pregnancy, during a primary HSV-2 infection, by an ascending in utero infection, or most likely, because of excretion of HSV-2 from the cervix during vaginal delivery. Perinatal infection and neonatal infection have similar morbid outcomes.

Initial infection with HSV-2 occurs later in life than HSV-1 and correlates with sexual activity. Seropositivity

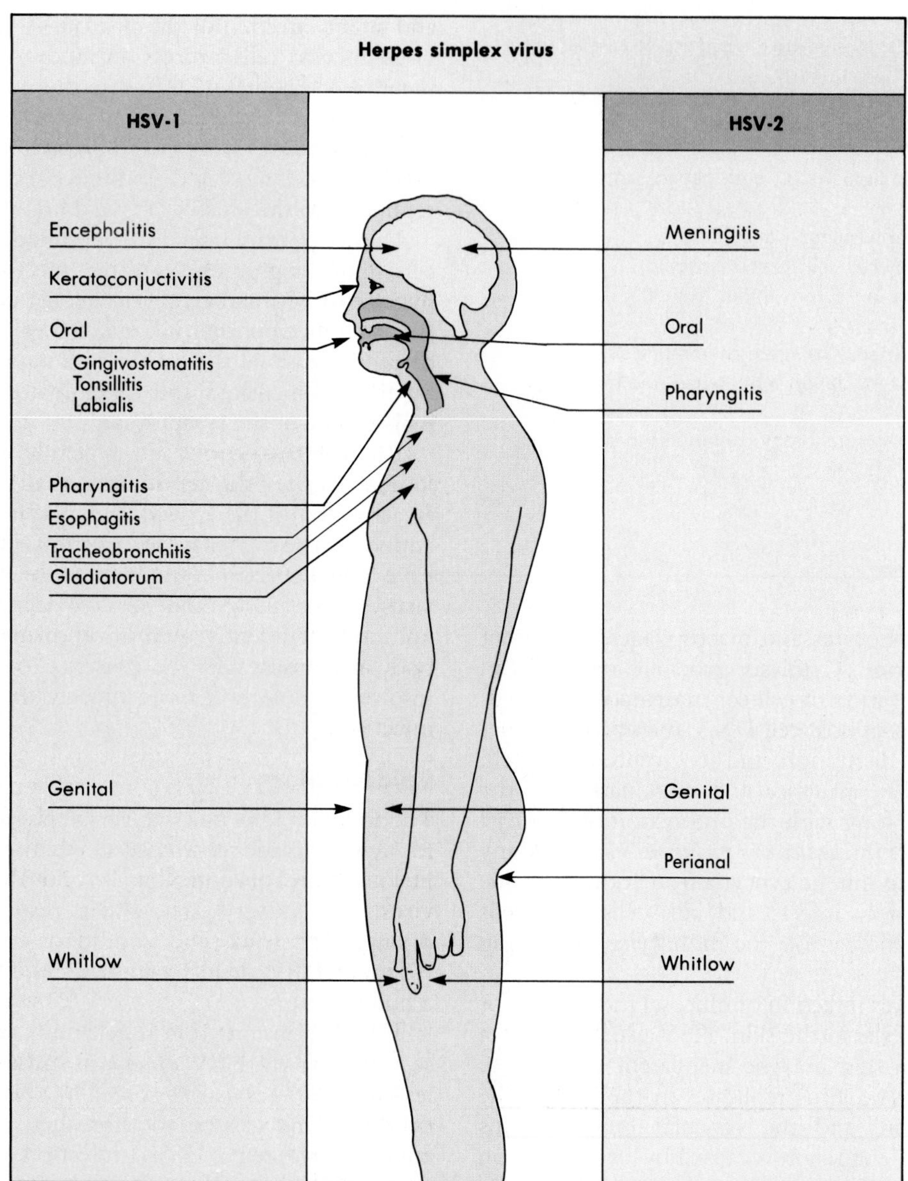

FIGURE 56-3. Disease syndromes of herpes simplex viruses. HSV-1 and HSV-2 can infect the same tissues and cause similar diseases but have a predilection for the sites and diseases indicated.

to HSV-2 ranges from less than 1% for college freshmen to 15% to 20% for the middle and higher socioeconomic population of adults, 40% to 60% for lower socioeconomic groups, and 80% for prostitutes.

HSV-2 is seroepidemiologically associated with human cervical cancer, possibly as a cofactor with human papillomavirus or other agent. Partial inactivation of the HSV-2 genome with UV light will allow the virus to immortalize cells in tissue culture.

Clinical Syndromes

Both HSV-1 and HSV-2 are common human pathogens that can cause painful but benign presentations and recurrent disease. The classical presentation is a clear vesicle on an erythematous base (dew drop on a rose petal), which progresses to pustular lesions, ulcers, and crusted lesions. However, both viruses can cause significant morbidity and mortality upon infection of the eye, brain, and disseminated infection of an immunosuppressed individual or neonate (Figure 56-4).

Oral herpes can be caused by HSV-1 or HSV-2. Primary **herpetic gingivostomatitis** in toddlers and children is almost always caused by HSV-1, whereas young adults may be infected with either type 1 or type 2. Lesions begin as clear vesicles but rapidly become ulcerated. These whitish areas may be widely distributed throughout the mouth, involving the palate, pharynx, gingivae, buccal mucosa, and tongue (Figure 56-5).

BOX 56-3 Epidemiology of Herpes Simplex Virus Infection

DISEASE/VIRAL FACTORS

Causes lifelong infection
Recurrent disease is a source of contagion
May cause asymptomatic shedding

TRANSMISSION

Transmitted in saliva, vaginal secretions, and by contact with lesion fluid
Transmitted orally, sexually, and by placement into eyes and breaks in skin
HSV-1 is generally transmitted orally; HSV-2 by sexual transmission

WHO IS AT RISK?

Children and sexually active individuals for classic presentations of HSV-1 and HSV-2, respectively
Physicians, nurses, dentists, and others in contact with oral and genital secretions are at risk for infections of fingers (herpetic whitlow)
Immunocompromised and neonates at risk to disseminated, life-threatening disease

GEOGRAPHY/SEASON

Worldwide
No seasonal incidence

MODES OF CONTROL

Acyclovir, adenosine arabinosine, iododeoxyuridine, trifluridine
No vaccine is available
Health care workers: wear gloves to prevent herpetic whitlow
Patients with active genital lesions should refrain from intercourse until lesions are completely reepithelialized

Individuals may experience recurrent mucocutaneous herpes simplex infection (**cold sores**; Figure 56-6) even though they never had clinically apparent primary infection. Virus is generally activated from the trigeminal ganglia. The symptoms for a recurrent episode are less severe, more localized, and have a shorter course than a primary episode. **Herpes pharyngitis** is becoming a prevalent diagnosis for viral sore throats in young adults. Severe HSV **stomatitis**, resembling a primary gingivostomatitis, may occur in patients who are immunosuppressed by disease or therapy.

Herpetic keratitis is almost always limited to one eye. It can cause recurrent disease, leading to permanent scarring, corneal damage, and blindness.

Herpetic whitlow is an infection of the finger, and **herpes gladiatorum** is an infection of the body. The virus establishes infection through cuts or abrasions in the skin. Herpetic whitlow often occurs in nurses or physicians who attend to patients with HSV infections, in thumb-sucking children (Figure 56-7), and in individuals who have genital HSV infection. Herpes gladiatorum is often acquired during wrestling.

Eczema herpeticum is acquired by children with active eczema. The underlying disease promotes the spread of the infection along the skin and potentially to the adrenal glands, liver, and other organs.

Genital herpes can be caused by HSV-1 (responsible for 10% of genital infections) or HSV-2. Most primary genital infections are asymptomatic. When present, lesions vary in number and are usually painful. In males, lesions typically are found on the glans or shaft of the penis and occasionally in the urethra. In females, lesions may be seen on the vulva, vagina, cervix, perianal area, or inner thigh and are frequently accompanied by itching and mucoid vaginal discharge. In both sexes a primary infection may be accompanied by fever, malaise, myalgia, and inguinal adenitis, symptoms related to a transient viremia. The presence of antibody to HSV-1 will lessen the symptoms. The symptoms and time course of primary and recurrent genital herpes are compared in Figure 56-4.

Recurrent genital HSV disease is shorter and less severe than primary episodes. Recurrences result from reactivation of latent virus in a sacral ganglion. Almost all genital recurrences are caused by HSV-2. In approximately half the patients, recurrences may be preceded by a characteristic prodrome of burning or tingling in the area in which the lesions will erupt. Episodes of recurrence may be as frequent as every 2 to 3 weeks or may occur infrequently. Unfortunately, any infected patient may shed virus asymptomatically. These individuals may be important vectors for the spread of this virus.

HSV proctitis can occur in homosexual men. It is a painful disease in which lesions may be found in the lower rectum and anus.

HSV meningitis is most often a complication of genital HSV-2 infection. It occurs within 10 days of a primary infection. Patients develop extreme nuchal rigidity, as well as other signs of meningitis, such as headache, photophobia, and nausea. Symptoms resolve promptly on their own.

Herpes encephalitis is an acute febrile disease usually caused by HSV-1. The lesions are generally limited to one of the temporal lobes. Viral pathology and immunopathology cause the destruction of the temporal lobe and give rise to erythrocytes in the cerebrospinal fluid, seizures, focal neurological abnormalities, and other characteristics of viral encephalitis. Herpes encephalitis is the most common fatal sporadic encephalitis and is lethal in 50% of patients. The disease occurs at all ages and at any time of the year. Fortunately, there are only 300 to 1000 cases per year.

HSV infection in the neonate and newborn is a devastating and usually fatal disease, caused most often by HSV-2. It may be acquired in utero but more frequently is contracted during passage through the genital canal

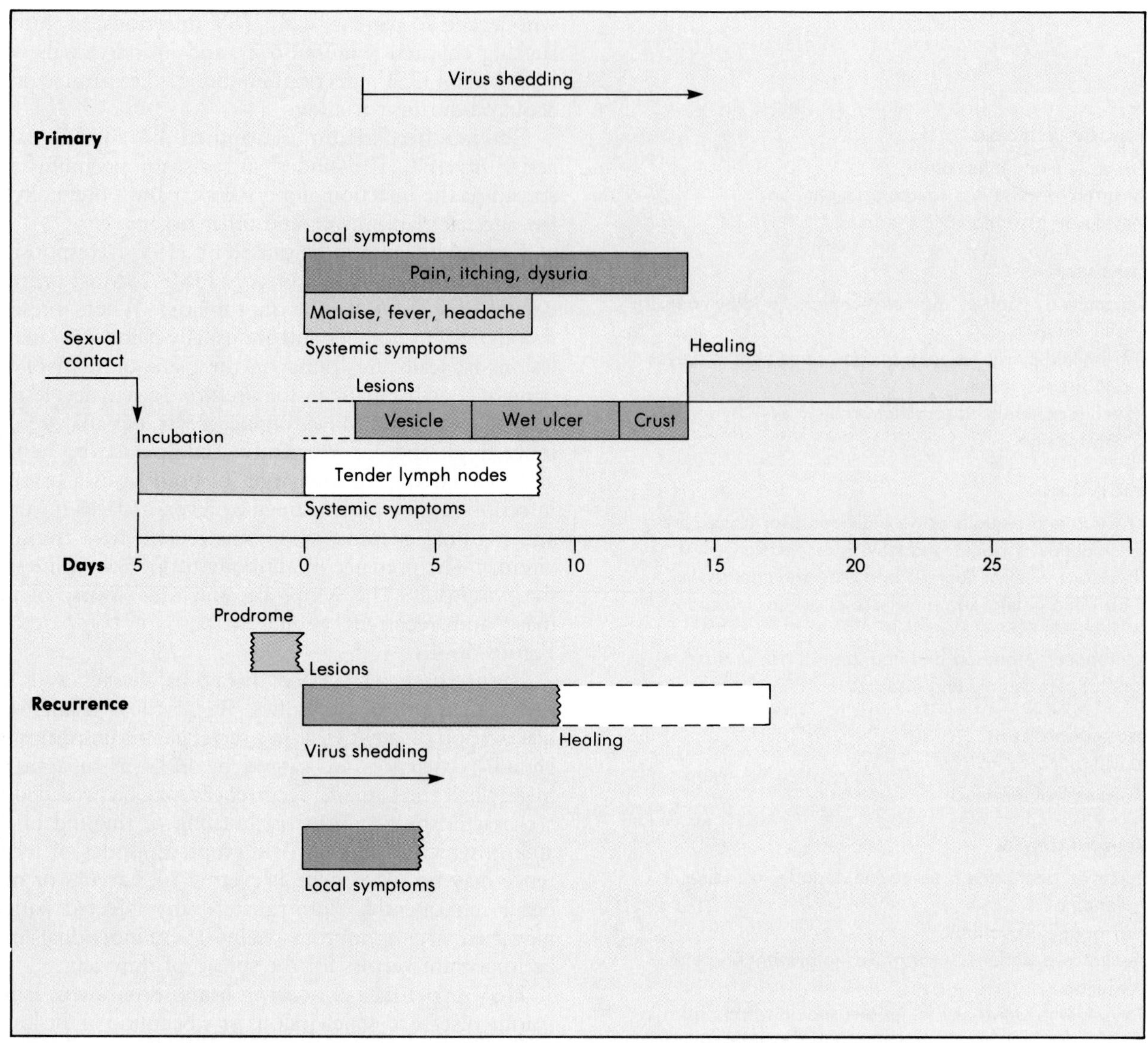

FIGURE 56-4 Clinical course of genital herpes infection. The time course and symptoms of primary and recurrent genital infection with HSV-2 are compared. *Top,* Primary infection. *Bottom,* Recurrent disease. (Data from Corey L et al: *Ann Intern Med* 98:958-973, 1983.)

when the mother is shedding herpesvirus at the time of delivery. In the absence of a developed cell-mediated immune response, HSV disseminates to the liver, lung, and other organs, as well as the central nervous system.

Laboratory Diagnosis

Cytology/Histology

The **Tzanck test** has been used to examine cells scraped from the base of herpes-like lesions (Table 56-2). The cells are smeared onto a slide, fixed, and stained with Wright or Giesma preparations. Syncytia, "ballooning" cytoplasm, and Cowdry's type A intranuclear inclusions are characteristic of HSV or VZV infection (see Figure 53-2). Cytologic examination is indicative but not definitive. A rapid definitive determination of HSV can be made by demonstrating virus antigen (immunofluorescence or immunoperoxidase) or DNA (in situ hybridization) in a Tzanck smear or biopsy.

Virus Isolation

Virus isolation is the most definitive assay for HSV infection. The highest rates of virus recovery are from, in order, vesicular lesions, pustular lesions, ulcers, and crusted lesions. Specimens are collected by aspiration of the lesion fluid or with a cotton swab and then inoculated directly into cell cultures.

HSV produces a cytopathic effect (CPE) within 1 to 3 days in HeLa, HEp-2, human embryonic fibroblasts, or rabbit kidney cells. HSV CPE begins with cytoplasmic granulation, after which the cells become enlarged and appear ballooned. The enlarged cells become rounded and then die (see Figure 53-4). Some isolates will induce

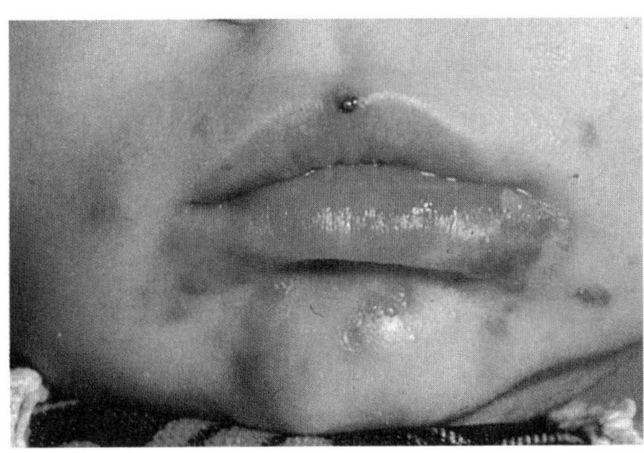

FIGURE 56-5 Primary herpes gingivostomatitis. (From Hart CA, Broadhead RL: *A color atlas of pediatric infectious diseases*, London, 1992, Mosby.)

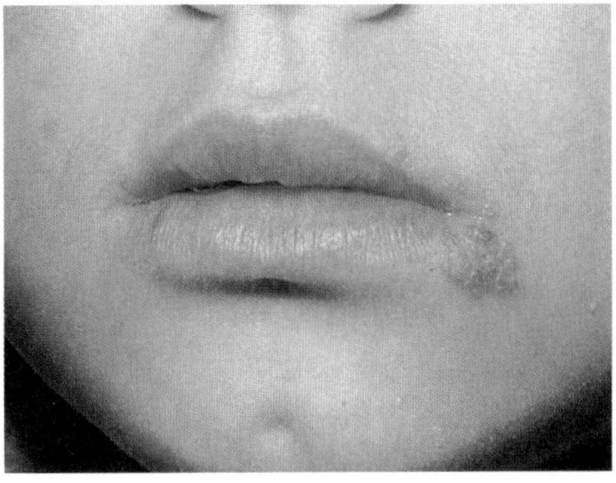

FIGURE 56-6 Cold sore of recurrent herpes labialis. (From Hart CA, Broadhead RL: *A color atlas of pediatric infectious diseases*, London, 1992, Mosby.)

fusion of neighboring cells, giving rise to multinucleated giant cells (syncitia).

Typing of HSV isolates can be performed by biochemical, biological, or immunological methods. The restriction endonuclease cleavage patterns of the DNA of HSV-1 and HSV-2 are unique and allow unequivocal typing of isolates. HSV type-specific DNA probes and antibodies are also available for detecting and differentiating HSV-1 and HSV-2.

Serology

Serologic procedures are useful only for diagnosing a primary HSV infection and for epidemiological studies. Serology is not useful for diagnosing recurrent disease because a significant rise in antibody titers does not usually accompany recurrent disease.

Treatment, Prevention, and Control

HSV encodes several target enzymes for antiviral drugs (Box 56-4). Most antiherpes drugs are nucleotide analogues or inhibitors of the viral DNA polymerase, an essential enzyme for virus replication and the best antiviral drug target. FDA-approved antiherpes compounds include acyclovir (ACV), foscarnet (phosphonoformic acid), vidarabine (adenosine arabinoside), idoxuridine (iododeoxyuridine), and trifluridine.

Acyclovir (ACV) is currently the most effective anti-HSV drug. ACV is activated by the viral thymidine kinase and then used as a substrate by the viral DNA polymerase. ACV is incorporated into, and prevents elongation of, the viral DNA. Acyclovir is effective in treating serious presentations of HSV disease, first episodes of genital herpes, and for prophylactic treatment. ACV is indicated for severe HSV syndromes such as neonatal disease, encephalitis, and extensive disease in the immunosuppressed patient. The drug is relatively nontoxic and can be administered prophylactically. The most prevalent form of resistance to ACV results from mutations that inactivate the thymidine kinase, thereby reducing conversion of the drug to its active form. Fortunately, resistant strains appear to be less virulent.

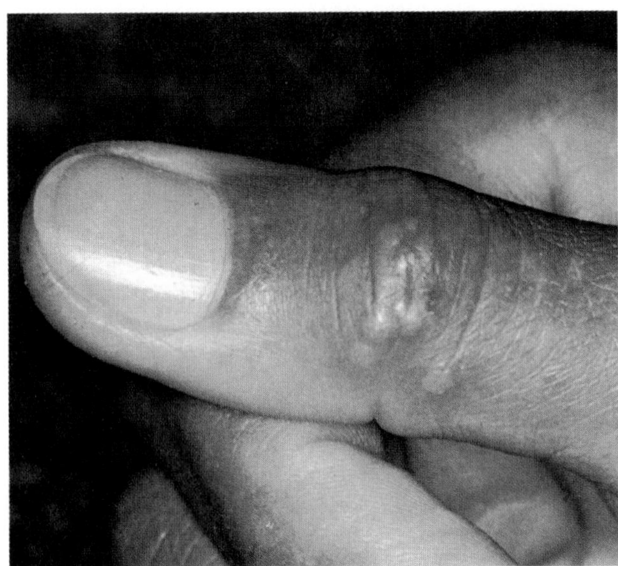

FIGURE 56-7 Herpetic whitlow. (From Emond RTD, Rowland HAK: *A color atlas of infectious diseases*, ed 2, London, 1987, Mosby.)

Adenine arabinoside (Ara A) is also approved for treatment of HSV infection. However, Ara A is less soluble, less potent, and more toxic than ACV. Trifluridine and acyclovir have replaced iododeoxyuridine as topical treatments of herpetic keratitis. Tromantadine, an amantadine derivative, is approved for topical use in countries other than the United States and inhibits penetration and syncytia formation. Topical interferon may also be effective against HSV. None of the treatments will prevent establishment or eliminate a latent infection.

HSV-1 is transmitted most often from an active mucocutaneous lesion, so avoidance of direct contact

TABLE 56-2 Laboratory Diagnosis of HSV Infections

Approach	Test/Comment
Direct microscopic examination of cells from base of lesion	Tzanck smear showing multinucleated giant cells and Cowdry's type A inclusion bodies
Cell culture	HSV replicates and causes identifiable CPE in most cell cultures
Assay of tissue biopsy, smear, or vesicular fluid for HSV antigen	Enzyme immunoassay, immunofluorescent stain, in situ DNA probe analysis
HSV type distinction (HSV-1 vs. HSV-2)	Type-specific antibody, DNA maps of restriction enzyme digests, SDS-gel protein patterns, DNA probe analysis
Serology	Epidemiology

BOX 56-4 FDA-Approved Antiviral Treatments for Herpesvirus Infections

HERPES SIMPLEX VIRUS 1 AND 2

Acyclovir
Adenosine arabinoside
Iododeoxyuridine
Trifluridine

VARICELLA ZOSTER VIRUS

Acyclovir
Varicella zoster immune globulin (VZIG)
Zoster immune plasma (ZIP)

EPSTEIN-BARR VIRUS

None

CYTOMEGALOVIRUS

Ganciclovir*
Foscarnet*

*Also inhibits HSV and VZV.

with these will reduce infection. Unfortunately, the symptoms may be inapparent, and thus the virus can be transmitted unknowingly.

Physicians, nurses, dentists, and technicians must be especially careful when handling potentially infected tissue or fluids. Gloves can prevent acquisition of infections of the fingers (herpetic whitlow). Individuals with recurrent herpetic whitlow disease are very contagious and can spread infection to patients. Virus is readily disinfected by washing with soap.

Patients who have a history of genital HSV infection must be instructed to refrain from sexual intercourse when prodromal symptoms or lesions occur. They can resume sexual intercourse only after lesions are completely reepithelialized because virus can be isolated from lesions even when crusted. Condoms may be useful and undoubtedly better than nothing but may not be fully protective.

If a pregnant woman has active genital HSV at term and the membranes are not ruptured, cesarean section provides a means of preventing contact of the infant with the virus-infected lesions. Unfortunately, as mentioned previously, the virus may be asymptomatically present in genital secretions, and a vaginally delivered infant may be exposed to virus during the delivery.

Killed, subunit, and vaccinia hybrid vaccines have been developed and are still being evaluated. Vaccination might prevent acquisition or establishment of latency or may ameliorate recurrences.

VARICELLA ZOSTER VIRUS

Varicella zoster virus (VZV) causes chickenpox (varicella) and with recurrence causes herpes zoster, or shingles. VZV shares many characteristics with HSV, including (1) the ability to establish latent infection of neurons and recurrent disease at the innervated dermatome, (2) the importance of cell-mediated immunity in controlling and preventing serious disease, and (3) the characteristic blister-like lesions of the disease. Unlike HSV, the predominant means of spreading VZV is by the respiratory route. After local replication in the respiratory tract, viremia occurs, leading to skin lesions over the entire body.

Structure and Replication

VZV has the smallest genome of the human herpesviruses, 124,900 base pairs, but each gene in VZV is represented by a counterpart in HSV. VZV replicates slower and in fewer types of cells than HSV. Human diploid fibroblasts in vitro and epithelial cells in vivo will support VZV replication. VZV establishes latent infection of neurons, as does HSV.

Pathogenesis and Immunity

Primary VZV infection begins in the mucosa of the respiratory tract and then progresses via the bloodstream and lymphatics to cells of the reticuloendothelial system

(Box 56-5; Figures 56-8 and 56-9). After 11 to 13 days, a secondary viremia spreads the virus through the body and to the skin. The virus causes a dermal vesiculopustular rash that develops in successive crops. Fever and systemic symptoms occur with the rash.

Following primary infection, the virus becomes latent in the dorsal root or cranial nerve ganglia. Reactivation occurs in older adults or in patients with impaired cellular immunity. On reactivation, the virus migrates along neural pathways to the skin, where a vesicular rash known as herpes zoster, or shingles, develops.

Antibody is important in limiting the viremic spread of VZV, but cell-mediated immunity is essential for limiting the progression and resolving the disease. The overzealous cell-mediated immune response of adults causes more extensive cell damage and a more severe presentation (especially in the lung) upon primary infection than for children. In the absence of cell-mediated immunity (CMI), the virus causes more disseminated serious disease.

BOX 56-5 Disease Mechanisms of VZV

- Initial replication in respiratory tract
- Tissue tropism includes most epithelial and fibroblast cells
- VZV can form syncytia and spread directly from cell to cell
- Latent infection of neurons occurs, usually dorsal root and cranial nerve ganglia
- Systemic spread of virus through viremia to the skin causes lesions in successive crops
- VZV can escape antibody clearance, and cell-mediated immune response is essential to control infection. Disseminated life-threatening disease can occur in immunocompromised individuals. Recurrence (herpes zoster) can be prompted by immunosuppression
- Herpes zoster may result from depression of cell-mediated immunity, although other mechanisms of viral activation may come into play.

Epidemiology

VZV is extremely communicable, with rates of infection greater than 90% among susceptible household contacts (Box 56-6). The disease is spread principally by the respiratory route but may also be spread by contact with skin vesicles. Primary VZV infection occurs throughout childhood, and more than 90% of adults in developed countries have VZV antibody. Herpes zoster results from reactivation of a patient's latent endogenous virus and not as an epidemic outbreak. Approximately 10% to 20% of the population infected with VZV develop zoster; the incidence parallels advancing age. Zoster lesions contain viable virus and therefore may be a source of varicella infection in a nonimmune individual (child).

Clinical Syndromes

Varicella (chickenpox) results from a primary infection with VZV; it is usually a mild disease of childhood and is usually symptomatic, although asymptomatic infection may occur (Figure 56-9). Varicella is characterized by fever and a maculopapular rash after an incubation period of about 14 days (Figure 56-10). Within hours, each maculopapular lesion forms a thin-walled vesicle on a maculopapular base (dew drop on a rose petal) that measures approximately 2 to 4 mm in diameter. This vesicle is the hallmark of varicella. Within 12 hours the vesicle becomes pustular and begins to crust, and then scabbed lesions appear. Successive crops of lesions appear for 3 to 5 days, and at any given time all stages of skin lesions can be observed.

The rash is generalized, more severe on the trunk than on the extremities, and notably present on the scalp, which distinguishes it from many other diseases. The

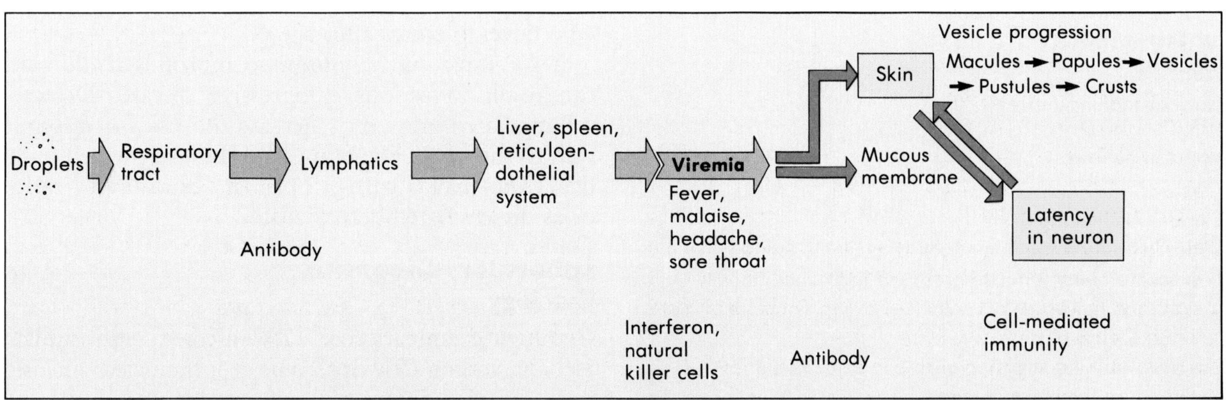

FIGURE 56-8 Mechanism of spread of VZV within the body. VZV initially infects the respiratory tract and is spread by the reticuloendothelial system and by viremia to other parts of the body. The spread can be blocked by the immune response at the stages indicated below the progression.

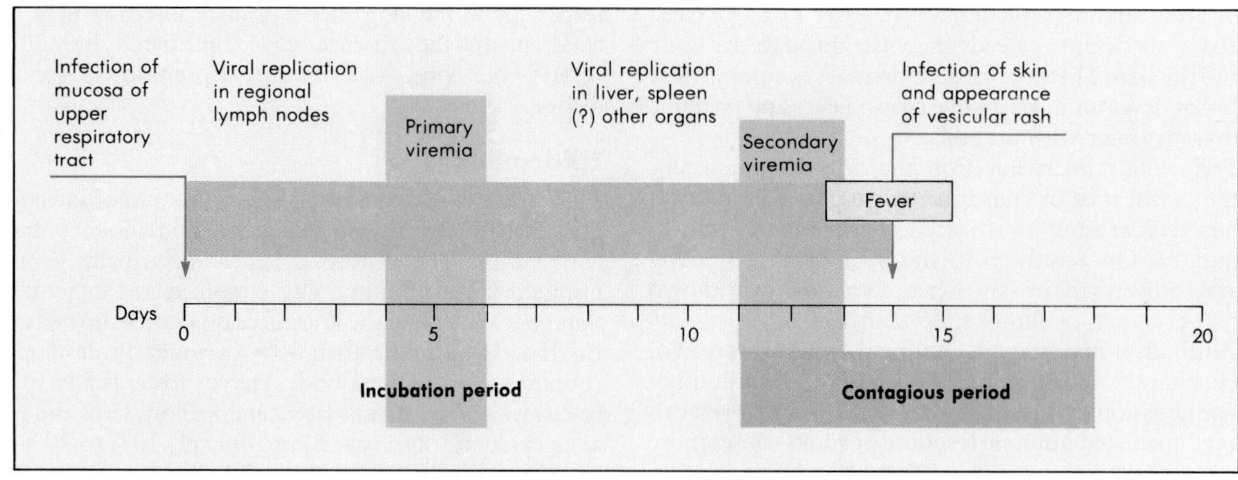

FIGURE 56-9 Time course of varicella (chickenpox). The course of disease in young children, as presented in this figure, is generally shorter and less severe than in adults.

BOX 56-6 Epidemiology of Varicella Zoster Virus Infection

DISEASE/VIRAL FACTORS

Causes lifelong infection
Recurrent disease is a source of contagion

TRANSMISSION

Mainly by respiratory droplets but also by direct contact

WHO IS AT RISK?

Children (age 5-9): mild classic disease
Teens and adults: more severe disease with potential pneumonia
Immune compromised and newborns: life-threatening pneumonia, encephalitis, and progressive-disseminated varicella
Elderly and immunocompromised: recurrent disease (zoster [shingles])

GEOGRAPHY/SEASON

Worldwide
No seasonal incidence

MODES OF CONTROL

Acyclovir
Immunity is lifelong
Varicella zoster immunoglobulin is available following exposure of immunocompromised individual, house staff, and newborns of mothers showing symptoms within 5 days of birth
Live vaccine (Oka strain) available in some countries other than the United States

lesions cause itching and scratching, which may lead to bacterial superinfection and scarring. Mucous membrane lesions in the mouth, conjunctivae, and vagina typically occur. Thrombocytopenia may also develop occasionally; in this case the rash may be hemorrhagic in nature.

Primary infection of adults is usually more severe than for children. **Interstitial pneumonia** may occur in 20% to 30% of adult patients and may be fatal. Extremely severe disseminated infection occurs in immunocompromised individuals.

Herpes zoster is a recurrence of a latent varicella infection acquired earlier in life. The appearance of chickenpox-like lesions is usually preceded by severe pain in the area innervated by the nerve. The rash is usually limited to a dermatome. It appears as small closely spaced maculopapular lesions on an erythematous base in contrast to the more diffuse pattern of vesicles characteristic of varicella (Figure 56-11). A chronic pain syndrome referred to as **postherpetic neuralgia**, which can persist for months to years, occurs in as many as 30% of patients who develop zoster after age 65.

VZV infection of immunocompromised individuals can result in serious, progressive disease. Defects in cell-mediated immunity increase the risk for dissemination to the lungs, the brain, and the liver, which may be fatal. This may occur with primary exposure to varicella or as disseminated herpes zoster.

Laboratory Diagnosis

Cytology

Cytologic examination of VZV-infected cells is similar to HSV including Cowdry's type A intranuclear inclusions and syncytia. These cells may be seen in skin lesions, respiratory specimens, or organ biopsies. Syncytia may also be seen in Tzanck smears of scrapings of a vesicle's base. Skin lesion scrapes or biopsies can also be analyzed by direct fluorescent antibody examination for membrane

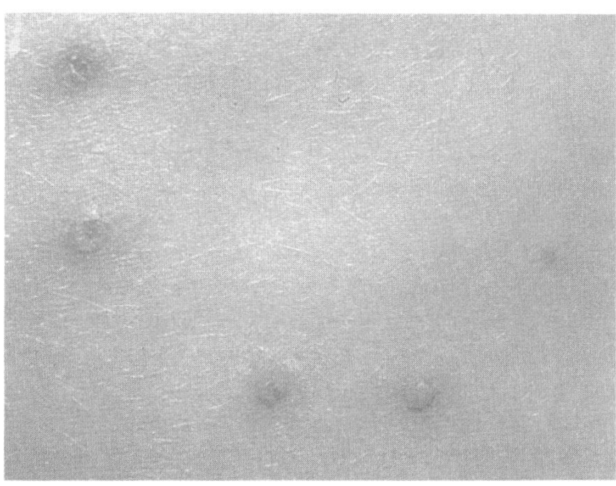

FIGURE 56-10 Characteristic skin rash of varicella demonstrating all of the stages of evolution of the rash. (From Hart CA, Broadhead RL: *A color atlas of pediatric infectious diseases*, London, 1992, Mosby.)

antigens (FAMA). Antigen detection is a more sensitive diagnostic technique for VZV infection than virus isolation.

Virus Isolation

Isolation of VZV in cell culture is difficult because the virus is labile during transportation to the laboratory and replicates poorly in vitro. Once skin lesions are crusted (5 or more days after onset), cultures are usually negative, but antigen can still be detected by FA or other immunological tests. Human diploid fibroblasts will support VZV replication and exhibit CPE similar to HSV but after a longer incubation period.

Serology

Serologic tests to detect antibodies to VZV are used to screen for immunity to VZV and document active VZV infection. Antibody levels are normally low and require analysis by sensitive tests, such as immunofluorescence or enzyme linked immunosorbent assay (ELISA). IgM and a significant antibody increase can be detected in individuals experiencing herpes zoster.

Treatment, Prevention, and Control

No treatment is indicated for varicella in children. Acyclovir has been approved as a possible means for treating serious VZV infections. However, the VZV DNA polymerase is much less sensitive to ACV, requiring large doses of drug and intravenous treatment (see Box 56-4).

As with other respiratory viruses, limiting transmission of VZV is difficult. Since VZV infection of children is generally mild and induces lifelong immunity, exposure to VZV early in life is often encouraged. High-risk individuals (e.g., immunosuppressed children) should be protected from exposure to VZV.

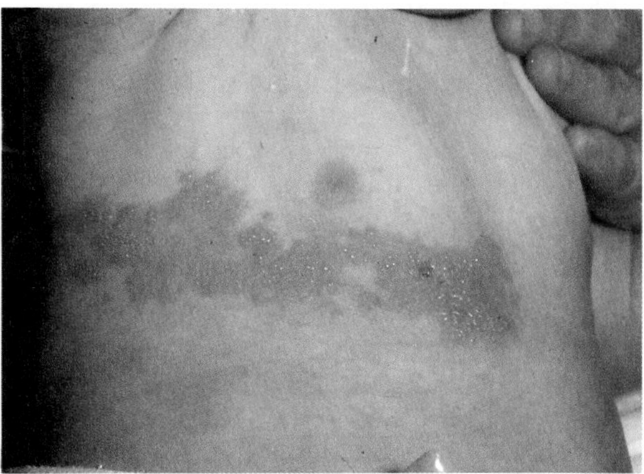

FIGURE 56-11 Herpes zoster in a thoracic dermatome.

VZV disease may be prevented or ameliorated in immunosuppressed patients susceptible to severe disease by administration of **varicella zoster immunoglobulin (VZIG)**. VZIG is prepared by pooling plasma from seropositive individuals. VZIG is ineffective as a therapy for patients suffering active varicella or herpes zoster disease.

A live attenuated vaccine for VZV (Oka strain) has been developed and licensed in several countries other than the United States. The vaccine induces protective or ameliorating antibody and is effective as a prophylactic treatment even after exposure to VZV. Most significantly, it promotes protection in immunodeficient children.

EPSTEIN-BARR VIRUS

Epstein-Barr virus (EBV) was discovered by electron microscopic observation of characteristic herpes virions in biopsies of an African Burkitt's lymphoma. Discovery of its association with infectious mononucleosis was accidental when serum collected from a laboratory technician during her convalescence from infectious mononucleosis demonstrated antibody that recognized African Burkitt's lymphoma cells. This finding was later confirmed in a large serologic study performed on college students.

EBV causes heterophile antibody positive infectious mononucleosis and has been causally associated with African Burkitt's lymphoma (endemic BL) and nasopharyngeal carcinoma. EBV has also been associated with B-cell lymphomas in patients with acquired or congenital immunodeficiencies. EBV is a mitogen for B lymphocytes and immortalizes B cells in tissue culture.

Structure and Replication

Epstein-Barr virus is a gamma-herpesvirus with a genome of 172,000 base pairs. EBV has a very limited host range and tissue tropism defined by the limited cellular expression of its receptor. This receptor is also the receptor for the C3d component of the complement system (also called CR2 or CD21). It is expressed on B lymphocytes of humans and New World monkeys and epithelial cells of the oropharynx and nasopharynx.

EBV infection has three potential outcomes: replication in epithelial cells permissive for EBV replication; latent infection of B lymphocytes in the presence of competent T lymphocytes; or stimulation and immortalization of B cells. B cells are semipermissive for EBV replication.

Different viral transcription programs are initiated for the latent and lytic infections. During latent infection, cells contain a small number of circular plasmid-like EBV genomes that replicate only during cell division. Select immediate early genes are expressed including Epstein-Barr virus nuclear antigens (EBNA) 1, 2, 3A, 3B, and 3C; LP; latent membrane protein-1 (LMP-1); LMP-2; and two small RNA molecules: EBER 1 and EBER 2. The EBNA and LP proteins are DNA-binding proteins that are essential for establishing an infection (EBNA 1), immortalization (EBNA 2), and other purposes. The LMP proteins are membrane proteins with oncogene-like activities.

Permissive cells allow the transcription and translation of the ZEBRA peptide, which activates the early genes of the virus and the lytic cycle. Following synthesis of the DNA polymerase and DNA replication, the viral capsid and glycoproteins of the virus are synthesized. These include the gp350/220 (related glycoproteins of 350,000 d and 220,000 d), which is the viral attachment protein, and gp85 (85,000 d).

BOX 56-7 Disease Mechanisms of Epstein-Barr Virus

- Virus in saliva initiates infection of oral epithelia and spreads to B cells in lymphatic tissue
- Productive infection in epithelial cells
- Promotes growth of B lymphocytes (immortalizes)
- T cells kill/control B-cell outgrowth and promote latency in B cells. *Required for controlling infection.* Antibody role is limited.
- T-cell response (lymphocytosis) contributes to **infectious mononucleosis** symptoms
- Causative association with lymphoma/leukemia in T-cell deficient individuals and African children living in malarial regions (African Burkitt's lymphoma) and nasopharyngeal carcinoma in China

Pathogenesis and Immunity

The virus establishes a productive infection in the epithelial cells of the oropharynx (Box 56-7; Figure 56-12). The virus is shed into the saliva and accesses B lymphocytes in lymphatic tissue and blood. Lytic infection leads to the production of EBV proteins, including the early antigens (EA), viral capsid antigen (VCA), and the glycoproteins of the membrane antigen (MA) (Table 56-3). A characteristic lymphocyte-defined membrane antigen (LYDMA) is an antigen recognized by T lymphocytes.

Infection of B cells in cell culture generally causes no visible change in the histology of the cell. However, EBV is a B-cell mitogen that will stimulate growth, prevent apoptosis (programmed cell death) and immortalize the cells. B cells isolated from a patient with infectious mononucleosis are also immortalized and grow into cell lines in the absence of T-cell suppression.

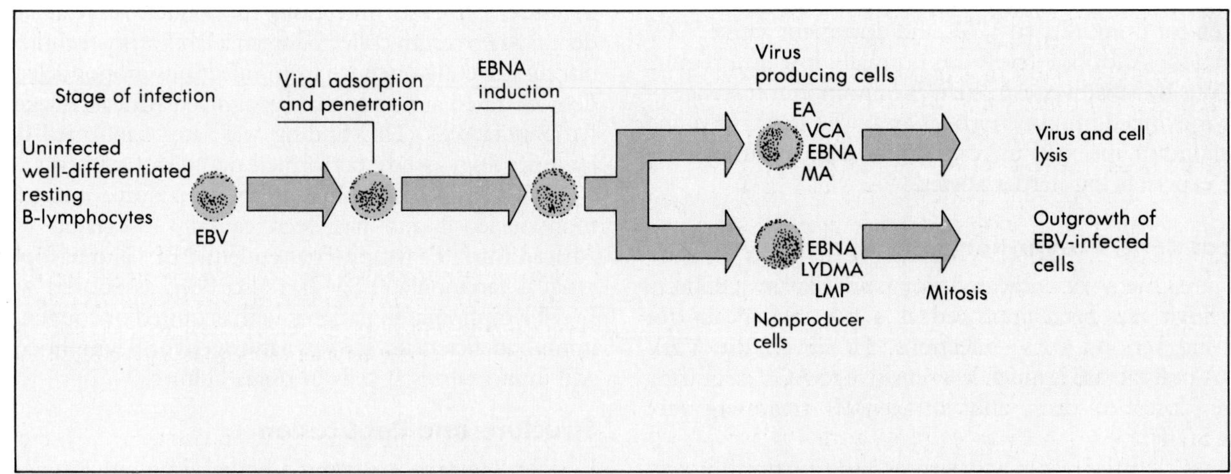

FIGURE 56-12 Progression of EBV infection. EBV infection may result in lytic or immortalizing infection, which can be distinguished by the production of virus and the expression of different viral proteins and antigens. T lymphocytes limit the outgrowth of the EBV-infected cells. *EBNA*, Epstein-Barr nuclear antigen; *EA*, early antigen; *VCA*, viral capsid antigen; *MA*, membrane antigen; *LMP*, latent membrane protein; *LYDMA*, lymphocyte defined membrane antigen.

TABLE 56-3 Cellular Antigens Associated With EBV-Infected Cells

Antigen				
Name	**Abbreviation**	**Cellular location**	**Biological association**	**Clinical association**
EBV nuclear antigen	EBNA	Nuclear	Nonstructural antigens; first antigens to appear; seen in all infected and transformed cells; binds to cell DNA	Anti-EBNA develops late in infection
Early antigen	EA-R	Restricted to cytoplasm	EA-R appears before EA-D; first sign that infected cell has entered lytic cycle	Anti–EA-R seen in Burkitt's lymphoma; anti–EA-D seen in infectious mononucleosis
	EA-D	Diffuse in cytoplasm and nucleus		
Viral capsid antigen	VCA	Cytoplasmic	Late antigen; found in virus producer cells	Anti-VCA IgM transient; anti-VCA IgG persistent
Lymphocyte-defined membrane antigen	LYDMA		Not found on Burkitt's lymphoma cells; found on cells infected in vitro and transformed; found on nonproducer cells	Not detectable by antibody
Membrane antigen	MA	Cell surface	Envelope glycoproteins	Same as VCA

EBV infection of the B cell alters its interaction with the rest of the immune system, as well as stimulating its growth. EBV enhances the expression of cell surface proteins such as HLA, adhesion proteins and the CD23 blast antigen. EBV also encodes an analogue of interleukin-10 (BCRF-1), which promotes immune escape by inhibiting γ-interferon secretion and early T-cell responses to the virus and by promoting B cell growth and IgG synthesis. EBV also promotes B-cell secretion of interleukin-5 and interleukin-6.

Infectious mononucleosis results from a civil war between the EBV-infected B cells and the protective T cells. The classical lymphocytosis (increase in mononuclear cells) associated with infectious mononucleosis is mainly due to activation and proliferation of suppressor (CD8) T cells. These appear as atypical lymphocytes (also called *Downey cells*; Figure 56-13). They increase in the peripheral blood during the second week of infection, accounting for 10% to 80% of the total white cells. The large T-cell response causes the swollen lymph glands, spleen, and liver, which occur later in the disease.

T cells limit the proliferation of EBV-infected B cells in tissue culture and are essential in controlling the disease (Figure 56-14). Individuals with impaired cell-mediated immunity have difficulty resolving an EBV infection, and chronic infections may result. The absence of effective T-cell control allows EBV-induced B-cell proliferation. Continued B-cell proliferation in conjunction with other cofactors may result in lymphoma.

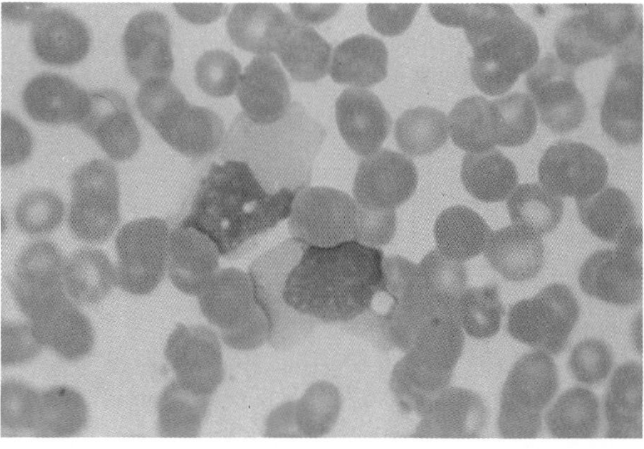

FIGURE 56-13 Atypical T-lymphocyte (Downey cells) characteristic of infectious mononucleosis. The cells have a more basophilic and vacuolated cytoplasm than normal lymphocytes, and the nucleus may be oval, kidney shaped, or lobulated. The cell margin may seem to be indented by neighboring red blood cells.

Epidemiology

EBV infection is transmitted in saliva (Box 56-8). More than 90% of EBV-infected individuals intermittently shed the virus for life, even when totally asymptomatic.

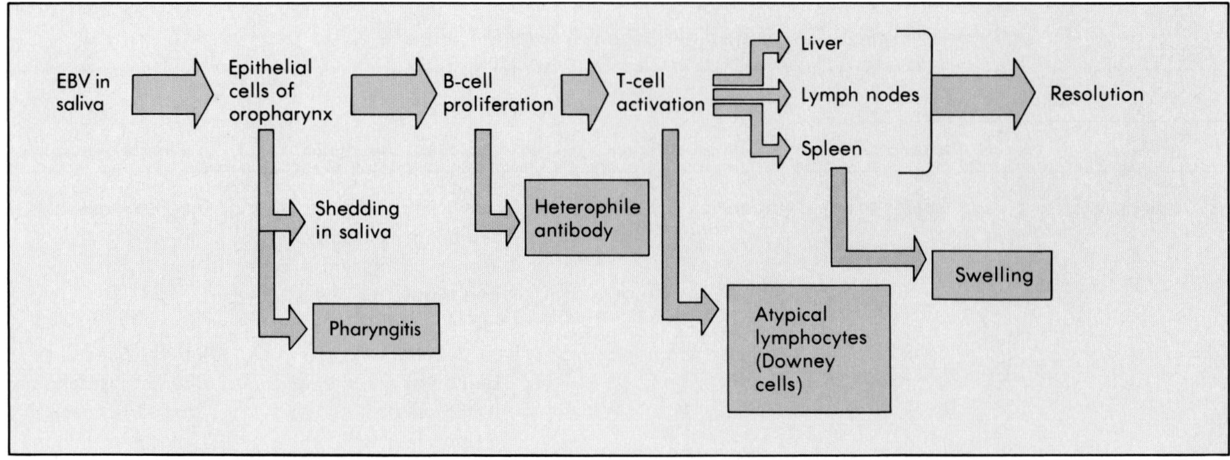

FIGURE 56-14 Pathogenesis of EBV. EBV is acquired by close contact between persons through saliva and infects the B lymphocytes. The resolution of the EBV infection and many of the symptoms of infectious mononucleosis result from activation of T lymphocytes in response to the infection.

BOX 56-8 Epidemiology of Epstein-Barr Virus Infection

DISEASE/VIRAL FACTORS

Causes lifelong infection
Recurrent disease is a source of contagion
May cause asymptomatic shedding

TRANSMISSION

Via saliva, close oral contact (kissing disease), or sharing toothbrushes, cups, etc.

WHO IS AT RISK?

Children may be asymptomatic or have mild symptoms
Teenagers and adults have infectious mononucleosis
Immunocompromised individuals at highest risk to life-threatening neoplastic disease

GEOGRAPHY/SEASON

Worldwide distribution of infectious mononucleosis
Causative association with African Burkitt's lymphoma in malarial belt of Africa
Causative association with nasopharyngeal carcinoma in China
No seasonal incidence

MODES OF CONTROL

None

Children can acquire the virus at an early age by sharing contaminated drinking glasses and generally undergo subclinical disease. Saliva sharing between adolescents and young adults often occurs by kissing, thus the nickname the "kissing disease." Disease in these individuals may be unnoticed or present in varying degrees of severity as infectious mononucleosis. Approximately 70% of the population of the United States has been infected by age 30.

The geographical distribution of EBV-associated neoplasms suggests an association with potential co-factors. The immunosuppressive potential of malaria has been suggested as a cofactor in the progression of chronic or latent EBV infection to African Burkitt's lymphoma. The restriction of nasopharyngeal carcinoma to certain regions of China has suggested a genetic predisposition to the cancer or possibly the presence of co-factors in the food or environment.

Transplant patients, AIDS patients, and genetically immunodeficient individuals are at high risk for lymphoproliferative disorders initiated by EBV. These may appear as polyclonal and monoclonal B-cell lymphomas. These individuals are also at high risk for a productive infection presenting as hairy oral leukoplakia.

Clinical Syndromes

Infectious Mononucleosis (IM)

As with other herpesviruses, EBV infection of a child is much milder than infection of adolescents or adults. Infection of children is usually subclinical. Infectious mononucleosis is characterized by fever, malaise, pharyngitis, lymphadenopathy, and often hepatosplenomegaly. The major complaint of persons with infectious mononucleosis is fatigue (Figure 56-15). The disease is rarely fatal in normal individuals but can cause serious complications resulting from neurological disorders, laryngeal obstruction, or rupture of the spleen. Neurological complications can include meningoencephalitis and the Guillain-Barré syndrome. Heterophile-negative "mononucleosis" is likely to be caused by CMV if the patient is 25 years of age or older.

Chronic EBV Disease

EBV can cause cyclical recurrent disease in some individuals. These patients have chronic tiredness and may also have low-grade fever, headaches, and sore throat. This is different from chronic fatigue syndrome, which has another etiology.

EBV-Induced Lymphoproliferative Disease

Individuals lacking T-cell immunity are likely to suffer life-threatening polyclonal leukemia-like B-cell proliferative disease and lymphoma upon EBV infection instead of IM. Individuals with congenital deficiency of T-lymphocyte function are likely to suffer life-threatening **X-linked lymphoproliferative disorder (XLP)**. Transplant patients undergoing immunosuppression are at high risk for **post-transplant lymphoproliferative disorder (PTLD)** instead of IM or following reactivation of latent virus. Similar diseases are observed for AIDS patients.

African (endemic) Burkitt's Lymphoma (AfBL)

African Burkitt's lymphoma is a poorly differentiated monoclonal B-cell lymphoma of the jaw and face that is endemic to children of the malarial regions of Africa. The tumors contain EBV DNA sequences but express only the EBNA 1 viral antigen. Virions can occasionally be seen by electron microscopy. In addition to EBV DNA, the tumor cells contain chromosomal translocations that juxtapose the c-myc oncogene to a very active promotor (e.g., immunoglobulin gene promotor [t(8;14), t(8;22), t(8;2]). The tumor cells are also relatively invisible to immune control. How malaria acts to promote EBV involvement with AfBL is not known. EBV is associated with Burkitt's lymphomas in other parts of the world, but to a much lesser extent.

Nasopharyngeal Carcinoma

This tumor is endemic to the Orient, occurs in adults, and also contains EBV DNA within tumor cells. Unlike Burkitt's lymphoma, where the tumor cells are derived from lymphocytes, the nasopharyngeal carcinoma tumor cells are of epithelial origin.

Hairy Oral Leukoplakia

Hairy oral leukoplakia is an unusual presentation of a productive EBV infection that causes lesions of the mouth. It is an opportunistic presentation in AIDS patients (Figure 56-16).

Laboratory Diagnosis

EBV-induced infectious mononucleosis is usually documented by the demonstration of atypical lymphocytes, heterophile antibody, and positive serologic findings. Virus isolation is not practical. DNA probe analysis and immunofluorescent detection of virus antigens are used to detect evidence of virus.

Atypical lymphocytes are probably the earliest detectable indication of an EBV infection, although they are not specific for EBV. These cells are present with the onset of symptoms and disappear with resolution of the disease.

Heterophile antibody is produced by the nonspecific, mitogen-like activation of B cells by EBV and production of a wide repertoire of antibodies. These antibodies include an IgM heterophile antibody that recognizes the Paul-Bunnell antigen on sheep and bovine erythrocytes but not guinea pig kidney cells. The heterophile antibody response can usually be detected by the end of the first week of illness and lasts for as long as several months. It is an excellent indication of EBV in adults but is not as reliable for children or infants. The **monospot** and other tests are more rapid and widely used for heterophile antibody.

Serologic tests are useful when EBV infections cannot be diagnosed by the usual clinical criteria and heterophile antibody tests (see Figure 56-15 and Table 56-4). Recent EBV infection is suggested by any of the following: (1) IgM antibody to VCA, (2) presence of VCA antibody and absence of EBNA, (3) rising titer of EBNA, or (4) presence of elevated VCA and EA antibodies. Presence of *both* VCA and EBNA antibody in an acute- or convalescent-phase serum suggests a past infection.

Treatment, Prevention, and Control

No effective treatment is available for EBV disease (see Box 56-4). The ubiquitous nature of EBV makes control of infection difficult. Quarantine of infected individuals is also difficult because of asymptomatic shedding of virus. Infection elicits lifelong immunity. The best means of preventing infectious mononucleosis is exposure to the virus early in life because the disease is more benign in children. An anti-EBV vaccine is being developed that may prevent African Burkitt's lymphoma and infectious mononucleosis.

CYTOMEGALOVIRUS

CMV is a common human pathogen, infecting 0.5% to 2.5% of all newborns and approximately 50% of the adult population in developed countries. It is the most common viral cause of congenital defects. CMV becomes particularly prominent as a pathogen in immunocompromised patients.

Structure and Replication

CMV is a member of the beta-herpesviruses. It has the largest genome of the human herpesviruses. Human CMV replicates only in human cells. Fibroblasts and macrophages are permissive for CMV replication. CMV establishes latent infection in mononuclear lymphocytes, stromal cells of the bone marrow, and other cells.

Pathogenesis and Immunity

In general the pathogenesis of CMV is similar to that of other herpesviruses (Box 56-9). CMV shares the capacity for (1) cell-to-cell spread in the presence of circulating antibody, (2) establishment of a latent state in the host,

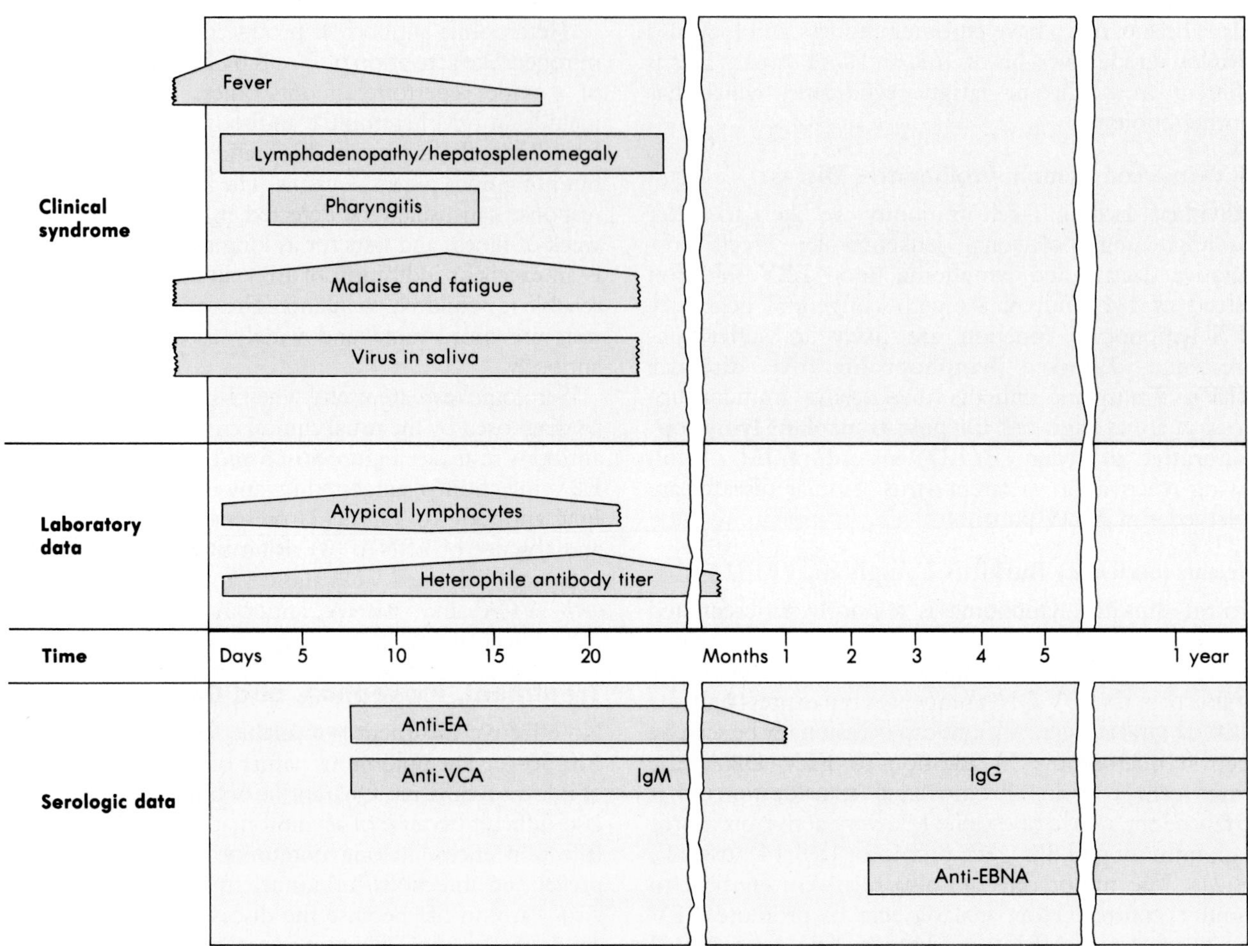

FIGURE 56-15 Clinical course and laboratory findings of infectious mononucleosis. EBV infection may be asymptomatic or produce the symptoms of mononucleosis. The incubation period can be as long as 2 months.

TABLE 56-4 Serologic Profile for EBV Infections

Patient's clinical status	Heterophile antibodies	EBV-specific antibodies: VCA-IgM	VCA-IgG	EA	EBNA	Comment
Susceptible	–	–	–	–	–	
Acute primary	+	+	+	±	–	
Chronic primary	–	–	+	+	–	
Past infection	–	–	+	–	+	
Reactivation infection	–	–	+	+	+	EA restricted or diffuse
Burkitt's lymphoma	–	–	+	+	+	EA restricted only
Nasopharyngeal carcinoma	–	–	+	+	+	EA diffuse only

Modified from Balows A, Hausler WJ Jr, and Lennette EH, editors: *Laboratory diagnosis of infectious diseases: principles and practices,* New York, 1988, Springer-Verlag.

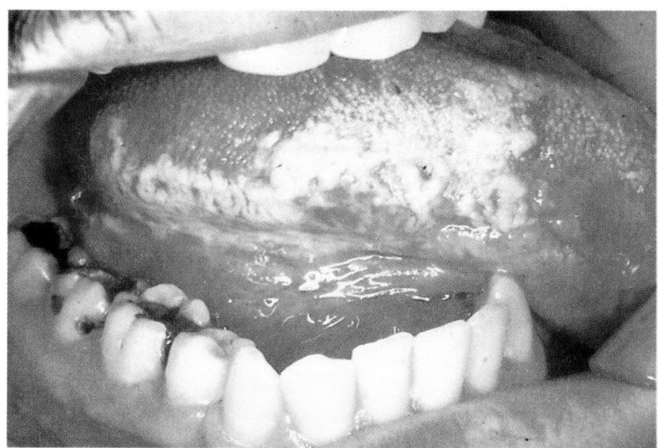

FIGURE 56-16 Hairy leukoplakia caused by EBV.

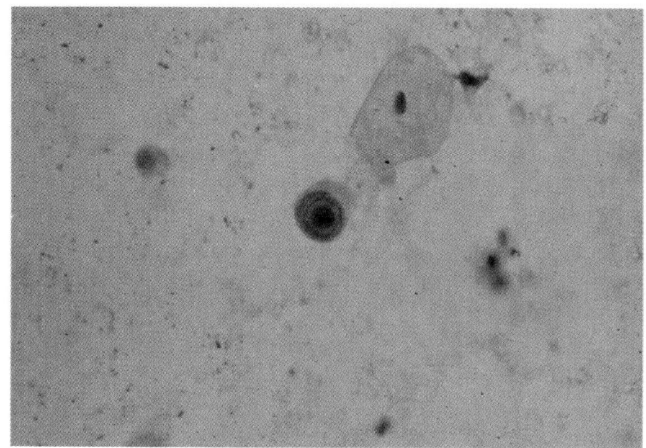

FIGURE 56-17 CMV-infected cell with basophilic nuclear inclusion.

BOX 56-9 Disease Mechanisms of CMV

CMV is acquired from blood, tissue, and most body secretions
Causes productive infection of epithelial and other cells
Establishes latency in T cells, macrophage, and other cells
Cell-mediated immunity is required for resolution and contributes to symptoms. Antibody role is limited
Suppression of CMI allows recurrence
Generally causes subclinical infection

TABLE 56-5 Asymptomatic Shedding of CMV

Source	Neonates	Children	Adults
Urine	0.5% to 2.5%	10% to 29%	0% to 2%
Oral secretions	0.5% to 2.5%	10% to 29%	0% to 2%
Cervical secretions			10% to 28%*
Semen			5% to 10%
Breast milk			13% to 27%

* Potential for CMV secretion increases in the third trimester of pregnancy.

and (3) reactivation under conditions of immunosuppression. However, CMV induces transient immunosuppression in the recipient and usually establishes asymptomatic infection.

CMV is highly cell associated and is predominantly transmitted by infected cells, including lymphocytes and leukocytes, which also spread the virus throughout the body (Figure 56-17). This close cell association protects the virus from antibody-mediated inactivation. In most cases the virus replicates and can be shed without causing symptoms (Table 56-5).

The virus establishes latency in mononuclear leukocytes and in organs such as the kidneys and heart. Latent CMV infection appears to be reactivated by immunosuppression (e.g., corticosteroids, HIV infection) and possibly by allogeneic stimulation (i.e., the host response to transfused or transplanted cells). Virus can be transmitted in cells by blood transfusion and organ transplants. Activation and replication of virus in the kidney and secretory glands promotes secretion in urine and bodily secretions.

Cell-mediated immunity is essential for resolving and controlling the outgrowth of CMV infection. Interestingly, CMV infection is immunosuppressive. This may help the virus establish latency and also prevent immunopathogenesis and symptoms. Primary CMV infection causes an increase in T-suppressor cells, which causes a decrease in the helper/suppressor (CD4/CD8) T-cell ratio. Lymphocyte function (e.g., proliferative responses to CMV antigens and mitogens) is also diminished during the acute infection but returns to normal during convalescence.

Epidemiology and Clinical Syndromes

CMV can be isolated from urine, blood, throat washings, saliva, tears, milk, semen, stool, amniotic fluid, vaginal and cervical secretions, and tissues taken for transplantation (Table 56-6 and Box 56-10). The major means of CMV transmission are by the congenital, oral, and sexual routes and by blood transfusion or tissue transplantation.

Congenital Infection

CMV is the most prevalent viral cause of congenital disease. A significant percentage (0.5% to 2.5%) of all newborns in the United States are infected with CMV at birth. Approximately 10% of these newborns show clinical evidence of disease, such as microcephaly, intracerebral calcification, hepatosplenomegaly, and rash. From 6000 to 7000 newborns each year may have unilateral or bilateral hearing loss and mental retardation

TABLE 56-6 CMV Syndromes

Tissue	Children/Adults	Immunosuppressed patients
Predominant nature of disease	**Inapparent infection**	**Disseminated disease, severe**
Eyes	–	Chorioretinitis
Lungs	–	Pneumonia
Gastrointestinal tract	–	Esophagitis, colitis
Nervous system	Polyneuritis, myelitis	Meningitis/encephalitis, myelitis
Lymphoid system	Mononucleosis syndrome, post-transfusion syndrome	Leukopenia, lymphocytosis
Major organs	Carditis,*, hepatitis*	Hepatitis
Neonates	Deafness, mental retardation	

*Complications of mononucleosis or postperfusion syndrome.

BOX 56-10 Epidemiology of Cytomegalovirus Infection

DISEASE/VIRAL FACTORS

Causes lifelong infection
Recurrent disease is a source of contagion
May cause asymptomatic shedding

TRANSMISSION

Via blood, organ transplants, and all secretions: urine, saliva, semen, cervical secretions, breast milk, tears
Transmitted orally, sexually, in blood transfusions, tissue transplants, in utero, at birth, and by nursing

WHO IS AT RISK?

Babies
Babies of mothers who seroconvert during term are at high risk for congenital defects
Sexually active individuals
Blood and organ recipients
Burn patients
Immunosuppressed individuals have symptomatic and recurrent disease

GEOGRAPHY/SEASON

Worldwide
No seasonal incidence

MODES OF CONTROL

None
Antiviral drugs available for AIDS patients
Use of condoms or abstinence from anal intercourse limits spread
Screening potential blood and organ donors for CMV reduces transmission of virus

resulting from congenital CMV infection. Mothers of almost all infants with these stigmata had a primary infection during pregnancy.

Fetuses are infected by virus in the mother's blood (primary infection) or by virus ascending from the cervix (following a recurrence). The symptoms of congenital infection are less severe or prevented in a seropositive mother. Congenital CMV infection is best documented by isolating the virus from the infant's urine during the first week of life.

Perinatal Infection

In the United States as many as 20% of pregnant women at term harbor CMV in their cervix and are likely to experience reactivation of virus during pregnancy. Approximately half the neonates born through an infected cervix acquire CMV infection and become excretors of the virus at 3 to 4 weeks of age. Neonates may also acquire CMV from maternal milk or colostrum. In healthy full-term infants perinatal infection causes no clinically evident disease.

Another means of CMV acquisition by neonates is through blood transfusions. If seronegative babies are exposed to blood from seropositive donors, 13.5% acquire CMV infection in the immediate postnatal period. If premature infants acquire CMV from transfused blood, significant clinical infection may occur, with pneumonia and hepatitis the major manifestations.

Infection in Adults

In low socioeconomic populations and in underdeveloped countries, postneonatal CMV infection is prevalent, apparently as a result of crowded living conditions. If such conditions are not present, only 10% to 15% of adolescents are infected, increasing to 50% by age 35. The virus may be spread in saliva, but the delay in seroconversion to older years indicates the importance of sexual and close personal contact for transmission. CMV has been isolated from the cervix of 13% to 23% of women

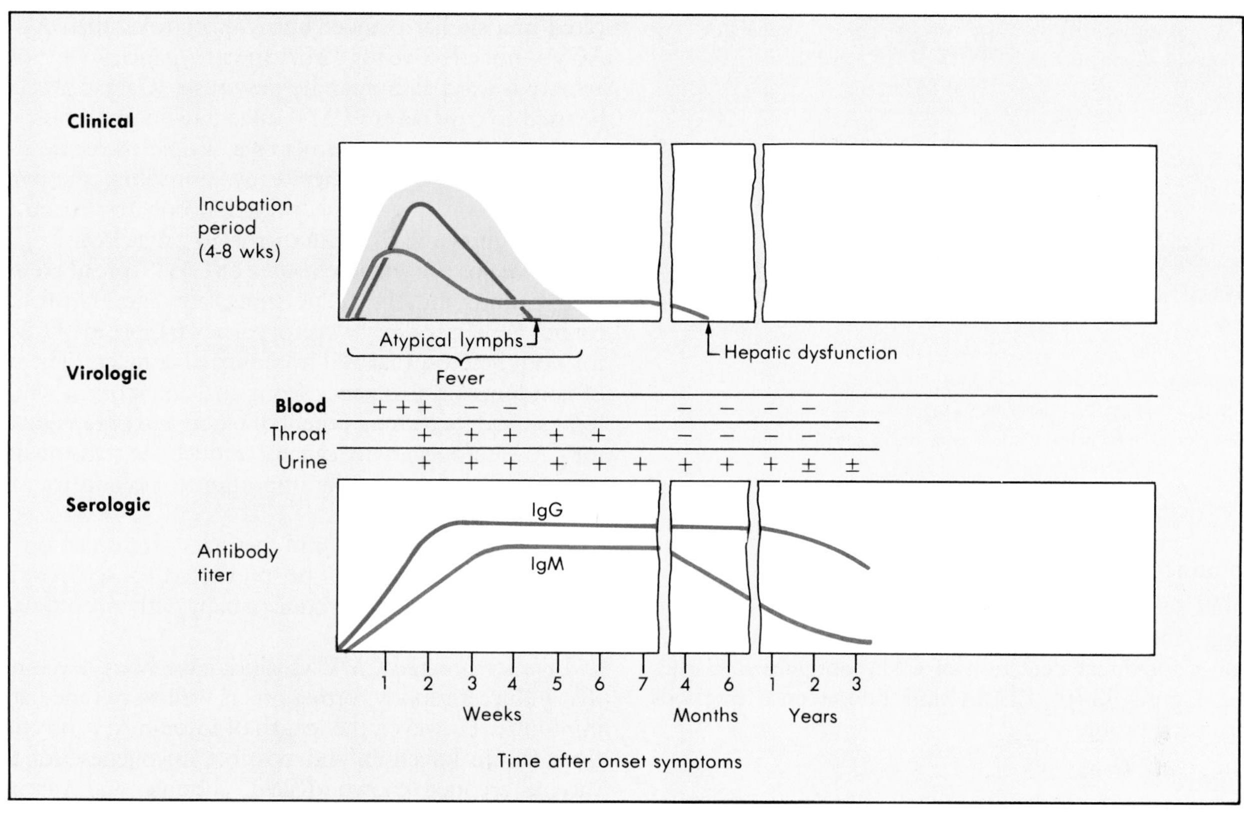

FIGURE 56-18 Clinical course of CMV infection. CMV infection is usually asymptomatic but may produce a mononucleosis syndrome, which can be distinguished from EBV infection.

at venereal disease clinics and is present in semen in the highest titer of any body secretion.

Although most CMV infections acquired in young adulthood are asymptomatic, patients may develop clinical illness resembling infectious mononucleosis caused by EBV, but with less severe pharyngitis and lymphadenopathy (Figure 56-18). Although CMV infection promotes T-cell outgrowth (atypical lymphocytosis) similar to EBV infection, heterophile antibody is not present. This reflects differences in the target cell and virus action on the target cell between CMV and EBV.

Transfusion and Transplantation Transmission

Transmission of CMV by blood most often results in an asymptomatic infection; if symptoms are present, they typically resemble infectious mononucleosis. Fever, splenomegaly, and atypical lymphocytosis usually begin 3 to 5 weeks after transfusion. Pneumonia and mild hepatitis may also occur. CMV may also be transmitted by organ transplantation (e.g., kidneys or bone marrow), and transplant recipients may reactivate CMV during periods of intense immunosuppression.

Infection in the Immunocompromised Host

CMV is a characteristic opportunistic infectious agent for immunocompromised individuals. Primary infection with CMV may also occur in these patients, and this form is more likely to cause symptomatic illness.

CMV often causes **retinitis** in patients with severe immunodeficiency (e.g., in as many as 10% to 15% of patients with AIDS). Interstitial pneumonia and encephalitis may also be caused by CMV but may be difficult to distinguish from other opportunistic infectious agents. As many as 10% of AIDS patients may develop CMV **colitis** or **esophagitis**. A lesser percentage of other immunocompromised patients may experience CMV infection of the gastrointestinal tract. Patients with CMV colitis usually have diarrhea, weight loss, anorexia, and fever. CMV esophagitis may mimic candidal esophagitis.

Laboratory Diagnosis

Histology

The histological hallmark of CMV infection is the cytomegalic cell, which is enlarged (25 to 35 mm) and contains a dense central "owl's eye" basophilic intranuclear inclusion (Table 56-7; see Figure 56-17). These infected cells may be found in any tissue of the body and in urine and are thought to be epithelial in origin. These inclusions are readily seen with Papanicolaou or hematoxylin and eosin (H and E) stains.

TABLE 56-7 Laboratory Tests for Diagnosis of CMV Infection

Test	Finding
Cytology/Histology*	"Owl eye" inclusion body
	Antigen detection
	In situ DNA probe hybridization
Cell culture	CPE in human diploid fibroblasts
	Immunofluorescence detection of early antigens
Serology	Primary infection

*Samples taken for analysis include urine, saliva, blood, bronchoalveolar lavage, and tissue biopsies.

Immune and DNA Probe Techniques

Rapid sensitive histological diagnosis can be obtained using antibodies (especially monoclonal) and DNA probes for direct detection of CMV antigens in tissues (see Figure 53-9). ELISA and fluorescence methods detect the probes.

Culture

Culture has been generally regarded as the definitive method for detecting CMV infection. It is especially reliable in immunocompromised patients because they often have high titers of virus in their secretions. For example, AIDS patients may have titers with greater than 10^6 viable virus in their semen.

CMV grows only in diploid fibroblast cell cultures and must be maintained for at least 4 to 6 weeks because the characteristic CPE develops very slowly in specimens with very low titers of the virus. More rapid results may be achieved by **culture amplification** of a specimen. In this procedure, specimens are inoculated by centrifuging them in a shell vial seeded with diploid fibroblast cells. Specimens are examined after 1 to 2 days of incubation by indirect immunofluorescence for either immediate early (IE) antigen or a combination of IE and early antigen (EA).

Serology

Seroconversion is usually an excellent marker for primary CMV infection. IgG titers to CMV antigen may be very high in AIDS patients, but a high titer level is not diagnostically useful. CMV-specific IgM antibody may also develop during reactivation of CMV and is not a dependable indication of primary infection.

Treatment, Prevention, and Control

Ganciclovir (dihydroxypropoxymethyl guanine [DHPG], Cytovene) and foscarnet (phosphonoformic acid) have been approved for treatment of CMV infections and are especially useful for immunosuppressed patients (see Box 56-4). Ganciclovir is structurally similar to ACV, is activated in a similar manner but is more toxic than ACV. ACV is not effective for CMV. In vitro, ganciclovir shows activity toward all human herpesviruses. Ganciclovir can be used to treat severe CMV infections in immunocompromised patients. Foscarnet is a simple molecule that inhibits the DNA polymerase by mimicking the pyrophosphate portion of nucleotide triphosphates. Foscarnet has been approved as an alternative to ganciclovir.

The major preventable routes of CMV spread are the sexual route and the tissue transplant and transfusion routes. Semen is a major vector for sexual spread of CMV for both heterosexual and homosexual contacts. The use of condoms or abstinence from anal intercourse would limit spread. Screening potential blood and organ donors for CMV seronegativity can also reduce the transmission of virus. This is especially important for blood transfusions for infants.

Although congenital and perinatal transmission of CMV cannot effectively be prevented, a seropositive mother is least likely to produce a baby with symptomatic CMV disease.

Live attentuated CMV vaccines have been developed that induce antibody formation, as well as cell-mediated immunity. However, the length of immunity, protection from future infection, and possible oncogenesis of the vaccine are not known. Killed, subunit, and vaccinia hybrid vaccines are being considered as alternatives. The prime targets for vaccination against CMV would be similar to those for rubella vaccine—children and seronegative women of childbearing age.

HUMAN HERPESVIRUS 6 AND 7

HHV6 was first isolated from the blood of AIDS patients and grown in T-lymphocyte cultures. HHV6 was identified as a herpesvirus by observation of the characteristic morphology in electron micrographs of infected cells. It is not serologically related and does not hybridize with the other human herpesviruses. As with EBV and CMV, it is lymphotropic and is ubiquitous. At least 45% of children are seropositive for HHV6 by age 2. In 1988 HHV6 was serologically associated with a common disease of children, **exanthem subitum**, commonly known as **roseola**. No other disease association has yet been made for this virus.

HHV7 was isolated in a similar manner as HHV6 from T cells of an AIDS patient also infected with HHV6. HHV7 remains an "orphan" virus with no disease association.

Pathogenesis and Immunity

The finding that HHV6 infection occurs very early in life suggests that it must be shed and spread readily. It is most likely spread by close contact or respiratory means.

The only target cell that has been identified is the T lymphocyte. HHV6 establishes a latent infection in T cells but may be activated and replicate on mitogen stimulation of the cells. Cells replicating the virus appear large and refractile with occasional intranuclear and intracytoplasmic inclusion bodies. T-cell leukemia cell lines also support the replication of the virus. Resting lymphocytes and lymphocytes of normal immune individuals are resistant to infection.

As with EBV and CMV, HHV6 replication is controlled by cell-mediated immunity. The virus is likely to become activated in AIDS patients and others with lymphoproliferative and immunosuppressive disorders. Activation of HHV6 initiates a lytic infection of T cells, which may contribute to the depression of the number of T cells observed in patients with AIDS. However, no known consequence of HHV6 activation has yet been found.

Clinical Syndromes

Exanthem subitum, or **roseola**, is a common benign exanthematous disease of children. It is characterized by rapid onset of high fever for a few days, followed by a generalized rash that lasts only 24 to 48 hours. The presence of infected T cells or activation of delayed type hypersensitivy T cells in the skin may account for the production of the rash. The disease is effectively controlled and resolved by cell-mediated immunity, but the virus establishes a lifelong latent infection of T cells.

HHV6 may also cause a mononucleosis syndrome and lymphadenopathy and may be a cofactor in the pathogenesis of AIDS.

HERPESVIRUS SIMIAE – B VIRUS

B virus (Herpesvirus simiae) is indigenous to Asian monkeys but can cause a highly lethal central nervous system infection in humans. The virus is transmitted by monkey bites or saliva or even by tissues and cells widely used in virology laboratories.

B virus is the simian counterpart of HSV and causes subclinical infections, as well as dermal, oral, or eye lesions in monkeys. Once infected, a human may have pain, localized redness, and vesicles at the site of the virus' entrance. Vesicles on the mucous membranes, pneumonia, diarrhea, abdominal pain, and pharyngitis have been reported. However, patients develop an encephalopathy that is frequently fatal; most who survive have serious brain damage. The diagnosis of B virus infections can be established by virus isolation or by serologic tests.

CASE STUDIES AND QUESTIONS

A 2-year-old child with fever for 2 days was not eating and crying often. Upon examination, the physician noted that the inside of the mouth was covered with numerous shallow pale ulcerations over the gums, tongue, and wall of the mouth. A few red papules and blisters were also observed around the border of the lips. The symptoms continued to worsen over the next 5 days and then slowly resolved with complete healing after 2 weeks.

1. The physician suspects that this is a herpes simplex virus infection. How would the diagnosis be confirmed?
2. How could you determine whether the infection is due to HSV-1 or HSV-2?
3. What immune responses are most helpful in the resolution of this infection, and when are they activated?
4. HSV escapes complete immune resolution by causing latent/recurrent infections. What would the site of latency be for this child, and what might promote future recurrences?
5. What are the most probable means by which the baby was infected by HSV?
6. Which antiviral drugs are available for HSV infections? Which drugs are effective, and what are their targets? Are they indicated for this child? If not, why not?

A 17-year-old high school student has several days of low-grade fever and malaise, followed by sore throat, swollen cervical lymph nodes, and increasing fatigue. The patient also notes some discomfort in the left upper quadrant of the abdomen. The sore throat, lymphadenopathy, and fever gradually resolve over the next 2 weeks, but full energy level does not return for another 6 weeks.

1. What laboratory tests would confirm the diagnosis of EBV-induced infectious mononucleosis and distinguish it from CMV infection?
2. What characteristic diagnostic feature of the disease does "mononucleosis" refer to?
3. What causes the swollen glands and fatigue symptoms?
4. Who is at greatest risk for a serious outcome from EBV infection? What is it? Why?

Bibliography

Belshe RB: *Textbook of human virology*, ed 2, St. Louis, 1991, Mosby.

Fields BN, Knipe DM. *Virology*, ed 2, New York, 1990, Raven Press.

Garcia-Blanco MA, Cullen BR: Molecular basis of latency in pathogenic human viruses, *Science* 254:815-820, 1991.

McGeoch DJ. The genomes of the human herpesviruses: contents, relationships and evolution, *Ann Rev Microbiol* 43:235-265, 1989.

Herpes simplex virus

Arbesfeld DM, Thomas I: Cutaneous herpes simplex infections, *Am Fam Physician* 43:1655-1664, 1991.

Croen KD, Strauss SE: Varicella zoster latency, *Ann Rev Microbiol* 45:265-282, 1991.

Current topics in microbiology and immunology, vol 179, 1992.

Dawkins BJ: Genital herpes simplex infections, *Prim Care* 17:95-113, 1990.

Grose C, Zaia JA: Varicella-Zoster Virus in Infectious Diseases.

In Gorbach SL, Bartlett JG, Blacklow NR, editors: *Infectious diseases*, Philadelphia, 1992, WB Saunders.
J Infect Dis 166(suppl 1): 1992.
Landy HJ, Grossman JH III: Herpes simplex virus, *Obstet Gynecol ClinNorth Am* 16:495-515, 1989.
Ostrove JM: Molecular biology of varicella zoster virus, *Adv Vir Res* 38:45-98, 1990.
Oxman MN: Herpes simplex viruses and human herpesvirus 6. In Gorbach SL, Bartlett JG, Blacklow NR, editors: *Infectious diseases*, Philadelphia, 1992, WB Saunders.

Varicella zoster virus

Rev Infect Dis 13(suppl 11): 1991.

Epstein-Barr virus

Englund JA: The many faces of Epstein-Barr virus, *Postgrad Med* 83:167-179, 1988.
Ooka T and Sixbey JW, editors: Epstein-Barr virus immunopathology, *Springer Semin Immunopathol*:13(2), 1991.
Spring SB, Schluederberg A, Allen WP, and Gruber J: Pathogenic diversity of Epstein-Barr virus, *J Natl Cancer Inst* 81:13-20, 1989.
Sugden B: EBV's open sesame, *Trends Biochemical Sci* 17:239-240, 1992.
Thorley-Lawson DA: Basic virologic aspects of Epstein-Barr virus infection, *Semin Hematol* 25:247-269, 1988.
Tomkinson BE, Sullivan JL: Epstein-Barr virus (infectious mononucleosis). In Gorbach SL, Bartlett JG, Blacklow NR, editors: *Infectious diseases*, Philadelphia, 1992, WB Saunders.

Cytomegalovirus, HHV6 and 7

Ablashi DV, Salahuddin SZ, Josephs SF, Balachandran N, Krueger GRF, and Gallo RC: Human Herpesvirus-6 (HHV6) (short review) in vivo 5:193-200, 1991.
Current topics in microbiology and immunology, volume 154, 1990.
Pellet PE, Black JB, Yamamoto Y: Human herpesvirus 6: the virus and the search for its role as a human pathogen, *Adv Virol* 41:1-52, 1992.
Transplant Proc 23 (suppl 3):1991.
Wyatt LS, Frenkel N: Human herpesvirus 7 is a constitutive inhabitant of adult human saliva, *J Virol* 66:3206-3209.
Yamanishi K et al.: Identification of human herpesvirus-6 as a causal agent for exanthem subitum, *Lancet* 1:1065-1067, 1988.

CHAPTER 57

Poxviruses

THE poxviruses include the human viruses **variola (smallpox)** (Orthopoxvirus), **molluscum contagiosum** (Molluscipoxvirus) and poxviruses in other genera that naturally infect animals but can cause incidental infection of humans (zoonosis). Many of these viruses share antigenic determinants with smallpox, allowing the use of an animal poxvirus for a human vaccine.

Smallpox was one of the major infectious diseases. In eighteenth century England it accounted for 7% to 12% of all deaths and the deaths of one third of children. Development of the first live vaccine in 1796 and a worldwide distribution program led to the eradication of smallpox by 1980.

Several lessons can still be learned from studying the poxvirus family for the following reasons: (1) the mechanisms of spread of variola virus within the body represent a model for other virus infections; (2) poxviruses other than variola virus cause human disease; and (3) vaccinia virus (a laboratory altered poxvirus) has become an excellent vector for the development of hybrid vaccines containing the genes of other infectious agents.

STRUCTURE AND REPLICATION

Vaccinia virus structure and replication are representative of other poxviruses and will be used as a prototype poxvirus. Poxviruses are the largest viruses, barely visible by light microscopy (Box 57-1). They measure 230 × 300 nm in size and are ovoid to brick shaped (Figure 57-1). An outer membrane and envelope enclose the core and core membrane, which are flanked by two lateral bodies and contain many enzymes and other proteins. The viral genome consists of a large double-stranded linear DNA, which is fused at both ends and for vaccinia virus consists of 86,000 base pairs (molecular weight approximately 120×10^6 d).

Replication of poxviruses is unique among DNA-containing viruses because the entire multiplication cycle takes place within the host cell cytoplasm (Figure 57-2). As a result, poxviruses must encode the enzymes that are required for mRNA and DNA synthesis, as well as activities that other DNA viruses normally obtain from the host cell.

Viral penetration occurs within phagocytic vacuoles. The outer membrane is removed in the vacuole and early gene transcription is initiated. The virion core contains a specific transcriptional activator and all the enzymes necessary for transcription, including a multi-subunit RNA polymerase, and enzymes for polyA addition and capping. Among the early proteins produced is an uncoating protein that removes the core membrane, liberating viral DNA into the cell cytoplasm. Replication of viral DNA follows in electron-dense cytoplasmic inclusions (Guarnieri's inclusion bodies) referred to as "factories." Late viral mRNA is translated into structural and virion proteins. Unlike other viruses, the poxvirus membranes assemble around the core factories. About 10,000 viral particles are produced per infected cell and are released upon cell lysis.

Vaccinia virus is being used as an expression vector to produce live recombinant/hybrid vaccines for more virulent infectious agents (Figure 57-3). The foreign gene, which encodes the immunizing molecule, and specific vaccinia gene sequences are added to a plasmid. This recombinant plasmid is inserted into a host cell that is then infected with vaccinia virus. The foreign gene is directed into the "rescuing" vaccinia virus genome because of the homologous vaccinia sequences included on the plasmid. Immunization with the recombinant vaccinia virus results in expression of the foreign gene and its presentation to the immune response almost as if by infection with the other agent. Vaccines for HIV, hepatitis B, influenza, and other agents have been prepared by these techniques. The potential for producing other vaccines in this manner is unlimited.

BOX 57-1 Unique Properties of Poxviruses

Largest most complex virus
Complex brick-shaped morphology with internal structure
Linear double-stranded DNA genome with fused ends
DNA virus that replicates in the cytoplasm
Virus encodes and carries all the proteins necessary for mRNA synthesis
Virus also encodes proteins for DNA synthesis, nucleotide scavenging, immune escape mechanisms, etc.
Virus is assembled in inclusion bodies (Guarnieri's bodies) where it acquires its envelope (does not bud)

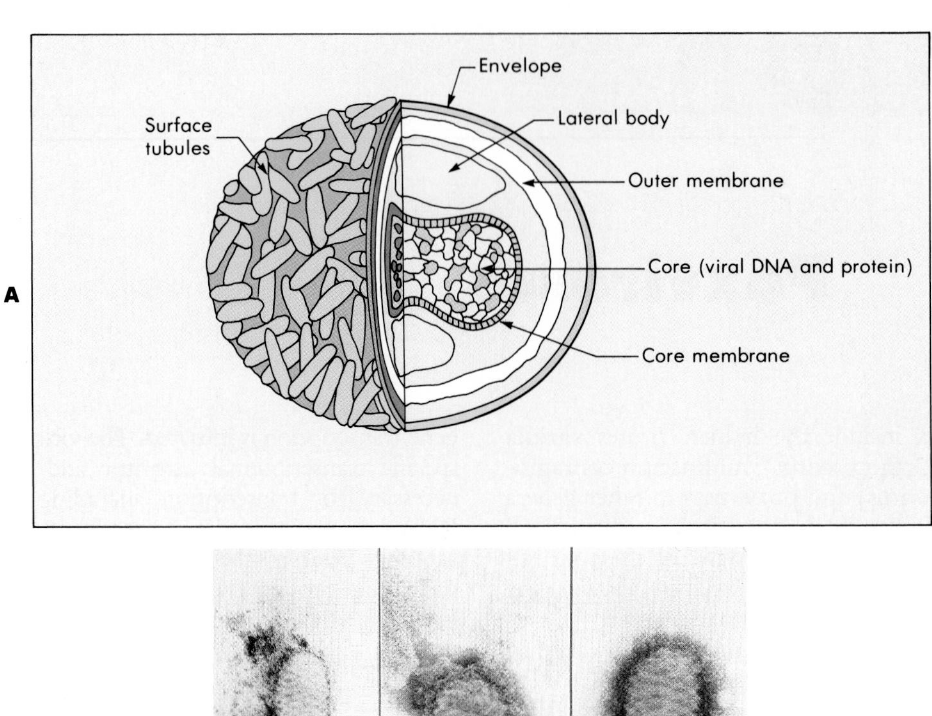

FIGURE 57-1 A, Structure of the vaccinia virus. The viral DNA and several proteins within the core are organized as a "nucleosome." Within the virion, the core assumes the shape of a dumbbell because of the large lateral bodies. Virions released through the cytoplasmic membrane are enclosed within an envelope that contains host cell lipids and several virus-specific polypeptides, including the hemagglutinin; they are infectious. Most virions remain cell associated and are released by cellular disruption. These particles lack an envelope, so the outer membrane constitutes their surface; like the enveloped particles, they are also infectious. **B,** Electron micrograph of orfvirus. Notice its complex structure. (Courtesy Centers for Disease Control.)

PATHOGENESIS AND IMMUNITY

Smallpox virus is inhaled and replicates in the upper respiratory tract (Box 57-2 and Figure 57-4). Dissemination occurs via lymphatic and cell-associated viremic spread. Internal and dermal tissues are inoculated following a second, more intense, viremia. Molluscum contagiosum and the other poxviruses are acquired by man by direct contact with lesions and do not spread extensively.

The poxviruses encode many proteins that facilitate their replication and pathogenesis in the host. These include proteins that initially stimulate host cell growth and then lead to cell lysis and virus spread. Molluscum contagiosum causes a tumor-like lesion rather than a lytic infection.

Cell-mediated immunity is essential for resolving a poxvirus infection. However, poxviruses encode proteins that help the virus evade immune control. These include cell-to-cell spread to avoid antibody and proteins that impede the interferon, complement, and inflammatory responses.

EPIDEMIOLOGY

Most of the poxviruses of current human importance are primary pathogens in vertebrates rather than humans (e.g., cow, sheep, goats) and infect humans only through "accidental" occupational exposure (zoonosis). The exception is molluscum contagiosum.

Smallpox (variola) was very contagious and was spread primarily by respiratory transmission or, less efficiently, by close contact with dried virus on clothes or other materials. Despite the severity of the disease and its tendency to spread, several factors contributed to the elimination of smallpox (Box 57-3).

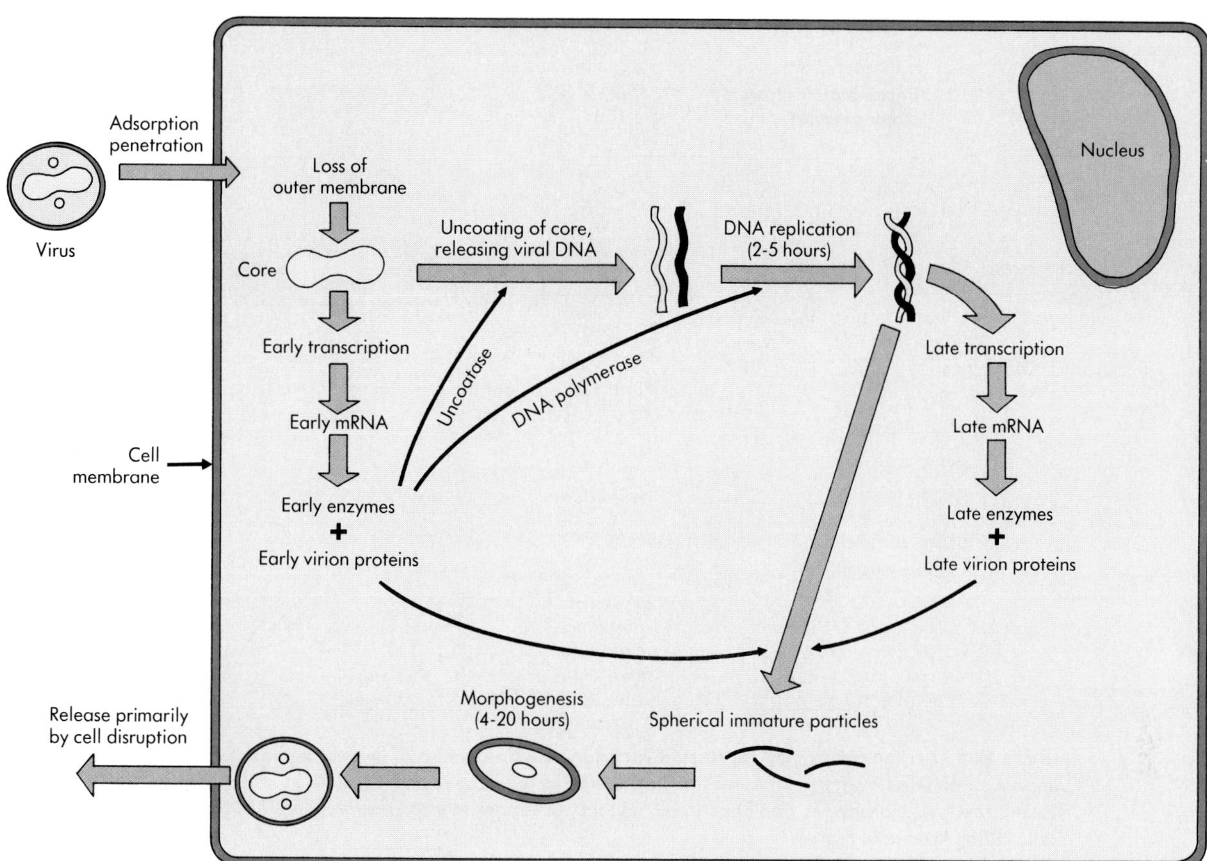

FIGURE 57-2 Replication of vaccinia virus. (Modified from Fields BN, Knipe DM et al., editors: *Virology*, ed 2, New York, 1990, Raven Press.)

CLINICAL SYNDROMES

See Table 57-1 for a list of diseases associated with poxviruses.

Smallpox

Two variants of smallpox existed: variola major, with a mortality of 15% to 40%, and variola minor, with a mortality of 1%. Smallpox was usually initiated by infection of the respiratory tract with subsequent involvement of local lymph glands, leading to viremia. Viremia was associated with fever, headache, backache, and later seeding of the skin with development of a characteristic vesiculopustular, virus-containing rash (Figure 57-5). The rash (pox) had two characteristics that distinguished it from other exanthems: (1) lesions were virtually all at the same stage of development as they progressed from macules to vesicles to pustules to crusting and healing, and (2) the rash was centrifugal (i.e., began centrally on the face, shoulders, chest, and later involved more distal sites.) In addition to skin involvement, visceral organs (especially the spleen, liver, and lungs) were also involved. The incubation period ranged from 5 to 17 days, with an average of 12 days (Figure 57-6).

Vaccinia

When smallpox was eradicated, the necessity for vaccination against this disease disappeared. The virus used for vaccination was the vaccinia virus, which was probably derived from an animal poxvirus such as horsepox. The vaccination procedure consisted of scratching live virus into the skin and observing for the development of vesicles and pustule(s) to confirm a "take." Revaccination at periodic intervals was necessary to maintain immunity. As smallpox waned, it became apparent that there were more complications related to vaccination than there were cases of smallpox. Several of these complications were severe and even fatal, including encephalitis and progressive infection **(vaccinia necrosum);** the latter occurred occasionally when immunocompromised patients were inadvertently vaccinated. The relative ease of person-to-person spread of vaccinia virus infections among unvaccinated individuals posed a threat to immunocompromised contacts of vaccinees.

Orf, Cowpox, and Monkeypox

The poxvirus of animals such as sheep or goats (orf) and cows (cowpox) can infect humans, usually as a result of accidental direct contact. Nodular lesions are usually on

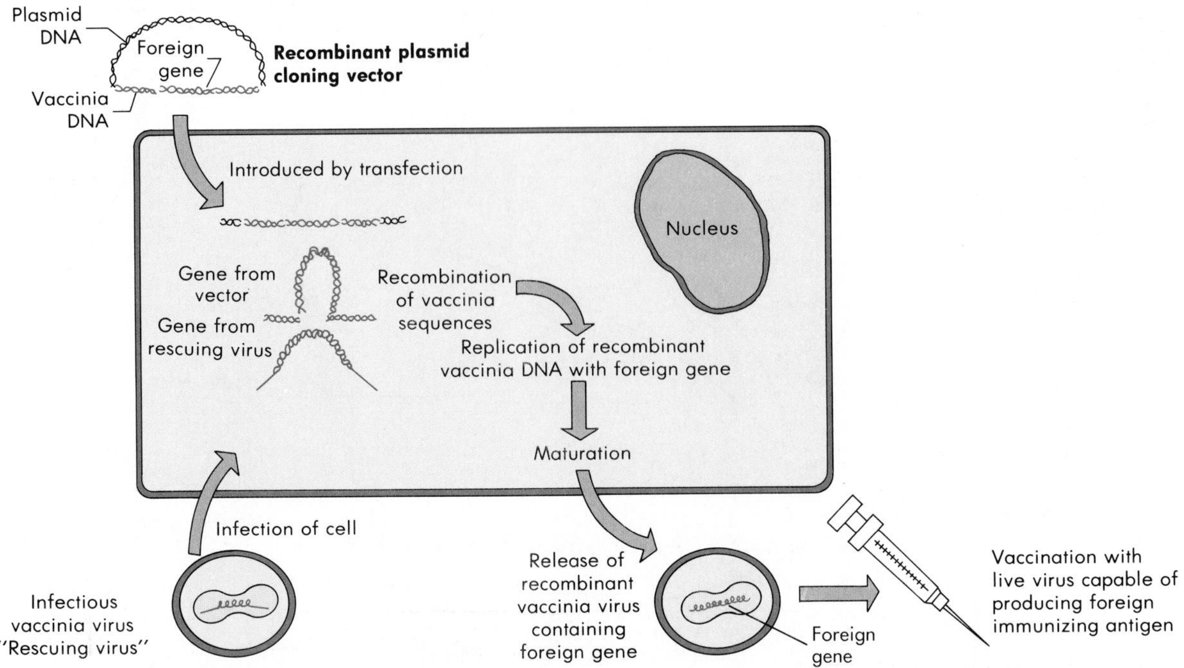

FIGURE 57-3 Vaccinia virus as an expression vector for the production of live recombinant vaccines. (Modified from Piccini A and Paoletti E: Vaccinia: virus, vector, vaccine. In Maramorosch K, Murphy FA, and Shatkin AJ, editors: *Advances in virus research*, vol 34, New York, 1988, Academic Press.)

BOX 57-2 Disease Mechanisms of Poxviruses

Smallpox initiated by respiratory infection and spread mainly by lymphatics and cell-associated viremia; molluscum contagiosum and zoonoses transmitted by contact
Virus may cause initial stimulation of cell growth and then cell lysis
Virus encodes immune escape mechanisms
Cell-mediated and humoral immunity are both important for resolution

the fingers or face and are hemorrhagic (cowpox) or granulomatous (orf or pseudocowpox; Figure 57-7). Vesicular lesions frequently develop and then regress in 25 to 35 days, generally without scar formation. The lesions may be mistaken for anthrax. The etiological viruses can be grown in culture or seen directly with electron microscopy.

More than 100 cases of illnesses resembling smallpox have been attributed to the monkeypox virus. All have occurred in western and central Africa, especially Zaire.

BOX 57-3 Properties of Smallpox That Led to Its Eradication

VIRUS CHARACTERISTICS

Exclusive human host range (no animal reservoirs or vectors)
Single serotype (immunization protects against all infections)
Animal and human poxviruses share antigenic determinants ("safe" live vaccines can be prepared from animal poxviruses)

DISEASE CHARACTERISTICS

Smallpox disease *always* presents with visible pustular disease (identification of sources of contagion allows quarantine and vaccination of contacts)

VACCINE

Stable, inexpensive, easy to administer vaccine
Presence of a scar indicates successful vaccination

PUBLIC HEALTH SERVICE EFFORTS

Successful WHO worldwide program combining vaccination and quarantine

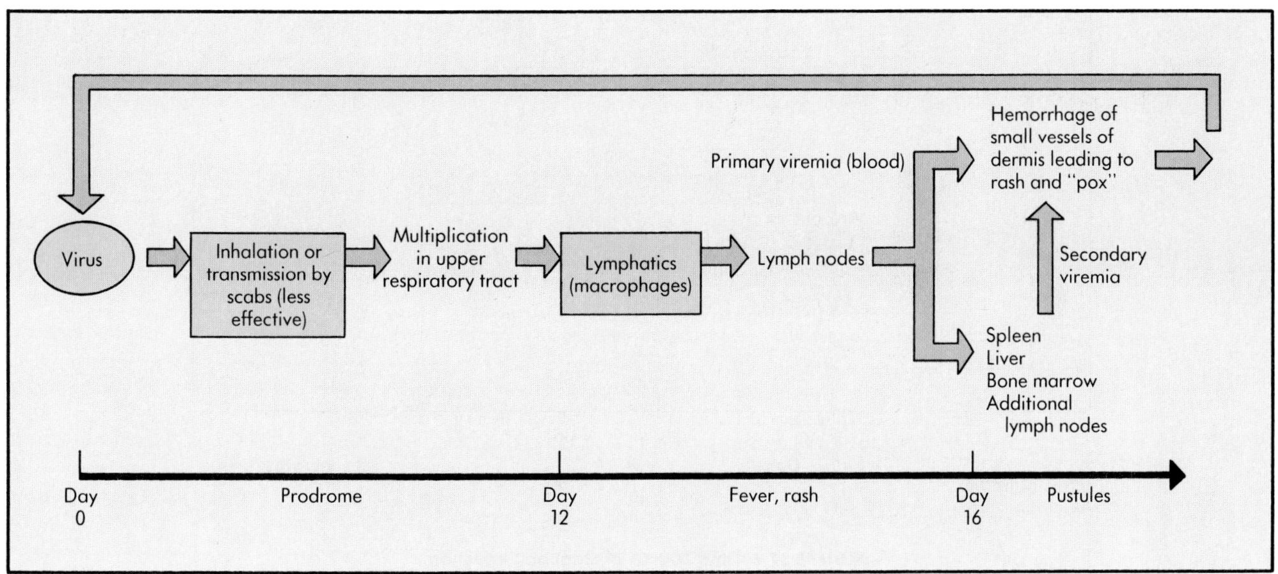

FIGURE 57-4 Spread of smallpox within the body. Virus enters and replicates in the respiratory tract without causing symptoms or contagion. The virus infects macrophages, which enter the lymphatics and carry the virus to regional lymph nodes. The virus replicates and intitiates a viremia, spreading the infection to the spleen, bone marrow, lymph nodes, liver, and all organs followed by the skin (rash). A secondary viremia causes additional lesions throughout the host and death or recovery with or without sequelae. Recovery was associated with prolonged immunity and lifelong protection.

TABLE 57-1 Diseases Associated with Poxviruses

Virus	Disease	Source	Location
Variola	Smallpox (now extinct)	Humans	Extinct
Vaccinia	Used for smallpox vaccination	Laboratory product	—
Orf	Localized lesion	Zoonosis—sheep, goats	Worldwide
Cowpox	Localized lesion	Zoonosis—rodents, cats, cows	Europe
Pseudocowpox	Milker's nodule	Zoonosis—dairy cows	Worldwide
Monkeypox	Generalized disease	Zoonosis—monkeys, squirrels	Africa
Bovine papular stomatitis virus	Localized lesion	Zoonosis—calves, beef cattle	Worldwide
Tanapox	Localized lesion	Rare zoonosis—monkeys	Africa
Yabapox	Localized lesion	Rare zoonosis—monkeys, baboons	Africa
Molluscum contagiosum	Many skin lesions	Humans	Worldwide

Modified from Balows A, Hausler WJ Jr, and Lennette EH, editors: *Laboratory diagnosis of infectious diseases: principles and practice*, vol 2, New York, 1988, Springer-Verlag.

Molluscum contagiosum

The lesions of molluscum contagiosum are caused by a poxvirus that is unclassified because it does not grow in cell cultures. The lesions differ significantly from pox lesions in that they are nodular to wartlike (Figure 57-8). They begin as papules and progress to pearly, umbilicated nodules, 2 to 10 nm in diameter, with a central caseous plug that can be readily expressed (squeezed out). They are most common on the trunk, genitalia, and proximal extremities and usually occur in a cluster of 5 to 20 nodules. The incubation period for molluscum contagiosum is 2 to 8 weeks, and the disease spreads by direct contact (e.g., sexual contact or wrestling) or fomites (e.g., towels).

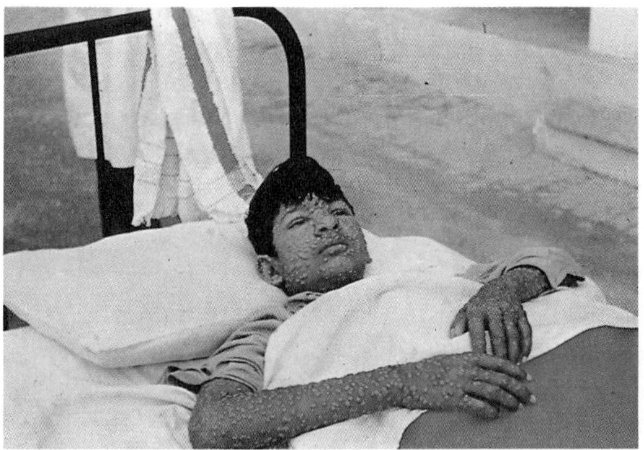

FIGURE 57-5 Child with smallpox. Note characteristic rash.

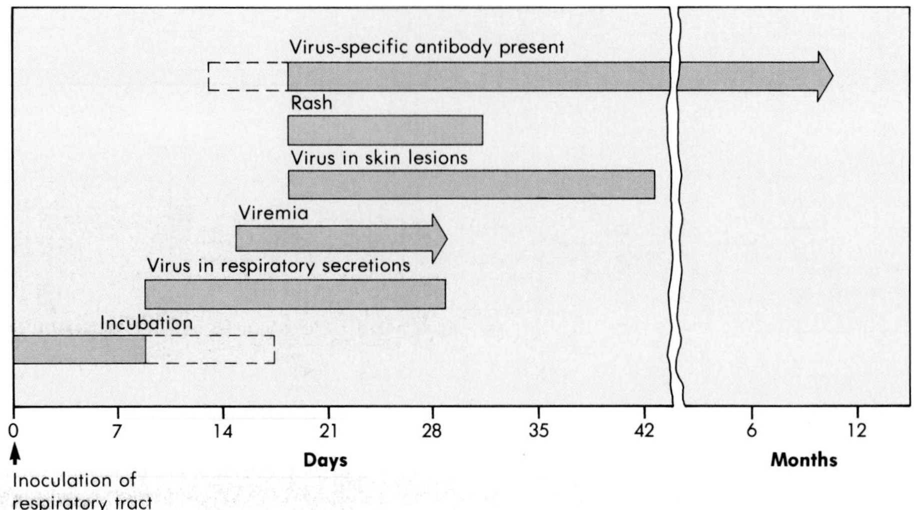

FIGURE 57-6 Time course of smallpox infection.

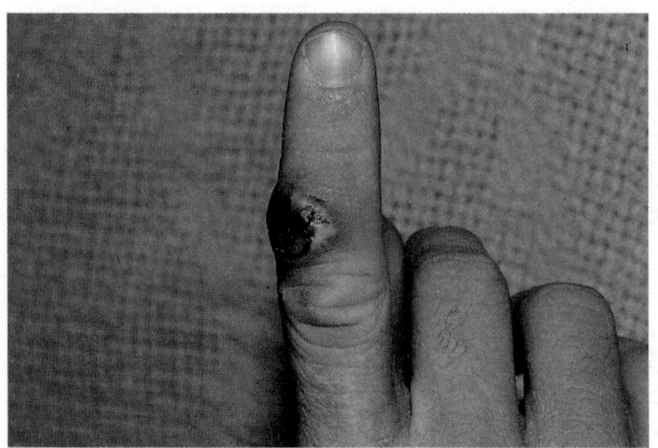

FIGURE 57-7 Orf lesion on finger of taxidermist. (Courtesy Joe Meyers, MD.)

LABORATORY DIAGNOSIS

The diagnosis of smallpox was usually made clinically but confirmed by growth of the virus in embryonated eggs or cell cultures. Characteristic lesions (pocks) appeared on the chorioallantoic membrane of embryonated eggs.

The diagnosis of molluscum contagiosum is confirmed histologically by the presence of very characteristic large eosinophilic cytoplasmic inclusions **(molluscum bodies)** in epithelial cells (see Figure 57-8). These can be seen in biopsy specimens or in the expressed caseous core.

TREATMENT, PREVENTION, AND CONTROL

Smallpox was the first disease to be controlled by immunization. The eradication of smallpox is one of the greatest triumphs of medical epidemiology. It resulted from a massive World Health Organization (WHO) campaign to vaccinate all susceptible individuals, especially those exposed to anyone with the disease, and thereby interrupt the chain of human-to-human transmission. This campaign, which began in 1967, succeeded, with the last case of naturally acquired infection reported in 1977 and the eradication of the virus acknowledged in 1980. Reference stocks of smallpox virus are being stored in only two World Health Organization Labs.

The initial attempt at immunization was **variolation** (i.e., the use of virulent smallpox pus to inoculate susceptible individuals). Variolation began in the Far East, was later used in England, and then Cotton Mather introduced it to the United States. This practice was associated with fatality in approximately 1%, a better risk than for smallpox itself. In 1796 Jenner developed and popularized the vaccination procedure using a less virulent virus that shares antigenic determinants with smallpox, cowpox, or horsepox. These were the precursor to the vaccinia virus used in more modern vaccines.

As eradication of smallpox approached, it became apparent that in the developed world the rate of serious reactions to vaccination (see discussion of vaccinia) exceeded the risk of infection. Therefore discontinuation of smallpox vaccination began in the 1970s, and its use was eliminated after 1980.

The lesions of molluscum contagiosum disappear in 2 to 12 months, presumably as a result of acquired immune responses. Treatment, if required, consists of curettage, liquid nitrogen, or iodine solutions.

QUESTIONS

1. Poxviruses have a more complex structure than most viruses. What problems does this create for virus replication?

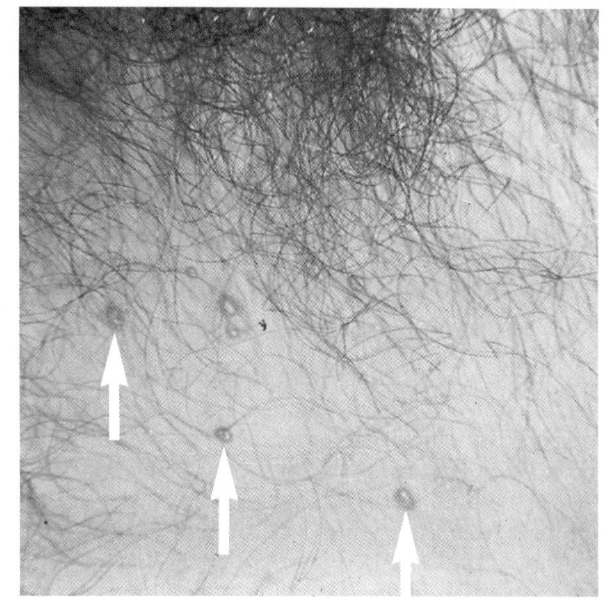

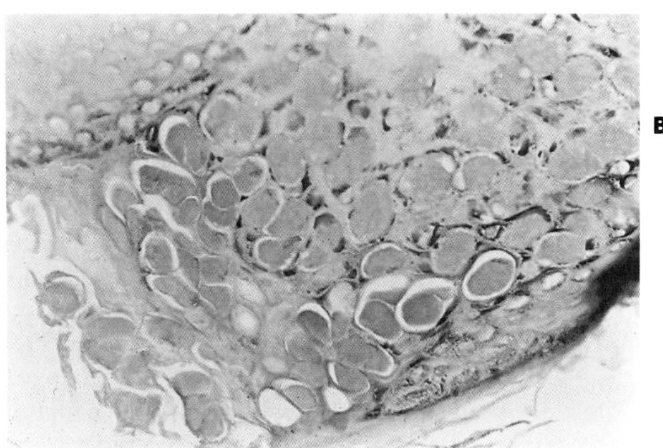

FIGURE 57-8 A, Skin lesion of molluscum contagiosum. **B,** Microscopic view of molluscum contagiosum; epidermis filled with molluscum bodies (×100).

2. Poxviruses replicate in the cytoplasm. What problems does this create for virus replication?
3. How does the immune response to smallpox infection differ for an immunologically naive person versus a vaccinated individual? When is antibody present in each case? What stage(s) of virus dissemination are blocked in each case?
4. What characteristics of smallpox facilitated its elimination?
5. Vaccinia virus is being used as a vector for development of hybrid vaccines. Why is vaccinia virus well suited for this task? Which infectious agents would be appropriate for a vaccinia hybrid vaccine and why?

Bibliography

Baxby D: Poxviruses. In Belshe RB, editor: *Textbook of human virology*, ed 2, St. Louis, 1991, Mosby.

Fenner F: A successful eradication campaign: global eradication of smallpox, *Rev Infect Dis* 4(5):916-930, 1982.

Fenner, F: Poxviruses. In Fields BN, Knipe DM, editors: *Virology*, ed 2, New York, 1990, Raven Press.

Moss B: Poxviridae and their replication. In Fields BN, Knipe DM, editors: *Virology*, New York, 1990, Raven Press.

Moyer RW, Turner PC: Poxviruses, *Curr Top Microbiol Immunol* 163:1990.

Piccini A, Paoletti E: Vaccinia: virus, vector, vaccine. In Maramorosch K, Murphy FA, and Shatkin AJ, editors: *Advances in virus research*, vol 34, New York, 1988, Academic Press.

CHAPTER 58

Parvoviruses

THE Parvoviridae are the smallest of the DNA viruses (Box 58-1). Their small size and limited genetic repertoire make them dependent on the host cell or a helper virus to replicate, more so than any other DNA virus.

Only one member of the Parvoviridae, **B19**, a member of the **parvovirus genera**, is known to cause human disease. B19 normally causes **erythema infectiosum (fifth disease)**, a mild febrile exanthematous disease in children, but is also responsible for episodes of aplastic crises in patients with chronic hemolytic anemia. It is also associated with rheumatic disease in adults. Intrauterine infection of a fetus may cause abortion. Other parvoviruses such as RA-1 (isolated from an individual with rheumatoid arthritis) and fecal parvoviruses have not been shown to cause human disease. The diseases caused by the feline and canine parvoviruses are preventable by vaccine.

Adeno-associated viruses, members of the **dependovirus genera**, commonly infect humans but only in association with a second "helper" virus, usually an adenovirus. Dependoviruses do not appear to cause illness nor do they modify infection by their helper viruses. A third genus of the family, densovirus, infects only insects.

STRUCTURE AND REPLICATION

The parvoviruses are extremely small (18 to 26 nm in diameter) with a nonenveloped, icosahedral virion (Box 58-2 and Figure 58-1). The B19 virus genome contains one linear single-stranded DNA molecule with a molecular weight of 1.5 to 1.8 × 10^6(5.5 kb in length) (Box 58-3). Plus and minus DNA strands are packaged separately into virions. At least two structural and one nonstructural proteins are encoded by overlapping reading frames on the plus-stranded genome. Only one serotype of B19 is known to exist.

B19 virus replicates in mitotically active cells and prefers cells of the erythroid lineage, such as fresh human bone marrow cells, erythroid cells from fetal liver, and erythroid leukemia cells (Figure 58-2). Following binding and internalization, the virion is uncoated and the single-stranded DNA genome is delivered to the nucleus. Factor(s) available only during the S phase of the cell's growth cycle and cellular DNA polymerase(s) are required to generate a complementary DNA strand. A double-stranded DNA version of the virion genome is required for transcription and replication. Inverted repeat

BOX 58-1 The Parvoviridae

Parvovirus (e.g., B19, RA-1)
Dependovirus
Densovirus

BOX 58-2 Unique Properties of Parvoviruses

Smallest DNA virus
Naked icosahedral capsid
Single-stranded DNA genome
Requires growing cells (B19) or helper virus (dependovirus) for replication

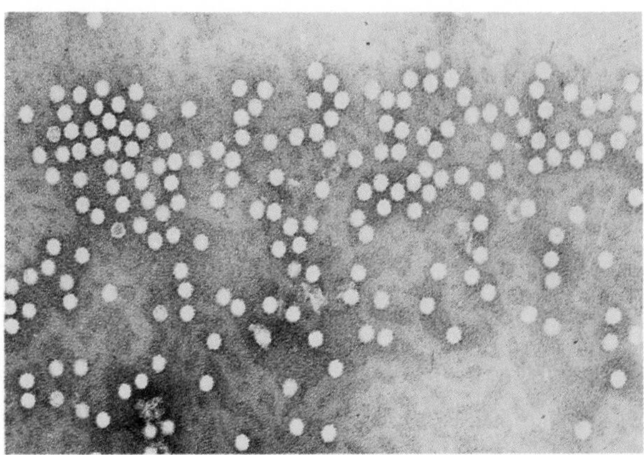

FIGURE 58-1 Electron micrograph of parvovirus. Parvoviruses are small (18-26 nm), nonenveloped, single-stranded DNA viruses. (Courtesy Centers for Disease Control.)

sequences of DNA at both ends of the genome facilitate viral DNA synthesis. These ends fold back and hybridize with the genome to create a primer for the cell's DNA polymerase. mRNA for the nonstructural (NS) regulatory and structural (VP) capsid proteins are generated from the same promotor by differential splicing of the primary transcript. Viral proteins synthesized in the cytoplasm return to the nucleus where the virion is assembled. Nuclear and cytoplasmic membrane degeneration occurs, and the virus is released upon cell lysis.

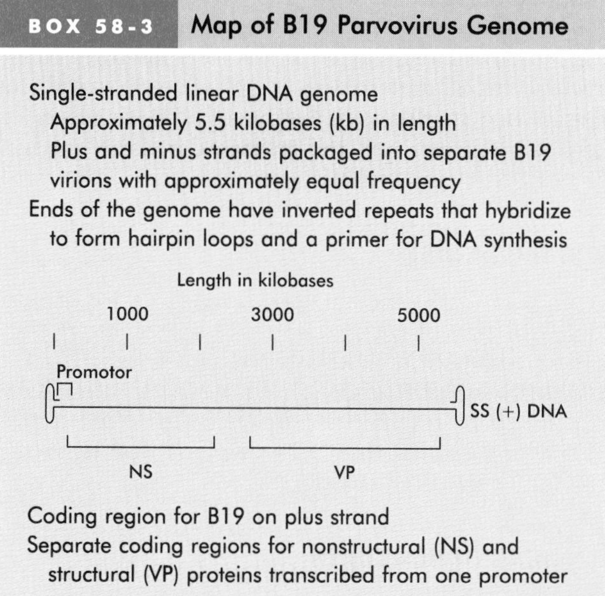

BOX 58-3 Map of B19 Parvovirus Genome
Single-stranded linear DNA genome
Approximately 5.5 kilobases (kb) in length
Plus and minus strands packaged into separate B19 virions with approximately equal frequency
Ends of the genome have inverted repeats that hybridize to form hairpin loops and a primer for DNA synthesis
Length in kilobases
1000
3000
5000
Promotor
SS (+) DNA
NS
VP
Coding region for B19 on plus strand
Separate coding regions for nonstructural (NS) and structural (VP) proteins transcribed from one promoter

PATHOGENESIS AND IMMUNITY

B19 targets erythroid cells and requires growing/cycling cells for replication, such as fetal or hematopoietic stem cells (Box 58-4). These basic requirements define the susceptible target cells and, with the immune response to the infection, determine the nature of its disease.

Studies on volunteers suggest that B19 virus first replicates in the upper respiratory tract. It then spreads by viremia to the bone marrow and elsewhere, where it replicates and kills or inhibits the growth of erythroid precursor cells (Figure 58-3). The disease course for B19 is biphasic. The **initial febrile stage** is the infectious stage.

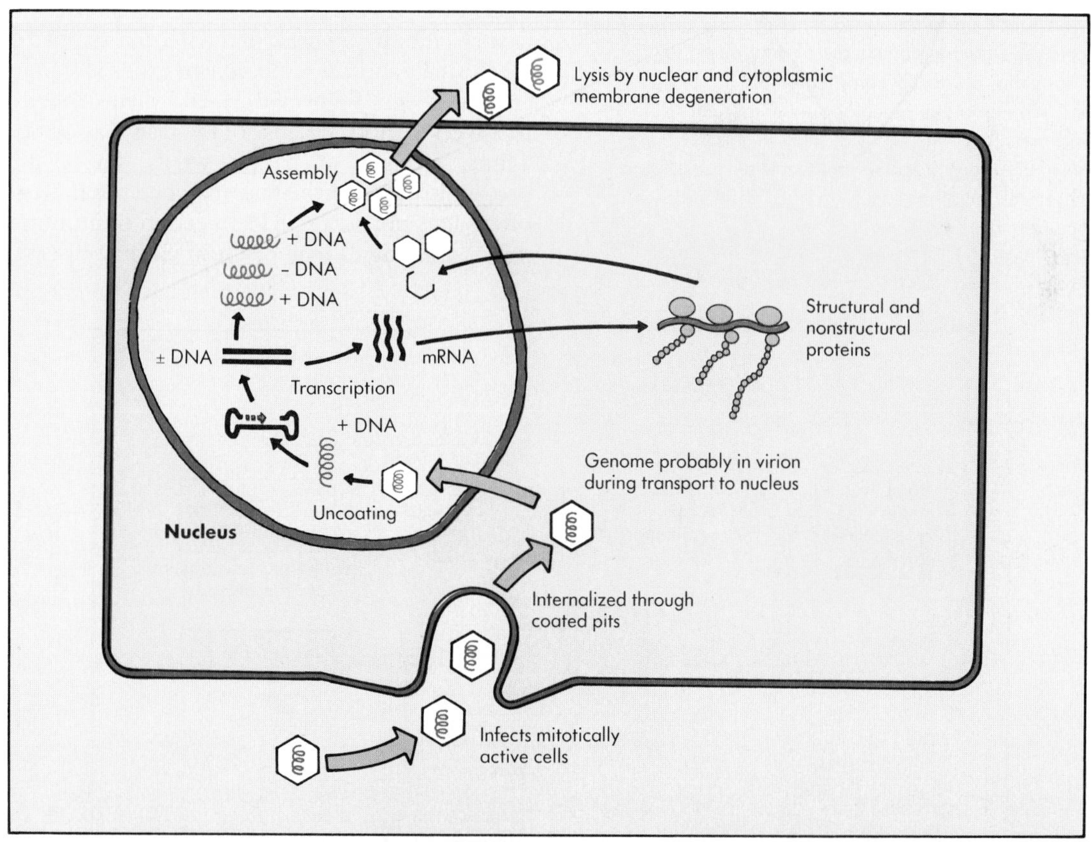

FIGURE 58-2 Postulated replication of parvovirus (B19) based on information from related viruses (minute virus of mice). The internalized parvovirus delivers its genome to the nucleus where the single stranded (+ or -) DNA is converted to double-stranded DNA by host factors and DNA polymerases present only in growing cells. Transcription, replication, and assembly occur in the nucleus. Virus is released by cell lysis.

The virus lytically infects erythroid precursor cells, depleting these cells and halting erythrocyte production. Viremia occurs within 8 days of infection, accompanied by nonspecific viral symptoms. High titers of virus are released into oral and respiratory secretions. The **second symptomatic stage** characteristic of the disease appears to be immune mediated. The rash and arthralgia associated with erythema infectiosum coincides with the appearance of virus-specific IgM and the disappearance of detectable B19 virus. Antibody presumably confers lifelong immunity.

B19 infection of a normal host may cause no noticeable symptoms or may cause fever and nonspecific symptoms such as sore throat, malaise, and myalgia, and a slight decrease in hemoglobin levels followed by a rash 2 to 3 weeks later (Figure 58-4).

B19 infection of hosts with chronic hemolytic anemia (e.g., sickle cell anemia) are at risk for a life-threatening reticulocytopenia referred to as **aplastic crisis**. Aplastic crisis is due to the combination of B19 depletion of red-cell precursors and the shortened red-cell survival time caused by the underlying anemia.

BOX 58-4 Disease Mechanisms of B19 Parvovirus

- Virus is spread by respiratory and oral secretions
- Virus infects mitotically active erythroid precursor cells in bone marrow and establishes a lytic infection
- Virus establishes a large viremia and can cross the placenta
- Antibody is important for resolution and prophylaxis
- Virus causes biphasic disease:
  - Initial phase related to viremia
    - Flu-like symptoms and virus shedding
  - Later phase related to immune response
    - Circulating immune complexes of antibody and virions that do not fix complement
    - Result: erythematous maculopapular rash, arthralgia, and arthritis
- Depletion of erythroid precursor cells and destabilization of erythrocytes initiate aplastic crisis in individuals with chronic anemia

EPIDEMIOLOGY

As much as 65% of the adult population are infected with B19 by 40 years of age (Box 58-5). Erythema infectiosum is most common in children from ages 4 to 15, and it tends to occur in late winter and spring. B19 is most likely transmitted by respiratory droplets and oral secretions. Parenteral transmission of B19 by blood-clotting factor concentrate has been described.

CLINICAL SYNDROMES

B19 virus is the cause of **erythema infectiosum** (fifth disease) (Box 58-6). Infection starts with an unremarkable prodrome period during which the individual is infectious. This is followed by a distinctive rash on the face resembling a cheek that has been slapped. The rash then usually spreads, especially to exposed skin such as the arms and legs (Figure 58-5), and then subsides over a 1 to 2 week period. Relapse of the rash may occur often. In adults, arthritis of hands, wrists, knees, and ankles predominates, and the rash may precede the arthritis but often does not occur. B19 infection of immunocompromised individuals may result in chronic disease.

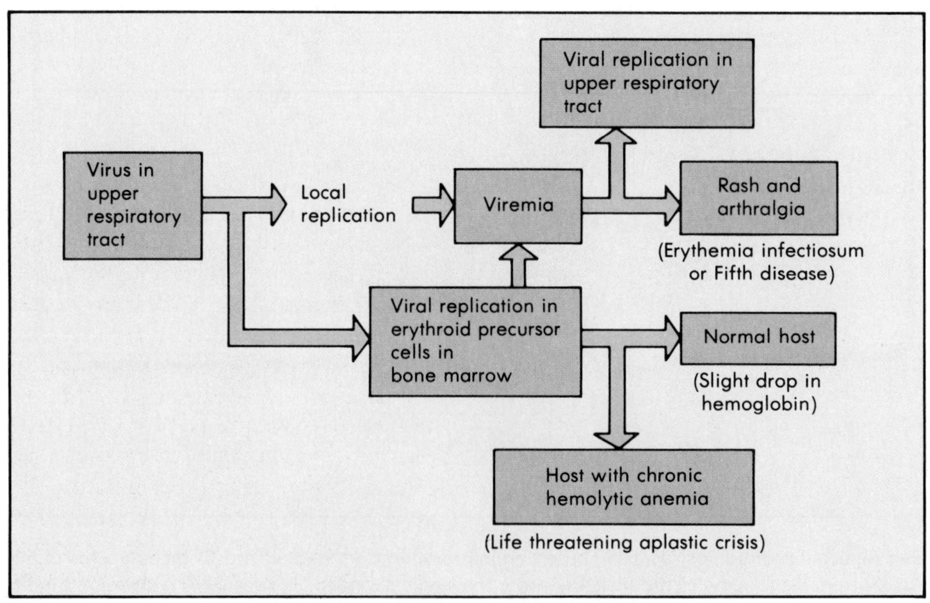

FIGURE 58-3 Mechanism of spread of parvovirus within the body.

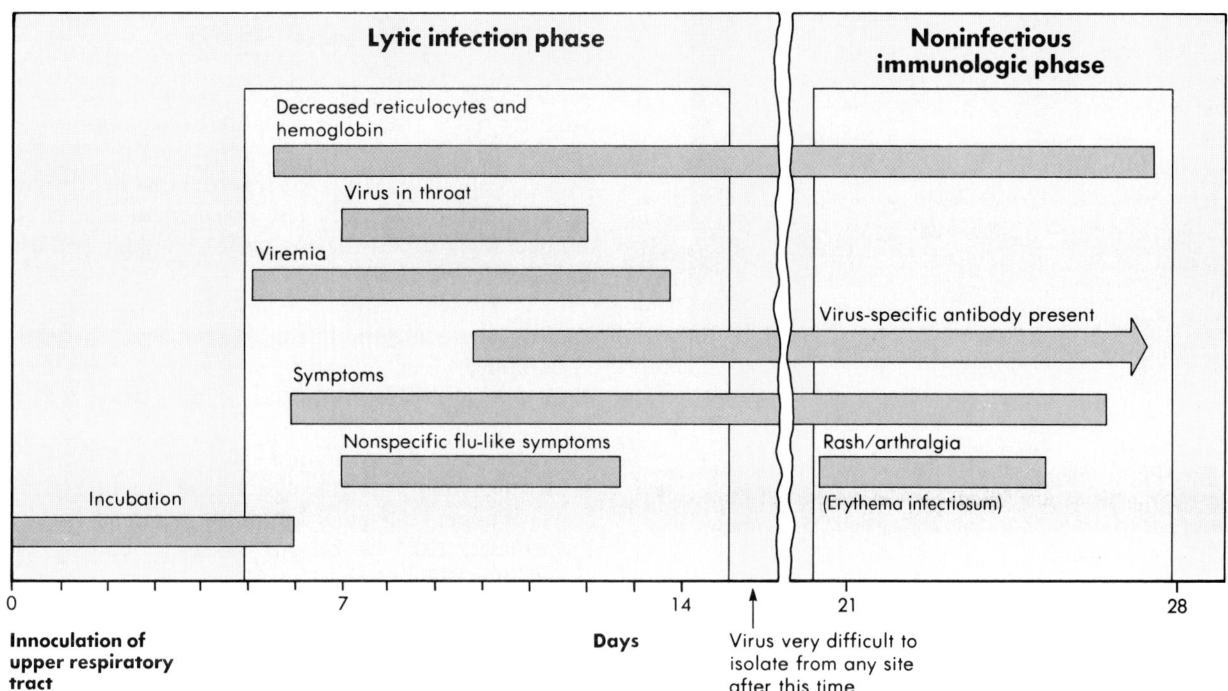

FIGURE 58-4 Time course of parvovirus (B19) infection. B19 causes biphasic disease, an initial lytic infection phase, characterized by febrile, flu-like symptoms, followed by a noninfectious immunological phase characterized by a rash and arthralgia.

BOX 58-5 Epidemiology of B19 Parvovirus Infection

DISEASE/VIRAL FACTORS

Capsid virus resistant to inactivation
Contagious period precedes symptoms
Virus crosses the placenta and infects fetus

TRANSMISSION

Respiratory droplets

WHO IS AT RISK?

Children, especially elementary-school age: erythemia infectiosum (fifth disease)
Pregnant women: fetal infection and disease
Individuals with chronic anemia: aplastic crisis

GEOGRAPHY/SEASON

Worldwide
Fifth disease more common in late winter and spring

MODES OF CONTROL

None

BOX 58-6 Clinical Consequences of Parvovirus (B19) Infection

Mild flu-like illness (fever, headache, chills, myalgia, malaise)
Erythema infectiosum (fifth disease)
Aplastic crisis in people with chronic anemia
Arthropathy (rheumatoid arthritis–like symptoms)
B19 virus crosses placenta, causing risk of fetal loss due to anemia-related pathology, but does not appear to cause congenital abnormalities

The most serious complication of parvovirus infection is the aplastic crisis that occurs in patients with chronic hemolytic anemia (sickle cell anemia). In these individuals the infection causes a transient reduction of erythropoiesis in the bone marrow. This results in a transient reticulocytopenia (7 to 10 days) and a decrease in hemoglobin levels. Aplastic crisis is accompanied by fever and nonspecific symptoms of malaise, myalgia, chills, and itching. A maculopapular rash with arthralgia and some joint swelling may also be present.

B19 infection of a seronegative mother increases the risk for fetal death. The virus can infect the fetus and kill erythrocyte precursors, causing anemia and congestive heart failure (hydrops fetalis). Infection of pregnant women often occurs without any adverse effect on the

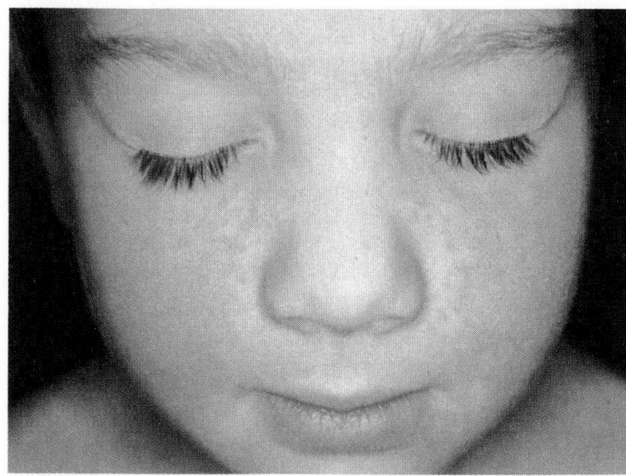

FIGURE 58-5 A "slapped cheek" appearance is typical of the rash for erythema infectiosum. (From Hart CA, Broadhead RL: *A color atlas of pediatric infectious diseases*, London, 1992, Mosby.)

fetus. There is no evidence that B19 causes congenital abnormalities (Box 58-5).

LABORATORY DIAGNOSIS

Routine laboratory diagnosis of B19 infection is not readily available. B19 virus can be detected in serum or throat washes during the prodromal period or aplastic crisis by immune electron microscopy, enzyme and radioimmunoassay, polymerase chain reaction, and nucleic acid hybridization. The polymerase chain reaction is a very sensitive method for detecting the B19 genome in clinical samples but requires adequate controls. Detection of virus-specific IgM or viral DNA sequences in blood is sufficient for the diagnosis. No cell culture system is available for tissue culture isolation of the virus.

TREATMENT, PREVENTION, AND CONTROL

No specific antiviral treatment is available. Control of respiratory spread could decrease transmission of B19 virus; however, infectivity precedes the clinically apparent immunological phase (erythema infectiosum). Transmission therefore would occur before preventive measures (e.g., isolation) would be enacted.

CASE STUDY AND QUESTIONS

Mrs. Doe calls the pediatrician, complaining that her daughter has a rash. The daughter's face appears as if slapped. She has no fever or other notable symptom. Upon questioning, Mrs. Doe reported that her daughter had a mild cold within the last 2 weeks and that she (the mother) was currently having more joint pain than usual and is very tired.

1. What features of this history suggest a parvovirus B19 etiology?
2. Is the child infectious, and, if not, when was she contagious?
3. What causes the symptoms?
4. Are the symptoms of the mother and daughter related?
5. What underlying condition would put the daughter at increased risk for serious disease following B19 infection? The mother?
6. Why is quarantine a poor means of limiting the spread of B19 parvovirus infection?

Bibliography

Anderson LJ: Human parvoviruses, *J Infect Dis* 161:603-608, 1990.

Anderson MJ: Parvoviruses. In Belshe RB, editor: *Textbook of human virology*, ed 2, St. Louis, 1991, Mosby.

Balows A, Hausler WJ Jr, and Lennette EH, editors: *Laboratory diagnosis of infectious diseases: principles and practice*, vol 2, New York, 1988, Springer-Verlag.

Berns KI: *The parvoviruses*, New York, 1984, Plenum Press.

Chorba T et al.: The role of parvovirus B19 in aplastic crisis and erythema infectiosum (fifth disease), *J Infect Dis* 154:383, 1986.

Berns KI: Parvovirus replication, *Microbiol Rev* 54:316-329, 1990.

Török TJ: Parvovirus B19 and Human Disease. In Stollerman GH et al.: *Advances in internal medicine*, vol 37, St. Louis, 1992, Mosby.

Naides SJ, Scharosch LL, Foto F, and Howard EJ: Rheumatologic manifestations of human parvovirus B19 infection in adults, *Arthritis Rheum* 33:1297-1309, 1990.

Ware RE: Parvovirus infections. In Krugman SK, Katz SL, Gersho AA, Wilfert CM: *Infectious diseases of children*, ed 9, St. Louis, 1992, Mosby.

CHAPTER 59

Picornaviruses

PICORNAVIRIDAE is one of the largest families of viruses and includes some of the most important human and animal viruses (Box 59-1). As the name indicates, these viruses are small (pico) ribonucleic acid (RNA) viruses that have a naked capsid structure. The family includes more than 230 members divided into four genera: enterovirus, rhinovirus, cardiovirus, and aphthovirus. Of these, only enterovirus and rhinovirus cause human disease. The enteroviruses and rhinoviruses can be distinguished by the stability of the capsid at pH 3, optimum temperature for growth, mode of transmission, and the diseases they cause (Box 59-2).

At least 72 serotypes of human enteroviruses exist, including the polio, coxsackie, and echo viruses. Hepatitis A virus is also classified in this group (enterovirus 72) but is discussed separately in Chapter 68. The capsids of these viruses are very resistant to harsh environmental conditions (sewage systems) and the gastrointestinal tract, which facilitates their transmission by the fecal-oral route. Although they may initiate their infection in the gastrointestinal tract, the enteroviruses rarely cause enteric disease, and infections are usually asymptomatic. Several different disease syndromes may be caused by a specific enterovirus serotype. Likewise, several different serotypes may cause the same disease, depending on the target tissue affected. The most well-known and well-studied picornavirus is poliovirus, of which there are three serotypes.

Coxsackieviruses are named after the town of Coxsackie, N.Y., where the first isolation was made. They are divided into two groups, A and B, on the basis of certain biological and antigenic differences and further subdivided into numerical serotypes by additional antigenic differences.

The name *echovirus* is an abbreviation of *e*nteric *c*ytopathic *h*uman *o*rphan, since these agents were not thought to be associated with clinical disease. The lack of pathogenicity in mice was used to distinguish echoviruses from coxsackieviruses. Now 32 serotypes are recognized. Since 1967, newly isolated enteroviruses are distinguished numerically.

The human rhinoviruses include at least 100 serotypes and are the major cause of the common cold. The rhinoviruses are sensitive to acidic pH and replicate poorly at temperatures above 33° C. This sensitivity usually limits rhinoviruses to upper respiratory infections.

STRUCTURE

The plus-strand RNA of the picornaviruses is surrounded by an icosahedral capsid approximately 30 nm in diameter. The icosahedral capsid has 12 pentameric vertices, each of which is composed of five protomeric units of proteins. The protomers are made of four virion polypeptides (VP_{1-4}). VP_2 and VP_4 are generated by cleavage of a precursor, VP_0. The presence of VP_4 in the virion solidifies the structure. VP_4 is not generated until the genome is incorporated into the capsid, and it is released on binding to the cellular receptor. The capsids are stable

BOX 59-1 Picornaviridae

- Enterovirus
  - Poliovrius types 1, 2, and 3
  - Coxsackie A virus types 1-22, 24
  - Coxsackie B virus types 1-6
  - Echovirus (ECHO virus) types 1-9, 11-27, 29-34
  - Enterovirus 68-72 (72 is hepatitis A virus)
- Rhinovirus Types 1-100+
- Cardiovirus
- Aphthovirus

BOX 59-2 Unique Properties of Human Picornaviruses

- Naked, small (25 to 30 nm), icosahedral capsid enclosing a single-strand positive (+) RNA genome
  - Enteroviruses: resistant to pH 3 to 9, detergents, mild sewage treatment, and temperature
  - Rhinoviruses: labile at acidic pHs; optimum growth temperature: 33° C
- Genome is a mRNA
- Virus replicates in the cytoplasm
- Viral RNA is translated into a polyprotein, which is then cleaved into enzymatic and structural proteins
- Most viruses are cytolytic

in heat and detergent, and, except for the rhinoviruses, are also stable in acid. The capsid structure is so regular that paracrystals of virions often form in infected cells (Figure 59-1 and Figure 59-2).

The genome of the picornaviruses resembles a messenger RNA (mRNA) (Figure 59-3). It is a single strand of plus-sense RNA of approximately 7400 bases that has a polyA at the 3′ end and a small protein called VPg (22 to 24 amino acids) attached to the 5′ end. The genome by itself is infectious and can initiate virus replication. The polyA sequence enhances the infectivity of the RNA, and the VPg may be important in packaging the genome into the capsid and initiating viral RNA synthesis.

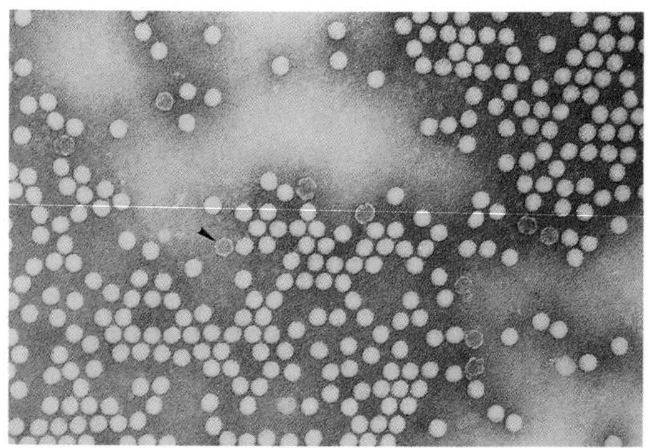

FIGURE 59-1 Electron micrograph of poliovirus. (Courtesy Centers for Disease Control.)

The genome encodes a polyprotein that is proteolytically cleaved to produce the enzymatic and structural proteins of the virus. In addition to the capsid proteins and VPg, the picornaviruses encode at least one protease and an RNA-dependent RNA polymerase. Poliovirus also produces a protease that degrades the 200,000 d cap-binding protein of eukaryotic ribosomes blocking translation of cellular mRNA.

REPLICATION

The specificity of picornavirus interaction for cellular receptors is the major determinant of their target tissue tropism and disease (see Figure 7-7). The VP_1 proteins at the vertices of the virion contain a canyon structure into

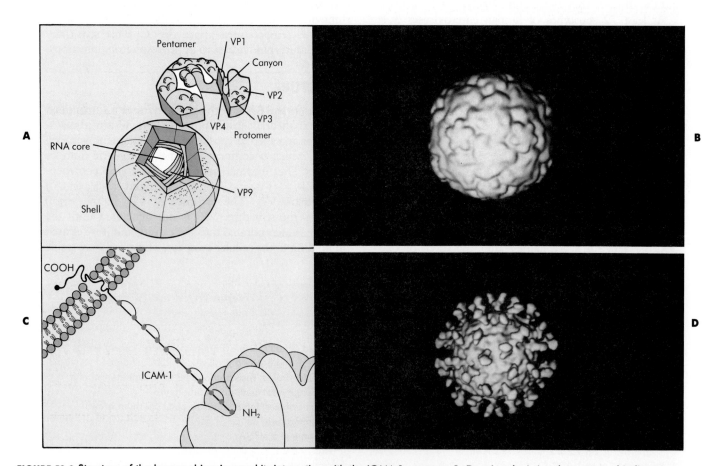

FIGURE 59-2 Structure of the human rhinovirus and its interaction with the ICAM-1 receptor. **A,** Drawing depicting the receptor-binding canyon surrounding the starlike structure at the vertices. **B,** Cryoelectron microscopy computed-generated reconstruction of human rhinovirus 16 (HRV 16). **C,** The terminal portion of the ICAM-1 molecule interacts with the virion. **D,** Cryoelectron microscopy reconstruction of ICAM-1 (terminal portion) interacting with HRV 16. (Computer reconstructions courtesy Tim Baker, Purdue University.)

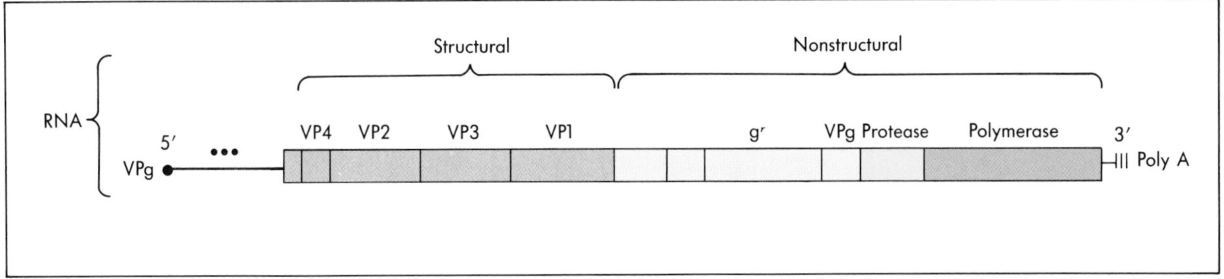

FIGURE 59-3 Structure of the picornaviral genome. The genome is translated as a polyprotein, which is successfully cleaved by virus encoded and cellular proteases to individual proteins. g^r represents the guanidine resistance marker, a genetic locus involved in initiation of RNA synthesis.

which the receptor binds. The site of binding is protected from antibody neutralization. Arildone and other antiviral compounds contain a 3-methylisoxazole group that binds to the floor of this canyon and alters its conformation to prevent the uncoating of the virus.

The picornaviruses have been categorized into several receptor families. The receptors for polioviruses and rhinoviruses have recently been identified as tissue-specific cellular adhesion molecules. These molecules are members of the immunoglobulin gene superfamily. Their function is to promote normal and immunological cell-to-cell interactions. At least 80% of the rhinoviruses and several serotypes of coxsackievirus recognize intercellular adhesion molecule 1 (ICAM-1). ICAM-1 is expressed on epithelial cells, fibroblasts, and endothelial cells. Poliovirus binds to a molecule of similar structure and presumably of similar function. The cells in which the poliovirus receptor is expressed correlate directly with the limited range of poliovirus infection.

On binding to the receptor, the VP_4 is released and the virion weakened. The virus is internalized by receptor-mediated endocytosis, and the virions dissociate in the acidic environment of the endosome, releasing the genome into the cytoplasm. The genome binds directly to ribosomes despite the lack of a 5′ cap structure. The ribosomes recognize a unique internal RNA loop in the genome. A polyprotein containing all the viral protein sequences is synthesized within 10 to 15 minutes of infection. The polyprotein is initially cleaved by cellular proteases until a viral protease is released to cleave the rest of the polyprotein. The RNA-dependent RNA polymerase generates a negative-strand RNA template from which the new mRNA/genome and templates can be synthesized. The amount of viral mRNA increases rapidly in the cell, with the number of viral RNA molecules reaching 400,000 per cell.

Several picornaviruses inhibit cellular RNA and protein synthesis during infection. Cleavage of the 200,000d cap-binding protein of the ribosome by a poliovirus protease prevents most cellular mRNA binding to the ribosome. Permeability changes induced by picornaviruses reduce the ability of cellular mRNA to bind to the ribosome. Viral mRNA can also outcompete cellular mRNA for the factors required in protein synthesis. These activities contribute to the cytopathic effect of the virus on the target cell.

As the viral genome is being replicated and translated, the structural proteins VP_0, VP_1, and VP_3 are cleaved from the polyprotein and assembled into subunits. Five subunits associate into pentamers, and 12 pentamers associate to form the procapsid. After insertion of the genome, VP_0 is cleaved into VP_2 and VP_4 proteins to complete the capsid. The virion is released upon cell lysis.

BOX 59-3 Disease Mechanisms of Picornaviruses

Enteroviruses enter via the upper respiratory tract, oropharynx, or intestinal mucosa and infect the underlying lymphatic tissue; rhinoviruses are restricted to the upper respiratory tract.
In the absence of serum antibody, Enterovirus spreads by viremia to cells of a receptor-bearing target tissue
Different serotypes of picornaviruses bind to different receptors, many of which are members of the immunoglobulin super gene family (e.g., ICAM-1)
The infected target tissue determines the subsequent disease
Viral, rather than immune, pathology is usually responsible for disease symptoms
Secretory antibody response is transient but can prevent initiation of infection
Serum antibody blocks viremic spread to target tissue, preventing symptoms
Enterovirus is shed into feces for long periods
Infection is usually asymptomatic or causes mild "flu-like" or upper respiratory disease

ENTEROVIRUSES

Pathogenesis and Immunity

Enterovirus infections are usually asymptomatic but can range from coldlike symptoms to paralytic disease (Box

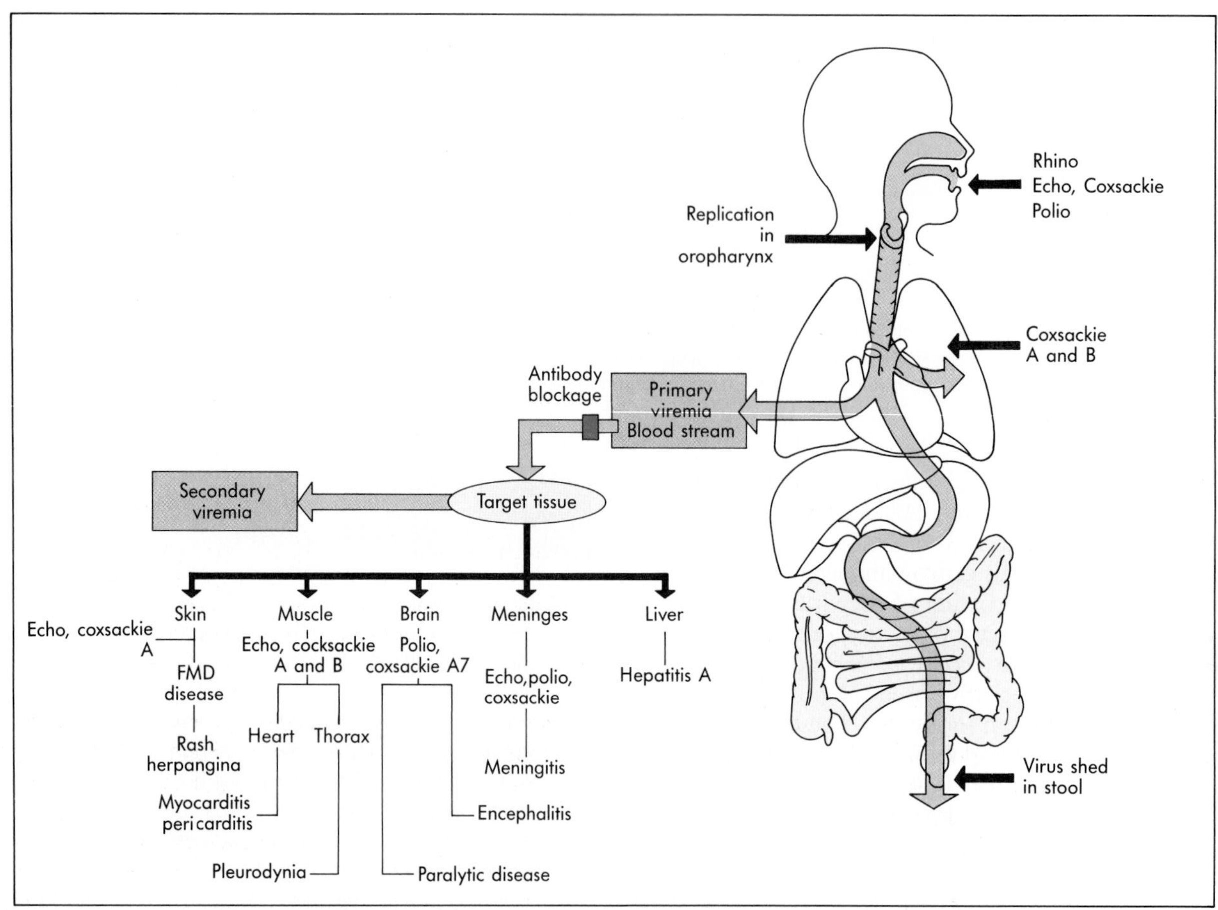

FIGURE 59-4 Pathogenesis of enteroviruses. The target tissue infected by the enterovirus determines the predominant disease caused by the virus.

59-3). Differences in pathogenesis for the enteroviruses mainly result from differences in tissue tropism and cytolytic capacity of the virus (Figure 59-4). Poliovirus has been studied extensively and is the prototype for the pathogenesis of the enteroviruses.

The upper respiratory tract, the oropharynx, and the intestinal tract are the portals of entry for the enteroviruses. The virions are impervious to stomach acid, proteases, and bile. The virus initiates replication in the mucosa and lymphoid tissue of the tonsils and pharynx and later infects lymphoid cells of Peyer's patches underlying the intestinal mucosa. Primary viremia spreads the virus to receptor-bearing target tissues, where a second phase of viral replication may occur, resulting in symptoms and a secondary viremia. Recent studies with transgenic mice suggest an alternate route for poliovirus infection of the brain. Viremia may spread poliovirus to skeletal muscle, from where the virus accesses the innervating nerves and then travels to the brain, somewhat like rabies (see Chapter 65). Virus shedding from the oropharynx can be detected for a short time before symptoms begin, whereas virus production and shedding from the intestine may last for 30 days or longer, even in the presence of a humoral immune response.

Poliovirus has one of the narrowest tissue tropisms, recognizing a receptor expressed on anterior horn cells of the spinal cord, dorsal root ganglia, motor neurons, skeletal muscle, and lymphoid and few other cells. Coxsackieviruses and echoviruses recognize receptors expressed on more cell types and tissues and cause a broader repertoire of diseases (Table 59-1). These and other enteroviruses recognize receptors on cells of the central nervous system, heart, lung, pancreas, and other tissues.

Most enteroviruses are cytolytic, replicating rapidly and causing direct damage to the target cell. Hepatitis A is the exception. It is not very cytolytic, and the kinetics of the immune response to hepatitis A correlate with the appearance of symptoms.

Antibody is the major protective immune response to the enteroviruses. Secretory antibody can prevent the initial establishment of infection in the oropharynx and gastrointestinal tract, and serum antibody prevents viremic spread to the target tissue and therefore disease. Serum antibody is generally observed 7 to 10 days after infection. The time course for antibody development following vaccine administration is presented in Figure 59-10.

TABLE 59-1 Summary of Clinical Syndromes Associated With Major Enterovirus Groups

Syndrome	Occurrence	Polioviruses	Coxsackie A viruses	Coxsackie B viruses	Echoviruses
Paralytic disease	Sporadic	+	+	+	+
Encephalitis, meningitis	Outbreaks	+	+	+	+
Carditis	Sporadic		+	+	+
Neonatal disease	Outbreaks			+	+
Pleurodynia	Outbreaks			+	
Herpangina	Common		+		
Hand-foot-mouth disease	Common		+		
Rash disease	Common		+	+	+
Acute hemorrhagic conjunctivitis	Epidemics		+		
Respiratory infections	Common	+	+	+	+
Undifferentiated fever	Common	+	+	+	+
Diarrhea, gastrointestinal disease	Uncommon				+
Diabetes, pancreatitis	Uncommon			+	
Orchitis	Uncommon			+	
Disease in immunodeficient patients	—	+	+		+
Congenital anomalies	Uncommon		+	+	

Cell-mediated immunity is not usually involved in protection but may play a role in pathogenesis. Hepatitis A virus is the exception. T cells appear to contribute to coxsackie B virus–induced myocarditis in mice.

Epidemiology

The enteroviruses are exclusively human pathogens (Box 59-4). As the name implies, these viruses are primarily spread by the fecal-oral route. Asymptomatic shedding can occur for up to a month. Poor sanitation and crowded living conditions foster transmission of enteroviruses (Figure 59-5). Sewage contamination of water supplies can result in enterovirus epidemics. Outbreaks of enterovirus disease are seen in schools and day-care settings. Summer is the major season for enterovirus disease. The coxsackieviruses and echoviruses may also be spread in aerosol droplets to cause respiratory infections.

Poliomyelitis occurs throughout the world, and polioviruses are spread most often during the summer and fall. With the success of the polio vaccines, the wild type poliovirus has been eliminated from the western hemisphere (Figure 59-6). However, in areas where the vaccine is not available or in communities where vaccination is contrary to religious beliefs or other teachings, paralytic polio still may occur.

Paralytic polio was once called a middle-class disease. Good hygiene would delay exposure to the virus until late childhood, the adolescent years, or adulthood, when infection would produce the most severe symptoms. Infection during early childhood generally results in asymptomatic or very mild disease.

As with poliovirus infection, coxsackie A virus disease in adults is generally more severe than in children. However, coxsackie B virus and some of the echoviruses (especially echo 11) can be particularly harmful to infants. Differences in the susceptibility to and severity of poliovirus and coxsackievirus infection with age may be due to differences in distribution and amount of receptor expression or other factors.

The enteroviruses most frequently associated with disease are coxsackie A9, A16, B2 to B5, and echo 6, 9, and 11. These viruses are found worldwide. Disease caused by the other enteroviruses occurs as sporadic outbreaks.

Clinical Syndromes

The clinical syndromes of the enteroviruses are determined by several factors, including the viral serotype, infecting dose, tissue tropism, portal of entry, age, sex, pregnancy, and state of health. The incubation period for enterovirus disease varies from 1 to 35 days, depending on the virus, the target tissue, and the age of the individual. The shortest incubation periods are for the viruses that affect oral and respiratory sites.

Poliovirus Infections

"Wild" polio infections are becoming rarer because of the success of the polio vaccines (Figure 59-6). However, vaccine-associated cases of polio do occur, and some populations remain unvaccinated. Poliovirus may cause one of four outcomes in unvaccinated individuals depending on the progression of the infection (Figure 59-7):

Asymptomatic illness results if the virus is limited to infection of the oropharynx and the gut. At least 90% of poliovirus infections are of the asymptomatic type.

Abortive poliomyelitis, the **minor illness**, is a nonspecific febrile illness occurring in approximately 5% of infected individuals. Symptoms of fever, headache, malaise, sore throat, and vomiting occur within 3 to 4 days of exposure.

BOX 59-4 Epidemiology of *Enterovirus* Infections

DISEASE/VIRAL FACTORS

Virion is resistant to environmental conditions (detergents, acid, drying, mild sewage treatment, and temperature)
Infection is often asymptomatic

TRANSMISSION

Fecal-oral route: poor hygiene, dirty diapers (especially in day-care settings)
Ingestion via contaminated food and water
Contact with infected hands and fomites
Inhalation of infectious aerosols

WHO IS AT RISK?

Polio: young children: asymptomatic or mild disease
Older children and adults: asymptomatic to paralytic disease
Coxsackievirus and echovirus: the nature of the disease correlates with specific enterovirus types and the age of the individual. Newborns and neonates are at highest risk to serious disease

GEOGRAPHY/SEASON

Worldwide distribution; wild type polio virtually eradicated in developed countries because of vaccine program
Disease more common in summer

MODES OF CONTROL

Polio: Live oral vaccine (trivalent OPV) or inactivated trivalent vaccine (IPV)
Other enteroviruses: no vaccine; good hygiene limits spread

Nonparalytic poliomyelitis or **aseptic meningitis** occurs in 1% to 2% of patients with poliovirus infections. The virus progresses into the central nervous system and the meninges, causing back pain and muscle spasms in addition to the symptoms of minor illness.

Paralytic polio, the **major illness**, occurs in 0.1% to 2.0% of persons with poliovirus infections and is the most severe outcome. Major illness follows 3 to 4 days after minor illness has subsided, thereby producing a biphasic illness. In this disease the virus spreads from the blood to the anterior horn cells of the spinal cord and the motor cortex of the brain. The severity of the paralysis is determined by the extent of the neuronal infection and the neurons affected. Spinal paralysis may involve one or more limbs, whereas bulbar (cranial) paralysis may involve a combination of cranial nerves and even the medullary respiratory center.

Paralytic poliomyelitis is characterized by an asymmetric flaccid paralysis with no sensory loss. Poliovirus type 1 affects 85% of patients with paralytic disease. Types 2 or 3 may cause vaccine-associated disease because of reversion from attenuated virus to virulence.

The degree of paralysis may vary from involving only a few muscle groups (e.g., one leg) to complete flaccid paralysis of all four extremities. The paralysis may progress over the first few days and result in complete recovery, residual paralysis, or death. Most recoveries occur within 6 months, but as long as 2 years may be required for complete remission.

Bulbar poliomyelitis can be more severe and may involve the muscles of the pharynx, vocal cords, and respiration and result in death in 75% of patients. Iron lungs, chambers providing external respiratory compression, were used to assist the breathing of polio patients during the 1950s. Before vaccination programs, iron lungs filled the wards of children's hospitals.

Post-polio syndrome is a sequelae of poliomyelitis that may occur much later in life (30 to 40 years) for 20% to 80% of the original victims. These individuals suffer a deterioration of the originally affected muscles. Poliovirus is not present, but the syndrome is believed to be due to a loss of neurons in the initially affected nerves.

Coxsackievirus and Echovirus

Several clinical syndromes may be caused by either coxsackievirus or echovirus (e.g., aseptic meningitis), but certain illnesses are especially associated with coxsackieviruses. For example, coxsackie A viruses are highly associated with herpangina, whereas myocarditis and pleurodynia are most frequently caused by coxsackie B serotypes (B for body). These viruses can also cause polio-like paralytic disease. The most common results of infection are no symptoms, mild upper respiratory or "flu-like" disease.

Herpangina is inappropriately named because it has no relation to herpesvirus. Rather, it is caused by several types of coxsackie A virus. Fever, sore throat, pain on swallowing, anorexia, and vomiting characterize herpangina. The classic finding is vesicular ulcerated lesions around the soft palate and uvula (Figure 59-8). Less typically the lesions may affect the hard palate. The virus can be recovered from the lesions or from feces. The disease is self-limited and requires only symptomatic management.

Pleurodynia (Bornholm disease), also known as the "devil's grip," is an acute illness in which patients have sudden onset of fever and unilateral low thoracic, pleuritic, chest pain, which may be excruciating. Abdominal pain and even vomiting may also occur. Muscles on the involved side may be extremely tender. Pleurodynia lasts an average of 4 days but may relapse after the patient has been asymptomatic for several days. Coxsackie B virus is the causative agent.

Viral, or **aseptic**, **meningitis** is an acute febrile illness accompanied by headache and signs of meningeal irritation, including nuchal rigidity. Petechiae or skin rash may occur in patients with enteroviral meningitis. Recovery is

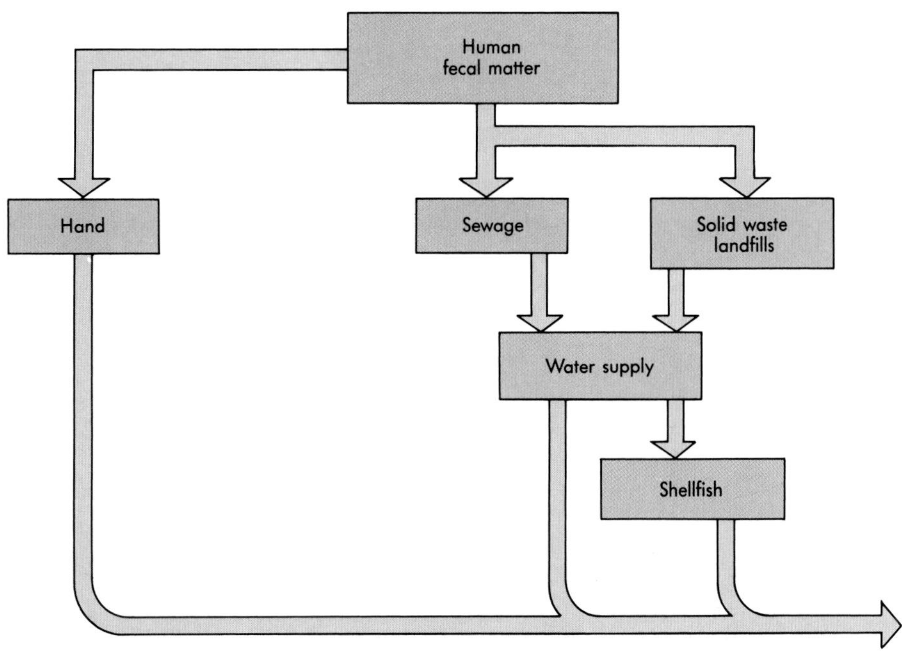

FIGURE 59-5 Transmission of enteroviruses. The capsid structure is resistant to mild sewage treatment, salt water, detergents, and temperature changes, allowing these viruses to be transmitted by fecal/oral routes and on hands.

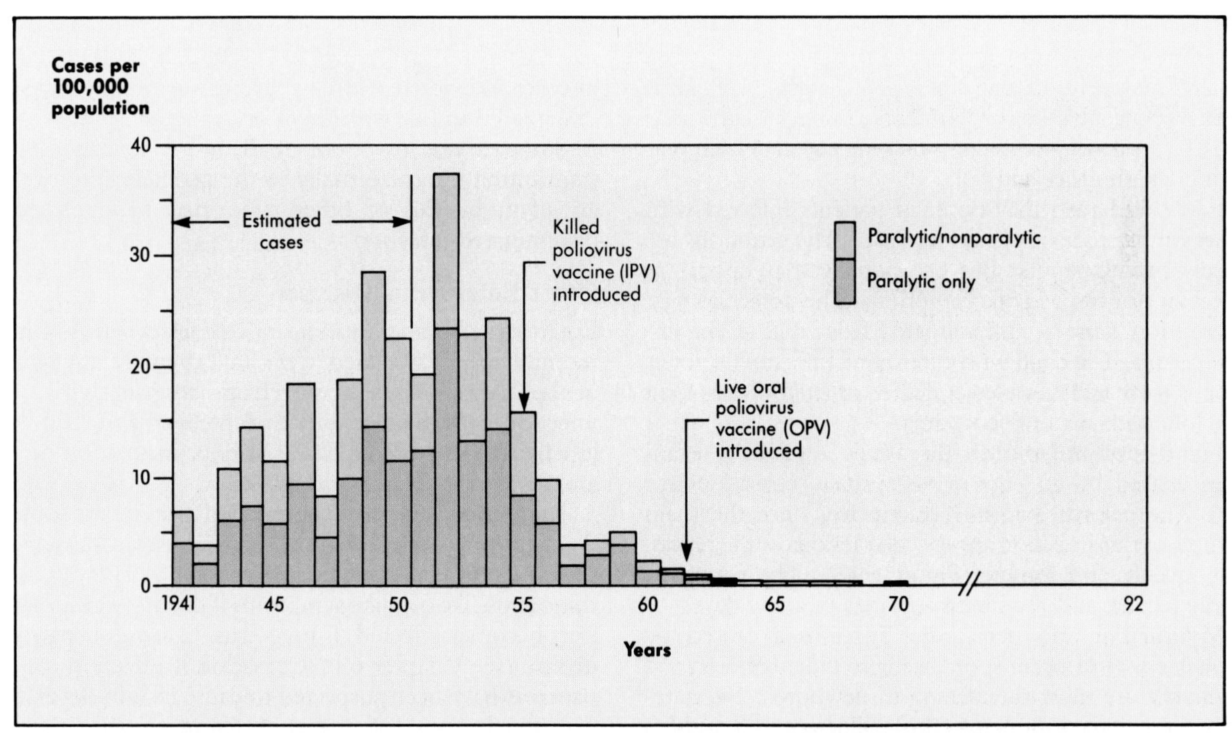

FIGURE 59-6 Polio incidence in the United States. Killed (inactivated) poliovirus vaccine was introduced in 1955 and live (oral) poliovirus vaccine in 1961-1962. (Courtesy Centers for Disease Control: Immunization against disease—1972, Washington, DC, 1973, US Government Printing Office.)

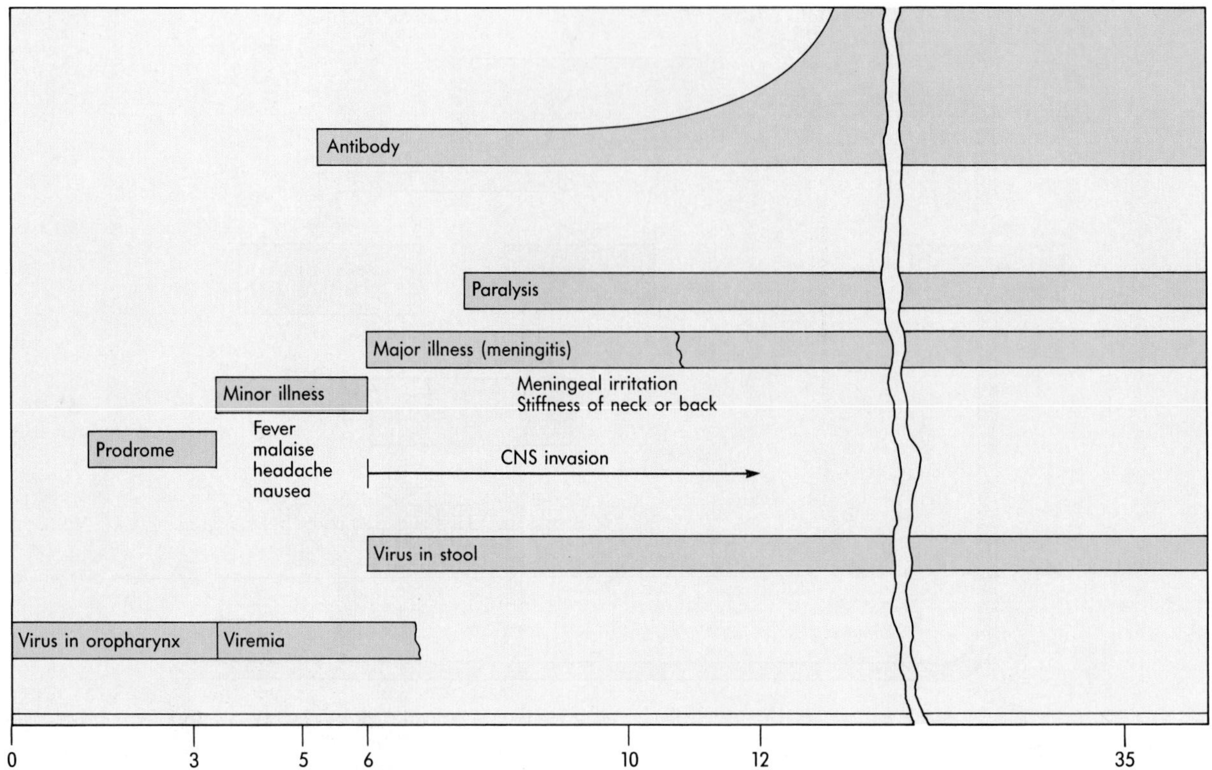

FIGURE 59-7 Progression of poliovirus infection. Polio infection may be asymptomatic or progress to either minor or major disease.

usually uneventful except if associated with encephalitis (meningoencephalitis) or in infants younger than 1 year old. Outbreaks of picornavirus meningitis occur each year during the summer and fall.

Fever and rash may occur in patients infected with either echoviruses or coxsackieviruses. The eruptions are usually maculopapular but occasionally may appear as petechial or even vesicular eruptions. The petechial type of eruption must be differentiated from that of meningococcemia. The child with enteroviral infection is not as ill or as toxic and has a lesser degree of leukocytosis than the child with meningococcemia.

Hand-foot-and-mouth disease is a vesicular exanthem caused by an enterovirus, usually coxsackievirus A16. The colorful name is descriptive, since the main features of this infection are vesicular lesions of the hands, feet, mouth, and tongue (Figure 59-9). The patient is mildly febrile, and the illness subsides in a few days.

Myocardial and pericardial infections caused by coxsackie B virus occur sporadically to older children and adults but are most threatening in newborns. Neonates with these infections have febrile illnesses and sudden unexplained onset of heart failure. Cyanosis, tachycardia, cardiomegaly, and hepatomegaly occur. Electrocardiographic changes are found in patients with myocarditis. Mortality is high, and autopsy reveals other involved organ systems, including brain, liver, and pancreas. **Acute benign pericarditis** affects young adults but may be seen in older individuals with symptoms resembling myocardial infarction but with more severe fever.

Some strains of coxsackie B and echovirus can be transmitted transplacentally to the neonate. Infection of an infant by this or other route may produce severe disseminated infection.

Other Enterovirus Diseases

Enterovirus 70 and a variant of coxsackievirus A24 have recently been associated with an extremely contagious ocular disease, **acute hemorrhagic conjunctivitis**. The infection causes subconjunctival hemorrhages and conjunctivitis. The disease has a 24-hour incubation period and resolves within 1 or 2 weeks.

Respiratory disease, hepatitis, and diabetes are some of the syndromes attributed to enteroviruses. Coxsackieviruses A21 and A24 and echoviruses 11 and 20 can cause rhinovirus-like coldlike symptoms if the upper respiratory tract becomes infected. Enterovirus 72 causes hepatitis A disease (see Chapter 68). Coxsackie B infections of the pancreas have been suspected to cause insulin-dependent diabetes because of the destruction of the islets of Langerhans.

Laboratory Diagnosis

Clinical Chemistry

Cerebrospinal fluid (CSF) from poliovirus or enterovirus aseptic meningitis reveals a predominantly lymphocytic

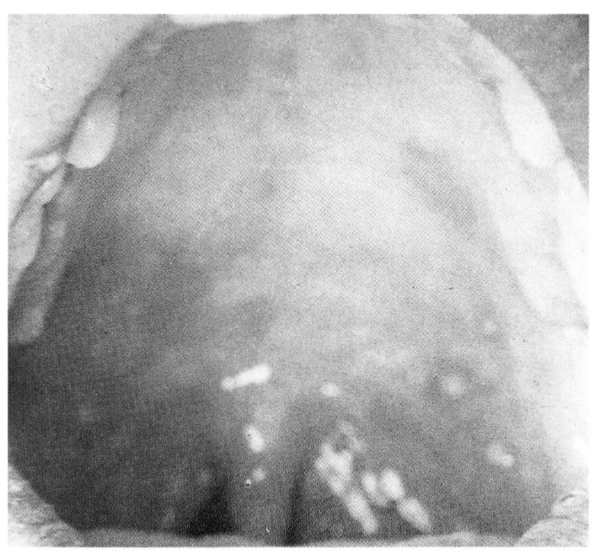

FIGURE 59-8 Herpangina. Characteristic discrete vesicles are seen on the anterior tonsillar pillars. (Courtesy Dr. GDW McKendrick; From Lambert HP et al.: *Infectious diseases illustrated*, London, 1982, Gower Medical Publishing.)

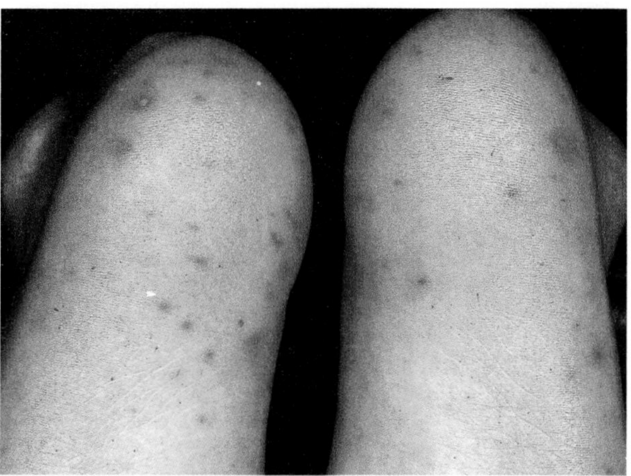

FIGURE 59-9 Hand-foot-and-mouth disease caused by coxsackie A virus. Lesions initially appear in the oral cavity and then develop within 1 day on the palms and, as seen here, soles. (From Habif TP: *Clinical dermatology: a color guide to diagnosis and therapy*, St Louis, 1985, Mosby.)

pleocytosis (presence of 25 to 500 cells). In contrast to bacterial meningitis, the CSF glucose level is usually normal or slightly low. CSF protein level is normal to slightly elevated. The CSF is rarely positive for the virus.

Culture

Polioviruses may be isolated from the pharynx during the first few days of illness and from the feces for as long as 30 days but rarely from the CSF. The virus grows well in monkey kidney tissue culture. Coxsackieviruses and echoviruses can usually be isolated from the throat and stool during infection and often from CSF in patients with meningitis. Virus is rarely isolated in myocarditis, since the symptoms occur several weeks after the initial infection. The coxsackie B viruses can be grown on primary monkey or human embryo kidney cells. Many coxsackie A virus strains do not grow in tissue culture and must still be grown in suckling mice. The specific enterovirus type can be determined only by using specific antibody and assays (e.g., neutralization, immunofluorescence).

Serology

Serologic confirmation of enterovirus infection can be made by detection of specific IgM or a fourfold increase in antibody titer between acute illness and convalescence. The many serotypes of echovirus and coxsackievirus make this approach difficult, but it may be useful in documenting poliovirus infection.

TREATMENT, PREVENTION AND CONTROL

No specific antiviral therapy is available for enterovirus infections. Supportive therapy is extremely important for patients with paralytic disease to assist in their potential recovery. Historically the iron lung was used to support patients with bulbar paralysis and impaired breathing.

The prevention of paralytic poliomyelitis is one of the triumphs of modern medicine. Infection with wild type poliovirus disappeared from the United States in 1979. The number of cases of polio decreased from 21,000 in the pre-vaccine era to 18 in 1977, in unvaccinated individuals. Unfortunately, health care delivery systems are not sufficient to provide adequate vaccine administration in underdeveloped countries, and wild type virus disease still exists in Africa, the Middle East, and Asia.

Two types of poliovirus vaccine exist, the *inactivated polio vaccine (IPV)*, developed by Jonas Salk and a *live attenuated oral vaccine (OPV)*, developed by Albert Sabin. Both vaccines incorporate the three strains of polio, are stable, are relatively inexpensive, and induce a protective antibody response (Figure 59-10).

The IPV was proved effective in 1955 but has generally been replaced by the oral vaccine because of ease of delivery and its capacity to elicit lifelong immunity (Box 59-5). The oral vaccine was attenuated (i.e., rendered less virulent) by passage in human or monkey cell cultures. Attenuation yields a virus capable of replicating in the oropharynx and intestinal tract and of being shed in feces for weeks. The live vaccine strain may spread to close contacts and (re)immunize them (a virtue in achieving mass immunization). The remote potential for causing paralytic disease is the major drawback of the live vaccine and is estimated to occur in 1 per 4 million doses administered (vs. 1 in 100 of those infected with "wild" poliovirus). The risk of vaccine-associated paralytic poliomyelitis is increased in immunocompromised individuals and is more likely to occur in susceptible adults than susceptible children. Vaccine-associated poliomyelitis may occur in contacts in addition to the actual vaccine recipient.

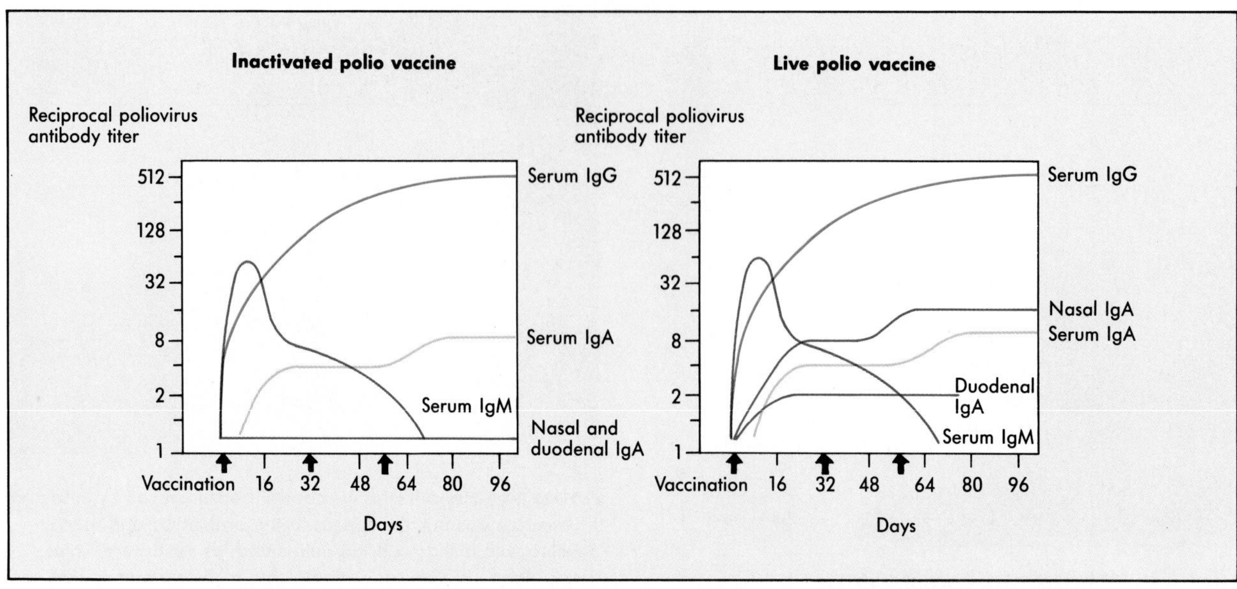

FIGURE 59-10 Serum and secretory antibody response to intramuscular inoculation of inactivated polio vaccine (IPV) and to orally administered, live attenuated polio vaccine (OPV). (Redrawn from Ogra P et al.: *Rev Infect Dis* 2:352-369, 1980.)

Children should receive the OPV at 2, 4, and 15 months and at 4 to 6 years of age. The inactivated polio vaccine instead of the OPV is administered in several European countries, with good results.

No vaccines exist for coxsackieviruses or echoviruses. Transmission can presumably be reduced by improvements in hygiene and living conditions.

RHINOVIRUSES

Rhinoviruses are the most important cause of the common cold and upper respiratory infection (URI). Infections are self-limited and do not cause serious disease. At least 100 serotypes of rhinovirus have been identified. At least 80% of the rhinoviruses share a common receptor, which is also used by some of the coxsackieviruses. This receptor has been identified as ICAM-1, as discussed earlier. ICAM-1 is a member of the immunoglobulin supergene family and is expressed on epithelial, fibroblast, and B-lymphoblastoid cells. The function of the molecule is to promote immune interactions, and its expression is stimulated by cytokines released during inflammation.

Pathogenesis and Immunity

In contrast to enteroviruses, rhinoviruses are unable to replicate in the gastrointestinal tract (see Box 59-3). The rhinoviruses are labile to acidic pH and grow best at 33° C, which may partly account for their predilection for the cooler environment of the nasal mucosa. Infection can be initiated by as little as one infectious viral particle. During the peak of illness, concentrations of 500 to 1000 infectious virions per ml are reached in nasal secretions. The virus enters through the nose, mouth, or eyes and initiates infection of the upper respiratory tract, including the throat. Most viral replication occurs in the nose, and the onset and severity of symptoms correlates with the time and quantity (titer) of virus shedding. Infected cells release bradykinin and histamine, which causes the "runny nose." Biopsies of nasal mucosa taken during a "cold" reveal severe edema of the subepithelial tissue but minimal inflammatory cell response. Infected ciliated epithelial cells may be sloughed from the nasal mucosa.

Immune protection to rhinoviruses is transient and cannot compensate for the large number of serotypes. Both nasal secretory (IgA) and serum (IgG) antibody are induced by primary rhinovirus infection and can be detected within a week of infection. The secretory IgA response dissipates quickly; and immunity begins to wane approximately 18 months after infection.

Interferon, generated in response to the infection, may both limit the progression of the infection and contribute to the symptoms. Interestingly, the release of cytokines during inflammation can promote the spread of the virus by enhancing the expression of ICAM-1 viral receptors. Cell-mediated immunity is not likely to play an important role in controlling rhinovirus infections.

Epidemiology

Rhinoviruses cause at least half of all upper respiratory tract infections (Box 59-6). Enteroviruses, coronaviruses, parainfluenza viruses, and other agents also cause a sizable proportion of colds. Rhinoviruses can be transmitted by two mechanisms: aerosols and on fomites (e.g., by hands or contaminated inanimate objects). Surprisingly, aerosols are probably not the major route, despite being an

BOX 59-5 Advantages and Disadvantages of Polio Vaccines

LIVE

ADVANTAGES

Effective
Lifelong immunity
Induces secretory antibody response similar to that of natural infection
Attenuated virus may circulate in community by spread to contacts (indirect immunization)
Easily administered
Repeated boosters not required

DISADVANTAGES

Vaccine-associated poliomyelitis in vaccine recipients or contacts
Spread of vaccine to contacts without their consent
Unsafe for immunodeficient patients

KILLED

ADVANTAGES

Effective
Can be incorporated into routine immunizations (with DPT)
Good stability in transport and storage
No risk of poliomyelitis in vaccines or contacts
Safe in immunodeficient patients

DISADVANTAGES

Does not induce local (gut) immunity
Booster vaccine required for lifelong immunity
Injection less acceptable than oral administration
Must achieve higher community immunization levels than with live vaccine

apparently efficient mode of transmission. Hands appear to be the major vector, and direct person-to-person contact is the predominant method of spread. Rhinoviruses can be recovered from the hands of 40% to 90% of persons with colds and from 6% to 15% of inanimate objects around them. These nonenveloped viruses are extremely stable and can survive on these objects for many hours.

Rhinoviruses produce clinical illness in only half those persons infected. Asymptomatic individuals are capable of spreading the virus even though they may produce less virus.

Rhinovirus "colds" affect persons most frequently in the early fall and the late spring in temperate climates. These peaks may reflect social patterns (e.g., return to school and day care) rather than any change in the virus itself.

Rates of infection are highest in infants and children. Children under 2 years of age are considered the primary vector that introduces colds into a family. Secondary infections occur in approximately 50% of family members, especially other children.

BOX 59-6 Epidemiology of Rhinovirus Infections

DISEASE/VIRAL FACTORS

Virion resistant to drying and detergents
Optimal replication at 33° C and cooler

TRANSMISSION

Direct contact via infected hands and fomites
Inhalation of infectious droplets

WHO IS AT RISK?

All ages

GEOGRAPHY/SEASON

Worldwide
Disease more common in early fall and late spring

MODES OF CONTROL

None
Washing hands and disinfecting contaminated objects helps prevent spread

Although many different rhinovirus serotypes may be found in a given community simultaneously, only a few predominate during a specific cold season. The major viruses are usually the newly categorized serotypes, suggesting that a gradual antigenic drift exists, similar to the pattern with influenza viruses.

Clinical Syndromes

Common cold symptoms caused by rhinoviruses cannot readily be distinguished from other viral respiratory pathogens (e.g., enteroviruses, paramyxoviruses, or coronaviruses). Upper respiratory tract infection usually begins with sneezing, followed soon by rhinorrhea (runny nose) (Figure 59-11). The rhinorrhea increases and is then accompanied by symptoms of nasal obstruction. Mild sore throat also occurs, along with headache and malaise. The illness peaks in 3 to 4 days, but the cough and nasal symptoms may persist for 7 to 10 days or longer. Fever and rigors sometimes accompany rhinovirus URIs.

Laboratory Diagnosis

The clinical syndrome of the common cold is usually so characteristic that laboratory diagnosis is unnecessary unless the physician needs to establish which of the many respiratory viruses is causing a specific patient's illness. The diagnostic methods for rhinoviruses include culture and serology.

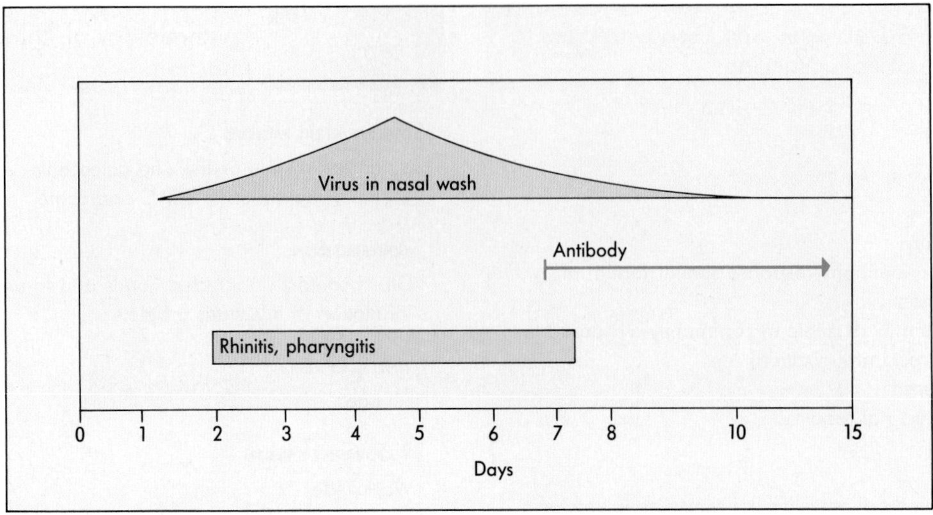

FIGURE 59-11 Time course of rhinovirus infection.

Culture

Nasal washings are the best clinical specimen for recovering the virus. Rhinoviruses grow in vitro only in cells of primate origin, with human diploid fibroblast cells, (e.g., WI-38) as the optimum system. As already stated, these viruses grow best at 33° C. Isolation in tissue culture occurs in 1 to 7 days, with an average of 4 to 5 days. Virus is identified by typical cytopathic effect and the demonstration of acid lability. Serotyping is rarely necessary but can be done by using pools of specific neutralizing sera.

Serology

Serologic testing to document rhinovirus infection is not practical. No antigen is common to all rhinoviruses, making it difficult to maintain virus stocks for testing. Furthermore, multiple serotypes of rhinovirus may circulate in the community simultaneously, increasing the difficulty of serologic testing.

Treatment, Prevention and Control

There are many over-the-counter remedies for the common cold, but no specific therapy has been found to be effective. Nasal vasoconstrictors may provide relief, but their use may be followed by rebound congestion and worsening symptoms. Rigorous studies of vitamin C therapy have not shown efficacy.

No antiviral drug has been proved therapeutically useful in controlling rhinovirus infections. Intranasal interferon will block infection for short-term use following a known exposure, but long-term use of intranasal interferon (e.g., throughout the "cold season") could cause symptoms at least as bad as the rhinovirus infection. Experimental antiviral drugs, such as arildone, rhodanine, disoxaril, and their analogues contain a 3-methylisoxazole group that inserts into the base of the receptor-binding canyon and blocks uncoating of the virus. Enviroxime inhibits the viral RNA-dependent RNA polymerase. A polypeptide receptor analogue based on the ICAM-1 protein structure may also have potential as an antiviral drug.

Rhinovirus is not a very good candidate for vaccine development. The multiple serotypes, apparent antigenic drift in rhinoviral antigens, requirement for secretory IgA production, and the transience of the antibody response pose major problems for the development of vaccines. In addition, the benefit-to-risk ratio would be very low since rhinoviruses do not cause significant disease.

Handwashing and disinfection of contaminated objects are the best means of preventing the spread of the virus. Impregnation of nasal tissue with antiviral chemicals has been attempted, but the product was not a commercial success.

CASE STUDY AND QUESTIONS

A 6-year-old girl was brought into the office at 4:30 PM for a sore throat, being unusually tired, and requiring excessive napping. She had a temperature of 39° C, an erythematous throat with enlarged tonsils, and a faint rash on her back. At 10:30 PM the patient's mother reports that the child vomited 3 times, continues to nap excessively, and complains of a headache when she is awake. At 11:30 PM you examine her and note that the child is lethargic and arouses only when her head is turned, complaining that her back hurts. Her cerebral spinal fluid contained RBC 0%, WBC 28: 50% poly, 50% lymphocytes. Normal glucose and protein; Gram stain showed no bacteria.

1. What are the key signs and symptoms described in this case?
2. What is the differential diagnosis?
3. What signs and symptoms are suggestive of an enterovirus infection?

4. How would the diagnosis be confirmed?
5. What are the most likely sources and means of infection?
6. What is the target tissue and mechanism of pathogenesis?

Bibliography

Levandowski RA: Rhinoviruses. In Belshe RB, editor: *Textbook of human virology*, ed 2, St. Louis, 1991, Mosby.

McKinlay MA, Pevear DC, Rossmann MG: Treatment of the picornavirus common cold by inhibitors of viral uncoating and attachment, *Ann Rev Microbiol* 46:635-654, 1992.

Melnick JL: Live attenuated poliovaccines. In Plotkin SA and Martin EA, editors: *Vaccines*, Philadelphia, 1988, WB Saunders.

Moore M, Morens DM: Enteroviruses including polioviruses. In Belshe RB, editor: *Textbook of human virology*, ed 2, St. Louis, 1991, Mosby.

Racaniello VR: Picornaviruses, *Curr Top Microbiol Immunol* vol 161. A series of reviews.

Ren R, Racaniello VR: Human poliovirus receptor gene expression and poliovirus tissue tropism in transgenic mice, *J Virology* 66:296-304, 1992.

Robbins FC: Polio-historical. In Plotkin SA and Martin EA, editors: *Vaccines*, Philadelphia, 1988, WB Saunders.

Salk J and Drucker J: Noninfectious poliovirus vaccine. In Plotkin SA and Martin EA, editors: *Vaccines*, Philadelphia, 1988, WB Saunders.

Wilfert CM, Lehrman SN, and Katz SL: Enteroviruses and meningitis, *Pediatr Infect Dis* 2:333-341, 1983.

CHAPTER 60

Orthomyxoviruses

INFLUENZA A, B, and C are the only members of the Orthomyxoviridae, of which only influenza A and B cause significant human disease. The orthomyxoviruses are enveloped and have a segmented negative-sense RNA genome. The segmented genome of these viruses facilitates development of new strains by mutation and reassortment of the gene segments between different human and animal strains of virus. This genetic instability is responsible for the annual influenza **epidemics** (mutation:drift) and periodic **pandemics** (reassortment:shift) of influenza infection worldwide.

Influenza is one of the most prevalent and significant virus infections worldwide. Epidemics (local) of influenza appear to have been described in ancient times. Probably the most famous influenza pandemic is the one that swept the world in 1918-1919, killing 20 million persons. More people died of influenza than from the battles of World War I. Pandemics in recent years have occurred in 1947, 1957, 1968, and 1977. Fortunately, vaccine and antiviral drug prophylaxis is available for individuals at risk for serious influenza outcomes.

Influenza viruses are respiratory viruses that cause respiratory and classic flu-like symptoms of fever, malaise, headache, and myalgia (body aches). The term *flu* has been misused to describe many other respiratory and viral infections (e.g., "intestinal flu").

STRUCTURE AND REPLICATION

Influenza virions are pleomorphic, appearing spherical or tubular (Box 60-1 and Figure 60-1) and 80 to 120 nm in diameter. The envelope contains two glycoproteins, the **hemagglutinin (HA)** and **neuraminidase (NA)**, and is lined by the **matrix (M_1)** and **membrane (M_2)** proteins. The genome consists of 8 (influenza A and B) different helical nucleocapsid segments, each of which contains a negative-sense RNA associated with the **nucleoprotein (NP)** and the **transcriptase (RNA polymerase components)** (PB1, PB2, PA) (Table 60-1). Influenza C has only 7 genomic segments.

The genome segments range from 890 to 2340 bases in size for influenza A. All of the proteins are encoded on separate segments except the NS_1 and NS_2 and the M_1 and M_2 proteins, which are transcribed from one segment each.

The hemagglutinin forms a spike-shaped trimer that measures 10 to 40 nm in length and is activated by protease cleavage into two subunits held together by a disulfide bond (see Figure 7-6). The HA has several functions: it is the viral attachment protein, binding to sialic acid on epithelial cell surface receptors; it promotes envelope to cell membrane fusion; it hemagglutinates human, chicken, and guinea pig red blood cells; and it elicits the protective neutralizing antibody response. Mutation-derived changes in HA cause the antigenic changes of minor ("drift") or major ("shift") degree. "Shifts" occur only with influenza A, and the different hemagglutinins are designated H1, H2, etc.

The neuraminidase glycoprotein forms a tetramer and has enzyme activity. The NA cleaves the sialic acid on glycoproteins, including the cell receptor. Cleavage of the sialic acid on virion proteins prevents clumping and appears to facilitate the release of virus from infected cells. Neuraminidase of influenza A also undergoes antigenic changes, which, if major, are designated N1, N2, etc.

The matrix and nucleoprotein antigens are type specific and are therefore used to differentiate types A, B, or C. The matrix proteins line the inside of the virion and promote assembly. The M_2 of influenza A also forms a

BOX 60-1 Unique Features of the Influenza A and B Viruses

- Enveloped virion with a genome of 8 different (−)RNA nucleocapsid segments
- The hemagglutinin (HA) glycoprotein is the VAP, fusion protein, and elicits neutralizing, protective antibody responses
- Influenza transcribes and replicates its genome in the target cell nucleus but assembles and buds from the plasma membrane
- The antiviral drugs amantadine and rimantadine inhibit an uncoating step and most likely target the M_2 protein
- The segmented genome promotes genetic diversity caused by mutation and reassortment of segments upon infection with two different strains

proton channel in membranes, promotes viral release, and is a target for the antiviral drug, amantadine.

New influenza strains are generated by mutation and by reassortment. The genetic diversity of influenza A is fostered by its segmented genome structure and ability to infect and replicate in humans and also many animal species, including birds, pigs, etc. Upon co-infection by different strains of influenza A, even from different species, the genome segments will randomly associate into new virions, creating hybrid viruses. The only constraint on the generation of new strains is that they must be able to replicate in the host. A major change in the HA glycoprotein without loss of cell binding may allow a mutant virus to change its antigenicity and infect the immunologically naive population. For example, a highly pathogenic reassortant virus for seals was generated by simultaneous infection of a seal with two avian influenza viruses (Figure 60-2). Similar reassortment is postulated to be the source of pathogenic human strains. Because of the high population density and proximity of humans, pigs, and ducks in China, it is thought to be a breeding ground for new reassortant viruses and the source of many of the pandemic strains of influenza.

Viral replication begins with the interaction of specific sialic acid structures on cell surface glycoproteins and HA glycoproteins on the virion. The virus is internalized in a coated vesicle and transferred to an endosome. A major change in the conformation of the HA proteins attached to their receptors occurs upon acidification of the endosome. Acidification causes the HA to bend over and expose hydrophobic fusion-promoting regions of the protein. The viral envelope fuses with the endosome

A

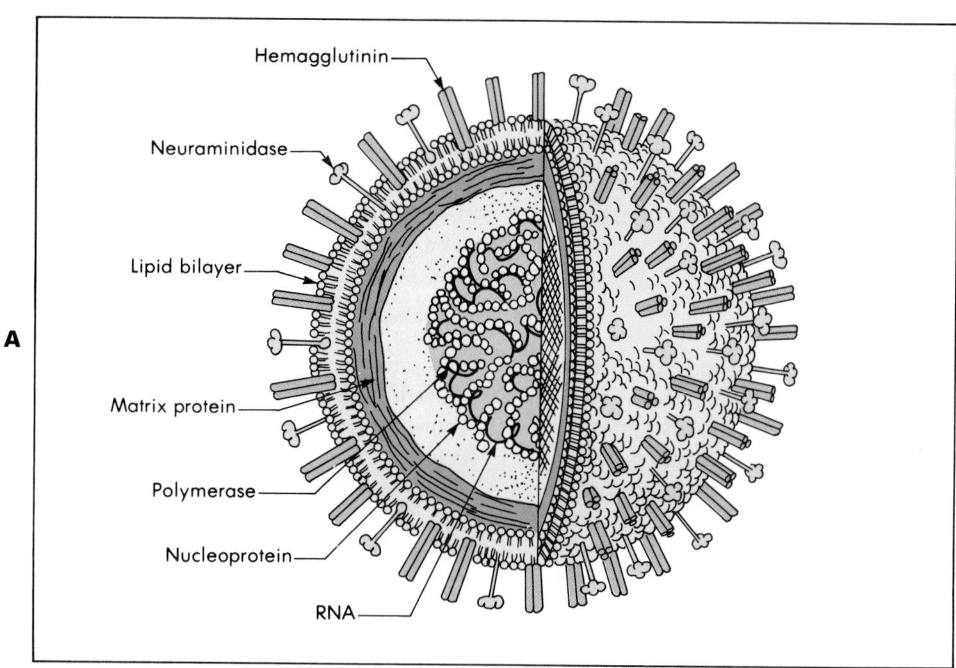

B

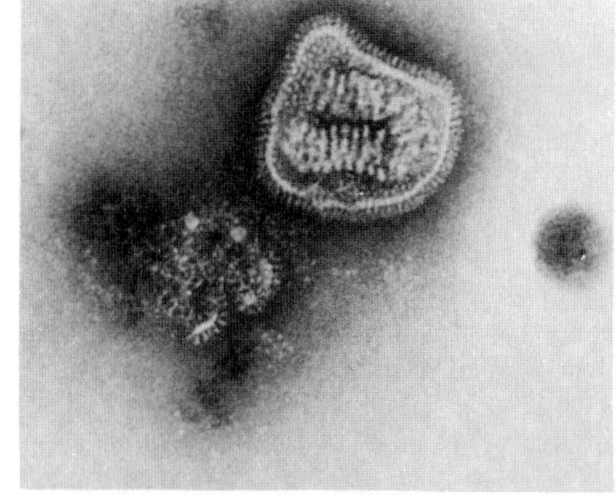

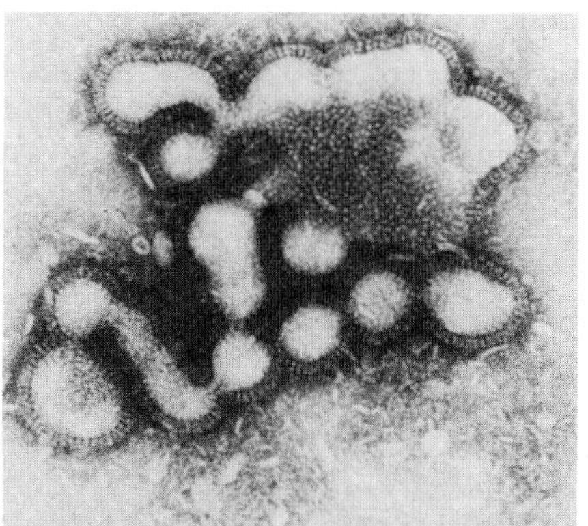

FIGURE 60-1 A, Model of influenza A virus. **B,** Electron micrograph of influenza A virus. (**A** redrawn from Tagawa SB. In Kaplan MM, Webster RG: The epidemiology of influenza, *Sci Am* December 1977. **B** from Balows A, et al., editors: *Laboratory diagnosis of infectious diseases: principles and practice*, vol 2, Heidelberg, 1988, Springer-Verlag.)

TABLE 60-1 Products of Influenza Gene Segments

Segment*	Proteins	Function
1	PB2	Polymerase component
2	PB1	Polymerase component
3	PA	Polymerase component
4	HA	Hemagglutinin, viral attachment protein, fusion protein, target of neutralizing antibody
5	NP	Nucleocapsid
6	NA	Neuraminidase: cleaves sialic acid and promotes virus release
7†	M_1	Matrix protein: virion structural protein, interacts with nucleocapsid and envelope, promotes assembly
	M_2	Membrane protein, forms membrane pore, target for amantadine, facilitates active HA production
8†	NS_1	Nonstructural protein, important but unknown function
	NS_2	Nonstructural protein, important but unknown function

*Listed in decreasing order of size.
†Encodes two mRNA.

membrane and delivers the nucleocapsid into the cytoplasm. The nucleocapsid travels to the nucleus where it is transcribed into mRNA. The influenza transcriptase (PA, PB1, PB2) uses host cell mRNA as primers for viral mRNA synthesis. In so doing, it steals the methylated cap region of the RNA required for efficient binding to ribosomes. All the genome segments are transcribed into 5′capped, 3′polyA containing mRNA for individual proteins, except the segments for the M and NS proteins, which are each differentially spliced to produce two different mRNA. The mRNAs are translated into protein in the cytoplasm. The HA and NA glycoproteins are processed by the endoplasmic reticulum and Golgi apparatus and displayed on the cell surface. M proteins bind to the cytoplasmic portion of the glycoproteins and line the inside of the membrane.

Later, positive-sense RNA templates for each segment, without cap or polyA, are produced and the negative-sense RNA genome is replicated in the nucleus. The genome segments are transported to the cytoplasm and associate with the nucleocapsid and polymerase proteins, which interact with the matrix protein (M) lining the plasma membrane. The genome segments are enveloped in a random manner, with approximately 11 segments per virion. This produces a small percentage of virions with a complete genome (and a large number of defective particles). These defective particles are antigenic and can cause interference, which may limit the progression of the infection. The virus buds from the cell and is released about 8 hours after infection (Figure 60-3).

PATHOGENESIS AND IMMUNITY

Influenza initially establishes a local upper respiratory tract infection (Box 60-2). The virus targets and kills mucus-secreting, ciliated, and other epithelial cells, causing the loss of this primary defense system. The neuraminidase (NA) facilitates the infection by cleaving sialic acid residues of the mucus and providing access to tissue. If the virus spreads to the lower respiratory tract, the infection can cause severe desquamation (shedding) of bronchial or alveolar epithelium down to a single-cell-thick basal layer or to the basement membrane. In addition to compromising the natural defenses of the respiratory tract, influenza infection promotes bacterial adhesion to epithelial cells. Pneumonia may result from viral pathogenesis or secondary bacterial infection. Influenza may cause a transient or low-level viremia with rare involvement of tissues other than the lung.

Histologically, influenza infection leads to an inflammatory cell response of the mucosal membrane, which consists primarily of monocytes and lymphocytes and few neutrophils. Submucosal edema is present. Lung tissue may reveal hyaline membrane disease, alveolar emphysema, and necrosis of alveolar walls (Figure 60-4).

Recovery is associated with interferon and cell-mediated immune responses. T-cell responses are important for both recovery and immunopathogenesis. However, influenza infection depresses macrophage and T-cell function, hindering immune resolution. Interestingly, recovery often precedes detection of antibody in serum or secretions.

Protection against reinfection is primarily associated with the development of antibodies to the hemagglutinin, but antibodies to NA are also protective. The antibody response is specific for each strain of influenza, but the cell-mediated immune response is more general and capable of responding to influenza strains of the same type (influenza A or B). Antigenic targets for T-cell responses include the nucleocapsid proteins (NP, PB2), matrix protein, and the HA.

The symptoms and time course of disease are related to the interferon and T-cell responses and the extent of epithelial tissue loss. Influenza is normally a self-limited disease with rare involvement of organs other than the lung. Many of the classic "flu" symptoms (e.g. fever, malaise, headache, and myalgia [body aches]) are associated with the interferon induction. Repair of the compromised tissue initiates within 3 to 5 days of symptoms but may take as long as a month. The time course of influenza virus infection is illustrated in Figure 60-5.

EPIDEMIOLOGY

The changing antigenic nature of influenza ensures the presence of a large population of immunologically naive,

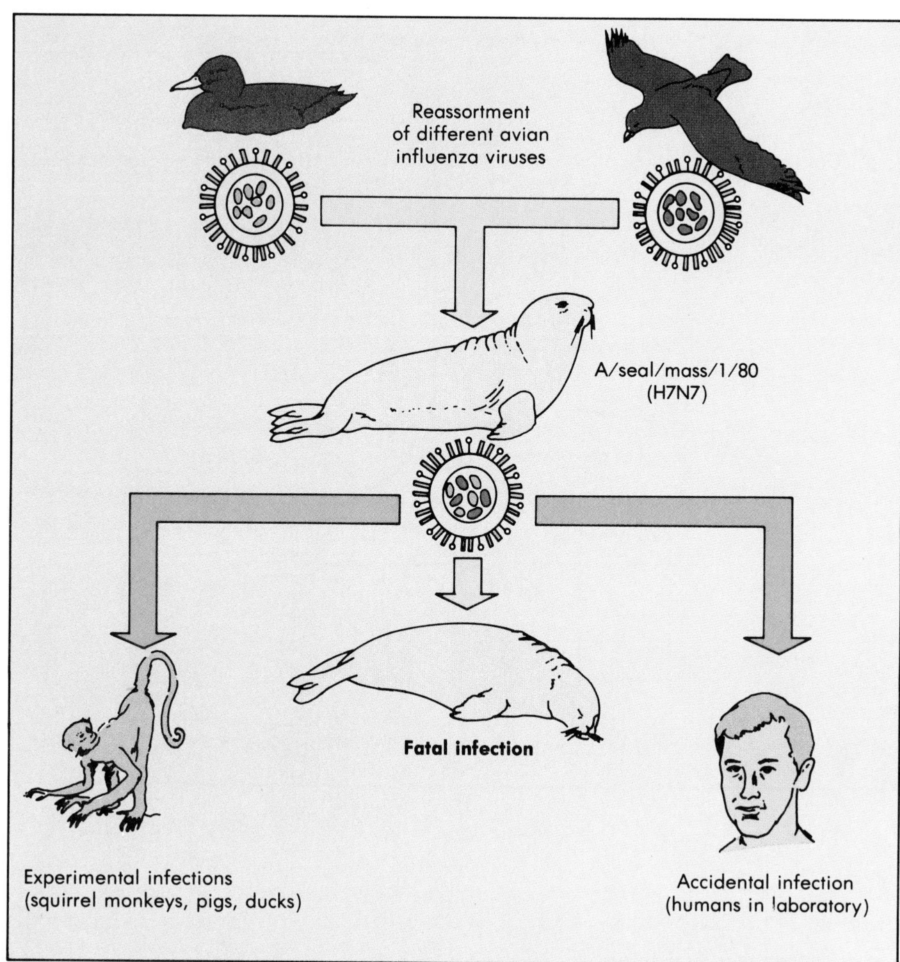

FIGURE 60-2 Reassortment of genome fragments of influenza A virus. Diagrammatic representation of the origin of seal influenza virus A/seal/Mass/1/80 (H7N7). Since all of the eight genes of seal influenza virus are most closely related to those in different avian viruses, it is proposed that seals were mixedly infected with influenza viruses by fecal contamination from birds. The resulting reassortant virus had the required gene constellation to replicate in seal tissues and caused high mortality. This virus has been accidentally transmitted to humans in the laboratory, causing conjunctivitis. Experimentally, the virus has been shown to replicate preferentially in mammalian species, causing systemic infection in some squirrel monkeys and asymptomatic infection of pigs. (Modified from Fields BN, editor: *Virology*, New York, 1985, Raven Press.)

susceptible individuals (especially children) (Box 60-3). An influenza outbreak can be readily detected by the increased absenteeism in schools and work and the number of emergency room visits. Influenza outbreaks occur annually, in temperate climates, during the winter months. Influenza virus is present in a community for only a short period (4 to 6 weeks).

Influenza infection is spread via small airborne droplets released during talking, breathing, and coughing etc. The virus can also sit on countertops for as long as a day.

The most susceptible population to influenza infection are children, and school-age children are most likely to spread the infection. Contagion precedes symptoms and lasts for long periods, especially in children. Children, immunosuppressed individuals (including pregnant women), the elderly, and individuals with heart and lung ailments (including smokers) are at highest risk to more serious disease, pneumonia, or other complications of infection.

Strains of influenza A virus are classified by type (A, B, C)/place of original isolation/date of original isolation/ and antigen (hemagglutinin and neuraminidase). For example, a current strain of influenza virus might be designated A/Bangkok/1/79 (H3N2). This designates an influenza A virus first isolated in Bangkok in January 1979, containing hemagglutinin (H_3) and neuraminidase (N_2) antigens. Strains of influenza B are designated by type, geography, and date of isolation (e.g., B/Singapore/ 3/64) without specific mention of H or N antigens.

Minor antigenic changes resulting from mutation of

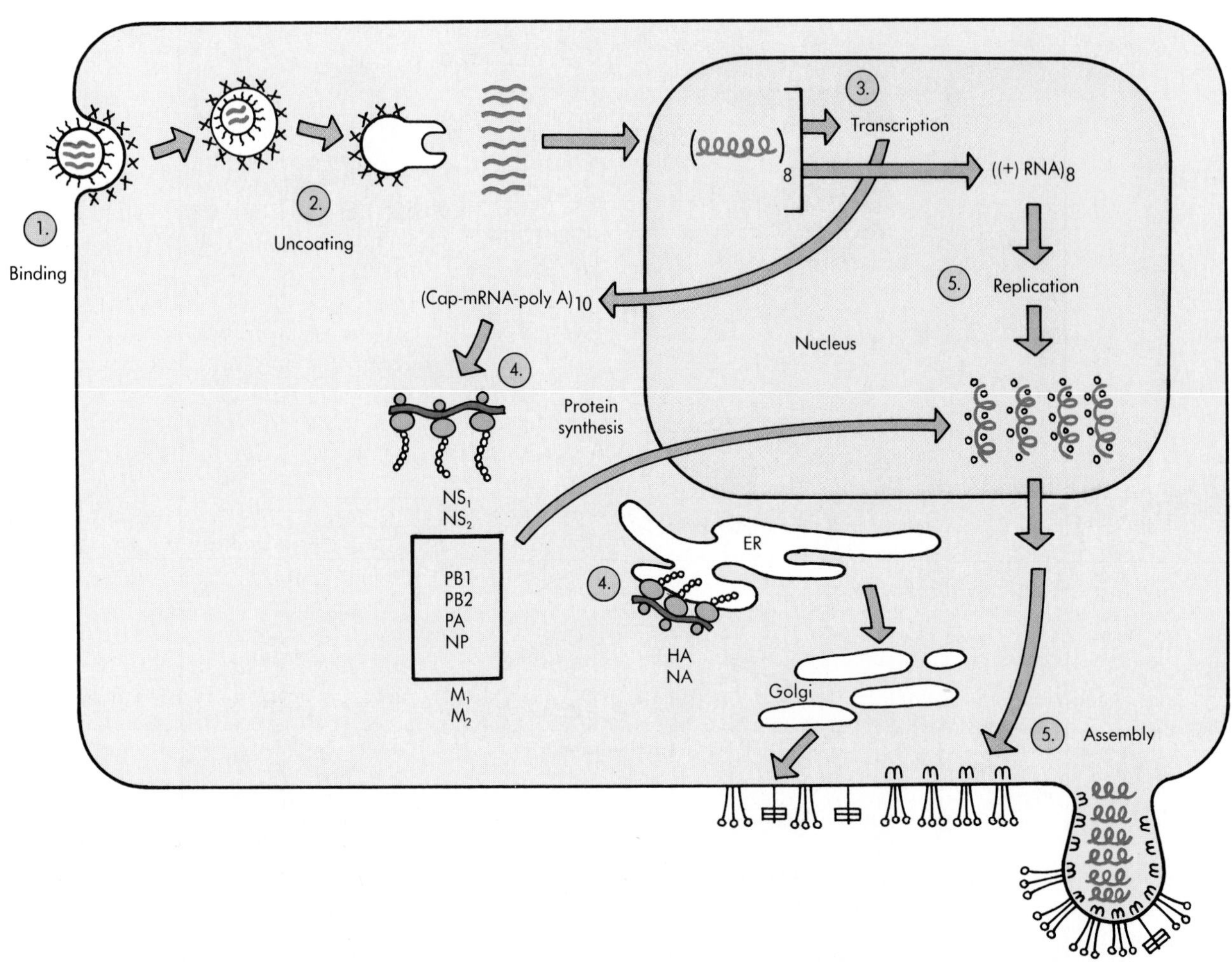

FIGURE 60-3 Replication of influenza A virus. After (*1*) binding to sialic acid containing receptors, influenza is endocytosed and (*2*) fuses with the vesicle membrane. Unlike most other RNA viruses, (*3*) transcription and (*5*) replication of the genome occurs in the nucleus. (*4*) Viral proteins are synthesized, helical nucleocapsids form and (*5*) associate with M-protein lined membranes containing HA and NA glycoproteins. The virus buds from the plasma membrane.

the viral genome are called **antigenic "drift."** Antigenic drift occurs every 2 to 3 years, causing local outbreaks of influenza A and B infection. Major antigenic changes (**"antigenic shift"**) result from genome reassortment between different virus strains, including animal strains, and occur only for influenza A. Many influenza A strains are animal viruses providing potential for reassortment. Major antigenic changes are often associated with pandemics. Antigenic shifts occur infrequently, recently averaging approximately every 10 years (Table 60-2). For example, the prevalent influenza A virus in 1947 was the H1N1 subtype. In 1957 there was a shift in both antigens, resulting in an H2N2 subtype. In 1968 H3N2 appeared, and in 1978 H1N1 reappeared. Presumably, the reappearance of H1N1 reflected the accumulation of a large population of susceptibles, all those younger than 30 years of age who lacked protective antibodies. The fact that those older than 30 years of age were protected despite the fact that H1N1 had not been present for 20 years is attributable to an anamnestic antibody response. In contrast to influenza A, influenza B is predominantly a human virus and does not undergo antigenic shift.

Surveillance of influenza A and B outbreaks is extensive to identify the new strains that should be incorporated into new vaccines. The prevalence of a particular strain of influenza A or B changes each year and reflects the presence of an immunologically naive population. Surveillance also extends into animal populations because of the possibility that recombinants responsible for influenza A pandemics arise from animal strains.

CLINICAL SYNDROMES

Depending on the degree of immunity to the infecting strain of virus and other factors, the infection may range from asymptomatic to severe. Patients with underlying

BOX 60-2 **Disease Mechanisms of Influenza A and B**

Virus can establish infection of upper and lower respiratory tract
Systemic symptoms are due to the interferon and lymphokine response to the virus. Local symptoms are due to epithelial cell damage, including ciliated and mucous-secreting cells
Interferon and cell-mediated immune responses (NK and T cell) are important for both immune resolution and immunopathogenesis
Infected individuals are predisposed to bacterial superinfection because of the loss of these natural barriers and induction of bacterial adhesion to epithelial cells
Antibody is important for future protection against infection and is specific for defined epitopes on HA and NA
The HA and NA of influenza A can undergo major (reassortment, shift) and minor (mutation, drift) antigenic changes to ensure the presence of immunologically naive, susceptible individuals
Influenza B undergoes only minor antigenic changes

cardiorespiratory disease or immune deficiency, even that associated with pregnancy, are more disposed to severe diseases.

After an incubation period of 1 to 4 days, the "flu" syndrome begins with a brief prodrome of malaise and headache lasting a few hours. This is followed by the abrupt onset of fever, severe myalgia, and usually a nonproductive cough. The illness persists for approximately 3 days, and then, unless a complication occurs, recovery is complete. In young children influenza resembles other severe respiratory infections causing bronchiolitis, croup, otitis media, and, rarely, febrile convulsions (Table 60-3). Complications of influenza include bacterial pneumonia, myositis, central nervous system involvement, and Reye's syndrome. Influenza B disease is similar to influenza A.

Influenza may directly cause pneumonia or more commonly promote a secondary bacterial superinfection leading to bronchitis or pneumonia. The tissue damage caused by progressive influenza virus infection of alveoli can be extensive, leading to hypoxia and bilateral pneumonia. Secondary bacterial infection usually involves *Streptococcus pneumoniae*, *Haemophilus influenzae*, or

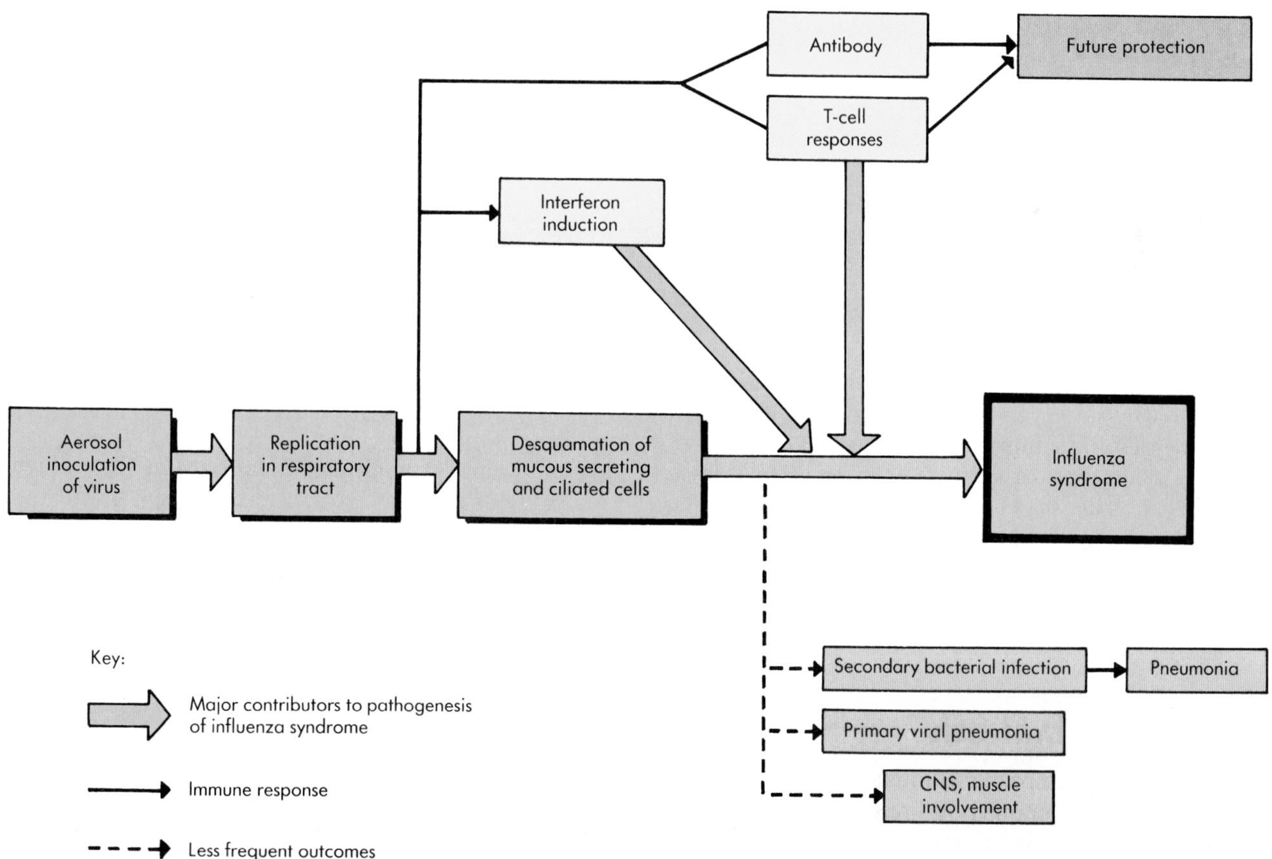

FIGURE 60-4 Pathogenesis of influenza A virus. The symptoms of influenza are caused by viral and immunopathology but the infection may promote secondary bacterial infection.

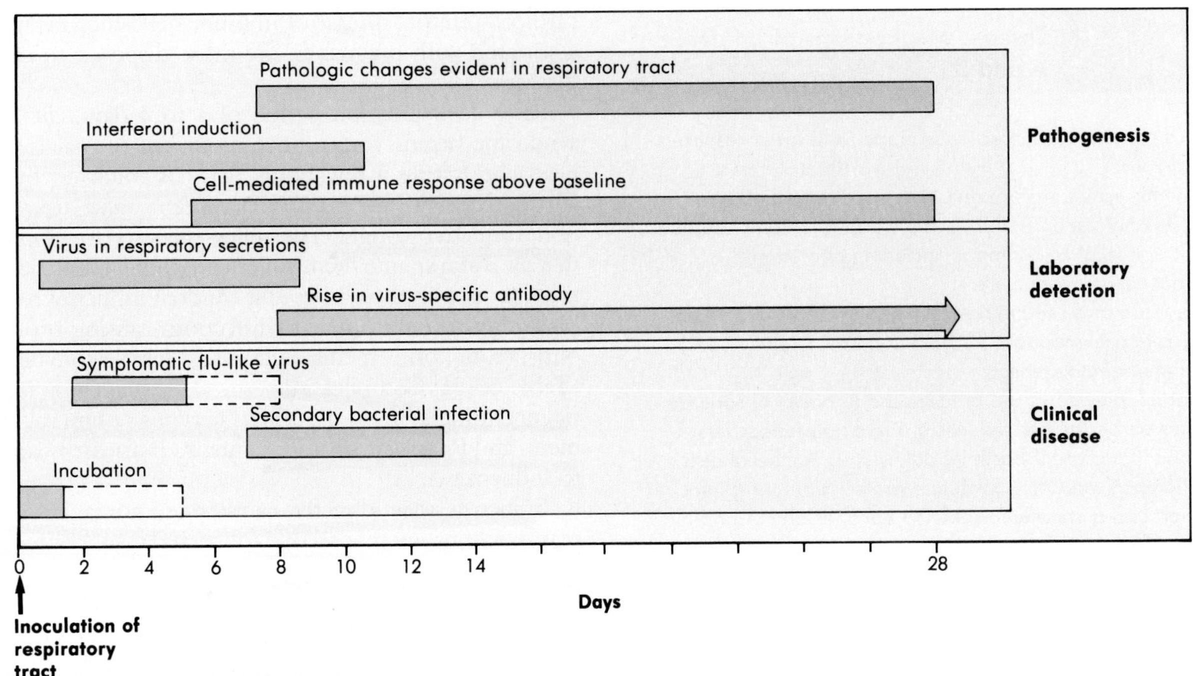

FIGURE 60-5 Time course of influenza A virus infection. The classic "flu syndrome" occurs early. Later, pneumonia may result from bacterial, viral or immuno-pathogenesis.

Staphylococcus aureus. In these instances sputum usually becomes productive and purulent.

Although generally limited to the lung, certain strains of influenza can spread to other sites in certain individuals. Myalgias may be the rule in influenza, but a true myositis (inflammation of muscle) with release of muscle enzymes is uncommon. It is most apt to occur in children and may be seen with influenza B, as well as influenza A.

Encephalopathy, although rare, may accompany acute influenza illness. It can be fatal and is associated with cerebral edema. Post-influenza encephalitis occurs 2 to 3 weeks following recovery from influenza, is associated with evidence of inflammation, and is rarely fatal.

Reye's syndrome is an acute encephalitis that occurs in children and follows a variety of acute febrile viral infections, including varicella, as well as influenza B and A. Salicylates (aspirin) increase the likelihood of developing this syndrome. In addition to encephalopathy, hepatic dysfunction is present. Mortality may be as high as 40%.

TABLE 60-2 Influenza Pandemics Resulting from Antigenic Shift

Year of pandemic	Influenza A subtype
1918	$H_{sw}N1$ Probable swine flu strain
1947	H1N1
1957	H2N2 Asian flu strain
1968	H3N2 Hong Kong flu strain
1978	H1N1

LABORATORY DIAGNOSIS

The characteristic symptoms of influenza combined with the presence of a community outbreak are often sufficient for a diagnosis. The laboratory can distinguish influenza from other respiratory viruses and define its type and strain (Table 60-4).

Influenza viruses from respiratory secretions can generally be isolated in primary monkey kidney cell cultures or the Madin Darby Canine Kidney (MDCK) cell line. Occasional strains may require chick embryo inoculation for primary isolation. Nonspecific cytopathic effects (CPE) may be noted in as few as 2 days (average 4 days). Before the development of CPE, the addition of guinea pig erythrocytes may reveal **hemadsorption** (the adherence of these erythrocytes to infected cells). Hemadsorption is not specific for influenza viruses and occurs with parainfluenza and other viruses.

Specific identification of the influenza virus requires immunological tests such as immunofluorescence or inhibition of hemadsorption or hemagglutination with specific antibody. Enzyme immunoassay or immunofluorescence can be used to detect viral antigen in exfoliated cells, respiratory secretions, or cell culture. Serology is too slow to aid the diagnosis and is generally used for epidemiological purposes.

BOX 60-3 Epidemiology of Influenza A and B

DISEASE/VIRAL FACTORS

Influenza is enveloped and is inactivated by detergents
Segmented genome facilitates major genetic strain changes, especially the targets of the humoral immune response, HA and NA
Influenza infects many vertebrate species including other mammals and birds
Co-infection with animal and human strains of virus can generate very different virus strains by genetic reassortment
Transmission of virus often precedes symptoms

TRANSMISSION

Inhalation of small aerosol droplets released by talking, breathing, coughing
Virus "likes cool," less humid atmosphere (e.g., winter heating season)
Spread extensively by school children

WHO IS AT RISK?

Seronegative individuals
Adults: Classic "flu syndrome"
Children: Asymptomatic to severe respiratory infections
High-risk groups: elderly, immunosuppressed individuals with underlying cardiac or respiratory problems including asthma and smokers

GEOGRAPHY/SEASON

Worldwide occurrence: epidemics local; pandemics worldwide
Disease more common in winter

MODES OF CONTROL

Amantadine approved for prophylaxis or early treatment
Killed vaccine containing the predicted yearly strains of influenza A and B

TREATMENT, PREVENTION, AND CONTROL

Hundreds of millions of dollars are spent to relieve the symptoms of influenza with acetaminophen, antihistamines, and similar drugs. The antiviral drugs, amantadine and its analogue, rimantadine, are effective for prophylactic use and for treatment during the first 24 to 48 hours after the onset of influenza A illness. These drugs inhibit an uncoating step of influenza A but not influenza B or C. The most likely target for their action is the M_2 protein. Treatment cannot prevent the later immunopathogenic stages of disease.

The airborn spread of influenza is almost impossible to limit. During periods of influenza activity, it is prudent to reduce interpersonal contact, especially with sick individuals. Omitting elective hospitalization for the elderly should be considered to reduce potential exposure during an influenza epidemic.

The best method for controlling the virus is immunization. Natural immunization, resulting from prior exposure, is protective for long periods. Protection is also available by immunization with a killed virus vaccine representing the "strain of the year" and by amantadine prophylaxis.

Killed (formalin inactivated) influenza vaccine is available each year. Killed vaccines may contain whole viruses, or they may be treated with detergents to fractionate the virus into subunits. Subunit vaccines are thought to be less immunogenic. Ideally, the vaccine incorporates antigens of the A and B influenza strains that will be prevalent in the community during the upcoming winter. In 1992 and 1993, the trivalent influenza vaccine consisted of inactivated A/Texas/91-like (H1N1), A/Beijing/89-like (H3N2), and B/Panama/90-like virus strains. Vaccination is routinely recommended for the elderly and those with chronic pulmonary disease and heart disease.

TABLE 60-3 Diseases Associated with Influenza Virus Infection

Disorder	Symptoms
Acute influenza infection in adults	Rapid onset of fever, malaise, myalgia, sore throat, and nonproductive cough
Acute influenza infection in children	Acute disease similar to adults but having higher fever, gastrointestinal symptoms (abdominal pain, vomiting), otitis media, myositis, and croup more frequently
Complications of influenza virus infection	Primary viral pneumonia Secondary bacterial pneumonia Myositis and cardiac involvement Neurological syndromes Guillain-Barré syndrome Encephalopathy Encephalitis Reye's syndrome

TABLE 60-4 Laboratory Diagnosis of Influenza Virus Infection

Test	Detects
Cell culture in primary monkey kidney cells (PMK) or MDCK cells	Presence of virus
Hemadsorption to infected cells	Presence of hemadsorbing virus
Antibody inhibition of hemadsorption	Presence of influenza, type, and strain
Immunofluorescence, ELISA	Influenza virus antigens in respiratory secretions or tissue culture
Hemagglutination	Presence of virus in secretions
Hemagglutination inhibition (HI)	Type and strain of influenza virus
Serology: Hemagglutination inhibition, hemadsorption inhibition, ELISA, immunofluorescence, complement fixation	Seroepidemiology

CASE STUDY AND QUESTIONS

In late December a 22-year-old man suddenly experienced headache, myalgia, malaise, dry cough, and a fever. He basically felt lousy. After a couple of days, he had a sore throat, and the cough got worse, and he started to feel nauseous and vomited. Several of his family members experienced similar symptoms during the previous 2 weeks.

1. In addition to influenza, what other agents could cause similar symptoms (differential diagnosis)?
2. How would the diagnosis of influenza be confirmed?
3. Amantadine is effective against influenza. What is its mechanism of action? Will it be effective for this patient? For uninfected family members or contacts?
4. When is/was the patient contagious, and how is the virus transmitted?
5. What family members are at greatest risk to serious disease and why?
6. Why is influenza so difficult to control even with a national vaccination program?

Bibliography

Kingsbury DW: Orthomyxoviridae and their replication. In Fields BN, Knipe DM, editors: *Virology*, New York, 1990, Raven Press.

Murphy BR, Webster RG: Orthomyxoviruses. In Fields BN, Knipe DM, editors: *Virology*, New York, 1990, Raven Press.

Hay AJ, Belshe RB, Anderson EL, Gorse GJ, and Westblom TU: Influenza viruses. In Belshe RB, editor: *Textbook of human virology*, ed 2, St. Louis, 1991, Mosby.

Helenius A: Unpacking the incoming influenza virus, *Cell* 69:577-578, 1992.

Stuart-Harris C: The epidemiology and prevention of influenza, *Am Sci* 69:166-172, 1981.

Webster RG, Bean WJ, Gorman OT, Chambers TM, Kawaoka Y: Evolution and ecology of influenza viruses, *Microbiol Rev* 56:152-179, 1992.

CHAPTER 61

Paramyxoviruses

THE family Paramyxoviridae consists of three genera: morbillivirus, paramyxovirus, and pneumovirus (Table 61-1). Human pathogens within the morbilliviruses include measles virus, within the paramyxoviruses are parainfluenza and mumps viruses, and within the pneumoviruses is respiratory syncytial virus. Their virions have similar morphologies, protein components, and the capacity to induce cell-cell fusion (syncytia formation/multinucleated giant cells). The genera can be distinguished by the gene order for the viral proteins and the biochemical properties of their viral attachment proteins.

The major diseases these agents cause are well known. Measles causes a potentially serious generalized infection characterized by a maculopapular rash (**rubeola**). Parainfluenza viruses cause upper and lower respiratory tract infections, primarily in children, including pharyngitis, croup, bronchitis, bronchiolitis, and pneumonia. Mumps virus causes a systemic infection, whose most prominent clinical manifestation is parotitis. Respiratory syncytial virus causes mild upper respiratory tract infections of children and adults but can cause life-threatening pneumonia in infants.

Measles and mumps have one serotype, which has allowed development of effective live vaccines. Successful vaccination programs using live attenuated measles and mumps vaccines in the United States and other developed countries have made measles and mumps rare diseases. The programs have led to the virtual elimination of the serious sequelae of measles infections. Measles remains a serious disease problem in the absence of vaccine-induced protection

TABLE 61-1 The Paramyxovirus Family

Genus	Human pathogen
Morbillivirus	Measles virus
Paramyxovirus	Parainfluenza viruses 1 to 4
	Mumps virus
Pneumovirus	Respiratory syncytial virus (RSV)

STRUCTURE AND REPLICATION

Paramyxoviruses consist of negative-sense, single-stranded RNA (5 to 8 × 10^6 d) in a helical nucleocapsid surrounded by a pleomorphic lipid-containing envelope of approximately 156 to 300 nm. (Figure 61-1). They are similar to orthomyxoviruses (influenza A to C) in many respects but are larger and do not have the unique segmented genome of influenza virus (Box 61-1). Although significant homology exists between paramyxovirus genomes, the order of the protein coding regions is different for each genera. The gene products of measles virus are shown in Table 61-2.

The nucleocapsid consists of the (−)ss RNA associated with the NP, P, and L proteins. The L protein is the RNA polymerase, the P protein facilitates RNA synthesis, and the NP protein helps maintain genome structure. The nucleocapsid associates with the matrix membrane pro-

BOX 61-1 Unique Features of the Paramyxoviridae

- Large virion consisting of a negative RNA genome in a helical nucleocapsid surrounded by an envelope containing a viral attachment protein (HN:paramyxovirus; H:morbillivirus; G:pneumovirus) and a fusion glycoprotein (F)
- The three genera can be distinguished by the activities of the viral attachment protein: HN of paramyxovirus has hemagglutin and neuraminidase activity; H of morbillivirus has hemagglutin activity; G of pneumovirus lacks these activities
- Virus replicates in the cytoplasm
- Virions penetrate the cell by fusion with the plasma membrane
- Viruses induce cell-cell fusion, causing multinucleated giant cells
- Paramyxoviridae are transmitted in respiratory droplets and initiate infection in the respiratory tract
- Cell-mediated immunity causes many of the symptoms but is essential for control of the infection

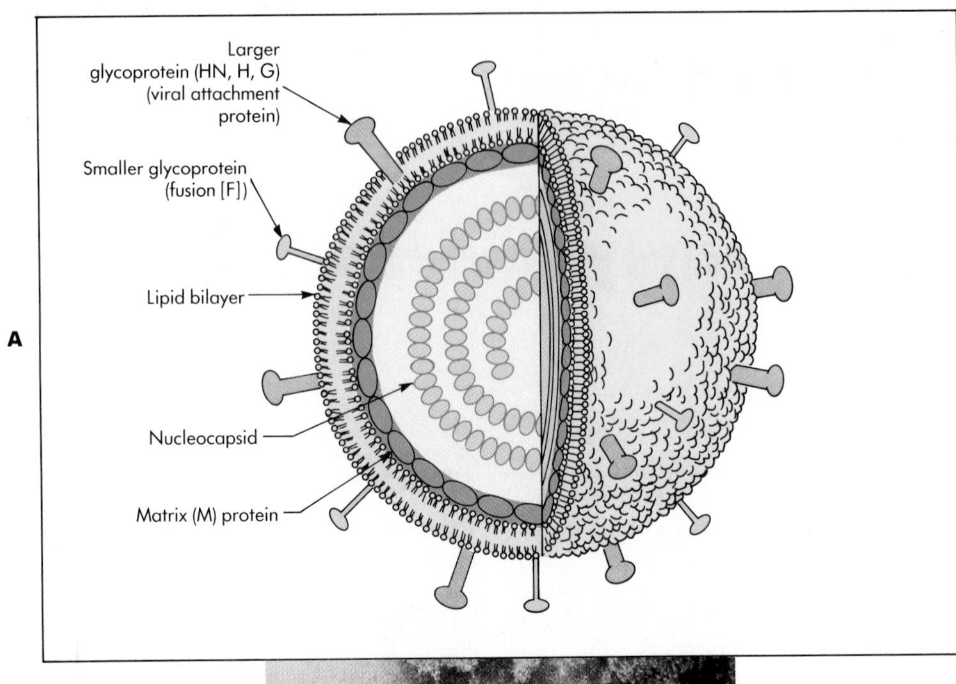

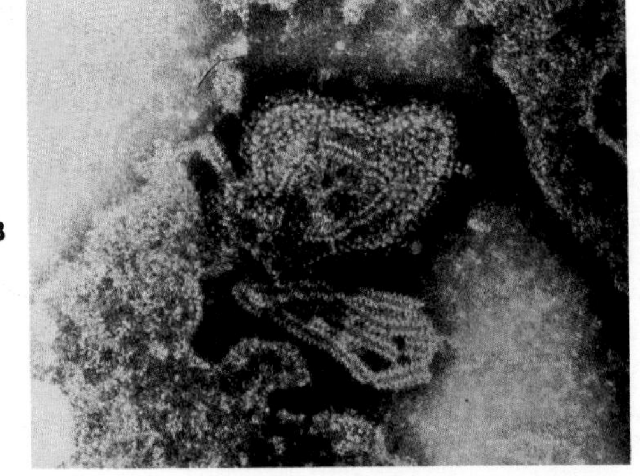

FIGURE 61-1 **A,** Model of paramyxovirus. The helical nucleocapsid, consisting of (−ss)RNA and the N, NP, and L proteins associate with the matrix protein (*M*) at the envelope inner membrane surface. The nucleocapsid contains RNA transcriptase activity. The envelope contains the viral attachment glycoprotein (HN, H, or G) and the fusion protein (*F*). **B,** Electron micrograph of a disrupted paramyxovirus showing the helical nucleocapsid. (**A** Redrawn from Jawetz E, Melnide JL, and Adelberg EA: *Review of medical microbiology*, ed 17, Norwalk, Conn, 1987, Appleton & Lange. **B** Courtesy Centers for Disease Control.)

TABLE 61-2 Virus Encoded Proteins of Measles Virus

Gene products*	Virion location	Function
Nucleoprotein (NP)	Major internal protein	Protects viral RNA
Polymerase phosphoprotein (P)	Associated with nucleoprotein	Possibly part of transcription complex
Matrix (M)	Inside virion envelope	Assembly of virions
Fusion factor (F)	Transmembraneous envelope glycoprotein	Active in fusion of cells, hemolysis, and virus entry
Hemagglutinin-neuraminidase (HN); hemagglutinin (H); G protein	Transmembraneous envelope glycoprotein	Adsorption to nucleated cells and erythrocytes
Large protein (L)	Associated with nucleoprotein	Polymerase

Modified from Fields BN, editor: *Virology*, New York, 1985, Raven Press.
*In order of transcription.

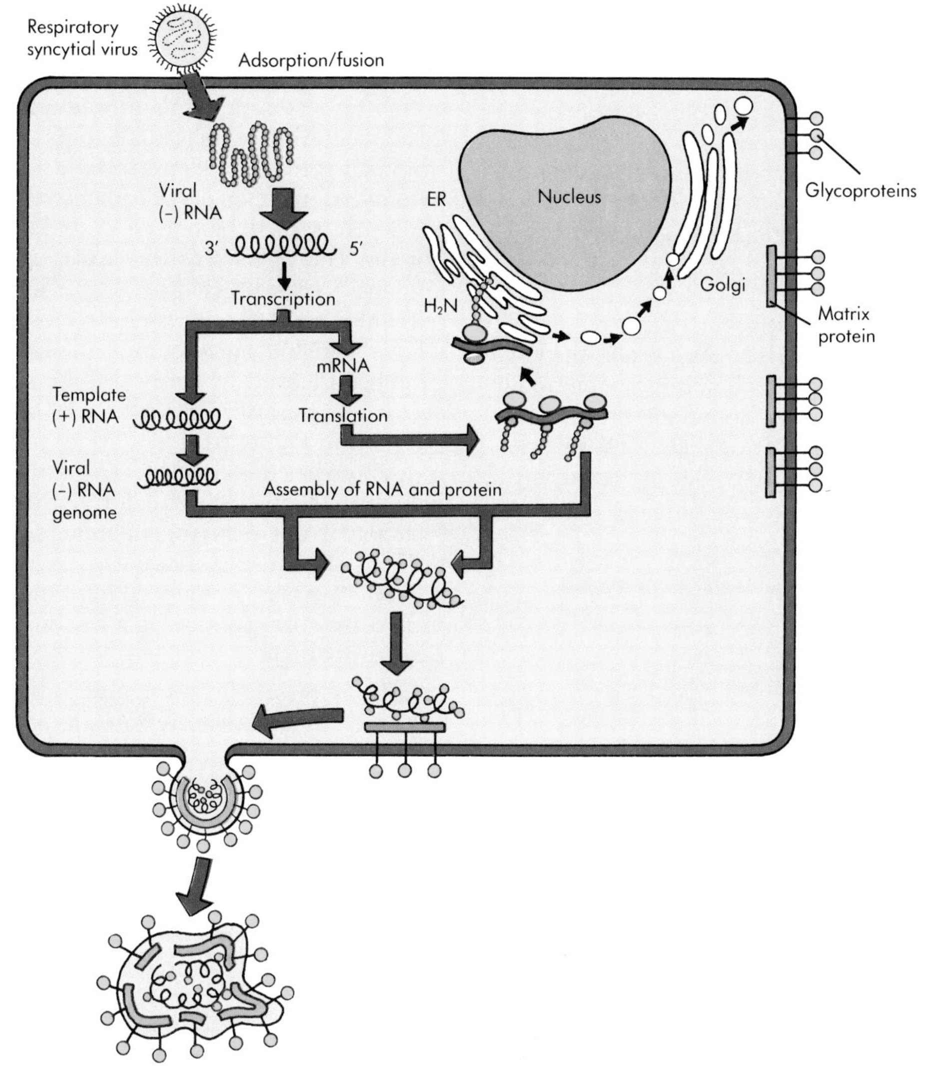

FIGURE 61-2 Replication of paramyxoviruses. The virus binds to glycolipids and fuses with the cell surface. Individual mRNAs for each protein and a full length template are transcribed from the genome. Replication occurs in the cytoplasm. The nucleocapsid associates with matrix and glycoprotein-modified plasma membranes and leaves the cell by budding. (Redrawn from Balows A et al.: *Laboratory diagnosis of infectious diseases: principles and practice,* New York, 1988, Springer-Verlag.)

tein (M) at the base of the lipid envelope. The virion envelope contains two glycoproteins, an **F** protein (fusion protein), which promotes fusion of viral and host cell membranes, and a viral attachment protein (**HN, H,** or **G**). The paramyxoviruses of the different genera can be distinguished by the activities associated with its viral attachment protein (see Box 61-1). The F protein must be activated by proteolytic cleavage, producing F_1 and F_2 glycopeptides held together by a disulfide bond, to express membrane-fusing activity.

Replication of the paramyxoviruses is similar to other negative-strand RNA viruses. The VAP (HN, H, G) protein on the virion envelope attaches to sialic acid on cell surface glycolipids and works with the F protein to promote fusion with the plasma membrane. Paramyxoviruses are also able to induce cell-cell fusion, creating multinucleated giant cells (syncytia).

The RNA polymerase activity carried in the nucleocapsid transcribes the genome into individual and full-length mRNA followed by translation and genome replication, which all occur in the cytoplasm. New genomes associate with the L, N, and NP proteins to form nucleocapsids, which associate with matrix proteins on viral glycoprotein–modified plasma membranes. The glycoproteins are synthesized and processed like cellular glycoproteins. Mature virions bud from the host cell plasma membrane and exit the cell. Replication of the paramyxoviruses is represented by the respiratory syncytial virus infectious cycle in Figure 61-2.

MEASLES VIRUS

Measles is the only virus of human importance in the morbillivirus genus. Historically, measles has been one of the most common viral infections and one of the most unpleasant. Virtually everyone born before the 1960s can vividly remember the high fever, excruciating headache, and malaise associated with measles infection.

Pathogenesis and Immunity

Measles is known for its propensity to cause cell fusion, resulting in giant cells (Box 61-2). As a result, the virus can pass directly from cell to cell and escape antibody control. Inclusions occur most commonly in the cytoplasm and are composed of incomplete viral particles. Infection usually leads to cell lysis, but persistent infections without lysis can occur in certain cell types (e.g., human brain cells).

BOX 61-2 Disease Mechanisms of Measles Virus

- Infects epithelial cells of respiratory tract
- Spreads systemically in lymphocytes and by viremia
- Replicates in cells of the conjunctiva, respiratory tract, gastrointestinal tract, urinary tract, lymphatic system, blood vessels, and central nervous system
- Rash is caused by T-cell response to virus-infected epithelial cell lining the capillaries
- Cell-mediated immunity is essential to control of infection, antibody is not sufficient due to measles' ability to spread cell to cell
- Sequelae in the central nervous system may result from immunopathogenesis (postinfectious measles encephalitis) or development of defective mutants (subacute sclerosing panencephalitis, SSPE)

Measles is highly contagious and transmitted from person to person by respiratory droplets (Figure 61-3). Local replication of virus in the respiratory tract precedes lymphatic spread and viremia. Wide dissemination of the virus causes infection of the conjunctiva, respiratory tract, urinary tract, small blood vessels, and the central nervous system. The characteristic measles rash is caused by immune T cells targeted to measles-infected endothelial cells lining small blood vessels. In most patients recovery follows, with lifelong immunity. In some, a postinfectious encephalitis, which is believed to be immune mediated, occurs after the rash. The time course of measles infection is shown in Figure 61-4.

Cell-mediated immunity is responsible for most of the symptoms and is essential for the control of measles infection. T cell–deficient children infected with measles have an atypical presentation of giant cell pneumonia without a rash. Immunocompromised patients with measles may have continuing infection, resulting in death.

Epidemiology

Measles is present in respiratory secretions before and after the onset of characteristic symptoms and is one of the most contagious infections known (Box 61-3). In a household approximately 85% of exposed susceptible persons will become infected, and 95% of these will develop clinical disease. Epidemics tend to occur in 1- to 3-year cycles when a sufficient number of susceptible individuals has accumulated. Many of these cases occur in preschool-age children who have not been vaccinated and who live in large urban areas. The peak seasons are in the winter and spring.

Measles has only one serotype and usually presents with symptoms. These properties allowed the development of an effective vaccine program. Since vaccination

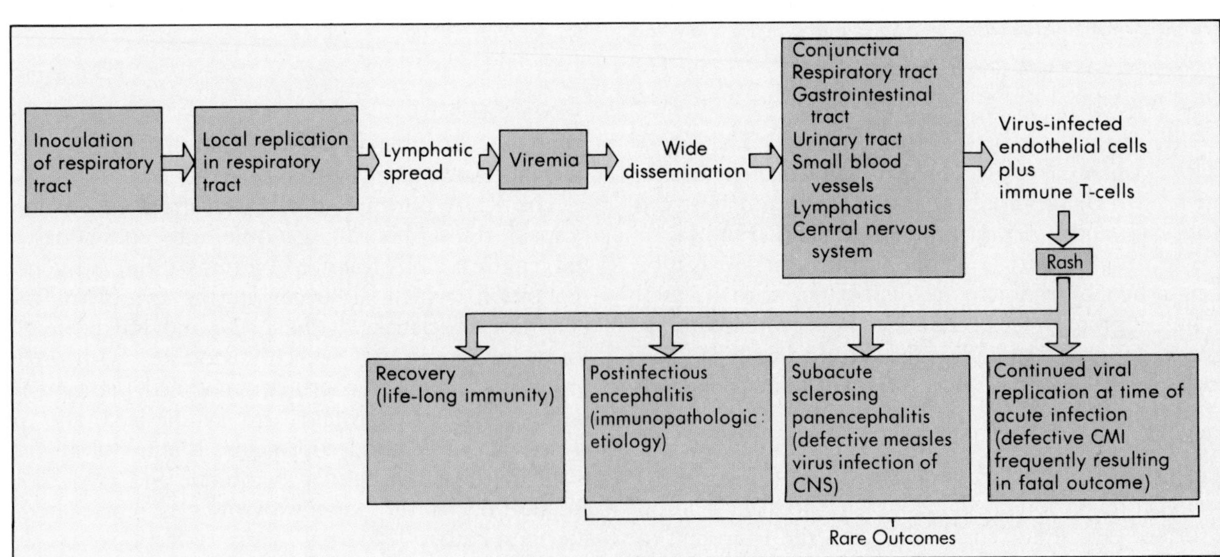

FIGURE 61-3 Mechanisms of spread within the body and pathogenesis of measles virus.

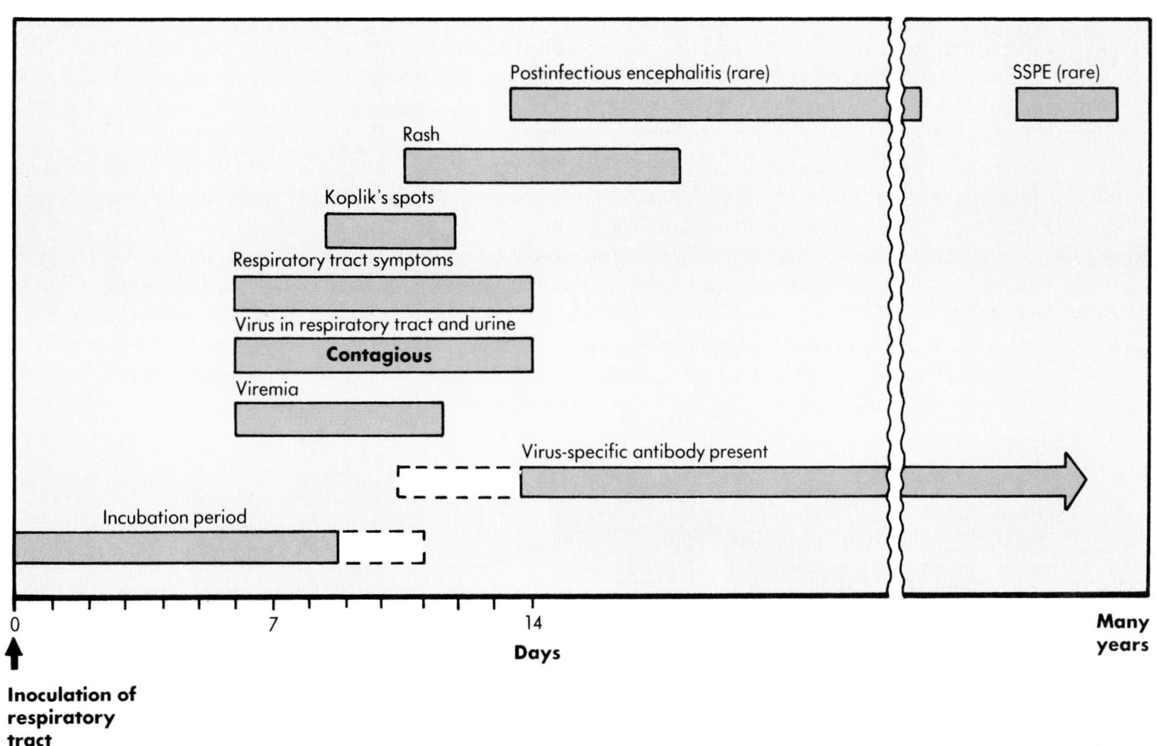

FIGURE 61-4 Time course of measles virus infection.

was introduced, the yearly incidence of measles has dropped dramatically, from 300 to 1.3 per 100,000 (U.S. statistics for 1981 to 1988). This represents a 99.5% reduction from the prevaccination period of 1955 to 1962. However, a fifteenfold increase in the incidence of measles was noted in 1989 to 1991 in the United States mainly because of poor compliance with vaccination programs. Measles is still common in developing countries and is the most important cause of death in children 1 to 5 years of age in several countries.

Clinical Syndromes

Measles is a serious febrile illness (Table 61-3). The incubation period is 7 to 13 days. The prodrome starts with high fever and the three "*c*'s"—cough, coryza, and conjunctivitis, in addition to photophobia. At this time the patient is most infectious.

After 2 days of illness, the typical mucous membrane lesions, known as **Koplik's spots** (Figure 61-5), appear. They are seen most commonly on the buccal mucosa across from the molars, but they may appear on other mucous membranes, including the conjunctiva and the vagina. The lesions, which last 24 to 48 hours, are usually small (1 to 2 mm) and are best described as grains of salt surrounded by a red halo. Their appearance in the mouth establishes with certainty the diagnosis of measles.

Within 12 to 24 hours after the appearance of Koplik's spots, the exanthem of measles starts below the ears and spreads over the body. The rash is maculopapular, usually very extensive, and often the lesions become confluent.

BOX 61-3 Epidemiology of Measles

DISEASE/VIRAL FACTORS

Large relatively unstable enveloped virion, easily inactivated
Contagion period precedes symptoms
Host range is limited to humans
Only one serotype
Immunity is lifelong

TRANSMISSION

Inhalation via large droplet aerosols

WHO IS AT RISK?

Unvaccinated individuals
Immunocompromised individuals: more serious outcome

GEOGRAPHY/SEASON

Worldwide
Endemic in fall to spring, possibly because of crowding indoors

MODES OF CONTROL

Live attenuated vaccine (Schwartz or Moraten variants of Edmonston B strain)
Immune serum globulin following exposure

TABLE 61-3 Clinical Consequences of Measles Virus Infection

Disorder	Symptoms
Measles	Characteristic maculopapular rash, coryza, cough and conjunctivitis, Koplik's spots; complications include otitis media, croup, bronchopneumonia, and encephalitis, the most severe complication (principal reason for vaccine)
Atypical measles	Rash is most prominent in distal areas Vesicles, petechiae, purpura, or urticaria may also be present
Subacute sclerosing panencephalitis	Central nervous system manifestations (e.g., personality, behavior, and memory changes, myoclonic jerks, spasticity, and blindness)

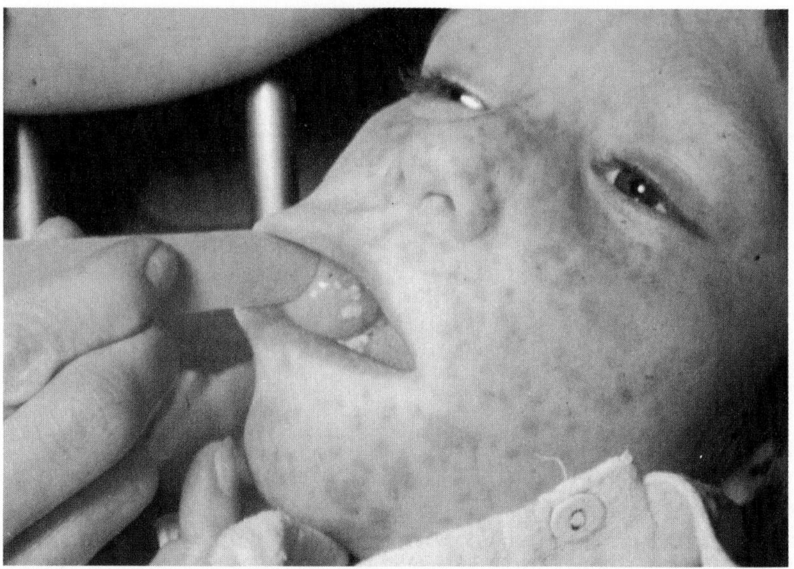

FIGURE 61-5 Koplik's spots in mouth and exanthem. Koplik's spots usually precede the measles rash and may be seen for the first day or two after the rash appears. (From Emond RTD, Rowland HAK: *A color atlas of infectious diseases, ed 2, London, 1987, Wolfe.)*

The rash, which takes 1 or 2 days to cover the body, fades in the same order it appeared. The fever is highest and the patient is sickest on the day the rash first appears (Figure 61-6).

One of the most feared complications of measles is the development of **encephalitis**, which may be fatal in 15% of cases. It may occur in as many as 0.5% of those infected and usually begins 7 to 10 days after onset of illness.

Pneumonia, which can also be a serious complication, accounts for 60% of reported deaths caused by measles virus infection. Mortality with pneumonia, as with other complications associated with measles, increases with malnutrition and is inversely proportional to age. **Giant cell pneumonia** without rash occurs in children lacking T-cell immunity. Bacterial superinfection is common in pneumonia caused by measles virus.

Atypical measles occurs in individuals who received the older inactivated measles vaccine and who subsequently were exposed to the wild measles virus. It may also rarely occur after vaccination with attenuated virus vaccine. This syndrome probably represents an enhanced immunopathology to wild measles virus because of prior sensitization but insufficient immune protection. The illness begins abruptly and is a more intense presentation of measles.

Subacute sclerosing panencephalitis (SSPE) is an extremely serious, very late neurological sequelae of measles that occurs in about 7 in 1,000,000 patients. In SSPE a defective measles virus persists in the brain and acts as a **slow virus**. The virus can replicate and spread directly from cell to cell but is not released. Many months or years after clinical measles the patient develops changes in personality, behavior, and memory. Myoclonic jerks, blindness, and spasticity follow. Unusually high levels of measles antibodies are found in the blood and spinal fluid. Eosinophilic inclusion bodies composed of paramyxovirus-like nucleocapsids are present in the brains of patients with SSPE. The

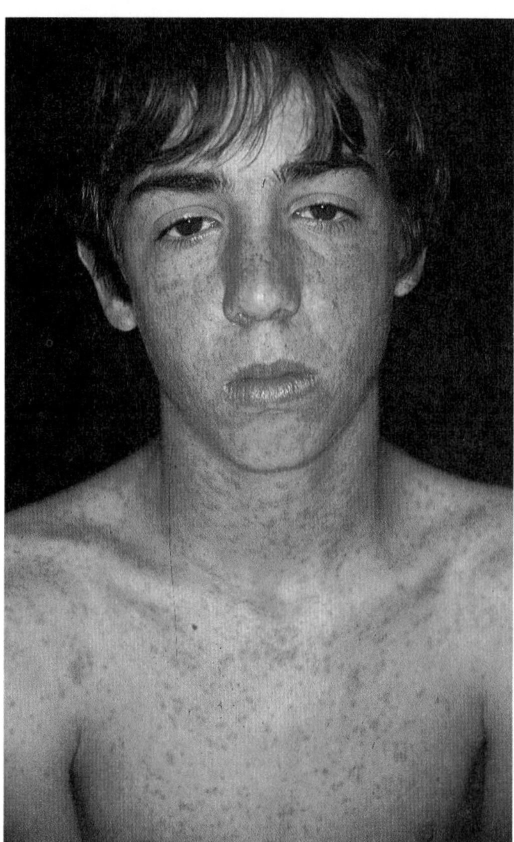

FIGURE 61-6 Measles rash. (From Habif TP: *Clinical dermatology: color guide to diagnosis and therapy*, St. Louis, 1985, Mosby.)

incidence of SSPE has decreased markedly with the success of measles vaccination.

Laboratory Diagnosis

Clinically, measles is usually so characteristic that it is rarely necessary to perform laboratory tests to make a diagnosis. Measles virus is difficult to isolate and grow. The virus can be grown in primary human or monkey cell cultures. Respiratory tract secretions, urine, blood, and brain tissue are recommended specimens. Respiratory and blood specimens are best collected during the prodromal stage up to 1 to 2 days after the appearance of the rash.

Measles antigen can be detected by immunofluorescence in pharyngeal cells or urinary sediment, but this test is not generally available. Characteristic cytopathologic effects including multinucleated giant cells with cytoplasmic and nuclear inclusion bodies can be seen in Giemsa-stained cells taken from the upper respiratory tract and urinary sediment.

Antibody, especially IgM, can be detected when the rash is present. Seroconversion or a fourfold increase in measles-specific antibodies between acute and convalescent sera represent the best method of confirming measles. Immune status testing to determine past infection or immunization is being used to document childhood immunization.

BOX 61-4 Measles, Mumps, Rubella Vaccine (MMR)

Composition: Live attenuated virus
- Measles: Schwartz or Moraten substrains of Edmonston B strain
- Mumps: Jeryl Lynn strain
- Rubella: RA/27-3 strain

Vaccination schedule: At 15 months and at 4 to 6 years or before junior high school

Efficiency: 95% lifelong immunization with a single dose

Data from MMWR 40 (RR-12), 1991.

Treatment, Prevention, and Control

A live attenuated measles vaccine in use since 1963 has significantly reduced the incidence of measles in the United States. The current Schwartz or Moraten attenuated strains of the original Edmonston B vaccine are currently being used in the United States. Live attenuated vaccine is given to all children after 15 months of age, in combination with mumps and rubella vaccine (**MMR vaccine**) (Box 61-4). Although successful vaccination results are greater than 95%, revaccination is being suggested for children before grade school or junior high school. A killed measles vaccine, introduced in 1963 and subsequently discontinued, provided only short-term immune protection. Recipients of killed vaccine were at risk for the more serious atypical measles presentation upon infection.

Hospitals in areas experiencing endemic measles may wish to vaccinate or check the immune status of their employees to decrease the risk of nosocomial transmission.

Exposed susceptible individuals who are immunocompromised should be given immune serum globulin to modify their measles infection. This product is most effective if given within 6 days of exposure. Inactivated "killed" vaccines are no longer available, even for the immunocompromised, because of the subsequent effect on naturally acquired measles virus infection (atypical measles). No specific antiviral treatment is available for measles.

PARAINFLUENZA VIRUSES

Parainfluenza viruses, discovered in the late 1950s, are respiratory viruses that usually cause mild coldlike symptoms but can also cause serious respiratory disease. Four serologic types within the parainfluenza genus are human pathogens. Types 1 to 3 are second only to respiratory syncytial virus as important causes of severe lower respiratory infection in infants and young children. They

BOX 61-5 Disease Mechanisms of Parainfluenza Viruses

Four serotypes of viruses
Infection is limited to respiratory tract; upper respiratory tract disease is most common, but significant disease can occur upon lower respiratory tract infection
Parainfluenza viruses are not systemic and do *not* cause viremia
Diseases include coldlike symptoms, bronchitis (inflammation of bronchial tubes), bronchiolitis (inflammation of bronchioles), croup (laryngotracheobronchitis)
Infection induces protective immunity of short duration

are especially associated with laryngotracheobronchitis (croup). Type 4 causes only mild upper respiratory infection in children and adults.

Pathogenesis and Immunity

Parainfluenza viruses infect epithelial cells of the upper respiratory tract (Box 61-5). The virus replicates more rapidly than measles and mumps viruses and can cause giant cell formation and cell lysis. Unlike measles and mumps viruses, the parinfluenza viruses rarely cause viremia. The viruses generally stay in the upper respiratory tract, causing only coldlike symptoms. In approximately 25% of cases the virus spreads to the lower respiratory tract and in 2% to 3% this may take the severe form of laryngotracheobronchitis.

The cell-mediated immune response is responsible for cell damage, as well as protection. IgA responses are protective but are short-lived. Multiple serotypes and the short duration of immunity following natural infection make reinfection common, but reinfection is milder, suggesting at least partial immunity.

Epidemiology

Paramyxoviruses are ubiquitous, and infection is common (Box 61-6). Transmission is by person-to-person contact and by respiratory droplets. Primary infections usually occur in infants and small children younger than 5 years of age. Reinfections occur throughout life, suggesting that immunity is short-lived. Infections with parainfluenza virus 1 and 2, the major causes of croup, tend to occur in the fall, whereas parainfluenza virus 3 infections occur throughout the year. All of these viruses spread readily within hospitals and can cause outbreaks in nurseries and pediatric wards.

Clinical Syndromes

Parainfluenza 1, 2, or 3 may cause respiratory syndromes ranging from mild coldlike upper respiratory infection (coryza, pharyngitis, mild bronchitis, and fever) to bronchiolitis and pneumonia. Older children and adults generally experience milder infections, although pneumonia may occur in the elderly. Parainfluenza infection of infants may be more severe, causing bronchiolitis, pneumonia, and most notably, croup (laryngotracheobronchitis). **Croup** results in subglottal swelling, which may close the airway. Clinically, after a 2- to 6-day incubation period the patient develops hoarseness, a "seal bark" cough, tachypnea, tachycardia, and suprasternal retraction. Most children recover within 48 hours. The principal differential diagnosis is epiglottitis caused by *Haemophilus influenzae*.

BOX 61-6 Epidemiology of Parainfluenza Virus Infections

DISEASE/VIRAL FACTORS
Large relatively unstable enveloped virion, easily inactivated
Contagion period precedes symptoms and may occur in the absence of symptoms
Host range is limited to humans
Reinfection later in life can occur

TRANSMISSION
Inhalation of large droplet aerosols

WHO IS AT RISK?
Children: mild disease, croup
Adults: reinfection with milder symptoms

GEOGRAPHY/SEASON
Ubiquitous and worldwide
Seasonal

MODES OF CONTROL
None

Laboratory Diagnosis

Parainfluenza virus isolated from nasal washings and respiratory secretions grow well in primary monkey kidney cells. However, like the other paramyxoviruses, the virions are labile during transit to the lab. Virus-infected cells in aspirates or in cell culture can be identified by immunofluorescence. In addition, virus-infected cells will show syncytia and can hemadsorb guinea pig erythrocytes. The hemagglutinin on the surface of infected cells attach the erythrocytes to the cell surface in a manner similar to influenza. The serotype of the virus can be determined using specific antibody to block hemadsorption or hemagglutination (hemagglutination inhibition [HI]).

Treatment, Prevention, and Control

Treatment includes nebulized cold or hot steam and careful monitoring of the upper airway. On rare occasions intubation may become necessary. No specific antiviral agents are available.

Vaccination with killed vaccines is ineffective possibly because they fail to induce local secretory antibody and appropriate cellular immunity. No live attenuated vaccine is presently available.

MUMPS VIRUS

Mumps virus is the cause of acute benign viral parotitis (swelling of the salivary glands). The disease produces obvious clinical symptoms resulting from a systemic infection with the potential for involvement of other organs.

Mumps virus was isolated in embryonated eggs in 1945 and in cell culture in 1955. Mumps virus is a member of the paramyxoviridae and is most closely related to parainfluenza virus 2, but there is no cross-immunity with the parainfluenza viruses.

Pathogenesis and Immunity

Mumps virus, of which only one serotype is known, causes a lytic infection of cells (Box 61-7). The virus replicates in the epithelial cells of the upper respiratory tract and either infects the parotid gland by way of Stensen's duct or by viremia. Mumps is spread throughout the body by viremia to the testes, ovary, pancreas, thryroid, and other organs. Infection of the CNS occurs with symptoms in as many as 50% of those infected (Figure 61-7). Inflammatory responses are mainly responsible for causing the symptoms. The time course of human infection is shown in Figure 61-8. Immunity is lifelong.

BOX 61-7 Disease Mechanisms of Mumps Virus

- Infects epithelial cells of respiratory tract
- Spreads systemically by viremia
- Systemic infection, especially of parotid gland, testes, and central nervous system
- Principal symptom is swelling of parotid glands because of inflammation
- Cell-mediated immunity is essential for control of infection and responsible for a portion of the symptoms. Antibody is not sufficient due to mumps' ability to spread cell to cell

Epidemiology

Mumps, like measles, is a very communicable disease with only one serotype and infects only humans (Box 61-8). In the absence of vaccination programs, infection is acquired in 90% of persons by age 15. The virus is spread by direct person-to-person contact and by respiratory droplets. The virus is present in respiratory secretions for as long as 7 days before clinical illness and often does not produce symptoms, so control of spread is virtually impossible. Spread of the virus is promoted by close quarters and particularly in the winter and spring.

Clinical Syndromes

Mumps infections are often asymptomatic. Clinical illness is manifested as a **parotitis** (painful swelling of the salivary glands) that is almost always bilateral and accompanied by fever. Onset is sudden. Oral examination reveals redness and swelling of the ostium of Stensen's duct. Submaxillary and submandibular glands may be involved, even in the absence of parotid involvement. Orchitis (usually unilateral), oophoritis, pancreatitis, and meningoencephalitis may occur a few days after the onset of the virus infection but can occur in the absence of parotitis. The swelling resulting from mumps orchitis may cause sterility. Mumps virus involves the central nervous system in approximately 50% of patients, and 10% may exhibit clinical evidence of infection. This is

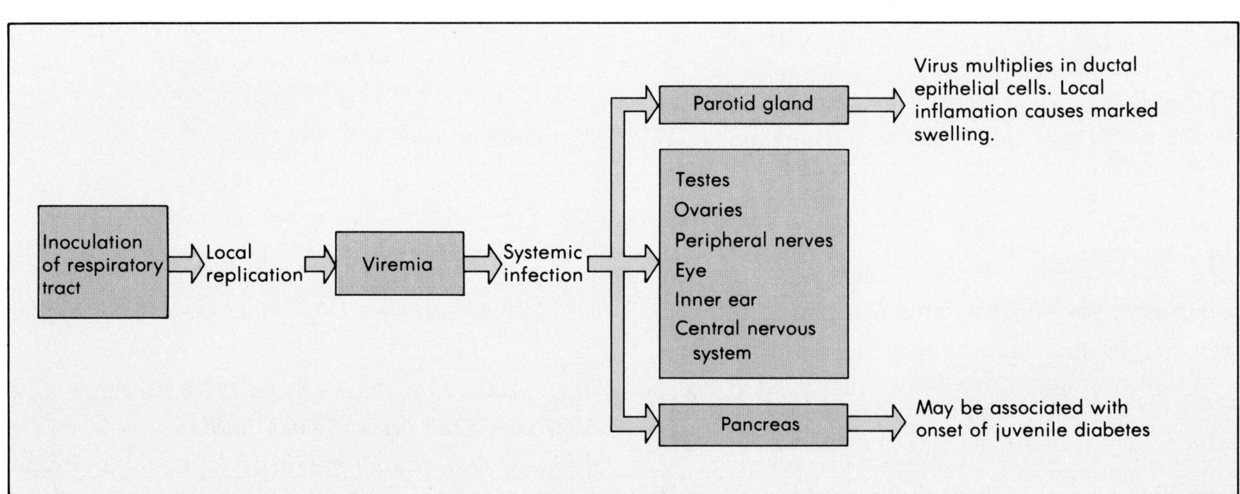

FIGURE 61-7 Mechanism of spread of mumps virus within the body.

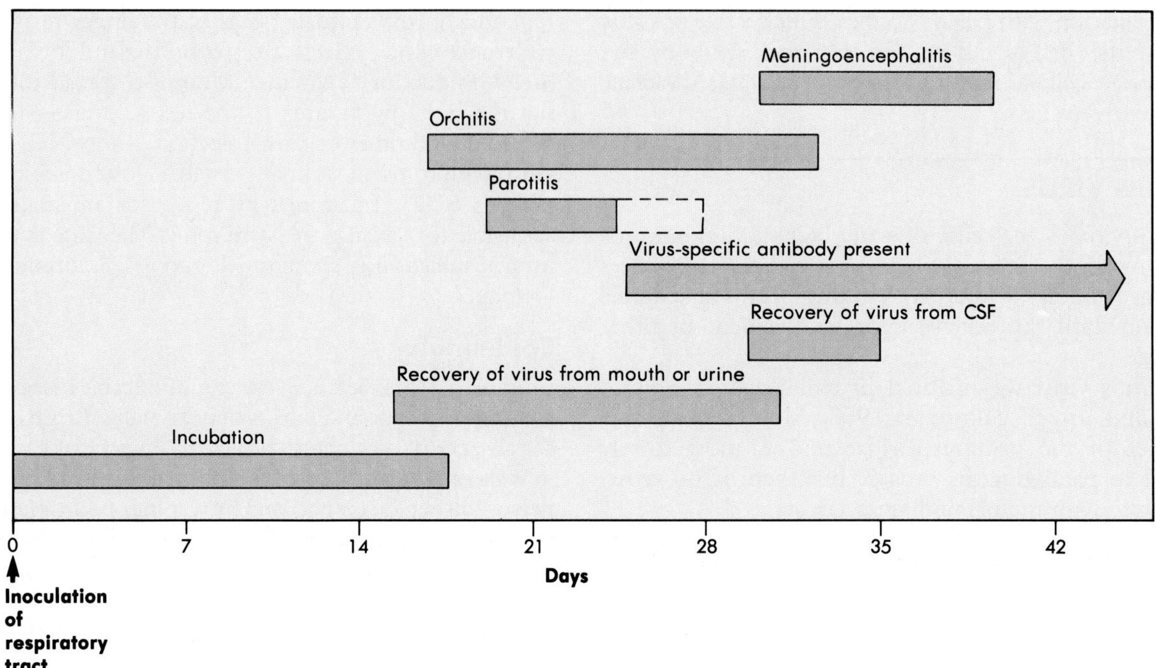

FIGURE 61-8 Time course of mumps virus infection.

usually a syndrome of "aseptic" meningitis, but encephalitis also occurs with involvement of the cerebellum. Because of the latter, children who have mumps encephaltis may be unsteady in standing or walking.

Laboratory Diagnosis

Virus can be recovered from saliva, urine, pharynx, secretions from Stensen's duct, and cerebrospinal fluid. Virus is present in saliva for approximately 5 days after the onset of symptoms and in urine for as long as 2 weeks. Mumps virus grows well in monkey kidney cells and can be recognized by the development of a cytopathogenic effect characterized by multinucleated giant cells. Hemadsorption of guinea pig erythrocytes also occurs on viral-infected cells.

A clinical diagnosis can be confirmed by serologic testing. A fourfold increase in virus-specific antibody level or the detection of mumps-specific IgM antibody indicates active infection. Hemagglutination inhibition (HI), ELISA, and immunofluorescence tests can be used to detect mumps virus, antigen, or antibody. Antibodies to specific mumps antigens provide hints to the course of the disease.

Treatment, Prevention and Control

Given the difficulties of controlling the spread of mumps, vaccines provide the only effective means for reducing infection. Since the introduction of the live attenuated vaccine (Jeryl Lynn vaccine) in the United States in 1967 and its administration as part of the MMR vaccine, the yearly incidence of cases has declined from 76 to 2 per 100,000. Unfortunately, use of this vaccine in the world is limited. Antiviral agents are not available.

BOX 61-8 Epidemiology of Mumps Virus

DISEASE/VIRAL FACTORS

Large relatively unstable enveloped virion, easily inactivated
Contagion period precedes symptoms
May cause asymptomatic shedding
Host range is limited to humans
Only one serotype
Immunity is lifelong

TRANSMISSION

Large droplet aerosols

WHO IS AT RISK?

Unvaccinated individuals
Immunocompromised individuals: more serious outcome

GEOGRAPHY/SEASON

Worldwide
Endemic in late winter and early spring

MODES OF CONTROL

Live attenuated vaccine (Jeryl Lynn strain)

RESPIRATORY SYNCYTIAL VIRUS

Respiratory syncytial virus (RSV), first isolated from a chimpanzee in 1956, is a member of the Pneumovirus genus. RSV is the most frequent cause of fatal acute respiratory infection in infants and young children. It

BOX 61-9 Disease Mechanisms of Respiratory Syncytial Virus

Localized infection of respiratory tract
Does not cause viremia or systemic spread
Pneumonia results from cytopathic effect of virus (including syncytia)
Bronchiolitis most likely mediated by host's immune response
Narrow airways of young infants readily obstructed by virus-induced pathology
Maternal antibody does not protect infant from infection
Natural infection does not prevent reinfection
Vaccination increases severity of disease

infects virtually everyone by 4 years of age, and reinfections occur throughout life, even among the elderly.

The major structural differences between RSV and the other paramyxoviruses are the smaller nucleocapsid and the lack of hemagglutinin and neuraminidase activities for RSV.

Pathogenesis and Immunity

Respiratory syncytial virus produces an infection localized to the respiratory tract (Box 61-9). As the name suggests, RSV induces syncytia, which provides a mechanism for the transmission of the virus to uninfected cells. Most of the pathologic effect of RSV is probably due to direct viral invasion of respiratory epithelium, but an additional component may result from immunologically mediated cell injury. Necrosis of bronchi and bronchioles leads to "plugs" of mucus, fibrin, and necrotic material within smaller airways. These in turn lead to air trapping and the appearance of hyperinflation that can be seen in chest x-ray films. Narrow airways of young infants are readily obstructed. Natural immunization does not prevent reinfection, and vaccination with killed vaccine appears to enhance the severity of subsequent disease.

Epidemiology

Respiratory syncytial virus is very prevalent in young children, with infection of 65% to 98% of children in day care occurring by age 3 (Box 61-10). As many as 25% to 33% of these cases involve the lower respiratory tract and are more serious. As many as 95,000 children are hospitalized for RSV infections in the United States each year.

RSV infections almost always occur in winter. Unlike influenza, which may occasionally "skip" a year, RSV epidemics occur every year.

The virus is very contagious with an incubation period of 4 to 5 days. The results of introducing the virus into a nursery, especially into an intensive care nursery, can be devastating. Virtually every infant becomes infected, with considerable morbidity; occasional fatalities occur. The virus is transmitted on hands, fomites, and to some degree by respiratory routes.

BOX 61-10 Epidemiology of Respiratory Syncytial Virus

DISEASE/VIRAL FACTORS

Large relatively unstable enveloped virion, easily inactivated
Contagion period precedes symptoms and may occur in the absence of symptoms
Host range is limited to humans

TRANSMISSION

Inhalation of large droplet aerosols

WHO IS AT RISK?

Infants: lower tract infection: bronchiolitis and pneumonia
Children: spectrum of disease: mild to pneumonia
Adults: reinfection with milder symptoms

GEOGRAPHY/SEASON

Ubiquitous and worldwide
Seasonal

MODES OF CONTROL

Vaccination may exacerbate future disease
Aerosol ribavarin available for infants with serious disease

Virtually all children are infected by RSV by the age of 4, especially in urban centers. Outbreaks may also occur among the elderly (e.g., in nursing homes). Virus is shed in respiratory secretions for many days, especially in infants.

Clinical Syndromes

Respiratory syncytial virus can cause any respiratory illness from a common cold to pneumonia. Upper respiratory infection with prominent rhinorrhea ("runny nose") is most common for older children and adults. In infants a more severe lower respiratory illness, bronchiolitis, may occur. Because of inflammation at the level of the bronchiole, there is air trapping and decreased ventilation. Clinically, the patient usually has low-grade fever, tachypnea, tachycardia, and expiratory wheezes over the lungs. Bronchiolitis is usually self-limited, but it can be a frightening disease to observe in an infant. In premature infants, those with underlying lung disease, and in the immunocompromised, it may be fatal (Table 61-4).

Laboratory Diagnosis

Respiratory syncytial virus is difficult to isolate in cell culture. Direct detection of viral antigen in infected cells and in nasal washings has been developed using immunofluorescence and enzyme immunoassay. Reagents for both tests are commercially available. Seroconversion or a fourfold or greater increase in antibody titer can substantiate the diagnosis.

TABLE 61-4 Clinical Consequences of Respiratory Syncytial Virus Infection

Disorder	Symptoms
Bronchiolitis and/or pneumonia	Fever, cough, dyspnea, and cyanosis in children younger than 1 year old
Febrile rhinitis and pharyngitis	Symptoms occur in children of all ages
Common cold	Upper respiratory infection in older children and adults who are being reinfected against a background of partial immunity

Treatment, Prevention, and Control

In otherwise healthy infants, treatment is supportive, with oxygen, intravenous fluids, and nebulized cold steam. Ribavarin, a guanosine analogue, is administered by inhalation (nebulization) and is approved for treatment of patients predisposed to a more severe course (e.g., premature or immunocompromised infants). Infected children must be isolated. Since hospital staff caring for infected children are known to transmit virus to uninfected patients, control measures, including gowns, goggles, masks, and handwashing, are essential.

Currently no vaccine is available for RSV prophylaxis. A previous vaccine containing inactivated RSV actually caused recipients to have more severe RSV infection when subsequently exposed to live virus. This is thought to have resulted from a heightened immunological response at the time of wild virus exposure.

CASE STUDY AND QUESTIONS

An 18-year-old freshman in college complains of a cough, runny nose, and conjunctivitis. The physician in the campus health center notices small white lesions inside the mouth. The next day, a confluent red rash covers his face and neck.

1. What clinical characteristics of this case are diagnostic for measles?
2. Are any laboratory tests readily available to confirm the diagnosis? If so, what are they?
3. Is there a possible treatment for this individual?
4. When is/was this individual contagious?
5. Why is this disease not common in the United States?
6. Provide several possible reasons why this individual was susceptible to measles at age 18.

A 13-month-old child has had a runny nose, mild cough, and low-grade fever for several days. The cough gets worse and sounds "barking." The child makes a wheezing sound when agitated. The child appears well except for the cough. A lateral x-ray examination of the neck shows a subglottic narrowing.

1. What is the specific and common name for these symptoms?
2. What other agents would cause a similar clinical presentation (differential diagnosis)?
3. Are there laboratory tests readily available to confirm the diagnosis? If so, what are they?
4. Is there a possible treatment for this individual?
5. When is/was this individual contagious and how is the virus transmitted?

Bibliography

Balows A, Hausler WJ Jr, and Lennette EH: *Laboratory diagnosis of infectious diseases: principles and practice*, New York, 1988, Springer-Verlag.

Belshe RB, editor: *Textbook of human viruses*, ed 2, St. Louis, 1991, Mosby.

Centers for Disease Control: Public-sector vaccination efforts in response to the resurgence of measles among preschool-aged children—United States, 1989-1991; *MMWR* 41:522-525, 1992.

Fields BN, Knipe DM, editors: *Virology*, ed 2, New York, 1990, Raven Press.

Galinski MS: Paramyxoviridae: transcription and replication, *Adv Vir Res* 40:129-163, 1991.

Hart CA, Broadhead RL: *Color atlas of pediatric infectious diseases*, St. Louis, 1992, Mosby.

Hinman AR: Potential candidates for eradication, *Rev Infect Dis* 4:933-939, 1982.

Krugman S, Katz SL, Gershon AA, Wilfert CM: *Infectious diseases of children*, St. Louis, 1992, Mosby.

White DO, Fenner F: *Medical virology*, Orlando, Fla, 1986, Academic Press.

CHAPTER 62

Reoviruses

THE **Reoviridae** include the orthoreoviruses, rotaviruses, and orbiviruses (Table 62-1). The name *reovirus* was proposed in 1959 by Albert Sabin for a group of respiratory and enteric viruses that were not associated with any known disease process, thus the name *r* (respiratory), *e* (enteric), *o* (orphan)—virus. The Reoviridae are nonenveloped viruses with double-layered protein capsids containing 10 to 12 segments of the double-stranded ribonucleic acid (RNA) genomes. These viruses are stable over wide pH and temperature ranges and in airborn aerosols. Previously, the **orbiviruses** had been classified as arboviruses.

The orthoreoviruses, also referred to as mammalian reoviruses or simply reoviruses, were first isolated in the 1950s from stools of children. They are the prototype of this virus family, and the molecular basis of their pathogenesis has been studied extensively. In general, these viruses cause asymptomatic infection of humans.

Rotaviruses cause human infantile gastroenteritis, a very common disease. Rotaviruses account for approximately 50% of all cases of diarrhea in children requiring hospitalization because of dehydration (70,000 cases per year in the United States). In underdeveloped countries rotaviruses may be responsible for as many as 1 million deaths each year.

TABLE 62-1 Reoviridae Responsible for Human Disease

Virus	Disease
Orthoreovirus*	Mild upper respiratory illness, gastrointestinal illness, biliary atresia
Orbivirus	Febrile illness with headache and myalgia
Rotavirus	Gastrointestinal illness, respiratory illness (?)

*Reovirus is a common name for the family Reoviridae and for the specific genus Orthoreovirus.

STRUCTURE

Rotavirus and reovirus share many structural, replicative, and pathogenic features. Reoviruses and rotaviruses have an icosahedral morphology with a double capsid (60 to 80 nm in diameter) (Box 62-1 and Figure 62-1). The name rotavirus is derived from the Latin *rota*, meaning wheel, referring to the virion appearance in negative-stain electron micrographs (Figure 62-2). Incomplete rotavirus particles are also seen in electron micrographs. These viruses lack the outer layer of the double-layered capsid and are often found in preparations from diarrheal stool and cell culture.

The virion serves three main purposes: packaging (nucleocapsid core), protection (outer capsid) and delivery (ISVP) (see the following). The virion must protect the nucleocapsid core from the environment, deliver the nucleocapsid core through the acidic environment of the G.I. tract and across the intestinal lumen to the target

BOX 62-1 Unique Features of Reoviridae

- Double capsid virion (60 to 80 nm) with icosahedral symmetry containing 10 to 12 double-stranded genome segments (depending upon the virus)
- Virion is resistant to environmental and G.I. conditions (e.g., detergents, acidic pH, drying)
- Rotavirus and orthoreovirus virions are activated by mild proteolysis to infectious subviral particles (ISVP) increasing their infectivity
- Inner capsid contains a compete transcription system, including enzymes for 5′capping and polyA addition
- Virus replication occurs in the cytoplasm. Double-stranded RNA remains in inner core
- Assembly of orthoreoviruses occurs on microtubules
- Rotavirus inner capsid aggregates in the cytoplasm and then buds into the endoplasmic reticulum, acquiring its outer capsid and a membrane, which is then lost
- Virus is released by cell lysis

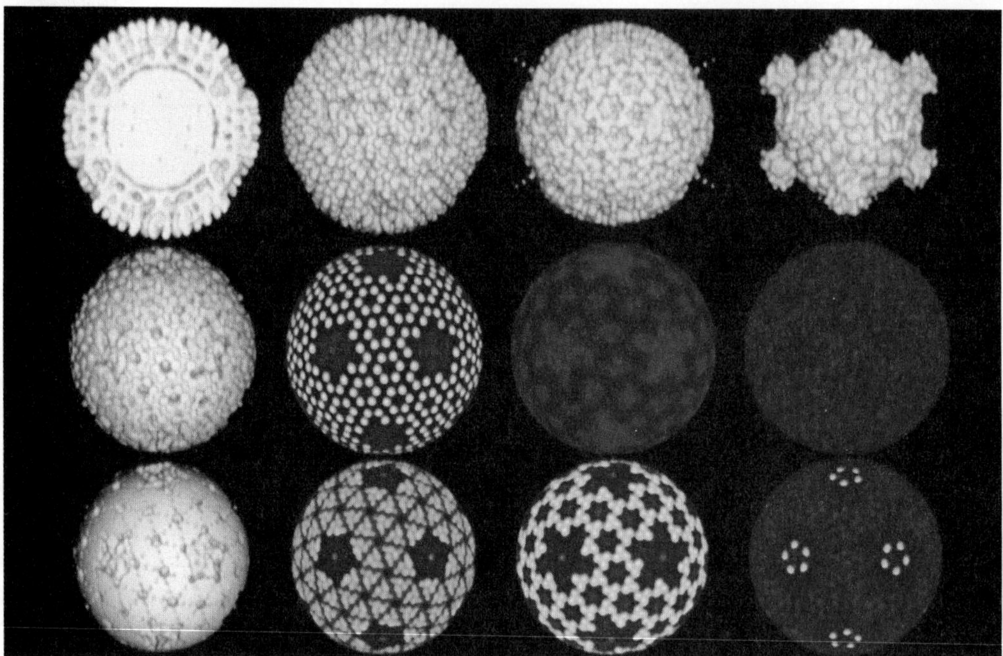

FIGURE 62-1 Computer reconstructions of cryoelectron micrographs of human reovirus Type 1 (Lang). *Top: left to right:* Cross-section of virion, virion, intermediate subviral particle (ISVP), and core particle. The ISVP and core particles are generated by proteolysis of the virion and play important roles in the replication cycle. *Second and Third Row:* Computer generated images of the virions at different radii after shaving off the outer layers of features. The colors help to visualize the symmetry and molecular interactions within the capsid. (Courtesy Tim Baker, Purdue University.)

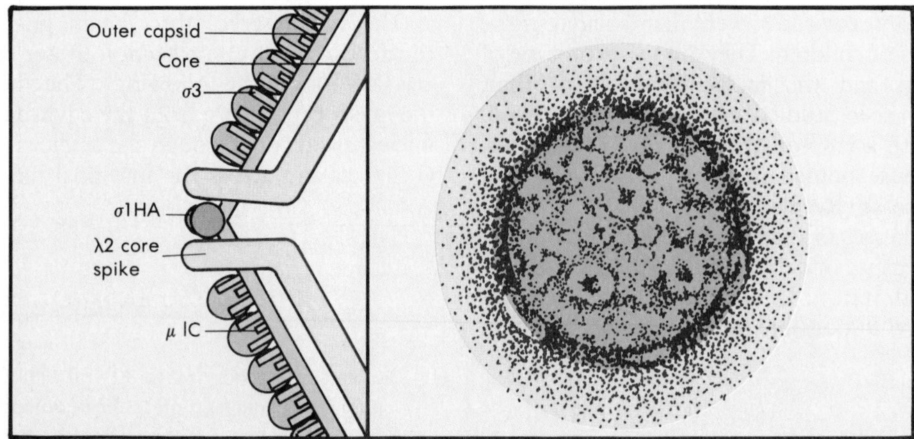

FIGURE 62-2 Structure of orthoreovirus core and outer proteins. (Redrawn from Sharpe AH and Fields BN: *N Engl J Med* 312:486-497, 1985.)

tissue, and deliver the nucleocapsid core into the cytoplasm of the target cells.

The outer capsid is composed of structural proteins (Figure 62-3), which surrounds a nucleocapsid core that includes enzymes for RNA synthesis and 10 (reo) or 11 (rota) different double-stranded RNA genome segments. Proteolytic cleavage of the virion (as in the G.I. tract) activates the virus for infection and produces an **intermediate/infectious subviral particle (ISVP)**. Interestingly, rotaviruses resemble enveloped viruses in that they have glycoproteins, acquire and then lose an envelope during assembly, and appear to have a fusion protein activity to promote direct penetration of the target cell membrane.

The genome segments of rotaviruses and reoviruses encode structural and nonstructural proteins. The genome segments, the proteins that they encode, and their functions are summarized in Table 62-2 for reovirus and Table 62-3 for rotavirus. As for influenza A, reassortment of gene segments can occur to create hybrid

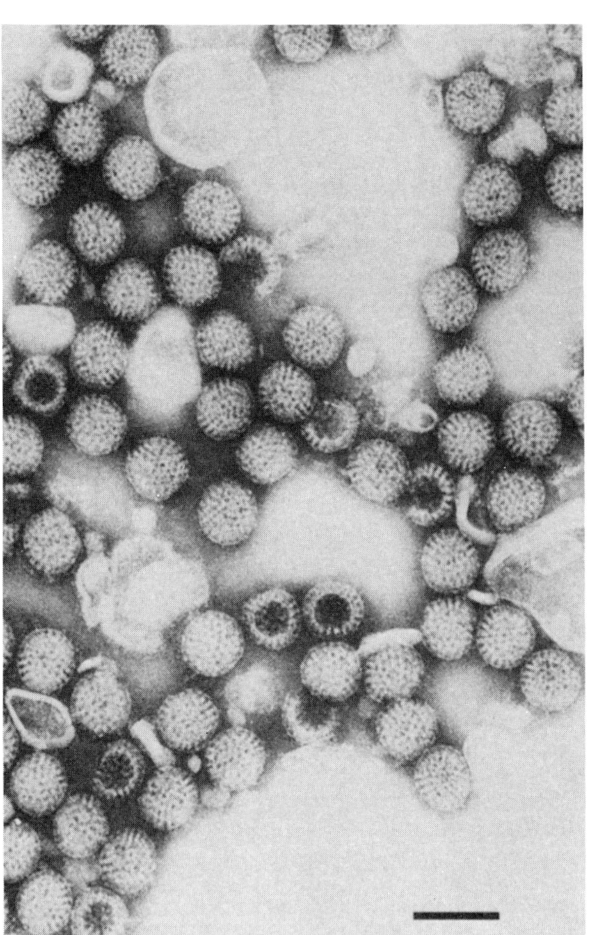

FIGURE 62-3 Electron micrograph of rotavirus. Bar = 100nm. (From Fields BN, editor: *Virology*, New York, 1985, Raven Press.)

viruses. The reovirus proteins are named as σ(1,2,3); μ(1,2); or λ(1,2,3), based on the size of the genome segment from which they were derived. Rotaviruses are numbered as virion protein (VP)(1-7) or nonstructural protein NS(1-4).

Core proteins include enzymatic activities required for transcription of mRNA. The σ1 protein and VP4 are located at the vertices of the capsid and extend from the surface like spike proteins. They have several functions including hemagglutination and virus attachment, and they elicit neutralizing antibodies. The VP4 is activated by protease cleavage, exposing a structure similar to the fusion proteins of paramyxoviruses. Its cleavage is required for productive entry into cells. The VP7 of rotaviruses also elicits neutralizing antibody and binds to a cell surface receptor.

REPLICATION

Replication of reovirus and rotavirus starts with ingestion of the virus (Figure 62-4). The complete virion is partially digested in the G.I. tract and presumably activated by protease cleavage of external capsid proteins (σ3/VP7) and loss of the σ3 and cleavage of the VP4 to produce the ISVP. The σ1/VP4 at the vertices of the ISVP binds to sialic acid–containing glycoproteins on epithelial and other cells, which include the beta-adrenergic receptor for reovirus. The ISVP of rotavirus penetrates the target cell membrane by an unknown mechanism. Whole virions of reovirus and rotavirus can be taken up by receptor-mediated endocytosis; however, this is a dead-end pathway for rotavirus.

Upon entry into the cell, the outer capsid releases the

TABLE 62-2 Orthoreovirus Genome Segments, Proteins, and Protein Functions

Genome segments (molecular weight)	Proteins	Functions (if known)
Large segments (2.8 × 10^6)		
1	λ1 (core)	Transcriptase component
2	λ2 (core, vertex spike)	Transcriptase component, capping enzyme*
3	λ3 (core)	Transcriptase component
Medium segments (1.4 × 10^6)		
1	μ2 (core)	–
2	μ1C (outer capsid)	Cleaved from μ1, complexes with σ3
3	μNS	Promotes viral assembly‡
Small segments (0.7 × 10^6)		
1	σ1 (outer capsid) (tetrameric)	Hemagglutinin, viral attachment protein, determines tissue tropism at vertices of capsid*
2	σ2 (core)	Transcriptase component
3	σNS	Transcriptase component
4	σ3 (outer capsid)	Complexes with μ1C, major component of outer capsid, controls viral and host RNA and protein synthesis

Modified from Fields BN, editor: *Virology*, New York, 1985, Raven Press.
*Elicits neutralizing antibodies.
‡NS proteins are not found in the virion.

TABLE 62-3 Functions of Rotavirus Gene Products

Genome segment	Protein/location	Function
1	VP1/central core	Transcriptase component
2	VP2/central core	Transcriptase component
3	VP3/central core	Transcriptase component
4	VP4/outer capsid spike protein at vertices of virion	Activated by cleavage to VP5 and VP8 in the ISVP, hemagglutinin, viral attachment protein
5	NS53	
6	VP6	Major structural protein of inner capsid, binds to NS28 at the ER to promote assembly of the outer capsid
7	NS34	
8	NS35	
9	VP7	Type-specific antigen, major outer capsid component, glycosylated in ER, and facilitates attachment and entry
10	NS28	Glycosylated and resident in the ER, promotes inner capsid binding to ER, transient envelopment, and addition of outer capsid
11	NS26	

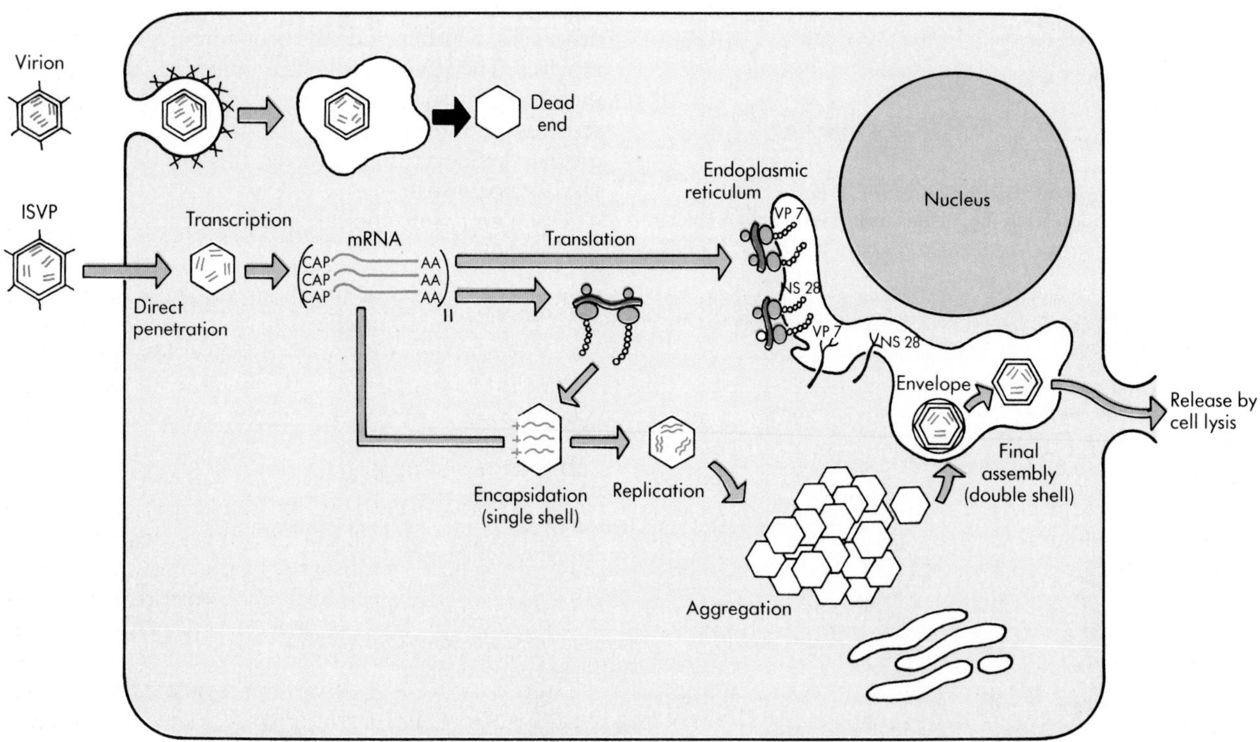

FIGURE 62-4 Replication of rotavirus. Rotavirus virions are activated by protease (e.g., in the G.I. tract) to an ISVP. The ISVP binds, penetrates the cell, and loses its outer capsid. The inner capsid contains the enzymes for mRNA transcription using the (−) strand as a template. Some mRNA segments are transcribed early, others later. The VP7 and NS28 are synthesized as glycoproteins and are expressed in the endoplasmic reticulum. (+)RNA are mRNA and also enclosed into inner capsids as templates to replicate the +/−, segmented genome. The capsids aggregate and then dock onto the NS28 protein in the ER, budding into the ER, acquiring VP7 and its outer capsid and an envelope. The virus loses the envelope and leaves the cell upon cell lysis.

core into the cytoplasm, and the enzymes in the core initiate mRNA production. The double-stranded RNA always remains in the core. Transcription of the genome occurs in two phases, early and late, but before genome replication. The (−)RNA strand is used as the template by virion core enzymes, which synthesize individual mRNAs complete with a 5′methyl guanosine cap and a 3′polyA tail. mRNA leaves the core and is translated. Virion proteins and (+)RNA segments associate together into corelike structures that aggregate into large cytoplasmic inclusions. The (+)RNA segments are copied to produce (−)RNAs in the new cores, which replicates the genome. The new cores can generate more (+)RNA or be assembled into virions.

The assembly processes for reovirus and rotavirus differ. For reovirus, the outer capsid proteins associate with the core, and the virion leaves the cell upon cell lysis. Rotavirus assembly resembles an enveloped virus. Rotavirus cores associate with the NS28 viral protein on the outside of the endoplasmic reticulum and acquire its outer capsid proteins and a membrane upon budding into the ER. The VP7 and NS28 proteins are glycosylated. The membrane is lost, and the virus leaves the cell upon cell lysis. Reovirus inhibits cellular macromolecular synthesis within 8 hours of infection.

BOX 62-2 Disease Mechanisms of Rotavirus

- Virus is spread by fecal-oral route and possibly respiratory route
- Cytolytic infection of the intestinal epithelium causes loss of electrolytes and prevents readsorption of water
- Disease can be significant in infants until 24 months of age and asymptomatic in adults
- Large amounts of virus are released during the diarrhea phase

ORTHOREOVIRUSES (MAMMALIAN REOVIRUSES)

The orthoreoviruses are ubiquitous, having been isolated in nearly all mammals worldwide. The virions are very stable and have been detected in sewage and river water. The mammalian reoviruses occur in three serotypes, referred to as reovirus types 1 to 3, based on neutralization and hemagglutination-inhibition tests. All three serotypes share a common complement-fixing antigen.

Pathogenesis and Immunity

Orthoreoviruses do not cause significant disease in humans. However, studies of reovirus disease in mice have advanced our understanding of virus pathogenesis. Depending on the reovirus strain, the virus can be neurotropic or viscerotropic in mice. The functions and virulence properties of the reovirus proteins were identified by comparing the activities of interstrain hybrid viruses differing in only one genome segment (encoding one protein). The new activity is attributable to the genome segment from the other virus strain.

Following ingestion and proteolytic production of the ISVP, the orthoreoviruses bind to M cells in the small intestine, which transfer the virus to the lymphoid tissue of Peyer's patches lining the intestines. The viruses replicate and initiate a viremia. Although the virus is cytolytic in vitro, it causes few if any symptoms before entering the circulation and producing infection at a distant site. In the mouse model the outer capsid protein responsible for hemagglutinin activity ($\sigma 1$) also facilitates viral spread to the mesenteric lymph nodes and determines whether the virus is neurotropic.

Mice, and presumably humans, elicit protective humoral and cellular immune responses to outer capsid proteins. Orthoreoviruses, although normally lytic viruses, are also capable of establishing persistent infection in cell culture.

Epidemiology

As mentioned, the orthoreoviruses have been detected worldwide. Seroprevalence studies suggest that most people are infected during childhood, and by adulthood approximately 75% have antibody. Immunizing infections are asymptomatic. Most animals, including chimpanzees and monkeys, also have detectable antibody. Whether animals are a reservoir for human infections is unknown.

Clinical Syndromes

Orthoreoviruses infect people of all ages, but linking specific diseases to these agents has been difficult. Most infections are thought to be asymptomatic or so mild that they go undetected. Thus far these viruses have been linked to mild upper respiratory illness (low-grade fever, rhinorrhea, pharyngitis), gastrointestinal disease, and biliary atresia.

Laboratory Diagnosis

Human orthoreovirus infection can be detected by assay of viral antigen or RNA in clinical material, virus isolation, or serologic assays for virus-specific antibody. Throat, nasopharyngeal, and stool specimens from patients with suspected upper respiratory or diarrheal disease are used as samples.

Human orthoreovirus can be isolated using mouse L-cell fibroblasts, primary monkey kidney cells, and HeLa cells. Cell cultures are incubated and observed for cytopathic effect (CPE) during a 3-week period. Early in the infectious cycle inclusions occur as small dots in the periphery of the host cell cytoplasm. Later, inclusions are larger and located adjacent to the nucleus. Hemagglutination, neutralization, and direct detection of viral antigen or RNA are used to confirm the presence of virus.

BOX 62-3 Epidemiology of Rotavirus

DISEASE/VIRAL FACTORS

Capsid virus is resistant to environmental and G.I. conditions
Large amounts of virus are released in fecal matter
Asymptomatic infection can result in virus release

TRANSMISSION

Transmitted in fecal material especially in day-care setting
Potential respiratory transmission

WHO IS AT RISK?

Rotavirus Type A

Infants until 24 months of age; infantile gastroenteritis with potential dehydration
Older children and adults: mild diarrhea
Undernourished individuals in underdeveloped countries: diarrhea, dehydration, and death

Rotavirus Type B

China: Severe gastroenteritis: infants, older children, and adults

GEOGRAPHY/SEASON

Worldwide
Disease more common in fall, winter, and spring

MODES OF CONTROL

Handwashing, isolation of known cases
Experimental live vaccines using bovine or monkey rotavirus

Serologic diagnosis of infection requires the documentation of a fourfold or greater increase in virus-specific antibody between an acute and convalescent specimen, since antibodies to orthoreoviruses typically are present in healthy children and adults. The techniques used to detect orthoreovirus antibody include hemagglutination inhibition, neutralization, complement fixation, and indirect immunofluorescence but are not routinely performed.

Treatment, Prevention, and Control

Orthoreovirus disease is mild and self-limited. For this reason treatment has not been necessary, and prevention and control measures have not been investigated.

ROTAVIRUSES

The rotaviruses are a large group of gastroenteritis-causing viruses found in many different mammals and birds. Although viruses have long been considered as a common cause of childhood diarrhea, it was not until 1973 that a rotavirus was first detected in humans. Since then rotaviruses have been implicated worldwide as common agents of infantile diarrhea.

Rotavirus virions are relatively stable at ambient temperature for 24 hours, following treatment with ether and other lipid solvents, or with repeated freeze-thawing. Infectivity is maintained at pH 3.5 to 10 and, importantly, is enhanced by proteolytic enzymes such as trypsin.

Human and animal rotaviruses are divided into serotypes, groups, and subgroups. Serotypes are determined by neutralization reaction and depend primarily on the VP7 outer capsid protein and, to a lesser extent, on the VP4 minor outer capsid protein. Groups are based primarily on the antigenicity of VP6 and on electrophoretic mobility of the genome segments. Subgroups are determined by complement fixation and depend on the VP6 inner capsid protein. Based on these reactions, seven serotypes (1 to 7), two subgroups (I and II), and at least five groups (A to E) have been described for human and animal rotaviruses.

Pathogenesis and Immunity

Rotaviruses are able to survive the acidic environment in a buffered stomach or in a stomach after a meal (Box 62-2). Viral replication follows adsorption to columnar epithelial cells covering the villi of the small intestine. Approximately 8 hours after infection, cytoplasmic inclusions are seen that contain newly synthesized proteins and RNA. The virus causes permeability changes and cell lysis.

Studies of biopsies of the small intestine from infants and of experimentally infected animals show shortening and blunting of the microvilli and mononuclear cell infiltration into the lamina propria. Infection prevents absorption of water, causing a net secretion of water and loss of ions resulting in a watery diarrhea. Loss of fluids and electrolytes can lead to severe dehydration and even death if therapy does not include electrolyte replacement. As many as 10^{10} virus particles per gram of stool may be released during disease.

Immunity to infection requires the presence of antibody, primarily IgA, in the lumen of the gut. Actively or passively acquired antibody (including antibody in colostrum and mother's milk) apparently lessens the severity of disease but does not consistently prevent reinfection. In the absence of antibody, inoculation of even small amounts of virus causes infection and diarrhea. Infection in infants and small children is generally symptomatic, whereas infection in adults is usually asymptomatic, possibly a result of preexisting immunity.

Epidemiology

Rotaviruses are found worldwide. Children are infected at an early age, as determined by the early acquisition of antibody (Box 62-3 and Figure 62-5). Rotaviruses are assumed to be passed from person to person by the fecal-oral route. Maximum shedding of virus occurs 2 to 5 days after initiation of diarrhea but can occur without symptoms. Virus survives well on inanimate objects, such

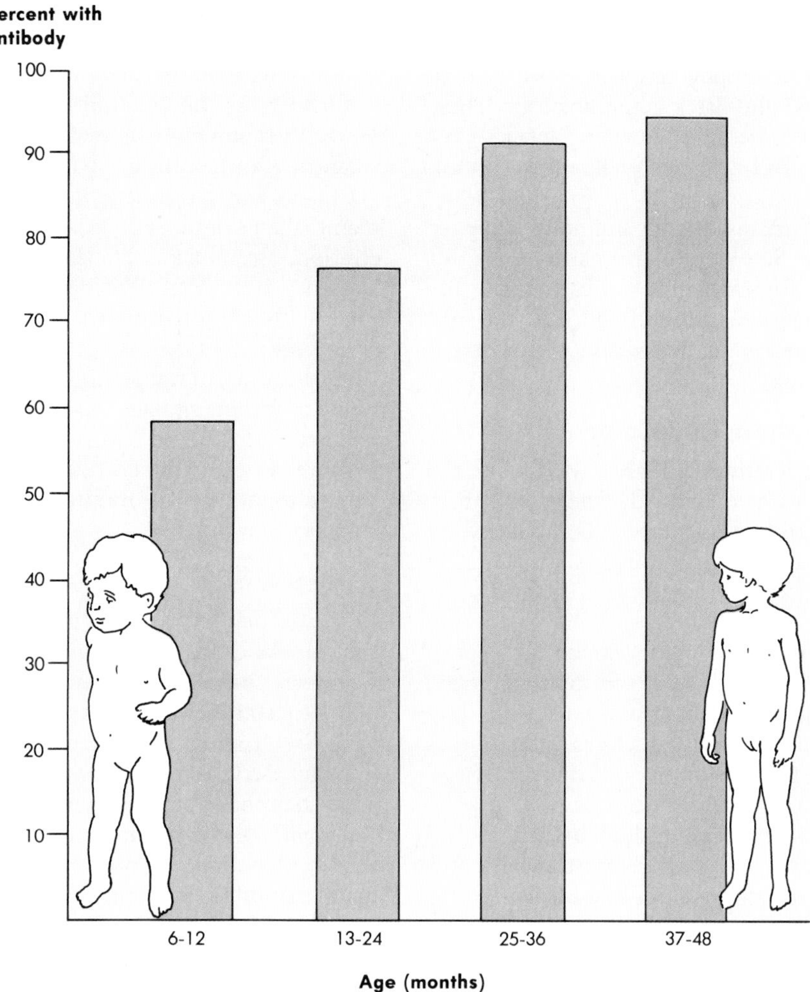

FIGURE 62-5 Prevalence of antibody to rotaviruses in children. (From Wyatt RG and Kapikian AZ: Viral gastrointestinal infections. In Feigin RD and Cherry JD, editors: *Textbook of pediatric infectious diseases*, ed 2, Philadelphia, 1987, WB Saunders.)

as hands, furniture, and toys, because it can withstand drying. Although domestic animals are known to harbor serologically related rotaviruses, they are not believed to be a common source of human infection. Outbreaks occur in preschool and day-care centers and among hospitalized infants.

Rotaviruses are one of the most common causes of serious diarrhea in young children worldwide. Most children have been infected by rotavirus by 4 years of age. In North America, outbreaks occur annually during the fall, winter, and spring. Serotype A is most common, whereas serotype B is associated with disease in older children and adults in China. More severe disease occurs in severely malnourished children. In developing countries rotavirus diarrhea is a severe life-threatening disease in infants that occurs year-round.

Clinical Syndromes

The incubation period for rotavirus diarrheal illness is estimated to be approximately 48 hours. The major clinical findings in hospitalized patients include diarrhea, vomiting, fever, and dehydration. Fecal leukocytes and blood in stool are not associated with rotavirus diarrhea. Rotavirus gastroenteritis is a self-limited disease. Recovery is generally complete and without sequelae. In rare instances severe untreated dehydration can lead to death.

The role of rotaviruses in respiratory infection is controversial. Human studies have detected virus in respiratory secretions of children with respiratory symptoms, and animal studies have documented that aerosol transmission can occur.

Laboratory Diagnosis

Clinical findings associated with rotavirus infection are not specific, making laboratory diagnosis essential. Available techniques include electron microscopy, direct antigen detection, and serodiagnosis.

Most infections are characterized by large quantities of virus in stool, making the direct detection of viral antigen the method of choice for diagnosis. Originally, the preferred method of diagnosis was the detection of viral particles in specimens by electron microscopy, but the availability of specific antibody has led to the use of enzyme immunoassay and latex agglutination. These methods are preferred because they are quick, easy, relatively inexpensive, and generally comparable to electron microscopy.

Cell culture of rotavirus is difficult and not reliable for diagnostic purposes. Serology is primarily used for research and epidemiological purposes. Because so many people have rotavirus-specific antibody, a fourfold rise in antibody titer is necessary for the diagnosis of recent infection or active disease.

Treatment, Prevention, and Control

No specific antiviral therapy is available. Morbidity and mortality in patients with rotavirus diarrhea result from dehydration and electrolyte imbalance. The purpose of supportive therapy is to replace fluids so that blood volume and electrolyte and acid-base imbalances are corrected.

Rotavirus vaccines are being developed to protect children, especially those in underdeveloped countries, from potentially fatal disease. Vaccines have been prepared from animal rotaviruses, such as the Rhesus monkey rotavirus and the Nebraska calf diarrhea virus. These vaccines share antigenic determinants with human rotaviruses, do not cause disease in humans, and afford some protection against infection. Unfortunately, they may not protect against all serotypes of rotavirus.

Acquisition of rotaviruses occurs very early in life. The ubiquitous nature of these viruses make prevention of spread and infection unlikely. Once hospitalized, however, diseased patients must be identified and isolated to limit spread of infection to other susceptible patients.

ORBIVIRUSES

The orbiviruses are a large group of viruses that infect both vertebrates and invertebrates. Disease caused by these viruses include Colorado tick fever of humans, bluetongue disease of sheep, African horse sickness, and epizootic hemorrhagic disease of deer.

Colorado tick fever, an acute disease characterized by fever, headache, and severe myalgia, was originally described in the nineteenth century and is now believed to be one of the most common tick-borne viral diseases in the United States. Although hundreds of infections occur annually, the exact number is not known because it is not a reportable disease. Other human pathogenic orbiviruses have been detected elsewhere in the world, but little is known about these viruses.

The structure and physiology of the orbiviruses is similar to other Reoviridae, with three major exceptions: (1) The outer capsid of the orbiviruses has no discernible capsomeric structure, even though the inner capsid is icosahedral; (2) The virus causes viremia, infects erythrocyte precursors, and remains in the mature red blood cells protected from the immune response; (3) The orbivirus life cycle includes both vertebrates and invertebrates (insects).

Orbiviruses contain double-stranded RNA with either 10 or 12 segments. Colorado tick fever viruses have 12 segments, and other orbiviruses have 10. Replication occurs in the cytoplasm of various cells of insect and mammalian origin. Specifics describing attachment, penetration, assembly, and release during cell lysis are not known.

Pathogenesis

Little is known of the pathogenesis of Colorado tick fever virus or other similar tick-borne viruses in humans. Colorado tick fever virus infects hematopoietic cells without severely damaging them. Viremia therefore can persist for weeks or months, even after symptomatic recovery.

Epidemiology

Colorado tick fever occurs in western and northwestern areas of the United States and western Canada where the wood tick *Dermacentor andersoni* is distributed (elevations 4000 to 10,000 feet) (Figure 62-6). Ticks acquire the virus by feeding on viremic hosts and subsequently transmit the virus in saliva when they feed on a new host. Many ticks have been shown to be infected; however, *D. andersoni* is the predominant vector and the only proven source of human disease. Natural hosts can be one of many mammals, including squirrels, chipmunks, rabbits, and deer. Exposure to ticks is the major risk factor. Human disease is reported during the spring, summer, and fall months.

Clinical Syndromes

Colorado tick fever virus generally causes mild or subclinical infection. Acute disease resembles dengue virus–like symptoms. After a 3- to 6-day incubation period, symptomatic infections start with sudden onset of fever, chills, headache, photophobia, myalgia, arthralgia, and lethargy (Figure 62-7). Characteristics of infection include a biphasic fever, conjunctivitis, and a possible lymphadenopathy, hepatosplenomegaly, and maculopapular or petechial rash. A leukopenia involving both neutrophils and lymphocytes is an important hallmark of the disease. Children occasionally have a more severe hemorrhagic disease. Colorado tick fever must be differentiated from Rocky Mountain spotted fever, a tick-borne bacterial infection characterized by rash.

Laboratory Diagnosis

Specific diagnosis can be made by direct detection of viral antigens, viral isolation, or serologic tests. Laboratory tests may be available through State Health Departments or the Centers for Disease Control. The best, most rapid method is detection of viral antigen on the surface of erythrocytes in a blood smear by immunofluorescence. Virus can be isolated from serum or plasma during the

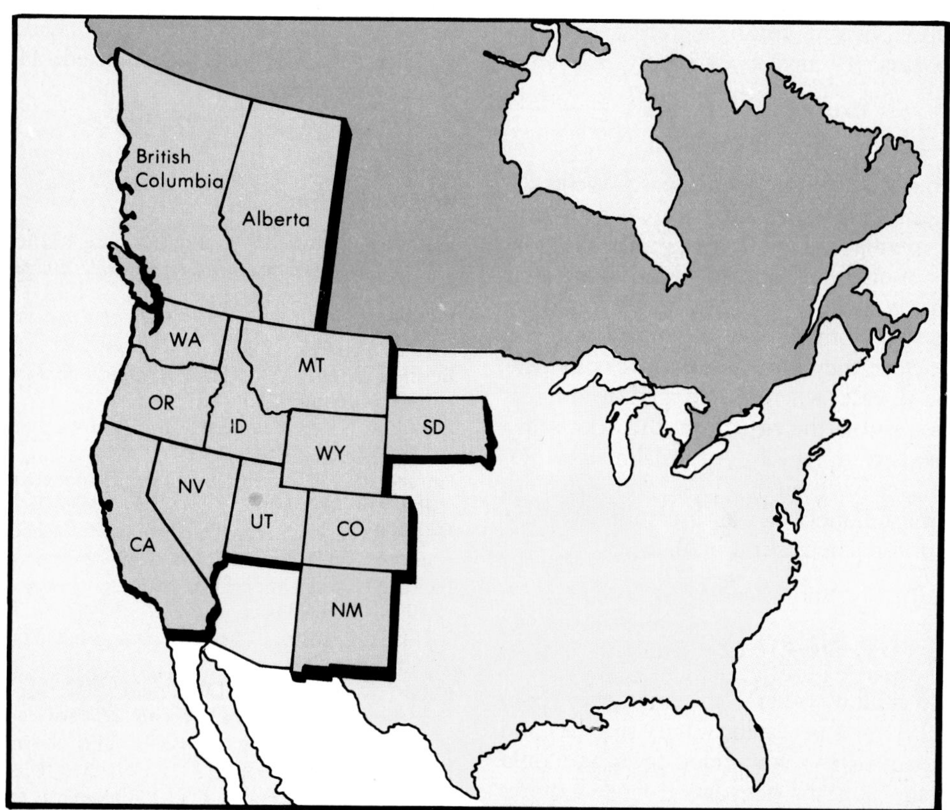

FIGURE 62-6 Geographical distribution of Colorado tick fever.

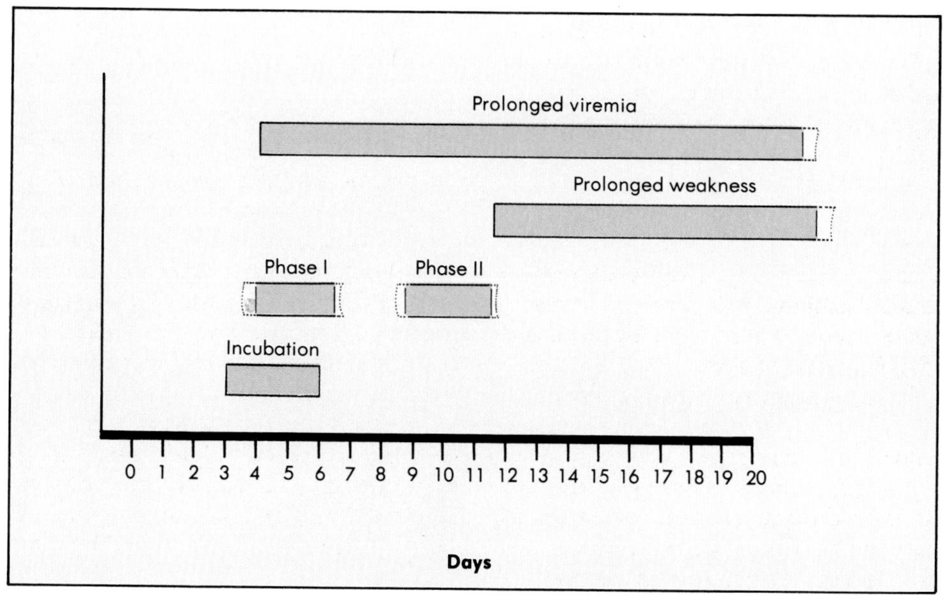

FIGURE 62-7 Time course of Colorado tick fever.

first few days of disease, before the appearance of neutralizing antibody, and later from a blood clot or washed erythrocytes. Virus can be grown in suckling mice or Vero cells.

Acute and convalescent specimens must be compared for serologic diagnosis because subclinical infections can occur and antibody may persist for a lifetime. Specific IgM is present for about 45 days after onset of illness and is also presumptive evidence of acute or very recent infection. Immunofluorescence is the best technique but complement fixation, neutralization, and enzyme immunoassy are also used to detect Colorado tick fever antibody.

Treatment, Prevention and Control

No specific treatment is available. The disease is generally self-limited, suggesting that supportive care is sufficient. As mentioned, viremia is long lasting, implying that infected patients should not donate blood soon after recovery. Prevention includes avoiding tick-infested areas, using protective clothing and tick repellents, and removing ticks before they bite. In contrast with tick-borne rickettsial disease where prolonged feeding is required for transmission, the virus from the tick's saliva can enter the bloodstream rapidly. A formalinized Colorado tick fever vaccine has been developed and evaluated, but because of the mildness of the disease it does not warrant distribution to the general public.

CASE STUDY AND QUESTIONS

A 6-month-old child was seen in the emergency room in January after 2 days of persistent watery diarrhea and vomiting accompanied by a low-grade fever and mild cough. The infant appears dehydrated and requires hospitalization. The patient attends a day-care center.

1. In addition to rotavirus, what other viral agents must be considered in the differential diagnosis of this infant? If the patient were a teenager or adult?
2. How would the diagnosis of rotavirus be confirmed?
3. How was the virus transmitted? How long is the patient contagious?
4. Who is at risk to serious disease?

Bibliography

Balows A, Hausler WJ, and Lennette EH, editors: *Laboratory diagnosis of infectious diseases: principles and practice*, New York, 1988, Springer-Verlag.

Bellamy AR and Both GW: *Molecular biology of rotaviruses*, *Adv Virol* 38:1-44, 1990.

Belshe RB, editor: *Textbook of human virology*, ed 2, St. Louis, 1991, Mosby.

Blacklow NR, Greenberg HB: Viral gastroenteritis, *N Engl J Med* 325:252-264, 1991.

Christensen ML: Human viral gastroenteritis, *Clin Microbiol Rev* 2:51-89, 1989.

Feigin RD and Cherry JD, editors: *Textbook of pediatric infectious diseases*, ed 2, Philadelphia, 1987, WB Saunders.

Fields BN and Knipe DM, editors: *Virology*, ed 2, New York, 1990, Raven Press.

Joklik WK, editor: *The Reoviridae*, New York, 1983, Plenum Publishing.

Nibert ML, Furlong DB, Fields BN: Mechanisms of viral pathogenesis. Distinct forms of reovirus and their roles during replication in cells and host, *J Clin Invest* 88:727-734, 1991.

Sharpe AH and Fields BN: Pathogenesis of viral infections: basic concepts derived from the Reovirus model, *N Engl J Med* 312:486-497, 1985.

Togaviruses and Flaviviruses

THE togaviruses and flaviviruses are enveloped, positive, single-stranded ribonucleic acid (RNA) viruses (Box 63-1). Until recently the flaviviruses were included in the togaviridae family. However, differences in size, morphology, gene sequence, and replication strategy have made it necessary to classify the flaviviruses as an independent virus family.

The togaviruses can be classified into four major groups (Table 63-1): Alphavirus, Rubivirus, Pestivirus, and Arterivirus. No known arteriviruses or pestiviruses cause disease in humans, so these are not discussed further. Rubella virus is the only member of the Rubivirus group; thus it is discussed separately because its disease presentation (German measles) and its means of spread differ from those of the alphaviruses. Alphavirus and Flavivirus are discussed together because of similarities in disease and epidemiology.

ALPHAVIRUSES AND FLAVIVIRUSES

The alphaviruses and flaviviruses are historically classified as **arboviruses** because they are usually spread by arthropod vectors. These viruses have a very broad host range, including vertebrates (e.g., mammals, birds, amphibians, reptiles) and invertebrates (e.g., mosquitos, ticks). Viruses spread by animals or with an animal reservoir are called **zoonoses**. Examples of pathogenic alphaviruses and flaviviruses are given in Table 63-2. The Hepatitis C virus was recently classified as a flavivirus based on its genome structure. It is not likely to be an arbovirus.

Structure

The alphaviruses are similar to the picornaviruses in that they have an icosahedral capsid and a plus-sense, single-strand RNA genome that resembles messenger RNA (mRNA). They differ by being slightly larger (45 to 75 nm in diameter) than picornaviruses and are surrounded by an envelope (Latin *toga*, meaning cloak). In addition, the togavirus genome encodes early and late proteins. The envelope consists of lipids obtained from the host cell membranes and glycoprotein spikes that protrude from the surface of the virion. Alphaviruses have two or three glycoproteins that associate to form a single spike. The COOH-terminus of the glycoproteins is anchored in the capsid, forcing the envelope to wrap tightly ("shrink-wrap") and take on the shape of the capsid (Figure 63-1).

The members of the alphaviruses share serologically definable, type-specific antigens. The capsid proteins of the alphaviruses are similar in structure and are the type-common antigens. The envelope glycoproteins express unique antigenic determinants that distinguish the different viruses and also antigenic determinants that are shared by a group, or "complex," of viruses.

The flaviviruses also have plus-strand RNA and an envelope. However, the virions are slightly smaller than those of the alphaviruses (37 to 50 nm in diameter), the RNA does not have a polyA sequence, and a capsid

BOX 63-1 Unique Features of Togaviruses and Flaviviruses

- Enveloped single-stranded plus RNA viruses
- Togavirus replication includes early (nonstructural) and late (structural) protein synthesis
- Togaviruses replicate in the cytoplasm and bud from the plasma membrane
- Flaviviruses replicate in the cytoplasm and bud from internal membranes

TABLE 63-1 Togaviruses and Flaviviruses

Virus group	Human pathogens
Togaviruses	
Alphavirus	Arboviruses
Rubivirus	Rubella virus
Pestivirus	None
Arterivirus	None
Flaviviruses	Arboviruses

TABLE 63-2 Alphaviruses and Flaviviruses

	Vector	Host	Distribution	Disease
ALPHAVIRUSES				
Sindbis*	*Aedes* and other mosquitos	Birds	Africa, Australia, India	Subclinical
Semliki Forest*	*Aedes* and other mosquitos	Birds	East and West Africa	Subclinical
Venezuelan equine encephalitis (VEE)	*Aedes, Culex*	Rodents, horses	North, South, and Central America	Mild systemic; severe encephalitis
Eastern equine encephalitis (EEE)	*Aedes, Culiseta*	Birds	North and South America, Caribbean	Mild systemic; encephalitis
Western equine encephalitis (WEE)	*Culex, Culiseta*	Birds	North and South America	Mild systemic; encephalitis
Chikungunya	*Aedes*	Humans, monkeys	Africa, Asia	Fever, arthralgia, arthritis
FLAVIVIRUSES				
Dengue*	*Aedes*	Humans, monkeys	Worldwide, especially tropics	Mild systemic; dengue hemorrhagic fever/shock syndrome (DHF/DSS)
Yellow fever*	*Aedes*	Humans, monkeys	Africa, South America	Hepatitis, hemorrhagic fever
Japanese encephalitis	*Culex*	Pigs, birds	Asia	Encephalitis
West Nile	*Culex*	Birds	Africa, Europe, Central Asia	Fever, encephalitis hepatitis
St. Louis encephalitis	*Culex*	Birds	North America	Encephalitis
Russian spring-summer encephalitis	*Ixodes* and *Dermacentor* ticks	Birds	Russia	Encephalitis
Powassan	*Ixodes* ticks	Small mammals	North America	Encephalitis

*Prototypical viruses.

structure is not visible within the virion. All the flaviviruses are serologically related, and antibodies to one virus may neutralize another virus.

Replication

As enveloped plus-strand RNA viruses, the general schemes for replication of the alphaviruses and flaviviruses are similar and can be discussed together (Figure 63-2). Differences will be noted in the text. The alphaviruses and flaviviruses attach to specific receptors expressed on many different cell types from many different species. The host range for these viruses includes vertebrates such as humans, monkeys, horses, birds, reptiles, and amphibians, and invertebrates such as mosquitos and ticks. However, the individual viruses have different tissue tropisms, which can account somewhat for their different disease presentations.

The virus enters the cell by receptor-mediated endocytosis (Figure 63-2, *A*). The viral envelope fuses with the membrane of the endosome on acidification of the vesicle to deliver the capsid and genome into the cytoplasm.

Once released into the cytoplasm, the alphavirus and flavivirus genomes bind to ribosomes as mRNA. Differences in the alphavirus and flavivirus genome structure dictate different translation programs.

The alphavirus genome is translated in early and late phases. The initial two thirds of the alphavirus RNA is translated into a polyprotein, which is subsequently cleaved by proteases into four nonstructural (Ns) proteins: Ns60, Ns89, Ns76, and Ns72. These proteins include an RNA-dependent RNA polymerase to transcribe the genome into a full-length 42S minus-sense RNA template and then replicate the genome to produce more 42S plus-sense mRNA. This results in a double-stranded RNA replicative intermediate.

The minus-sense RNA template is also used for transcription of the late structural genes of the virus. A 26S mRNA, corresponding to the other one third of the genome, encodes the capsid (C) and envelope (E_{1-3}) proteins. Late in the replication cycle, viral mRNA can account for as much as 90% of the mRNA in the infected

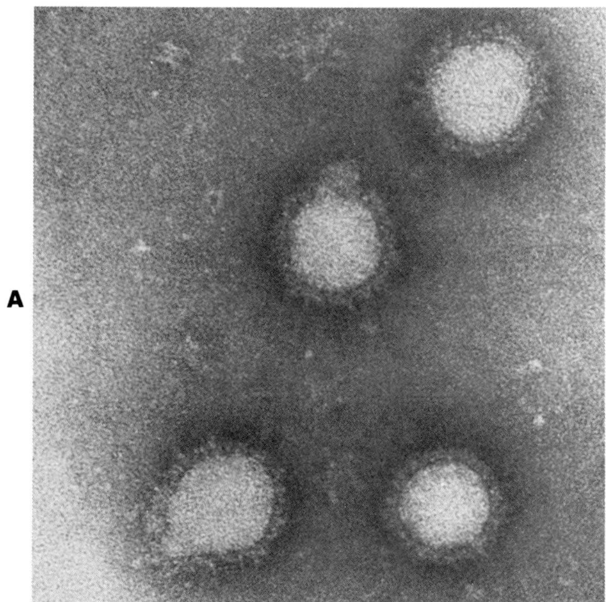

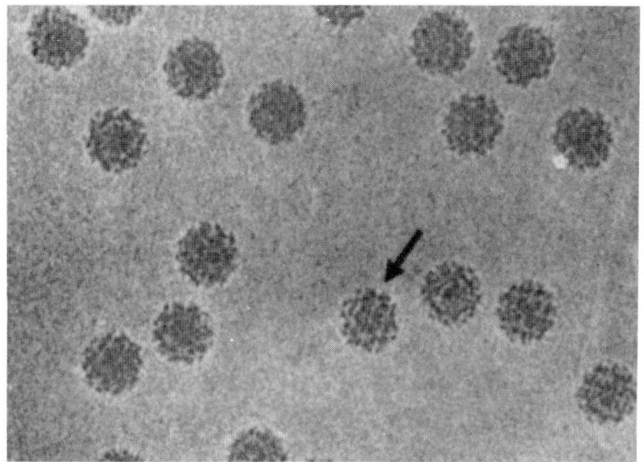

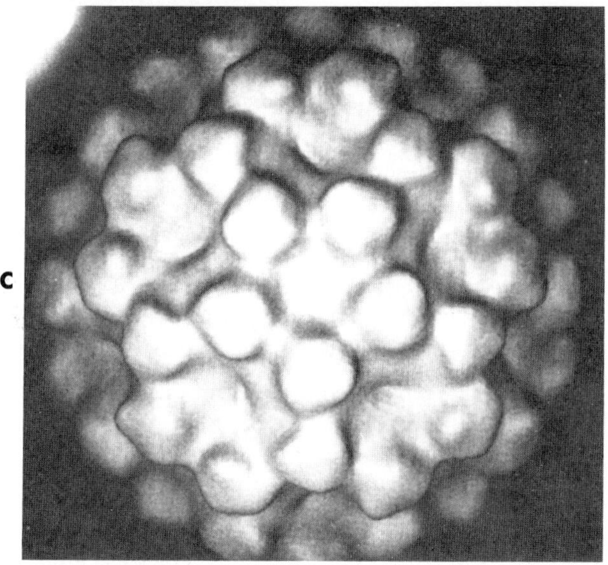

FIGURE 63-1 Alphavirus morphology. **A,** The outline of the envelope and the glycoprotein spikes of the sindbis virus are visualized by negative staining. **B,** More detail on the morphology of the virion is obtained from cryoelectron microscopy. **C,** Surface representation of the sindbis virus obtained by image processing of the cryoelectron micrographs indicates that the envelope is held tightly to and conforms to the shape and symmetry of the capsid. (From Fuller SD: *Cell* 48:923, 1987.)

cell. The abundance of late mRNAs allows production of a large amount of structural proteins required for packaging the virus.

The structural proteins are produced by protease cleavage of the late polyprotein produced from the 26S mRNA. The C protein is translated first and cleaved from the polyprotein (Figure 63-2, *B*). A signal sequence is then made that associates the nascent polypeptide with the endoplasmic reticulum. The envelope glycoproteins are then translated, glycosylated, and then cleaved from the remaining portion of the polyprotein to produce the E_1, E_2, and E_3 glycoprotein spikes. The E_3 remains associated with the Semliki Forest virus spikes but is released from other alphavirus glycoprotein spikes. The glycoproteins are processed by the normal cellular machinery in the endoplasmic reticulum and Golgi apparatus and are also acetylated and acylated with long-chain fatty acids (Figure 63-2, *C*). Alphavirus glycoproteins are transferred efficiently to the plasma membrane.

The C proteins associate with the genomic RNA soon after their synthesis and, for alphaviruses, form an

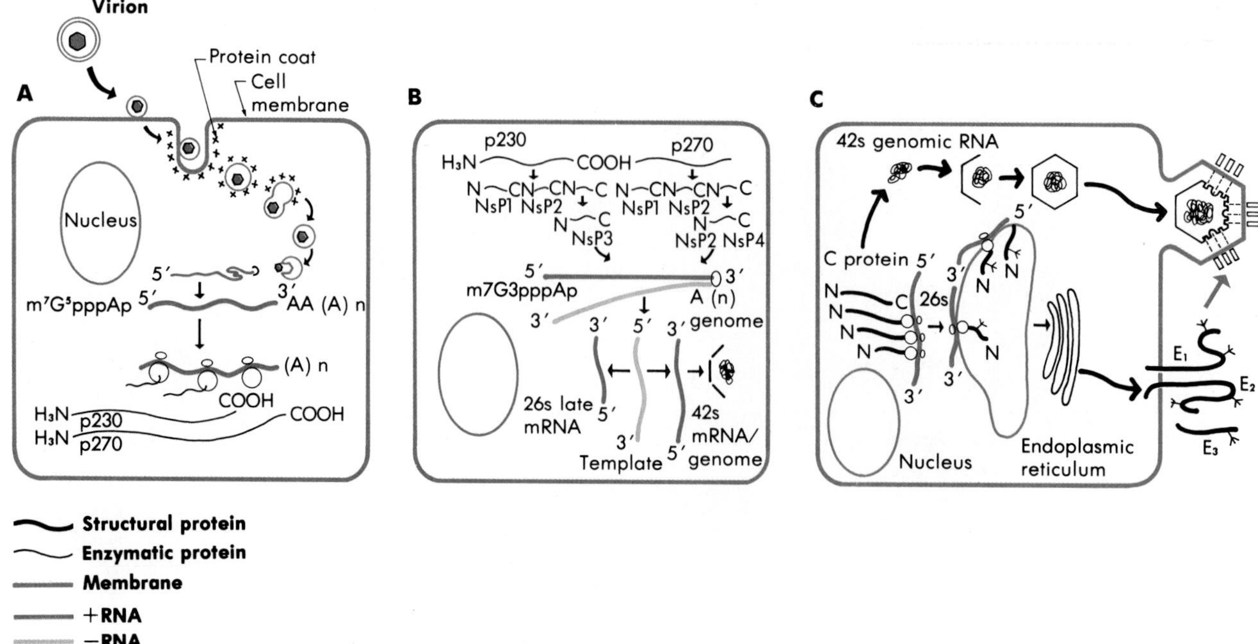

FIGURE 63-2 Replication of a togavirus: Semliki Forest virus. **A,** Semliki Forest virus binds to cell receptors, is shuttled into a coated pit, and is internalized in a coated vesicle. The virus is transferred to an endosome, and the viral envelope fuses with the endosomal membrane on acidification to release the nucleocapsid into the cytoplasm. Ribosomes bind to the plus-sense RNA genome, and the p230 or p270 (read-through) early polyproteins are made. **B,** The polyproteins are cleaved to produce nonstructural proteins 1 to 4 (NsP_{1-4}), which include a polymerase to transcribe the genome into a minus-sense RNA template. The template is used to produce a full-length 42S plus-sense mRNA genome and a late 26S mRNA. **C,** The *C* (capsid) protein is translated first, exposing a protease cleavage site and then a signal peptide for association with the endoplasmic reticulum. The E glycoproteins are then synthesized, glycosylated, processed in the Golgi apparatus, and transferred to the plasma membrane. The capsid proteins assemble on the 42S genomic RNA and then associate with regions of cytoplasmic and plasma membranes containing the E_{1-3} spike proteins. Budding from the plasma membrane releases the virus.

icosahedral capsid. Capsid structures for the flaviviruses may exist but have not been seen. Once completed, the capsid associates with portions of the membrane expressing the viral glycoproteins. The alphavirus capsid has binding sites for the C-terminus of the E glycoprotein spike, which pulls the envelope tightly around itself similar to a formfitting wrapper (see Figures 63-1 and 63-2, *C*). Alphaviruses are released on budding from the plasma membrane.

Attachment and penetration of the flaviviruses occurs as described for the alphaviruses, but the flaviviruses can also attach to the Fc receptors on macrophages, monocytes, and other cells when they are coated with antibody. The antibody actually enhances the infectivity of these viruses by providing new receptors for the virus and by promoting viral uptake into these target cells.

The major differences between alphaviruses and flaviviruses are in the organization of their genomes and their mechanisms of protein synthesis. In contrast to the alphaviruses, the entire flavivirus genome is translated into a single polyprotein (Figure 63-3). As a result, no temporal distinction exists in the translation of the different viral proteins. The polyprotein produced from the yellow fever genome contains 4 to 8 nonstructural proteins plus the capsid and envelope structural proteins. Unlike the alphaviruses, the structural genes are at the 5′end of the genome. As a result, the portions of the polyprotein containing the structural (not the catalytic) proteins are synthesized first and at the highest efficiency. This strategy may allow production of more structural proteins, but it decreases the efficiency of nonstructural protein synthesis and the initiation of virus replication. This may contribute to the long latent period that precedes detection of flavivirus replication.

Another distinction is that budding of flaviviruses occurs predominantly from intracellular membranes into the cytoplasm or into vesicles rather than at the cell surface, as for alphaviruses. The virus can be released by exocytosis, but the most efficient means of virus release requires lysis of the cell.

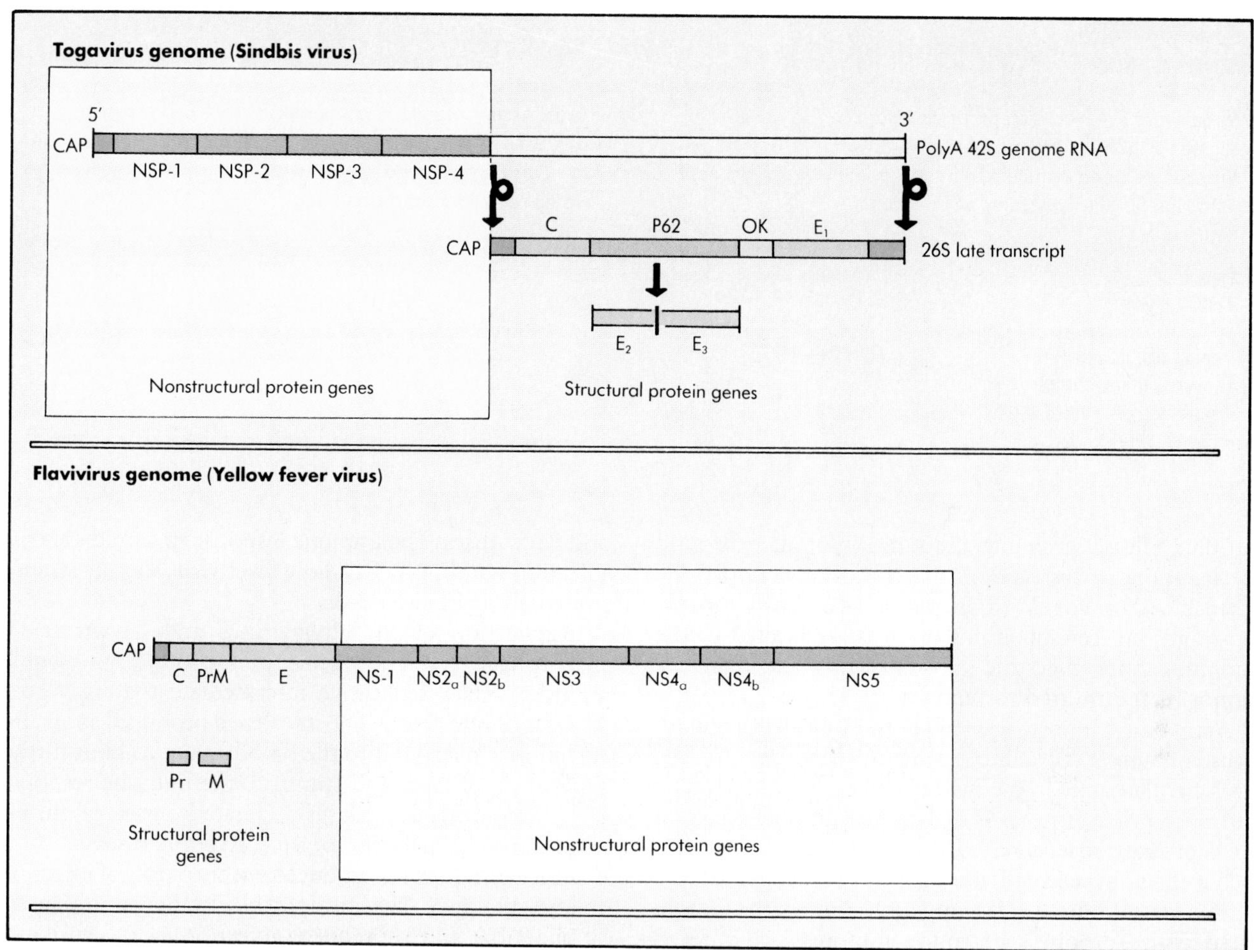

FIGURE 63-3 Comparison of the the togavirus (alphavirus) and flavivirus genomes. Alphavirus: The enzymatic activities are translated from the 5′end of the input genome, promoting their early rapid translation. The structural proteins are translated later from a smaller mRNA transcribed from the genome template. Flavivirus: The genes for the structural proteins of the flaviviruses are at the 5′ end of the genome/mRNA, and only one species of polyprotein is made, which represents the entire genome. (Redrawn from Hahn CS, Galler R, Rice CM: Flavivirus genome organization, expression, and replication, *Ann Rev Microbiol* 44:649-688, 1990.)

Pathogenesis and Immunity

The pathogenic characteristics of alphaviruses and flaviviruses are determined by their route of entry into the host, the concentration of virus within the individual, specific tissue tropisms of the individual virus type and the outcome of the infection. Since these viruses are acquired from the bite of an arthropod such as a mosquito, the course of infection in both the vertebrate host and the invertebrate vector are important to understanding the disease.

These viruses can cause lytic or persistent infections of both vertebrate and invertebrate hosts (Box 63-2). Infections of invertebrates are usually persistent, with continued virus production. Properties of both the virus and the cell determine whether infection will kill the cell.

The death of the cell results from a combination of virus-induced insults. The large amount of viral RNA produced on replication and transcription of the genome blocks cellular mRNA binding to ribosomes. In addition, an increase in permeability of the target cell membrane resulting from the virus infection produces alterations in sodium and potassium ion concentrations. These changes can alter enzyme activities and favors the translation of viral mRNA over cellular mRNA. The displacement of cellular mRNA from the protein synthesis machinery prevents rebuilding and maintenance of the cell and is a major cause for the death of the virus-infected cell. Some alphaviruses, such as western equine encephalitis (WEE) virus, make a nucleotide triphosphatase that degrades deoxyribonucleotides, depleting even the substrate pool for DNA production.

Female mosquitos acquire the alphaviruses and flaviviruses by taking a blood meal from a viremic vertebrate host. The virus infects the epithelial cells of the midgut of the mosquito, spreads through the basal lamina of the midgut to the circulation, and then infects the salivary glands. The virus sets up a persistent infection and replicates to high titers in these cells. The salivary glands

BOX 63-2 Disease Mechanisms of Togaviruses and Flaviviruses

Viruses are cytolytic, except for rubella
Viruses establish systemic infection and viremia
Viruses are good inducers of interferon, which can account for the flu-like symptoms of infection
Viruses, except rubella and hepatitis C, are arboviruses
Flaviviruses infect cells of the monocyte-macrophage lineage
Non-neutralizing antibody can enhance flavivirus infection via Fc receptors on macrophage

	Flu-like syndrome	Encephalitis	Hepatitis	Hemorrhage	Shock
Dengue	+		+	+	+
Yellow fever	+		+	+	+
St. Louis encephalitis	+	+			
Venezuelan encephalitis	+	+			
Western equine encephalitis	+	+			
Eastern equine encephalitis	+	+			
Japanese encephalitis	+	+			

can then release virus into the saliva. Not all arthropod species support this type of infection. For example, the normal vector for WEE virus is the *Culex tarsalis* mosquito, but certain strains of virus are limited to the midgut, cannot infect the salivary glands, and therefore cannot be transmitted to humans.

After biting a host, the female mosquito regurgitates virus-containing saliva into the victim's bloodstream. The virus circulates free in the plasma and comes into contact with susceptible target cells such as the endothelial cells of the capillaries, macrophages, monocytes, and the reticuloendothelial system (Figure 63-4).

The initial viremia, following replication of the virus in these tissues, produces systemic symptoms such as fever, chills, headaches, backaches, and flu-like symptoms within 3 to 7 days of infection. Some of these symptoms can be attributed to the interferon produced following infection of these target cells. This is considered a mild systemic disease, and most virus infections do not progress beyond this point.

Following replication in cells of the reticuloendothelial system, a secondary viremia may result. This viremia can produce sufficient virus to infect target organs such as the brain, liver, skin, and vasculature, depending on the tissue tropism of the virus (Figure 63-5). Access to the brain is provided by infection of the endothelial cells lining the small vessels of the brain or the choroid plexus.

The primary target cells of the flaviviruses are derived from the monocyte/macrophage lineage. Although these cells are found throughout the body and may have different characteristics, they express Fc receptors for antibody and release lymphokines upon challenge. Flavivirus infection is enhanced 200-fold to a thousandfold by non-neutralizing antiviral antibody that promotes binding of the virus to the Fc receptors and uptake into the cell.

Immune Response

Both humoral and cellular immunity are elicited and are important to the control of primary infection and prevention from future infections with the alphaviruses and flaviviruses. The immune response to a mild systemic infection with the 17D yellow fever virus vaccine strain is presented in Figure 63-6.

Replication of the alphaviruses and flaviviruses in macrophage and endothelial cells produces a double-stranded RNA replicative intermediate that is a good inducer of interferon. The interferon produced soon after infection is released into the bloodstream to limit further replication of virus and stimulate the immune response. The interferon also causes the rapid onset of flu-like symptoms characteristic of mild systemic disease.

Circulating IgM is produced within 6 days of infection, followed by IgG. The antibody blocks the viremic spread of the virus and subsequent infection of other tissues. Immunity to one flavivirus can protect against other flaviviruses by recognition of the type-common antigens expressed on all members of the viral family. One example of this may be occurring in the Far East, where Japanese encephalitis but not yellow fever virus is endemic despite the presence of the *Aedes aegypti* mosquito vector for yellow fever.

Cell-mediated immunity is also important in control of the primary infection. Natural killer cells, T cells, and macrophages are activated by interferon and can respond to the cell surface antigens displayed on the infected cells.

Immunity to these viruses is a double-edged sword. Inflammation resulting from the cell-mediated immune response can destroy tissue and significantly contribute to the pathogenesis of encephalitis. Prior immunity can promote hypersensitivity reactions such as delayed-type hypersensitivity, formation of immune complexes with virions and viral antigens, and activation of complement. This can weaken the vasculature and cause it to rupture, leading to hemorrhagic symptoms.

A non-neutralizing antibody can enhance uptake of the flaviviruses into macrophages and other cells that express Fc receptors. Such an antibody can be generated to a related strain of virus in which the neutralizing epitope is not expressed or is different. The consequences of such a partial immunity can be devastating. For example, prior infection by one strain of dengue virus will predispose an

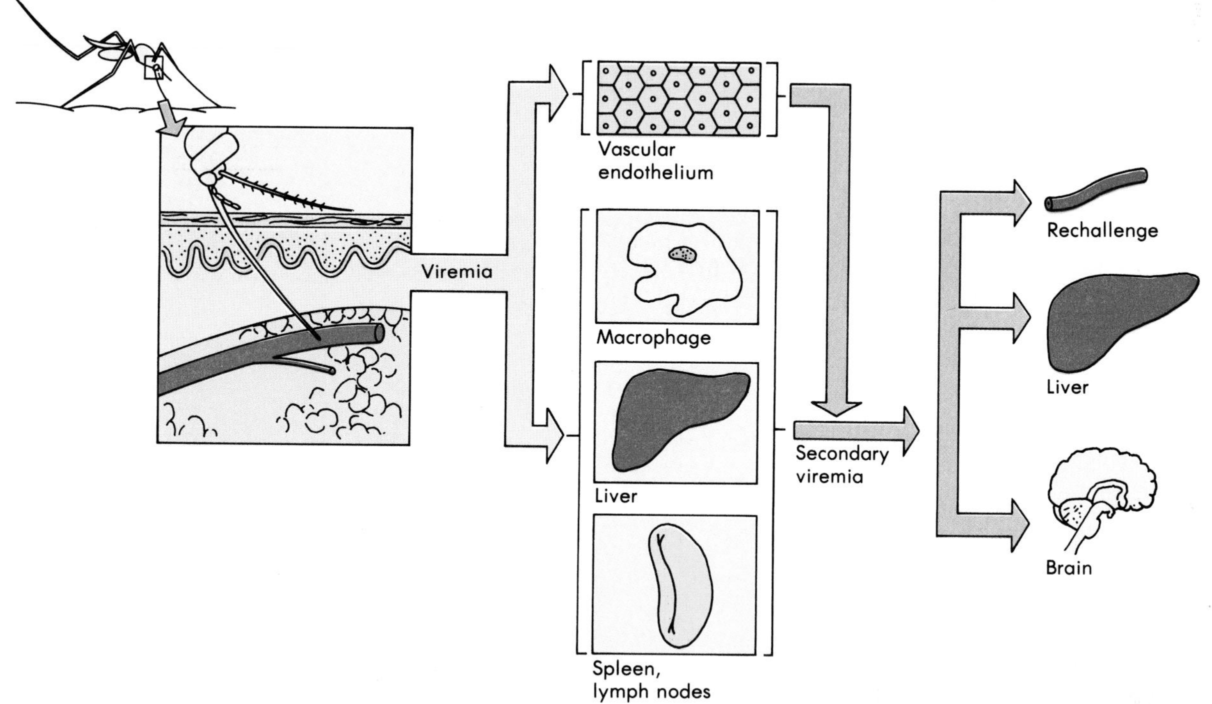

FIGURE 63-4 Spread of alphavirus and flavivirus infection within the host. The female mosquito regurgitates virus into a capillary after taking a blood meal. The virus infects the endothelial cells lining the vasculature and is taken up and replicates in cells of the reticuloendothelial system (*RES*). A secondary viremia can result to allow more extensive infection of the vasculature, the liver, other tissues, and the brain (encephalitis viruses).

individual to dengue hemorrhagic fever when infected by another strain of dengue. The weakening and rupture of the vasculature is believed to result from activation of complement and other hypersensitivity reactions. In 1981 an epidemic of dengue-2 virus in Cuba infected a population previously exposed to dengue-1 (between 1977 and 1980). More than 100,000 cases of dengue hemorrhagic fever/dengue shock syndrome (DHF/DSS) resulted, with 168 deaths.

Epidemiology

Alphaviruses and flaviviruses are prototypical arboviruses (*ar*thropod-*bo*rne viruses) (Box 63-3). To be an arbovirus, the virus must be able to (1) infect both vertebrates and invertebrates, (2) initiate a sufficient viremia in a vertebrate host for a sufficient time to allow acquisition by the invertebrate vector, and (3) initiate a persistent productive infection of the salivary gland of the invertebrate to provide virus for infection of other host animals. If the virus is not in the blood, the mosquito cannot pick it up. A full cycle of infection occurs when the virus is transmitted by the arthropod vector and amplified in a susceptible, immunologically naive host (**reservoir**) to allow reinfection of other arthropods (Figure 63-7). Table 63-2 lists vectors, natural hosts, and geographical distribution for representative alphaviruses and flaviviruses.

Humans are usually "dead-end" hosts that cannot spread the virus back to the vector because a persistent viremia is not maintained. Many more humans are infected than show significant symptoms. Incidence of arbovirus disease is sporadic. However, hundreds to thousands of cases of St. Louis encephalitis virus are noted per year in the United States.

These viruses are usually restricted to the ecological niche of a specific arthropod vector and its vertebrate host. The most common vector is the mosquito, but some arboviruses are also spread by ticks and sandflies. Even in a tropical region overrun with mosquitos, the spread of these viruses is still restricted to a specific genus of mosquitos. Not all arthropods can act as good vectors for each virus. For example, *Culex quinquefasciatus* is resistant to infection by WEE virus (alphavirus) but is an excellent vector for St. Louis encephalitis virus (flavivirus). As with mosquito-borne viruses, the life cycle of the tick dictates the pattern of spread of Russian spring-summer encephalitis virus and other tick-borne viruses (see Figure 63-7).

Birds and small mammals are the usual reservoir hosts for the alphaviruses and flaviviruses, but reptiles and amphibians can also act as hosts. A large population of viremic animals can develop in these species to continue the infection cycle of the virus.

During the summer months the arboviruses are cycled between a host (bird) and an arthropod (e.g., mosquito).

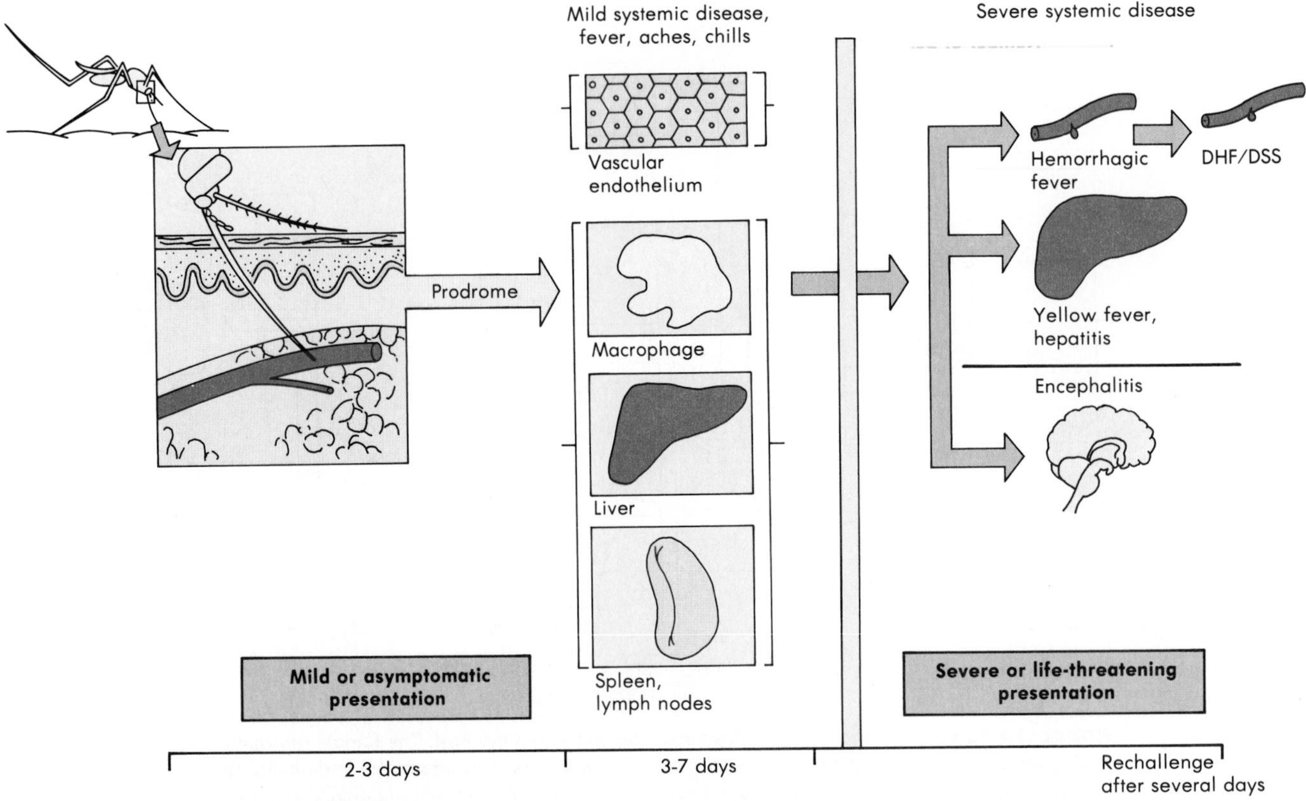

FIGURE 63-5 Disease syndromes of the alphaviruses and flaviviruses. Following a short prodrome period, a mild systemic disease can result. Most infections are limited to this extent. If sufficient virus is produced during the secondary viremia to escape immune protection and reach critical target tissue, severe systemic disease or encephalitis may result. For dengue virus, rechallenge with another strain can result in severe hemorrhagic disease (dengue hemorrhagic fever, DHF), which can cause shock (dengue shock syndrome, DSS) because of the loss of fluids from the vasculature.

This maintains and increases the amount of virus in the environment. In the winter neither the normal host nor the vector remain to maintain the virus. The virus may persist in arthropod larvae or eggs or in reptiles or amphibians that remain in the locale, or it may migrate with the birds and then return during the summer.

Most of the vectors relevant to the alphaviruses and flaviviruses are mosquitos, which are usually found in tropical forests or swamps. When humans travel into these environments, they risk being bitten by virus-bearing mosquitos. For example, as many as 50% of the Indians living in the Everglades have antibodies to Venezuelan equine encephalitis (VEE) virus. Pools of standing water, drainage ditches, and sumps in cities can also provide breeding grounds for mosquitos, such as *Aedes aegypti*, the vector for yellow fever and chikungunya. In endemic regions the risk for arbovirus infection increases during the rainy season.

Humans can be reservoir hosts for yellow fever, dengue, and chikungunya viruses (see Figure 63-7). These viruses are maintained by *Aedes* mosquitos in a **sylvatic** or **jungle cycle**, in which monkeys are the natural host, and also in an **urban cycle**, in which humans are the host. *A. aegypti* is a vector for each of these viruses and is a household mosquito. It breeds in pools of water, open sewers, and other accumulations of water in cities. St. Louis encephalitis virus can also establish an urban cycle of spread using its vector, *Culex* mosquitos, which prefer stagnant water such as sewage. Large numbers of inapparent infections in high-density populations provide sufficient viremic human hosts for continued spread of these viruses.

Clinical Syndromes

Infection by the alphaviruses usually causes a low-grade disease characterized by flu-like symptoms (chills, fever, rash, aches) that correlate with systemic infection during the initial viremia. Eastern equine encephalitis (EEE) virus, WEE virus, and VEE virus infection can progress to encephalitis (as the name implies) in humans and horses, with EEE causing the most severe disease. These viruses are usually more of a problem to livestock than to humans. Other alphaviruses such as sindbis and chikungunya generally cause only systemic disease.

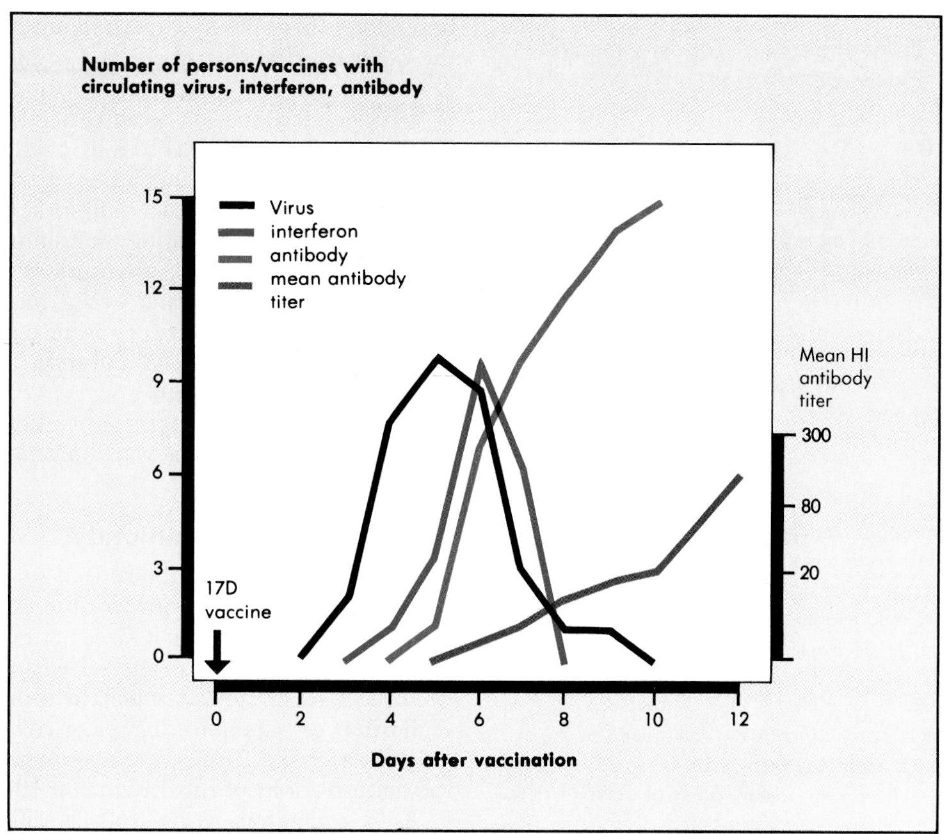

FIGURE 63-6 Immune response during mild systemic disease following vaccination with the 17D yellow fever vaccine. The number of individuals with circulating virus and interferon and their antibody titers (as measured by hemagglutination inhibition [HI]) following infection with the vaccine was determined for 15 volunteers. (Redrawn from Wheelock EF and Sibley WA: *N Engl J Med* 273:194, 1965.)

Most infections with flaviviruses are relatively benign, although encephalitic or hemorrhagic disease can occur. The encephalitis viruses include St. Louis, Japanese, Murray Valley, and Russian spring-summer. West Nile, dengue, and other viruses usually are limited to a mild systemic disease, possibly with a hemorrhagic rash. On rechallenge with a related strain, dengue can also cause severe hemorrhagic disease and shock (DHF/DSS). The hemorrhagic/shock symptoms are attributed to rupture of the vasculature, internal bleeding, and loss of plasma.

Yellow fever infections are characterized by severe systemic disease, with degeneration of the liver, kidney, and heart, and hemorrhage of blood vessels. Liver involvement leads to the jaundice from which the disease obtains its name, but massive gastrointestinal hemorrhages ("black vomit") may also occur. The mortality following yellow fever is as high as 50% during epidemics.

Laboratory Diagnosis

The alphaviruses and flaviviruses can be grown in both vertebrate and mosquito cell lines, but most are difficult to isolate. Infection can be detected by cytopathology, immunofluorescence, or by hemadsorption of avian erythrocytes. After isolation, the viruses can be distinguished by RNA "fingerprints" of the genomic RNA. Monoclonal antibodies to the individual viruses have become useful in distinguishing the individual species and strains of viruses.

A variety of serologic methods can be used to diagnose infections, including hemagglutination inhibition, ELISA, and latex agglutination. A fourfold increase in titer between acute and convalescent sera is used to indicate a recent infection. The serologic cross-reactivity between viruses in a group or complex limits identification of the actual viral species in many cases.

Treatment, Prevention, and Control

No treatments exist for arbovirus diseases other than supportive care.

The easiest means to prevent the spread of any arbovirus is elimination of its vector and breeding grounds. Following the discovery by Walter Reed and colleagues in 1900 that yellow fever was spread by *A. aegypti*, the number of cases was reduced from 1400 to 0 within 2 years by controlling the mosquito population. Avoidance of the breeding grounds of a mosquito vector is also good prevention.

Vaccination is one of the best means of protection. A

BOX 63-3 Epidemiology of Togaviruses and Flavivirus Infections

DISEASE/VIRAL FACTORS

Enveloped virus must stay wet and can be inactivated by drying, soap, and detergents
Can infect mammals, birds, reptiles, and insects
Rubella infects man and can be asymptomatic

TRANSMISSION

Rubella: respiratory route
Other togaviruses and flaviviruses: specific arthropods characteristic of each virus

WHO IS AT RISK?

Arboviruses: People who enter the ecological niche of the arthropod: usually flu-like symptoms.
fever and chills ± encephalitis or hemorrhagic fever or arthritis
Rubella: children: mild exanthematous disease
neonates (< 20 weeks): congenital defects

GEOGRAPHY/SEASON

Endemic regions for each arbovirus is determined by the habitat of the mosquito or other vector
Aedes: Dengue, Yellow fever: urban, pools of water
Culex: St. Louis encephalitis: forest/urban
Disease more common in summer
Rubella: worldwide

MODES OF CONTROL

Eliminate mosquito breeding sites and mosquitos
Live attenuated vaccine for Yellow fever virus, Japanese encephalitis virus, and rubella

live vaccine is available against yellow fever and Japanese encephalitis viruses and killed vaccines against EEE, WEE, and Russian spring-summer encephalitis viruses. These vaccines are for individuals working with the virus or at risk for contact. A live vaccine against VEE virus is available but only for use in domestic animals. A vaccine against dengue virus has not been developed because of the potential risk of immune enhancement of disease with subsequent challenge.

The yellow fever vaccine is prepared from the 17D strain isolated from a patient in 1927 and grown for long periods in monkeys, mosquitos, embryonic tissue culture, and embryonated eggs. The vaccine is administered intradermally and elicits lifelong immunity to yellow fever and possibly other cross-reacting flaviviruses (see Figure 63-6).

RUBELLA VIRUS

Rubella virus shares the structural properties and mode of replication with the other togaviruses discussed earlier, but it differs in its mode of spread and acquisition. Unlike the other togaviruses, rubella is a respiratory virus and does not cause readily detectable cytopathology.

Rubella infection usually causes a mild exanthematous childhood disease but has serious consequences for the neonate. Rubella, meaning "little red" in Latin, was first distinguished from measles and other exanthems by German physicians, providing the common name for the disease, **German measles**. An astute Australian ophthalmologist, Norman McAlister Gregg, recognized in 1941 that maternal rubella infection was the cause of congenital cataracts. Maternal rubella infection has since been correlated with several other severe congenital defects. This prompted the development of a unique program to vaccinate children to prevent infection of pregnant women and neonates.

Pathogenesis and Immunity

Rubella virus has more subtle effects on the cell than the alphaviruses. Lytic infections are observed only in certain cell lines, such as Vero or RK13, but even in these cells the cytopathic effect is very limited. Changes in the cell do occur, and replication of rubella will interfere with the replication of superinfecting picornaviruses. Heterologous interference with picornavirus replication allowed the first isolations of rubella virus in 1962.

As a respiratory virus, rubella differs from other togaviruses in the means of spread within the body, the prodrome period, the time course and symptoms of the disease, and the protective immune response (Figure 63-8). The virus first infects the upper respiratory tract and then spreads to local lymph nodes, which coincides with a period of lymphadenopathy. This is followed by establishment of viremia, which spreads the virus throughout the body. Infection of other tissues and the characteristic mild rash result. The prodrome period is approximately 2 weeks (Figure 63-9). The individual can shed virus in respiratory droplets during the prodrome period and for as long as 2 weeks after the onset of the rash.

Immune Response

The immune response generated against rubella infection is different from the response to alphaviruses and flaviviruses. As a respiratory virus, rubella penetrates the natural defenses of the nasopharynx and lung. Antibody generated soon after initiation of the viremia blocks viremic spread of the virus. Virus replication in the tissues can continue, however, until it can be cleared by cell-mediated immunity or limited by interferon. Only one serotype of rubella exists, and natural infection produces lifelong protective immunity. Immune complexes most likely cause the rash and arthralgia associated with rubella infection.

Unlike the alphaviruses and flaviviruses, secretory IgA in the respiratory tract plays an extremely important role in protection against a second challenge with rubella. Serum antibody limits the viremic spread and promotes

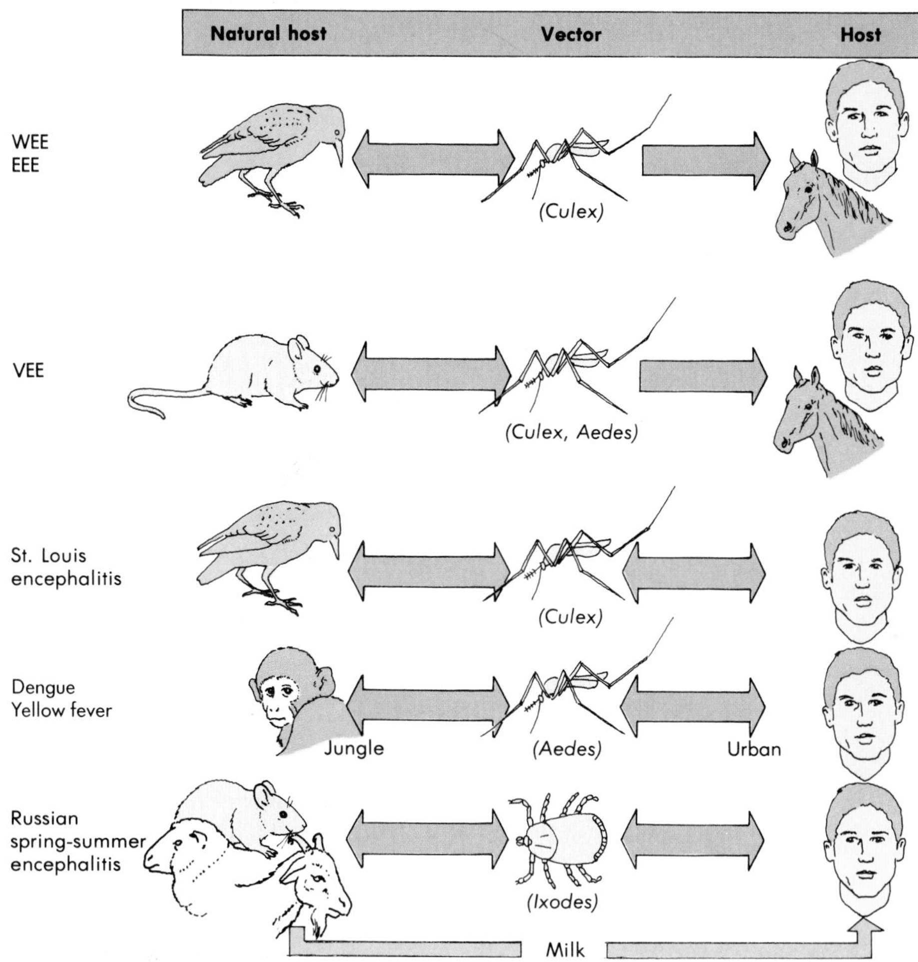

FIGURE 63-7 Patterns of alphavirus and flavivirus transmission. The cycle of arbovirus transmission maintains and amplifies the virus in the environment. Host-vector relationships that can provide this cycle are indicated by the double arrow. "Dead-end" infections with no transmission of the virus back to the vector are indicated by the single arrow. For St. Louis encephalitis, yellow fever, and dengue virus, humans are not dead-end hosts and support an urban cycle. The Russian spring-summer encephalitis virus can be transmitted to humans by a tick bite and in milk from infected goats.

elimination of the virus on reinfection. This action prevents infection of other tissues and the onset of disease. Most importantly, serum antibody in a pregnant woman prevents the spread of the virus to the fetus.

Congenital Infection

Rubella infection in a pregnant woman can result in serious congenital abnormalities. If the mother does not have antibody, the virus can replicate in the placenta and spread to the fetal blood supply and throughout the fetus. Rubella can replicate in most tissues of the fetus. The virus may not be cytolytic, but the normal growth, mitosis, and chromosomal structure can be altered by the infection. This can lead to improper development, small size of the infected baby, and the teratogenic effects associated with congenital rubella infection. The nature of the disorder is determined by the affected tissue and the stage of development that was disrupted. The virus may persist in tissues, such as the lens of the eye, for as long as 3 to 4 years and may be shed for up to a year after birth. The presence of the virus during the development of the baby's immune response may even have a tolerative effect on the system, preventing effective clearance following birth. Immune complexes may also form in the neonate or the infant to produce further clinical abnormalities.

Epidemiology

Humans are the only host for rubella (Box 63-3). The virus is spread by respiratory secretions and is generally acquired in childhood. The virus is less communicable than measles or varicella, but contagion is promoted in crowded conditions such as day-care centers.

Approximately 20% of women of childbearing age escape infection during childhood and are susceptible to infection unless previously vaccinated. Programs to

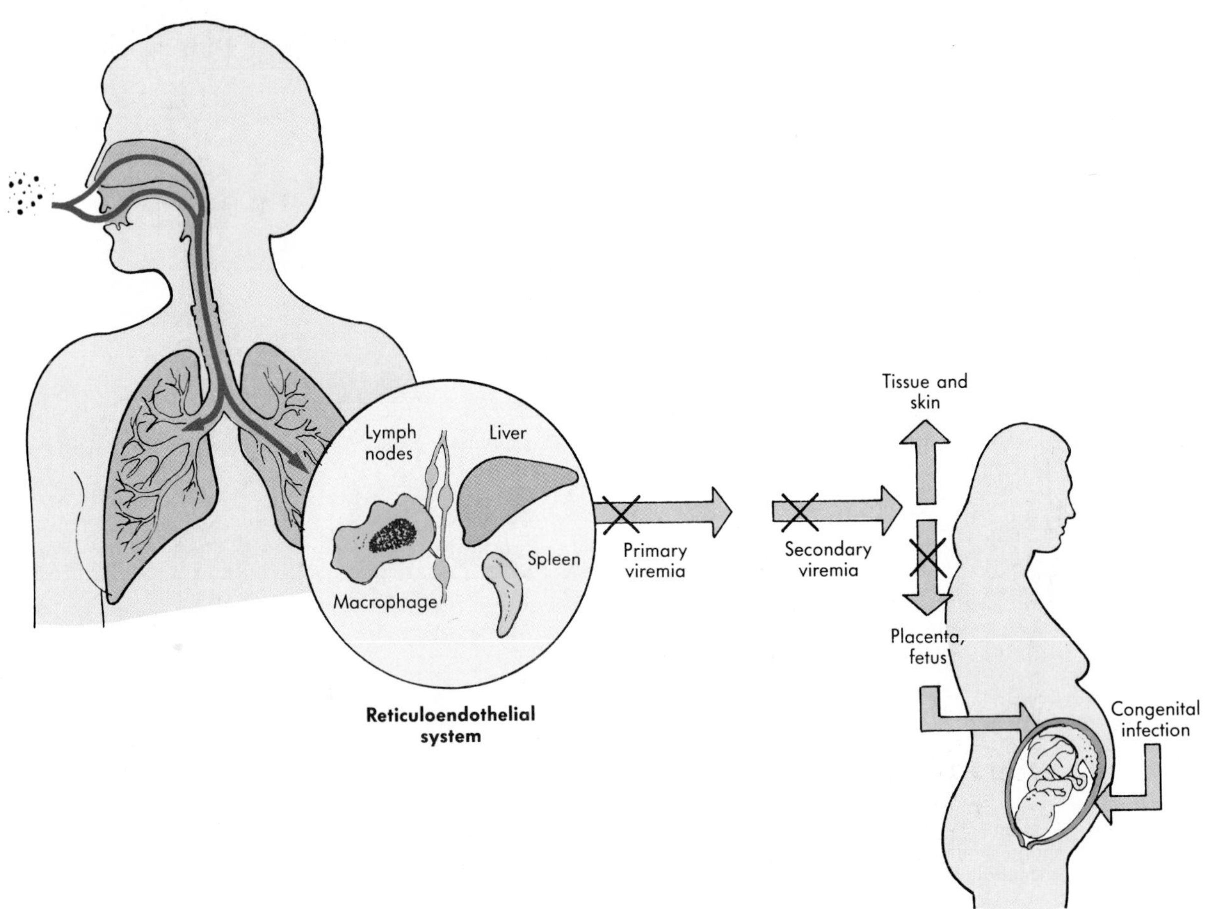

FIGURE 63-8 Spread of rubella virus within the host. Rubella enters and infects the nasopharynx and lung, then spreads to the lymph nodes and reticuloendothelial system. The resulting viremia spreads the virus to other tissues and the skin. Circulating antibody can block transfer of virus at the indicated points (denoted by *X*). In an immunologically deficient pregnant woman the virus can infect the placenta and spread to the fetus.

ensure that expectant mothers have antibodies to rubella are in effect in many U.S. states.

Before the development and use of the rubella vaccine, cases of rubella in school children would be reported every spring, and major epidemics of rubella occurred at regular 6- to 9-year intervals. The severity of the 1964 to 1965 epidemic in the United States is indicated in Table 63-3. The rate of congenital rubella in such cities as Philadelphia was as high as 1% of all pregnancies during this epidemic. Since the development of the vaccine, the incidence of rubella and congenital rubella is now less than 1 and 0.1 per 100,000 pregnancies, respectively.

Clinical Syndromes

Rubella infection is usually not cytolytic, and the disease is normally benign in children. The symptoms in children are a 3-day rash and swollen glands (Figure 63-9 and 63-10). Infection of adults can be more severe, leading to outcomes such as arthralgia, arthritis, and (rarely) thrombocytopenia, and a postinfectious encephalitis similar to postinfectious measles encephalitis. Immunopathology, resulting from cell-mediated immunity and hypersensitivity reactions, is a major cause of the more severe adult forms of rubella.

Congenital disease is the most serious outcome of rubella infection. The fetus is at major risk until the twentieth week of pregnancy. Maternal immunity to the virus resulting from prior exposure or vaccination prevents spread of the virus to the fetus. The most common manifestations of congenital rubella infection include cataracts, mental retardation, and deafness (Tables 63-3 and Box 63-4). Mortality in utero and within the first year of birth is high for these babies.

Laboratory Diagnosis

Isolation of rubella virus is difficult and rarely done. The diagnosis is usually confirmed by the presence of anti-rubella–specific IgM. A fourfold increase in specific IgG antibody titer between acute and convalescent sera is also used to indicate a recent infection. Antibodies to rubella are assayed early in pregnancy to determine the immune status of the woman. This test is required in many states.

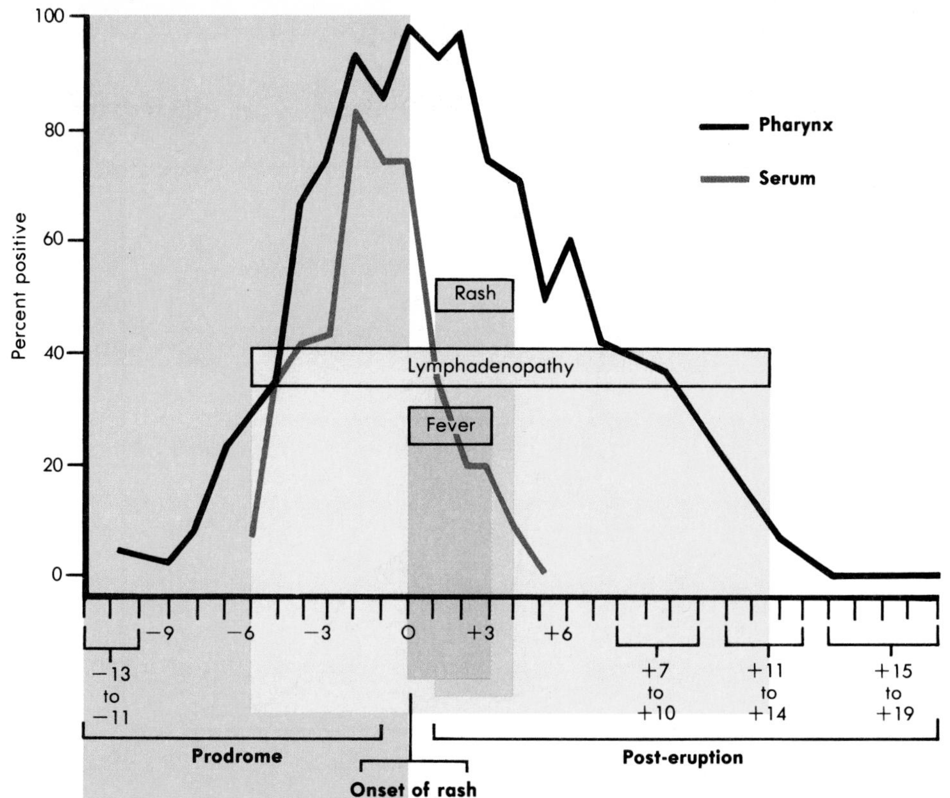

FIGURE 63-9 The time course of rubella disease. Rubella production in the pharynx precedes the appearance of symptoms and continues throughout the course of the disease. Onset of lymphadenopathy coincides with the viremia. Fever and rash are later symptoms. The individual is infectious as long as the virus is produced in the pharynx. (Redrawn from Plotkin SA: Rubella vaccine. In Plotkin SA and Mortimer EA, editors: *Vaccines*, Philadelphia, 1988, WB Saunders.)

TABLE 63-3 Estimated Morbidity Associated With the 1964-1965 U.S. Rubella Epidemic

Clinical events	Number affected
Rubella cases	12,500,000
Arthritis-arthralgia	159,375
Encephalitis	2,084
Deaths	
Excess neonatal deaths	2,100
Other deaths	60
Total deaths	2,160
Excess fetal wastage	6,250
Congenital rubella syndrome	
Deaf children	8,055
Deaf-blind children	3,580
Mentally retarded children	1,790
Other congenital rubella syndrome symptoms	6,575
Total congenital rubella syndrome	20,000
Therapeutic abortions	5,000

From National Communicable Disease Center: Rubella surveillance. US Department of Health, Education and Welfare, no. 1, June 1969.

FIGURE 63-10 A close-up of the rubella rash. Small erythematous macules are visible. (From Hart CA, Broadhead RL: *A color atlas of pediatric infectious disease*, London, 1992, Mosby.)

BOX 63-4 Prominent Clinical Findings in Congenital Rubella Syndrome

- Cataracts and other ocular defects
- Heart defects
- Deafness
- Intrauterine growth retardation
  - Failure to thrive
  - Mortality within the first year
- Microcephaly
  - Mental retardation

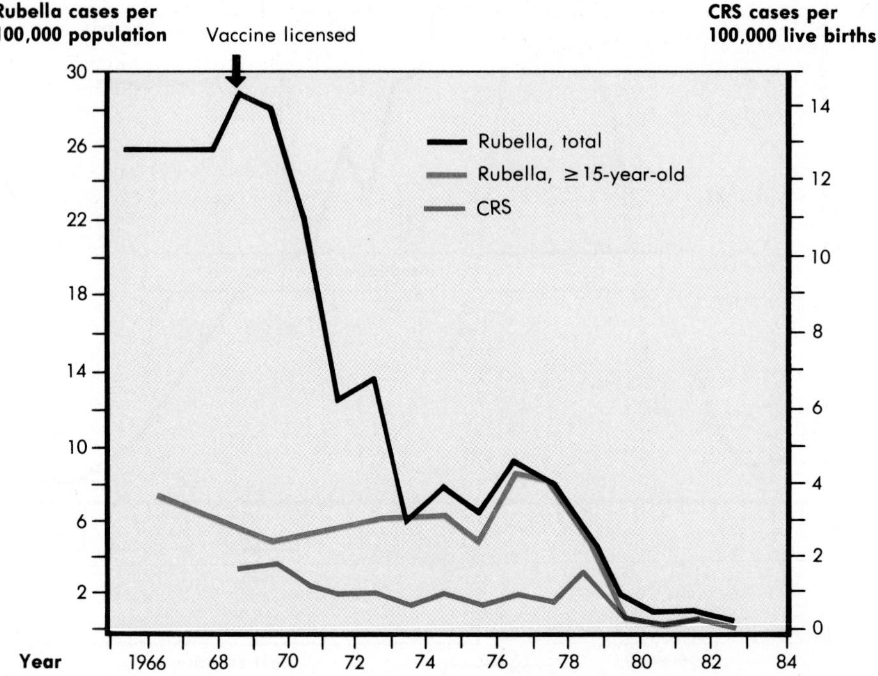

FIGURE 63-11 The effect of rubella virus vaccination on the incidence of rubella and congenital rubella syndrome. (Redrawn from Williams MN and Preblud SR: *MMWR* 33:1SS, 1984.)

When isolation is necessary, the virus is usually obtained from urine and is detected by interference with ECHO 11 virus replication in primary African green monkey kidney cell cultures.

Treatment, Prevention, and Control

No treatment has been found for rubella.

The best means of preventing rubella is vaccination with the live cold-adapted RA27/3 vaccine strain of virus (Figure 63-11). The live rubella vaccine is usually administered in conjunction with the measles and mumps vaccines (*MMR vaccine*). The triple vaccine is included routinely in well-baby care. Vaccination promotes both humoral and cellular immunity.

A major objective of the vaccination program is to decrease the number of susceptible individuals in the population, especially children. Since only one serotype for rubella exists and humans are the only reservoir, vaccination of a large proportion of the population can significantly reduce the chance of exposure to the virus. Unlike smallpox, vaccination programs will not eliminate rubella. The virus can be transmitted by persons with asymptomatic infections.

CASE STUDY AND QUESTIONS

A 27-year-old businessman experienced a high fever, serious retroorbital headache, and severe joint and back pain 5 days after he and his family returned from a trip to Malaysia. The symptoms lasted for 4 days, and then a rash appeared on the palms and soles for 2 days.

His 5-year-old son experienced mild flu-like symptoms and then collapsed after 2 to 5 days. His hands were cold and clammy, with a flushed face and warm body. There were petechiae on his forehead and ecchymoses elsewhere. He bruised very easily. He was breathing rapidly and had a weak rapid pulse. After 24 hours, he showed a rapid recovery.

1. What features of these cases contribute to the diagnosis of dengue virus infection?
2. Of what significance is the trip to Malaysia?
3. What is the source of infection for the father and son?
4. What is the significance and pathogenic basis for the development of petechiae and ecchymoses in the child?

A 25-year-old man returned from a trip to Mexico, and 2 weeks later he had arthralgia (joint aches) and a mild rash that started on his face and spread to his body. He recalled that he felt like he had the "flu" a few days before onset of the rash. The rash went away in 4 days.

1. What features of this case contribute to the diagnosis of rubella infection?
2. Why is it significant that the symptoms started after a trip outside the United States?
3. What precaution could he have taken to prevent this infection?
4. How is this infection transmitted?

5. Who is at risk for serious outcome of this infection?
6. If this disease is normally mild in children, why is immunization so important?

Bibliography

Belshe RB, editor: *Textbook of human virology*, ed 2, St. Louis, 1991, Mosby.

Fields BN, Knipe DM: *Virology*, ed 2, New York, 1990, Raven Press.

Freestone DS: Yellow fever vaccine. In Plotkin SA and Mortimer EA, editors: *Vaccines*, Philadelphia, 1988, WB Saunders.

Hahn CS, Galler R, Rice CM: Flavivirus genome organization, expression, and replication, *Ann Rev Microbiol* 44:649-688, 1990.

Johnson RT: *Viral infections of the nervous system*, New York, 1982, Raven Press.

Koblet H: The "merry-go-round": Alphaviruses between vertebrate and invertebrate cells, *Adv Vir Res* 38:343-403, 1990.

Plotkin SA: Rubella vaccine. In Plotkin SA and Mortimer EA, editors: *Vaccines*, Philadelphia, 1988, WB Saunders.

Stollar V: Approaches to the study of vector specificity for arboviruses—model systems using cultured mosquito cells. In Maramorosch K, Murphy FA, and Shatkin AJ, editors: *Advances in virus research*, vol 33, New York, 1987, Academic Press.

Tsai TF: Arboviral infections in the United States, *Inf Dis Clinics North Am* 5:73-102, 1991.

CHAPTER 64

Bunyaviridae

THE Bunyaviridae comprise a "supergroup" of at least 200 enveloped, segmented, negative-strand RNA viruses. The supergroup is further broken into five genera based on structural and biochemical features: Bunyavirus, Phlebovirus, Uukuvirus, Nairovirus, and Hantavirus (Table 64-1). Most of the Bunyaviridae are arboviruses (arthropod borne) that are spread by mosquitos, ticks, or flies and are endemic to the environment of the vector.

STRUCTURE

These viruses are roughly spherical particles 90 to 120 nm in diameter (Box 64-1). The envelope of the virus contains two glycoproteins (G1 and G2) and encloses three unique negative-strand RNAs associated with protein (nucleocapsids) (Table 64-2). The nucleocapsids include the large (**L**), medium (**M**), and small (**S**) RNA associated with the RNA-dependent RNA polymerase (L protein), and two nonstructural proteins (NS_s, NS_m) (Figure 64-1). Unlike other negative-strand RNA viruses, the Bunyaviridae do not have a matrix protein. Differences in the sizes of the virion proteins, the lengths of the L, M, and S strands of the genome, and their transcription distinguish the five genera of Bunyaviridae.

REPLICATION

Bunyaviridae follow the rules for replication of enveloped, negative-strand viruses. The G1 glycoprotein of the virus interacts with cell surface receptors, undergoes endocytosis, and fuses with endosomal membranes upon acidification of the vesicle. Release of the nucleocapsid into the cytoplasm allows mRNA and protein synthesis to begin.

The M strand encodes the NS_m nonstructural protein and the G1 (viral attachment protein) and G2 glycoproteins, and the L strand encodes the L protein (polymerase) (see Table 64-2). The S strand of RNA encodes two nonstructural proteins, N and NS_s. The S strand of the phleboviruses is "ambisense," meaning that the N protein mRNA is transcribed directly from the genome and the NS_s protein mRNA is transcribed from the replicative intermediate.

Replication of the genome by the L protein also

TABLE 64-1 Notable Bunyaviridae Genera

Genus	Members	Vector	Pathological conditions	Vertebrate hosts
Bunyavirus	Bunyamwera virus, California encephalitis virus, LaCrosse virus, Oropouche virus; 150 members	Mosquito	Febrile illness, encephalitis, febrile rash	Rodents, small mammals, primates, marsupials, birds
Phlebovirus	Rift Valley fever virus, Sandfly fever virus; 36 members	Fly	Sandfly fever Hemorrhagic fever Encephalitis Conjunctivitis, myositis	Sheep, cattle, domestic animals
Nairovirus	Crimean-Congo hemorrhagic fever virus; 6 members	Tick	Hemorrhagic fever	Hares, cattle, goats, seabirds
Uukuvirus	Uukuniemi virus; 7 members	Tick	—	Birds
Hantavirus	Hantaan virus; 1 member	None	Hemorrhagic fever with renal syndrome, adult respiratory distress syndrome	Rodents

*An additional 35 viruses possess several common properties with Bunyaviridae but are as yet unclassified.

provides new templates for transcription, increasing the rate of mRNA synthesis. The glycoproteins are synthesized and glycosylated in the endoplasmic reticulum. They are transferred to the Golgi apparatus where budding of the virus occurs. The G1 and G2 are not translocated to the plasma membrane. Virions are released by cell lysis or exocytosis.

BOX 64-1 Unique Features of Bunyaviruses

At least 200 related viruses, in 5 genera, which share common morphology and basic components
Virion is enveloped with 3 (L, M, S) negative RNA nucleocapsids but no matrix protein
Virus replicates in the cytoplasm
Virus can infect humans and arthropods
Virus in arthropods can be transmitted to its eggs

TABLE 64-2 Genome and Proteins of California Encephalitis Virus

Genome (negative-strand RNA)		Proteins
L (2.9 × 10⁶)	L	RNA polymerase, 170 kd
M (1.6 × 10⁶)	G1	Spike glycoprotein, 75 kd
	G2	Spike glycoprotein, 65 kd
	NS_m	Nonstructural protein, 15 to 17 kd
S (0.4 × 10⁶)	N	Nucleocapsid protein, 25 kd
	NS_s	Nonstructural protein, 10 kd

PATHOGENESIS

As arboviruses, Bunyaviridae share many of the pathogenic mechanisms of the togaviruses and flaviviruses (Box 64-2). The virus is spread by the arthropod vector and is injected into the blood to initiate a viremia. Progression past this stage to secondary viremia and further dissemination of the virus can deliver the virus to target organs characteristic of the individual viral disease such as the CNS, major organs (liver and kidney), and the vascular endothelium.

Bunyaviridae cause encephalitis by neuronal and glial damage, as well as cerebral edema. Lesions are concentrated in cortical gray matter of the frontal, temporal, and parietal lobes, basal nuclei, midbrain, and pons. In certain of the viremic infections (e.g., Rift Valley fever), hepatic necrosis may occur. In others (e.g., Crimean hemorrhagic fever and Hantaan virus infection), the primary lesion is leakage of plasma and erythrocytes through the vascular endothelium. In the latter infection these changes are most prominent in the kidney and are accompanied by hemorrhagic necrosis of the kidney.

EPIDEMIOLOGY

These viruses are transmitted by infected mosquitos, ticks, or phlebotomus flies to rodents, birds, and larger animals (Box 64-3). The animals become the reservoir for continuing the cycle of infection. Humans are infected when they enter the environment of the insect vector (Figure 64-2). Unlike many other arboviruses, many of the Bunyaviridae can survive a winter in the ova of the mosquito and stay in a locale. The Hantavirus group does not have an arthropod vector but spreads from mammal to mammal, usually rodents, and can spread directly to humans by aerosols.

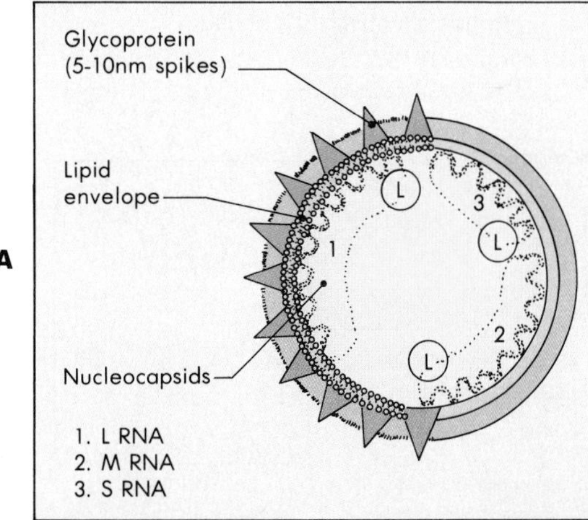

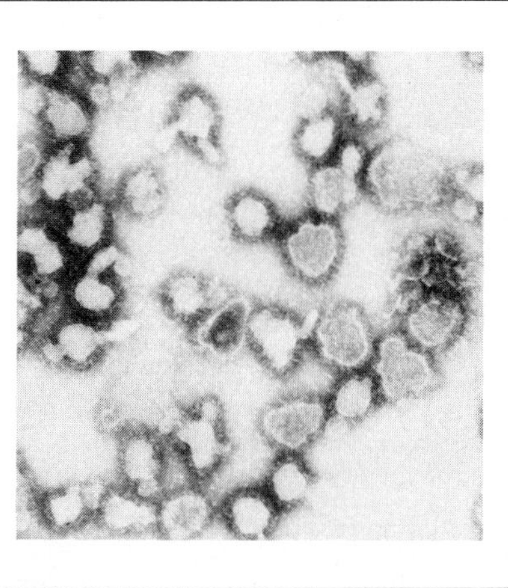

FIGURE 64-1 **A,** Model of bunyavirus particle. **B,** Electron micrograph of LaCrosse variant of bunyavirus. Note the spike proteins at the surface of the virion envelope. (**A,** Redrawn from Fraenkel-Conrat H and Wagner RR, editors: *Comprehensive virology,* New York, 1979, Plenum Press; **B,** Courtesy Centers for Disease Control.)

Many of the members of this virus family are found in South America, Southeast Europe, Southeast Asia, and Africa and share the exotic names of their ecological niche. Viruses of the California encephalitis virus group (e.g., LaCrosse virus) are found in the forests of North America and cause human encephalitis in the United States (Figure 64-3). An outbreak of adult respiratory distress syndrome in the southwestern United States in 1993 was attributed to a hantavirus. These viruses are spread mainly by *Aedes* mosquitos principally in the summer months.

CLINICAL SYNDROMES

Bunyaviridae (mosquito-borne) usually cause a nonspecific febrile illness related to the viremia (Table 64-1) that is indistinguishable from those caused by other viruses. The incubation period for these illnesses is approximately 48 hours, and the fevers last approximately 3 days. Most patients with infections have mild illness, even those infected by agents known to cause severe illness (e.g., Rift Valley fever virus or the LaCrosse virus). Onset of encephalitis illnesses (e.g., LaCrosse virus) is sudden following an incubation period of approximately 1 week with fever, headache, lethargy, and vomiting. Seizures occur in 50% of patients with encephalitis, usually early in the illness. Signs of meningeal irritation are present in only one third of cases. On average, illness lasts 7 days. Fatalities occur in less than 1%, but seizure disorders may occur as sequelae in as many as 20% of patients. Hemorrhagic fevers such as Rift Valley fever are characterized by petechial hemorrhages, ecchymosis, epistaxis, hematemesis, melena, and bleeding of gums. Death occurs in as many as 50% of cases with hemorrhagic phenomena.

BOX 64-2 Disease Mechanisms for Bunyaviruses

Virus is acquired from an arthropod bite (e.g., mosquito)
Initial viremia may cause flu-like symptoms
Establishment of secondary viremia may allow virus access to specific target tissues: CNS, organs, and vascular endothelium
Antibody is important in controlling viremia; interferon and cell-mediated immunity may prevent outgrowth of infection

BOX 64-3 Epidemiology of Bunyavirus Infections

DISEASE/VIRAL FACTORS

Able to replicate in mammalian and arthropod cells
Able to pass into the ovary and infect the arthropod eggs, allowing the virus to survive during winter

TRANSMISSION

Via arthropods through break in skin
California encephalitis group: carried by *Aedes* mosquitos
Aedes mosquitos are daytime feeders living in the forest
Aedes lay eggs in small pools of water trapped in trees, tires, etc.

WHO IS AT RISK?

Persons in the habitat of the arthropod vector
California encephalitis group: campers, forest rangers, woodsmen

GEOGRAPHY/SEASON

Disease incidence correlates with distribution of vector
Disease more common in summer

MODES OF CONTROL

Elimination of vector or vector's habitat
Avoidance of vector's habitat

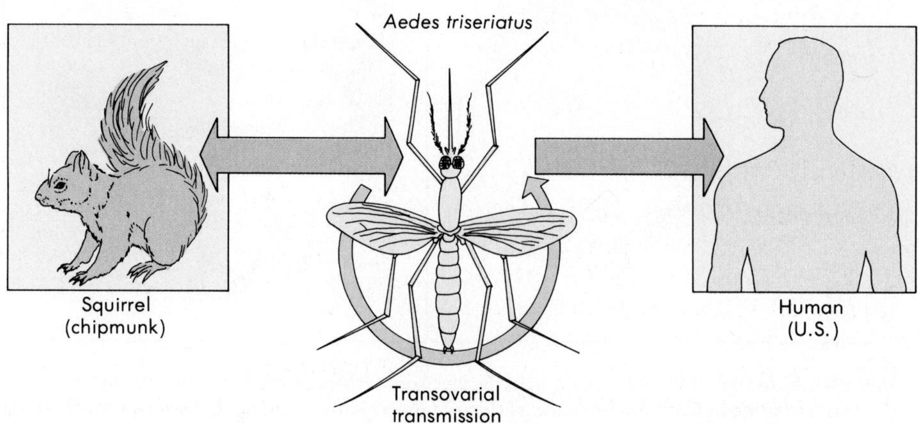

FIGURE 64-2 Transmission of LaCrosse (California) encephalitis virus.

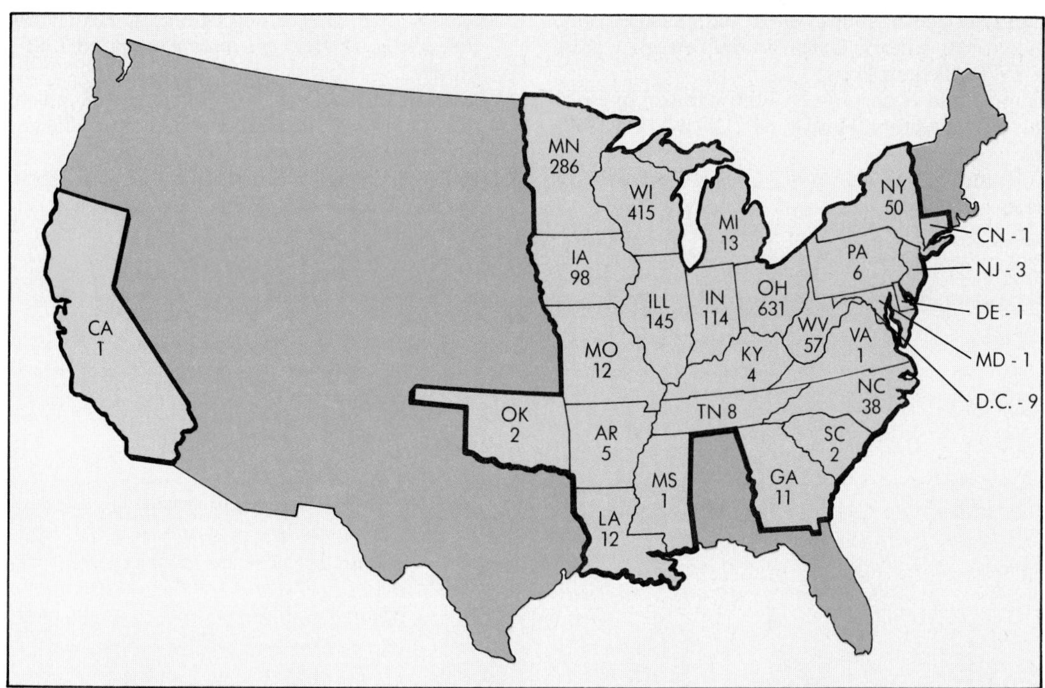

FIGURE 64-3 Distribution of California encephalitis, 1964 to 1989. (From Tsai TF: Arboviral infections in the United States, *Infect Dis Clin North Am* 5:73-102, 1991.)

LABORATORY DIAGNOSIS

Diagnosis of bunyaviruses is generally performed serologically. Virus neutralization assays, if appropriate cell cultures are available, are the assay of choice, but other serologic assays are also used. IgM-specific assays are useful to document acute infection. Seroconversion or a fourfold increase in IgG antibody is useful to document recent infection, but cross-reactions within viral genera are common.

ELISA techniques may detect antigen in clinical specimens from patients with high levels of viremia (e.g., Rift Valley fever, hemorrhagic fever with renal syndrome, and Crimean hemorrhagic fever). ELISA tests have been developed to detect viral antigen in mosquitos.

Isolation of the virus from routine specimens may be difficult and may require special cell cultures or inoculation of suckling mice.

TREATMENT, PREVENTION, AND CONTROL

No specific therapy is available for Bunyaviridae infections. Human disease is prevented by interrupting the contact between humans and the vector, whether arthropod or mammal. Arthropod vectors are controlled by eliminating the growth conditions for the vector, insecticide spraying and by netting or window and door screening, protective clothing, and control of tick infestation of animals. Rodent control minimizes transmission of many viruses, especially Hantaan virus. Rift Valley fever vaccines for use in humans and animals (sheep and cattle) have been developed.

CASE STUDY AND QUESTIONS

A 15-year-old summer camp counselor in Ohio suddenly complains of a headache, nausea, and vomiting and has a fever and develops a stiff neck. She was admitted to the hospital where a spinal tap showed inflammatory cells. She became lethargic over the next day but regained her alertness after 4 to 5 days.

1. The physician suspected LaCrosse encephalitis virus as the agent. What hints from the case suggest LaCrosse virus?
2. What other agents would also be considered in the differential diagnosis?
3. How was the patient infected?
4. How would the transmission of this agent be prevented?
5. How can the local public health department determine the prevalence of LaCrosse virus in the environment of the summer camp? What samples would they obtain, and how would they test them?

Bibliography

Bishop DHL, Schmaljohn CS, and Patterson JL: Bunyaviruses and their replication. In Fields BN and Knipe DM, editors: *Virology*, ed 2, New York, 1990, Raven Press.

Bishop DHL and Shope RE: Bunyaviridae. In Fraenkel-Conrat H and Wagner RR, editors: *Comprehensive virology*, vol 14, New York, 1979, Plenum Press.

Gonzalez-Scarano F and Nathanson N: Bunyaviruses. In Fields BN and Knipe DM, editors: *Virology*, ed 2, New York, 1990, Raven Press.

Kolakofsky D: Bunyaviridae, *Curr Top Microbiol Immunol* 169, 1991. A series of reviews.

McKee KT, LeDuc JW, and Peters CJ: Hantaviruses. In Belshe RB, editor: *Textbook of human virology*, ed 2, St. Louis, 1991, Mosby.

Peters CJ and LeDuc JW: Bunyaviruses, phleboviruses and related viruses. In Belshe RB, editor: *Textbook of human virology*, ed 2, St. Louis, 1991, Mosby.

Tsai TF: Arboviral infections in the United States, *Inf Dis Clin North Am* 5:73-104, 1991.

CHAPTER 65

Rhabdoviruses

THE members of the family Rhabdoviridae (Greek *rhabdos*, meaning rod) include pathogens for a variety of mammals, fish, birds, and plants. The rhabdoviruses include (1) Vesiculovirus (vesicular stomatitis viruses, or VSV), (2) Lyssavirus (rabies and rabies-like viruses), (3) an unnamed genus comprising the plant rhabdovirus group, and (4) other ungrouped rhabdoviruses of mammals, birds, fish, and arthropods (Box 65-1).

Rabies virus is the most significant pathogen of the rhabdoviruses. Until Louis Pasteur's development of one of the earliest killed virus vaccines, a bite from a "mad dog" led to the characteristic symptoms of hydrophobia and almost certain death.

PHYSIOLOGY, STRUCTURE, AND REPLICATION

Rhabdoviruses are bullet shaped, enveloped virions, 50 to 95 nm in diameter and 130 to 380 nm in length (Box 65-2 and Figure 65-1). Spikes composed of a trimer of the glycoprotein (G) cover the surface of the virus (see Figure 7-9). The G protein is the viral attachment protein and will generate neutralizing antibodies. The G protein of vesicular stomatitis virus (VSV) is a simple glycoprotein with *N*-linked glycan. This G protein has been used as the prototype for studying glycoprotein processing and cell surface expression.

Within the envelope, the helical nucleocapsid is coiled symmetrically into a cylindrical structure, giving the appearance of striations (see Figure 65-1). The nucleocapsid is composed of one molecule of single-stranded ribonucleic acid (RNA) and the nucleoprotein (N), large (L), and nonstructural (NS) proteins. The matrix (M) protein lies between the envelope and the nucleocapsid. The N protein is the major structural protein of the virus. It protects the RNA from ribonuclease digestion and maintains the RNA in a configuration for transcription. The N protein of rabies virus is phosphorylated, whereas the N protein of VSV is not. The L and NS proteins comprise the RNA-dependent RNA polymerase.

The replicative cycle of VSV is the prototype for the rhabdoviruses and other negative-strand RNA viruses (see Figure 65-2). The viral glycoprotein G attaches to the host cell and is internalized by endocytosis. The viral envelope fuses with the membrane of the endosome upon acidification of the vesicle. This releases the nucleocapsid into the cytoplasm where replication takes place.

The RNA-dependent RNA polymerase associated with the nucleocapsid transcribes the viral genomic RNA (ss[−]RNA), producing five individual mRNAs. These mRNAs are then translated into the five viral proteins. The viral genomic RNA is also transcribed into a full length (+)RNA template that is used to generate new genomes. The G protein is synthesized by membrane-bound ribosomes, processed by the Golgi apparatus, and delivered to the cell surface in membrane vesicles. The matrix protein associates with the G protein–modified membranes.

Assembly of the virion occurs in two phases: assembly of the nucleocapsid in the cytoplasm and envelopment and release at the cell plasma membrane. The genome associates with the N protein, and then with the polymerase proteins L and NS to form the nucleocapsid. Association with the M protein at the plasma membrane induces coiling of the nucleocapsid into its condensed form. The virus then buds through the plasma membrane and is released when the entire nucleocapsid is enveloped. Cell death and lysis follow infection by most rhabdovi-

BOX 65-1 Rhabdoviridae

Vesiculovirus
Lyssavirus
Plant rhabdovirus group
Ungrouped rhabdoviruses

BOX 65-2 Unique Features of Rhabdoviruses

Bullet-shaped, enveloped, negative single-stranded RNA virus
Prototype for replication of the negative-stranded enveloped viruses
Replicates in the cytoplasm

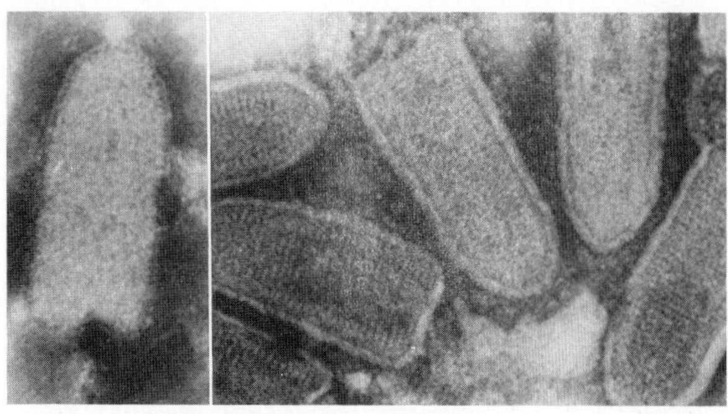

FIGURE 65-1 Rhabdoviridae seen by electron microscopy: rabies virus (*left*) and vesicular stomatitis virus (*right*). (From Fields BN: *Virology*, New York, 1985, Raven Press.)

ruses, with the important exception of rabies virus, which produces little discernible cell damage.

PATHOGENESIS AND IMMUNITY

Only the pathogenesis of rabies virus will be discussed (Box 65-3). Rabies infection usually results from the bite of a rabid animal. Rabies infection of the animal causes secretion of the virus in its saliva and promotes aggressive behavior ("mad dog") that promotes its transmission. Other routes of infection, such as inhalation of aerosolized virus, transplantation of infected tissue (e.g., cornea), or inoculation through intact mucous membranes, have been documented.

Virus multiplies at the site of inoculation, usually in striated muscle, and remains localized for days to months (Figure 65-2) before infecting the peripheral nerves. The following factors determine the time course for virus progression to the central nervous system (CNS) and onset of symptoms: virus concentration in the inoculum, proximity of the wound to the brain, severity of the wound, host's age, and host's immune status.

Rabies virus travels by retrograde axoplasmic transport to the dorsal root ganglia and to the spinal cord. Once the virus gains access to the spinal cord, rapid infection of the brain follows. The affected areas include the hippocampus, brain stem, ganglionic cells of pontine nuclei, and Purkinje's cells of the cerebellum. Virus then disseminates centrifugally from the CNS via afferent neurons to highly innervated sites, such as the skin of the head and neck, salivary glands, retina, cornea, nasal mucosa, adrenal medulla, renal parenchyma, and pancreatic acinar cells. Invasion of the virus into the brain and spinal cord causes an encephalitis and neuronal degeneration. Despite extensive CNS involvement, few gross or histopathologic lesions are seen in patients with rabies. With rare exception, rabies is fatal once clinical disease is apparent.

In contrast to other viral encephalitis syndromes, inflammatory lesions are rarely observed for rabies. Neutralizing antibodies are not apparent until after clinical disease is well established. Little antigen is released, and the infection probably remains hidden from the immune response. Cell-mediated immunity appears to play little or no role in protection from rabies virus infection.

Antibody can block the spread of virus to the CNS and to the brain if administered or generated during the incubation period. The incubation period is usually long enough to allow generation of a protective antibody response following active immunization with the rabies vaccine.

BOX 65-3 Disease Mechanisms of Rabies Virus

- Rabies is usually transmitted in saliva and acquired from the bite of a rabid animal
- Rabies virus is not very cytolytic and seems to remain cell associated
- The virus replicates in the muscle at the site of the bite with minimal or no symptoms (*incubation phase*)
- The length of the incubation phase is determined by the infectious dose and the proximity of the infection site to the CNS and brain
- After weeks to months, the virus infects the peripheral nerves and travels up the CNS to the brain (*prodrome phase*)
- Infection of the brain causes classical symptoms, coma, and death (*neurological phase*)
- During the neurological phase, the virus spreads to the glands, skin, etc. including the salivary glands, from where it is secreted and transmitted
- Rabies infection does not elicit an antibody response until the late stages of disease when the virus has spread from the CNS to other sites
- Antibody can block the progression of the virus
- The long incubation phase allows *active immunization* as a postexposure treatment

EPIDEMIOLOGY

Rabies is the classical zoonotic infection, spread from animals to humans (Box 65-4). It is endemic worldwide in a variety of animals. Rabies is maintained and spread in two ways: urban rabies, with the dog serving as the primary transmitter, and sylvatic (forest) rabies, involving many species of wildlife. The principal reservoir for rabies in most of the world is the dog. In Latin America large numbers of stray unvaccinated dogs and the absence of rabies control programs are responsible for thousands of rabies cases in dogs each year. Because of the excellent vaccination program in the United States, sylvatic rabies accounts for the majority of animal rabies. Statistics for animal rabies are collected by the Centers for Disease Control, and in 1992 more than 8000 cases were documented for skunks, raccoons, bats, and farm animals, in addition to dogs and cats (Figure 65-3). Badgers and foxes are also major carriers of rabies in Western Europe. In South America vampire bats transmit rabies to cattle, resulting in millions of dollars in losses each year.

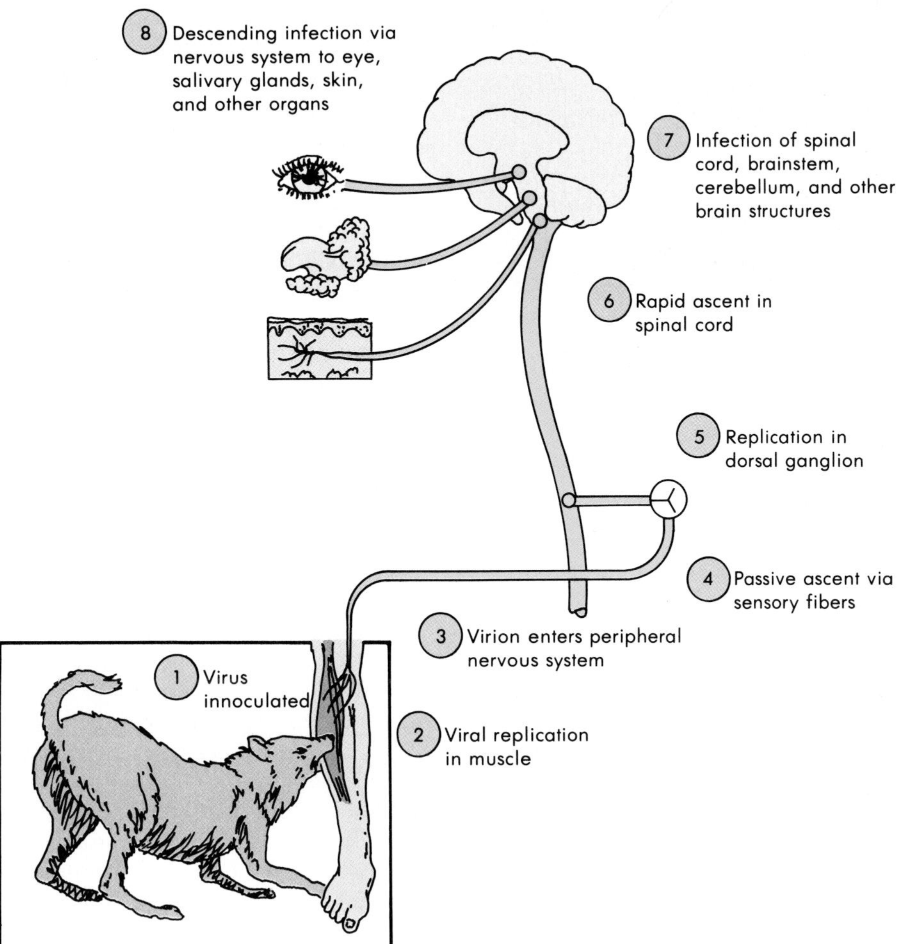

FIGURE 65-2 Schematic representation of pathogenesis of rabies virus infection. Numbered steps describe sequence of events. (Redrawn from Belshe RB, editor: *Textbook of human virology*, ed 2, St. Louis, 1991, Mosby.)

The distribution of human rabies generally follows the distribution of animal cases in each country. It is estimated that rabies accounts for at least 25,000 deaths annually in India, of which 96% are transmitted by dogs. In Latin America cases of human rabies are transmitted primarily by dogs in urban areas. In the United States, because of effective dog vaccination programs and limited contact with skunks, raccoons, and bats, the incidence of human rabies is 0 to 1 case per year (Figure 65-4). Even so, annual costs for rabies prevention are greater than $300 million.

CLINICAL SYNDROMES

Rabies is almost always a fatal disease unless treated by vaccination. Following a long but highly variable incubation period, the prodrome phase of rabies ensues (Figure 65-5). Symptoms such as fever, malaise, headache, pain or paresthesia (itching) at the site of the bite, gastrointestinal symptoms, fatigue, and anorexia typically occur. After a prodrome of 2 to 10 days, neurological symptoms specific for rabies appear. Hydrophobia (fear of water), the most characteristic symptom of rabies, occurs in 20% to 50% of patients. The symptom is triggered by the pain associated with the patient's attempts to swallow water. Focal and generalized seizures, disorientation, and hallucinations also frequently occur during the neurological phase. From 15% to 60% of patients exhibit paralysis as the only manifestation of rabies, which may lead to respiratory insufficiency.

Following the neurological phase, which lasts from 2 to 10 days, the comatose phase develops. This phase almost universally leads to death resulting from neurological and pulmonary complications.

LABORATORY DIAGNOSIS

An occurrence of an animal bite and neurological symptoms generally provide the diagnosis of rabies. Laboratory tests are usually performed to confirm the diagnosis and to determine whether a suspected animal is rabid (postmortem). Unfortunately, evidence of infection, including symptoms and antibody, does not occur until it is too late for intervention.

Diagnosis of rabies is made by histopathology, detection of viral antigen in the CNS or skin, virus isolation,

BOX 65-4 Epidemiology of Rabies

DISEASE/VIRAL FACTORS

Enveloped virus must stay wet but can be inactivated by soap and detergents
Disease has long incubation period

TRANSMISSION

Zoonosis: Reservoir: Wild animals
Vector: Wild animals and unvaccinated dogs and cats
Source of virus: Major: Saliva in a rabid animal bite
Minor: Aerosols in bat caves containing rabid bats

WHO IS AT RISK?

Veterinarians, animal handlers
Person bitten by a rabid animal
Inhabitants of countries with no pet vaccination program

GEOGRAPHY/SEASON

Worldwide, except some island nations
No seasonal incidence

MODES OF CONTROL

Vaccination program for pets
Vaccination for high-risk personnel
Future vaccination program for control of rabies in forest mammals

and serology. The hallmark of rabies diagnosis has been the detection of intracytoplasmic inclusions consisting of matrices of viral nucleocapsids (**Negri bodies**) in affected neurons (see Figure 53-3). Although diagnostic of rabies, Negri bodies are seen in only 70% to 90% of infected human brain tissue.

Antigen detection by immunofluorescence has become the most widely used method for rabies diagnosis. Brain biopsy or autopsy material, impression smears of corneal epithelial cells, and skin biopsy material from the nape of the neck are the most frequently used specimens to detect viral antigen by direct immunofluorescence. The test has a high degree of sensitivity and specificity in experienced hands.

Rabies can also be grown in cell culture or by intracerebral inoculation of infant mice. Inoculated cell cultures or brain tissues are subsequently examined by direct immunofluorescence.

Rabies antibody titers in serum and cerebrospinal fluid (CSF) can be measured by a rapid fluorescent focus inhibition test, by mouse infection neutralization, or by plaque reduction. Antibody usually is not detectable until the late stages of infection and disease.

TREATMENT AND PROPHYLAXIS

With the exception of three documented human survivors of rabies, clinical rabies is invariably a fatal infection unless treated. Once the onset of symptoms has begun, little other than supportive care is possible.

Postexposure prophylaxis currently is the only hope for preventing overt clinical illness in the affected individual.

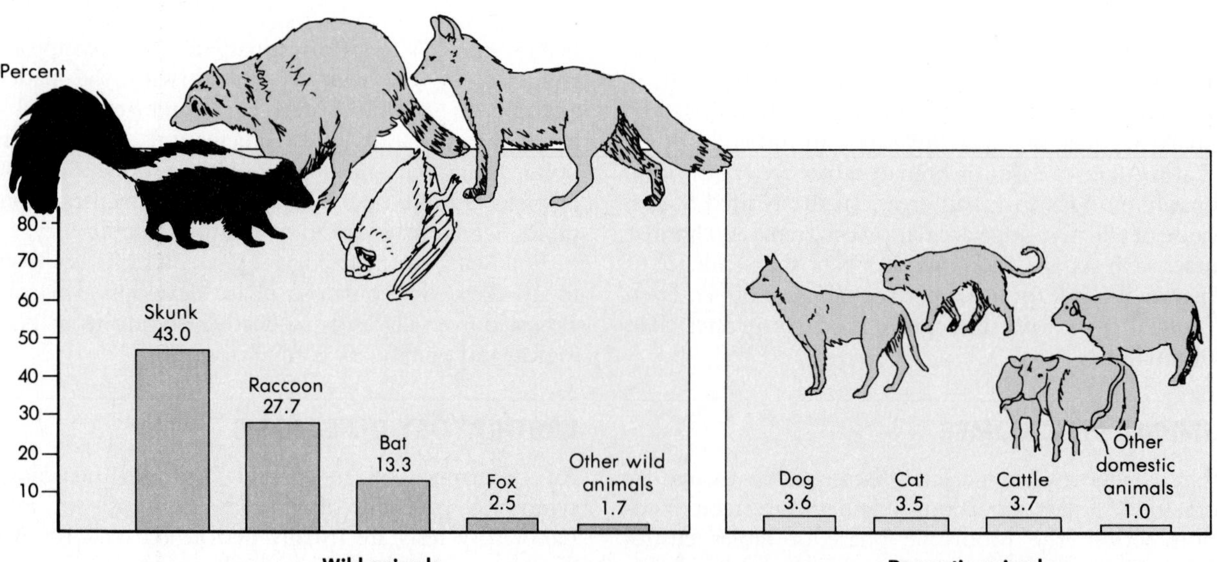

FIGURE 65-3 Distribution of animal rabies in the United States, 1987. The percentages relate to the total number of cases of animal rabies. (Redrawn from Centers for Disease Control: Rabies surveillance, United States, 1987. In CDC surveillance summaries, *MMWR* 37(SS-4) September 1988.)

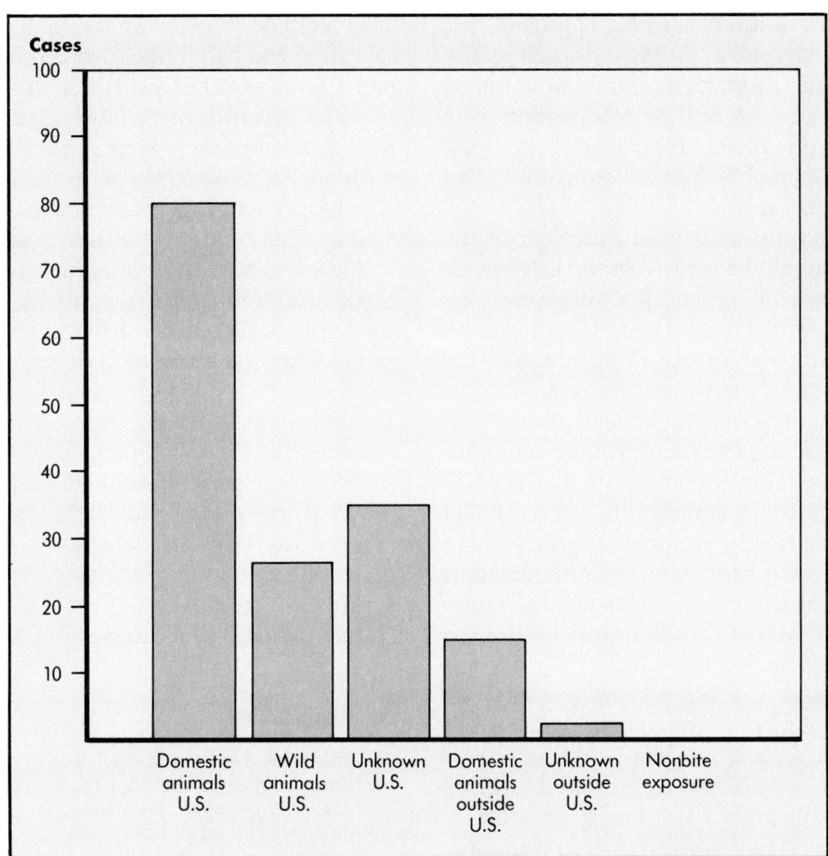

FIGURE 65-4 Human rabies cases reported in the United States from 1950 to 1987 by location and source of exposure. (Redrawn from Centers for Disease Control: Rabies surveillance, United States, 1987. In CDC surveillance summaries, *MMWR* 37(SS-4), September 1988.)

Disease phase	Incubation Phase	Prodrome Phase	Neurological Phase	Coma	
Symptoms	Asymptomatic	Fever, nausea, vomiting Loss of appetite Headache Lethargy Pain at site of bite	Hydrophobia, pharyngeal spasms Hyperactivity, anxiety, depression CNS symptoms: loss of coordination, paralysis, confusion, delirium	Coma: Cardiac arrest Hypotension Hypoventilation Secondary infections	Death
Time	60-365 days after bite	2-10 days	2-7 days	0-14 days	
Viral status	Low titer Virus in muscle	Low titer Virus in CNS and brain	High titer Virus in brain and other sites	High titer Virus in brain and other sites	
Immunological status			Detectable antibody in serum and CNS		

FIGURE 65-5 Progression of rabies disease.

Although human cases of rabies are rare, approximately 20,000 individuals receive rabies prophylaxis each year in the United States alone. Prophylaxis should be initiated for individuals exposed by bite or by contamination of an open wound or mucous membrane to saliva or brain tissue of a suspected animal, unless the animal is tested and shown not to be rabid.

The first protective measure is local treatment of the wound. The wound should be washed immediately with soap and water, detergent, or another substance that inactivates the virus. The World Health Organization Expert Committee on Rabies also recommends the instillation of antirabies serum around the wound.

Subsequently, immunization with vaccine in combination with administration of one dose of equine antirabies serum (ARS) or human rabies immune globulin (HRIG) is recommended. Passive immunization with HRIG provides antibody until the patient produces antibody in response to the vaccine. A series of five immunizations over a month is administered. The slow course of rabies disease allows generation of an active immunity in time for protection.

The rabies vaccine is a killed vaccine prepared by chemical inactivation of rabies-infected tissue culture cells (e.g., VERO, human diploid [HDCV] or fetal rhesus lung cells [RHV]). These vaccines have replaced vaccines (Semple or Fermi) prepared in the brains of adult or suckling animals. The HDCV is administered intramuscularly on days 0, 3, 7, 14, and 28 following exposure.

Preexposure vaccination of animal workers, laboratory workers who handle potentially infected tissue, and individuals traveling to areas where rabies is endemic should be performed. HDCV administered intramuscularly or intradermally in three doses is recommended and provides 2 years of protection.

Ultimately, prevention of human rabies hinges on effective control of rabies in domestic and wild animals. Control of domestic animal rabies depends on removal of strays and unwanted animals and vaccination of all dogs and cats. A variety of attentuated oral vaccines has been used successfully to immunize foxes. A live recombinant vaccinia virus vaccine expressing the rabies virus glycoprotein has been developed and is being tested.

CASE STUDY AND QUESTIONS*

An 11-year-old boy was brought to a hospital in California after falling; the symptoms were treated, and he was released. The following day he refused to drink water with his medicine, and he became more anxious. That night he began to act up and hallucinate. He also was salivating and had difficulty breathing. Two days later, he had a fever of 40.8° C (105.4° F) and experienced two episodes of cardiac arrest. Although rabies was suspected, no remarkable data were obtained from a computer tomography of the brain or cerebrospinal fluid analysis. A skin biopsy from the nape of the neck was negative for viral antigen on day 3 but was positive for rabies on day 7. He continued to deteriorate and died 11 days later. Upon questioning the parents, it was learned that the child had been bitten on the finger by a dog 6 months earlier while on a trip to India.

1. What clinical features of this case are suggestive of rabies?
2. Why does rabies have such a long incubation period?
3. What treatment should have been given immediately after the dog bite? As soon as the diagnosis was suspected?
4. How do the clinical aspects of rabies differ from other neurological viral diseases?

*Modified from *MMWR* 41:461-463, 1992.

Bibliography

Anderson LJ, Nicholson KG, Tauxe RV, and Winkler WG: Human rabies in the United States, 1960-1979: epidemiology, diagnosis, and prevention, *Ann Intern Med* 100:728-735, 1984.

Baer GM, Bellini WJ, and Fishbein DB: Rhabdoviruses. In Fields BN, Knipe DM, editors: *Virology*, New York, 1990, Raven Press.

Centers for Disease Control: Rabies surveillance, United States, 1987. In CDC surveillance summaries, *MMWR* 37(SS-4), 1988.

Centers for Disease Control: Rabies vaccine, adsorbed: a new rabies vaccine for use in humans, *MMWR* 37:217-218, 223, 1988.

Fishbein DB: Rabies, *Infect Dis Clin North Am* 5:53, 1991.

Immunization Practices Advisory Committee: Rabies prevention: supplementary statement on the preexposure use of human diploid cell rabies vaccine by the intradermal route, *MMWR* 35:767-768, 1986.

Robinson PA: Rabies virus. In Belshe RB, editor: *Textbook of human virology*, ed 2, St. Louis, 1991, Mosby.

Steele JH: Rabies in the Americas and remarks on the global aspects, *Rev Infect Dis* 10(suppl 4):S585-S597, 1988.

Wagner RR: Rhabdoviridae and their replication. In Fields BN, Knipe DM, editors: *Virology*, New York, 1990, Raven Press.

Warrell DA, Warrell MJ: Human rabies and its prevention: an overview, *Rev Infect Dis* 10(suppl 4):S726-S731, 1988.

Winkler WG and Böel K. Control of rabies in wildlife, *Sci Am* June, 1992.

Wunner WH, Larson JK, Dietzschold B, and Smith CL: The molecular biology of rabies viruses, *Rev Infect Dis* 10(suppl 4):S771-S784, 1988.

CHAPTER 66

Miscellaneous Viruses

CORONAVIRUSES

Coronaviruses are named for their solar corona–like appearance when viewed with the electron microscope (Figure 66-1) because of the surface projections on the virion. Coronaviruses are the second most prevalent cause of the common cold (rhinovirus is first). Electron microscopy studies link coronaviruses to gastroenteritis in children and adults. Only two strains of virus have been isolated from humans; however, other strains are believed to exist.

Structure and Replication

Coronaviruses are enveloped virions, with long helical nucleocapsids that measure 80 to 160 nm (Box 66-1). The glycoproteins on the surface of the envelope appear as club-shaped projections that are 20 nm in length and 5 to 11 nm wide. The virion is normally sensitive to acid, ether, and drying, but some strains are capable of traversing the G.I. tract.

The genome is composed of plus-stranded, unsegmented RNA (27,000 to 30,000 bases; 7×10^6 d). Upon infection, the genome is translated to produce an RNA-dependent RNA polymerase (**L** [225,000 d]). Virions contain glycoproteins **E1** (20,000 to 30,000 d) and **E2** (160,000 to 200,000 d), a core nucleoprotein (**N** [47,000 to 55,000 d]), and some strains also contain a hemagglutinin-neuraminidase (**E3** [120,000 to 140,000 d]) (Table 66-1). The E2 glycoprotein is responsible for viral attachment, membrane fusion, and is the target of neutralizing antibodies. The E1 glycoprotein is a transmembrane matrix protein. The replication scheme for coronaviruses is presented in Figure 66-2.

Pathogenesis and Clinical Syndromes

Coronaviruses inoculated into the respiratory tracts of human volunteers infect epithelial cells. Infection remains localized to the upper respiratory tract because the *optimum temperature for viral growth is 33° C to 35° C.* After infection an increase in coronavirus-specific serum antibody can be detected; however, serum antibody does not prevent reinfection (Box 66-2).

The virus is most likely spread by aerosols and in large droplets (e.g., sneezes). Coronaviruses cause upper respiratory infection, similar to "colds" caused by rhinoviruses, but with a longer incubation period (average 3 days). The infection may exacerbate chronic pulmonary disease such as asthma and bronchitis. Although the infection is usually mild, pneumonia may occur in children and adults.

Infections, which occur mainly in infants and children, appear either sporadically or in outbreaks with a winter and a spring pattern. Usually, one strain will predominate in an outbreak. Based on serologic studies, coronaviruses cause approximately 10% to 15% of the upper respiratory tract infections and pneumonias in humans. Antibodies to coronaviruses are uniformly present by adulthood, but reinfections are common despite the preexisting serum antibodies.

Coronavirus-like particles have been seen by electron microscopy in stools of adults and children with diarrhea and gastroenteritis and infants with neonatal necrotizing enterocolitis. However, improved cell culture methods and serologic studies are needed to prove the association of coronaviruses with human gastroenteritis.

Laboratory Diagnosis

Laboratory diagnosis of coronaviruses is not routinely done. Coronaviruses will grow only in human embryonic trachea organ cultures, and serologic assays are not routinely available. Electron microscopy has been used to detect coronavirus-like particles in stool specimens.

Treatment, Prevention and Control

Control of respiratory transmission of coronaviruses would be difficult and probably unnecessary because of the mildness of the infection. No vaccine or specific antiviral therapy is available.

CALICIVIRUS (NORWALK AGENT) AND OTHER SMALL ROUND GASTROENTERITIS VIRUSES

Norwalk agent was discovered by electron microscopy in stool from adults suffering from epidemic acute gastroenteritis in Norwalk, Ohio. Norwalk agent and other small round gastroenteritis viruses include the caliciviruses, astroviruses, and unclassified viruses bearing the names of the geographical locations where they were identified (Box 66-3).

A

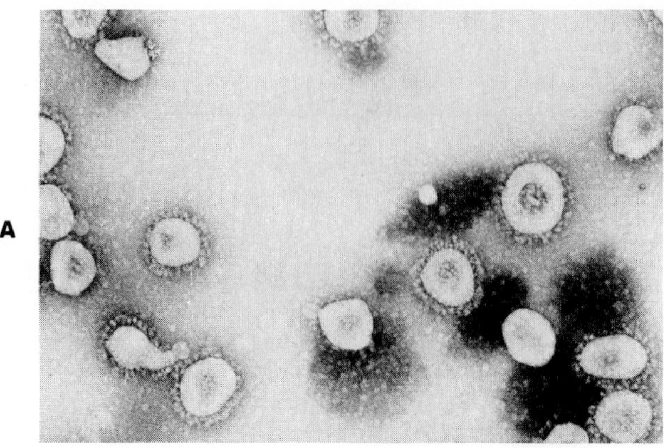

B

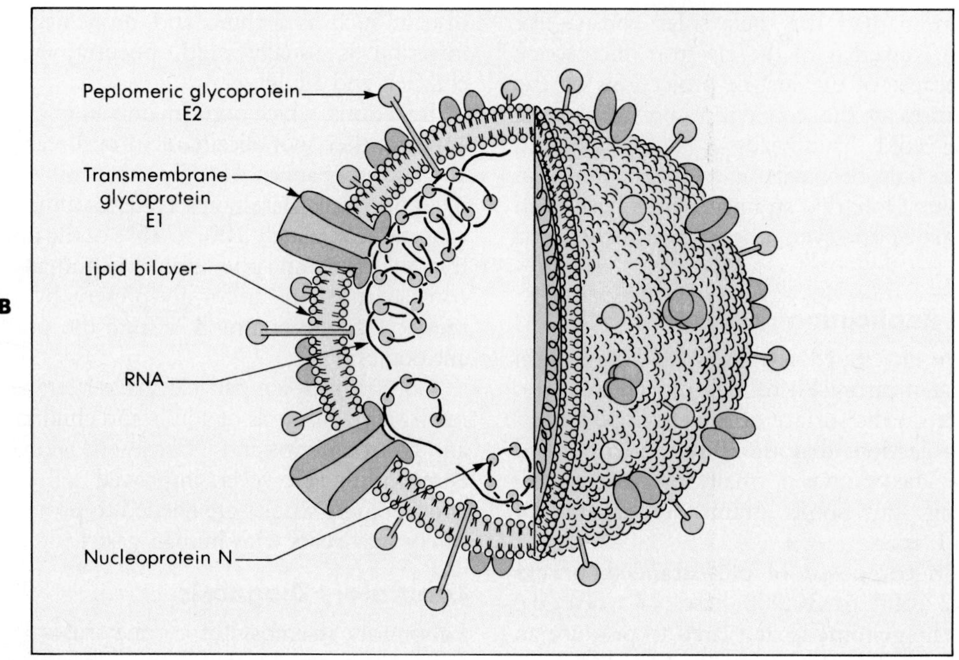

FIGURE 66-1 **A,** Electron micrograph of human respiratory coronavirus (×90,000). **B,** Model of a coronavirus. The viral nucleocapsid is a long flexible helix composed of the plus-strand genomic RNA and many molecules of the phosphorylated nucleocapsid protein *(N)*. The viral envelope includes a lipid bilayer derived from intracellular membranes of the host cell and two viral glycoproteins (*E1* and *E2*). (**A,** Courtesy Center for Disease Control. **B,** Redrawn from Fields BF and Knipe DM, editors: *Virology*, New York, 1985, Raven Press.)

BOX 66-1 Unique Features of Coronaviruses

- Medium-sized virions with solar corona-like appearance
- Single-stranded (+)RNA genome enclosed in an envelope containing the E2 viral attachment protein, E1 matrix protein, and N nucleocapsid protein
- Translation of genome occurs in two phases; early phase produces an RNA polymerase (L), late phase from (−)RNA template yields structural and nonstructural proteins
- Virus assembles at the rough endoplasmic reticulum
- Difficult to isolate and grow in routine cell culture

Structure and Replication

These viruses are 20 to 30 nm capsid viruses and can be distinguished by their size, the morphology of their capsid, and antigenic epitopes. Caliciviruses, including Norwalk agent, are single-strand plus RNA viruses (approximately 7500 bases) with a 27 nm capsid consisting of one 60,000 d capsid protein. Norwalk virions are round with a ragged outline, whereas calicivirions have cup-shaped indentations and a six- pointed star image. The astroviruses have a five- or six-pointed star image on the surface of the virions but no indentations. Antibodies from seropositive individuals can also be used to distinguish these viruses.

Caliciviruses and astroviruses can be grown in cell

TABLE 66-1 Major Human Coronavirus Proteins

Proteins	Molecular weight (k)	Location	Functions
E2 (peplomeric glycoprotein)	160-200	Envelope spikes (peplomer)	Binding to host cells; fusion activity
H1 (hemagglutinin protein)	60-66	Peplomer	Hemagglutination
N (nucleoprotein)	47-55	Core	Ribonucleoprotein
E1 (matrix glycoprotein)	20-30	Envelope	Transmembrane proteins
L (polymerase)	225,000	Infected cell	Polymerase activity

Modified from Balows A et al., editors: *Laboratory diagnosis of infectious diseases: principles and practice*, Heidelberg, 1988, Springer-Verlag.

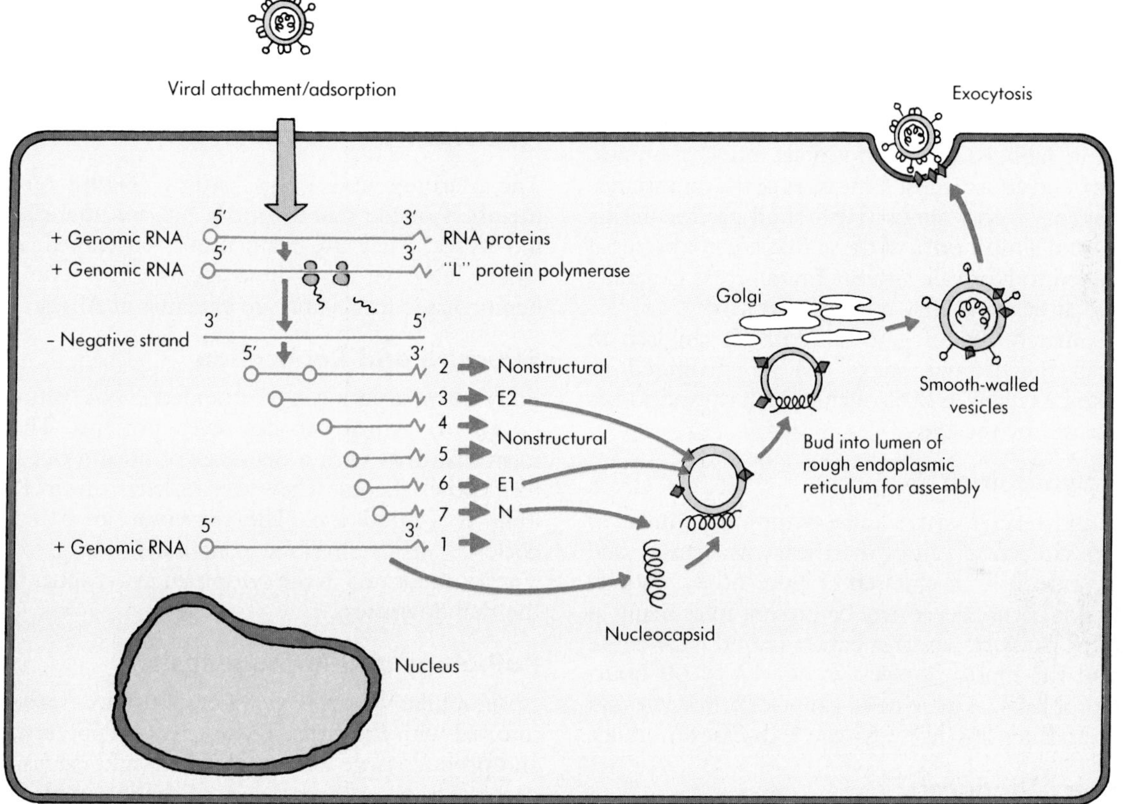

FIGURE 66-2 Replication of human coronaviruses. The E2 glycoprotein interacts with receptors on epithelial cells, the virus fuses or is endocytosed into the cell, and the genome is released into the cytoplasm. Protein synthesis is divided into early and late phases similar to togaviruses. The genome binds to ribosomes, and an RNA-dependent RNA polymerase is translated. This enzyme generates a full-length (−) RNA template for production of new virion genomes and six individual mRNAs for the other coronavirus proteins. The genome associates with rough endoplasmic reticulum membranes modified by virion proteins and buds into the RER lumen. Vesicles that contain virus migrate to the cell membrane and are released by exocytosis. (Redrawn from Balows A et al., editors: *Laboratory diagnosis of infectious diseases: principles and practice*, New York, 1988, Springer-Verlag.)

culture, but the Norwalk viruses cannot. These viruses replicate in the cytoplasm, with release of viral particles upon cell destruction.

Pathogenesis

Jejunal biopsy of human volunteers infected with caliciviruses reveals blunting of villi, cytoplasmic vacuolation, and infiltration with mononuclear cells, but virus particles are not detected by EM of epithelial cells. The virus compromises the function of the brush border, which prevents proper absorption of water and nutrients. Although no histological changes occur in gastric mucosa, gastric emptying may be delayed.

Epidemiology

Norwalk and related viruses typically cause outbreaks of gastroenteritis such as those that occur on cruise ships or in communities as a result of common source contami-

BOX 66-2 Disease Mechanisms of Human Coronaviruses

- Infects epithelial cells of upper respiratory tract
- Replicates best at 33° C to 35° C; therefore restricted to upper respiratory tract
- Reinfection occurs in the presence of serum antibodies
- Enveloped virus that may be able to survive the G.I. tract

nation (e.g., water, shellfish, food service). These viruses are transmitted by the fecal-oral and possibly airborne routes.

Exposure to Norwalk agent in developed countries occurs later in life than in underdeveloped countries, presumably as a result of good sanitation. In developed countries outbreaks may occur year-round and have been described in schools, resorts, hospitals, nursing homes, restaurants, and cruise ships. A measure of the importance of these agents is that almost 10% of all gastroenteritis outbreaks and almost 60% of those that are nonbacterial are attributed to Norwalk viruses. Immunity is generally short-lived at best and may not be protective.

Approximately 3% of gastroenteritis in children in day-care in the United States can be attributed to caliciviruses. As many as 70% of children have antibodies to astroviruses by the age of 7.

Clinical Syndromes

Norwalk and related viruses cause symptoms similar to rotaviruses. Infection causes diarrhea with nausea and vomiting, especially in children (Figure 66-3). Bloody stools do not occur. Fever may be present in as many as one third of patients. The incubation period is 24 to 48 hours, and the illness resolves within 12 to 60 hours without problems. Astroviruses cause diarrhea without vomiting and are less likely to cause disease in adults.

Laboratory Diagnosis

Laboratory diagnosis of the small round gastroenteritis viruses is limited to electron microscopy and serology. Immune electron microscopy can be used to concentrate and identify the virus from stool. The addition of an antibody directed against the suspected agent causes the virus to aggregate, facilitating recognition. The viruses are difficult or do not grow in tissue culture.

Serology is the method used to identify most infections. Antibody to the Norwalk agent may be detected by radioimmunoassay (RIA) or ELISA. Antibodies to the other calici-like agents are more difficult to detect.

Treatment, Prevention, and Control

No specific treatment is available. Bismuth subsalicylate may reduce gastrointestinal symptoms. Outbreaks may be minimized by handling food carefully and maintaining the purity of the water supply.

BOX 66-3 Characteristics of Norwalk Agent, Calicivirus, and Other Small Round Gastroenteritis Viruses

- Very small capsid viruses distinguishable by capsid morphology
- Resistant to environmental pressure: detergents, drying, acid
- Transmitted by fecal-oral route in contaminated water and food
- Causes outbreaks of gastroenteritis
- Disease resolves after 48 hours without serious consequences

FILOVIRUSES

The Marburg and Ebola viruses (Figure 66-4) were members of the rhabdoviridae but are now classified as filoviruses. They are filamentous, enveloped, negative-strand RNA viruses. These agents cause severe or fatal hemorrhagic fevers and are endemic in Africa.

Structure and Replication

Filoviruses have a single-stranded RNA genome (4.5×10^6 d), which encodes seven proteins. The virions form filaments with a diameter of 80 nm but may also form other shapes. They vary in length from 800 to as long as 14,000 nm. The nucleocapsid is helical and enclosed in an envelope containing one glycoprotein. Virus is replicated in the cytoplasm in a manner similar to the rhabdoviruses.

Pathology and Pathogenesis

Eosinophilic cytoplasmic inclusions are seen in cells infected with the virus. These viruses replicate efficiently and produce large amounts of virus and extensive tissue necrosis in parenchymal cells of the liver, spleen, lymph nodes, and lungs. Widespread hemorrhage causes edema and hypovolemic shock.

Epidemiology

Marburg virus infection was first detected among laboratory workers in Marburg, Germany, who had been exposed to tissues from apparently healthy African green monkeys. Rare cases of Marburg virus infection have been reported in Zimbabwe and Kenya.

Ebola virus has caused disease only in Africans in Zaire and the Sudan. In rural areas of central Africa as much as 18% of the population have antibody to this virus, suggesting that subclinical infections do occur. Travelers in or residents of central Africa (e.g., Zaire or the Sudan) may be exposed to the Ebola virus.

The mechanisms of natural transmission are unknown. These viruses may be endemic in wild monkeys and can

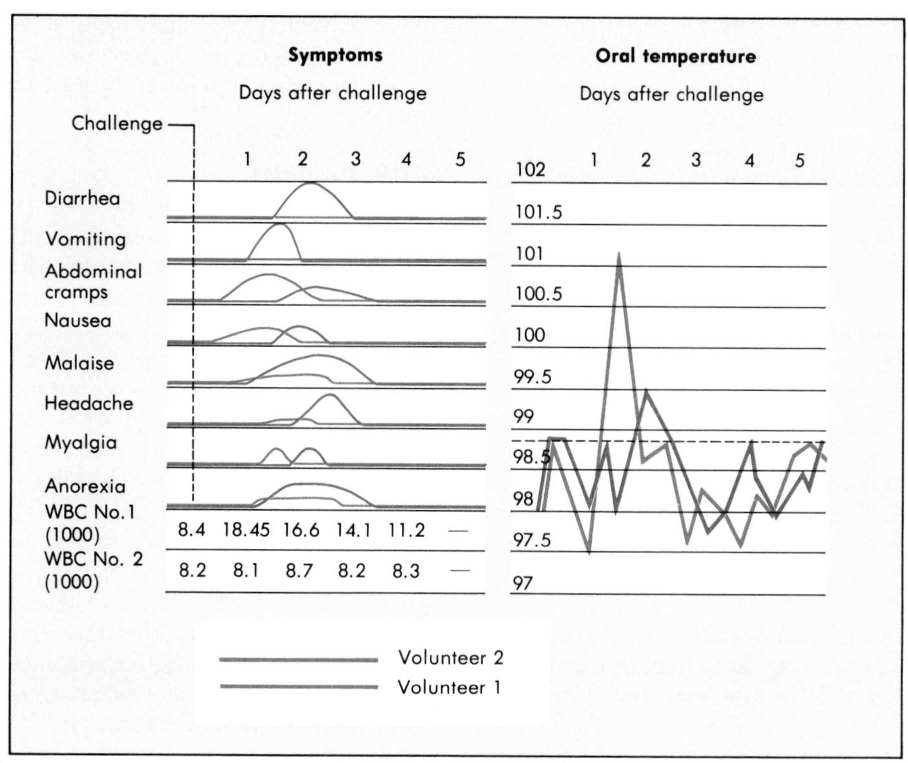

FIGURE 66-3 Response of two volunteers to oral administration of stool filtrate derived from volunteers who received original Norwalk rectal swab specimen. The height of the curve is directly proportional to the severity of the sign or symptom. Volunteer 1 had severe vomiting without diarrhea, whereas volunteer 2 had diarrhea without vomiting, although both received the same inoculum.

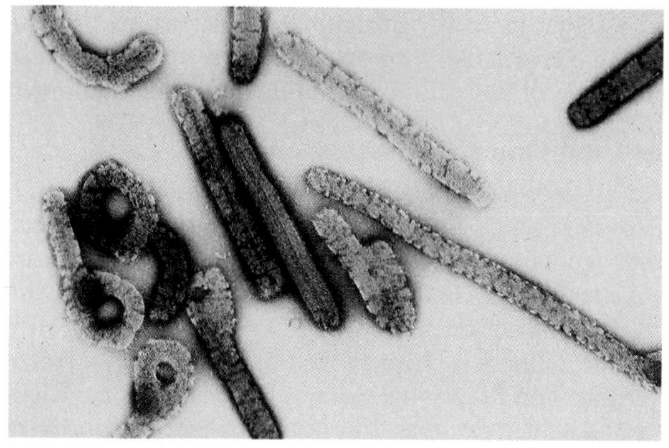

FIGURE 66-4 Electron micrograph of Ebola virus. (Courtesy Centers for Disease Control.)

be spread from monkey to human and between humans. Laboratory contact with infected monkeys obtained from a questionable source was a source of human infection and death. These viruses have been transmitted by accidental injection and by the use of contaminated syringes. Virus may also be passed by close contact with body fluids.

Clinical Syndromes

Marburg and Ebola viruses are the most severe causes of viral hemorrhagic fevers. Illness usually begins with flu-like symptoms such as headache and myalgias. Within a few days nausea, vomiting, and diarrhea occur; a rash also may develop. Subsequently, hemorrhage from multiple sites and death occur in as many as 90% of patients with clinically evident disease.

Laboratory Diagnosis

All specimens for filovirus diagnosis must be handled with extreme care to prevent accidental infection. Handling of these viruses requires level 4 isolation procedures that are not routinely available. Marburg virus may grow rapidly in tissue culture (Vero cells), although Ebola virus recovery may require animal (e.g., guinea pig) inoculation.

Infected cells have large eosinophilic cytoplasmic inclusion bodies. Viral antigens in tissues can be detected by direct immunofluorescence analysis.

IgG and IgM antibody to filovirus antigens can be detected by IFA, enzyme linked immunosorbent assay (ELISA), or RIA. Seroconversion or a fourfold increase of IgG antibody levels may be diagnostic of active infection, as may the detection of specific IgM antibody.

Treatment, Prevention, and Control

Antibody-containing serum and interferon therapies have been tried for these infections. Infected individuals should be quarantined, and contaminated animals should be sacrificed. Handling of the viruses or contaminated materials requires very stringent isolation procedures (level 4).

ARENAVIRUSES

The arenaviruses include lymphocytic choriomeningitis (LCM) and hemorrhagic fever viruses such as Lassa fever, Junin, and Machupo. These viruses are zoonoses, which cause persistent infections of specific rodents. The rodents become the reservoir for the viruses and, although asymptomatic or minimally diseased, will excrete the virus in their secretions. The virus becomes endemic in the habitat of the rodent.

Structure and Replication

Arenaviruses are pleomorphic enveloped viruses (120 nm diameter), which have a sandy appearance (arenosa, Greek, meaning sandy) in the electron microscope because of the ribosomes in the virion (Box 66-4). Although functional, the ribosomes do not seem to serve a purpose. Virions contain a beaded nucleocapsid with two single-stranded RNA circles ("S" 3.2 and "L" 4.8 $\times 10^6$ d) and a transcriptase. The L strand is negative-sense RNA and encodes the polymerase. The S strand encodes the nucleoprotein (N) and the glycoproteins but is ambisense. Whereas the mRNA for the N protein is transcribed directly from the ambisense S strand, the mRNA for the glycoprotein is transcribed from a full-length template of the genome. As a result, the glycoproteins are produced as late proteins after genome replication. Arenaviruses replicate in the cytoplasm and acquire their envelope by budding from the host cell plasma membrane.

Arenaviruses readily cause persistent infections. This may result from inefficient transcription of the glycoprotein genes.

Pathogenesis

Arenaviruses are able to infect macrophages and possibly cause the release of mediators of cell and vascular damage. Tissue destruction is significantly exacerbated by T-cell immunity. However, persistent infection of rodents results from neonatal infection and induction of immune tolerance.

BOX 66-4 Characteristics of Arenaviruses

Enveloped virion with two circular negative RNA genome segments (L, S) appearing sandy because of ribosomes
S genome segment is ambisense
Arenaviruses are zoonoses, establishing persistent infections in rodents
Pathogenesis of arenavirus infections is largely attributed to T-cell immunopathogenesis

Epidemiology

Arenaviruses are mainly found in the tropics of Africa and South America. The arenaviruses infect specific rodents and are endemic to their habitat. LCM, for example, infects hamsters and house mice (*Mus musculus*) and in Washington, D.C., was present in 20% of mice. LCM disease in the United States correlates with contact with pet hamsters and rodent breeding facilities. Lassa fever virus infects *Mastomys natalensis*, an African rodent. Chronic infection is common in these animals and leads to chronic viremia and virus shedding in saliva, urine, and feces. Infection of humans may occur by way of aerosols, contamination of food, or fomites. Bites are not a usual mechanism of spread. Persistently infected rodents do not usually exhibit illness. Human-to-human infection occurs with Lassa fever virus through contact with infected secretions or body fluids, but this mode of spread rarely if ever occurs with LCM or other hemorrhagic fevers. The incubation period for arenavirus infections averages 10 to 14 days.

Clinical Syndromes

Lymphocytic Choriomeningitis

The name of the virus suggests that meningitis is a typical clinical event, but actually a febrile illness with myalgia (influenza-like) occurs more often. Current estimates show that approximately 25% of infected persons exhibit clinical evidence of CNS infection. The meningeal illness, if it occurs, may be subacute and persist for several months. Perivascular mononuclear infiltrates may be seen in neurons of all sections of brain and in the meninges.

Lassa and Other Hemorrhagic Fevers

Lassa fever, with its focus of endemicity in west Africa, is the best known of the arenavirus hemorrhagic fevers. Other agents, however, such as Junin and Machupo, cause similar syndromes in different geographical areas (Argentina and Bolivia, respectively).

Clinical illness is characterized by fever, coagulopathy, petechiae, and occasional visceral hemorrhage, as well as liver and spleen necrosis, but not vasculitis. Hemorrhage and shock occur, as well as occasional cardiac and liver damage. In contrast to LCM, no lesions are present in the central nervous system (CNS) of patients with hemorrhagic fevers. Pharyngitis, diarrhea, and vomiting may be prevalent, especially in patients with Lassa fever. Death occurs in as many as 50% of those with Lassa fever and in a smaller percentage among those infected with the other arenaviruses that cause hemorrhagic fevers. The diagnosis is suggested by recent travel to endemic areas.

Laboratory Diagnosis

The diagnosis of arenavirus infection is usually made through serologic tests. These viruses are too dangerous for routine isolation. Arenaviruses can be isolated by inoculation of blood or cerebrospinal fluid into suckling mice or Vero monkey cells. Throat specimens can yield arenaviruses; urine is often positive for the Lassa fever virus but negative for the LCM virus. Substantial risk is present for laboratory workers handling body fluids. Therefore if the diagnosis is suspected, laboratory personnel should be warned and specimens processed only in facilities specialized for the isolation of contagious pathogens (level 3 for LCM and level 4 for Lassa fever and other arenaviruses).

Treatment, Prevention, and Control

The antiviral drug, ribavirin, has limited activity toward arenaviruses and can be used to treat Lassa fever virus infections. However, supportive therapy is usually all that is available for patients with arenavirus infections.

Prevention of these rodent-borne infections depends on limiting contact with the vector. Improved hygiene to limit contact with mice reduced the incidence of LCM in Washington, D.C. In the geographical areas where hemorrhagic fever occurs, trapping of rodents and careful storage of food may decrease contact.

Laboratory-acquired cases can be reduced by processing samples for arenavirus isolation in at least Type 3 or 4 biosafety facilities and *not* in the usual clinical virology laboratory.

CASE STUDY AND QUESTIONS*

A 58-year-old woman complained of "flu-like" symptoms, severe headache, stiff neck, and photophobia. She was lethargic and had a mild fever. Her cerebrospinal fluid contained 900 white blood cells, mostly lymphocytes and LCMV. She recovered after a week. Her home was infested with grey mice (*Mus musculus*).

1. What are the significant symptoms for this disease?
2. How is the virus transmitted?
3. What type of immune response is most important in controlling this infection?

Several adults complained of serious diarrhea, nausea, vomiting, and a mild fever 2 days after visiting The Cafe Grease. The symptoms were too severe to be food poisoning or routine gastroenteritis but lasted only 24 hours.

1. What characteristics distinguish this disease from rotavirus infection?
2. What is the most likely means of virus transmission?
3. What physical characteristics of the virus allow this means of transmission?
4. What public health measures can be followed to prevent such outbreaks?

* Modified from *MMWR* 33:290-291, 1984.

Bibliography

Balows A, Hausler WJ Jr, and Lennette EH: *Laboratory diagnosis of infectious diseases: principles and practice*, New York, 1988, Springer-Verlag.

Belshe RB, editor: *Textbook of human virology*, ed 2, St. Louis, 1991, Mosby.

Bishop RF: Other small virus-like particles in humans. In Tyrrell DAJ and Kapikian AZ, editors: *Virus infections of the gastrointestinal tract*, New York, 1982, Marcel Dekker.

Blacklow NR, Greenberg HB: Viral gastroenteritis, *N Engl J Med* 325:252-264, 1991.

Christensen ML. Human viral gastroenteritis, *Clin Microbiol Rev* 2:51-89, 1989.

Fields BN and Knipe DM, editors: *Virology*, ed 2, New York, 1990, Raven Press.

Oldstone MBA: Arenaviruses, *Curr Top Microbiol Immunol*, vol 133 and 134, A series of reviews.

ter Meulen V, Siddell S, and Wege H, editors: *Biochemistry and biology of coronaviruses*, New York, 1981, Plenum Press.

Xi JN, Graham DY, Wang KN, Estes MK. 1990. Norwalk virus genome cloning and characterization, *Science* 250:1580-1583, 1990.

CHAPTER 67

Retroviruses

THE retroviruses are enveloped, positive-strand RNA viruses with a unique morphology and means of replication. In 1970 Baltimore and Temin showed that the retroviruses encode an RNA-dependent DNA polymerase (reverse transcriptase) and replicate through a DNA intermediate. The DNA copy of the viral genome is integrated into the host chromosome to become a cellular gene. This discovery, which earned the Nobel Prize, contradicted the central dogma of molecular biology that stated that genetic information passed from DNA to RNA and then to protein.

Three subfamilies of retrovirus exist. These subfamilies and their human members are the **oncornavirus**, or oncovirus (human T-lymphotropic virus 1, 2, and 5; HTLV-1, HTLV-2, HTLV-5), **lentivirus** (human immunodeficiency virus 1 and 2; HIV-1, HIV-2), and **spumavirus** (Table 67-1). Spumavirus was the first human retrovirus to be isolated, but no spumavirus has been associated with human disease. **Endogenous retroviruses**, the ultimate parasite, have integrated and are transmitted vertically as part of the host chromatin. Although they may not replicate, their gene sequences have been detected in many animal species and humans.

The first retrovirus to be isolated was the Rous sarcoma virus, shown by Peyton Rous to produce solid tumors (sarcomas) in chickens. As with most retroviruses, the Rous sarcoma virus proved to have a very limited host and species range. Cancer-causing retroviruses have been isolated from other animal species and are classified as RNA tumor viruses or oncornaviruses. Many of these viruses alter cellular growth by expressing analogues of cellular growth-controlling genes (**oncogenes**).

The retroviruses are probably the most studied group of viruses in molecular biology. Not until 1981, however, was a human retrovirus isolated and associated with human disease. HTLV-1 was isolated from an individual with adult human T-cell leukemia by Robert Gallo and associates.

In the late 1970s and early 1980s, it was noted that an unusual number of young homosexual men, Haitians, heroin addicts, and hemophiliacs (the initial "4H club" of risk groups) were dying of normally benign opportunistic infections. Their symptoms defined a new disease, **acquired immunodeficiency syndrome (AIDS)**. AIDS is not limited to these groups, and more than a million men, women, and children around the world currently have AIDS. Montagnier and associates in Paris and Gallo and co-workers in the United States reported the isolation of a retrovirus, **human immunodeficiency virus (HIV-1)**, from patients with lymphadenopathy and AIDS. A variant of HIV-1, designated **HIV-2**, was isolated later

TABLE 67-1 Classification of Retroviruses

Subfamily	Characteristics	Examples
Oncovirus	Associated with cancer and neurological disorders	
A	Intracytoplasmic precursor of B-type virus; double-membrane particles	
B	Eccentric nucleocapsid core in mature virion	Mouse mammary tumor virus
C	Centrally located nucleocapsid core in mature virion	Human T-lymphotropic virus (HTLV-1, HTLV-2, HTLV-5), Rous sarcoma virus (chickens)
D	Nucleocapsid core with cylindric form	Mason-Pfizer monkey virus
Lentivirus	Slow disease onset: causes neurological disorders and immunosuppression; virus with D-type, cylindrical, nucleocapsid core	Human immunodeficiency virus (HIV-1, HIV-2), visna virus (sheep), Caprine arthritis/encephalitis virus (goats)
Spumavirus	Causes no clinical disease but characteristic vacuolated "foamy" cytopathology	Human foamy virus

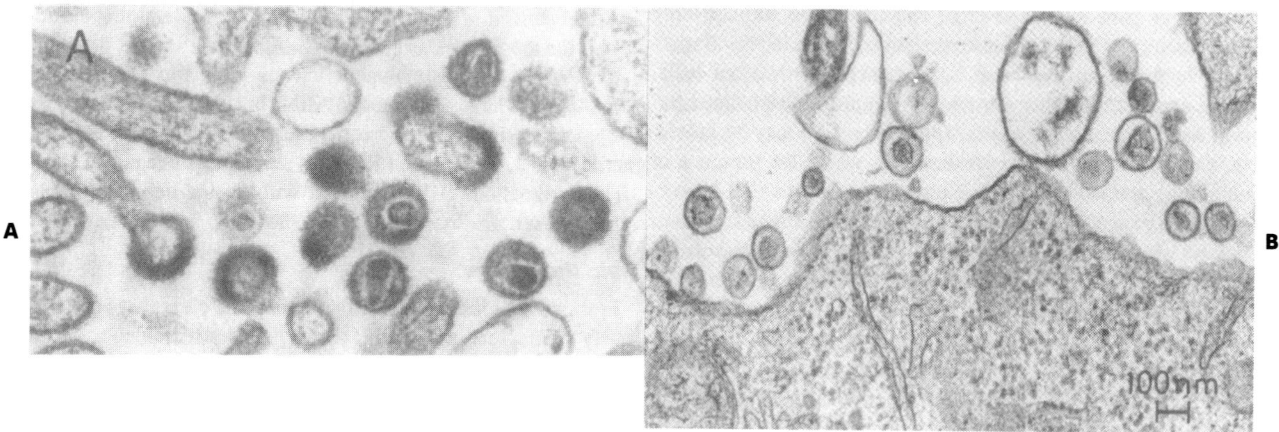

FIGURE 67-1 Electron micrographs of two retroviruses. **A,** Human immunodeficiency virus-1. Note the cone-shaped nucleocapsid in several of the virions. **B,** Human T leukemia virus. Note the C-type morphology characterized by a central symmetrical nucleocapsid. (Reprinted from Belshe RB, editor: *Textbook of human virology*, ed 2, St. Louis, 1991, Mosby.)

and is prevalent in West Africa. Understanding this disease and its agents has become the infectious disease challenge of the 1990s.

Our understanding of the retroviruses has paralleled progress in molecular biology. Newer technologies were and are still required to advance our knowledge of the retroviruses and their association with human disease. Their limited host range and tissue tropism has made it difficult to establish appropriate cell systems for their growth. Their ability to integrate into host chromosomes and remain latent has made them difficult to detect, study, and treat. However, the retroviruses have provided a major tool for molecular biology, the reverse transcriptase enzyme, and have advanced our understanding of cell growth, differentiation, and oncogenesis through the study of viral oncogenes.

The pathogenic human retroviruses include HTLV-1 and HTLV-2, which are oncoviruses, and HIV-1 and HIV-2, which are lentiviruses. HTLV-1 and HIV-1 both infect CD4 T lymphocytes, are spread by similar means, and have long latent periods. Nonetheless they cause very different diseases because of the nature of their interaction with the infected host cell.

BOX 67-1 Unique Characteristics of Retroviruses

- Enveloped spherical virion; 80 to 120 nm enclosing a capsid containing two copies of the positive-strand RNA genome (approximately 9 kilobases for HIV and HTLV)
- RNA-dependent DNA polymerase (reverse transcriptase) and integrase enzymes are carried in the virion
- Cell-specific expression of the virus receptor is the initial determinant of tissue tropism
- Replication proceeds through a DNA intermediate, termed the *provirus*
- The provirus integrates randomly into the host chromosome and becomes a cellular gene
- Transcription of the genome is regulated by the interaction of host transcription factors with promotor and enhancer elements in the LTR portion of the genome
- Transcription of the genome replicates the virus and also produces mRNA for the gag, pro, and pol genes, and then singly spliced for the env gene and doubly spliced for the tax/rex (HTLV-1) or tat/rev (HIV-1)
- Virus assembles and buds from the plasma membrane

CLASSIFICATION

The retroviruses are classified by disease, tissue tropism and host range, and virion morphology (see Table 67-1). The oncoviruses include the only retroviruses that can immortalize or transform target cells. The oncoviruses are also categorized by the morphology of their core and capsid in electron micrographs as type A, B, C, or D (see Table 67-1). The lentiviruses are slow viruses associated with neurological and immunosuppressive disease. The spumaviruses, represented by a foamy virus, cause a distinct cytopathologic effect but do not seem to cause clinical disease.

STRUCTURE

The retroviruses are roughly spherical, enveloped RNA viruses with a diameter of 80 to 120 nm (Figure 67-1 and Box 67-1). The envelope contains viral glycoproteins and is acquired by budding from the plasma membrane. The envelope surrounds a capsid that contains two identical copies of the positive-strand RNA genome inside an electron-dense core. The virion also contains 10 to 50 copies of the reverse transcriptase and integrase enzymes

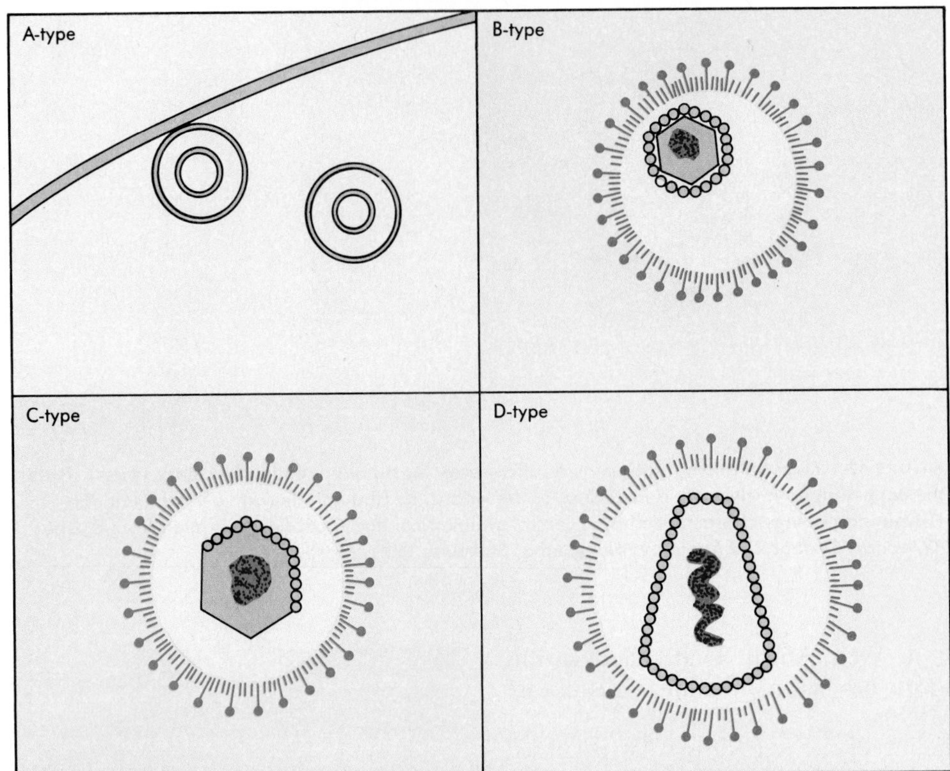

FIGURE 67-2 Morphological distinction of retrovirions. The morphology and position of the nucleocapsid core are the means of classification. A-type particles are immature intracytoplasmic forms that bud through the plasma membrane into mature B-type particles. C-type and D-type particles are mature virion forms that are completely assembled at the plasma membrane.

and two cellular transfer RNAs (tRNA). These tRNAs are base paired to each copy of the genome to be used as a primer for the reverse transcriptase. The morphology of the core differs for different viruses and is used as a means of classifying the retroviruses (Figure 67-2). The HIV virion core resembles a truncated cone (Figure 67-3).

The retrovirus genome has a 5′ cap and is polyadenylated at the 3′ end (Figure 67-4 and Table 67-2). Although the genome resembles a messenger RNA (mRNA), it is not infectious because it does not encode a polymerase that can directly generate more mRNA. The genome consists of at least three major genes that encode polyproteins for the enzymatic and structural proteins of the virus: **gag** (group-specific antigen), **pol** (polymerase), and **env** (envelope). At each end of the genome are **long terminal repeat (LTR)** sequences. The LTR contains promoters, enhancers, and other gene sequences for binding different cellular transcriptional factors. Oncogenic viruses may also contain a growth-regulating oncogene at the expense of other sequences. HTLV and the lentiviruses, including HIV, also encode several regulatory proteins.

The capsid is composed of several proteins cleaved from a polypeptide encoded by the gag gene. The viral enzymes are encoded by the pol gene, including the protease, reverse transcriptase, and integrase. These proteins are cleaved as part of the nucleocapsid assembly process.

The viral glycoproteins are produced by proteolytic cleavage of the polyprotein encoded by the env gene. Their size differs for each group of viruses. For HTLV-1, the gp62 is cleaved into a gp46 and p21, and for HIV, the gp160 is cleaved into the gp41 and gp120. These glycoproteins form lollipop-like spikes visible on the surface of the virion. The larger of the glycoproteins is responsible for the tissue tropism of the virus and is recognized by neutralizing antibody. The smaller subunit (gp41 in HIV) forms the lollipop stick and promotes cell-to-cell fusion. The gp120 of HIV is extensively glycosylated, and its antigenicity can drift during the course of a chronic HIV infection. Both of these factors impede immune clearance of the virus. Detection of these glycoproteins is a useful marker of infection.

REPLICATION

Replication of the retroviruses is initiated by the binding of the viral glycoprotein spikes to specific cell surface receptor proteins (Figure 67-5). *The presence of virus receptors is the initial determinant of the tissue and host tropism of the virus.*

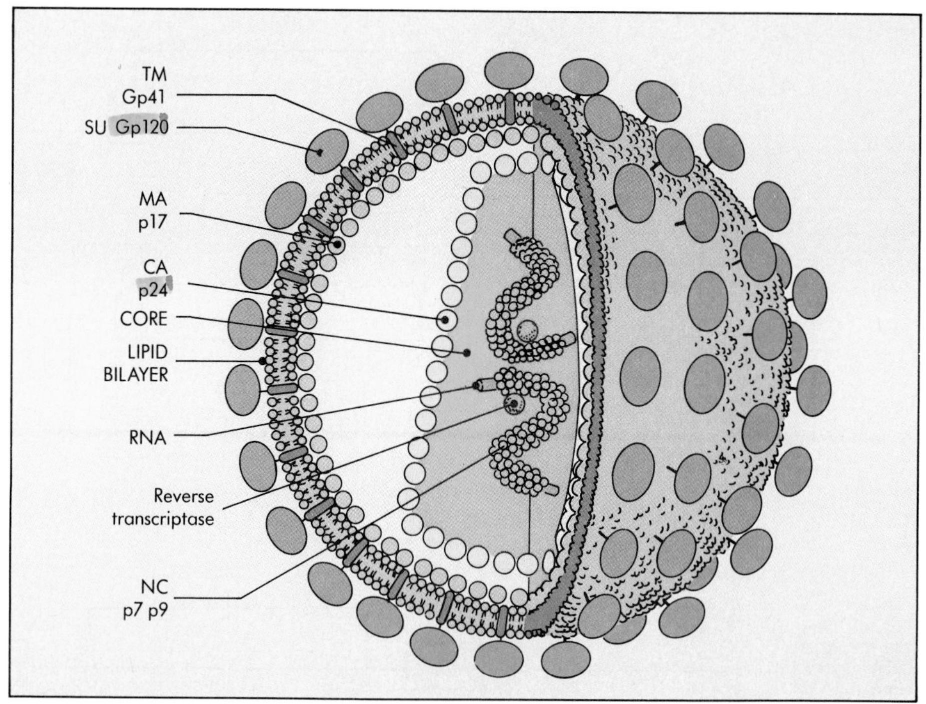

FIGURE 67-3 Cross-section of HIV. The enveloped virion contains two identical RNA strands, RNA polymerase, integrase, and two tRNAs base paired to the genome within the protein core. This is surrounded by proteins and a lipid bilayer. The envelope spikes are made of the gp120 attachment protein and gp41 fusion protein. (Redrawn from Gallo RC and Montagnier L: *Sci Am* 259:41-51, 1988.)

The gp120 of HIV interacts with a specific epitope of the CD4 surface molecule expressed on T-helper lymphocytes and cells of the macrophage lineage (e.g., macrophage, dendritic cells, microglial cells). HIV enters the cell by fusion of the envelope with the cellular plasma membrane; other retroviruses may enter the cell by receptor-mediated endocytosis.

Once released into the cytoplasm, the reverse transcriptase uses the virion tRNA as a primer and synthesizes a complementary negative-strand DNA. The reverse transcriptase also acts as an RNase, degrades the RNA genome, and then synthesizes the positive strand of DNA (Figure 67-6). During the synthesis of the virion DNA (**provirus**), sequences from each end of the genome (U3 and U5) are duplicated, which juxtaposes the long terminal repeats (LTR) to both ends. This process creates sequences that are required for integration and also enhancer and promoter sequences to regulate transcription. The DNA copy of the genome is larger than the original RNA.

The reverse transcriptase enzyme is very error prone. The error rate for the reverse transcriptase from HIV is 1 per 2000 base pairs or approximately 5 per genome (HIV−9000 bp). This genetic instability for HIV generates new strains of virus during the course of an individual's disease, a property that may alter the pathogenicity of the virus and promote immune escape.

The double-strand cDNA is then delivered to the nucleus and spliced randomly into the host chromosome with the aid of a viral-encoded, virion carried–integrase. HIV and other lentiviruses produce a large amount of nonintegrated circular DNA, which is not transcribed efficiently but may contribute to the cytopathogenesis of the virus.

Once integrated, the viral DNA is transcribed as a cellular gene by the host RNA polymerase II. Transcription of the genome produces a full-length RNA, which is processed to produce several mRNA containing either the gag, gag-pol, or env gene sequences. The full-length transcripts of the genome can also be assembled into new virions.

As a cellular gene, retroviral replication depends on the efficiency of its transcription. The efficiency of viral transcription is the second major determinant of retroviral tissue tropism and host range. The efficiency of viral genome transcription and whether the virus remains latent depend on the ability of the cell to use the enhancers and promoter sequences encoded in the LTR region, the extent of methylation of the DNA region, and the cell's growth rate. Stimulation of the cell by mitogens, certain lymphokines, or infection with exogenous viruses (e.g., herpesviruses) produces transcription factors that also bind to the LTR and can activate transcription of the virus.

Viral oncogenes (if present) promote cell growth and as a result also stimulate transcription and virus replication. Replication of HTLV and HIV are more complex and are regulated further by other viral proteins.

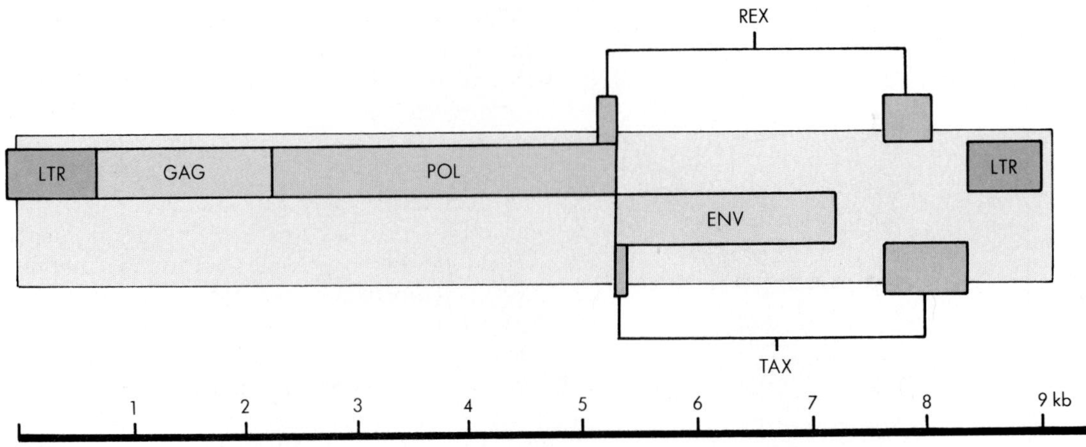

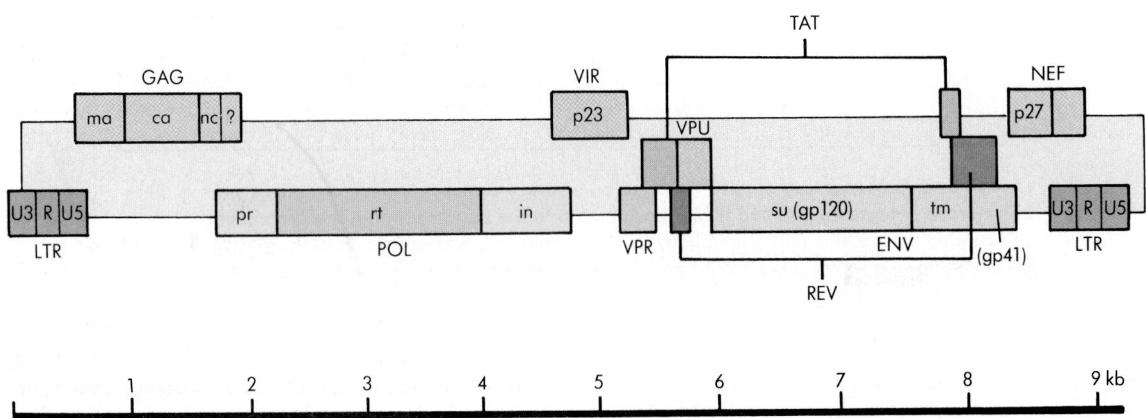

FIGURE 67-4 Genomic structure of human retroviruses. **A,** HTLV-1. The genes are defined in Table 67-2 and Figure 67-6. Unlike the other genes of these viruses, production of the mRNA for *tax* and *rex* (HTLV-1), and *tat* and *rev* (HIV) require excision of two intron units. Protein nomenclature for HIV: *ma*, matrix protein; *ca*, capsid protein; *nc*, nucleocapsid protein; *pr*, protease; *rt*, reverse transcriptase; *in* integrase; *su*, surface glycoprotein component; *tm*, transmembrane glycoprotein component. (Redrawn from Belshe RB, editor: *Textbook of human virology,* ed 2, St. Louis, 1991, Mosby.)

HTLV-1 encodes two proteins that regulate virus replication, **tax** and **rex**. Unlike the other viral mRNA, the mRNA for tax and rex requires more than one splicing step. The rex gene encodes two proteins that bind to a structure on the viral mRNA, preventing further splicing and promoting its transport to the cytoplasm. The doubly spliced tax/rex mRNA is expressed early (low concentration of rex), and structural proteins are expressed late (high concentration of rex). As a result, rex regulates the extent of mRNA processing, selectively enhancing the expression of the singly spliced structural genes late in infection. The tax protein is a transcriptional activator (*in trans*). Tax enhances transcription of the viral genome from the promotor gene sequence in the 5′LTR, as well as other genes including the lymphokine genes for IL2, IL3, and GM-CSF and the receptor for IL2. Activation of these genes leads to activation and growth of the infected T cell.

The expression of HIV proteins is regulated by as many as six gene products (see Table 67-2). The **nef**, **tat**, and **rev** genes produce proteins that create a network of regulatory factors that control their own synthesis and the synthesis of the virion's proteins. The tat, like tax, is a *t*rans*a*ctivator of *t*ranscription of viral and cellular genes. The rev acts like the rex protein. The nef protein represses expression of all the viral genes that may play a role in inducing latency. HIV is also under cellular control, and activation of the T cell by a mitogen or antigen also activates the virus.

The proteins translated from the gag, gag-pol, and env mRNAs are synthesized as polyproteins and are subsequently cleaved to functional proteins (see Figure 67-6). The viral glycoproteins are synthesized, glycosylated, and processed by the endoplasmic reticulum and Golgi apparatus. The glycoprotein is cleaved into a membrane spanning and an extracellular region and associates to

TABLE 67-2 Retrovirus Genes and Their Function

Gene	Virus	Function
gag	All	Group-specific antigen: core and capsid proteins
pol	All	Polymerase: reverse transcriptase, protease, integrase
env	All	Envelope: glycoproteins
tax	HTLV	Transactivation of viral and cellular genes
tat	HIV-1	Transactivation of viral and cellular genes
rex	HTLV	Regulation of RNA splicing and promotion of export to cytoplasm
rev	HIV-1	Regulation of RNA splicing and promotion of export to cytoplasm
nef	HIV-1	Negative early factor, down-regulates virus expression, promotes latency
vif	HIV-1	Virus infectivity, helps to initiate replication
vpu		Facilitates release of virus
vpr		Transactivator carried in virion
LTR		Long terminal repeats: promoter, enhancer elements

form dimers or trimers that migrate to the plasma membrane.

The gag and the gag-pol polyproteins are acylated and then bind to the plasma membrane. The association of two copies of the genome and cellular tRNA molecules with this aggregate triggers the release of the viral protease and cleavage of the gag polyproteins. This action releases the reverse transcriptase and forms the virion core, which remains associated with the virion glycoprotein-modified plasma membrane.

The virus buds from the plasma membrane and simultaneously acquires its envelope and is released from the cell. Cell-to-cell spread of HIV is further enhanced by its ability to form multinucleated giant cells, or syncytia. Syncytia are fragile, and their formation enhances the cytolytic activity of the virus.

HUMAN IMMUNODEFICIENCY VIRUS

Pathogenesis and Immunity

The major determinant in the pathogenesis and disease caused by HIV is the virus tropism for CD4 expressing T cells and macrophages. (Box 67-2 and Figure 67-7). The CD4 T cells are the helper and delayed type hypersensitivity (DTH) T cells.

After infection of these cells, the virus continues to replicate in lymph nodes but is latent in other T cells. The virus may remain latent for long periods, but when activated in CD4 T cells the virus kills the cell. This activation may occur after stimulation of the cell by an antigen or mitogen.

HIV induces several cytopathic effects that may kill the cell. These include accumulation of nonintegrated circular DNA copies of the genome, increased permeability of the plasma membrane, and syncytia formation. The ability of HIV to kill the target cell correlates with the amount of CD4 expressed by the cell. The gp120 binds tightly to CD4, can prevent its cell surface expression and immunological function, and promotes cell-cell fusion leading to cell lysis. Another theory for the cytolytic activity of HIV is binding of HIV virions or the gp 120 to CD4 molecules on T cells may trigger apoptosis (programmed cell death).

Macrophages are persistently infected with HIV. They may be spared the cytolytic action of gp120 because they express lesser amounts of CD4 than T cells. Monocytes and macrophages are probably the major reservoirs and means of distribution for HIV. Circulating macrophages, microglial cells of the brain, pulmonary alveolar macrophages, dendritic cells, and other cells of the monocyte-macrophage lineage can spread the virus and potentially contribute to HIV disease.

In addition to immunosuppressive disorders, HIV can also cause neurological abnormalities. The microglial cell and macrophage are the predominant cell type of the brain infected with HIV, but neurons and glial cells may also be infected. Infected monocytes and microglial cells may release neurotoxic substances or chemotactic factors to promote inflammatory responses in the brain. Direct cytopathic effects of the virus on neurons are also possible.

Neutralizing antibodies are generated against the gp120 protein and also participate in antibody-dependent cellular cytotoxicity (ADCC) responses. CD8+ cytotoxic T cells are also generated to the HIV-infected CD4+ cells. Other cell-mediated and cytokine responses may suppress the replication of HIV and promote latency following the initial acute phase of infection.

The ability of HIV to incapacitate the immune system, remain latent in lymphocytes, and alter its antigenicity allows the virus to escape immune clearance and prevents resolution of the disease (Table 67-3). The virus appears to establish a latent and low-level chronic infection in every infected individual. A slow progressive decrease in the levels of CD4 cells may precipitate immunodeficiency after long periods.

The central role of the CD4 helper T cell in the initiation of an immune response and for delayed type hypersensitivity (DTH) is indicated by the extent of immunosuppression induced by HIV infection (Figure 67-8, Table 67-4 and Box 67-3). Activation of the CD4

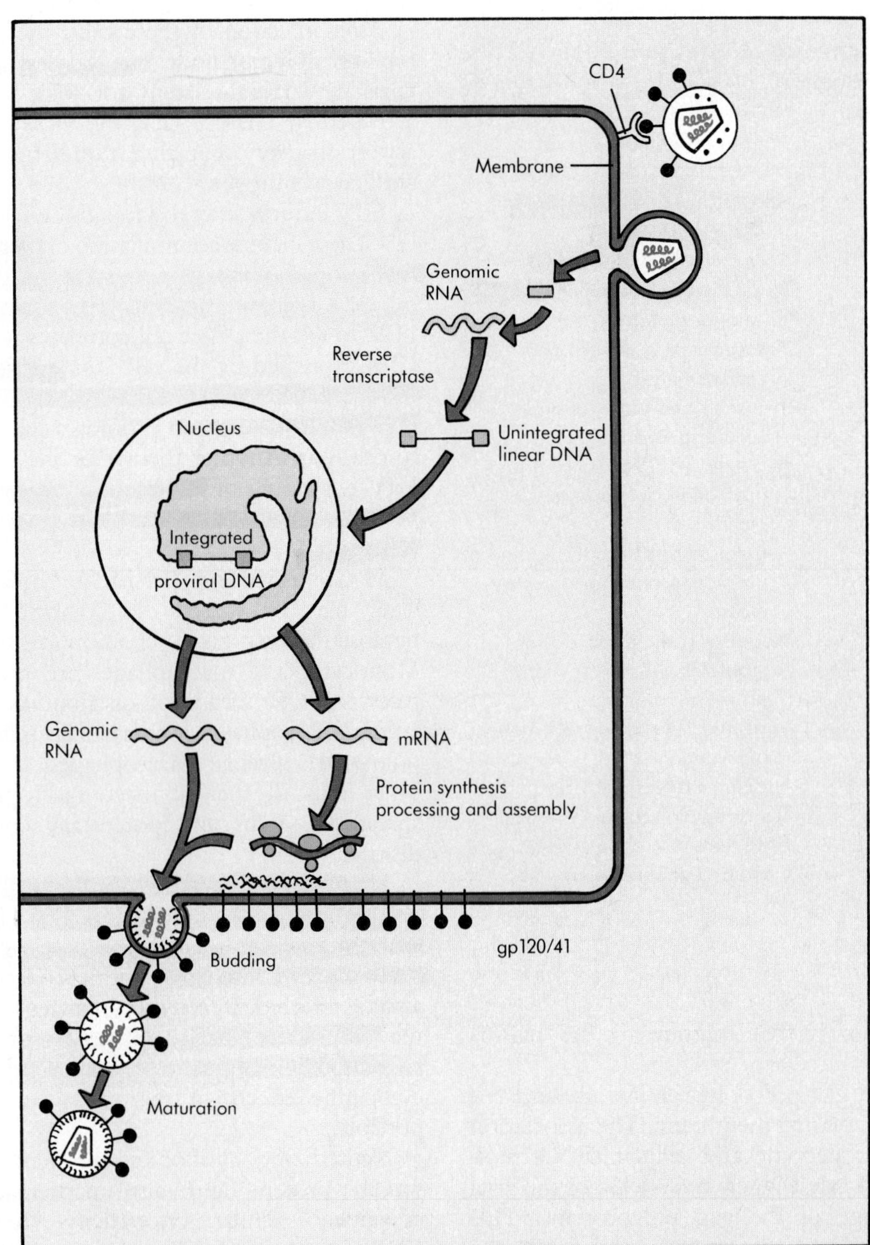

FIGURE 67-5 The life cycle of HIV. HIV binds to CD4 molecules and enters by fusion. The genome is reverse transcribed into DNA in the cytoplasm and integrated into the nuclear DNA. Transcription and translation of the genome occurs similar to HTLV-1 (see Figure 67-6). The virus assembles at the plasma membrane and matures after budding from the cell. (Redrawn from Fauci AS: *Science* 239:617-622, 1988.)

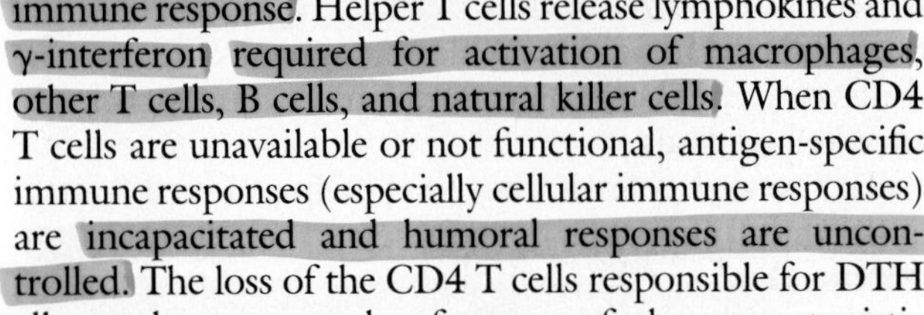

T cells is one of the first steps in the initiation of normal immune response. Helper T cells release lymphokines and γ-interferon required for activation of macrophages, other T cells, B cells, and natural killer cells. When CD4 T cells are unavailable or not functional, antigen-specific immune responses (especially cellular immune responses) are incapacitated and humoral responses are uncontrolled. The loss of the CD4 T cells responsible for DTH allows the outgrowth of many of the opportunistic infections characteristic of AIDS.

Epidemiology

AIDS was first described in male homosexuals in the United States but is spreading in epidemic proportions throughout the population (Box 67-4). An estimated 8 to 10 million people have been infected with HIV. As of mid-1992, more than 220,000 people are estimated to have AIDS in the United States (43,000 cases reported to the CDC for the entire year of 1992) and 500,000 worldwide as reported to WHO; these figures understate the estimated 1 million cases (Figures 67-9 and 67-10).

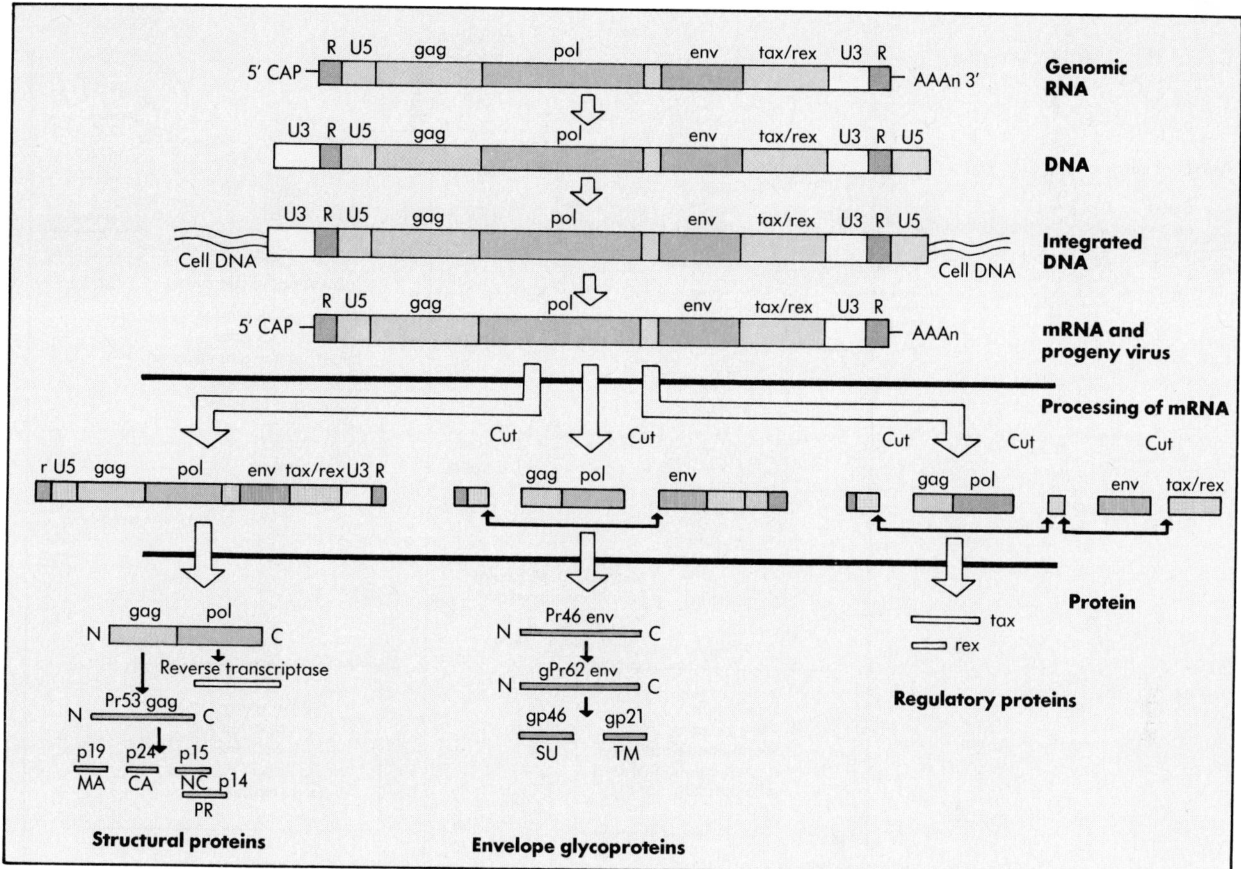

FIGURE 67-6 Transcription and translation of HTLV-1. The different mRNA for the env proteins are produced by one splice of the genome, whereas two splices are required for the tax/rex mRNA. Gene nomenclature: *gag*, group antigen gene; *pol*, polymerase; *env*, envelope glycoprotein gene; *tax*, transactivator; *rex*, regulator of expression of virion proteins. Protein nomenclature: *MA*, matrix; *CA*, capsid; *NC*, nucleocapsid; *PR*, protease; *SU*, surface component; *TM*, transmembrane component of envelope glycoprotein; *N*, N terminus; *C*, C terminus of peptide. Prefixes: *p*, protein; *Pr*, precursor polyprotein; *gp*, glycoprotein; *gPr*, glycosylated precursor polyprotein.

BOX 67-2 Disease Mechanisms of HIV

- HIV infects CD4+ T cells and cells of the macrophage lineage (e.g., monocytes, macrophages, alveolar macrophage of the lung, dendritic cells of the skin, and microglial cells of the brain)
- Causes lytic and subsequently latent infection of CD4 T cells and persistent low-level productive infection of macrophage lineage cells
- Causes syncytia formation with cells expressing large amounts of CD4 antigen (T cells) with subsequent lysis of the cells
- Alters T cell and macrophage cell function

All HIV-infected individuals whose disease has progressed to AIDS are expected to die of the complications of the disease.

HIV-1 is thought to be derived from a simian immunodeficiency virus. The initial human infection may have occurred in Africa relatively recently but went unnoticed in rural areas. The migration of infected individuals to the cities after the 1960s brought the virus into population centers, and the cultural acceptance of prostitution promoted its transmission through the population.

Transmission

The presence of HIV in blood, semen, and vaginal secretions of infected individuals and the long incubation period before symptoms promote the spread of the disease by sexual contact and exposure to contaminated blood and blood products (Table 67-5). The virus can also be transmitted perinatally to newborns. HIV is *not* transmitted by casual contact, touching, hugging, kissing, coughing, sneezing, insects, water, food, or utensils, toilets, swimming pools, or public baths.

Populations at Highest Risk

Sexually active individuals (homosexual *and* heterosexual), intravenous drug users and their sexual partners,

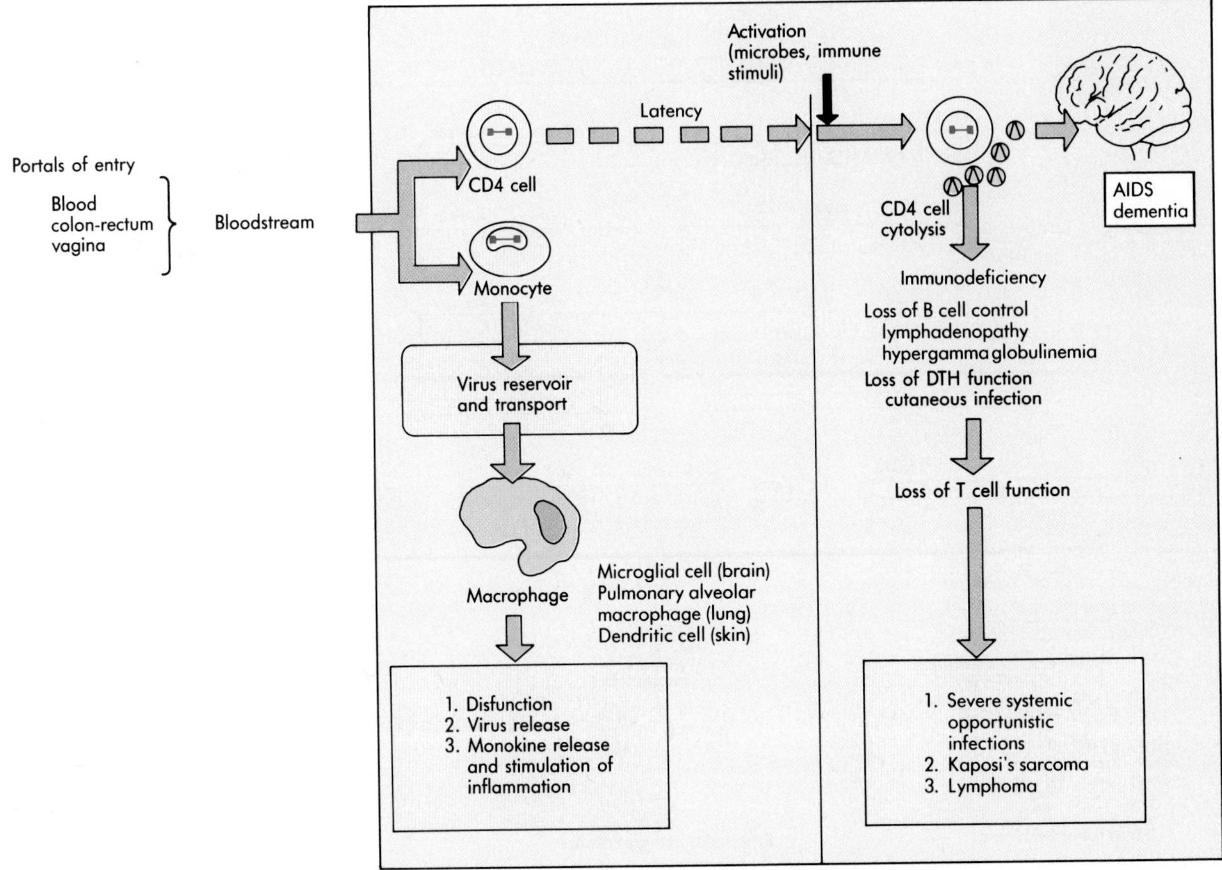

FIGURE 67-7 Pathogenesis of HIV. HIV causes lytic and latent infection of CD4 T cells, persistent infection of cells of the monocyte/macrophage family, and disrupts neurons. The outcomes of these actions are immunodeficiency and AIDS dementia. (Redrawn from Fauci AS: *Science* 239:617-622, 1988.)

TABLE 67-3 Means of HIV Escape from the Immune System

Characteristic	Function
Infection of lymphocytes and macrophages	Inactivates key elements of immune defense
Inactivation of CD4 helper cells	Loss of activator of the immune system and delayed type hypersensitivity response
Antigenic drift of the gp120	Evade antibody detection
Heavy glycosylation of gp120	Evade antibody detection
Latent infection	Evade immune resolution

and newborns of HIV-positive mothers are at highest risk to HIV infections. Blacks and Hispanics are disproportionally represented in the HIV-positive population. Health care workers who may come in contact with contaminated blood or blood products are also at increased risk to infection.

AIDS was initially observed in young promiscuous male homosexuals and is still prevalent in the gay community. Anal intercourse is an efficient means of transmission of the virus. However, heterosexual transmission by vaginal intercourse and intravenous drug abuse have become the major routes of spread of HIV in the population. Sharing of contaminated syringe needles is common practice in "shooting galleries." In New York City more than 80% of intravenous drug abusers are HIV antibody positive, and these individuals are the major source of heterosexual and congenital transmission of the virus.

Before 1985, individuals receiving blood transfusions, organ transplants, and hemophiliacs receiving clotting factors from pooled blood were at high risk to HIV infection. Screening of the blood supply has practically eliminated the incidence of transfusion-related transmission of HIV. Hemophiliac recipients of pooled clotting factors are protected further by proper handling of the factor (prolonged heating) to kill the virus. However, as many as 60% of hemophiliac individuals may be HIV antibody positive, reflecting prior exposure to HIV-contaminated factor VIII pooled from thousands of donors.

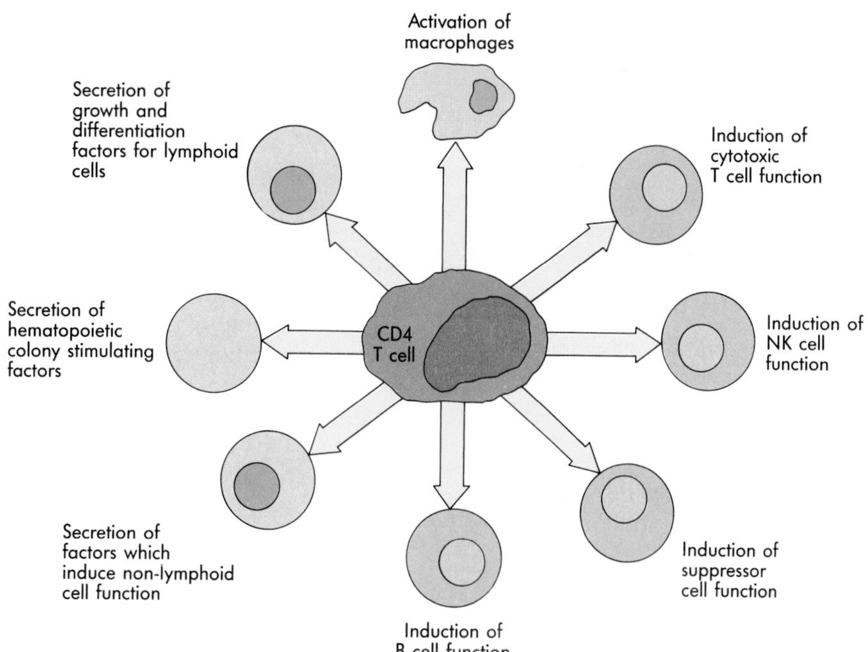

FIGURE 67-8 The CD4 T cell plays a critical role in the regulation of the human immune response by the release of soluble factors and the delayed type hypersensitivity response towards intracellular pathogens. Thus destruction of CD4 T cells by HIV has a dramatic impact. (Redrawn from Fauci AS: *Science* 239:617-622, 1988.)

TABLE 67-4 Immune Function Abnormalities Resulting from HIV Infection

Cells	Abnormalities
T helper (CD4) lymphocytes	Decreased proliferative responses
	Decreased T-cell help and control
	Decreased cytotoxic T-cell activity against virus-infected cells
	Decreased DTH response
Monocytes	Decreased chemotaxis
	Decreased IL-1 production
	Decreased microbiocidal activity
	Increased release of TNF and other cytokines
Natural killer cells	Decreased cytotoxic activity
B lymphocytes	Decreased antigen-specific humoral responses (antibody production)
	Uncontrolled production of antibody (hypergammaglobulinemia)

BOX 67-3 Mechanisms of HIV-Induced Immune Suppression

DIRECT

HIV cytocidal effect on CD4 lymphocytes
Syncytia formation
Functional defects in infected CD4 cells
Impaired antigen presentation or monokine production by macrophage

INDIRECT

Generation of suppressor T cells or factors
Induction of autoimmune phenomena
Cytotoxic cell activity against viral or self-proteins
Decreased humoral immune responses

Interestingly, HIV-seropositive hemophiliac persons are less prone to developing "full-blown AIDS" than are sexually active individuals and intravenous drug abusers. This has suggested that a cofactor may be required to activate the virus and cause AIDS. Co-infection or reactivation of latent viruses such as the herpesviruses (herpes simplex, Epstein-Barr, cytomegalovirus, HHV6) or hepatitis B may induce HIV replication from latently infected cells.

A small number of health care workers have contracted HIV infection from accidental needle sticks, cuts, or exposure of broken skin to contaminated blood. Prospective studies of needle stick recipients indicate that fewer than 1% of those exposed to HIV-positive blood experience seroconversion. Tattoo needles and contaminated inks are another potential vector of HIV transmission.

BOX 67-4 Epidemiology of HIV Infections

DISEASE/VIRAL FACTORS

Enveloped virus is easily inactivated and must be transmitted in body fluids
Disease has a long prodrome period
Virus can be shed before the development of identifiable symptoms

TRANSMISSION

Virus is present in blood, semen, and vaginal secretions
See Table 67-5 for modes of transmission

WHO IS AT RISK?

IV drug abusers, multipartner sexually active individuals (homosexual and heterosexual), prostitutes, newborns of HIV-positive mothers
Before 1985: blood and organ transplant recipients, hemophiliacs

GEOGRAPHY/SEASON

Expanding epidemic worldwide
No seasonal incidence

MODES OF CONTROL

Antiviral drugs: AZT, ddI, and ddC delay the onset and control the severity of symptoms and decrease the extent of virus production and shedding
Vaccines for prevention and treatment are in trials
Safe monogamous sex
Use of clean, sterile injection needles
Large-scale screening programs of the blood and organ supply used for transplants, transfusions, and production of clotting factors used by hemophiliacs

Geographical Distribution

The incidence of HIV-1 infections is spreading worldwide. The largest number of AIDS cases are reported in the Americas and Africa, with a growing number of cases from Asia (see Figure 67-10). HIV-2 is much more prevalent in Africa (especially West Africa) than in the United States. Heterosexual transmission is the major means of spread for both HIV-1 and HIV-2 in Africa, and both men and women are equally affected by these viruses. HIV-2 produces a disease similar to but less severe than AIDS.

Clinical Syndromes

HIV disease may be viewed as a continuum from asymptomatic infection to profound immunosuppression, sometimes referred to as "full-blown AIDS" (Figure 67-11). The diseases related to AIDS are mainly due to opportunistic infections, cancers, and direct effects of HIV on the central nervous system (Box 67-5).

Initial HIV infection is asymptomatic or resembles infectious mononucleosis with an "aseptic" meningitis or a rash. As in mononucleosis, the symptoms correspond to immune responses to a widespread infection of lymphoid cells. This illness subsides spontaneously and is followed by a latent period that may last many years before the symptoms of acquired immunodeficiency syndrome (AIDS). Current understanding is that at least 60% of HIV-infected individuals will become symptomatic, and the overwhelming majority of these will ultimately succumb to AIDS. AIDS is therefore one of the most devastating epidemics ever recorded.

The definition of AIDS is currently based on the presence of antibody to HIV, a reduction of CD4 T-cell levels to less than 500/mm^3, HIV wasting syndrome (weight loss and diarrhea for more than 1 month) and occurrence of Kaposi's sarcoma or specific opportunistic diseases, especially *Pneumocystis carinii* pneumonia. Some patients may progress through all the syndromes just mentioned, whereas others may have Kaposi's sarcoma or *Pneumocystis carinii* pneumonia without ever having earlier symptoms or signs.

AIDS may manifest in one of several different ways:

Lymphadenopathy and Fever (AIDS-Related Complex, or ARC)

This process develops insidiously and may be accompanied by weight loss and malaise. These findings may persist indefinitely or may progress. Symptoms may also include opportunistic infections, diarrhea, night sweats, and fatigue.

Opportunistic Infections

Normally benign infections by agents such as yeast and other fungi, DNA viruses capable of recurrent disease, parasites, and intracellular growing bacteria cause significant disease following HIV depletion of CD4+ T cells. *Pneumocystis carinii* pneumonia is a major sign of AIDS. Oral candidiasis (thrush), cerebral toxoplasmosis, and cryptococcal meningitis often occur, as well as prolonged and severe infections by the herpesviruses (e.g., herpes simplex virus; varicella-zoster virus; Epstein-Barr virus–induced hairy leukoplakia of the mouth; cytomegalovirus illnesses (especially retinitis, pneumonia, and gay bowel disease) and papovaviruses (JC: progressive multifocal leukoencephalopathy [PML]). Tuberculosis and other mycobacterial diseases and diarrhea caused by common pathogens (*Salmonella, Shigella, Campylobacter*) and uncommon agents (cryptosporidia, mycobacteria, *Amoeba*) occur frequently.

Malignancies

The most notable malignancy is the development of Kaposi's sarcoma, a previously benign skin cancer that disseminates to involve visceral organs in these immunodeficient patients. Non-Hodgkin's lymphoma and EBV-related lymphomas are also prevalent.

Wasting

The progressive development of "slim disease" is especially common in Africa.

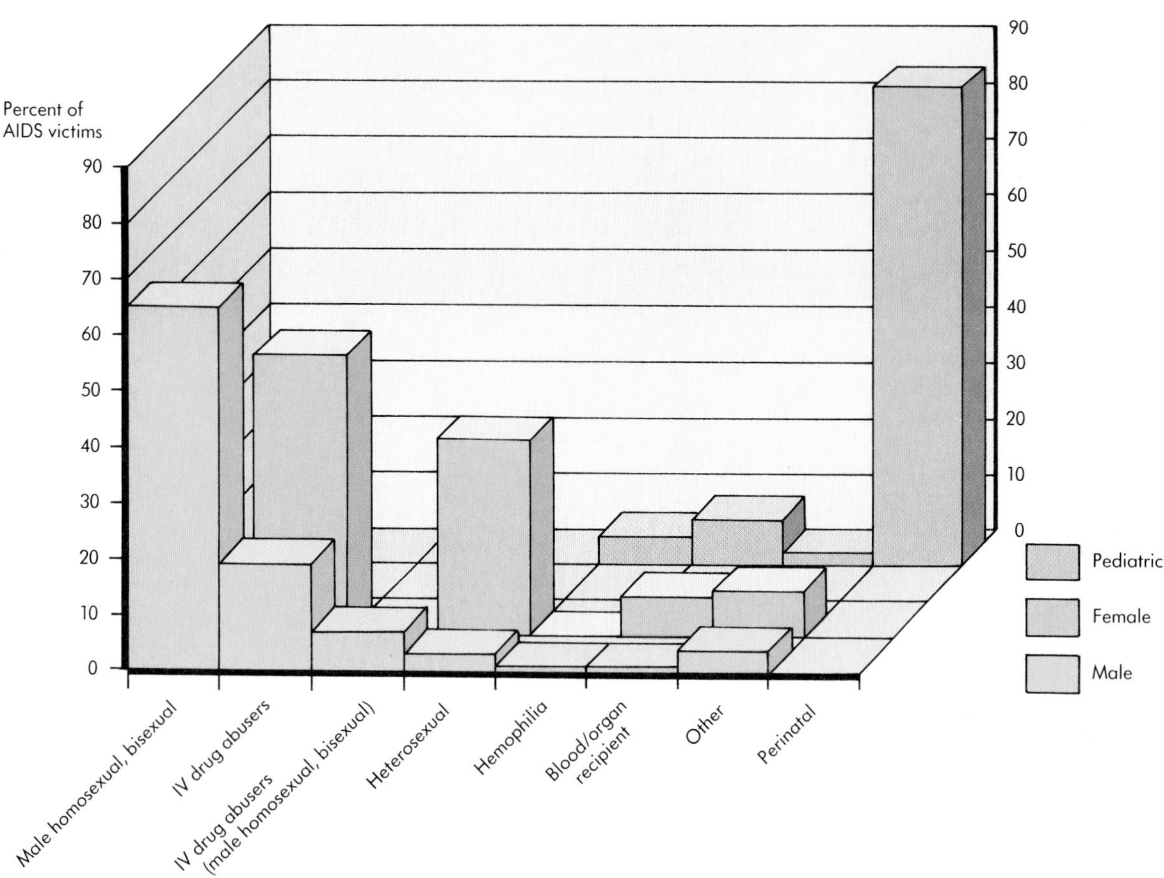

FIGURE 67-9 AIDS statistics for the United States as of June 1992. The percentages of AIDS cases are presented by exposure category for men, women, and children under 13. Unlike Africa and many other parts of the world, male homosexuals are the largest exposure category in the United States. However, intravenous drug abusers and heterosexual partners are becoming more prevalent. (Data reported by CDC and published in *AIDS 1992* vol 6:1229-1233).

AIDS-Related Dementia

This may result from HIV infection of the microglial cells and neurons of the brain. Patients may undergo a slow deterioration of intellectual abilities and other signs of neurological disorder, similar to those of the early stages of Alzheimer's disease.

Laboratory Diagnosis

Identification of HIV-positive individuals is performed to initiate antiviral drug therapy, to identify carriers who may transmit infection to others (specifically blood or organ donors, pregnant women, and sex partners), and to confirm the diagnosis of AIDS (Table 67-6). The chronic nature of the disease allows use of serology for documenting HIV infection. Unfortunately, serologic diagnosis cannot identify recently infected individuals. This is a big problem for screening HIV-positive individuals. The presence of the p24 viral antigen indicates recent infection. The virus cannot be routinely isolated.

Serology

Enzyme linked immunosorbent assay (ELISA) or agglutination procedures are used for routine screening. More specific procedures, such as Western blot and immunofluorescent assay (IFA), are subsequently used to confirm seropositive results. The ELISA test measures antibody to one or more envelope proteins (e.g., gp120) and can generate false positive data. The Western blot assay (see Figure 53-13) determines the presence of antibody to each of the viral antigens, including the core protein (p24). The presence of serum antibody does not label a patient as having AIDS; the latter is a clinical diagnosis that depends on symptomatology, signs, and other laboratory tests. HIV antibody may develop slowly, requiring 4 to 8 weeks in most patients but 6 months or more in as many as 5% of those infected (see Figure 67-11).

Reverse Transcriptase and Antigen Assays

Detection of HIV and other retroviruses is often accomplished by measuring the appearance of reverse transcriptase in serum or medium and, for HIV, detecting viral antigen (p24) in the medium. The p24 antigen can be detected in the lymphocytes of as many as 60% of patients with HIV infection and indicates that active viral replication is occurring. This antigen is detectable during the initial acute phase of HIV disease and then disappears as the virus enters the latent state (see Figure 67-11), only

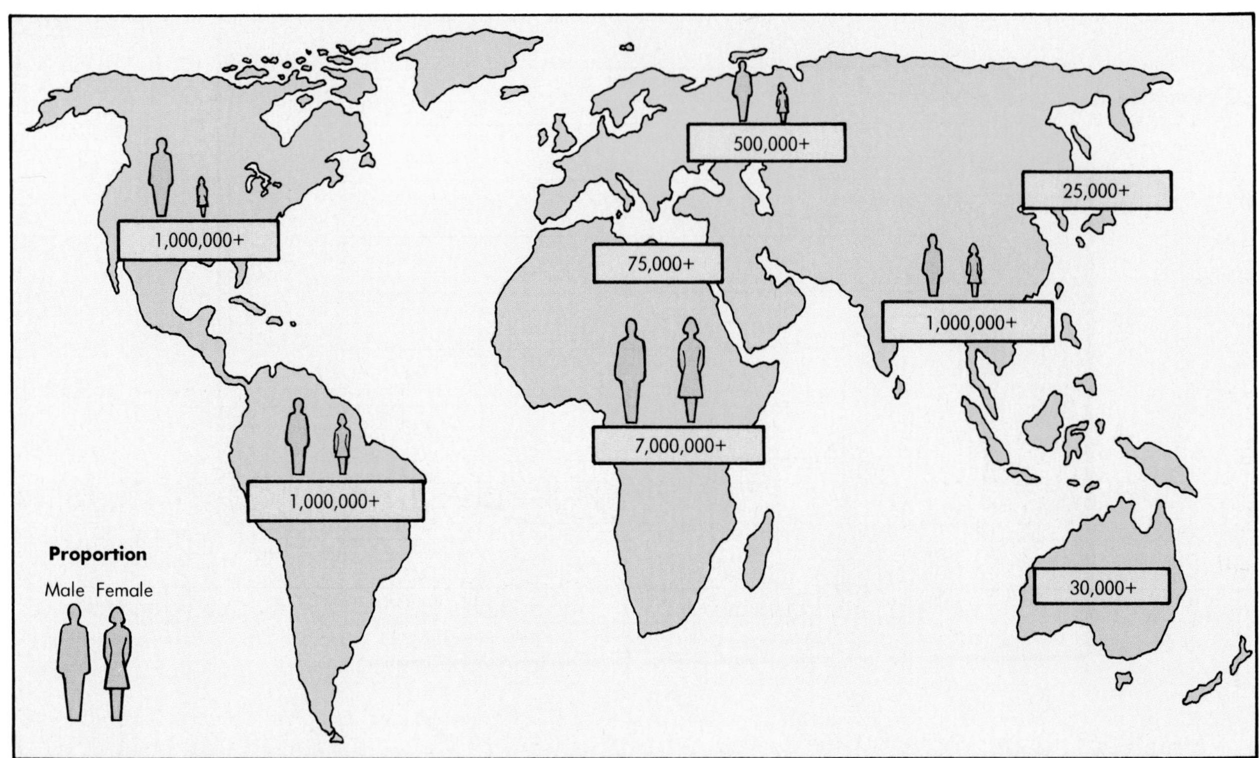

FIGURE 67-10 Estimated cumulative global distribution of adult HIV infections, July 1992. The estimated cumulative global total of HIV-infected adults in 1992 is about 10 million, which means that, for the world population, 1 in every 250 adults has been infected with HIV. Infection rates vary widely in different regions of the world. The highest rates are in sub-Saharan Africa, where 1 in 40 men and 1 in 40 women are estimated to be infected, with an estimated cumulative total of more than 6.5 million. (Modified from Global programme On AIDS: current and future dimensions of the HIV/AIDS pandemic; a capsule summary, [WHO/GPA/RES/SFI/92.1] Geneva, July 1992, World Health Organization.)

to reappear years after infection when widespread replication resumes.

Culture

Culture of HIV is more difficult than for many other viruses of human importance and is not done routinely. The virus is cell associated and requires co-culture of patient peripheral blood mononuclear cells (PBMCs) with PBMCs from non–HIV-infected donors in the presence of IL-2 to promote the growth of T cells in culture. Culture appears to detect even latent virus. Characteristic CPE includes syncytia formation and cytolysis.

Immunological Studies

Indication of an HIV infection can be obtained from analysis of T-lymphocyte subsets. The absolute number of CD4 lymphocytes and the ratio of helper to inducer lymphocytes (CD4/CD8 ratio) are abnormally low in HIV-infected individuals. The stage of AIDS disease is defined by the concentration of CD4 lymphocytes.

Treatment, Prevention, and Control

Treatment

An extensive program to develop antiviral drugs and vaccines against HIV has been initiated worldwide (Table 67-7). Azidothymidine (AZT), dideoxyinosine (ddI) and

TABLE 67-5 Transmission of HIV Infection

Routes	Specific transmission
Known routes of transmission	
Inoculation of blood	Transfusion of blood and blood products
	Needle sharing among intravenous drug users
	Needle stick, open wound, and mucous membrane exposure in health care workers
	Tattoo needles
Sexual	Anal and vaginal intercourse
Perinatal	Intrauterine
	Peripartum
	Breast milk
Routes investigated and shown *not* to be involved in transmission	
Close personal contact	Household members
	Health care workers not exposed to blood

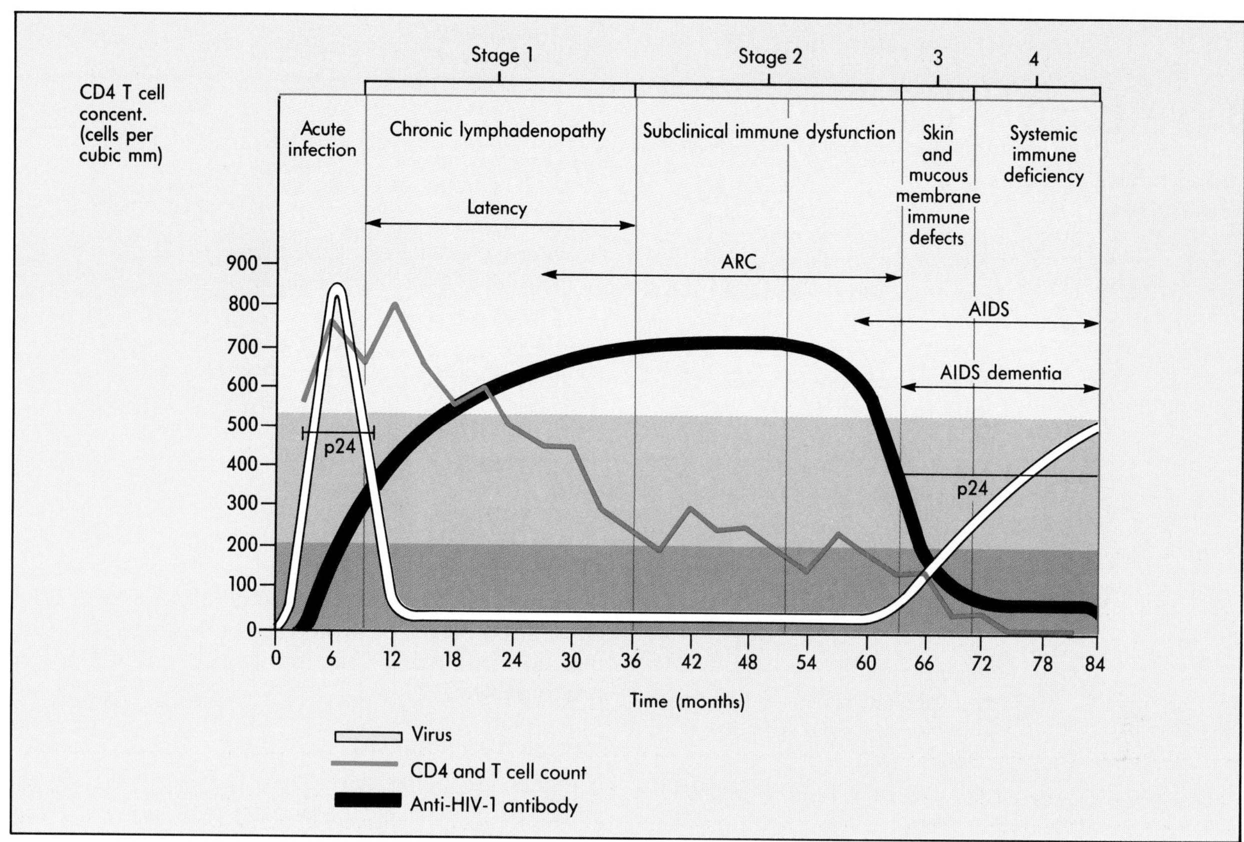

FIGURE 67-11 Time course and stages of HIV disease. A long latent period follows the initial mononucleosis-like symptoms. The progressive decrease in CD4 T lymphocytes, even during the latency period, allows opportunistic infections. The stages (World Health Organization [WHO] and Centers for Disease Control [CDC]) in HIV disease are defined by the CD4 T-cell levels and opportunistic diseases. (Redrawn from Redfield RR and Buske DS: *Sci Am* 259:90-98, 1988.)

dideoxycytidine (ddC) are the only anti-HIV drugs approved by the U.S. Food and Drug Administration (FDA), but several others are currently in clinical trials. Antiviral drug therapy cannot cure an HIV infection but can delay or possibly prevent the onset of symptoms.

AZT, ddI, and ddC inhibit the reverse transcriptase and, after incorporation into DNA, cause chain termination. These drugs produce significant toxic side effects that must be monitored. However, administration of AZT earlier in the infection allows use of lower doses with less toxicity and better outcomes. Current guidelines allow AZT treatment for asymptomatic or mildly symptomatic individuals with CD4 counts less than 500.

Other approaches to anti-HIV drug development include other nucleotide analogues and other inhibitors of reverse transcriptase, receptor antagonists (CD4 and gp120 analogues), protease inhibitors, inhibitors of tat function (Ro 24-7429), glycoprotein glycosylation inhibitors, interferon and interferon inducers, and antisense RNA to essential genome sequences (see Chapter 16).

Education

The principal method for control of HIV infection is to alert the population to the methods of transmission and measures that may curtail virus spread. Monogamous relationships, practice of safe sex, and the use of condoms reduce the possibility of exposure. Contaminated needles are a major source of HIV in intravenous drug abusers and must not be shared. Reuse or contaminated needles in clinics were the source of outbreaks in former Soviet Bloc and other countries. In some locations efforts are being launched to provide sterile equipment to intravenous drug abusers.

Blood and Blood Product Screening

Individuals and blood products are screened before use. Individuals testing positive for HIV must not donate blood. Methods to encourage this must be improved. Individuals who anticipate the need for blood, such as those awaiting elective surgery, should consider donating blood beforehand. To limit the worldwide epidemic, blood screening must be initiated in underdeveloped nations.

Infection Control

The infection control procedures for HIV are the same as for hepatitis B virus. Universal blood and body fluid precautions should be taken. Universal precautions mean that all patients should be assumed to be infectious for HIV and other blood-borne pathogens. Protective cloth-

BOX 67-5 Indicator Diseases of Acquired Immunodeficiency Syndrome (AIDS)*

Opportunistic infections	
Protozoal	Toxoplasmosis of the brain Cryptosporidiosis with diarrhea Isosporiasis with diarrhea
Fungal	Candidiasis of the esophagus, trachea, lungs *Pneumocystis carinii* pneumonia Cryptococcosis, extrapulmonary Histoplasmosis, disseminated Coccidioidomyocosis, disseminated
Viral	Cytomegalovirus disease Herpes simplex virus infection, persisting or disseminated Progressive multifocal leukoencephalopathy
Bacterial	*Mycobacterium avium* complex, disseminated Any "atypical" mycobacterial disease Extrapulmonary tuberculosis *Salmonella* septicemia, recurrent Multiple or recurrent pyogenic bacterial infections
Opportunistic neoplasias	
Kaposi's sarcoma	
Primary lymphoma of the brain	
Other non-Hodgkin's lymphomas	
Others	
HIV wasting syndrome	
HIV encephalopathy	
Lymphoid interstitial pneumonia	

From Belshe RB, editor: *Textbook of human virology*, ed 2, St. Louis, 1991, Mosby.
*Manifestations of human immunodeficiency virus (HIV) infection defining AIDS according to criteria of Centers for Disease Control.

ing (e.g., gloves, mask, and gown) and other barriers should be used to prevent exposure to blood products. Contaminated surfaces should be disinfected with either 10% household bleach, 70% ethanol or isopropanol, 2% glutaraldehyde, 4% formaldehyde, or 6% hydrogen peroxide. Laundry washing in hot water with detergent should be sufficient to inactivate the virus.

TABLE 67-6 Laboratory Analysis for HIV

Test	Detects
Serology	Initial screening
ELISA	
Latex agglutination	
Western blot analysis	Confirmation test
Immunofluorescence	Confirmation test
p24 antigen	Early marker of infection
Isolation of virus	Not readily available
CD4/CD8 T cell ratio	Correlate of HIV disease

Immunization

Unlike many other viruses, natural infection with HIV is not a good means of protecting individuals from future infection or disease since recurrence and AIDS seems unavoidable.

Vaccine Development

Vaccines are being developed and evaluated for their ability to protect and potentially treat HIV infections. A successful vaccine would prevent acquisition of virus by adults and transmission of virus to infants by HIV-positive mothers and block the progression of the disease.

Most approaches to an HIV vaccine utilize gp120 or its precursor, gp160, as immunogen. The gene for this protein has been cloned and expressed in different eukaryotic cell systems (e.g., yeast, baculovirus) and developed as a subunit vaccine. The env gene has also been incorporated into vaccinia virus to create a hybrid vaccine. Inoculation with this virus should mimic vaccination with a live virus and elicit both humoral and cellular responses to the viral antigen. Specific epitopes and T-cell antigens are also being investigated.

The development of a vaccine against AIDS is fraught with several problems unique to the virus. Initial protection would require secretory antibody to prevent sexual transmission of the virus. Antibody alone may be insufficient to protect against HIV infection; a cellular immune response may also be necessary. The antigenicity of the virus changes through mutation. The virus can be spread through syncytia and also remains latent in an individual, hiding from antibody. HIV also infects and inactivates those cells required to initiate an immune response.

In addition to the problems of the virus and the vaccine development, the efficacy of the vaccines must be tested in human trials and a proper regimen of vaccination developed to elicit protective immunity. Finally, evaluating the success of the vaccine in limiting the spread and morbidity of HIV infection will be difficult. Long-term

TABLE 67-7 Potential Antiviral Therapies for HIV Infection

Drug	Target	Status
ANTIVIRAL DRUGS		
Azidothymidine (AZT)	Reverse transcriptase	FDA approved
Dideoxycytidine (ddC)	Reverse transcriptase	FDA approved
Dideoxyinosine (ddI)	Reverse transcriptase	FDA approved
VACCINES		
gp160/120 subunit vaccines	Genetically engineered, elicits antibody	Trials
gp120/vaccinia hybrid	Genetically engineered, elicits antibody and cell-mediated immunity	Trials
Killed vaccine	Nucleic acid inactivated	Trials

follow-up will be required to monitor efficacy, and unlike the hepatitis B virus vaccine, serologic responses may not be sufficient to indicate success.

HUMAN T-LYMPHOTROPIC VIRUS AND OTHER ONCOGENIC RETROVIRUSES

The oncoviruses were originally called the RNA tumor viruses and have been associated with leukemias, sarcomas, and lymphomas in many different animals. These viruses are not cytolytic. The members of this family are distinguished by the mechanism of cell transformation and thus the length of the latency period between infection and development of disease (Table 67-8).

A large group of oncoviruses, the sarcoma/acute leukemia viruses, have incorporated into their genome cellular genes (**proto-oncogenes**), which encode growth-controlling factors into their genome, such as growth hormones, growth hormone receptors, protein kinases, guanosine triphosphate(GTP)-binding proteins, and nuclear DNA-binding proteins. These viruses can cause transformation and are highly oncogenic. At least 35 different viral oncogenes have been identified (Table 67-9). The mutations from the original cellular proto-oncogene present in the viral oncogene, or the overproduction of the oncogene, promote the transformation of an infected cell.

Incorporation of the oncogene into many of these viruses replaces coding sequences for the gag, pol, or env genes such that these viruses are defective and require helper viruses for replication. Many of these viruses remain endogenous and are transmitted vertically through the germ line.

TABLE 67-8 Mechanisms of Retrovirus Oncogenesis

Disease	Speed	Effect
Acute leukemia/sarcoma	Fast: oncogene	Direct effect Provision of growth-enhancing proteins
Leukemia	Slow: transactivation	Indirect effect Insertion mutagenesis Proximity of viral promoters and enhancers to growth genes

The leukemia viruses, including HTLV-1, are replication competent but cannot transform cells in vitro. They cause cancer after a long latent period, at least 30 years. The virus may promote the outgrowth of the cell in two ways. First, by integrating near and juxtaposing the viral enhancer and promoter gene sequences of the LTR region to cellular growth-controlling genes, the virus may activate their expression. Second, a transcriptional regulator, tax, is produced that is capable of activating promotors in the LTR region and specific cellular genes (including growth-controlling and lymphokine genes such as interleukin-2 and GM-CSF) to promote the outgrowth of that cell. Uncontrolled cell growth may be sufficient to transform the cell neoplastically or may promote other genetic aberrations over a long period. These viruses are also associated with nonneoplastic neurological disorders and other diseases. HTLV-1 causes **adult acute T-cell lymphocytic leukemia (ATLL)** and also **tropical spastic paraparesis**, a nononcogenic neurological disease.

The human oncoviruses include HTLV-1, HTLV-2, and HTLV-5, but only HTLV-1 has been definitively associated with disease (ATLL). HTLV-2 was isolated from atypical forms of hairy cell leukemia, and HTLV-5 was isolated from a malignant cutaneous lymphoma. HTLV-1 and HTLV-2 share as much as 50% homology.

Pathogenesis and Immunity

HTLV-1 is cell associated and is spread in cells following blood transfusion, sexual intercourse, or breast-feeding. The virus enters the bloodstream and infects the CD4 helper and DTH T lymphocytes. These T cells have a tendency to reside in the skin, which contributes to the symptoms of ATLL. Neurons also express a receptor for HTLV-1.

HTLV is competent for replication, and the gag, pol, and env genes are transcribed, translated, and processed, as described earlier. In addition to its action on viral

TABLE 67-9 Representative Examples of Oncogenes

Function	Oncogene	Virus
Tyrosine kinase		
	src	Rous sarcoma virus
	abl	Abelson murine leukemia virus
	fes	ST feline sarcoma virus
Growth factor receptors		
	erb-B (EGF receptor)	Avian erythroblastosis virus
	erb-A (thyroid hormone receptor)	Avian erythroblastosis virus
GTP-binding proteins		
	Ha-ras	Harvey murine sarcoma virus
	Ki-ras	Kirsten murine sarcoma virus
Nuclear proteins		
	myc	Avian myelocytomatosis virus MC29
	myb	Avian myeloblastosis virus
	fos	Murine osteosarcoma virus FBJ
	jun	Avian sarcoma virus 17

Modified from Jawetz E, Melnick JL, Adelberg EA et al.: *Medical microbiology*, ed 18, Los Altos, Calif, 1989, Appleton & Lange.

genes, the tax protein transactivates the cellular genes for the T-cell growth factor, IL-2 and its receptor, which activates growth in the infected cell. The virus may remain latent or replicate slowly for many years but may also induce the clonal outgrowth of particular T-cell clones.

Although the virus can induce a polyclonal outgrowth of T cells, the HTLV-1–induced **adult T-cell leukemia (ATL)** is usually monoclonal. Chromosomal aberrations and rearrangements in the T-cell antigen receptor beta gene may accumulate in the HTLV growth-stimulated cells and produce the leukemia.

Antibodies are elicited to the gp46 and other proteins of HTLV-1. The presence of these antibodies in infected individuals may down-regulate the expression of viral antigens. This would prevent cell-mediated immune clearance of virally infected cells. HTLV-1 infection also causes immune suppression.

Epidemiology

HTLV-1 is endemic in southern Japan and is also found in the Caribbean and among Blacks in the southeastern United States. In the endemic regions of Japan, children obtain HTLV-1 from their mothers in breast milk, whereas adults are infected sexually. The seroconversion rate on some southern Japanese islands may be as high as 13%, with a mortality resulting from leukemia double that of other regions. Transmission of HTLV-1 by illicit intravenous drug use and blood transfusion is becoming more prominent in the United States.

Clinical Syndromes

HTLV infection is usually asymptomatic but can progress to ATLL in approximately 1 in 20 persons over a 30- to 50-year period. ATLL caused by HTLV-1 is a neoplasia of CD4 helper T cells that can be acute or chronic. The malignant cells have been termed "flower cells," are pleomorphic, and contain lobulated nuclei. In addition to an elevated white blood cell count, this form of ATLL is characterized by skin lesions similar to another leukemia, Sézary syndrome. Acute ATLL is usually fatal within 1 year of diagnosis regardless of treatment.

Laboratory Diagnosis

HTLV-1 infection is detected immunologically by the presence of viral-specific antigens in blood.

Treatment, Prevention and Control

No treatment has been proved effective against HTLV-1 infection. Presumably AZT and other inhibitors of reverse transcriptase would be effective against HTLV-1, but controlled studies are needed to prove the benefit of this approach.

The means for limiting the spread of HTLV-1 are the same as for HIV. Sexual precautions, screening the blood supply, and increased awareness of the potential risks and diseases will help block transmission of the virus. Maternal infection of children is very difficult to control. Routine screening procedures for HTLV-1 in the blood supply are likely to be instituted in the near future.

ENDOGENOUS RETROVIRUSES

Different retroviruses have integrated into and become a part of the chromosomes of humans and animals. Complete and partial provirus sequences can be detected in humans with gene sequences similar to HTLV, mouse mammary tumor virus, and other retroviruses. These endogenous viruses generally lack the ability to replicate because of deletions, insertion of termination codons, or are poorly transcribed. Retrovirus sequences may make up as much as 0.1% of the human genome. They may represent integration sites for other retroviruses or serve an unknown function.

CASE STUDY AND QUESTIONS

A 28-year-old male has several complaints. He has a bad case of thrush (oral candidiasis), serious bouts of diarrhea, low-grade fever, has lost 20 pounds in the last year without dieting, and most seriously, complains of difficulty breathing. His lungs show bilateral infiltrate on x-ray examination, characteristic of *Pneumocystis pneumoniae*. A stool sample is positive for giardia. He is a heroin addict and admits to sharing needles at a "shooting gallery."

1. What laboratory tests should be done to support and confirm a diagnosis of HIV infection and AIDS?
2. How did this individual acquire the HIV infection? What are other high-risk behaviors for HIV infection?
3. What is the immunological basis for the increased susceptibility of this patient to opportunistic infections?
4. What precautions should be taken in handling samples from this patient?
5. Several forms of HIV vaccines are being developed. What are possible components of an HIV vaccine? Who would be appropriate recipients of an HIV vaccine?

Bibliography

AIDS articles, *Science* 239(4840), Feb. 5, 1988.

AIDS '91 Summary: a practical synopsis of The VII International Conference, Richmond, Va, 1992, Philadelphia Sciences Group.

AIDS: Ten years later, *FASEB J* 5:2338-2455, 1991. A series of reviews.

Allain J-P, Gallo RC, and Montagnier L, editors: *Human retroviruses and disease they cause*, Symposium Highlights, Chicago, 1988, Excerpta Medica.

Anderson RM: Understanding the AIDS pandemic, *Sci Am*, May 1992

Cann AJ and Chen ISY: Human T-cell leukemia virus type I and II. In Fields BN and Knipe DM, editors: *Virology*, ed 2, New York, 1990, Raven Press.

Coffin JM: Retroviruses and their replication. In Fields BN and Knipe DM, editors: *Virology*, ed 2, New York, 1990, Raven Press.

Curr Top Microbiol Immunol 160: A series of reviews.

Fauci AS: The human immunodeficiency virus: infectivity and mechanisms of pathogenesis, *Science* 239:617-622, 1988.

Guidelines for prevention of transmission of human immunodeficiency virus and hepatitis B virus to health-care and public-safety workers, *MMWR* 38 (S-6) 1989.

Hehlmann R: Human retroviruses. In Belshe RB, editor: *Textbook of human virology*, ed 2, St. Louis, 1991, Mosby.

Hehlmann R and Erfle V: Introduction to Retroviruses. Human Retroviruses. In Belshe RB, editor: *Textbook of human virology*, ed 2, St. Louis, 1991, Mosby.

Hirsch MS and Curran J: Human immunodeficiency viruses. In Fields BN and Knipe DM, editors: *Virology*, ed 2, New York, 1990, Raven Press.

Levy JA: Pathogenesis of human immunodeficiency virus infection, *Microbiol Rev* 57:183-289.

Ng VL and McGrath MS: Human T-cell leukemia virus involvement in adult T-cell leukemia, *Cancer Bull* 40:276-280, 1988.

Oldstone MBA and Koprowski H. Retrovirus Infections of the Nervous System, 1990. Schüpbach J. 1989. Human Retrovirology, *Curr Top Microbiol Immunol* 142:1989. A series of reviews.

The Science of AIDS 1989: readings from *Sci Am*, Scientific American Books.

Williams AO: AIDS: an African perspective, Boca Raton, Fla, 1992, CRC Press.

What science knows about AIDS, *Sci Am* Oct. 1988.

Wong-Staal F: Human immunodeficiency viruses and their replication. In Fields BN and Knipe DM, editors: *Virology*, ed 2, New York, 1990, Raven Press.

CHAPTER 68

Hepatitis Viruses

THERE are at least five viruses, A through E, that are called hepatitis viruses (Table 68-1). Although the target organ for each of these viruses is the liver, they differ greatly in their structure, mode of replication, course of disease, and mode of transmission. The hepatitis A and B viruses are the best known, but in recent years two non-A, non-B viruses (C and E) have been described, as has hepatitis D, the delta agent. Additional non-A, non-B agents may also exist.

Each of the hepatitis viruses infects and damages the liver, causing classic icteric symptoms of jaundice and release of liver enzymes. The specific course, nature, and serology of the disease are different for each virus. These viruses are readily spread since infected individuals are contagious before, or even without, showing symptoms.

Hepatitis A (1) is caused by a picornavirus that contains ribonucleic acid (RNA) and is sometimes known as *"infectious hepatitis,"* (2) is spread by the fecal-oral route, (3) has an incubation period of approximately 1 month, (4) does not cause chronic liver disease, and (5) rarely causes fatal disease.

Hepatitis B, previously known as *"serum hepatitis,"* (1) is produced by a deoxyribonucleic acid (DNA) virus, (2) is spread parenterally by blood or needles, by sexual contact, and perinatally, (3) has a median incubation period of approximately 3 months, (4) is followed by chronic hepatitis in 5% to 10% of patients, and (5) is causally associated with primary hepatocellular carcinoma. An estimated 300,000 cases of hepatitis B occur in the United States each year, with 4000 fatalities caused by this agent.

Non-A, non-B hepatitis viruses (**NANBHV**) include the newly described hepatitis C, E, and possibly other undefined hepatitis viruses. Hepatitis C virus (HCV) is spread by the same routes as HBV and can also cause chronic disease, but is a flavivirus and differs in mode of replication and general course of disease. Hepatitis E virus (HEV) is an enteric virus.

Delta hepatitis, or hepatitis D virus (HDV), is unique in that it occurs only in patients who have active hepatitis B virus infection. HDV replicates only in the presence of actively replicating hepatitis B virus. HBV acts as a "helper" agent for hepatitis D by providing an envelope for delta virus RNA and its antigen(s). Acute and chronic hepatitis may be caused by the delta agent.

HEPATITIS A VIRUS

Hepatitis A virus (HAV) causes infectious hepatitis and is spread by the fecal-oral route. HAV infections often result from consumption of contaminated shellfish or other food and water. HAV is a picornavirus and has been renamed **Enterovirus 72**.

Structure

HAV has the structural characteristics of a picornavirus (Figure 68-1). It has a 27 nm naked icosahedral capsid surrounding a positive single-stranded RNA genome of approximately 7470 nucleotides. The HAV genome has a VPg protein attached to the 5′end and polyadenosine attached to the 3′end. The capsid is extremely stable (Box 68-1).

Replication

Replication of HAV has not been studied as extensively as that of other picornaviruses (see Chapter 59). HAV interacts specifically with a receptor expressed on liver cells and establishes a slow steady-state infection with little or no cytopathology in the cells. Laboratory isolates of HAV have been adapted to growth in continuous monkey kidney cell lines, but clinical isolates are very difficult to grow in cell culture.

Pathogenesis

The details of the pathogenesis of HAV can be determined only by analogy with other enteroviruses and limited numbers of animal studies. HAV is ingested, probably replicates in the oropharynx and the epithelial lining of the intestines, initiates a transient viremia, and is targeted to parenchymal cells of the liver (Figure 68-2). The virus can be localized by immunofluorescence in hepatocytes and Kupffer's cells. Virus is produced in these cells and is released into the bile and from there into the stool. Virus is shed into the stool approximately 10 days before symptoms or antibody can be detected.

HAV replicates slowly in the liver without apparent cytopathic effect (CPE). Replication of the virus elicits interferon production, which works to limit virus replication to some extent but also activates natural killer cells. Antibody, complement, and antibody-dependent cellular cytotoxicity also facilitate the clearance of the virus and

TABLE 68-1 Comparative Features of Hepatitis Viruses

	Hepatitis A	Hepatitis B	Hepatitis C	Hepatitis D	Hepatitis E
Common name	"Infectious"	"Serum"	"Non A Non B–post-transfusion"	"Delta"	"Enteric Non A Non B"
Virus structure	Picornavirus Capsid, RNA	Hepadnavirus Envelope, DNA	Flavivirus Envelope, RNA	Viroid-like Envelope, circular RNA	Calicivirus-like Capsid, RNA
Transmission	Fecal-oral	Parenteral, sexual	Parenteral, sexual	Parenteral, sexual	Fecal-oral
Onset	Abrupt (varies)	Insidious (varies)	Insidious (varies)	Abrupt (varies)	Abrupt (varies)
Incubation period	15-50 days	45-160 days	14-180 days	15-64 days	15-50 days
Severity	Mild	Occasionally severe	Usually subclinical	Co-infection with HBV occasionally severe; superinfection with HBV often severe	Normal patients: mild; pregnant patients: severe
Mortality	<0.5%	1%-2%	0.5%-1%	High to very high	Normal patients: 1%-2%; pregnant patients: 20%
Chronicity/carrier state	No	Yes	Yes	Yes	No
Other disease associations	None	Primary hepatocellular carcinoma, cirrhosis	Primary hepatocellular carcinoma, cirrhosis	Cirrhosis, fulminant hepatitis	None
Laboratory diagnosis	Symptoms and anti-HAV IgM	Symptoms and serum levels of HBsAg, HBeAg, and anti-HBc IgM	Symptoms and anti-HCV ELISA	Anti-HDV ELISA	—

the induction of immunopathology. Icterus resulting from damage to the liver occurs simultaneously with detection of antibody to the virus. Mononuclear cell infiltrates are also observed in areas affected by HAV at the same time as liver enzymes are noted in the serum.

The liver pathology caused by HAV infection is indistinguishable histologically from that caused by HBV. Liver damage is most likely caused by immunopathology instead of virus-induced cytopathology. However, unlike HBV, HAV cannot initiate a chronic infection and is not associated with hepatic cancer.

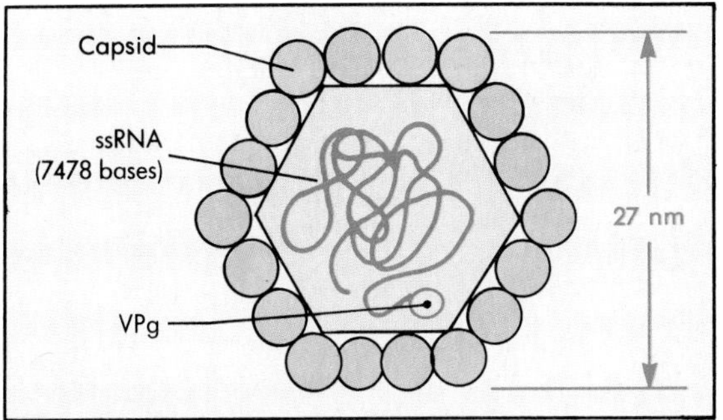

FIGURE 68-1 Diagram of the picornavirus structure of the hepatitis A virus (HAV). The icosahedral capsid is made up of four viral polypeptides (VP1 to VP4). Inside the capsid is a single-strand positive sense RNA that has a genomic viral protein (VPg) on the 5′end.

Epidemiology

Approximately 40% of acute hepatitis cases are caused by HAV (Box 68-2). Spread is by person-to-person contact, usually via a fecal-oral route, or by exposure to contaminated food or water. Close personal contact facilitates spread. The virus is transiently present in blood, but high concentrations of virus are present in feces for several weeks, especially in the 2 weeks before the onset of jaundice. Virus is not present in urine or other body fluids, and a chronic carrier state does not occur. The virus spreads readily in a community since most individuals are contagious before symptoms and 90% of children and 25% to 50% of adults have inapparent but productive infections.

HAV is spread by the fecal-oral route—in contaminated water, in foods, and by dirty hands. HAV is resistant to detergents, acid, temperatures elevated as high as 60° C, and can survive for many months in fresh and salt water. Raw or improperly treated sewage can taint the water supply and contaminate shellfish. Shellfish are very efficient filter feeders and can concentrate the viral particles, even from dilute solutions.

HAV outbreaks usually originate from a common source (e.g., water supply, restaurant, day-care center). Day-care settings are a major source of spread of the virus. HAV can spread among classmates and to their parents. Since the children and personnel in day-care centers may be transient, the number of contacts at risk for HAV infection from a single day-care center can be great.

The incidence of HAV infection is directly related to poor hygienic conditions and overcrowding. Most individuals infected with HAV in developing countries are children who have mild illness and then lifelong immune protection to reinfection. In more highly developed countries, infection occurs later in life. The seropositivity rate of adults ranges from a low 13% of the adult population in Sweden to 88% in Taiwan and 97% in Yugoslavia, with a 41% to 44% rate in the United States.

BOX 68-1 Characteristics of Hepatitis A Virus

Stable to
- Acid at pH 3
- Solvents (ether, chloroform)
- Detergents
- Saltwater, groundwater (months)
- Drying (stable)
- Temperature:
  - −20° C to −70° C: years
- 4° C: weeks
- 56° C for 30 minutes: stable
- 61° C for 20 minutes: partial inactivation

Inactivated by
- Chlorine treatment of drinking water
- Formalin (0.35%, 37° C, 72 hours)
- Peracetic acid (2%, 4 hours)
- B-propiolactone (0.25%, 1 hour)
- Ultraviolet radiation (2 $\mu W/cm^2/min$)

Clinical Syndromes

The symptoms caused by hepatitis A are very similar to those for hepatitis B and are caused by immune-mediated damage to the liver. The disease in children is generally milder than for adults and usually asymptomatic. HAV symptoms occur abruptly 15 to 50 days after exposure and increase for 4 to 6 days before the icteric (jaundice) phase (Figure 68-3). Jaundice is observed in 2 of 3 adults but only 1 or 2 of 10 children. Symptoms generally wane during the jaundice period. Virus shedding in the stool precedes the onset of symptoms by approximately 14 days

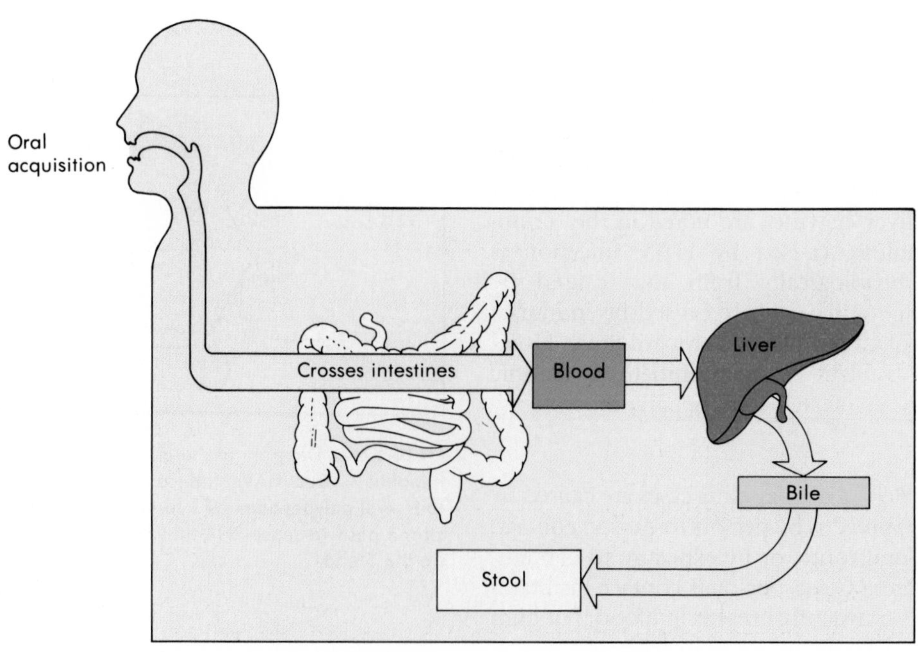

FIGURE 68-2 Spread of HAV within the body.

BOX 68-2 Epidemiology of Hepatitis A and Hepatitis E Virus Infections

DISEASE/VIRAL FACTORS

Capsid viruses very resistant to inactivation
Contagious period extends from before to after symptoms
May cause asymptomatic shedding

TRANSMISSION

Fecal-oral transmission
Ingestion of contaminated food and water
Hepatitis A virus in shellfish from sewage-contaminated water
Transmitted by food handlers, day-care workers, children

WHO IS AT RISK?

Persons in overcrowded, unsanitary areas
Children: mild disease, possibly asymptomatic; day-care centers a major source of spread of hepatitis A virus
Adults: abrupt onset hepatitis
Pregnant women: high mortality with hepatitis E virus

GEOGRAPHY/SEASON

Worldwide
No seasonal incidence

MEANS OF CONTROL

Good hygiene
HAV: Passive antibody protection for contacts
Active vaccine in development

but ceases before the cessation of symptoms. Complete recovery occurs 99% of the time.

Fulminant hepatitis in HAV infection occurs in 1 to 3 persons per 1000, with an 80% mortality. Unlike HBV, immune complex–related symptoms (e.g., arthritis, rash) rarely occur in HAV disease.

Laboratory Diagnosis

The diagnosis of hepatitis A is generally made from the time course of the clinical symptoms, identification of a known infected source, and most reliably by specific serologic tests. The best means for demonstrating acute HAV infection is the presence of anti-HAV IgM, measured by an enzyme linked immunosorbent assay (ELISA) or radioimmunoassay (RIA). Detection of HAV antigen or infectious virus in the stool is possible but difficult, because efficient tissue culture systems for growing the virus are not available and virus may be shed before symptoms are observed.

Treatment, Prevention, and Control

Spread of hepatitis A is reduced by interrupting the fecal-oral spread of the virus. Potentially contaminated water or food, especially uncooked shellfish, must be avoided. Proper handwashing, especially in day-care centers, mental hospitals, and other care facilities, is very important. Chlorine treatment of drinking water is generally sufficient to kill the virus.

Prophylaxis with immune serum globulin (ISG) given before or early in the incubation period (i.e., less than 2 weeks after exposure) is 80% to 90% effective in preventing clinical illness.

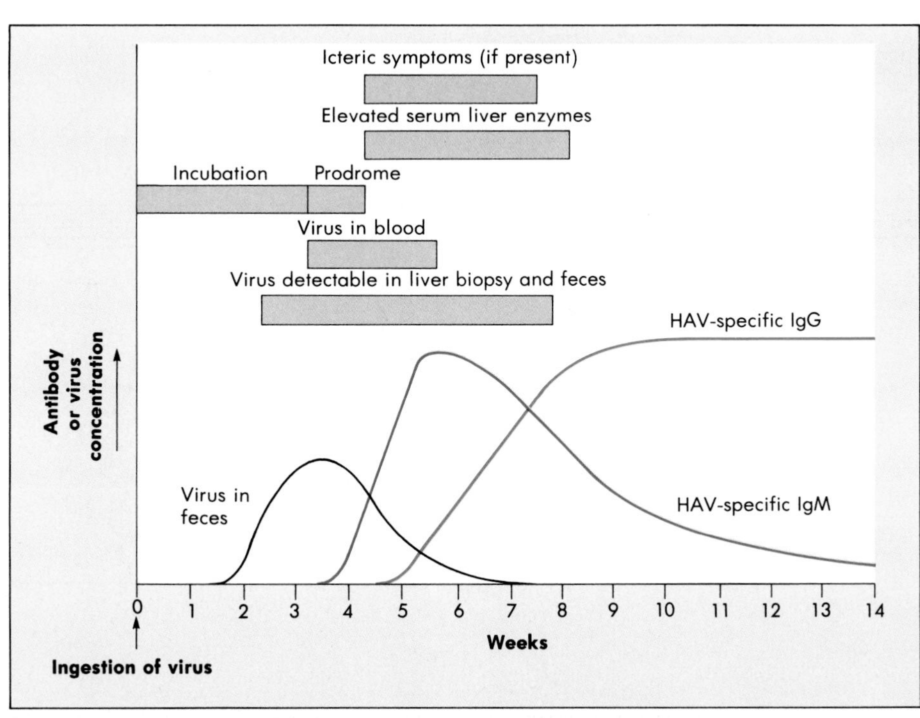

FIGURE 68-3 Time course of HAV infection.

Hepatitis A is a candidate for vaccine development because only one serotype has been identified. A vaccine for HAV has become a reality since the development of tissue culture systems for cultivation of the virus. Initial clinical trials of a killed virus vaccine were encouraging.

BOX 68-3 Unique Features of Hepadnaviruses

Enveloped virion containing partial double-stranded circular DNA genome
Replicates through a circular RNA intermediate
Virus encodes and carries a reverse transcriptase
Virus encodes several proteins (HBsAg (1,m,s); HBe/HBc) that share genetic sequences but with different mRNA or in-frame start codons (AUG)
HBV has a strict tissue tropism to the liver
HBV-infected cells produce and release large amounts of HBsAg particles lacking DNA
The HBV genome can integrate into the host chromosome

HEPATITIS B VIRUS

Hepatitis B virus (HBV) is the major member of the hepadnaviruses, a small family of enveloped DNA viruses. Other members of this family (Box 68-3) include woodchuck, ground squirrel, and duck hepatitis viruses. These viruses have very limited tissue tropisms and host ranges. HBV infects the liver and possibly the kidney and pancreas of only humans and chimpanzees. Molecular biological advances have allowed study of HBV despite the limited host range and the lack of a cell culture system for growing HBV.

Structure

HBV is a small enveloped DNA virus with several unusual properties (Figure 68-4). The genome is a small circular, partly double-stranded DNA of only 3200 bases. Although a DNA virus, it encodes a reverse transcriptase and replicates through an RNA intermediate.

The virion, also called the **Dane particle**, is 42 nm in diameter. The virions are unusually stable for an enveloped virus. They resist treatment with ether, low pH, freezing, and moderate heating. This assists trans-

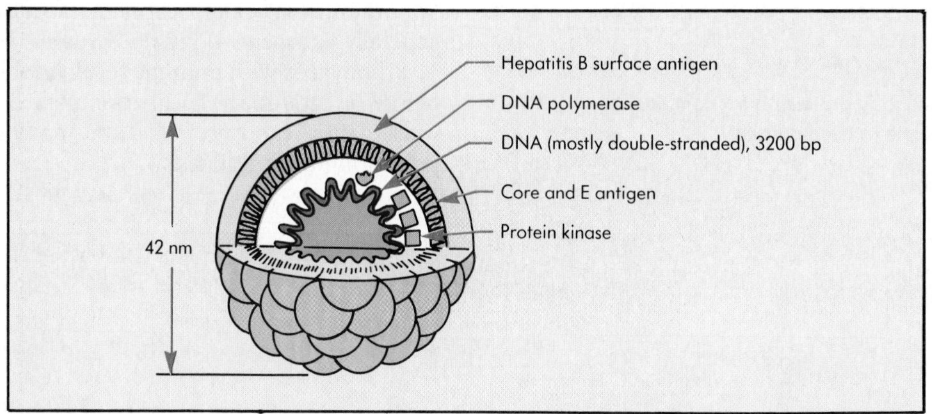

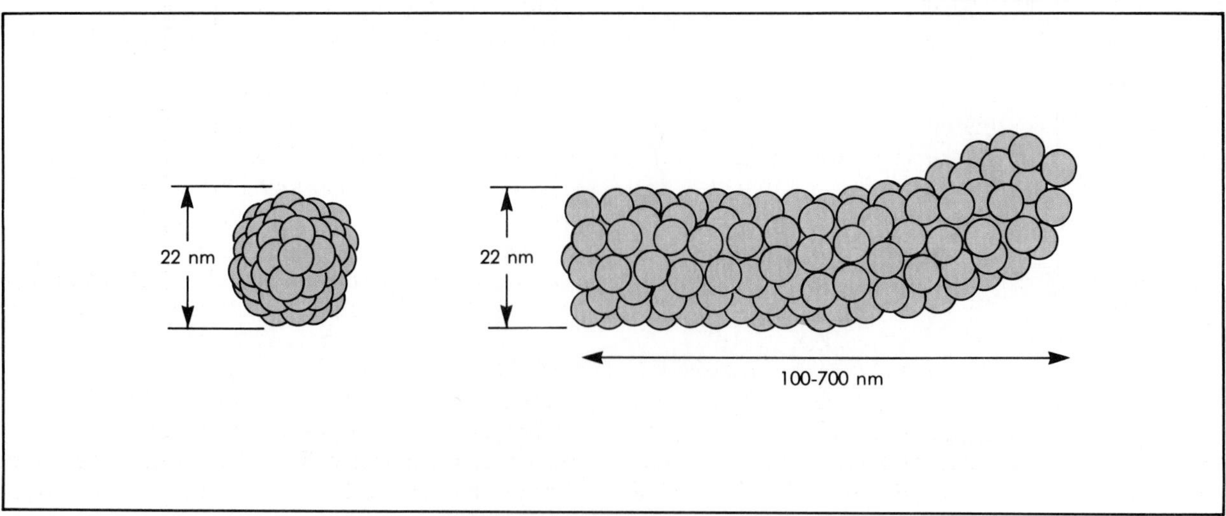

FIGURE 68-4 Hepatitis B virus (Dane particle) and HBsAg particles.

mission from one individual to another and hampers disinfection.

The HBV virion includes a polymerase with reverse transcriptase activity and a protein kinase surrounded by the core antigen **(HBcAg)** and an envelope containing the glycoprotein surface antigen **(HBsAg)**. An **HBeAg** protein is a minor component of the virion. The HBeAg and HBcAg proteins share most of their protein sequence. However, the HBeAg is processed differently by the cell, is primarily secreted into serum, does not self-assemble like a capsid antigen, and expresses different antigenic determinants.

HbsAg-containing particles are released into serum of infected individuals and outnumber the actual virions. These particles can be spherical (but smaller than the dane particle) or filamentous (Figure 68-4). These particles are immunogenic and were processed into the first commercial vaccine against HBV.

The HBsAg, originally termed the **Australia antigen,** is found in the envelope, on the surface of the virion, and on the **spherical** and **filamentous particles**. The HBsAg include three glycoproteins (L, M, S) encoded by the same gene, read in the same frame, but translated into protein from different AUG start codons. The **S** protein is completely contained in the **M** protein, which is contained in the **L**; all share the same C-terminal amino acid sequences. The three forms of HBsAg are found in equimolar amounts in the virion. The **S** or small glycoprotein (gp27; 24 to 27 kd) is the major component of HBsAg particles. The **S** glycoprotein self-associates into 22 nm spherical particles that are released from the cells. The filamentous particles of HBsAg found in serum contain mostly S but also small amounts of the **M** (gp36; 33 to 36 kd) and **L** (gp42; 39-42 kd) glycoproteins and other proteins and lipids. The L glycoprotein is an essential component for virion assembly and promotes filament formation and retention of these structures in the cell. The glycoproteins of HBsAg contain the group- (termed a) and type-specific determinants of HBV (termed d or y and w or r). Combinations of these antigens (e.g., ady, adw) result in eight subtypes of HBV that are useful epidemiological markers.

Replication

Replication of HBV is unique for several reasons (see Box 68-1). HBV has a very defined tropism for the liver. Its small genome necessitates economy as illustrated by the pattern of its transcription and translation. In addition, HBV replicates through an RNA intermediate and produces and releases antigenic decoy particles (HBsAg) (Figure 68-5).

HBV attachment to hepatocytes is mediated by the HBsAg glycoproteins. The actual receptor and mechanism of entry are not known. However, HBsAg binds to polymerized human serum albumin and other serum proteins, and this interaction may target the virus to the liver.

On penetration into the cell, the partial DNA strand of the genome is completed to form a complete double-strand DNA circle and delivered to the nucleus. Transcription of the genome is controlled by cellular transcription elements found in hepatocytes. The DNA is transcribed into three major classes (2100, 2400, and 3500 bases) and two minor classes (900 bases) of overlapping mRNAs (Figure 68-6). The 3500 base mRNA is larger than the genome. It encodes the HBc and HBe antigens, the polymerase, and a protein primer for DNA replication and also acts as the template for replication of the genome. The HBe and HBc are related proteins that are translated from different in-phase start codons of closely related mRNA. This causes differences in their processing, structure, and distribution in the cell and virion. Similarly, the 2100 base mRNA encodes both the small and medium glycoproteins from different in-phase start codons. The 2400 base mRNA overlaps the 2100 base mRNA and also encodes the large glycoprotein. The 900 base mRNA encodes the X protein, which promotes virus replication as a transactivator of transcription and protein kinase.

Replication of the genome occurs in the cytoplasm. The 3500 base mRNA is packaged into the nucleocapsid that contains the RNA-dependent DNA polymerase. This polymerase has **reverse transcriptase** and riboendonuclease H activity but lacks the integrase activity of the retrovirus enzyme. Negative-strand DNA is synthesized on a protein primer, also included in the core using the 3500 base RNA as template. The RNA is degraded by the polymerase as the DNA is synthesized. The positive-strand DNA is then synthesized from the negative DNA template. The nucleocapsid is enveloped within HBsAg-containing membranes, capturing genomes containing RNA-DNA circles with different lengths of RNA. Continued degradation of the remainder of the RNA in the virion yields a partly double-strand DNA genome. The virion is probably released from the hepatocyte by exocytosis and not by cell lysis.

The entire genome can also be integrated into the host chromatin. HBsAg, but not other proteins, can often be detected in the cytoplasm of cells containing integrated HBV DNA. The significance of the integrated DNA to replication of the virus is not known, but integrated viral DNA has been found in hepatocellular carcinomas.

Pathogenesis and Immunity

HBV can cause acute or chronic, symptomatic, or asymptomatic, hepatitis. Which of these occurs seems to be determined by the individual's immune response to the infection. Detection of both the HBsAg and the HBeAg components of the virion in the blood indicates ongoing active infection (Figure 68-7). HBsAg particles will continue to be released into the blood even after virion release has ended and until the infection is resolved.

The major source of infectious virus is blood, but HBV can be found in semen, saliva, milk, vaginal and menstrual secretions, and amniotic fluid. The most efficient means of acquiring HBV is by injection into the bloodstream. Common but less efficient routes of infection are sexual contact and birth.

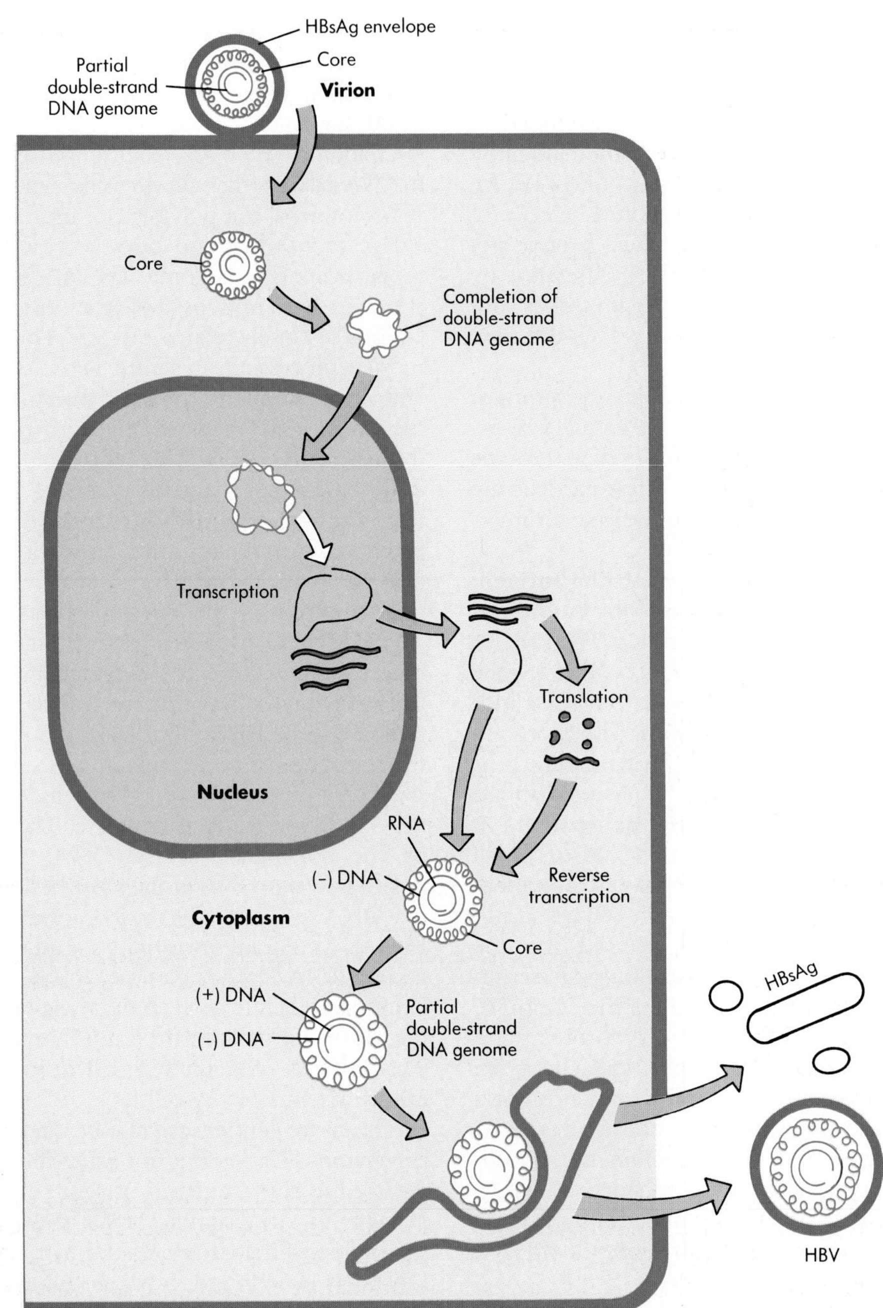

FIGURE 68-5 Proposed pathway for replication of hepatitis B virus. Following entry into the hepatocyte and uncoating of the nucleocapsid core, the partially double-stranded DNA genome is completed by enzymes in the core and then delivered to the nucleus. Transcription of the genome produces four mRNA including a mRNA larger than the genome (3500 bases). The mRNA moves to the cytoplasm and is translated into protein. Core proteins assemble around the 3500 base mRNA and (-) sense DNA is synthesized by a reverse transcriptase activity in the core. The RNA is then degraded as a (+)DNA is synthesized. The core is enveloped before completion of the (+)DNA and then released by exocytosis.

Initiation of virus replication may occur within 3 days of acquisition. Symptoms may not be observed for 45 days or longer, depending on the infecting dose of virus, the route of infection, and the individual. The virus replicates in hepatocytes with minimal cytopathic effect and proceeds for relatively long periods without causing liver damage (i.e., elevation of liver enzymes) or symptoms. During this time, copies of the HBV genome integrate into the hepatocyte chromatin and remain latent. Intracellular buildup of filamentous forms of HBsAg can produce the ground glass hepatocyte cytopathology characteristic of HBV infection.

Cell-mediated immunity and inflammation are responsible for both the symptomatology and the resolution of

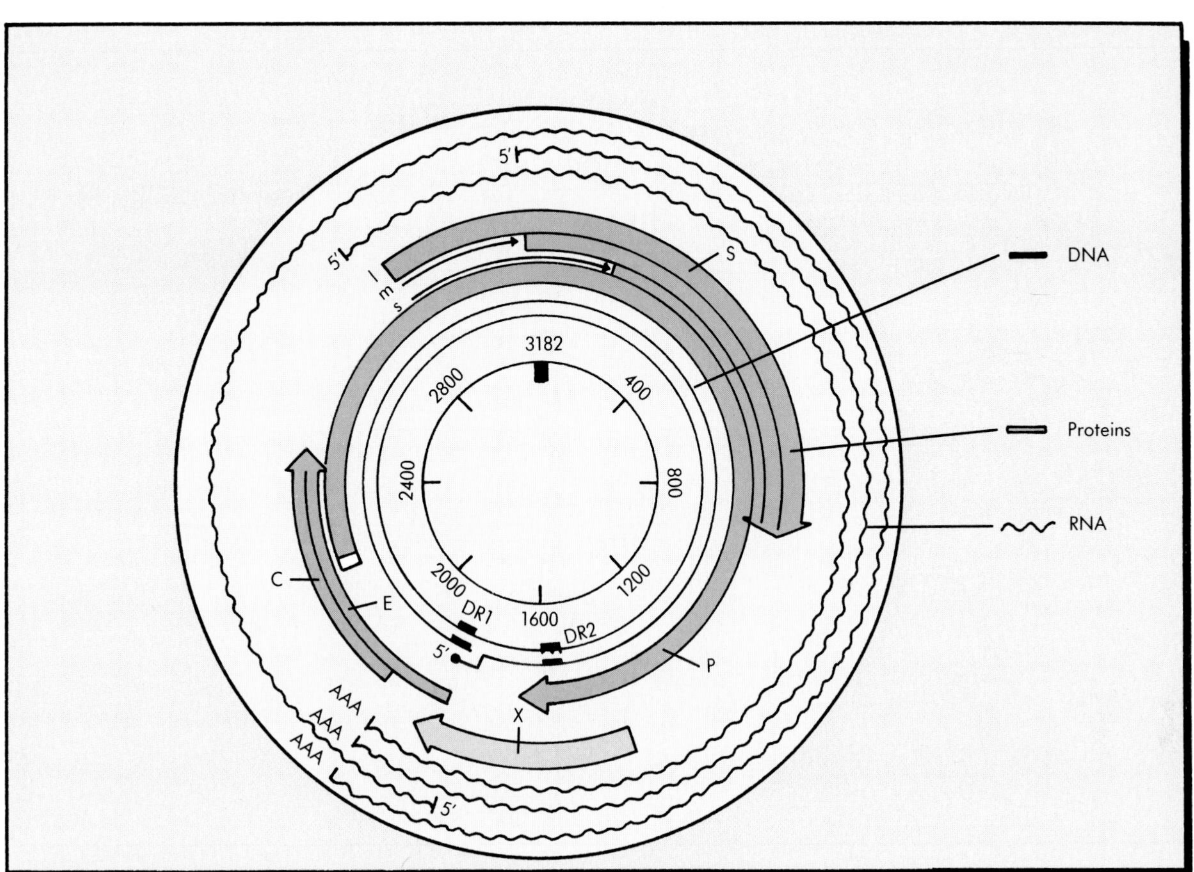

FIGURE 68-6 mRNA transcripts and proteins of HBV. Diagram depicts the mRNA and proteins encoded by the HBV genome. Note that several proteins share the same coding sequences but start at different AUG codons and different mRNAs overlap. The 3500 base transcript is larger than the genome and is the template for replication of the genome. DR1 and DR2 are direct repeat sequences of DNA important for replication and integration of the genome. The genome is in black with the nucleotide map length in the central circle. *E,* E protein (HBeAg); *C,* C protein (HBcAg); *P,* polymerase-protein primer for replication; *S,* S protein (HBsAg); *l, m, s,* large, medium, or small glycoproteins. (Redrawn from Blum HE, Gevok W, Vyas GN: *Trends Gen* 5:154-158, 1989.)

the HBV infection. Interferon most likely initiates the response by enhancing MHC antigen expression and display of peptides from the HBs, HBc, and HBe antigens to cytotoxic T-killer cells. An insufficient T-cell response to the infection generally results in mild symptoms, an inability to resolve the infection, and chronic hepatitis (Figure 68-8). Antibody (as generated by vaccination) will protect against infection. Serum HBsAg binds and blocks the action of neutralizing antibody, which limits its capacity to resolve an infection. Immune complexes formed between HBsAg and anti-HBs contribute to the symptoms causing hypersensitivity reactions, leading to such problems as vasculitis, arthralgia, rash, or renal damage.

Infants have an immature cell-mediated immune response and exhibit less tissue damage and milder symptoms. As many as 90% of infants infected perinatally become chronic carriers. Virus replication persists in these individuals for long periods.

During the acute phase of infection, the liver parenchyma shows degenerative changes consisting of cellular swelling and necrosis, especially in hepatocytes surrounding the central vein of a hepatic lobule. The inflammatory cell infiltrate is mainly composed of lymphocytes. Resolution of the infection allows the parenchyma to regenerate. Fulminant infections, activation of chronic infections, or co-infection with the delta agent can lead to permanent liver damage and cirrhosis.

Epidemiology

In the United States more than 300,000 persons are infected by HBV each year. Even more people are infected in underdeveloped nations, with as much as 15% of the population infected during birth or childhood. High rates of seropositivity are observed in Italy, Greece, Africa, and Southeast Asia (Figure 68-9). In some areas of the world (southern Africa and southeastern Asia) the seroconversion rate of the population is as high as 50%. Primary hepatocellular carcinoma is also endemic in these regions.

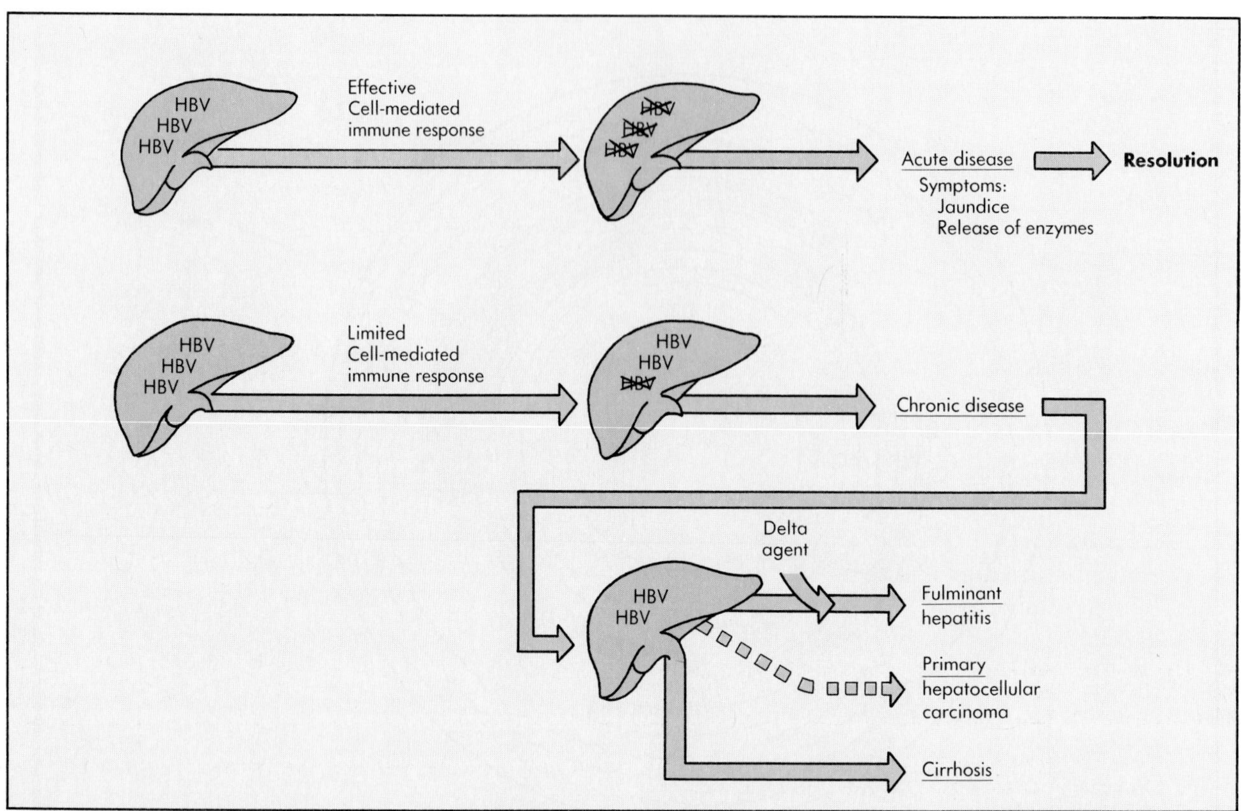

FIGURE 68-7 Major determinants in acute and chronic HBV infection. Hepatitis B virus infects the liver but does not cause direct cytopathology. Cell-mediated immune lysis of infected cells, potentially triggered by interferon action, produces symptoms and resolves the infection. Insufficient immunity can lead to chronic disease. Chronic HBV disease predisposes an individual to more serious outcomes. *Solid arrows* indicate symptoms; *broken arrows* indicate a possible outcome.

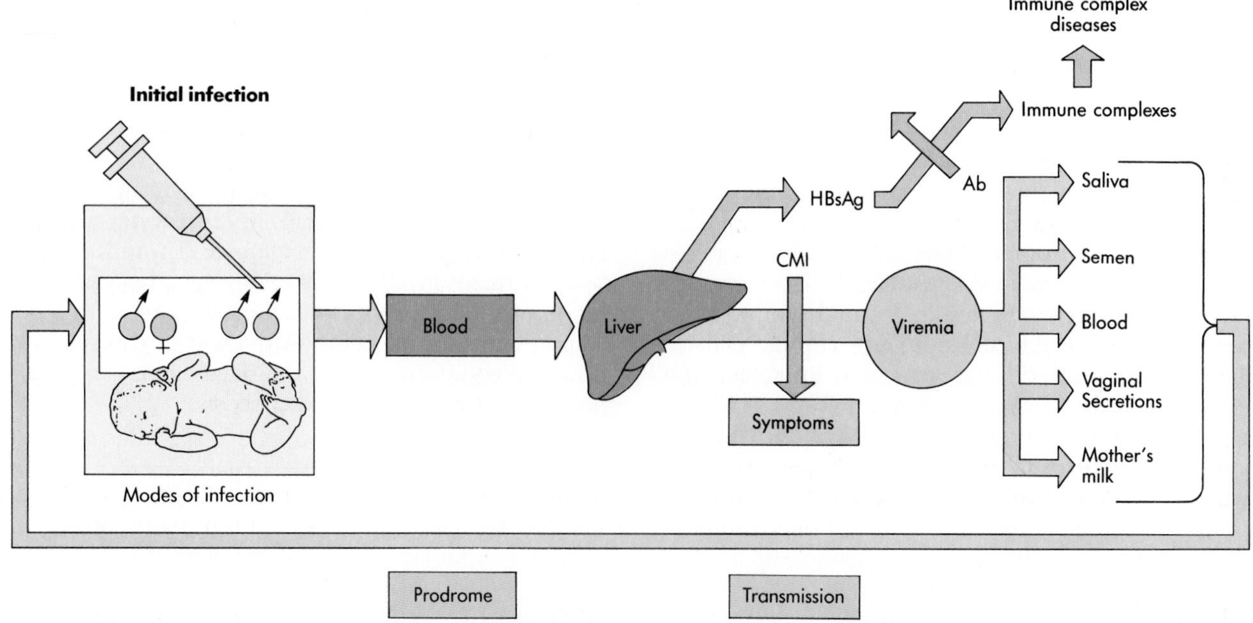

FIGURE 68-8 Spread of HBV in the body. Initial infection by HBV occurs by injection, heterosexual and homosexual sex, and birth. The virus spreads to the liver, replicates, induces a viremia, and is transmitted in various body secretions in addition to blood to start the cycle again. Symptoms are caused by cell-mediated immunity and immune complexes between antibody and HBsAg.

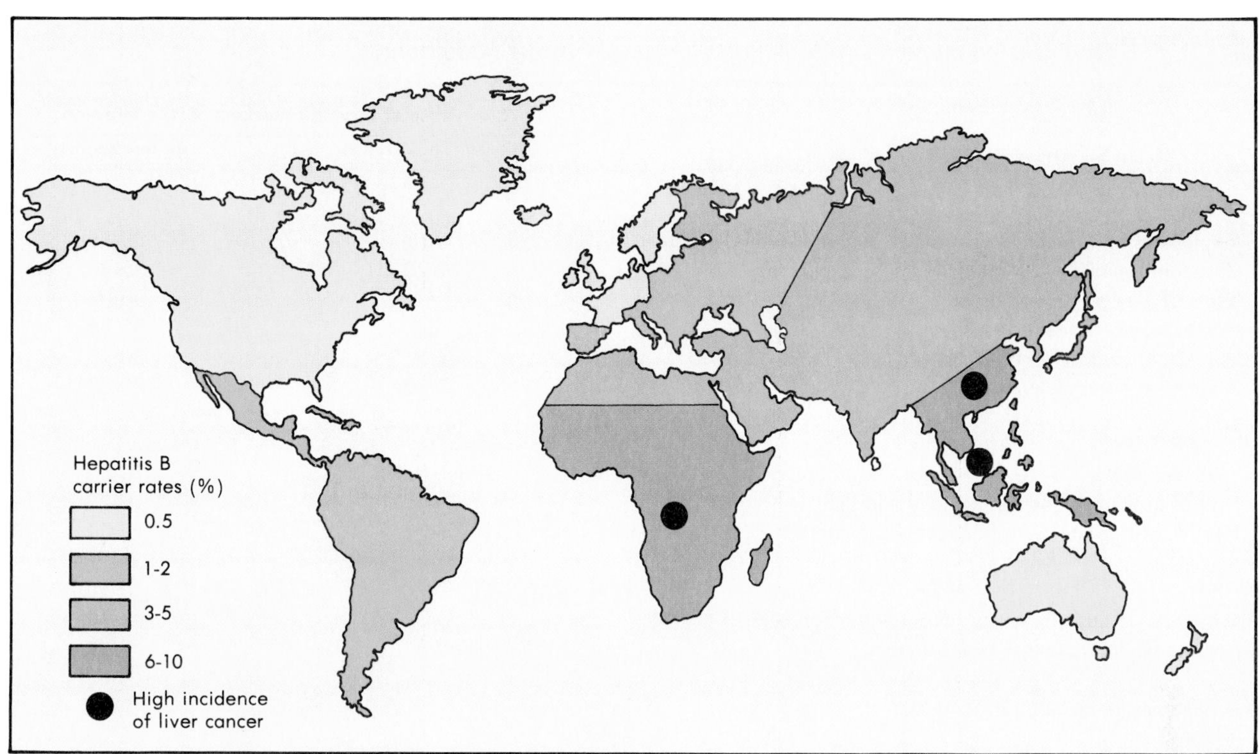

FIGURE 68-9 Worldwide prevalence of hepatitis B carriers and primary hepatocellular carcinoma. (Redrawn from Szmuness W et al: *J Med Virol* 8:123, 1981.)

The large number of asymptomatic chronic carriers capable of secreting virus in blood and other body secretions fosters the spread of the virus. A chronic carrier is defined as an individual who is HBsAg positive on two occasions at least 6 months apart. Overall, in the United States 0.1% to 0.5% of the general population are chronic carriers. Carrier status may be lifelong.

The virus is spread mainly by percutaneous routes (e.g., needle sharing, acupuncture, ear piercing, tatooing) and by very close personal contact with exchange of secretions (e.g., sex, childbirth). HBV also can be transmitted to babies in mother's milk. The virus can be transmitted by contaminated blood or blood products, but serologic screening of donor units in blood banks has greatly reduced this risk. Mosquitos and other blood-eating insects have also been suggested but are limited transmitters of HBV. Given the modes of transmission, groups at high risk for infection have been identified (Table 68-2). Babies born to chronic HBV positive mothers are at highest risk for infection. Sexual promiscuity and drug abuse are major risk factors for HBV. Screening the blood supply and safer sex habits for prevention of HIV transmission have decreased the transmission of HBV.

One of the major concerns about HBV is its association with **primary hepatocellular carcinoma** (PHC). This type of carcinoma probably accounts for 250,000 to 1 million deaths per year worldwide; in the United States approximately 5000 deaths per year are attributed to PHC.

Clinical Syndromes

Acute Infection

The clinical presentation of HBV in children is less severe than in adults and may be asymptomatic. Clinically apparent illness occurs in as many as 25% of those infected with HBV (Figures 68-10 to 68-12).

Hepatitis B infection is characterized by a long incubation period and an insidious onset. Symptoms during the prodromal period may include fever, malaise, and anorexia. This is followed by nausea, vomiting, abdominal discomfort, fever, and chills. The classic icteric symptoms of liver damage (e.g., jaundice, dark urine, pale stools) follow soon thereafter. Recovery is indicated by a decline of fever and renewed appetite.

Fulminant hepatitis occurs in approximately 1% of icteric patients and may be fatal, with much more severe symptoms and indications of severe liver damage, such as ascites and bleeding.

Chronic Infection

Chronic hepatitis occurs in 5% to 10% of HBV infections, usually after mild or inapparent initial disease. Chronic hepatitis may be detected only by elevated liver enzyme levels on a routine blood chemistry profile, but as many as 10% of patients with chronic hepatitis may

TABLE 68-2 Expected Hepatitis B Virus Prevalence in Various Population Groups

Group	Prevalence of serologic markers of HBV infection: HBsAg (%) (Chronic)	All markers (%)
HIGH RISK		
Immigrants and refugees from areas of high HBV endemicity	13	80-85
Clients in institutions for mentally retarded persons	10-20	35-80
Users of illicit parenteral drugs	7	60-80
Homosexually active males	6	35-80
Household contacts of HBV carriers	3-6	30-60
Patients on hemodialysis units	3-10	20-80
INTERMEDIATE RISK		
Prisoners (male)	1-8	10-80
Staff of institutions for the mentally retarded	1	10-25
Health care workers with frequent blood contact	1-2	15-30
LOW RISK		
Health care workes with no (or infrequent) blood contact	0-3	3-10
Healthy adults (volunteer blood donors)	0-3	3-5

From Hoofnagle JH: *Lab Med* 14:705, 1983.

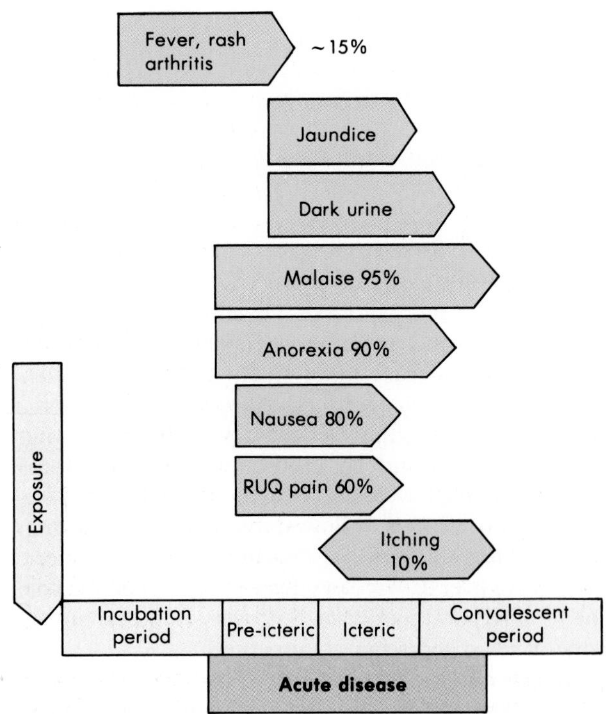

FIGURE 68-10 Symptoms of typical acute viral hepatitis B infection are correlated with the four clinical periods of this disease. (Redrawn from Hoofnagle JH: *Lab Med* 14:705, 1983.)

develop cirrhosis and liver failure. Chronically infected individuals are the major source for spread of the virus and are at risk for fulminant disease if co-infected with the delta hepatitis virus (HDV).

Primary Hepatocellular Carcinoma (PHC)

The World Health Organization estimates that 80% of all cases of PHC can be attributed to chronic hepatitis B infections. The HBV genome is integrated into these PHC cells, and the cells express HBV antigens. PHC is usually fatal and is one of the three most common causes of cancer mortality in the world. In Taiwan at least 15% of the population are HBV carriers, and nearly half of the individuals die of either PHC or cirrhosis. PHC may become the first vaccine-preventable human cancer.

HBV may induce PHC by promoting continued liver repair and cell growth in response to tissue damage or by integrating in the host chromosome and stimulating cell growth directly. Integration could stimulate genetic rearrangements or juxtapose viral promotors next to cellular growth controlling genes. Alternatively, a protein encoded by the HBV X-gene may transactivate (turn on) transcription of cellular proteins and stimulate cell growth. The presence of the HBV genome may allow a subsequent carcinogenic event to promote development of the carcinoma. The latency period between HBV infection and PHC may be as short as 9 years or as long as 35 years.

Laboratory Diagnosis

The initial diagnosis of hepatitis can be made from the clinical symptoms and the presence of liver enzymes in the blood (see Figure 68-12). However, the serology of HBV infection describes the course and the nature of the disease (Table 68-3). Acute and chronic HBV infections can be distinguished by the presence of HBsAg and HBeAg in the serum and the pattern of antibodies to the individual

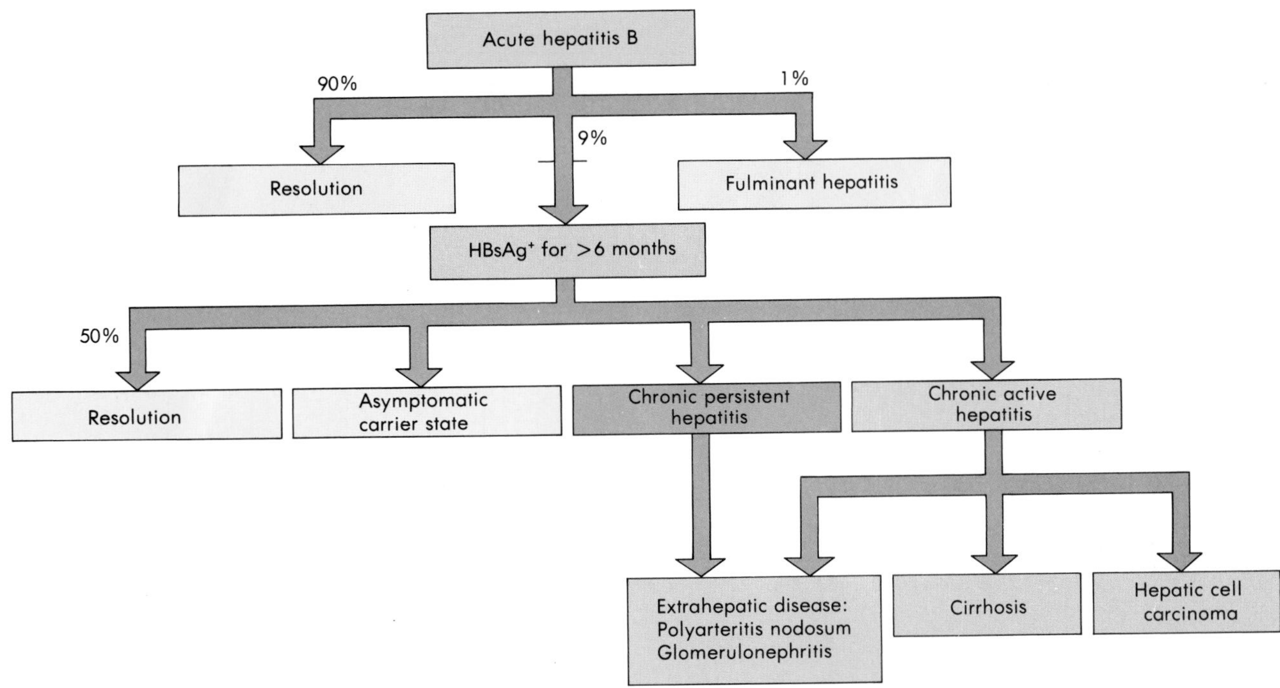

FIGURE 68-11 Clinical outcomes of acute hepatitis B infection. (Redrawn from White DO and Fenner F: *Medical virology*, ed 3, New York, 1986, Academic Press.)

HBV antigens. The serologic pattern of HBV infection is better understood by remembering that antibody bound into an antibody-antigen complex cannot be detected in routine laboratory tests.

HBsAg, HBcAg, and HBeAg are secreted into the blood during virus replication. Although HBc and HBe share protein sequences, the differences in processing, secretion, and tertiary structure make them useful as distinct serologic markers. No test is readily available for HBcAg, but HBsAg and HBeAg can be detected in clinical laboratory assays. Detection of HBeAg is the best correlate to the presence of infectious virus. A chronic infection can be distinguished by the continued presence of HBeAg and/or HBsAg and a lack of detectable antibody to these antigens.

During the symptomatic phase of infection, detection of antibodies to HBeAg and HBsAg is obscured because the antibody is complexed with antigen in the serum. Indication of recent acute infection, especially during the period when neither HBsAg nor anti-HBs can be detected (the window), is best established by measurement of IgM anti-HBc.

Treatment, Prevention, and Control

No specific treatment exists for hepatitis B infection, although limited studies suggest that interferon, adenine arabinoside, corticosteroids, and azathioprine alone or in certain combinations may have a role in the treatment of different types of chronic active hepatitis.

Transmission of HBV by blood or blood products has been greatly reduced by screening of donated blood for the presence of HBsAg and anti-HBc. Additional efforts to prevent hepatitis B consist of avoiding intimate personal contact with a carrier of HBV and avoiding the life-styles that facilitate spread of the virus. Household contacts and sexual partners of HBV carriers are at increased risk, as are hemodialysis patients, recipients of pooled plasma products, health care workers exposed to blood, and babies born of HBV-carrier mothers.

Vaccination is recommended for infants, children, and especially individuals in high-risk groups who are known to be anti-HBsAg negative (see Table 68-2). Vaccination is useful even after exposure for newborns of HBsAg-positive mothers and persons with accidental percutaneous or permucosal exposure to blood or secretions from an HBsAg-positive individual. Immunization of mothers should decrease transmission to babies and older children, which will also reduce the number of chronic HBV carriers. Prevention of chronic HBV will, most likely, prevent PHC.

The HBV vaccines are subunit vaccines. The initial HBV vaccine was derived from the 22 nm HBsAg particles in human plasma from chronically infected individuals. The current vaccine is genetically engineered and is produced by the insertion of a plasmid containing the **S** gene for HBsAg into a yeast, *Saccharomyces cerevisiae*.

The vaccine must be given in a series of three injections, with the second and third given 1 and 6 months after the first. More than 95% of individuals receiving the full 3-dose course will develop protective antibody.

A

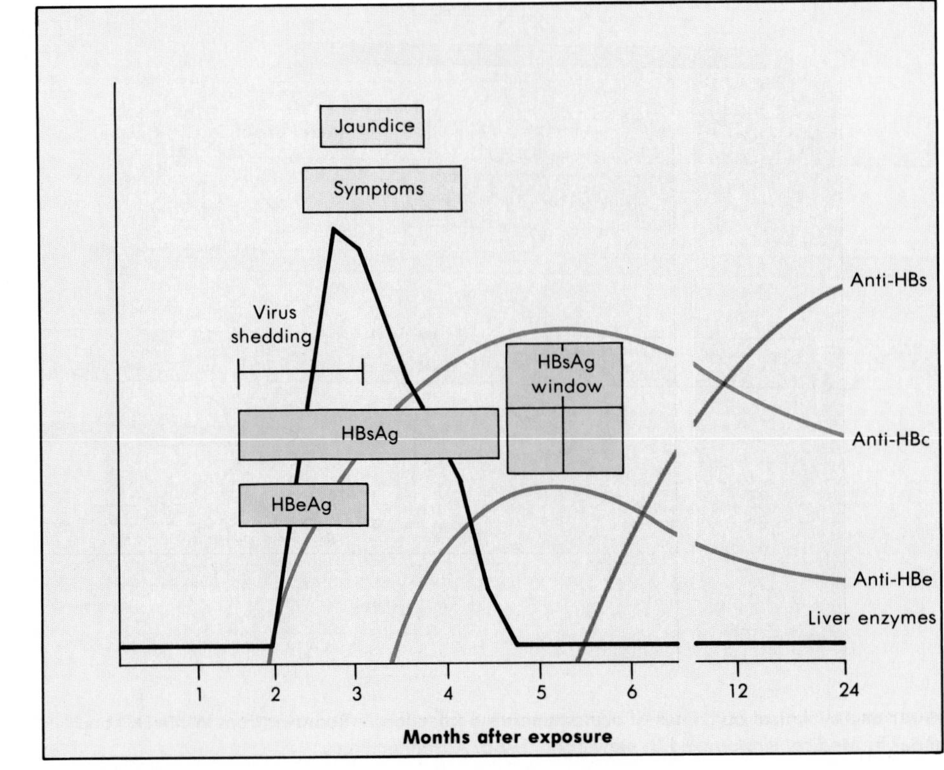

B

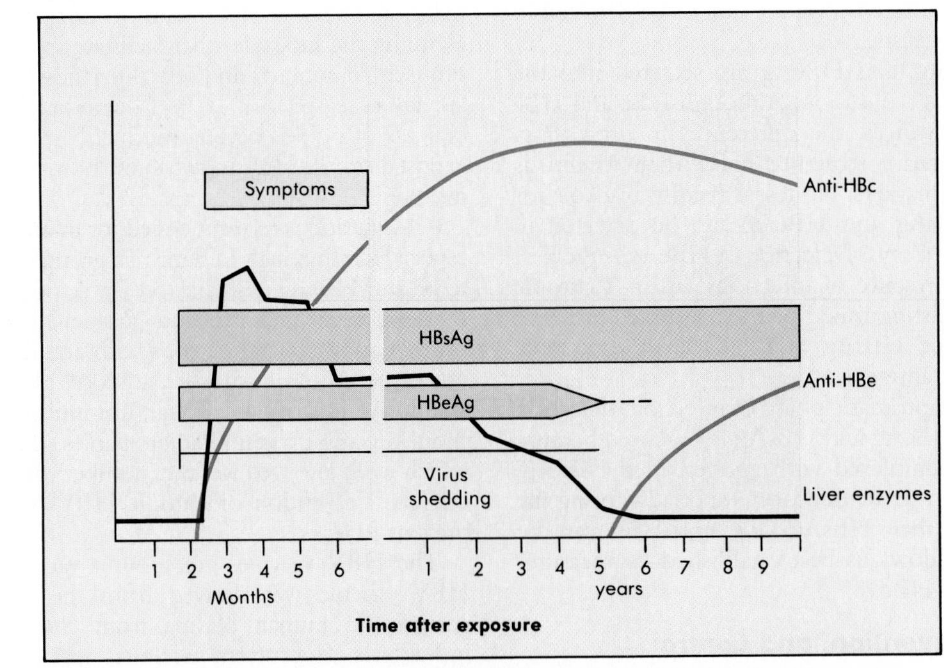

FIGURE 68-12 A, The serologic events associated with the typical course of acute hepatitis B disease. **B,** Development of the chronic hepatitis B virus carrier state. *HBsAg*, Hepatitis B surface antigen; *HBeAg*, hepatitis B e antigen; *anti-HBs*, antibody to HBsAg; *anti-HBc*, antibody to hepatitis B core antigen; *anti-HBe*, antibody to HBeAg. The HBsAg window occurs with a decrease in HBsAg but before anti-HBs detection. **A** and **B** redrawn from *Ann Rev Med*, vol 32, 1981.

C

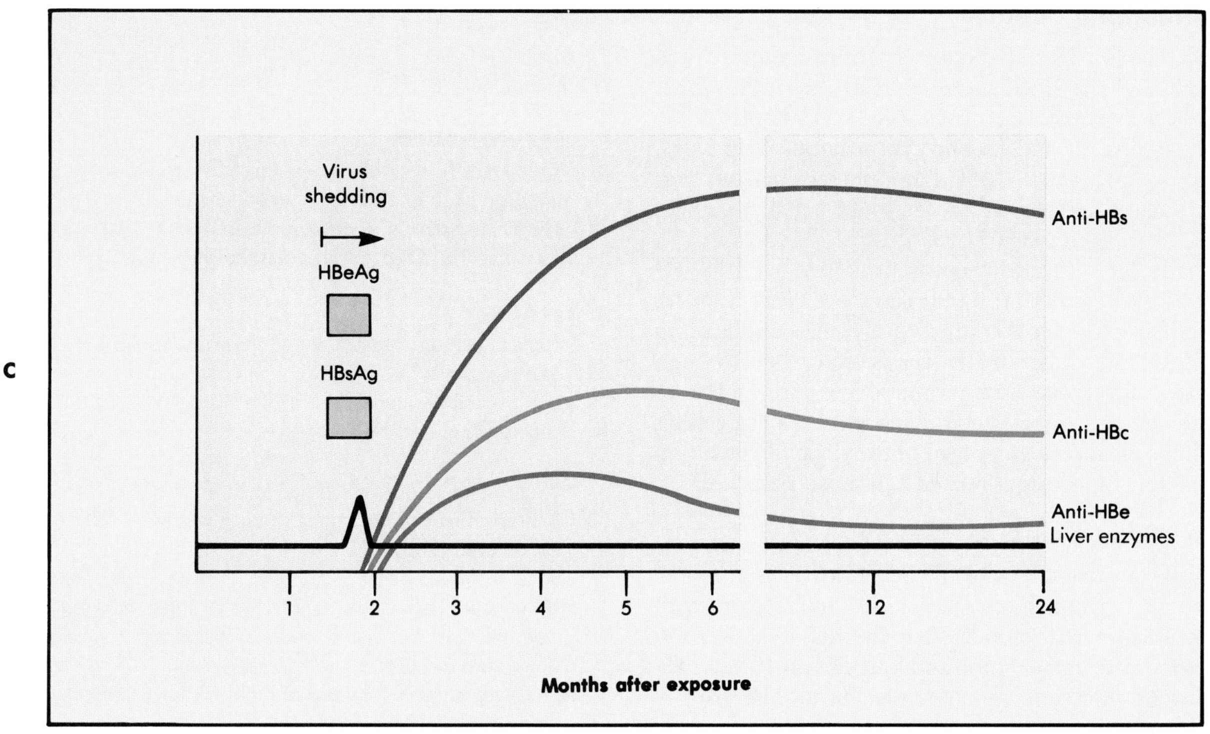

FIGURE 68-12—cont'd **C,** Clinical, serologic, and biochemical course of a subclinical asymptomatic hepatitis B virus infection. **C** redrawn from Hoofnagle JH: *Lab Med* 14:705, 1983.)

TABLE 68-3 Interpretation of Serologic Markers of HBV Infection

	Disease state						
					Resolved		
Serologic reactivity	**Early (presymptomatic)**	**Early acute**	**Acute***	**Chronic**	**Late Acute**	**Acute**	**Vaccinated**
Anti HBc	+/−	−	−	+	+/−	+	−
Anti HBe	−	−	−	−	−	+/−†	−
Anti HBs	−	−	+	−	−	+	+
HBeAg	−	+	+	+	−	−	−
HBsAg	+	+	+	+	+	−	−
Infectious virus	+	++	++	++	+	−	−

*Anti-HBc IgM should be present.
†AntiHBe may be negative following chronic disease.

Hepatitis B immune globulin (HBIG) is prepared from plasma selected for a high titer of anti-HBV. HBIG is indicated in postexposure prophylaxis for newborn infants of HBsAg-positive mothers and for persons with accidental percutaneous or permucosal exposure to blood or secretions from individuals who are HBsAg positive.

HEPATITIS C

Hepatitis C accounts for 90% of the cases of NANBH infection and is the major cause of post-transfusion hepatitis. HCV is a flavivirus with a (+) RNA genome and is enveloped. The genome of HCV (9500 nucleotides) has been cloned and sequenced.

Epidemiology

The existence of NANB hepatitis viruses in serum was indicated by the incidence of HBV-negative, post-transfusion hepatitis (see Box 68-4). Hepatitis C is spread parenterally and sexually. Intravenous drug users, transfusion recipients, and hemophiliac persons receiving factor *VIII* or *IX* are at highest risk to infection.

Hepatitis C infection occurs in 5% to 10% of transfusion recipients (150,000 cases per year), causing chronic hepatitis in half of these individuals and leading to cirrhosis in at least 20% of the acute cases. The high incidence of chronic asymptomatic infections (1% of American blood donors) and the inadequacy of screening procedures promotes the spread of the virus via the blood supply. Non-transfusion–related cases also occur.

Clinical Syndromes

HCV can cause acute or chronic infections. A viremia can be detected within 1 to 3 weeks of transfusion with HCV-contaminated blood. The viremia lasts 4 to 6 months for an acute infection and longer than 10 years for a persistent infection. In its acute form, NANBH is similar to acute hepatitis A and B, but the inflammatory response is less and the symptoms are usually milder. Chronic infection is even more prevalent than for HBV, often leading to acute disease and cirrhosis. The continual liver repair and induction of cell growth during chronic HCV infection has been suggested as a predisposing factor in primary hepatocellular carcinoma. Antibody to HCV is not protective and experimental infection of chimpanzees suggests that immunity to HCV may not be lifelong.

BOX 68-4 Epidemiology of Hepatitis B, C, and D Viruses

DISEASE/VIRAL FACTORS

Enveloped viruses labile to drying. HBV less sensitive to detergents than other enveloped viruses
Virus is shed during asymptomatic periods
Cause chronic disease with potential shedding

TRANSMISSION

In blood, semen, vaginal secretions (HBV: saliva and mother's milk)
Via transfusion, needle stick, shared drug paraphernalia, sex, and nursing babies

WHO IS AT RISK?

Children: mild asymptomatic disease with establishment of chronic infections
Adults: Insidious onset of hepatitis
HBV-infected individuals co-infected or super-infected with HDV: abrupt more severe symptoms with possible fulminant disease
Adults with chronic HBV are at high risk for primary hepatocellular carcinoma

GEOGRAPHY/SEASON

Worldwide
No seasonal incidence

MODES OF CONTROL

Avoidance of high-risk behavior
HBV: Vaccine
Screening of blood supply

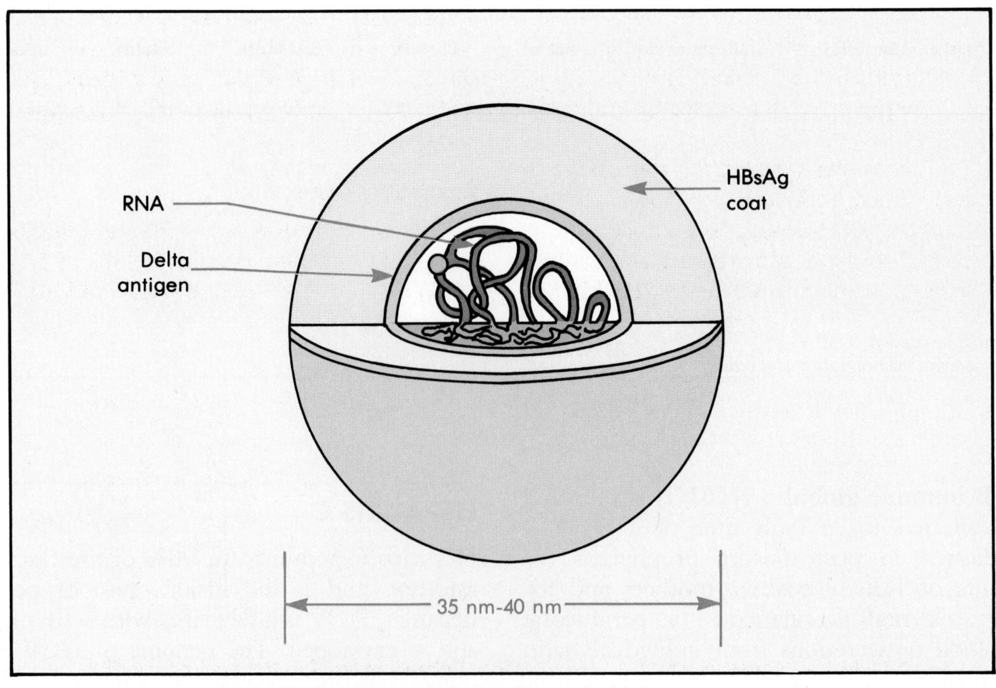

FIGURE 68-13 The delta hepatitis virion.

Laboratory Diagnosis

Diagnosis of HCV is based on ELISA detection of antibody. Antibody may be detected within 6 to 8 weeks of infection, but antibody is not always present in viremic individuals. This suggests that serologic assays may be useful to identify only chronic rather than acute HCV disease. The presence of the virion RNA in serum is a better determinant of disease. A variation of the polymerase-chain-reaction (PCR) technique, based on the known sequence of HCV, can detect the presence of HCV RNA in seronegative individuals and may become a key tool in the diagnosis of HCV infection.

Treatment, Prevention, and Control

Recombinant alpha-interferon is the only effective treatment identified for HCV. No other treatments except supportive therapy are available for HCV and the other NANBH.

Illicit drug abuse and transfusion are the most identifiable source of NANBH viruses. Unlike HBV, the tests available for HCV cannot detect a current acute case of HCV, and tests for other NANBH viruses are not available. This has frustrated the development of effective screening procedures for protection of the nation's blood supply.

HEPATITIS D VIRUS (DELTA AGENT)

Structure and Replication

Approximately 15 million people in the world are infected with hepatitis D virus, and the virus is responsible for 40% of fulminant hepatitis infections. Hepatitis D virus is a defective satellite virus that can replicate only in HBV-infected cells. It is a viral parasite, proving that "even fleas have fleas." The HBsAg is essential for packaging the virus. The delta agent resembles plant virus satellite agents and viroids in size, genome structure, and requirement for a helper virus for replication (Figure 68-13).

The HDV RNA genome is very small (approximately 1700 nucleotides) single stranded, and circular, an unusual RNA structure. The virion, approximately 35 to 37 nm in diameter, consists of the genome and a small (predominant) or large form of the delta antigen (22,000 and 24,000 d) surrounded by an HBsAg-containing envelope.

The delta agent binds to and is internalized by hepatocytes in the same manner as HBV because of the presence of HBsAg in its envelope. Once inside the cells, the genome is transcribed and replicated in the nucleus. The small delta antigen protein is an RNA-binding protein and is essential for these processes. The mechanisms and polymerases involved in these processes are not known. The gene for the delta antigen is prone to mutation during infection, allowing production of the large delta antigen. Production of the large delta antigen limits replication of the virus and hence cell destruction. The genome, delta antigen, and HBsAg associate together and are then released from the cell.

Pathogenesis

The delta agent is spread in blood, semen, and vaginal secretions, similar to HBV. It can replicate and cause disease only in individuals with active HBV infections. Since the two agents are transmitted by the same routes, an individual can be **co-infected** with HBV and delta agent at the same time, or a person with chronic HBV can be **superinfected** with delta agent to cause disease. A more rapid, severe progression occurs after superinfection of an HBV carrier than during co-infection since HBV must first establish its infection for HDV to replicate (Figure 68-14). Superinfection of an individual allows the delta agent to replicate immediately.

Replication of the delta agent results in cytotoxicity and liver damage. A persistent delta agent infection is often established in HBV carriers even after symptoms have ended. Antibodies are elicited against the delta agent. However, protection probably relates to the immune response to HBsAg since it is the external antigen and viral attachment protein for HDV. Unlike hepatitis B, damage to the liver occurs by the direct cytopathic effect of the delta agent combined with the underlying immunopathology of the HBV disease.

Epidemiology

The delta agent infects children and adults with underlying HBV infection (see Box 68-4). Individuals who are persistently infected by both HBV and HDV are a source

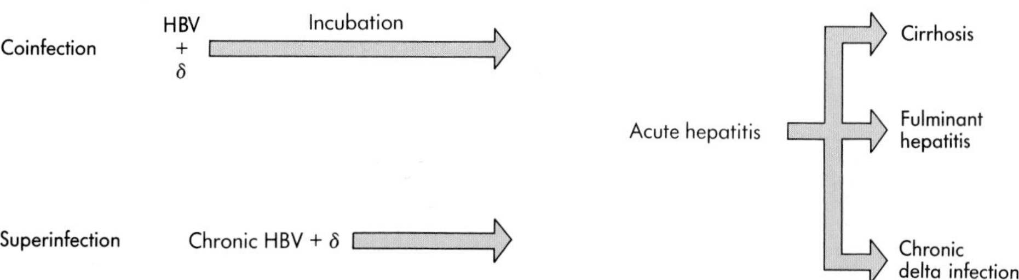

FIGURE 68-14 Consequences of delta virus infection. Delta virus requires the presence of HBV infection. Superinfection of an individual already infected with HBV (HBV carrier) causes a more rapid severe progression than co-infection.

for the virus. The agent has a worldwide distribution and is endemic in southern Italy, the Amazon basin, parts of Africa, and the Middle East. Epidemics of delta agent infection occur in North America and Western Europe, usually in illicit drug users.

HDV is spread by the same routes as HBV, and the same groups are at risk to infection. Parenteral drug abusers and hemophiliacs are at highest risk to infection.

Clinical Syndromes

The delta agent increases the severity of hepatitis B infections. Individuals infected with delta agent are much more likely to develop fulminant hepatitis than are those with the other hepatitis viruses. Chronic infection with delta agent can occur in individuals with chronic HBV.

Laboratory Diagnosis

Detection of the delta antigen or antibodies is the only way to determine the presence of the agent. ELISA and RIA procedures are available. The presence of the delta antigen in the blood during the acute phase of disease can be detected on detergent treatment of the serum.

Treatment, Prevention, and Control

No known specific treatment exists for delta hepatitis. Since the delta agent depends on HBV for replication and is spread by the same routes, prevention of infection with HBV will prevent hepatitis D infection. Immunization with hepatitis B vaccine protects against subsequent delta virus infection. If an individual has already acquired hepatitis B, delta agent infection may be prevented by reducing exposure to illicit intravenous drugs, carriers of this virus, or HDV-contaminated blood products.

HEPATITIS E

Hepatitis E virus (ET-NANBH) is predominantly spread by the fecal-oral route, especially in contaminated water (see Box 68-2). It resembles the calicivirus or Norwalk agent in size (27 to 34 nm) and structure. Although HBE is found throughout the world, it is most problematic in developing countries. Epidemics have been reported in India, Pakistan, Nepal, Burma, North Africa, and Mexico.

The symptoms and course of HEV are very similar to HAV, causing only acute disease. However, the onset of symptoms for HEV may occur later and with a poor serum IgG response. The mortality for HEV is 1% to 2%, approximately 10 times that of HAV. HEV infection is especially serious for pregnant women (mortality of approximately 20%).

CASE STUDY AND QUESTIONS

Patient A. A 55-year-old man is admitted to the hospital with fatigue, nausea, and abdominal discomfort. He has a slight temperature, his urine is dark yellow, and his abdomen is distended and tender. He returned from a trip to Thailand within the last month.

Patient B. A 28-year-old woman was admitted to the hospital complaining of vomiting, abdominal discomfort, nausea, anorexia, dark urine, and jaundice. She admits to having shared needles as a former heroin addict and is 3 months pregnant.

Patient C. A 65-year-old man is admitted with jaundice, nausea, and vomiting 6 months after undergoing coronary bypass surgery.

1. What clinical or epidemiological clues would assist in the diagnosis of hepatitis A, B, and C, respectively?
2. What laboratory tests would be helpful in distinguishing the different hepatitis infections?
3. What is the most likely means of virus acquisition in each case?
4. What personal and public health precautions should be taken to prevent transmission of virus in each case?
5. Which of the patients are susceptible to chronic disease?
6. What laboratory tests would distinguish acute from chronic hepatitis B disease?
7. How can hepatitis B disease be prevented? Treated?

Modified from Marx JF: Viral hepatitis: unscrambling the alphabet, *Nursing* 93:34-42, 1993.

Bibliography

Blum HE, Gerok W, and Vyas GN: The molecular biology of hepatitis B virus, *Trends Genetics* 5:154-158, 1989.

Bradley DW, Krawczynski K, Kane MA: Hepatitis E. In Belshe RB, editor: *Textbook of human virology*, ed 2, St. Louis, 1991, Mosby.

Fields BN and Knipe DM, editors: *Virology*, ed 2, New York, 1990, Raven Press.

Frosner G: Hepatitis A virus. In Belshe RB, editor: *Textbook of human virology*, ed 2, St. Louis, 1991, Mosby.

Hadler SC and Fields HA: Hepatitis delta virus. In Belshe RB, editor: *Textbook of human virology*, ed 2, St. Louis, 1991, Mosby.

Hoofnagle JH: Type A and type B hepatitis, *Lab Med* 14: 705-716, 1983.

Lennette EH, Halonen P, Murphy FA, editors: *Laboratory diagnosis of infectious diseases: principles and practice*, New York, 1988, Springer-Verlag.

Lutwick LI. Hepatitis B virus. In Belshe RB, editor: *Textbook of human virology*, ed 2, St. Louis, 1991, Mosby.

Mason WS and Seeger C, editors: Hepadnaviruses: molecular biology and pathogenesis, *Curr Top Microbiol Immunol* 168, New York, 1991, Springer-Verlag.

Plageman PGW: Hepatitis C virus, *Arch Virol* 120:165-180, 1991.

Reyes GR and Baroudy BM: Molecular biology of non-A, non-B hepatitis agents: hepatitis C and hepatitis E viruses, *Adv Vir Res* 40:57-102, 1991.

Robinson W, Koike K, and Will H, editors: *Hepadna virus*, New York, 1987, Alan R. Liss.

Tam AW, Smith MM, Guerra ME, Huang C-C, Bradley DW, Fry KE, Reyes GR: Hepatitis E virus: molecular cloning and sequencing of the full-length viral genome, *Virol* 185:120-131, 1991.

CHAPTER 69

Unconventional Slow Viruses: Prions

THE unconventional slow viruses cause spongiform encephalopathy, slow neurodegenerative diseases. These include the human diseases of kuru, Creutzfeldt-Jakob disease (CJD), Gerstmann-Straussler-Scheinker disease (GSS), and the animal diseases scrapie, bovine spongiform encephalopathy, chronic wasting diseases in mule deer and elk and transmissible mink encephalopathy (Box 69-1). *CJD and GSS are also genetic human disorders.*

Slow virus agents are filterable and can transmit disease but otherwise do not conform to the standard definition of a virus (Table 69-1). Unlike conventional viruses, no virion structure or genome has been detected; no immune response is elicited; and the agents are extremely resistant to inactivation by heat, disinfectants, and radiation. The slow virus agent appears to be a modified host protein, a **prion** (small proteinaceous infectious particle), which can transmit the disease.

After long incubation periods these agents cause damage to the central nervous system (CNS), which leads to subacute spongiform encephalopathies. The long incubation period, which can extend to 30 years in humans, has made study of these agents difficult. Carlton Gajdusek won the Nobel Prize for showing an infectious etiology for kuru and the means for initial analysis of the agent. The major breakthroughs came when the kuru agent was transmitted to monkeys and when it was recognized that the scrapie agent induced a characteristic cytopathology in hamsters considerably before the disease was evident. These studies provided a useful means for assaying this agent and its biological properties.

BOX 69-1 Slow Virus Diseases

HUMAN

Kuru
Creutzfeldt-Jakob disease (CJD)
Gerstmann-Straussler-Scheinker syndrome (GSS)

ANIMAL

Scrapie (sheep and goats)
Transmissible mink encephalopathy
Bovine spongiform encephalopathy
Chronic wasting diseases (mule deer and elk)

STRUCTURE AND PHYSIOLOGY

The slow virus agents were suspected to be viruses because they pass through filters that block the passage of particles greater than 100 nm and still transmit disease. Isolates diluted as much as 10^{11} can still induce disease in susceptible individuals. The agents are resistant to a wide range of chemical and physical treatments, such as formaldehyde, ultraviolet radiation, or heat to 80° C.

The prototype of these agents is scrapie, which has been adapted to infect hamsters. Scrapie-infected ham-

TABLE 69-1 Comparison of Classical Viruses and Prions

	Virus	Prion
STRUCTURE		
Filterable, infectious agents	Yes	Yes
Presence of nucleic acid	Yes	No?
Defined morphology (electron microscopy)	Yes	No
Presence of protein	Yes	Yes
Disinfected by		
Formaldehyde	Yes	No
Proteases	Some	No
Heat (80° C)	Most	No
Ionizing and UV irradiation	Yes	No
DISEASE		
Cytopathic effect	Yes	No
Incubation period	Depends on virus	Long
Immune response	Yes	No
Interferon production	Yes	No
Inflammatory response	Usually	No

TABLE 69-2 Comparison of PrP^{Sc} and PrP^{c}*

	PrP^{Sc}	PrP^{c}
Structure	Globular	Extended
Protease resistance	No	Yes
Presence in scrapie fibrils	Yes	No
Location on/in cells	Cytoplasmic vesicles	Plasma membrane
Turnover	Days	Hours

*PrP^{Sc} is the prion scrapie agent and PrP^{c} is the natural cellular homologue.

BOX 69-2 Pathogenic Characteristics of Slow Viruses

No cytopathologic effect in vitro
Long doubling time of at least 5.2 days
Long incubation period
Causes vacuolation of neurons (spongiform), amyloid-like plaques, gliosis
Symptoms include loss of muscle control, shivering, tremors, and dementia
No antigenicity
No inflammation
No immune response
No interferon production

sters have scrapie-associated fibrils (SAF) in their brain. The SAF are infectious and contain the prion.

The prion lacks detectable nucleic acids and consists of aggregates of a protease-resistant, hydrophobic glycoprotein, which for scrapie is termed **PrP^{Sc}** (scrapie prion protein) (27,000 to 30,000 d). Humans and other animals encode a protein **PrP^{C}** (cellular prion protein), which is closely related to PrP^{Sc} in protein sequence but differs in many of its properties (Table 69-2). Differences in posttranslational modifications cause the two proteins to behave very differently. The PrP^{Sc} is protease resistant, aggregates into amyloid rods (fibrils), is found in cytoplasmic vesicles in the cell, and is secreted. The normal cellular PrP is protease sensitive and appears on the cell surface.

Many theories have been developed to describe how an aberrant protein could cause disease. One model suggested by Stanley Prusiner is that the PrP^{Sc} binds to the normal PrP^{c} on the cell surface and causes it to be processed into PrP^{Sc}, which then aggregates as amyloid-like plaques in the brain. The cell replenishes the PrP^{c}, and the cycle continues. The fact that these plaques consist of host protein might explain the lack of an immune response to these agents in the spongiform encephalopathies.

Although the evidence is strong to indicate that the prion is infectious and can cause scrapie and that similar proteins are responsible for CJD and kuru, other possibilities remain. The protein may be a component of an undiscovered virus or may be induced by a virus infection.

PATHOGENESIS

The term **spongiform encephalopathy** is derived from the characteristic degeneration of neurons and axons of gray matter (Box 69-2). Vacuolation of the neurons, amyloid-containing plaques, fibrils, a proliferation and hypertrophy of astrocytes, and fusion between neurons and adjacent glial cells are observed (Figure 69-1). Prions accumulate to high concentrations in the brain, contributing to the tissue damage. Prions can also be isolated from tissue other than the brain, but only the brain shows any pathology. No inflammation or immune response is generated to the agent, which distinguishes the disease from a classical viral encephalitis.

The incubation period for CJD and kuru may be as long as 30 years, but once the symptoms are evident, the patient dies within a year.

EPIDEMIOLOGY

The predominant means for transmission of CJD are by injection, transplantation of contaminated tissue (e.g., corneas), or contact with contaminated medical devices (e.g., brain electrodes) (Box 69-3). CJD and GSS are also inheritable, and families have been identified with genetic histories of these diseases. These diseases are rare but occur worldwide.

In contrast, kuru was limited to a very small area of the New Guinea highlands. Transmission of kuru was related to the cannibalistic ceremonies of the Fore tribe of New Guinea. Kuru means shivering or trembling. Before Gajdusek intervened, the custom of these people was to eat the bodies of their deceased kinsmen. When Gajdusek began his study, he noted that women and children were most susceptible to the disease. The women and children prepared the food and were given the less desirable viscera and brains to eat. Their risk for infection, therefore, was increased by handling the contaminated tissue. Potential acquisition occurred through the conjunctiva or cuts in the skin and also by ingesting the neural tissue, which should contain the highest concentrations of the kuru agent. Cessation of this cannibalistic custom has stopped the spread of kuru.

CLINICAL SYNDROMES

The slow virus agents cause a progressive, degenerative neurological disease with a long incubation period but with rapid progression to death after onset of symptoms (Figure 69-2). The spongiform encephalopathies are

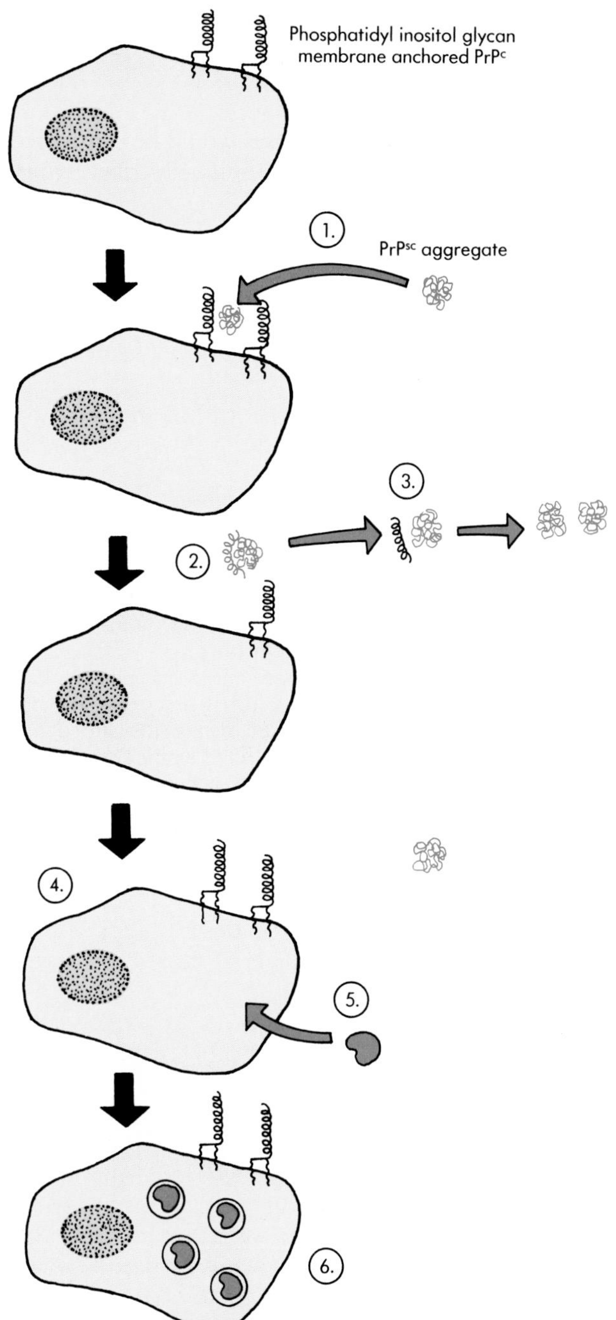

FIGURE 69-1 A model for proliferation of prions. The PrP[c] is a normal cellular protein that is anchored in the cell membrane by phosphatidyl inositol glycan. PrP[Sc] is a hydrophobic globular protein that (*1*) aggregates with itself and with PrP[c] on the cell surface. (*2*) This causes the release of PrP[c] and (*3*) its conversion to PrP[Sc]. (*4*) The cell synthesizes new PrP[c], and the cycle is repeated. (*5*) A form of PrP[Sc] are internalized by neurons and (*6*) accumulate, giving the cell a spongiform appearance. Other models have been proposed.

characterized by loss of muscle control, leading to shivering, myoclonic jerks, tremors, loss of coordination, and rapidly progressive dementia.

LABORATORY DIAGNOSIS

There are no methods for direct virus detection in tissue using electron microscopy, antigen detection, or nucleic acid probes. There are also no serologic tests to detect viral antibody. The diagnosis must be made clinically, with confirmation by pathologic examination of brain revealing the histological changes described previously in the section on pathogenesis.

BOX 69-3 Epidemiology of Disease Caused by Slow Viruses

DISEASE/VIRAL FACTORS

Agents are impervious to standard viral disinfection procedures

Diseases have very long incubation periods, as long as 30 years

TRANSMISSION

Via infected tissue, or the syndrome may be inherited

Infection occurs through cuts in the skin, transplant of contaminated tissues (e.g. cornea), use of contaminated medical devices (e.g., brain electrodes), and potentially ingestion of infected tissue

WHO IS AT RISK?

Kuru: women and children of the Fore tribe of New Guinea

CJD and GSS: Surgeons, transplant and brain surgery patients, others??

GEOGRAPHY/SEASON

GSS and CJD: Sporadic occurrence worldwide

Kuru: New Guinea

No seasonal incidence

MODES OF CONTROL

No treatments available

Kuru: Cessation of ritual cannabolism has led to the disappearance of Kuru

GSS and CJD: Disinfection of neurosurgical tools and electrodes in 5% hypochlorite, 1.0 M NaOH or autoclaving at 15psi for 1 hour.

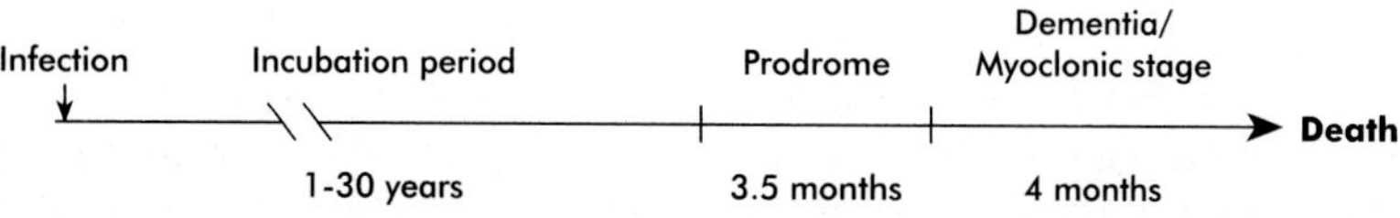

FIGURE 69-2 Progression of transmissible Creutzfeldt-Jakob disease.

TREATMENT, PREVENTION, AND CONTROL

No treatment exists for kuru or CJD. The causative agents are impervious to disinfection procedures used for other viruses, including formaldehyde, detergents, or ionizing radiation. Autoclaving at 15 psi for 1 hour instead of 20 minutes, or 5% hypochlorite solution, or 1.0 M sodium hydroxide, can be used for decontamination. Instruments and brain electrodes are a means of transmission for these agents and should be carefully disinfected before reuse.

CASE STUDY AND QUESTIONS

A 70-year-old woman complained of severe headaches and appeared dull and apathetic with a constant tremor in the right hand. One month later, she appeared to have memory loss and experienced moments of confusion. The patient continued to deteriorate, and an abnormal electroencephalogram was obtained 2 months later (periodic biphasic and triphasic slow-wave complexes). By 3 months, the patient was in a coma-like state with occasional spontaneous clonic twitching of the arms and legs with a startle myoclonic jerking response elicited by a loud noise. The patient died of pneumonia 4 months after the symptoms were originally noted.

No gross abnormalities were obtained upon autopsy. Astrocytic gliosis of the cerebral cortex with fibrils and intracellular vacuolation were observed microscopically throughout the cerebral cortex. There was no swelling and no inflammation.

1. What viral neurological diseases would be considered in the differential diagnosis from the described symptoms? Other diseases?
2. What key features of the postmortem are characteristic of the unconventional slow virus disease agents (spongiform encephalopathies, prions)?
3. What key features distinguish the unconventional slow virus diseases from more conventional neurological viral diseases?
4. What precautions should the pathologist take for protection against infection during the postmortem examination?

Bibliography

Chesebro B: Spongiform encephalopathies: the transmissible agents. In Fields BN and Knipe DM, editors: *Virology*, ed 2, New York, 1990, Raven Press.

Chesebro BW: Transmissible spongiform encephalopathies, *Curr Top Microbiol Immunol* 172, 1991. A series of reviews.

Gajdusek DC: Unconventional viruses causing subacute spongiform encephalopathies. In Fields BN and Knipe DM, editors: *Virology*, ed 2, New York, 1990, Raven Press.

Prusiner SB: Molecular biology and genetics of neurodegenerative diseases caused by prions, *Adv Vir Res* 41:241-280, 1992.

CHAPTER 70

Role of Viruses in Disease

MOST viral infections cause mild or no symptoms and do not require extensive treatment. The common cold, influenza, "flu-like" syndrome, and gastroenteritis are common viral diseases. Other viral infections that cause significant tissue damage or that target essential tissues and organs can cause serious and even life-threatening disease. In general, the symptoms and severity of a viral infection are determined by two things: the victim's ability to prevent or rapidly resolve the infection before the virus can reach important organs or cause significant damage; and the ability of the body to repair the damage. Previous chapters stressed the viral characteristics that promote disease. In this chapter, viral diseases will be discussed with respect to their symptoms, organ system, and the host factors that influence their presentation.

VIRAL DISEASES

The major sites of viral disease are the respiratory tract; the gastrointestinal tract; the epithelial, mucosal, and endothelial linings of the skin, mouth, and genitalia; lymphoid tissue; liver and other organs; and the central nervous system (Figure 70-1).

Oral and Respiratory Tract Infections

The oropharynx and respiratory tract are the most common sites of virus infection and disease (Table 70-1). The viruses are spread in respiratory droplets and aerosols, food and water, saliva, by close contact, and on hands. Similar respiratory symptoms may be caused by several different viruses. For example, bronchiolitis may be caused by respiratory syncytial or parainfluenza virus. Alternatively, one virus may cause different symptoms in different people. For example, influenza virus may cause a mild upper respiratory tract infection in one person or life-threatening pneumonia in another.

The symptoms and severity of a respiratory viral disease depend on the nature of the virus, the site of infection (upper or lower respiratory tract), and the immune status and the age of the individual. Conditions such as cystic fibrosis and smoking, which compromise the ciliated and mucoepithelial barriers to infection, increase the risk of serious disease.

Pharyngitis is a common viral presentation. Most enteroviruses infect the oropharynx and then progress by way of a viremia to other target tissues. Symptoms such as acute onset pharyngitis, fever, and oral **vesicular lesions** are characteristic of coxsackie A virus (**herpangina, hand-foot-mouth disease**) and some coxsackie B and echovirus infections. Herpesviruses cause local primary infections of the oropharynx. Latent neuronal infection follows HSV **gingivostomatitis** with recurrence as **herpes labialis** (cold sores, fever blisters). HSV is also a common cause of pharyngitis. Epstein-Barr virus and HHV6 initiate and may cause symptoms in the oropharynx and then establish infection of lymphocytes. Vesicular lesions on the buccal mucosa (**Koplik spots**) are an early diagnostic feature of measles infection.

Upper respiratory tract viral infections, including the **common cold** and pharyngitis, are generally benign but still account for at least 50% of absenteeism from schools and the workplace. Rhinoviruses and coronaviruses are the predominant causes of upper respiratory tract infections. A runny nose (rhinitis) followed by congestion, cough, sneezing, conjunctivitis, headache, and sore throat are typical symptoms of the common cold. Other causes of the common cold and pharyngitis include specific serotypes of echoviruses and coxsackieviruses, adenoviruses, influenza, parainfluenza, and respiratory syncytial virus.

Tonsillitis, laryngitis, and **croup (laryngotracheobronchitis)** may accompany certain respiratory virus infections. Adenovirus and the early stages of Epstein-Barr virus disease are characterized by sore throat and tonsillitis with an exudative membrane. HSV and group A coxsackieviruses may also involve the tonsils but with vesicular lesions. Laryngitis (adults) and croup (children) are caused by inflammatory responses to the virus infection that narrow the trachea below the vocal cords (subglottic area). This causes loss of voice, a hoarse, barking cough, and the risk, especially in younger children, for a blocked airway and choking. Children infected with parainfluenza viruses are especially at risk for developing croup.

Lower respiratory tract viral infections can result in more serious disease. Symptoms of lower respiratory tract viral infections include **bronchiolitis** (inflammation of

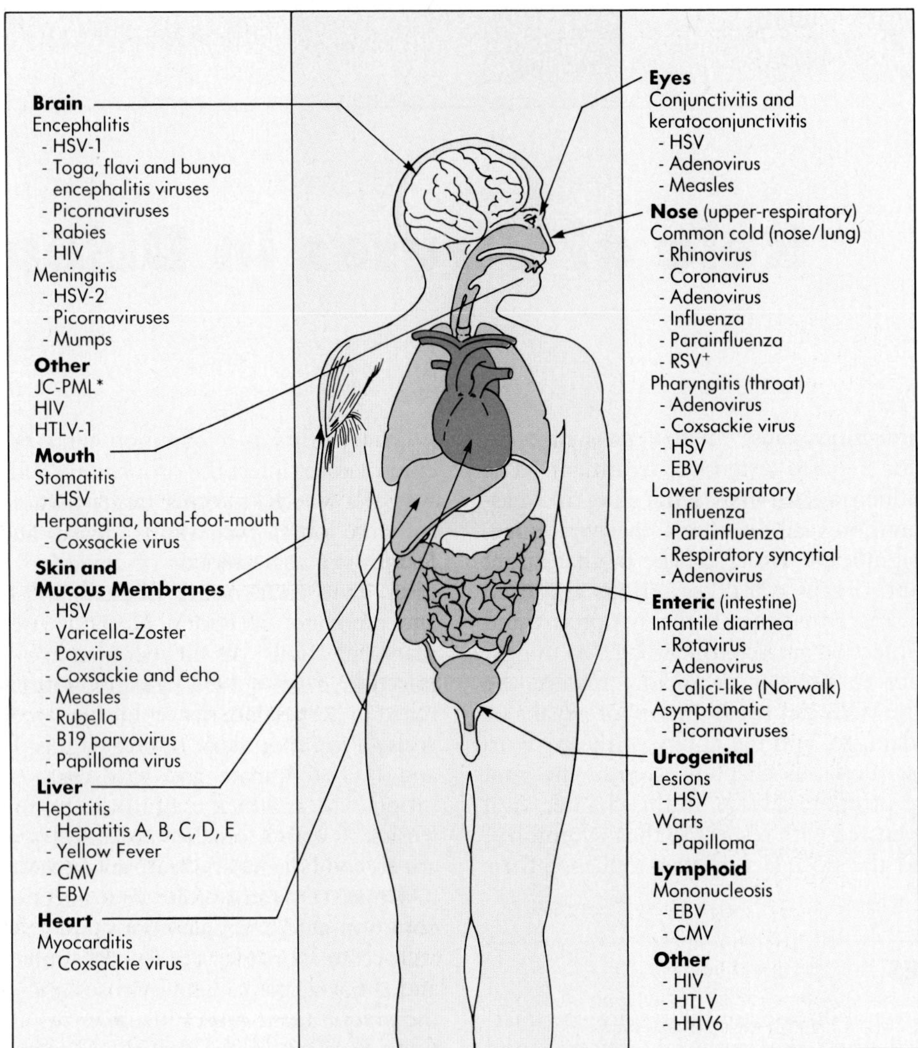

FIGURE 70-1 Major target tissues of viral disease. *Progressive multifocal leukoencephalopathy; †respiratory syncytial virus.

the bronchioles), pneumonia, and related diseases. The parainfluenza and respiratory syncytial viruses are major problems for infants and children but cause only asymptomatic infections or common cold symptoms in adults. Infection early in life does not necessarily prevent rechallenge since protection of the lung requires secretory antibody and this is a transient response. Parainfluenza 3 and especially respiratory syncytial virus infections are major causes of life-threatening pneumonia or bronchiolitis in infants younger than 6 months.

Influenza is probably the best known and most feared of the common respiratory viruses. The annual introduction of new strains of virus ensures the presence of immunologically naive victims. Children are universally susceptible to new strains of virus, whereas older individuals may have been immunized by a prior outbreak of the annual strain. The elderly are especially susceptible to new strains of virus since they may not be able to mount a sufficient primary immune response to the new strain of influenza or be able to repair the tissue damage caused by the disease. Other possible viral agents of pneumonia include adenovirus, paramyxoviruses, and primary varicella-zoster virus infections of adults.

Many viral infections start in the respiratory tract, infect the lung, and spread without significant symptoms. Varicella-zoster and measles virus initiate infection in the lung and can cause pneumonia but generally cause systemic infections resulting in an **exanthem** (rash). Other viruses that establish primary infection of the oropharynx or respiratory tract and then progress to other sites include rubella, mumps, enteroviruses, and the other human herpesviruses (HSV, EBV, CMV, and HHV6).

Flu-like and Systemic Symptoms

Many viral infections cause classic flu-like symptoms (fever, malaise, anorexia, headache, and bodyaches) during a viremic phase of disease because of the release of interferon and lymphokines. In addition to the respira-

TABLE 70-1 Oral and Respiratory Diseases

Disease	Etiological agent
Common cold (including pharyngitis)	Rhinovirus* Coronavirus* Influenza Parainfluenza Respiratory syncytial virus Adenovirus Enteroviruses
Pharyngitis (in addition to the common cold viruses)	Herpes simplex virus* Epstein-Barr virus* Adenovirus* Coxsackie A virus* (herpangina, hand-foot-mouth disease) and other Enteroviruses
Croup, tonsillitis, laryngitis, and bronchitis (children <2 years)	Parainfluenza 1* Parainfluenza 2 Influenza Adenovirus Epstein-Barr virus
Bronchiolitis	Respiratory syncytial virus* (infants) Parainfluenza 3* (infants and children) Parainfluenza 1, 2
Pneumonia	Respiratory syncytial virus* (infants) Parainfluenza virus* (infants) Influenza virus* Adenovirus Varicella-zoster (primary infection of adults or immunocompromised hosts) Cytomegalovirus (infection of immunocompromised host)

*Most common causal agents.

tory viruses, flu-like symptoms may accompany infections by arbo-encephalitis viruses, HSV-2, and other viruses.

Arthritis and other inflammatory diseases may also be specific symptoms of a virus challenge. B19 and RA-1 parvovirus infection of adults, rubella, and several other togaviruses elicit an arthritis symptom. Immune-complex disease associated with chronic hepatitis B virus can result in various presentations, including arthritis and nephritis.

Gastrointestinal Tract Infections

Infections of the gastrointestinal tract can result in gastroenteritis and diarrhea but frequently produce few or no symptoms (Box 70-1). Norwalk virus, caliciviruses, astroviruses, adenoviruses, reoviruses, or rotaviruses infect the small intestine, but not the colon, damaging the epithelial lining and the absorptive villi. This results in malabsorption of water and electrolyte imbalance. The resultant diarrhea in older children and adults is generally self-limited and can be treated by rehydration and restoration of the electrolyte balance. These viruses are major problems for adults and children in regions of drought and starvation.

BOX 70-1 Gastroenteritis Viruses

Infants
- Rotavirus A*
- Adenovirus 40, 41
- Coxsackie A24

Infants, children, and adults
- Norwalk virus
- Calicivirus
- Astrovirus
- Rotavirus B: outbreaks in China
- Reovirus

*Most common cause.

Viral gastroenteritis has a much more significant effect on infants and may require hospitalization. Rotavirus and adenovirus serotypes 40 and 41 are the major causes of infantile gastroenteritis. The extent of tissue damage and consequent loss of fluids and electrolytes is a more significant problem for infants.

Fecal-oral spread of enteric viruses is promoted by poor hygiene and is especially prevalent in day-care centers. Norwalk virus and calicivirus outbreaks affecting older children and adults are generally linked to a common contaminated food or water source. Vomiting usually accompanies diarrhea upon infection with Norwalk virus. Enteroviruses (picornaviruses) are spread by the fecal-oral route; however they usually cause little or no gastrointestinal symptoms. These viruses establish a viremia and spread to other target organs and then cause clinical disease.

Exanthems and Hemorragic Fevers

Virus-induced skin disease (Table 70-2) can result from infection through the mucosa, through small cuts or abrasions in the skin (herpes simplex virus), as a secondary infection following establishment of a viremia (varicella-zoster virus and smallpox), or through the inflammatory response mounted against viral antigens (measles rash). The major forms of skin lesions are classified as maculopapular, vesicular, nodular, and hemorrhagic rashes. **Macules** are flat colored spots. **Papules** are slightly raised areas of the skin and may result from immune or inflammatory responses rather than the virus. **Vesicular lesions** are blisters and are likely to contain virus. Papillomaviruses alter the growth patterns of skin cells, causing **warts**.

The classic childhood exanthems include roseola infantum (exanthem subitum [HHV6]), fifth disease (erythema infectiosum [B19 parvovirus]), and, in unvaccinated children, measles and rubella. The rash follows a viremia and is accompanied by fever. Except for measles, exanthems are not serious diseases. Rashes are also

TABLE 70-2 Viral Exanthems

Disease	Etiological agent
Rash	
Rubeola	Measles
German measles	Rubella
Roseola infantum	Human herpesvirus 6
Erythema infectiosum	B19
Boston exanthem	Echovirus 16
Infectious mononucleosis	Epstein-Barr virus, cytomegalovirus
Vesicles	
	Herpes simplex virus*
	Varicella-zoster virus*
Hand-foot-mouth disease, herpangina	Coxsackie A virus*
Papillomas	
Wart	Papilloma virus*
	Molluscum contagiosum

*Most common cause.

BOX 70-2 Infections of the Organs and Tissues

Liver
- Hepatitis A*, B*, C, D, E
- Yellow fever
- Epstein-Barr virus

Hepatitis in the neonate or immunocompromised individual
- Cytomegalovirus
- Herpes simplex virus
- Varicella
- Rubella (congenital rubella syndrome)

Heart
- Coxsackie B

Kidney
- Cytomegalovirus

Muscle
- Coxsackie B (pleurodynia)

Glands
- Cytomegalovirus
- Mumps

Eye
- Herpes simplex virus
- Adenovirus*
- Measles
- Rubella
- Enterovirus 70
- Coxsackie A24

*Most common cause.

associated with enterovirus, dengue, and other flaviviruses and alphaviruses and are occasionally seen with infectious mononucleosis.

Yellow fever virus, dengue virus, and other **hemorrhagic fever** viruses establish a viremia and infect the endothelial cell lining of the vasculature, which may compromise the structure of the blood vessel. Viral or immune cytolysis may lead to increased permeability or rupture of the vessel, producing a **hemorrhagic rash** with **petechiae** (pinpoint hemorrhages under the skin) and **ecchymoses** (massive bruises) and may lead to internal bleeding, loss of electrolytes, and shock.

Infections of the Eye

Infections of the eye result from direct contact with virus or from viremic spread (Box 70-2). **Conjunctivitis** (pinkeye) is a normal feature of many childhood infections and is a characteristic of specific adenovirus serotypes (3, 4a, and 7), measles, and rubella. **Keratoconjunctivitis** caused by adenovirus (8, 19a, and 37), herpes simplex virus or varicella-zoster, involves the cornea and can cause severe damage. Enterovirus 70 and coxsackie A24 viruses can cause an **acute hemorrhagic conjunctivitis. Cataracts** are classic features of babies born with congenital rubella syndrome. **Chorioretinitis** is associated with congenital cytomegalovirus infection and CMV infection of immunosuppressed individuals (e.g., AIDS).

Infections of the Organs and Tissues

Infection of the major organs may cause significant disease or result in further spread or secretion of the virus (Box 70-2). The symptoms may result from tissue damage or inflammatory responses.

The liver is a prominent target for many viruses that reach the liver by either viremia or the mononuclear phagocyte (reticuloendothelial) system. The liver acts as a source for secondary viremia but can also be damaged by the infection. The classic symptoms of **hepatitis** result from infections with hepatitis A, B, C, D, and E viruses and yellow fever virus and are often associated with EBV infectious mononucleosis and CMV infections. The liver is also a major target following disseminated herpes simplex virus infection of neonates and infants.

The heart and other muscles are also susceptible to viral infection and damage. Coxsackievirus can cause either **myocarditis** or **pericarditis** in newborns, children, and adults. Coxsackie B virus can infect muscle and cause **pleurodynia** (Bornholm disease). Other viruses (e.g., influenza virus, cytomegalovirus, and Epstein-Barr virus) may also infect the heart.

Infection of the secretory glands, accessory sexual organs, and mammary glands results in contagious spread of the virus (cytomegalovirus). An inflammatory response to the infection, as for mumps (**parotitis, orchitis**), may be the cause of the symptoms. Cytomegalovirus infection of the kidney and reactivation are problems for immunosuppressed individuals and a predominant cause for kidney transplant failure.

BOX 70-3 Central Nervous System Infections

Meningitis
- Enteroviruses*
  - ECHO
  - Polio
  - Coxsackie
- HSV-2
- Adenovirus
- Mumps
- Lymphocytic choriomeningitis virus
- Epstein-Barr virus
- Arbo-encephalitis viruses

Paralysis
- Polio
- Enteroviruses 70, 71
- Coxsackie A7

Encephalitis
- HSV-1*
- VZV
- Arbo-encephalitis viruses*
- Rabies
- Coxsackie A and B
- Polio

Post-infectious encephalitis (immune-mediated)
- Measles
- Mumps
- Rubella
- Varicella
- Influenza

Other
- JC (PML [in immunosuppressed individuals])
- Measles variant (SSPE)
- Prion (encephalopathy)
- HIV (AIDS dementia)
- HTLV-1 (tropical spastic paraparesis)

*Most common cause.

Infections of the Central Nervous System

Infections of the brain and central nervous system may cause the most serious of viral diseases because of the importance of the CNS and its very limited capacity to repair damage (Box 70-3). Tissue damage is usually caused by a combination of viral and immunopathogenesis. However, most neurotropic virus infections do not result in disease because the virus either does not reach the CNS or does not cause sufficient tissue damage to exhibit symptoms.

Virus may spread to the central nervous system in blood (arboviruses), macrophages (HIV), or following peripheral infection of neurons (olfactory) or by first infecting skin (herpes simplex virus) or muscle (rabies) and then progressing to the innervating neuron. The virus then infects those neuronal cells that express a viral receptor. The temporal lobe is targeted in HSV encephalitis, Ammon's horn in rabies, and the anterior horn of the spinal cord and motor neurons in paralytic poliomyelitis.

Viral infections of the CNS are usually distinguished from bacterial infections by the presence of monocytes, low numbers of polymorphonuclear leukocytes, and normal levels of glucose in the cerebrospinal fluid. Specific antigen detection by immunoassay or virus isolation from CSF or a biopsy confirms the diagnosis and identifies the viral agent. The season of the year also facilitates the diagnosis since enteroviral and arboviral diseases generally occur during the summer, whereas HSV encephalitis and other viral syndromes may be observed all year.

The type of CNS disease depends on the specific part of the brain (central nervous system and/or meninges) infected. Aseptic meningitis is caused by an inflammation and swelling of the meninges enveloping the brain and spinal cord in response to infection with enteroviruses, HSV-2, mumps, or lymphocytic choriomeningitis virus. The disease is usually self-limited and, unlike bacterial meningitis, resolves without sequelae unless the virus gains access and infects neurons or the brain (meningoencephalitis). The viruses gain access to the meninges from a viremia.

Encephalitis and myelitis result from a combination of viral and immune pathogenesis in brain and neurons and are either fatal or cause significant damage and permanent neurological sequelae. Herpes simplex virus, varicella-zoster virus, and RNA viruses such as rabies virus, California encephalitis viruses, St. Louis encephalitis virus, and measles virus are potential causes of encephalitis. Polio virus and several other enteroviruses cause paralytic disease.

HSV and VZV are ubiquitous and usually cause asymptomatic latent infections of the central nervous system but can also cause encephalitis. Most arbo-encephalitis virus infections result in flu-like symptoms rather than encephalitis. Post-measles encephalitis and subacute sclerosing panencephalitis were rare sequelae of measles infection in the pre-vaccine era.

Other viral-induced neurological syndromes include HIV dementia, HTLV-1 tropical spastic paraparesis, JC papovavirus, progressive multifocal leukoencephalopathy (PML) in immunosuppressed individuals, and the spongiform encephalopathies (Kuru, Creutzfeldt-Jakob disease) that are postulated to be caused by prions.

Hematological Diseases

Lymphocytes and macrophages are not very permissive for virus replication but are targets for several viruses that establish persistent infections. Transient virus replication of EBV, HIV, or CMV elicits a large T-cell response, resulting in mononucleosis-like syndromes. In addition, CMV, measles, and HIV infections of T cells are immunosuppressive. HIV reduces the numbers of CD4 helper and DTH T cells, which further compromises the immune system. HTLV-1 infection causes little disease

BOX 70-4 Sexually Transmitted Viruses

Papillomavirus HPV 6, 11, 42
HPV 16, 18 (associated with human cervical carcinoma)
Herpes simplex virus (predominantly HSV-2)
Cytomegalovirus
Hepatitis B virus
HIV
HTLV-1

upon infection but may lead to adult T-cell leukemia or tropical spastic paraparesis much later in life.

Macrophages and cells of the macrophage lineage are infected by many viruses. Macrophages act as vehicles for spreading the virus through the body. Viruses replicate inefficiently in macrophages, and the cells are generally not lysed by the infection. This promotes persistent/chronic infections. The macrophage is the primary target cell for dengue virus. Nonneutralizing antibody can actually promote dengue infection of the cell through Fc receptors. HIV infection of macrophages and cells of the macrophage lineage provide a reservoir for the virus and access to the brain. AIDS dementia is thought to result from the actions of HIV-infected microglial cells in the brain.

Sexually Transmitted Viral Diseases

Sexual transmission is not a very efficient route of virus spread, yet it is a major route for papillomavirus, HSV, CMV, HIV, HTLV-1, and HBV (Box 70-4). These viruses establish chronic and latent-recurrent infections with asymptomatic shedding. These viral properties foster dissemination via a route of transmission that is relatively infrequent and would be avoided during symptomatic disease. These viruses can also be transmitted neonatally or perinatally to infants. Papillomaviruses and HSV-2 establish local primary infections with recurrent disease at the same site. Lesions or asymptomatic shedding are sources for sexual transmission and perinatal transmission to the newborn. CMV and HIV enter the bloodstream and infect lymphoid cells, whereas HBV is delivered to the liver. These viruses are present in blood, semen, and vaginal secretions, which can transmit the virus to sexual partners and neonates.

Viruses Spread by Transfusion and Transplantation

Hepatitis B virus (HBV), hepatitis C virus (HCV), human immunodeficiency virus (HIV), human T lymphotropic virus (HTLV-1), and cytomegalovirus are transmitted in blood and organ transplants. The chronic nature, persistent asymptomatic virus release, or infection of macrophages and lymphocytes promote transmission by these routes. Screening of the blood supply for HBV and HIV has controlled transmission of these viruses by transfusion. Large scale screening procedures for the other viruses have not been developed, and the risk remains for spreading HCV, HTLV, and CMV by these routes.

Syndromes of Possible Viral Etiology

Several diseases have symptoms, epidemiology, or other characteristics that resemble viral infections or may be sequelae of viral infections (e.g., inflammatory responses to a persistent virus infection). These include multiple sclerosis, Kawasaki disease, arthritis, diabetes, and chronic fatigue syndrome.

CHRONIC AND POTENTIALLY ONCOGENIC INFECTIONS

Chronic infections occur when the immune system has difficulty resolving the infection. The DNA viruses (except parvovirus and poxvirus) and the retroviruses cause latent infections with the potential for recurrence. Cytomegalovirus and other herpesviruses, hepatitis B, C, and D virus, and retroviruses cause chronic productive infections.

Hepatitis B virus, Epstein-Barr virus, papillomavirus, and HTLV-1 are associated with human cancers. Cofactors and/or chromosomal aberrations enable a clone of virus-containing cells to grow out into a cancer. Immunosuppression, during AIDS, cancer chemotherapy, or transplant procedures also promotes lymphomagenesis by EBV.

Epstein-Barr virus normally causes infectious mononucleosis but is associated with African Burkitt's lymphoma and nasopharyngeal carcinoma; HTLV-1 is associated with human adult T-cell leukemia. Many papillomaviruses induce a simple hyperplasia characterized by a wart; however several other strains of papillomaviruses have been associated with human cancers (e.g., type 16 and 18 with cervical carcinoma). Chronic hepatitis B virus infection has been associated with primary hepatocellular carcinoma. HSV-2 has been associated with human cervical carcinoma, most likely as a cofactor.

Development of a worldwide vaccine program for hepatitis B virus would not only reduce the spread of viral hepatitis but should also prevent the occurrence of primary hepatocellular carcinoma. Epstein-Barr virus and papillomavirus associated cancers should also be preventable by vaccination.

INFECTIONS OF THE IMMUNOCOMPROMISED HOST

Patients deficient in cell-mediated immunity are generally more susceptible to infection by enveloped viruses (especially the herpesviruses, measles, and even the vaccinia virus used for smallpox vaccinations) and recurrences of latent viruses (herpesviruses and papovaviruses). Severe T-cell deficiencies also affect the antiviral antibody response. Cell-mediated immunodeficiencies can be congenital or acquired. They may result from genetic defects (e.g., Duncan's disease, DiGeorge syndrome, Wiskott-Aldrich syndrome), leukemia or lymphoma, infections (e.g., AIDS), or immunosuppressive therapy.

Viruses cause atypical and more severe presentations in immunosuppressed individuals. Herpesvirus (herpes simplex virus, cytomegalovirus, varicella-zoster virus) infections, normally benign and localized, can progress locally or disseminate and cause visceral and neurological infections that may be life threatening. Measles infection can cause a giant-cell (syncytial) pneumonia rather than the characteristic rash.

IgA-deficient and hypogammaglobulinemic individuals (antibody deficient) have more problems with respiratory and gastrointestinal viruses. Hypogammaglobulinemic individuals are more likely to suffer significant disease following infection by the live polio vaccine, echovirus, and varicella-zoster virus.

CONGENITAL, NEONATAL, AND PERINATAL INFECTIONS

Development and growth in the fetus are so ordered and rapid that viral infection may damage or prevent the appropriate formation of important tissues, leading to miscarriage or congenital abnormalities. Infection may occur in utero (**prenatal**) (rubella, parvovirus B19, CMV, HIV), upon traversing the birth canal (**neonatal**) (HSV-2, HBV, CMV), or soon after birth (**postnatal**) (HIV, CMV, HBV, HSV, coxsackie B and echovirus).

Neonates depend on the mother's immunity to protect them from viral infections. Neonates receive maternal antibodies through the placenta and then through the mother's milk. This type of passive immunity can remain effective for 6 months to a year after birth. Maternal antibody can protect against virus spread to the fetus by viremia (e.g., rubella, B19), protect against many enteric and respiratory viral infections, and reduce the severity of other viral diseases after birth. The cell-mediated immune system is not mature at birth. As a result, newborns are susceptible to syncytia-forming viruses such as herpes simplex virus or other viruses that spread by cell-to-cell contact (e.g., VZV, cytomegalovirus, HIV).

Rubella virus and cytomegalovirus are examples of teratogenic viruses that can cause congenital infection and severe congenital abnormalities. HIV infection, in utero or from mother's milk, initiates a chronic infection that leads to lymphadenopathy, failure to thrive, or encephalopathy within 2 years of birth. Herpes simplex virus can be acquired on passage through an infected birth canal and result in life-threatening disseminated disease. Nosocomial infection of newborns can result in a similar outcome. B19 is acquired in utero and can cause spontaneous abortion.

INFECTION CONTROL

Infection control is essential in hospital and health care settings. Respiratory virus spread is the most difficult to prevent. Virus spread can be controlled by:

1. Limiting contact with sources of infection (i.e., wearing gloves, mask, goggles, using quarantine)
2. Improving hygiene, sanitation, and disinfection
3. Ensuring that all personnel are immunized against common diseases
4. Educating all personnel on points 1, 2, and 3, and how to decrease high-risk behaviors

Methods for disinfection differ for each virus and depend on the structure of the virus. Most viruses are inactivated by 70% ethanol, 10% chlorine bleach, 2% glutaraldehyde, 4% formaldehyde, or autoclaving (as per CDC guidelines for HIV and HBV: *MMWR* 38:S-6, 1989). Most enveloped viruses are deactivated by soap and detergents. Other means of disinfection are also available.

Special precautions are required for handling human blood. All blood should be assumed to be contaminated with HIV or HBV and handled with caution. In addition to the disinfection and protection procedures mentioned, special care must be taken with syringe needles and surgical tools contaminated with blood to prevent needle sticks or cuts. Specific guidelines are available from the Centers for Disease Control.

Control of a viral outbreak usually requires identification of the viral source or reservoir, followed by cleanup, quarantine, and/or immunization. The first step in controlling an outbreak of gastroenteritis or hepatitis A virus is identification of the food, water, or possibly a day-care center that may be the source of the outbreak.

Education programs can promote compliance with immunization programs and help change those life-styles that promote virus transmission. Such programs have made a significant impact in reducing the prevalence of vaccine-preventable diseases such as smallpox, polio, measles, mumps, and rubella. Educational programs will hopefully also promote changes in life-styles and habits that will restrict the spread of the blood-borne and sexually transmitted hepatitis B virus and HIV.

QUESTIONS

1. What disinfection procedures are sufficient for inactivating the following viruses: hepatitis A virus, hepatitis B virus, herpes simplex virus, and rhinovirus?
2. What precautions should health care workers take to protect themselves from infection by the following viruses: hepatitis B virus, influenza A virus, herpes simplex virus (whitlow), and HIV?
3. What predisposing conditions would exacerbate infection by influenza A virus, varicella-zoster virus, or rotavirus?

4. Describe and compare the nature and mechanism of exanthem development for measles, varicella-zoster virus, herpes simplex virus (primary and recurrence), and yellow fever.
5. A kidney transplant recipient undergoing immunosuppressive therapy had a lymphoma that regressed with reduction of the immunosuppressive therapy. The lymphoma cells contained EBV. How might EBV be involved in this lymphoma? Why did the lymphoma regress upon reduction of immunosuppressive therapy? What other virus infections would this individual be at increased risk for during the immunosuppressive therapy?

References

Belshe RB, editor: *Textbook of human virology*, ed 2, St. Louis, 1991, Mosby.

Ellner PD, Neu HC: *Understanding infectious disease*, St. Louis, 1992, Mosby.

Emond RTD and Rowland HAK: *Color atlas of infectious diseases*, ed 2, St. Louis, 1987, Mosby.

Gorbach SL, Bartlett, JG, Blacklow NR: *Infectious diseases*, Philadelphia, 1992, WB Saunders.

Hart CA, Broadhead RL: *Color atlas of pediatric infectious diseases*, St. Louis, 1992, Mosby.

Haukenes G, Haaheim LR, Pattison JR: *A practical guide to clinical virology*, New York, 1989, John Wiley & Sons.

Krugman S, Katz SL, Gerson AA, Wilfert CM: *Infectious diseases of children*, ed 9, St. Louis, 1992, Mosby.

Mandell GL, Douglas RG Jr, Bennett JE: *Principles and practice of infectious disease*, ed 3, New York, 1990, Churchill Livingstone.

Mims CA and White DO: *Viral pathogenesis and immunology*, Oxford, 1984, Blackwell Scientific Publications.

Shulman ST, Phair JP, Sommers HM: *The biologic and clinical basis of infectious diseases*, ed 4, Philadelphia, 1992, WB Saunders.

White DO and Fenner FJ: *Medical virology*, ed 3, Orlando, Fla, 1986, Academic Press.

Index

B

C

O